New Concise Medical Dictionary

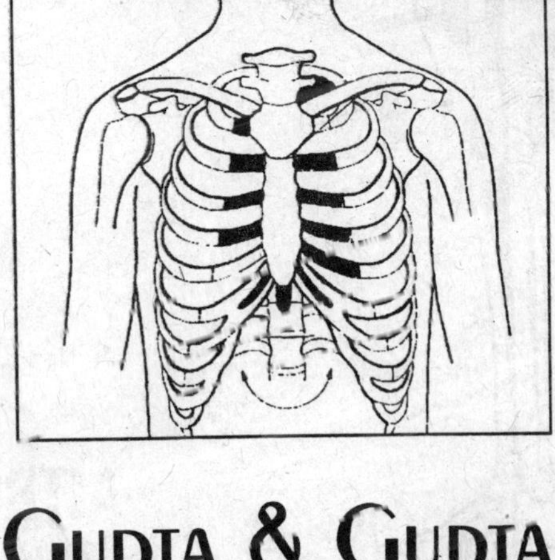

Gupta & Gupta

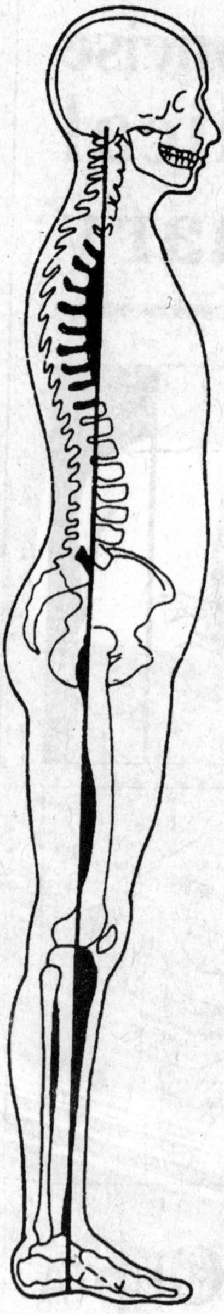

New Concise Medical Dictionary

Fifth Edition

Dr. L.C. Gupta
MD (PSM), MD (RAD)
DMRE, DSc (HON)

- World Record of writing 111 Medical Books - 2010
- B.C. Roy National Award - 1988
- Presidents Police Medal for Distinguished Services - 1993

Dr. Kusum Gupta
MA (Eng Lit) LLB, PhD (Hon)
New Delhi

Dr. Abhitabh Gupta
M.D. (Physician) DMRE
Paramount Health Care Management, New Delhi

Dr. Abhishek Gupta
M.D. (Physician) DRM
SGPGI, Lucknow

Dr. Sujata
M.S., M.Ch. (Plastic Surgery)
Safdarjung Hospital, New Delhi

A.I.T.B.S.

AITBS Publishers, India
(MEDICAL PUBLISHERS)

Our valued contributors

- **Dr ASMT Hossain**
  M.D. (Bern) DSc (Warsaw)
  MPhil (London) DTM & H (Edinburgh)
  DV (Liverpool) DIH (St Andrews)
  DPH (Edinburgh)
  Medical Author of Eminence
  DHAKA (Bangladesh)
- **Dr N C Shah,** MD
  Paramount Health Care Management,
  Mumbai
- **Dr V Maheswari,** MS
  Maheswari Nursing Home
  Gwalior-2
- **Col J K Bhagat,** MD, DRM
  INHS ASHIWINI
  Mumbai
- **Dr Vikas Dhikav,** MBBS
  New Delhi
- **Dr Vandana Mangal,** MD
  SMS Medical College, Jaipur
- **Dr Daya B. Dayal,** MD (FMT)
  New Delhi
- **Dr L R Lodha,** MD
  Medical College, Jodhpur
- **Dr A K Dube,** MS
  Leading Eye Surgeon, Gwalior
- **Mrs Mani Raj Sharma**
  Mr Raj Kumar Sharma
  New Delhi
- **Dr Anurag Gupta,** MBBS
  Manipal
- **Dr Pradeep Dhar,** MBBS
  PHM, New Delhi
- **Dr S K Acharya,** MS
  BSF HQS., New Delhi
- **Dr B K Das**
  Prof/Head Nuclear Medicine
  SGPGI, Lucknow
- **Dr T N Rao,** DTM & H
  New Delhi
- **Prof Dr Arun Malhotra,** DRM, PhD
  AIIMS, New Delhi
- **Dr A K Saxena**
  New Delhi
- **Dr Ajay Gupta,** MS
  Jhansi
- **Mr S K Mishra,** LL B
  HUDCO, Calcutta

Mr Pradeep K. Gupta Advocate
Mr Sanjay Gupta Advocate
Mr Atul Gupta Gwalior
Mrs Rakhi Gupta Indore

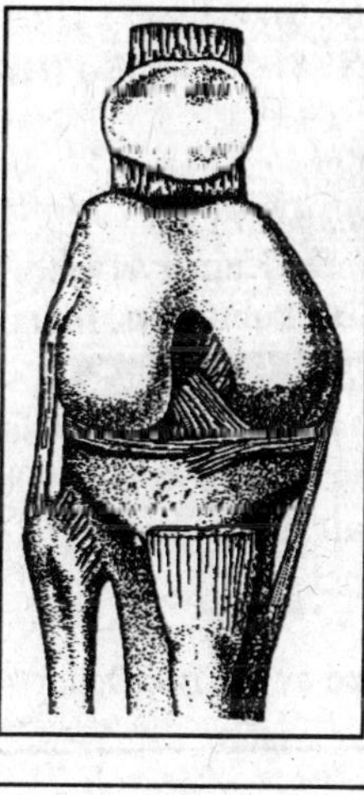

First Edition : 2002
Second Edition : 2003
Third Edition : 2004
Fourth Edition : 2006
Fourth Revised Edition : 2008
Fifth Edition : 2014

ISBN : 978-81-7473-178-4 (Paper Back) (13 Digit)
ISBN : 81-7473-178-4 (Paper Back) (10 Digit)
ISBN : 978-81-7473-353-5 (Hard Bound) (13 Digit)
ISBN : 81-7473-353-1 (Hard Bound) (10 Digit)

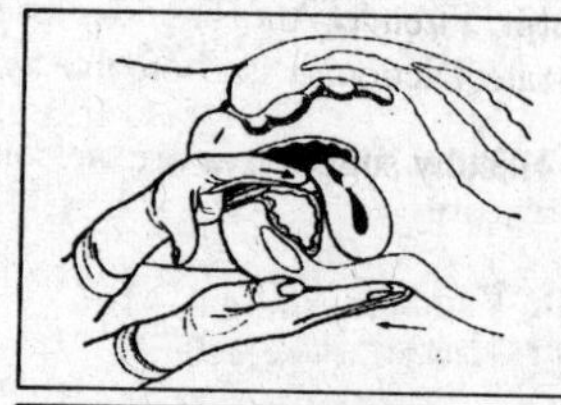

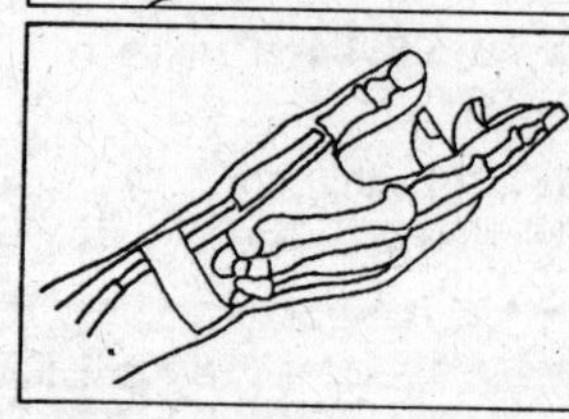

Published by :
Virender Kumar Arya for
AITBS Publishers, India
Medical Publishers
J-5/6 Krishna Nagar, Delhi - 110051 (INDIA)
Phone: 22009096, 22009084, Fax: 011-22009074
E-mail: aitbs@bol.net.in & aitbsindia@gmail.com

Printed by AITBS, Delhi

Preface

Present dictionary will help in knowing about the "word" its meaning and reference. Certain important clinical features have also been mentioned wherever needed to explain the term clearly making dictionary a little different than others.

We are deeply obliged to our valued contributors specially our friend, guide and philosopher Dr. ASMT Hossain who is pillar of our strength from Bangladesh. We owe to many unknown authors, medical artists and medical publishers for permitting us to use their creation just for the benefit of students and for some permission is still awaited. Whatever is in this dictionary credit goes to them first and then to us. We salute them from the core of our heart.

We have been encouraged by three dynamic brothers of Modern Book Depot chain of book shops Mr. Jiwan Ram, Mr. Diwan Chand and Mr. Kanwar Bhan.

We are thankful to the Officers of Medical Council of India for their support and encouragement.

Mr. Virender Arya has done his best to bring the dictionary in presentable form at a cheaper rate. Dictionary is affordable by every one, either to have personally or to gift to dear one.

Healthy suggestions are welcome.

L.C. Gupta
Kusum Gupta
Abhitabh Gupta
Abhishek Gupta
Sujata

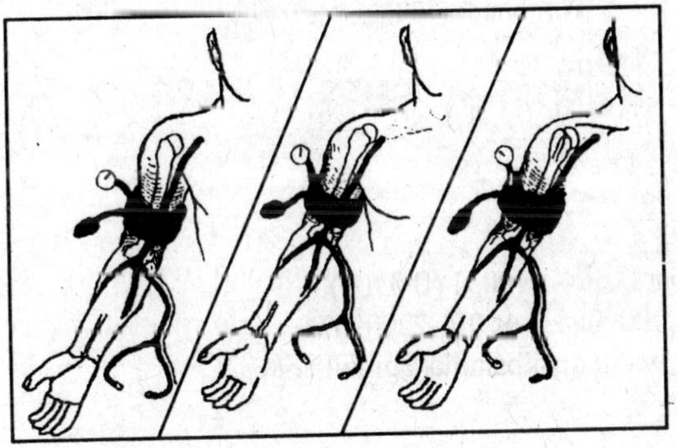

Dedicated

to

INDIAN MEDICAL ASSOCIATION

(Madhya Pradesh Branch)

Serving the society effectively

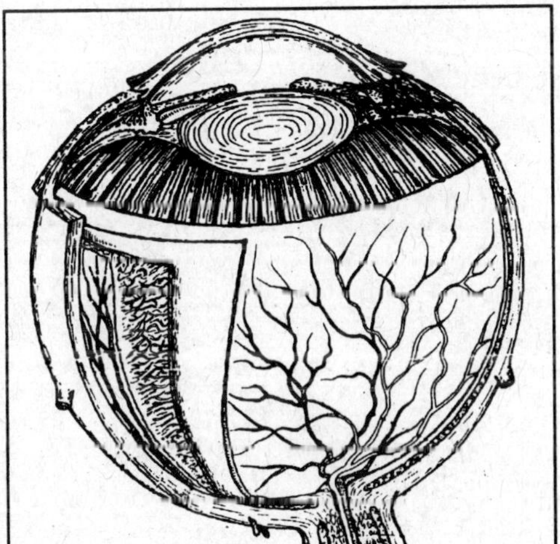

Section-1

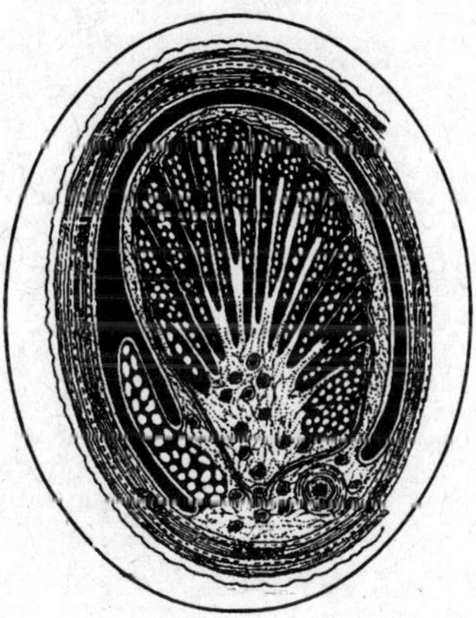

A

A cultural nursing care Care that lacks concern for cultural differences.

A wave The rise in the atrial pressure curve caused by the contraction of the atria during atrial systole.

A/G ratio Albumin globulin ratio.

Aaron's sign Continuous firm pressure of the finger over Mc Burney's point (about 2" above the antero-superior iliac spine on the line drawn between the spine and the umbilicus) elicits a referred pain or feeling of distress in the epigastrium or precordial region. It is present in the cases of acute appendicitis.

Abacterial Free from bacteria.

Abandonment Withdrawing a patient from treatment without giving reasonable notice or providing a competent replacement.

Abatement Decrease in severity of symptoms.

Abbreviations Chapter containing main reference.

ABC protein A protein that contains the widely conserved ATP-binding cassette, a motif that couples energy from ATP (adenosine triphosphate) binding and hydrolysis to various transport processes (ABC transport).

ABCs of emergency care Levels of emergency care to determine airway, breathing, and circulation.

Abdomen This is the area bounded above by ribs and by pelvis at lower end. The contents of abdomen are separated from thorax by diaphragm. It contains digestive system, urinary system and contents of pelvis.

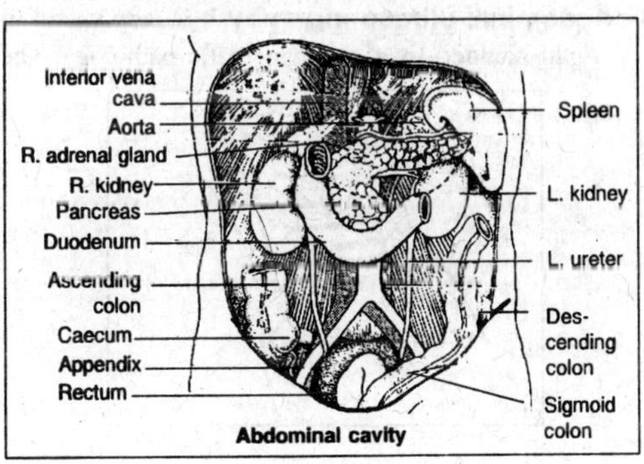

Abdominal cavity

Abdomen in acute hydraminos The abdomen becomes tense, tender and disproportionately large due to rapid and excessive increase in size of uterus. Fluid thrill is present. Fetus may not be recognised by palpation or auscultation. External and internal ballotment can be elicited. Malpresentations are common.

Abdomen, acute This is persistent, severe abdominal pain of sudden onset. There may be vomiting and fever. Abdominal muscles will be

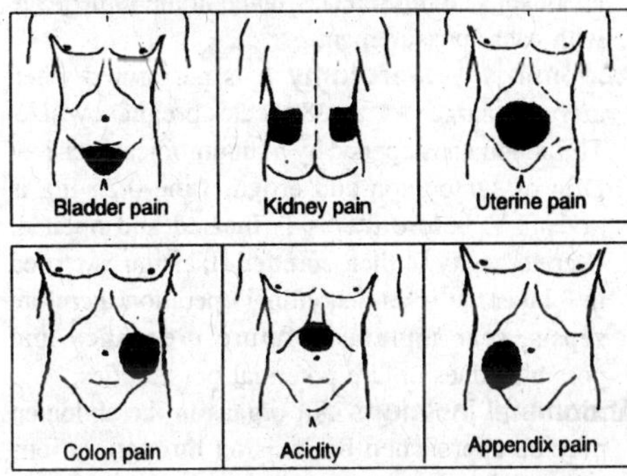

rigid. Most important causes are inflamed appendix, salpingitis, perforated peptic ulcer and peritonitis. Urinary stone will also cause severe pain.

Abdominal aortic aneurysmectomy Localized area of increased aortic diameter in abdominal area; usually atherosclerotic, but may be an extension of a dissection from above in the aorta.

Abdominal apoplexy There is massive intraperitoneal haemorr-hage. It is prevalent in arteriosclerosis. There develops severe abdominal pain, and shock. Peritoneal irritation develops. Spontaneous rupture of intra-abdominal vessels takes place. Prognosis is better if suture of bleeding point is performed in time.

Abdominal circumference A parameter used in the diagnosis of IUGR, in which the size of the fetus is estimated based on the measurement of the abdomen at the level of the liver and the left portal vein.

Abdominal cocoon There develops intestinal obstruction. Causes of it include subacute peritoneal infections, and fibrin deposit. There develops large fibrotic sac wrapping the small bowel.

Abdominal enlargement After 16 weeks abdomen start enlarging. Other causes of abdominal distension are full bladder, tumors and ascites.

Abdominal field block Technique using 100-200 ml local anesthetic agent involving infiltration of skin, subcutaneous tissue, abdominal muscles and fascia. It provides analgesia of abdominal wall and anterior peritoneum but not viscera. Now it is not very much in use.

Abdominal girth The measurement of the abdomen's circumference, taken at the same place with each measurement.

Abdominal hysterotomy It is performed when uterus is large, 14 to 28 weeks pregnancy size. The abdomen is opened by a subumbilical incision. Drip of syntocinon and erogmetrine 0.25 mg is given I.V. before uterus is incised and opened. Uterine cavity is then curetted. Incision is closed in 3 layers. It is an abdominal operation therefore sepsis, scar rupture in future pregnancy and possible adhesion are potential possibilities.

Abdominal incisions All organs in the abdomen may be approached by incision through various parts of the abdominal wall. Incision should give the surgeon free access. After operation the wound should heal well. A good example of a planned incision is the so-called 'grid iron' incision for removal of the vermiform appendix. The skin and superficial fasciae are incised by a downward and medially curving line which crosses the junction of the lateral and middle thirds of a line joining the umbilicus to the anterior superior iliac spine.

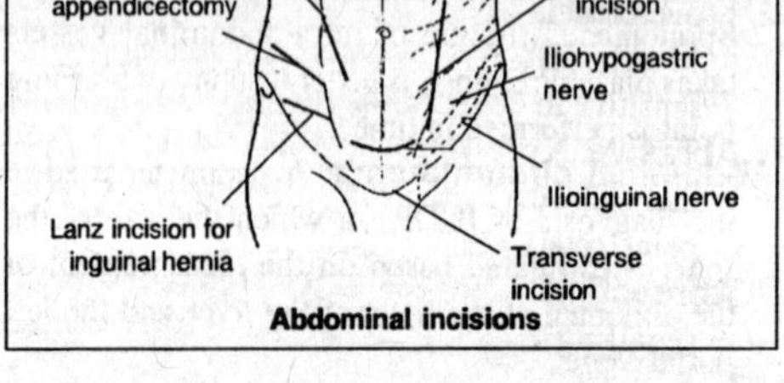

Abdominal incisions

Abdominal muscles Muscles supporting the anterior aspect of the abdomen.

Abdominal pain Other symptoms include nausea, belching, gurgling sounds and flatulence. It may be caused by acidity. Inflammation and distension of viscera. Girls may have pain during menstruation. Occasionally pain may be due to endometriosis, pyelonephritis and volvulus

Abdominal paracentasis It is the procedure of puncturing the peritoneal cavity in order to drain out fluid of ascites. It relieves pressure on the organs of abdomen. Usual puncture site is below umbilicus in midline. Tighten abdominal binder when fluid starts flowing out. In one sitting not more than half of fluid is to be removed. Rapid withdrawal is avoided. Seal the puncture site with tincture benzoin and cover with sterile pad. Tighten the abdominal binder.

Abdominal pregnancy Ectopic pregnancy occurring in the cavity of the abdomen.

Abdominal quadrants Health professionals divide the abdomen (through the navel) into four areas to help locate specific organs.

Abdominal regions Anatomists have divided the abdomen into nine regions to identify the location of organs.

Abdominal swelling Abdominal distension may be due to obesity, ascites or after 14 weeks of pregnancy, kidney or liver disease.

Abdominal thrust maneuver A first-aid procedure for choking. Employs a quick, upward thrust against the diaphragm that forces air out of the lungs with sufficient force to expel any lodged material. Also called the Heimlich maneuver.

Abdominal ultrasonography It is very useful in gall bladder, liver and pancreatic pathology. The

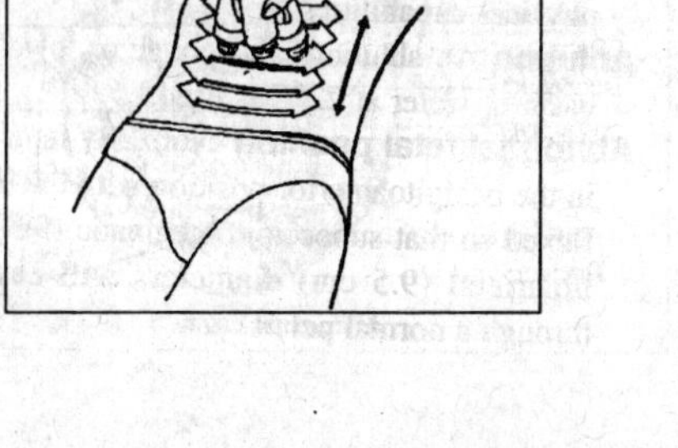

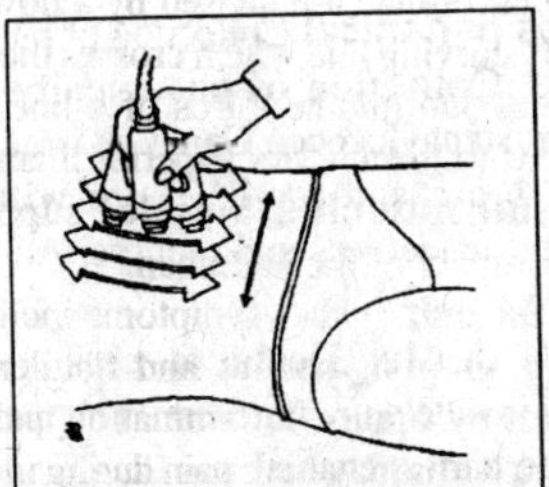
Abdominal ultrasonography

transducer moves in a rock and slide motion in transverse as well as sagittal plane.

Abdominopelvic cavity Inferior component of the ventral body cavity that is subdivided into a superorior abdominal cavity and an inferior pelvic cavity.

Abduce Abduct.

Abducent nerve Abducent nerve is the 6th cranial nerve. It supplies one muscle of each eye required for moving eye outwards. It originates from pons. Damage of this nerve can cause double vision or conver-gent strabismus.

Abduction Movement away from the midline.

Abductor pommel An upholstered block or wedge placed on the front of the upholstered block or wedge placed on the front of the wheelchair seating surface; used to maintain abduction of the lower extremities.

Ability Present skill, as in riding a bicycle or reciting a poem. Con-trasted with aptitude, which refers to what an individual can do rather than what one might do if given appropriate training.

Abiotic Not living; relating to the nonliving aspects of the environ ment.

Ablation It is a removal or excision of dead or diseased part of body. The ablation may be done with radiation or ablation therapy.

Ablation procedure Cauterization of the area in the heart that is inducing the arrhythmia.

Ableism Prejudice against those without full physical capabilities.

Ablution An ablution is a sponge or towel bath. A basin of water at 22°C is used.

Abnormal fetal position Normally fetus delivers in the occipitoanterior position with the head well flexed so that suboccipitobregmatic (9.5 cm) and biparietal (9.5 cm) diameters will easily pass through a normal pelvis.

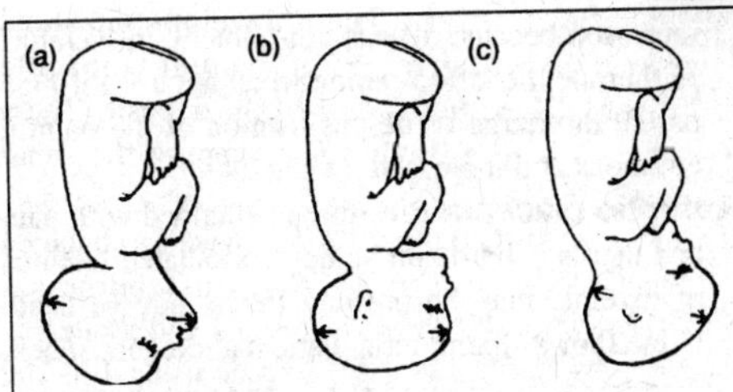

(a) Mentovertical
(b) Occipitofrontal diameter
(c) Suboccipito-bregmatic

Abnormal uterine contractions Contractions can be monitored by means of external to codynanometry or by means of intrauterine catheter to measure pressure dirctly. Care should be taken that in between contractions uterus should be relaxed.

ABO isoimmunization Group 'O' women have serum antibody which can pass through placenta. She has anti A and anti B agglutinins which may be augmented by pregnancy by a secretor fetus of group A or B or AB. This immunization will particularly occur if mother is group 'O' and baby belongs to group 'A'.

Abortifacient An agent producing an abortion.

Abortion It is known as mis-carriage. Prostaglandins are known as abortifacient. It causes softening and widening of cervix and muscular contractions of uterus. Therapeutic abortion is carried out to save life or health of mother and child.

Abrade To wear away by friction.

Abrasion It is a skin injury caused by scrapping which results in oozing of blood and serum. These are easily infected and treatment includes removal of foreign matter, cleaning and applying dressings. To avoid tetanus and secondary infection antitetanus injection may be given along with antibiotics.

Abrasions dental Enamel of tooth along with dentin is weared out. It may be caused by overbrushing the teeth.

Mostly affected canine and premolars become sensitive to cold and hot food.

Abrasive A substance used for grinding or polishing that will wear away a material or tissue. It can be of point, rotary or strip type.

Abreaction Emotional release or discharge after recalling a painful experience that has been repressed because it was consciously intolerable. A therapeutic effect sometimes occurs through partial discharge or desensitisation of the painful emotions and increased insight.

Abruptio placenta Bleeding is attended with pain and uterus is hard and tender. Associated features of toxemia may be present. Fetus may be dead. Urine shows albuminuria. Patient undergoes shock.

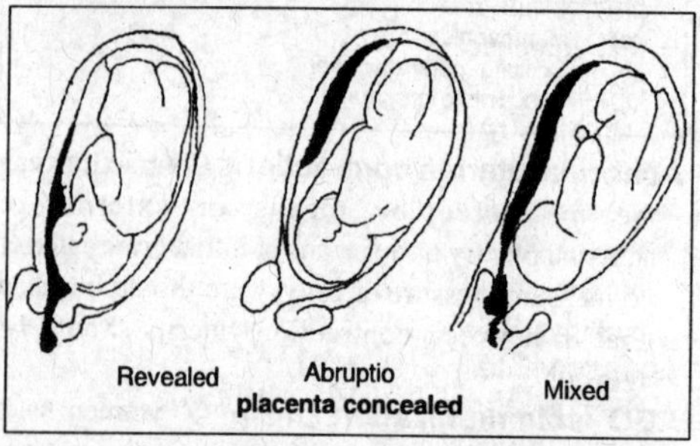

Abruptio placental haemorrhage It is a bleeding occurring by accident or chance and refers to bleeding related to placenta which is normally situated in upper segment of uterus. It is the condition present when bleeding occurs from decidua behind the placenta. Partial detachment

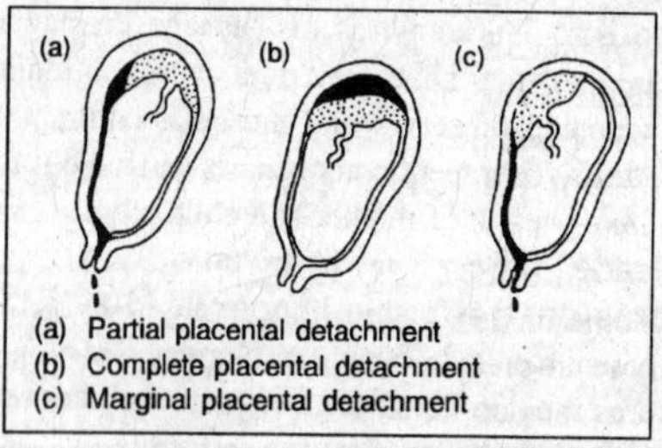

(a) Partial placental detachment
(b) Complete placental detachment
(c) Marginal placental detachment

following retroplacental haemorrhage followed by external blood loss. Complete detachment follows retroplacental haemorrhage near the centre of placental attachment site and there is no external blood loss. In marginal detachment early little loss is seen.

Abruption of placenta It is also known as abruptio placentae. It is associated with a raised blood pressure and is found in essential hypertension, pre eclampsia and eclampsia. It may be concealed, revealed or mixed type. Some blood seeps down the vagina the remainder being trapped inside the uterus.

Absccess periapical Collection of pus at root tip.

Abscess Collection of pus usually caused by bacteria, staphylococci. Common occurrence is in breast, brain and tooth. There will be fever, sweating, tenderness and redness. Antibiotics are effective.

Abscess, dental Dental abscess results when bacteria invade pulp. It generally happens in dental caries. In caries, enamel and dentin are destroyed and pulp is exposed to bacteria. The affected tooth aches and bites become painful. Gum around tooth becomes red and swollen. An antibiotic may be given. When infection is subsided then cavity is filled up with dental cement.

Absolute reliability The extent to which a score varies on repeated measurements; it is quantified by the standard error of measurement.

Absolutely refractory Refers to the period in an action potential during which a new action potential cannot be elicited, because of the closing of gate 2 of voltage-sensitive sodium channels.

Absorption The taking in or reception of gases, liquids, light, heat, or solutes, such as the movement of digested molecules across the intestinal wall and into the blood stream, the movement of substances through the skin, and the movement of fluid into the lymphatics from the interstitial fluid.

Abstinence Voluntarily denying oneself some kind of gratification; in the area of alcohol or drug dependence, being without the substance on which the subject is dependent. The abstinence syndrome is equivalent to withdrawal symptoms and its appearance suggests the presence of physiologic dependence or addiction.

Abstinence syndrome Group of symptoms that occur when a person addicted to drug withdraws.

Abstract attitude (categorial attitude) Cognitive functioning that includes assuming a mental set voluntarily; shifting voluntarily from one aspect of a situation to another, keeping in mind simultaneously various aspects of a situation; grasping the essentials of a whole, breaking it into its parts and isolating them voluntarily; planning ahead; and/or thinking or performing symbolically. A characteristic of many psychiatric disorders is the inability to assume the abstract attitude or to shift readily from the concrete to the abstract and back again as demanded by circumstances.

Abstraction Teeth or other maxillary and mandibular structures to their normal position away from occlusal plane.

Abulia Lack of will or motivation, often expressed as inability to make decisions.

Abutment Teeth adjacent to an empty space in the mouth that will be used to support the prosthetic device that will fill the space.

Acanthor The stage in acanthocephalan life history that results from embryogenesis in the egg shells within the female worm, adapted for the infection of the intermediate host.

Acarines Represents their second most successfull group of terrestrial arthropods. These have two major body regions but are wingless and possess four pairs of walking appendages. Segmentation is indistinct.

Acceleration The rate of change of velocity with respect to time. Body acceleration has been defined as the rate of change of velocity of a point posterior to the sacrum. Acceleration is usually measured in meters per second per second (m/s^2).

Accelerometer A device used to measure the vertical, anterior-posterior, and medial-lateral accelerations of body segments.

Acceptability of medical care A measure of the patients' satisfaction with available medical care.

Access victims Individuals who offer support and human assistance to survivors and families of victims such as mental health professionals and nurses.

Accessibility of medical care The degree to which patients can receive care without undue geographic or financial obstacles.

Accessory Subordinate, attached or added for convenience.

Accessory atrioventricular tracts or bundles The fine terminal branches of the internodal tracts that are postulated to "bypass" the atrioventricular node; their existence and function are controversial.

Accessory fertilization cells In chaetognaths, paired somatic cells in the ovary to which eggs are attached and which sperm must pass through in order to fertilize the eggs.

Accessory fluid In arthropods, the liquid part of the ejaculate accom-panying and surrounding the spermatozoa or earlier develop-mental stages of sperm cells.

Accessory movement Movement within a joint and surrounding soft tissues that is necessary for normal range of motion but cannot be voluntarily performed.

Accessory organ An organ that assists other organs in accom-plishing their functions.

Accessory pigments Visible light-absorbing pigments carote-noids, xanthophyll, and phycobilins in plants and photosynthetic bacteria that complement chlorophylls in trapping energy from sunlight.

Accessory root canal A lateral branching of root canal usually occuring in apical third of root.

Accessory sex glands In males, a collective term for the prostate gland, the seminal vesicles, the bulbourethral glands, the vas deferens, and the epididymis.

Accessory teeth This is a tooth excess of normal complement. The term accessory is sometimes used for teeth that do not resemble the normal form whereas super-numerary is used for teeth that mimic the normal shape. An accessory tooth between the maxillary central incisors is called mesiodens, whereas one located to the arch is a peridens. An accessory tooth distal to the third molar is a distomolar and one located at buccal or lingual to the molar is a paramolar. These are more common in maxilla than mandible and most frequent sites are between the maxillary central incisor and distal to the molars.

Accident An unusual event or one that happens without known cause. In transportation, it means any out of course event that may cause injury to people or damage to property. Because many of these are predictable, they are increasingly referred to as incidents, crashes or collisions.

Accidental choking Choking is usually accidental. It occurs when food enters accidentally into larynx. Occasionally vomitus may be inhaled. Piece of meat or fish, false teeth may result in asphyxia. Suicidal choking is rare while homicidal choking as infanticide is common.

Accidental hemorrhage It is the bleeding from the site of a normally implanted placenta between 28th week of pregnancy and the birth of the baby.

Accidental hypothermia This may occur during intra-or extradural block or vascular surgery with massive blood transfusion. It can also occur in newborn and aged and secondary to myxoedema, hypo-pituitarism, adrenal failure, drug overdose, drowning and as a result of coma. Management includes warm water bath at 37°C, intra-venous fluid infusion, steroids and glucose.

Acclimatization Autonomic or behavioral changes occuring with in an organism that reduces the strain caused by stressful changes in the natural climate.

Accommodating resistance exercise A term used synonymously with isokinetic exercise.

Accommodation In a person with normal vision, the eye is so constituted that the parallel rays coming from distance beyond 6 metres are brought to focus on the retina. The near object emits divergent rays and obviously these rays cannot form a focus on the retina.

These divergent rays need convergence to form a focus on the retina. Accommodation is a phenomenon in which there is an increase in refractive power of lens due to increase in curvature of lens. Lens has a considerable degree of plasticity, i.e. it can mould in any shape.

Accountability of medical care The degree to which the health care system takes public responsibility for its actions.

This involves public representation on the board of directors of the health care facility, regular review of financial records by certified public accountants, and appropriate public disclosure of financial records and of quality of care studies.

Accracy The ability of a test to obtain the correct measure, on average.

Accretions Accumulation of foreign material such as mucinous plaque and calculus on teeth.

Acculturation Process by which a society is influenced culturally by another society.

Accurate empathy Communication technique used by nurse to show understanding of client's feelings and experiences.

ACE inhibitors These are the prime mode of therapy in heart failure with systolic dysfunction. These reduce afterload and ventricular filling pressure without affecting BP or heart rate. Cardiac output is significantly increased.

ACE inhibitors should not be given in bilateral renal artery stenosis. Potassium sparing diuretics should be used with caution during ACE inhibitor therapy. Nowadays mild heart failure is treated with ACE inhibitor displacing digoxin and diuretics.

Acebutolol It is beta-blocker used in hypertension and angina pectoris and in irregular heart beats. By reducing production of angiotensin it reduces constriction of blood vessels. Side effects include headache, dizziness and dry cough.

Acellular hyaline membrane A layer of nearly translucent material formerly eosinophilic that lines the bronchioles, alveolar ducts, and alveoli of premature infants with respiratory distress.

Acetabulum Shallow vinegar vessel or cup. Cup-shaped depression on the lateral surface of the coxa, where the head of the femur articulates.

Acetaminophen It is used to treat mild pain and fever. It does not cause stomach irritation or bleeding. Overdose and continuous use damage liver, otherwise it is much safer than aspirin.

Acetate A molecule that, when combined with choline, forms acetylcholine.

Acetazolamide It is a carbonic anhydrase inhibitor. It thus reduces the formation of aqueous humour. Tablets of 500 mg shall produce effect in two hours and effect lasts about six hours.

So it is to be repeated every 6 hours. It should be used for short term to control the intraocular pressure. It produces fatigue and tingling sensation of extremities.

Acetest A test that measures the presence of ketone bodies in the urine. A large quantity of acetone causes rapid change in the color of the Acetest tablet.

Acetogenesis The process of forming acetate by a linear combi-nation of two molecules of CO_2 or CO.

Acetogenic Of microorganisms, carrying out or capable of aceto-genesis.

Acetone Dimethyl ketone, a colourless, volatile, inflammable liquid, miscible with water useful as a solvent and having sweet, fruity, ethereal odour. Found in urine and blood in diabetes. Its presence indicates metabolic acidosis.

Acetone-butanol fermentation A bacterial fermentation carried out by certain sugar-metablozing species of Clostridium. The typical endproducts include acetone, n-butanol, and acetic acid.

Acetyl coenzyme A important intermediate byproduct in metabolism formed the breakdown of glucose, fatty acids, and certain amino acids.

Acetyl CoA Acetyl coenzyme A, formed by the combination of the two-carbon acetyl group with coenzyme A; the molecule that combines with a four-carbon molecule to enter the citric acid cycle.

Acetylcholine Chemical neuro-transmitter

Acetylcholinesterase An enzyme in the membrane of postsynaptic cells that catalyzes the conversion of Ach into choline and acetic acid. This enzymatic reaction inactivates the neurotransmitter.

Acetylsalicylic acid Aspirin was introduced in 1899. It is rapidly hydrolysed to salicylic acid in plasma. It has anti-inflammatory effect. Analgesic effect is mild, less than codeine because prostaglandin G/H synthase is readily regenerated. Aspirin is most effective against somatic as opposed to visceral origin. Its antiplatelet effect is due to permanent inactivation of prostaglandin G/H synthase in platelets. Being non-nucleated platelets cannot regenerate. Aspirin acts in hypothalamus and lowers the level of temperature. It does not affect temperature raised by exercise or heat and neither lowers normal temperature. Respiratory stimulation is characteristic of aspirin intoxication and occurs both by directly stimulating the respiratory centre and indirectly through increased CO_2 production. Aspirin relieves mild to moderate pain of non-visceral origin such as headache, dysmenorrhoea, osteoarthritis, myalgia and painful body metastases. Anti-inflammatory action is useful in rheumatoid arthritis and acute rheumatic fever. Side effects of aspirin includes heartburn, epigastric distress and vomiting.

It causes superficial gastric erosion and results in occult blood loss. A rapidly dispersing tablet which is swallowed as liquid is less likely to cause problem.

ACH index Arm, chest, hip index to assess status of nutrition.

Achalasia It is a disorder of oesophagal motility caused by degeneration of nerve cells in mysenteric plexus or vagal nuclei. It results in dysphagia and esophageal dilatation.

Achalasia cardia In this condition sphincter between oesophagus and stomach fail to relax and does not permit food to enter stomach. It results in difficulty and pain while swallowing and pain in lower chest. Barium swallow shows dilatation of barium above narrowing.

Achard's syndrome Clinical features include mandibulofacial dysostosis, skeletal anomalies, arachnodactyly, high arched palate and heart disease. Ocular symptoms include myopia, lens dislocation and spherophakia.

Achievement motive The desire to accomplish difficult tasks and overcome obstacles. More specifi-cally, when failure in a given task with attaining a certain standard set for himself or herself.

Achievement test A test which, as distinguished from aptitude and intelligence tests, measures what has been accomplished, as in mathe-matics, history, or French.

Achilles tendon Common tendon of the calf muscles that attaches to the heel (calcaneus); named after a mythical Greek warrior who was vulnerable only in the heel.

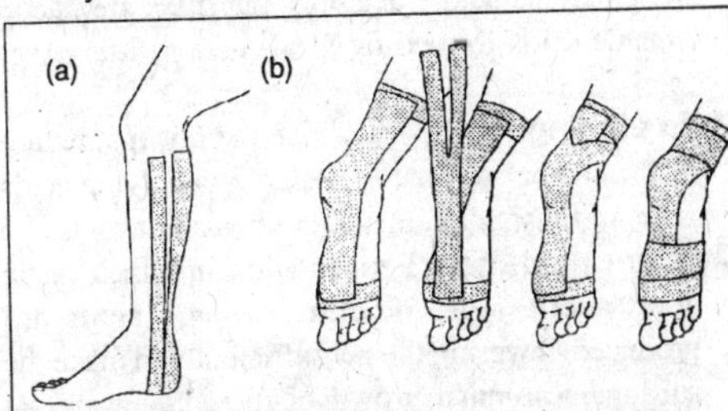

(a) Bandage for immobilization of foot, (b) bandages for support of Achilles

Achlorhydria There is an absence of normal acid secretion of stomach. It may be due to pernicious anaemia or chronic atrophic gastritis. Vitamin B_{12} may help.

Acholuric jaundice In it symp-toms may be absent and patient may go on doing work as usual. There is jaundice, weakness, anaemia or splenomegaly. Lately as jaundice deepens general malaise may be associated with fever. Gall stones composed of bile pigment may form. Red cells are small in diameter but more globular and are abnormally fragile. Constant leucocytosis is present. Colour of faeces is normal.

Achondroplasia Person is dwarf. Clinical features include osseous impingement upon cranial nerves, rhizomelic short stature, frontal bossing, depressed nasal bridge, relative mandibular prognathism, connective tissue dysplasia and hypotonia in infancy. Ocular features include strabismus, optic atrophy and hypermetropia.

Achylia gastrica A condition in which, secretion of gastric juice is diminished.

Acid A chemical substance which in aqueous solution undergoes dissociation with the formation of hydrogen ions; pH less than 7.0. It is a compound that releases hydrogen ions in solution and is of sour taste. Strong acids are corrosives causing burn to skin. Hydrochloric acid is a component of digestive juice and lactic acid is a breakdown product of glucose. Acid in stomach may produce epigastric pain getting relief on ingesting antacids. Any substance that is a proton donor; or any substance that releases hydrogen ions.

Acid dyspepsia It is due to causes which bring about directly or reflexly excessive secretion of gastric juice or retention with pyloric spasm. There may be nervous strain and worry. In achylia gastrica there may be acid eructations but these are due to organic acids formed by fermentation. It is never fatal.

Acid etching Process by which the prism structure of the enamel surface is altered by applying acids such as phosphoric, lactic, or chelating agents.

Acid fermentation Fermentation in which lactic acid, acetic acid, or other organic acids are produced, lowering the pH sufficiently to make the substrate resistant to growth of microorganisms that might otherwise spoil the food.

Acid forming foods Foods that have acid-ash residue after burning. Examples are meat, fish, cereal and some nuts.

Acid reflux There is regurgitation of acidic fluid from stomach into the oesophagus. There develops burning pain in chest which may be due to inflammation of oesophagus. Mild regurgitation takes place in pregnancy and in overweight people. It takes place due to inefficiency of muscular valve of lower end of oesophagus.

Acid resistance The ability of a microbial strain to exist for an extended period at pH values too acidic for growth, retaining the ability to be cultured after the acidity is neutralized.

Acid shock A sudden decrease of the pH level of a growth medium to a level of acidity at or below the limit for growth.

Acid-base equilibrium It is the balance between the amount of acidic and alkaline substances in the olood. Normally blood is slightly alkaline substance in blood. Plasma contains dissolved carbon dioxide which is acidic. Kidneys and lungs maintain this balance. Acidosis develops when respiration is impaired and lungs cannot remove sufficient CO_2 from blood.

Acidemia A condition of increased hydrogen ion concentration (decreased pH) in the blood.

Acid-etch technique Treatment of tooth enamel with an acid to produce a microscopic roughening by dissolving the top layer, exposing the enamel rods and prisms.

Acid-fast staining This method was discovered by Paul Ehrlich and modified by Ziehl and Neelsen. Tubercle bacilli and lepra bacilli when stained and heated, strong reagent resists decolourisation on subsequent treatment with dilute sulphuric acid are known as acid-fast bacilli. These bacilli are stained red.

Acidic corrosion The loss of elemental constituents to the adjacent environment as the result of the influence of a solution with a pH £ 7.0.

Acidic solution Solution with more hydrogen ions than hydroxide ions; has a pH of less than 7.

Acidifers Acids are used as flavour enhancing agent. As preservative these inhibit growth of micro-organisms and autoxidants to prevent discolouration or rancidity. Malic acid is used.

Acidogenic Acid-forming or producing.

Acidophile Literally acid lover an organism whose optimal external pH for growth is in the acidic range, generally below pH 6. Hyper-acidophiles may grow below pH-3.

Acidophilic Growing optimally in an acidic setting.

Acidophilus milk Milk fermen-ted by several bacteria such as lactobacillus acidophilus.

Acidosis In it there is accumulation of acid or loss of alkalies. In metabolic acidosis increased amount of acid is produced. Ketoacidosis occurs in uncontrolled diabetes mellitus, in starvation and diarrhoea. In kidney failure there is insufficient excretion of acid in urine.

Respiratory acidosis occurs when breathing fails to remove enough carbon dioxide from lungs causing increased blood acidity. Condition characterised by a lower than normal blood pH (pH of 7.35 or lower).

Acidosis in exercise Intense exercise of a short duration increases the lactate concentration in muscle and marked development of interacellular acidosis. It is considered responsible for muscle fatigue.

Acilitation The state of a nerve in which it is stimulated but not to the point of threshold, the point at which it transmits a nerve signal.

Acini Masses of cells in the pancreas that secrete digestive enzymes.

Acinic cell carcinoma This tumour occurs primarily in parotid gland and clinically resembles a benign neoplasm. Rarely lesions of minor salivary glands of the tongue, palate and floor of mouth may be seen. It usually occurs in third decade. Tumour is of low grade and may metastasise to regional lymph nodes. Distant metastases are rare.

Acitivity analysis The process of analyzing a given acitivity by breaking it down into its component parts.

ACLS Advanced cardiac life support; process that includes BLS, plus the use of adjunctive equipment to support ventilation, establishment of an IV fluid lifeline, drug administration, cardiac monitoring, defibrillation, control of cardiac arrhythmias, and postresuscitation care.

Acme The time of greatest intensity. In obstetrics, the period when the intensity of a contraction is at its height.

Acne Mostly occur in young people who are having oily skin. Inflammation of hair follicles and sebaceous glands results in acne vulgaris. Chemical acne is caused by exposure to certain chemicals and oils. Chloracne is a form of acne caused by exposure to chlorinated hydrocarbon chemicals.

Acne spots are caused by obstruction of the follicle and sebum. Corti-costeroids and androgens, barbiturates increase incidence of acne. As one spot heals others tend to appear. Healing spots fade and form a pink mark. In some cases acne appears as small, depressed pits while in some keloid may form. Retinoids help because these reduce oil production. Proper wash and hygiene helps.

Aconite Its roots are stout and dark and contain maximum poison. It has sweetish taste. It is used to enhance the intoxication properties of alcoholic liquors and is used by addicts. Clinical manifestations develop within an hour. Ingestion produces a feeling of warmth in mouth changing into prickly sensations extending to skin. There is salivation and muscle weakness. Intelligence and pupils are not affected till death. Heart becomes slow and irregular. Large doses may produce arrhythmias.

Acosta's syndrome Cause is cerebral hypoxia at high altitude. There will be restlessness and irritability, headache, impaired judgement at 1500 feet, confusion, cyanosis, muscular incoordination and possible loss of consciousness at 18,000 to 20,000 feet. Ocular features include blurred vision, difficulties in colour discrimination, impaired light adaptation, retinal haemorrhage. In chronic cases there will be lid oedema, bluish colouration of sclera and decreased visual acuity.

Acoustic beam The beam of ultrasound produced by probe.

Acoustic enhancement The increased echogenicity of tissues that lie behind a structure which causes little or no attenuation such as fluid-filled cyst.

Acoustic microscopy It is the use of ultra high-frequency ultrasound to produce images of biological structures with a resolution approaching that of light microscopy. Ultrasound frequency of 10 MHz to 2GHz is used. It has a transmitting and receiving ultrasound transducer. The specimen is placed between the two transducers. The specimen areas of 250 mm are scanned in about one second with highly focused ultrasound. The pixel size in final image is 1 mm.

Acoustic nerve neuroma This is called auditory nerve tumour and is part of vestibular nerve, concerned with hearing. These tumours develop between the age of 40 and 60 years. It can cause deafness and noises in ear, loss of balance and pain in affected ear. Enlarging tumour can press cerebellum and cause ataxia. MRI is a good diagnostic tool and surgical resection is the treatment.

Acoustic shadowing The decreased echogenicity lying behind structure. It is equal to the product of density of tissue and speed of ultrasound.

Acoustic window A tissue that offers little obstruction to ultrasound waves. It can be used as a route to obtain images of a deeper structure.

Acquintance rape Rape invol-ving a perpetrator who is known to victim.

Acquired A disorder which develops after birth at any time.

Acquired characteristics Those obtained after birth, as a result of environment.

Acquired drive Any learned rather than interited predisposition to behave in a certain manner.

Acquired dylexia A lesion in the dominant angular gyrus. It results in inability to comprehend written symbols. It is often associated with posterior aphasia.

Acquired dyslexia Difficulty in reading caused by postnatal damage to brain.

Acquired immunity Immunity that is obtained after birth through the use of injections or exposure to a harmful agent.

Acquired lymphoedema It is due to obstruction, due to removal of axillary lymphatics as in radical mastectomy. Repeated acute infection and chronic infection of cervix, uterus and filariasis may also result it.

Acquired motives Motivation which is not inborn in the organism. For example, the desire for a certain set of golf clubs or to receive a passing grade in school. Also called secondary motivation.

Acquisition In learning, the process by which an association is formed in classical or operant conditioning; in memory, the stage at which information is stored in memory.

Acquisition time The time taken to acquire single or multiple cross-sections in cross-sectional imaging modalities. The acquisition time T is intimately linked to the spatial resolution of image characterised by voxel size V. The quantitative formula states that S/N ratio is proportional to V and square root of T.

Acrasy Pathological absance of self control.

Acrocinesia Escessive monements as seen in hysteria.

Acrocyanosis Cyanosis of the extremities, especially of the hands and feet, seen in the newborn for the first few hours after birth.

Acrocynosis Bluish discolouration of hands and feets due to reduced peripheral circulation.

Acrodermatitis chronica atrophicans It is a rare familial skin disorder, occurs in infants and zinc deficiency is found. There develops vesiculobullous eruption around body orifices, skin of knees, elbows and paronychial areas. There will be complete alopecia, ocular features include scarring of conjunctiva, recurrent iridocyclitis, photophobia, blepharitis and corneal opacification.

Acrodermatitis enteropathica It is an inherited recessive disorder which presents in infancy as an erythematous eruption with vesicles, pustules and crusting. It affects particulary the skin around the mouth and anogenital region, fingers and scalp. Diarrhoea and alopecia occur. It is due to zinc deficiency.

Acrodynia A disease of children in which manifestations occur at the time of eruption of teeth. Syndrome includes superficial sensory loss, photophobia muscular hypotonia, periodontitis.

Acrodysostosis Onset is prenatal. There develops growth deficiency. Middle ear infection results brachycephaly, flat nasal bridge, hypoplastic maxilla, shortness of extremities are more pronounced. Mental deficiency and hypogonadism are found. Deformities are slow progressing.

Acrohypothermy Abnormal coolness of skin of extremities found in certain patients of schizophrenia.

Acromania Violent incurable insanity.

Acromegaly It is caused by excessive secretion of growth hormone from anterior pituitary gland. It includes enlargement of hands, specially fingers, feet, coarsening of facial features, enlargement of ears and nose. Face becomes longer. Voice becomes husky. There may be headache and visual disturbances.

Acromicria A body type earth amall head and limbs than rest of body.

Acromioclavicular ligament It is injured in collision sports. Grade I involves disruption on only

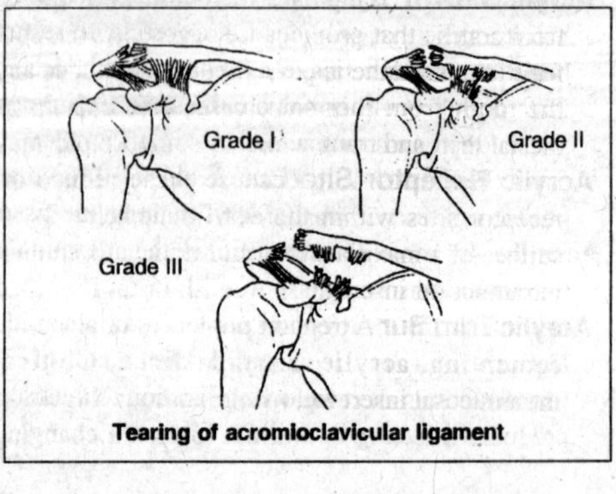

Tearing of acromioclavicular ligament

the capsular ligament of joint. There is sharp local pain. Grade II injury involves complete capsular disruption and partial tearing. Pain is severe and movements are restricted. Total rupture of coracoclavicular ligament signifies a grade III injury.

Acro-osteolysis syndrome It is a hereditary disorder with autosomal involvement. Clinical features include abnormal nails, corneal opacities, skin xanthoma, sub-cutaneous nodules and nephropathy.

Acroparaesthesia It is known as nocturnal arm dysaesthesia also. Paraesthesia, anaesthesia pain in arm while lying on bed. Muscles innervated by ulnar nerve are mostly affected. Numbness also develops. It always affects the dominant arm. In the morning hand becomes stiff and can be used properly once it is massaged.

Acrophobia Fear of heights.

Acroscentism Deprivation.

Acrosclerosis Scleroderma which affect extremities, head, face associated with Raynaud's phenomenon. There may be significant thickening of periodontal membrane.

Acrosome A dense lysosome-like body in the head of a sperm cell that contains enzymes that facilitate the penetration of a sperm cell into a secondary oocyte.

Acrosome reaction An exocytotic event that is an absolute pre-requisite to successful fertilization and that occurs following sperm binding to the zona pellucida of the egg.

Acrylic These are used as provisional crown and bridge resins. The powder is composed of small beads of PMMA polymer with small amounts of peroxide initiator and oxide particles as pigments.

Acrylic crown Temporary restoration constructed from acrylic that provides full coverage to restore function and esthetics to a prepared tooth, protect the tooth from thermal changes, and eliminate mesial drift and trauma.

Acrylic Receptor Site Bur A bur used to create receptor sites within the acrylic along the tissue surface of a maxillary denture for the affixation of intramucosal inserts.

Acrylic Trim Bur A trephine bur that removes excess cementing acrylic around the base of an intramucosal insert following fixation to the tissue surface of a maxillary denture.

Acta Official acts or recorded proceedings of a scientific group or organization.

Actatic Not cordinated.

Actatic speech Uncordinated verbal communication, noticeable gaps between words are seen.

ACTH Adrenocorticotropic hormone is produced by anterior part of pituitary gland. It stimulates adrenal cortex to produce other hormones too. Its production is controlled by hypothalamus. ACTH level increases in response to stress, emotion, injury, infection, burns and decrease in blood pressure. Tumour of pituitary gland causes excess of ACTH production resulting in Cushing's syndrome. ACTH is used to treat inflammatory disorders such as arthritis, ulcerative colitis and severe hepatitis. In multiple sclerosis also it has been used.

Actin A protein making up the thin filments of muscle; also an important component of the cytoskeleton of many eukaryotic cells.

Actin myofilament One of the two major kinds of protein fibres that make up a sarcomere; thin filaments resemble two minute strands of pearls twisted together.

Acting out Expressions of unconscious emotional conflicts or feelings in actions rather than words. The person is not consciously aware of the meaning of such acts. Acting out may be harmful or, in controlled situations, therapeutic (e.g. children's play therapy). Refers especially to acting out of transference wishes and emotions.

Actinic These are changes caused by ultraviolet rays in sunlight due to over exposure. It results in thickening of skin with roughness.

Actinic cheilosis It is a premalignant lesion of the lips that occurs almost exclusively on the lower lip. It may be due to radiation from sun. The typical early lesions are filmy white or even striated. Continued exposure may result tissues slightly elevated, crusted or red and ulcerated. Lesion may be localised or whole of lip may be involved.

Actinic rays Radiant energy of short wave visible and of the ultra violent region of spectrum.

Actinomycetes Widespread gram-positive bacteria that ranges morphologically from cocci-like fragments to mycelium which may form complex spore structures.

Actinomycosis This is caused by actinomyces bacteria. These becteria resemble fungi and affects mouth and jaw. It develops painful swelling over jaw. Yellow openings discharge yellow pus granules. It results due to poor dental hygiene. In women when pelvis is involved it may result in abdominal pain, fever, and in between menstrual bleeding. Penicillin is an effective treatment. It is a noncommunicable chronic suppurative disease caused by filamentous bacteria found in normal flora of mouth. Condition produces abscess formation with central necrosis surrounded by granulation tissue and fibrous tissue. Pus of the lesion contains sulphur granules. The swelling develops slowly, becomes fluctuating, points to the surface and finally breaks down to form chronic sinus with little tendency of healing. There may be large woody swelling, procaine penicillin G is useful.

Actinomycosis, liver It may be mistaken for abscess of liver and starts as one or more foci in the liver substance which slowly enlarges and undergo suppuration. Liver enlarges uniformly, then becomes prominent at one place. It responds to penicillin.

Action Potential nerve impulse.

Action cue Non verbal communication that consist of body momements, such as nodding of head to agree.

Action patterns Relatively stableand predictable ways of behaving.

Action potential A rapid change in electrical charges across a neuron's cell membrane, with depolarization followed by repolarization, leading to a nerve impulse moving down an axon; associated with nerve and muscle activity.

Action therapy Behaviour modification therapy.

Activating effect of hormones The actions of hormones on cells in the adult organism that usually last only while the hormone is present.

Activation It is the process of inducing radiopacity by irradiation. All radionuclides used in nuclear imaging are produced by activation or if radionuclide products are parent nuclide is produced by activation.

Activation energy Energy required to initiate a chemical reaction. Activation energy is less for mixture with O_2 than with air.

Activation gate The manner in which flux is controlled through an ionic channel in a cell membrane; as the membrane potential becomes less negative, this "gate" opens, allowing ions to pass along the channel,

Activator Acatalyst.

Activators These increase the activity of a complete enzyme (protein + co-enzyme). In the absence of activator enzyme may be inactive or sluggish. Activators are usually inorganic ions. Typical activating ions are 'cl' for ptylin, 'Mg' for plasma phosphatase and 'Ca' for thrombase. Activators which are enzymes are called kinases.

Active acquired immunity It is the resistance developed by an individual as a result of an antigenic stimulus and this involves the active involvement of the person's own immune apparatus leading to synthesis of antibodies. Active immunity appears only after a latent period. In whooping cough, measles and mumps the immunity is long lasting.

Active algolagnia Sadism

Active assisted movement Movement of a joint in which both the client and the therapist produce the motion.

Active avoidance To learn to perform spatial motor patterns in order to avoid deleterious consequences of stressors such as painful foot.

Active cycle of breathing A series of maneuvers performed by the patient to clear secretions and increases thoracic expansion.

Active euthanasia Absisted suicide.

Active exercise Therapeutic activity performed independently.

Active insufficiency The inability of a two-joint. or multi-joint muscle to generate an effective force when placed in a fully shortened position. The same meaning is implied by the expression "the muscle has been put on a slack."

Active joint movement Movement of a joint through its range of movement by the patient.

Active listening Understanding another person by watching, as well as listening. Empathising, nodding and sending other signals that one is listening.

Active memory Short term memory.

Active negativism Resistamce to demands.

Active phase of delivery It starts when patient reaches 3 cm dilatation and is completed when it is fully dilated. Total duration of labour in primigravida is 12 hours while in multigravide it is 7 hours. Primigravida progresses 1.5 cm/hour during active phase while in multigravida it progresses more than 2 cms/hour.

Active range of motion The amount of joint motion obtained with unassisted voluntary joint motion.

Active resistive movement Movement of a joint by the client against resistance provided by the therapist.

Active site The region of an enzyme surface that binds the substrate molecule and catalytically transforms it; also known as the catalytic site.

Active surveillance Occurs when public health officials initiate contact with physicians, laboratories, or hospitals to obtain information about diseases of nterest.

Active touch The perception of objects by touching them.

Active transport The movement of materials across a cell membrane from low to high concentration in combination with membrane-bound carrier molecules and requiring a source of energy.

Active vitamin D Fat-soluble vitamin produced from precursor molecules in skin exposed to ultraviolet light; increases calcium and phosphate uptake from the intestines.

Active zone Site of release of neurotransmitter through the presynaptic membrane.

Activin A protein hormone produced widely with effects on development, the pituitary, gonads, and other organs.

Activist movements Fromation of groups in support of or opposition to social or political policies.

Aotivity coefficient The factor by which the numerical value of the concentration of a solute must be multiplied to give its true thermodynamic activity.

Activity configuration The process of selecting specific activities to use during intervention.

Activity group A group of people engaged in a common acitivity or task.

Activity program A planned program of activities intended to promote the general health and well-being of residents in long-term care facilities.

Activity quotient Measure of person's emotionality as determined by the ratio of verbs to adjectives the perosn uses while communicating.

Activity tolerance Kind and amount of exercise or work that a person is able to perform.

Actone A specific action.

Actual diagnosis Problem that currently exists.

Actual self The totality of self at any instant in time including unconcious elements.

Actualising tendency According to the person-centred approach to personality, an inborn human tendency to develop and use all our capabilities to the fullest degree possible.

Actuarial method of life table analysis A method of life table analysis in which proportionate survival is assessed at fixed intervals, such as months, that have been established prior to data accrual. See also Life table analysis.

Acuity Sharpness or clearness, especially of the special senses.

Acuity charting Documentation that quantifies the level of care required by a client in health care setting.

Acupressure It uses manual pressure to stimulate the energy points on the body. Therapist applies light or medium pressure with fingers to the same points used in acupuncture. Aim is to stimulate the body's electromagnetic energy to assist body's own recuperative powers to remove energy blockages. These blockage may be the result of build up of lactic acid and carbon monoxide in muscle tissue causing musculature to stiffen, putting pressures on nervous and circulatory system. Removal of blockage relaxes the whole body and restore harmony of systems.

Acupuncture It is a branch of Chinese system in which needles are inserted into patient's skin to treat diseases and give effective anaesthesia. Chinese think that life force flows through the body along meridians. Blockage of one or more meridians causes disease. Doctors aim to restore health by inserting needles at specific sites. These are specific acupressure and acupuncture points. Acupuncture causes release of endorphins which act as natural analgesics within nerves. Acupuncture has shown successful results in dental surgery and during labour. Arthritis responds favourably. There are 14 meridian lines, each considered to affect a particular part of body and each meridian has many acupuncture points. Treatment depends on temperature of needle used, angle of insertion,

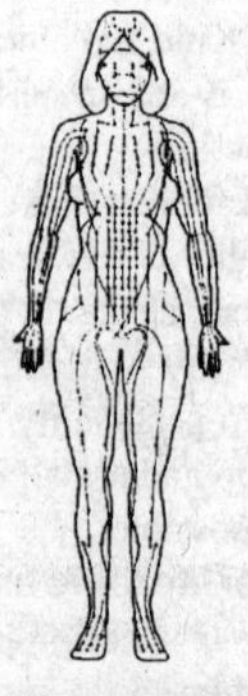

Basic meridians acupuncture points

twisting or vibration of needle while inserted, speed of insertion, withdrawal and length of time for which needle is to be left in body. On some occasions symptoms may increase temporarily.

Acupuncture anesthesia Pain relief derived by the insertion and tursting of needles in various parts of body.

Acure rosaçea An excessive flushing of blood vessels in nose and check. Nervous factor and drinking alcohol may encourage the reflex.

Acusector An electric needle used like a scalpel in dividing tissues.

Acute Having rapid onset, short, severe course, and pronounced symptoms; opposite of chronic.

Acute anaemia It develops when considerable amount of blood is lost. Loss of one and half litre of blood at once may be dangerous. Woman sustains blood loss more easily than man. Loss of 250 ml below the age of one year is very serious. In acute anaemia victim complains of general malaise, thirst, giddiness and everything dark in front of eyes. Skin and mucous membrane of lips and eyelids become pale, eyes become shunken, yawning begins and cold sweats break out. Pulse becomes faster. External bleeding must be stopped early. Foot end is to be raised.

Acute and conclescent sera Acute sera are the first serum samples collected soon after symptoms of an infectious disease occur. Convalescent sera are follow-up samples collected after a period of time that is sufficient to allow for antibody titers to rise. A significant increase in the titers is taken as proof of recent infection.

Acute antibiotic stomatitis It can follow over use or topical use of antibiotics speically tetracycline suppressing normal competing oral flora. Clinically whole mucosa is sore and red. Topical antifungal treatment increases it.

Acute anxiety attact A sudden feeling of morbid dread and apprehension stimulated by a threatening position.

Acute appendicitis Chief symptom is pain, coming on acutely, first referred to umbilicus or epigastrium and later becoming localised to right iliac fossa. Vomiting may be urgent. There will be tenderness, rigidity and later a local swelling. There may be deep tenderness on palpation well marked at McBurney's point. There is rigidity or guarding of the muscle.

The pulse becomes quick and thready. Temperature is low. There is no rigor. Fever often falls and pain goes with the onset of gangrene or with spreading peritonitis. Pulse remains rapid. Tongue is always coated. Constipation is usually present. Urine is scanty. Leucocytosis develops.

Acute bronchiolitis Children are usually affected. Disease starts with coryza and may come at height of measles and whooping cough. There may be cough, severe breathlessness and hurried respiration. Central cyanosis, toxaemia, restlessness, insomnia and pallor are present.

Acute bronchitis It is the inflammation of bronchial tree caused by various organisms. Predisposing factors are whooping cough, common cold without expectoration or with mucoid or mucopurulent product. Fever is not a constant feature.

Acute care Health services provided to an individual whose illness has had a sudden onset with short but severe course.

Acute caseous pneumonia It is more common in children than in adults.It is caused by rupture of caseating TB focus into bronchus. This sets up tuberculous lobar pneumonia. Fever does not respond to penicillin. Physical signs cavity of breaking down in lung, purulent expectoration, night sweats, haemoptysis and finding TB bacilli in sputum.

Acute coryza It is common in temperate climate. First complaint is of sore throat and stuffiness in nose. A steadily increasing mucoid catarrhal secretion develops in nose within 24 hours. This becomes mucopurulent. Temperature rises to 99 to 100°F.

Acute delirious mania It may develop acutely. It is attended by pyrexia, usually running a fatal course. There may be outbreaks of great violence and refusal of food. Temperature ranges irrgularly from 100 to 104°F.

Acute distress order A mental disorder involving anxiety, dissociation and reexperiencing that leads to clearly impaired functioning arising after exposure to traumatic stressor in a month time frame.

Acute dry pericarditis Pain may be related to respiration, coughing and sneezing. Pain may be like myocardial infarction. Fever of low grade is usually present. Sometimes pericardial rub may be palpable on auscultation. Pericardial friction sound may be audible. Pericardial friction is of to and fro character. SGOT and LDH may be elevated.

Acute exercise A single session or bout of exercise.

Acute fatty liver of pregnancy Large doses of tetracycline 2.4 to 4 gm/day given I.V. have been reported to cause fatty liver of pregnancy.

Acute glomerulonephritis It is a terminal stage developing from membranous glomerulonephritis. The kidneys become granular and contracted from which capsule strips off with difficulty. Polyurea is due to less tubular reabsorption, high blood urea level acting as diuretic. Person will develop anorexia, weakness, palpitation and dimness of vision. Anaemia is present. Blood pressure (BP) becomes high and ophthalmoscopic examination may show papilloedema. Urine quantity is 3 litre in 24 hours. Specific gravity is low and fixed at 1010. Albuminuria is intermittent or absent. Blood urea is high and renal function test is impaired.

Acute haemorrhagic pancreatitis There develops haemorrhagic necrosis of pancreas, escape of pancreatic enzymes and formation of plaques of fat necrosis. 50 per cent cases have diseases of biliary tract. Exact cause is not clear. Onset is sudden and may occur during an alcoholic bout. There will be severe and persistent pain in epigastrium and left upper abdomen which is relieved by leaning forward. Pain is severe in first 24 hours and then passes off gradually. Patient looks severely ill. BP is low. Extremities are cold, sweating is present. Temperature is subnormal. It may be rarely high. Jaundice may be present. Serum amylase level is raised within 12 hours and remains raised for 3 to 5 days. Amylase is also present in ascitic fluid. Blood sugar level may be high. Ultrasound is a good tool of examination.

Acute herpetic conjunctivitis It occurs as a primary manifestation of herpes. It usually affects children who are infected by carriers of the virus. There will be large follicles on conjunctiva, preauricular adenopathy and reduced corneal sensation. Treatment is by application of acyclovir ophthalmic ointment six times a day.

Acute herpetic gingivostomatitis Inflammation of the gingivae and oral mucosa caused by the invasion of the herpes virus. Distinguished by red and swollen gingivae, red temperature. Common in childhood; duration about 14 days.

Acute illness One that comes on suddenly and lasts a short time.

Acute illness pattern The temporary alteration of daily routines to deal with the crisis of acute diseases and injuries, such as communicable diseases, bone fractures, and appendicitis. After disease treatment, families usually return to predisease family routines.

Acute intoxication, alcohol The rapid cousumption of large quantities of alcohol produces the syndrome of drunkenness, slurring of speech, unsteadiness, poor motor coordination, nystagmus and depression. Person who drinks daily develops some tolerance.

Acute intussusception Person gets a fit of screaming. There will be a curved sausage-shaped lump in line of colon with its concavity directed towards the umbilicus. Lump may not be felt when it is lying under costal margin. Child should be examined between two screaming, otherwise rigidity of abdomen muscles will be there. The *signe de dance*—a feeling of emptiness in right iliac fossa is usually of poor help. Barium enema will show pine-like peak.

Acute laryngitis Symptoms include disturbing rough feeling and dryness in the larynx. There will be dry cough and patient will develop habit of throat clearing. Hoarseness will increase, vocal cords appear red and sometimes swollen and cord adductions may be incomplete.

Acute leukaemia It may begin suddenly and adopts a rapid course in a few weeks or months. In the beginning there may be a leukaemic phase but later blood cells count become very high. There is anaemia and thrombocytopenia. Oral lesions are most constant finding in acute leukaemia. Enlargement, bleeding and necrosis of gingiva, bleeding and oozing of blood around teeth is seen. There may be ecchymosis and necrosis of oral mucosa. Tooth extraction is followed by profuse bleeding. The peripheral blood shows very high number of cells.

Acute leukemia and pregnancy It is a rapidly progressive fatal disease. Woman develops fever, easy fatigue, abnormal leukocytosis resembling acute infectious disease. There may be bleeding diathesis. There is characteristic immaturity and increased number of leukocytosis. Anemia and young red cells are present in peripheral blood. Thrombocytopenia is also characteristic. Pregnancy does not affect the course of leukemia. Chemotherapy is to be given.

Acute liver abscess Solitary or multiple collections may occur in liver. Onset is acute with pain and tenderness of liver accompanied by dry cough, shallow respiration and digestive disturbance. Pain is affected by respiration and when patient lies on left side. Liver is enlarged and enlargement may extend downwards. There may be fluctuation. Jaundice is rarely present. There will be high fever, rigors and sweating. Constitutional symptoms are severe.

Acute lupus erythematosus Acute form of LE usually occurs in young females. It is characterised by red oedematous macules, papules, vesicle and bullae over molar areas. There will be fever, leucopenia and splenomegaly. LE cells are seen. These are large circular, homogeneous basophilic inclusions probably a leucocyte, seen within a neutrophil. LE test is positive in 80% cases. Oral lesions may precede or follow skin lesions and are seen in 25% cases. These consist of multiple white plaques with dark reddish purple margin and may clinically resemble leucoplakia. In some patients ulceration of plaques may occur.

Acute lymphangitis It occurs when infection commonly by *Streptococcus pyogenes* spreads beyond a point of infection to the group of draining lymph nodes. There an abscess may form. Infection may bypass one group to another higher group at higher level of glands. It is seen as red blushes and streaks in skin corresponding to inflamed lymphatics. Elevation of limb with cloxacillin helps the patient.

Acute mastitis in pregnancy Infection occurs through cracked nipple. There will be fever with chill. Marked engorgement of breast appears before the onset of acute mastitis. Clinical features seldom appear before one week of puerperium. Full symptoms appear in 3-4th week after delivery.

Acute melancholia There is more marked psychomotor retardation. There is more profound misery. Delusional ideas are marked. Patient thinks they are most wicked individuals. Hypochondrial ideas are also prominent. Auditory hallucinations may be prominent. Food is refused and insomnia is marked.

Acute necrotising haemorrhagic encephalomyelitis It is an acute disease with extensive destruction and liquefaction of cerebral white matter accompanied by multiple small haemorrhages. There is myelin loss with dominant polymorphonuclear cell infiltration. Neurological signs are frequently unilateral. Clinical picture resembles encephalitis, bacterial cerebritis or brain abscess.

Acute necrotising ulcerative gingivitis ANUG is commonly referred as Vincent's gingivitis. The causative organisms are not known. However, spirochaetes are present in large number of cases. It has correlation with stress, smoking and poor oral hygiene. Patient has fever, cervical lymphadenopathy, malaise, swollen, red painful gingiva and necrosis of interdental papillae. Ulcerated area is covered by pseudomembrane. Patient has fetid breath. Treatment consists of rest, fluid, aspirin and debridement of area with hand scalers or an ultrasonic device.

Acute necrotising ulcerative gingivo-periodontitis This is also a very rare form of periodontal disease that is associated with repeated long-term episodes of acute necrotising ulcerative gingivitis. It is characterised by formation of deep intradental craters in some or all areas of mouth. Periods of exacerbation occur during which greyish pseudomembranes made up of necrotic tissue and bacteria form in the affected region and breath becomes fetid. Treatment consists of local therapy and tetracylines.

Acute nephritic syndrome It is a glomerulonephropathy associated with bilateral inflammation of kidney and usually presents with hypertension, heavy cellular exudate in urine, oedema and oliguria. It occurs most commonly as an immune reaction, after viral infection. There develops swelling of face particularly the eyelids and gradually whole body specially in early morning. Face is most commonly involved. Fever is of low grade. There is pain in abdomen. BP is raised in 50% cases. Heart may be mildly dilated and urine shows leucocytosis, amount is 300 to 600 cc in 24 hours. Specific gravity is high. Albumin is present and urea is raised. Also antibody titre in serum is raised. Recovery occurs in 80% cases. As complication hypertensive left ventricular failure may develop.

Acute noise trauma Hearing loss is noticed immediately after sensational noise exposure. It tends to improve markedly in hours or days. Hearing loss is symmetric but may be milder on the side away from noise source. There may develop tinnitus.

Acute nonspecific lymphadenitis It occurs most frequently in cervical area in association with infections of teeth or tonsils, when generalised it is characteristic of viral infection and bacteraemia. Microscopically the nodes become swollen, grey-red and engorged. Affected nodes are tender and when abscess formation is extensive become fluctuant. The overlying skin is frequently red and penetration or perforation of infection to the skin may produce draining sinuses. After treatment scar may remain.

Acute oral oedema Acute circumscribed oedema of oral tissue including the lips, palate, tongue and larynx can cause alarming symptoms. It may become life-threatening when it involves larynx. There will be massive paroxysmal oedematous swelling of oral mucosa and may involve lips. Burning pain or occasional itching may precede the oedema. Boundaries of oedema are ill defined.

Acute ouset Sudden occurence of a disorder.

Acute pain Discomfort that is of short duration.

Acute pancreatitis Acute pancreatitis is sudden causing substantial damage to the parenchyma. The triggering cause of acute pancreatitis is usually unknown. The mechanism seems to be that pancreatic enzymes, particulary lipases and elastase are activated and are toxic themselves or give rise to toxic compounds which cause destruction of parenchyma of gland. Biliary tract disease and alcohol are the common cause. Outstanding clinical feature is abdominal pain, the severity of which may be anything from mild to devastating. Pain is in epigastrium and may radiate to back, to the left shoulder tip or to the lower abdomen. In severe case pain may last for hours and days. Nausea and vomiting follow. Haematemesis is not uncommon. It may be due to erosive gastritis or duodenitis. There may be fever and dyspnoea and delirium, confusion or even coma. There is tenderness and rigidity. In severe attacks of haemorrhagic pancreatitis there may be discolouration around the umbilicus or in the flank. Serum amylase is raised. There may be transient hyperglycaemia.

Acute pancreatitis and pregnancy It is an uncommon complication of pregnancy and is seen in third trimester. Use of chlorthiazide for the control of oedema may cause. Chlorthiazide has been linked to fatal pancreatitis in pregnancy. Upper abdominal pain, nausea and vomiting, abdominal distension with absent bowel sound and low fever are clinical features. There is freqeuncy of dyspeptic disorder in pregnancy.

Acute pulpitis It results from heat and cold associated with deep or extensive fillings, sudden severe physical trauma, chemical injury such as application of irritants to exposed dentin and bacterial invasion such as seen in deep carious lesions. In rare cases inflammation of pulp may follow. Clinically there is severe pain which arises from throbbing type to intermittent attacks. Severity of pain changes when patient is lying down and with change of temperature. Products of inflammation and pressure act on nerve endings to produce pain. Microscopically pulpitis is characterised by oedema and moderate to dense infiltration by neutrophils. Area appears as space surrounded by neutrophils. Treatment includes removal of cause, pulp capping or root canal treatment. The cracked tooth syndrome is a condition in which pulpitis results from a crack in the tooth. Patients complain of ill-defined pain. Although crack in crown is invisible but it extends to the pulp and saliva and organism.

Acute pyelonephritis This is an acute inflammation of pelvis of ureter and adjoining part of renal parenchyma. *B. coli* infection is the most common cause. There will be frequency of micturition due to cystitis. Fever comes with chill and rigor. Pain in loin is due to stretching of renal capsule. Burning sensation develops during micturition. There is marked reduction in urine volume. Temperature is raised and renal angle becomes tender. There develops leucocytosis. Urine is turbid with flesh odour. Albumin is present in small amount. Microscopically pus cells are plenty, RBCs are moderate, epithelial cells are in moderate quantity.

Acute recurrent gingivitis It is a rare type of self-limiting, recurrent, painful gingivitis that involves interdental papilla. Regional lymphadenopathy is present and lesions spread to adjacent marginal and papillary areas. Ulceration is absent and there is no pseudomembrane formation or interdental cratering. Oral hygiene is gènerally good and lesion resolves in 10 days. It is related to stress.

Acute rejection Presence of preformed antibodies or infiltrates of mononuclear cells leading to myocyte necrosis in a transplanted organ.

Acute renal failure It indicates a clinicopathological condition which results when renal excretory function is temporarily lost due to renal tubular degeneration by renal ischaemia or toxic agents. It is mainly a complication due to hypotension resulting in renal arteriolar constriction leading to tubular necrosis. Incompatible blood transfusion, haemolytic crisis and severe infection may cause it. In oliguric phase urine volume is very scanty and contains RBC, epithelial cells and dirty brown granular cast. Specific gravity is 1010 to 1016. Gradually patient develops anorexia, vomiting, drowsiness, mental confusion, twitching and bleeding. It lasts for 1 to 3 weeks. ECG shows evidence of hyperpotassaemia. Hypertension frequently develops and may give rise to heart failure and encephalopathy. In polyuric phase mineral and salts are heavily wasted in urine. Urine specific gravity is low. Blood urea nitrogen (BUN) levels are high. Serum sodium, chloride and potassium levels become low. Patient is dehydrated soon.

Acute renal failure in pregnancy It is the gravest complication in pregnancy. It is found as acute renal failure in early pregnancy as in septic abortion and acute renal failure; in late pregnancy as in fatal cases of abruptio placentae, toxaemia of pregnancy and those complicated with severe infection.

Acute stress Changes in physiology and behavior that occurs during shortly after exposure to a stressor.

Acute stress reaction A severe emotional response to extreme environmental stress.

Acute toxic confusional psychosis Patient becomes confused with rise in temperature and state of muttering delirium. Complexion becomes pale and muddy with malar flush. Mouth and tongue become dirty and there is sores on the lips.

Acute transverse myelopathy In this condition a flaccid paralysis and sensory loss ascend from the feet to the midthoracic region or higher. There is spinal pain. It may develop as a manifestation of carcinoma of bronchus. Many are left with permanent residual deficit. MRI may be done to exclude an acute compressive lesion. Cord may appear swollen. CSF contains an excess of lymphocytes.

Acute tubular insufficiency There develops oliguria of variable degree, person develops anorexia, nausea, vomiting and dry mouth. In acute phase large oedematous kidney develops. Nephrotoxins, antipyretics and haemolytic crisis may cause. Specific gravity of urine will be lesser than 1020. Renal failure index is more than 2 or 3.

Acute tubular necrosis Sudden severe injury to renal tubule cells. Often resulting from transient hypoperfusion.

Acutenaculum An instrument for holding a surgical needle; a needle holder.

Acyclovir It is the drug used in the treatment of virus causing herpes simplex and herpes zoster. It reduces severity of infection. It may result in irritation or rash when used locally. When taken orally headache and dizziness may result.

Ad Lib At pleasure, as desired.

Adamite Obsolete term for a nudist.

Adaptability Capacity to make appropriate responses to changed or changing situation.

Adaptation Manner in which an organism responds to change.

Adaptation adjustment Sensory adaptation involves a change in the characteristics of experience as a result of prior stimulation, as when we gradually see more clearly in a darkened room or taste something as especially sour after eating sweets. Additive effect in a multifactor study, when the influence of all the factors together is the same as the sum of their separate influences. There are no interactions.

Adaptation syndrone The physiological changes that may occur in organism as a result of stress, exhaustion or mass be death.

Adaption time The time from the start of stimulus throngh the end of the effect in the sense organ stimulated.

Adaptive behavior scale A questionmark containing 242 items to be answered by parents and other adults about mental defectives to make care of themselves.

Adaptive family health model In this model, families are adaptive if they have the ability to change and grow and possess the capacity to rebound quickly after crisis.

Adaptive immunity Immune system response in which there is an ability to recognise, remember, and destroy a specific antigen.

Adaptive reaction The adjustment of eyes to varying intensity of light.

Adaptive shortening Tightness that occurs as a result of a muscle remaining in a shortened position.

Adaptive thermogenesis Energy used by the body to adjust to changing physical and bialogical environments.

Addict Pathologically habituated to a substance or practice.

Addison's anaemia In adult type it develops due to lack of intrinsic factor necessary for absorption of vitamin B_{12} is associated with gastric atrophy and deficiency of many other gastric secretions. Skin becomes pallor, with yellowish hue, heart dilates. Tongue and gastric mucosa atrophy.

Addison's disease It results due to deficiency of corticosteroids. It may be caused by any disease which destroys adrenal cortex. Auto-immune disease and tuberculosis are the main cause. Disease has slow onset of years together. Symptoms include excessive loss of sodium and water in the urine, extreme muscle weakness, dehydration, hypotension, confusion and coma. In chronic form person feels tiredness, weakness, vague abdominal pain and weight loss. Regular doses of cortisone is the treatment.

Addition silicone These are known as polyvinglsiloxanes containing silicone polymers and many vinyl groups. These are supplied in 3 different form one is two-paste system and second is gun and cartridge system.

Adducted aphonia Loss of voice as a result of contracture of muscles that move the vocal cord.

Adduction Movement towards the axis of midline of the body.

Adductor A muscle causing movement toward the midline.

Adductor cushion (lateral knee block) An upholstered block or pad placed on the lateral aspect of the wheelchair seating surface; used to control excessive adduction of the lower extremities.

Adelophagy A form of embryonic nutrition in which off spring feed on extraembryonic yolk.

ADEM Acute disseminated encephalomyelitis is a monophasic encephalitis or myelitis of abrupt onset with damage principally to the white matter of cerebrum or spinal cord. Pathologically there is perivenous mononuclear cell infiltration and demyelination. It may follow vaccination against rabies. Person may develop fever, meningeal sign, headache, delirium and convulsion. Hemiplegia, paraplegia and loss of bladder control may ensue. Some patients may show with pure spinal cord syndrome and cerebellar sign may predominate in others.

Adenalgia Pain in gland due to inflammation.

Adenine One of the bases in a DNA (deoxyribonucleic acid) strand that binds to a base (thymine) in another strand to form double stranded DNA.

Adenitis It is an inflammation of lymph glands. Glands enlarge if infection is in their specific area. Cervical lymphadenitis may be due to tuberculosis or any other bacterial infection. Inflammation

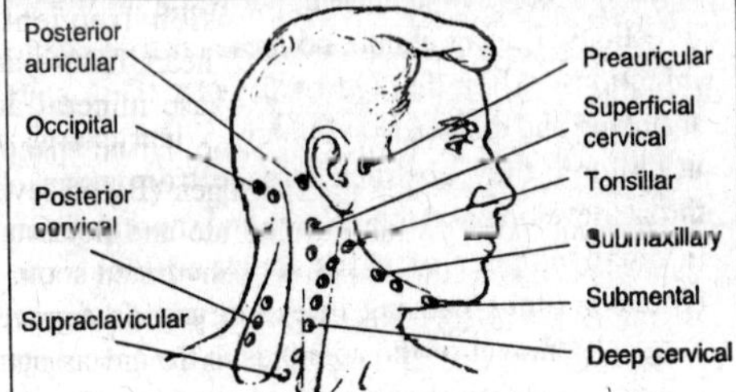

Lymph glands of neck

subsides within a fortnight after appropriate antibacterial treatment but antituberculous treatment takes months together.

Adenocarcinoma It is a cancer of glandular tissue and develops in pancreas, kidney and salivary glands. It arises from epithelium, layer of cells lining the inside of an organ.

Adenocystic carcinoma It constitutes 4 per cent of salivary gland tumours. It occurs in persons beyond 50 years of age. Parotid gland is generally involved. In major glands tumour may present with features of benign tumours with pain and neurological symptoms; lesions of palate are accompanied by toothache, loosening of tooth, radiolucencies and if tooth is extracted failure of socket to heal. It is a slow growing tumour. Tumour contains dark staining epithelial cells resembling basal cells of mucous membrane. It does not metastasise until late in life. It is locally aggressive and may cause death by local extension. Wide excision is the treatment.

Adenohypophysis The anterior, glandular lobe of the pituitary gland that secretes FSH (folliclestimulating hormone), LH (luteinizing hormone), ACTH (adrenocorticotropic hormone), TSH(thyroid-stimulating hormone), GH (growth hormone), and prolactin. Secretions of the adenohypophysis are controlled by hormones produced by the hypothalamus.

Adenoid cystic carcinoma It mostly involves minor salivary glands as well as sublingual gland, submandibular gland and parotid. Palpation may reveal a hard, nodulated mass that is fixed or poorly mobile. Growth is slow. The tumour tends to track along nerves and vessels and facial paralysis is common. Distant haematogenous spread is common.

Adenoids These are two swelling like structures above the tonsils made of lymph nodes. These act as body's defence against upper respiratory tract infections. During childhood these enlarge due to infections. After the age of 5 years these start shrinking and disappear at puberty. When enlarged in children they obstruct passage from nose to throat, develop nasal tone, voice and snoring. Even in small number of cases they can block the eustachian tube causing infection and deafness. Surgical removal of the adenoids is the treatment if it does not respond to medical treatment.

Adenolipoma Adenolipomas of adrenal gland are extremely rare fatty tumours that may show degeneration, haemorrhage, fibrosis and calcifications. These are usually asymptomatic but may cause pain if it is larger.

Adenolymphoma It is an epithelial tumour arising within periparotid lymph node. Epithelial cells later proliferate in an acinar form and give rise to swelling called adenolymphoma.

It is usually limited in the area of parotid gland because lymph node containing ectopic salivary tissue is usually found in the parotid gland and not in submaxillary salivary gland. It is common after the age of 40 in males. Patient presents with a slowly growing painless swelling of oval or circular shape.

It measures 1 to 3 cm in diameter. Surface is smooth with well-defined margin. Consistency is soft to cystic. It is not fixed to deeper structure and cervical lymph nodes are not enlarged.

Adenoma It is a benign, non-cancerous tumour of any gland. It may be cystic too. Adenoma of endocrine glands, i.e. pituitary, thyroid and adrenal gland can cause excessive hormone production.

Adenomatosis oris An enlargement of mucous gland of lip without inflammation.

Adenomatous Pertaining to adenoma or to nodular hyperplasia of a gland.

Adenopathy Enlargement of the glandular organs and tissues generally attributed to a disease process.

Adenosclerosis The hardening of a gland.

Adenosine It reduces oxygen consumption, increases coronary blood flow, causes vasodilatation and slows arterioventricular conduction.

Adenosine triphosphate (ATP) Adenosine, an organic base, with three phosphate groups attached to it; energy stored in adenosine triphosphate (ATP) is used in nearly all the energy-requiring reactions in the body. It is a compound which plays a central role in energy metabolism. ATP is sometimes described as universal currency of energy. Practically all energetic demands of cell are met by breakdown of ATP.

Adenotome An instrument for cutting glands.

Adenotomy The cutting or removal of a gland.

Adenovirus In 1962 Trentin showed that human adenovirus type 12 produced sarcomas when inoculated. Subsequent work has shown that several other adenoviruses of human and animal origin are also oncogenic. Human types 12, 18, and 31 have the highest oncogenic potential.

Adenylate-forming enzymes A large family of enzymes that activate short chain fatty acids or aminoacids as acyl adenylates.

Adequacy of medical care A sufficient volume of care to meet the needs of a community.

Adequate daily intake Amount of macronutrients, if taken daily are believed to be adequate for health.

Adequate intake (AI) The approximate level of an average nutrient intake determined by observation of a particular group or population that appears to maintain good health.

Adherend The surface with which an adhesive bonds.

Adhesin A molecute, typically a protein, that mediates bacterial attachment by interacting with specific receptors.

Adhesio A connecting band or structure.

Adhesion The property of remaining in close proximity, as the resulting from the physical or chemical attraction of atoms of a substance or molecular attraction existing between the surfaces of bodies in contract. The stable joining of parts to each other.

Adhesion molecules Molecules normally sited on the cell surfaces, involved in embryogenesis, cell growth and differentiation and repair of wound.

Adhesions Abnormal adherence of collagen fibers to surrounding structures during immobilization, following trauma or as a complication of surgery, which restricts normal elasticity of the structures involved.

Adhesiotomy The cutting or division of adhesions.

Adhesive capsulitis The inflammation of a joint capsule with adhesions.

Adhesive dressing These sterile dressings consist of a pad of absorbent gauge of cellulose held in place by a layer of adhesive material. These are of different sizes and shapes and are supplied in paper or plastic covers. The surrounding skin must be dry before application and edges of dressing pressed firmly down.

Adhesives These enhance the bonding between various materials and tooth structure or as sealants of the pits and fissures present on the occlusal surface.

Adhoc Devoloped or created for a specific purpose.

Adhoc theory Descriptive theory in which a nonexhaustive list of characteristsics is used to describe a phenomenon.

Adiabactic Occurring without gain or loss heat.

Adiabatic change Volume change of gas in which there is no transfer of heat to or from the system.

Adie's syndrome It is more common in females and manifests in second and third decade. There will be slightly enlarged pupils, delayed or diminished direct and consensual reaction to light. Consensual reflex is abolished on the affected side but normal on the other side. There will be loss of tendon reflexes particularly ankle and knee jerks.

Adifax It is structurally related to amphetamine but it causes release of serotonin from nerve store rather than noradrenaline. It is sedative rather than stimulant to CNS. It may induce satiety. There may be mood elevation at the onset of therapy. Blood pressure is reduced. In obese persons it is the drug of choice specially if hypertension is also there. Weight reduction starts in 2 weeks and lasts for 3 months. After that it becomes practically ineffective. Side effects include sleepiness, depression, diarrhoea, impotence and increased dreaming.

Adipocere This change occurs in bodies submerged in water or buried in moist graves. The substance formed is called adipocere on account of fat and waxy appearance. It is a soft, waxy looking substance, greasy to touch and varying in colour from dull white to dark brown. It has disagreeable rancid odour. On fracture it displays traces of fibres and blood vessels between which material is deposited. It melts at 200°F and is soluble in ether. The subcutaneous fat and bone marrow first undergo this change.

Adipocyte An animal cell specialized for the storage of fats.

Adipocytes Cells specialized for storage of fat.

Adipose Most people have a layer of adipose tissue beneath the skin and around kidneys. It acts as insulation against cold and serves as a storage of energy. Consumption of lot of fats will increase the amount of adipose tissue.

Adipose tissue It is a layer of fat beneath the skin and around various internal organs. Distribution of adipose tissue differs from part to part in males and females. In ladies it is more than males. Adipose tissue is made up of fat deposited, acting as energy store. The tissue acts as an insulator against loss of body heat. It is distributed in the subcutaneous areolar tissue except subcutaneous tissue of penis and scrotum. It is found between scapulae, in mesentery, yellow marrow and around kidney and heart. It is concerned with metabolism of tissue and nerves. It serves as a packing material and forms shock absorbing pads. It packs the orbital cavity and angles of joints. It gives roundness and beauty of figure.

Adipsia Absence of thirst.

Adjurant Supplementary.

Adjusted rates Same as standardized rates.

Adjustment Alignment of one's inner needs with the realities of personal capabilities, and/or environment; may be adaptive or maladaptive.

Adjustment level The degree of successful adaptation of a functioning organnism to its environment.

Adjuvant One of a heterogeneous group of substances that enhance the immune response to an antigen. Several mechanisms may be involved, but prolonging exposure of the antigen to immunocompetent cells is thought to be a major factor.

Adjuvant therapy The treatment of a disease with substances that enhance the action of drugs, especially drugs that promote the production of antibodies.

Adjuvants Drugs that assist in accomplishing the desired effect of a primary drug.

Adler, Alfred (1870-1937) Viennese psychiatrist, founder of the school of individual psychology.

Adler's dream theory That dreams foretell the future because dream is a kind of rehersal for location.

Adler's sign Abdominal tenderness remains unmovable and fixed even on changing the position of the patient. This sign is present in cases of ectopic pregnancy.

Admedial Situated near the median plane.

Administrative laws Legal provisions through which federal, state, and local agencies maintain self-regulation.

Admission Entering a health care agency for nursing care and medical or surgical treatment.

Adnerval Situated near a nerve.

Adolescence This is the period between childhood and adulthood. It is a time of much change of individual and the concerned family. During adolescence adult's self-identity is formed. This involves achieving independence and emotional separation from parents. It is the time to develop sexual attitudes and aggressive drive. During this period he or she may rebel against parents and his or her models may be some cine actor or actress, pop singer, teacher. Sexual experimentation may occur in fantasy. Homosexual behaviour develops occasionally. Child may become moody and there may be fluctuating school performance. They may feel nervous, depressed, withdrawn and may become conscious of their looks and personality. This may lead to outbursts of bad temper or other undesirable behaviour. Due to peer group pressures they may become involved in drug abuse for kicks. Most of these are temporary problems that resolve on their own. Parents should maintain communication with children during this period.

Adolescent crisis Emotional turmoil of adolescence.

Adolescent egocentrism The belief of some adolecents that they should be the focus of attention and their problems are unique.

Adoration An attitude of high and intense esteem for a person viewel as incomparably superior to adorer.

ADP (adenosine diphosphate) A ribonucleoside 5'-diphosphate serving as phosphate group acceptor in the cell energy cycle.

Adrenal biopsy It is the biopsy performed for the differential diagnosis between metastases and adenomas. Adrenal biopsy is performed under CT, ultrasound or MR guidance. This biopsy is not useful in differential diagnosis between adenoma and adrenal carcinoma or for the evaluation of endocrine active tumours.

Adrenal cortex The outer part of the adrenal gland, which secretes the following steroid hormones: glucocorticoids, mainly cortisol; mineralocorticoids, mainly aldosterone; and androgens.

Adrenal crisis Acute manifestation of adrenal insufficiency with symptoms including hypotension, hypovolemic shock, fever and hypogycemia. It is a medical emergency.

Adrenal gland One of a pair of flattened endocrine glands located above each kidney and composed in two parts, the cortex and the medulla. The cortex is derived from embryonic mesoderm. The medulla has an origin similar to that of the sympathetic nervous system. Cortex secretes corticosteroid hormones that have effect on body's metabolism. It is responsible for hairiness and body shape. Smaller inner part is medulla responsible of body's first line of response and defence against physical and emotional stress.

Adrenal medulla The inner part of the adrenal gland, which secretes mainly epinephrine but also small amount of norepinephrine.

Adrenalectomy Surgical removal of adrenal glands from body.

Adrenaline It stimulates both alpha and beta receptors. It is formed in adrenal medulla where it is stored in intracellular granules and is liberated by acetylcholine. It increases the stroke volume rate and cardiac output. The systolic blood pressure rises but the diastolic falls. Vessels of skin, mucosa, and kidney are relaxed with physiological doses and constrict after large doses. Angina pectoris may be precipitated. Peripheral venous pressure is increased. It is most potent drug to stimulate arrested heart but is not commonly used due to danger of ventricular dysrhythmia. Renal bloodflow is decreased so is urine. Bronchial tone is reduced. Pyloric sphincter is contracted. Glycogen is mobilised from liver giving rise to an increase in blood sugar level. It is used in anaphylactic shock, as bronchodilator, to produce vaso-constriction in local analgesia.

Adrenarche A condition of intensified secretion by the adrenal cortex, especially androgens, occurring in humans at about eight years of age in both sexes.

Adrenergic A term used to describe the actions of epinephrine, norepinephrine, or other molecules with similar activity as in adrenergic receptor and adrenergic stimulation.

Adrenergic fibers (FYE-bers) Axons whose terminals release norepinephrine and epinephrine.

Adrenergic neuron A neuron containing epinephrine; the term adrenergic derives from the term adrenaline.

Adrenergic receptors Membrane proteins activated by adrenaline.

Adrenergic system That system of organs and nerves in which perinephrine (adrenaline) is the neurotransmitter.

Adrenoceptors The sites on an effector organ innervated by postganglionic adrenergic fibers of the sympathetic division of the autonomic nervous system.

Adrenodontia The canines are large and sharp, and the occlusal surfaces of the teeth have a brownish coloration.

Adrenogenital syndrome Boys develop isosexual precocious puberty with laryngeal enlargement and a dark vocal timbre after 7 years of age and vocal change after 10 years of age. It is caused by increased adrenocortical androgen production. Urinary 17-ketosteroids are elevated.

Adrenoleucodystrophy This is a disorder of very long chain fattyacid metabolism, an X-linked disorder. Brain is also infiltrated by lymphocytes. Adrenal infiltration results in Addison's disease. MRI shows high signal around the occipital horns of lateral ventricles.

Adrenotropic Having specific affinity for or influence on the adrenal glands.

Adson's test It is a test to determine presence of subclavian artery compression. Feel the radial pulse of the seated patient. Then patient is asked to take a deep breath and hold it, then he is asked to turn his chin up and to the affected side as far as possible. If there is obliteration or diminution of the radial pulse, the sign is positive.

Adsorption A process believed to be physical in nature in which molecules of a gas or liquid condense or adhere on the surface of another substance.

Adult foster home Boarding home.

Adult periodontitis It is most common and is caused by subgingival plaque of which the unattached component plays a dominant role. Gram-negative bacteria of flagellated forms and spirochaetes are present in this plaque. In addition to these, medium-sized spirochaetes are also present in large numbers. Invasion of gingival tissue may also occur. It is usually bilateral and primarily interdental, Periodontitis in adults has short, rapid bursts of progression or disease activity, followed by periods of inactivity or even repair.

These periods may be months or years. Disease activity may not affect all the areas of mouth at one point of time. Clinically periodontitis is characterised by changes in gingival colour, loss of stippling oedema, hyperplasia, formation of clefts, presence of true pockets which may exude pus on pressure and tooth mobility. X-ray shows evidence of bone destruction. Loss of lamina dura on the alveolar crest gives the crest a concave or shaggy appearance. There may be vertical resorption of bone and narrowing of bony septa.

Adulteration The addition of any organism or substance that may make a consumer product harmful to users.

Adultery It differs from seduction because one or both partners are married but not to each other. Normally the adulterer is a married partner. On occasion it is committed with fraud, an unmarried female does not know that the other is already married.

Adulthood Period after adolescence aerobic respiration (air-O-bik res-pi-RAY-shun) the stage of cellular respiration requiring oxygen.

Adumbration A geometric lack of sharpness of X-Ray shadow.

Advance directive A written agreement established between a patient and a care provider to withhold heroic measures of life-sustaining treatment if their condition becomes irreversible. These agreements are usually written at a time when the individual is healthy or able to make conscious decisions about their welfare.

Advanced bell eruption Enamel organ formation creating the crown of the tooth.

Advanced cardiac life support The electrical, pharmacologic, vascular and airway access techniques used to resuscitate or sustain life in addition to those associated with the basic life support measures of cardiopulmonary resuscitation.

Advanced functions Duties delegated by a dentist allowing a dental auxiliary to perform specific intraoral tasks. Special restrictions and educational requirements are identified by individual state dental practice acts to define the delegations of advanced functions.

Advanced life support Intervention protocols applied to resuscitate or stabilize the condition of critically ill or critically injured patients.

Advanced practice Specialized areas of expertise, such as nurse practitioner and nurse midwifery.

Advanced trauma life support System of trauma management devised by Nebraska USA in 1978. It is based on concept of reducing morbidity and morbidity in first hour after trauma.

Adventitia Coming from abroad, foreign. Outermost covering of an organ that is continuous with the surrounding connective tissue.

Adventitious breath sounds Abnormal sounds heard during auscultation of the lung fields.

Adverse drug reactions Nontherapeutic effects of medications.

Advocacy Speaking or arguing in support of a policy or a person's right.

Advocate A person who speaks or acts on behalf of those who cannot protect or speak for themselves.

Aedeagus The extensible portion of the intromittent organ or penis of most insects.

Aerobic Growing only in the presence of molecular oxygen.

Aerobic bacteria Microorganisms that require oxygen to live at a moderate to slow speed without hindering the ability to breathe.

Aerobic exercise Any sustained exercise where the required energy is supplied by the available oxygen within the system.

Aerobic glycolysis The conversion of glucose to ATP for energy when oxygen is available.

Aerobic pathway A form of energy production that depends on oxygen.

Aerobic process A Physiological process that requires the presence of oxygen to proceed.

Aerobic re-conditioning Training programme designed to improve cardiovascular fitness and physical strength.

Aerobic respiration Breakdown of glucose in the presence of oxygen to produce carbon dioxide, water, and approximately 38 ATP molecules; includes glycolysis, the citric acid cycle, and the electron-transport chain.

Aerobic training Continuous vigorous exercise requiring the body to increase its consumption of oxygen and develop the muscles' ability to sustain activity over a long period of time.

Aerobics It means which require air to live. This is a exercise in which the body is able to meet the muscles increased demand of oxygen.

In swimming, jogging and cycling oxygen reaches the muscles at the rate at which it is used up. In it activity can be sustained for long periods. While in anaerobics there is different reaction to get energy from sugar and fats of muscles. The waste products of anaerobic exercises are lactic acid which accumulate in muscles, and muscles become fatigued so such exercises can be performed for a shorter period. When aerobic exercises are regularly done it improves your stamina and endurance.

Aerocele A tumor formed by air filling an adventitious pouch, such as a laryngocele or tracheocele.

Aerocyanosis Exposure to cold may cause vasospasm resulting in it. But it has no association with occlusive arterial disease. Condition involves the hands and feet but can also affect tip of nose and ears.

Following exposure to cold the affected part appears cold, clammy and cyanotic accompanied by hyperhidrosis. Symptoms subside once the part becomes warmer. Cyanosis is persistent and symmetrical in distribution and becomes more intensified on further exposure to cold. As part of prevention best is to protect hands and feet against exposure to cold. Condition does not require any treatment.

Aerodontalgia Pulpal pain with decreased barometric pressure.

Aerophilic Requiring air for proper growth.

Aerosol 1. A colloidal suspension of fine solid or liquid particles in air. 2. Specifically, a suspension of true air-borne particles; i.e., particles with a negligible settling tendency under average room conditions.

Aerosol infection An infection spread by airborne particles, as distinct from droplet-borne respiratory infections, which spread via larger respiratory droplets.

Aerosol mask A device used to facilitate the delivery of an aerosol to a patient.

Aerosol therapy Devices for providing aerosal therapy are metered dose inhaler, dry powder inhaler and nebulisers. MDI's and DPI's require the patient to inhale deeply which may not be possible in all asthmatics. These require accurate synchroni-sation of activation and inhalation which is difficult for young children and elderly to inhale.

AET Aquatic exercise therapy is the union of aquative exercise and physical therapy.

Aet-HC It contains tretinoin, hydroquinone and hydrocortisone and is most useful in melasma and other hyperpigmentation disorders.

Aetiology The science or study of the cause of disease; that which is known about the causes of a disease.

Afebrile Absence of a fever.

Affect Subjective experience of emotion accompanying an idea or mental representation. The word, affect is often used loosely as a generic term for feeling, emotion, or mood. Affect and emotion are commonly used interchangeably.

Affection Feeling and emotions of tenderness and attachment specially when fellings are nonsexual.

Affectional drive The compelling urge to give and to recieve offten.

Affective ambiance Stanifestation of occuring contradictory feelings towards an object or events.

Affective disorder A psychiatric disorder characterised by a severe emotional reaction, often depressive in nature, usually with a disruptive effect on the person's thinking and behaviour.

Affective domain An area of education concerned with the learning of attitudes and values. Educational objectives in the affective domain concern the development of positive feelings and attitudes in the learner.

Affective faillure An extreme deficiency or inadequacy of emotional reactions. Person with no feelings.

Affective rigidity Condition in which emotions, feelings or mood remains unchanged.

Affective state A psychological condition which underlies or involves feeling or emotion. The feeling aspects of emotion, as opposed to behavioural and physiological aspects.

Affective touch Touching that demonstrates concern or affection.

Afferent Carrying or conveying toward the center (for example, an afferent neuron carries nerve impulses toward the central nervous system).

Afferent arteriole A blood vessel within the kidney that supplies blood to the glomerulus .

Afferent fibre Nerve fibre going from the peripheral to the central nervous system; sensory or afferent fibre.

Afferent loop syndrome This syndrome occurs after partial gastrectomy with chronic or recurrent partial obstruction in afferent loop. There will be abdominal pain and epigastric fullness which will be relieved by vomiting. Stasis in afferent loop causes bacterial growth and distension. Anaemia usually develops. Distension and vomiting occur 15 to 30 minutes after food.

Afferent message Impulse message carried by afferent nerves toward the brain from peripheral areas.

Afferent stimuli Techniques of stimulation such as-stroking, brushing, icing, heating pressure, bone pounding, slow and quick muscle stretch, joint retraction and approximation are used to facilitate or inhibit motor response. Ontogenic developmental sequence is outlined and is strictly followed in the application of stimuli.

1. Total flexion or withdrawal pattern
2. Roll over
3. Pivot prone
4. Co-contraction neck
5. On elbow (prone and push backwards)
6. All fours (static, weight shift, crawl)
7. Standing upright
8. Walking.

Affiant A person who makes an affidavit.

Affidavit A voluntary, sworn statement of facts or a declaration in writing made before a person with the authority to administer on oath. These are usually prepared by an attorney in consultation with the affiant, then signed before a notary public.

Affiliation motive The motive to seek the company of others and to be with one's own kind, based on such things as cooperation, similarity, friendship, sex, and protection.

Affinity The degree of association between two entities.

Affirmative Defenses Arguments raised by a defendant in a civil lawsuit that indicate extenuating circumstances that negate the plaintiff's claim.

Affirmed Action of an appellate court in which it declares that a judgement, decree, or order of a lower court is valid and correct and must stand.

Affirming communication Family communication characterized by taking care not to hurt other members emotionally or physically, taking time to hear what others have to say, conveying respect for others' feelings, and ending conflicts on a positive note.

Afflux The rush of blood or liquids to a part.

Affusion An affusion is the procedure in which water is poured from a pail or pitcher or is thrown or falls on patient seated or standing in an empty bathtub.

AFIS Automated Fingerprint Identification Systems.

Aflatoxin This is a poisonous substance produced by *Aspergillus flavus* mold. Peanuts are generally affected by it. It may even cause liver cancer.

African eye worm disease Causative agent is *Loa loa* and it causes transient erythematous swelling, pruritus, eosinophilia, fever, urticaria and rarely neurologic involvement. There may develop conjunctivitis, keratitis, optic nerve atrophy, white cottony mass of vitreous, macular haemorrhages and paralysis of extraocular muscles.

After play Affectionate interaction following an orgasm.

Afterbirth The structures cast off after the expulsion of the fetus, including the membranes and the placenta with the attached umbilical cord; the secundines.

Aftercare Posthospitalisation programme of rehabilitation designed to reinforce the effects of therapy and to help the patient adjust to his or her environment.

Afterglow It is the stage of physical relaxation exhibiting emotional warmth following the successful completion of sexual intercourse. Pressure is released, heart rate is slowed down and muscular tension releases. Partners feel a sense of closeness.

Afterimage A sensory which appears after withdrawal of certain visual stimuli. A negative afterimage has a colour that is approximately complementary to the original stimulus. A positive afterimage is a momentary increase in the brightness of a colour experienced immediately after one ceases looking at that colour.

Afterload The resistance against which the ventricles must pump blood, it is increased in people who have hypertension.

Afterpains Those pains, that occur after the expulsion of the afterbirth; result from the contractile efforts of the uterus to return to its normal condition. Cramping pain following child birth, caused by alternating relaxation and contraction of uterine muscles.

Afterplay It is the continuation of erotic gratification after climax has been reached. It is as important as foreplay. During this period the couple should care for each other, play, talk, laugh or mediate.

Aftertaste A taste continuing after the substance producing it has been removed.

Afunctional A condition of being in nonfunction. In implant dentistry, existing in a state such that the forces that affect healing are negligible, such as when an endosteal implant is submerged or semi-submerged in a protocol to achieve osteointegration.

Agametic Asexual.

Agamogenesis Asexual reproduction.

Agar It is called reversible hydrocolloid because it can be changed from liquid solution or into a rubber like gel simply by raising or lowering its temperature. Transformation is a physical change and not a chemical reaction.

Agar hydrocolloids It is compounded from reversible agar gels. When heated they liquefy or go into solid state and on cooling they return to the gel state. Agar impressions are dimensionally unstable on standing so models should be made as soon as possible after the impression is taken.

Ago Time elapsed since birth.

Age adjustment A procedure for overall comparison of two or more populations in which background differences in the distribution of variables are removed.

Age of burns Immediately after the burn the skin becomes red, within 2 to 3 hours vesiccation starts and in 36 to 72 hours pus forms on the surface and under slough. In 96 hours red inflammatory zone recedes. In one week superficial slough starts separating and in 2 to 3 weeks slough is completed and red granulating surface is exposed.

Age of injury Colour changes in bruises start after 18 to 24 hours. Divided surface of an aseptic incised wound which are in opposition are covered with lymph in 36 hours. Edges will join together in 3 days and wound heals by seventh day. Pus appears in 26 to 48 hours in septic wound.

Age of scar Firm union occurs in 5 to 6 days producing reddish or bluish angry scar. By the end of 14 days the scar becomes pale, it is still soft and sensitive. In about 2 to 6 months scar becomes brown or copper red but does not wrinkle. After 6 months it becomes tough and wrinkled.

Age regression When a hypno-tised person behaves as he or she allegedly did at an earlier age; regarded as characteristic of some hypnotic behaviour.

Age verification Bone X-ray helps in age verification in case of medicolegal importance Lateral epicondyle unites between 10-12 years ; Medial epicondyle unites between 13-14 years; Tip of olecranon and ulna unites between 14 15 years ; Crest tuberosity ossifies between 18-20 years ; Neck of femur completely ossifies at 14 years ; Pisiform bone ossifies between 9-12 years.

Aged residue A term from pesticide that over time diffuses into the internal soil matrix and is no longer available for microbial attack.

Agency The legal term for the relationship in which one person either acts for or represents another. The person acting is the agent and the person for whom the agent acts is called the principal. Lawyers act as agents for their clients when they negotiate leases and other contracts with a third-party for their client. Physicians act as agents for their patients when they order medical tests for which a patient is legally obliged to pay a hospital.

Agenesis The failure of an organ to develop.

Age-prediotod maximal heart rate The highest heart rate attained during maximal exercise; generally considered 220 minus an individual's age in years.

Agerasia Appearing well preserved.

Age-specific rate A rate for a particular age group.

Agglutinate Antibodies causing antigens to clump or stick together.

Agglutination It is clumping together of suspended matter in solution such as blood cells or bacteria. It may occur when blood of different blood groups is mixed. Certain antibodies present in blood serum cause agglutination known as agglutinins. The process by which cells stick together to form clumps.

Aggregate effects Group effects.

Aggregate of people A group of people with similar characteristics, such as all people infected with HIV, all those diagnosed with juvenile onset diabetes, or all homeless families.

Aggregated lymphatic follicles Clusters of lymph nodules that are most numerous in the ileum. Also called Peyer's

Aggregation The process by which active platelets connect with vessel wall and each other to form a thrombus.

Aggression Behavior intended to harm or injure another person or thing.

Aggressive cues External or internal stimuli that elicit aggressive behavior by virtue of their learned association to it.

Aggressiveness Strong self assertiveness, social dominence and a tendency towards hostality.

Aging Progressive changes produced with the passage of time

Agining process The gradual degenerative changes that occur after young adulthood as a person ages.

Agism Systematic stereotyping of and discrimination against elderly people to create distance from their social plight and to avoid primitive fears of aging and death. It is distinguished from gerontophobia, a specific pathologic fear of old people and aging.

Agitographia Abnormally repid writing and unconcious omission and distortion words.

Aglossia Congenital anomaly in which a portion or all of tongue is absent.

Aglossostomia Congenital absence of the tongue and mouth opening.

Aglycemia Absence of sugar from the blood.

Aglycon An organic molecule that can be glycosylated.

Agnathia Failure of development of jaw is referred as agnatnia. Condition is rare. When it is seen it is associated with developmental disturbances and is usually incompatible with life.

Agnosia This is an inability to recognise objects. Most common cause is stroke and head injury. For an object to be recognised, the sensory information must be interpreted which involves recall of memorised information about similar objects. Agnosia is caused by damage to the areas of brain involved in these memory recall functions. There is no specific treatment for it.

Agnostic A person who doubts the existence of God because it can't be proved or disproved.

Agomphious Without teeth.

Agonadal Absence of gonads.

Agonal thrombi Person dying slowly often form a firm string like, but tough, pale yellow thrombus usually in the right side of heart. The process begins in atrial appendages and extends into the right auricle and to the right ventricle like a tree. On left side these are not big.

Agonist A contracting muscle whose action is opposed by another muscle. Muscles, or portions of muscles, so attached anatomically that when they contract, they develop forces that reinforce each other.

Agonists and antagonists Agonists have both receptor affinity and intrinsic activity. Competitive antagonists have receptor affinity but no intrinsic activity. Noncompetitive antagonists have receptor affinity but no intrinsic activity. Partial agonists have considerable receptor affinity and some intrinsic activity, thus may produce antagonist or agonist effect.

Agoraphobia An intense fear of being in places or situations in which help may not be available or escape could be difficult.

Agranulocyte Leucocytes with very small cytoplasmic granules that cannot be easily seen with the light microscope; lymphocytes and monocytes.

Agranulocytic angina It develops due to hypersensitivity reaction to chemicals and drugs or ionising radiation.

Agranulocytosis It is caused by deficiency of neutrophils caused by poisoning of bone marrow by drugs like chloromycetin. Symptoms include fever, ulcers in mouth and throat. It may prove to be fatal. Treatment includes withdrawal of drug causing it and transfusion of white blood cells.

Agraphia It is a loss of ability to write despite normal function of hand and muscle. But there is damage of cerebrum. There is no specific treatment. With the time some may recover partially.

Agression Behavior intended to cause psychological or physical harm to someone or to a surrogate target. The behavior may be verbal or physical.

Agrobacterium A genus of gram-negative, aerobic bacteria of the family Rhizobiaceae that are noted as plant pathogens; e.g., A. Tume-faciens, the inducer of crown gall tumors.

Agrophobia It is a fear of going into open spaces, while claustro-phobia is a fear for enclosed spaces. Agrophobia becomes house bound.

Ahedonia Inability to enjoy anything.

Ahypnia Pathological uisomnia.

Aicardi's syndrome Symptoms are present at birth which progress with age and cause is unknown. There will be infantile spasms, epileptic seizures, mental anomaly, vertebral anomalies, hypotonia, occipital flattening, defects of corpus callosum and microph-thalmia. Patient will have lid twitching, absent pupillary reflexes and funnel-shaped disc.

AIDS Acquired immune deficiency syndrome is caused by HIV virus and there is no specific treatment available. All HIV-infected people do not develop AIDS, but once it is developed there is no treatment. Individuals may not have any symptoms while others may have short-lived illness, resembling mononucleosis.

In severe cases there may be marked weight loss, diarrhoea, fever and oral candidiasis. When brain is infected it may cause dementia. Diagnosis is done by enzyme-linked immunoabsorbent assay (ELISA) test and confirmed by Western blot test. Prevention includes safe sex. Unprotected anal and vaginal sex should be avoided. Hugging, mutual masturbation and dry kissing are safe. Intravenous drug users should avoid sharing of needles. Donated blood, organs and semen should be screened for HIV antibodies. Several antiviral drugs such as zidovudine (AZT) and acyclovir are being used to treat patients with HIV infection. No vaccine could be prepared due to changing behaviour of HIV virus.

AIDS embryopathy There will be growth failure, microcephaly, hypertelorism, flat nasal bridge and box-like forehead.

Aim A relatively remote goal to be attained by voluntary activity.

Air embolism Causative factors include operations involving injury to veins in the neck, thorax, breast and pelvis. Diagnostic and therapeutic injection of air into peritoneal cavity, pleural cavity, large joints, perinephric area may also result it. Surgical emphysema and accidental entrance of air during IV drip may cause air embolism. If air enters in vein it will cause a hissing sound in the wound going to right heart and lung causing an air lock obstruction in the pulmonary artery. This may result in loud precordial murmur. There will be sudden cyanosis, hypotension, engorged neck veins, irregular gasping respiration.

Air inhibition The top layer of a dental composite or sealant, which is exposed to the air, does not polymerize completely because of an inhibiting effect of oxygen.

Air inversion Occurs when cooler air settles close to the surface of the earth an warmer air rises above, so that the natural mixing of air does not occur and pollution is concentrated.

Air leak Escaping air in closed chest drainage; may be client centered or within the chest tube system.

Air/water syringe Apparatus of metal, glass, or plastic material consisting of a nozzle, or needle, barrel, and plunger or rubber bulb, through which air, water, or a combination of the two may be delivered under pressure to the desired area.

Airborne precaution Measures that reduce the risk of transmitting airborne infectious agents.

Air-bubbles These are white spots appearing on film. It happens when air is trapped on the film surface after the film is placed in processing solution. Air-bubbles check the chemicals from affecting the emulsion in that area.

Airway Collective system of tubes in the upper and lower respiratory tract.

Airway clearance techniques Manual or mechanical procedures that facilitate clearance of secretions from the airways.

Airway management Skills that maintain the patency of natural or artificial airways.

Airway obstruction Obstruction may occur at mouth, pharynx, larynx, trachea and large bronchi. It may be caused by falling of tongue backwards, larynospasm, stricture or tumor.

Airway pressure Pressure within in the breathing system and trachea and large bronchi. It may be caused by falling of tongue backwards, laryngo-spasm, stricture or tumor.

Airway resistance The residence to the flow of air in the lungs offered by the bronchioles.

Akathisia It is a state of motor restlessness induced by antipsychotic drugs. It is characterised by feelings of tension and inability to tolerate inactivity. Feeling is relieved by tapping the feet, shifting the position on chair. 20 to 30% of patients on phenothiazines suffer from it. Disease settles on withdrawal of drug.

Akinesia There is almost complete loss of movement. It may be a result of loss of power in a group of muscles caused by damage to nerves supplying that group, may be after a stroke. In parkinsonism there is normal power with rigidity.

Ala Bulgar.

Alanine amino transferase An enzyme found in the liver and blood serum, the concentration of which is often elevated in cases of liver damage.

Al-Anon An organisation of relatives of alcoholics operating in many communities under the philosophic and organisational structure of Alcoholics Anonymous to facilitate discussion and resolution of common problems.

Alar collapse Visible indrawing of the nasal alae during forcible inspiration. Nasal breathing is significantly improved by placing a small cotton wade into dome of nasal vestibule to prevent alar collapse.

Alate A term for winged sexuals, especially in termites.

Alateen An organisation of teen-aged children of alcoholic parents operating in some communities under the philosophic and organisational structure of Alcoholics Anonymous. It provides a setting in which the children may receive group support in achieving a better understanding of their parents' problems and better methods for coping with them.

Ala-tragus line An imaginary line that intersects the ala of the nose and the tragus of the ear; used in positioning a patient for a panoramic film (ala is the tissue that surrounds the nostril; tragus is a cartilaginous projection anterior to the external opening of the ear).

Albation The act of whitening; bleaching.

Albefaction The process of making white or bleaching.

Albers-Schönberg syndrome It follows recessive inheritence. Prognosis in malignant form is poor with death usually in infancy. There will be cartilage and bone thickening, multiple fractures, hyperchromic anaemia, osteomyelitis and severe form of jaundice.

Person will develop lymphadenopathy and hydroce-phalus in infants. Serum calcium levels will be low while phosphorus levels will be high. Person may develop oculomotor paralysis, cranial nerve VII palsy, ptosis, congenital cataract and nystagmus.

Albinism It is a congenital disease. Black colour of skin or eyes or hair is due to melanin pigment. In albinism melanin is absent. Skin and hair are snowy white. Eyes become intolerant to bright light. There may be abnormal flickering movements of eyes and myopia. Gene defect is the cause. If a normally pigmented couple has an albino child, any subsequent children generally have a one in four chance of being affected. The skin ages prematurally and is prone to cancers on sun-exposed areas. It is an autosomal recessive disorder and is characterised by complete absence of melanin in the skin, hair and eyes. It occurs at birth and persist throughout life. In complete albinism the melanocytes are present but they cannot form melanin due to lack of enzyme tyrosinase.

The condition typically presents with white skin, pale yellow or white hair and pink or blue eyes. Person develops hypersensitivity to sunlight and develops photophobia, nystagmus and defective vision. Skin biopsy confirms the diagnosis and there is no effective treatment available to it.

Albino It results due to absence of melanin. Person develops white hair and pink eyes. It is a genetic condition inherited as recessive trait which results in absence of enzyme which normally controls the production of melanin pigment.

Albinotic eye Albinism is a conge-nital condition where pigment is deficient. The total albinism is due to an inborn error of metabolism characterised by lack of enzyme tyrosinase which converts the dopa into melanin. The criterion of ocular albinism is a lack of deficiency of pigment in the retinal pigment epithelium. The eyebrows and lashes become white and there is red reflex from pupil. Person becomes myopic and nystagmus is a constant feature due to defective macula. Visual acuity is subnormal and electroretino-gram is normal.

Albright's syndrome It is a disorder of dominant inheritance involving various organs like brain, bones, skin and pseudopara-thyroidism. Clinical features include bowing of tibia, deformity of femur and skin pigmentation of bony sites involved. Females may develop precocious puberty. There will be increased density of facial bones.

Albumen Egg white, a mixture of more than 40 proteins secreted by the oviduct.

Albumen gland A female sex gland concerned with the secretion of perivitelline fluid.

Albumin Albumin is made in the liver from amino acids that have been absorbed from digested protein. Albuminuria is the presence of protein albumin in urine. It indicates a failure of kidney's filtering mechanism due to glomerulo-nephritis or nephrotic syndrome.

Albumin index A measure of quality of an egg. The ratio between the height of the albumin and the width when broken on to a flat surface. As the egg deteriorates albumin index decreases i.e. egg white spreads.

Albumin-globulin These are typical proteins. These contain most of the amino acids more or less uniformly distributed and are neither, basic nor acidic. Albumins are soluble in water, globulins are not, but both are soluble in weak salt solutions. Both are coagulated by heat. Albumin and globulin are most frequently found together in serum, muscle, milk and egg white.

Albuminous Containing or of the nature of an albumin.

Alcaptonuria A rare in born error of metabolism of two amino acids phenylalanine and tyrosine. Urine turns black. It is harmless.

Alcohol It is produced from the fermentation of carbohydrates by yeast. Alcohol is used as an antiseptic and as a solvent. Recently its consumption has become a social problem. Alcohol is a depressant, depresses CNS activity thus reducing anxiety, tensions and inhibitions. It develops euphoria. Its consumption increases the lethal confidence of the vehicle driver.

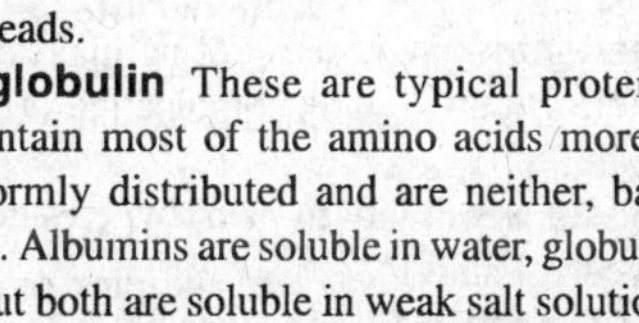
Alcoholic gait

Alcohol abuse The use of alcohol in a manner harmful to individual and/or others such as contributing to the failure to fulfill familial or work obligations but not a severe enough problem to meet crieteria for alcohol dependence.

Alcohol fermentation The ana-erobic conversion of glucose to ethanol via glycolysis.

Alcohol myopia The behavior displayed after imbibing alcohol in which local and immediate cues become prominent.

Alcoholic blackout Amnesia without loss of consciousness in which the intoxicated person retains the ability to perform certain automatised behaviors without any subsequent memory for the episode.

Alcoholic disinfectant Ethyl alcohol is best against both gram-positive and gram-negative organisms and also tubercle bacilli. Alcohol acts by protein denaturation and exhibits action only in the presence of water. Absolute alcohol has very little if any bactericidal property. It has no appreciable action on spores. Ethyl alcohol is extensively used for sterilisation of skin prior to operation.

Alcoholic fermentation Fermen-tation in which carbon dioxide flushes out residual oxygen, rendering the substrate anaerobic and producing ethanol at levels that make the substrate resistant to development of food poisoning and spoilage microorganisms.

Alcoholic hallucinosis Special diagnosis referring to an alcohol arthdrawl syndrome characterized by audiory hallucimations.

Alcoholic jealousy A from of jealousy experienced by chronic alcoholies.

Alcoholic myopathy An acute form of alcoholic myopathy occurs after being characterised by weakness, pain, tenderness and swelling in proximal muscles.

Serum phosphocreatine kinase is elevated and biopsy shows muscle fibre necrosis. Many chronic alcoholics show a pseudo-Cushing's syndrome with truncal obesity and wasted limbs.

Alcoholic neuropathy A distal sensorimotor neuropathy with painful burning feet and tender calves is very common in chronic alcoholics. It is not certain whether this is due to thiamine deficiency or direct toxic effect of alcohol.

Alcoholism It is a form of drug abuse, increased tolerance to alcohol, symptoms of alcohol withdrawl when intake is stopped and craving for alcohol develops.

Alcok's canal Pudendal canal.

Aldose A simple sugar in which the carbonyl carbon atom is an aldehyde; that is, the carbonyl carbon is at one end of the carbon chain.

Aldosterone A hormone secreted by the adrenal cortex that is important in the control of blood pressure and the regulation of sodium and potassium concentration. It acts on the kidney to decrease the amount of sodium lost in urine. Excessive production of aldosterone is known as aldosteronism.

It can be caused by a tumour of gland. Elevated blood pressure shows excesss of potassium in urine. It causes tiredness of muscle, weakness and impairs kidney function.

Aldosteronism An intrinsic disorder of the adrenal cortex that results in the excessive secretion of aldosterone.

Alernative hypothesis The hypothesis that there is in fact a real (true) difference between means or proportions of groups being compared or that there is a real association between two variables.

Alert inactivity period Time at which the infant's eyes are open and limb movements are quiet.

Alertness Being awake, attentive and ready to act.

Alexander's technique This technnique devised by F.M. Alexander is an educational process that promotes general re-education of the whole body. It can be beneficial in functional, structural and neurologic difficulties. The principle of technnigue involves inhibiting and unlearning habitual, unconscious control of the body and then learning a new conscious thinking process for control of the body.

Aleukia Absence of leukocytes from the blood; Leukopenia.

Alexia There is blindness of words. Person is not able to recognise the written words thus is unable to read.

Alexithymia A disturbance in affective and cognitive function which overlaps diagnostic entities but is common in psychosomatic, addictive, and post-traumatic stress disorders. The chief manifestation is difficulty in describing or recognising one's own emotions, with a limited fantasy life and general constriction in the affective life.

Alfa fetoprotein A protein produced by liver. It can bind circulating estrogen and sequester it from brain.

Alfalfa A leguminous plant chiefly used for animal forage.

Alfano syndrome The syndrome results from obstruction of superior vena cava from aortic aneurysmal tumours of mediastinum and fibrosing mediastinitis, carcinoma of lung, thyroid tumours, lymphoma and some idiopathic causes. Clinical features include non-pitting oedema of face, neck and upper trunk. There will be cyanosis and dilated veins over face, epistaxis and retinal haemorrhages.

Alganesthesia Absence of normal sense of pain.

Algedonics To study combination of pleasure and pain.

Algesia Sensitivity to pain; hyperesthesia.

Algesic Painful.

Algesic tooth Painful tooth.

Algesimeter An instrument used in measuring the sensitiveness to pain as produced by pricking with a sharp point.

Algesimetry The measurement of sensitiveness to pain.

Alginate A hydrated, viscous polysaccharide copolymer com-prising variable amounts of B-D-mannuronic acid and A-L-guluronic acid. Alginate is excreted from the cells of Azotobacter species, giving them a slimy glutinous appearance.

Alginate hydrocolloids Dental alginate impression materials change from solid phase to the gel phase as a result of chemical reaction. Once gelation is completed the material cannot be reliquefied to sol phase. The alginates have been useful in taking study impressions for orthodontic and other purposes. These have good elastic properties. Casts are made by pouring dental plasters into impression and no separating medium is necessary. Alginic acid is prepared from a marine plant. Fast-set materials have working times of 1.25 to 2 minutes. Disinfection of impressions is a concern with respect to viral diseases such as hepatitis B, AIDS and herpes simplex.

Algiomotor producing painful movement; such as spasm.

Algiomuscular Pertaining to muscular action resulting from painful stimulation.

Algometry The measurement of sensitivity to painful stimuli, as with an algometer.

Alienation The estrangement felt in a cultural setting one views as foreign, unpredictable, or unacceptable. For example, in depersonalisation phenomena, feelings of unreality or strangeness produce a sense of alienation from one's self or environ-ment. In obsessions, where there is fear of one's emotions, avoidance of situations that arouse emotions, and continuing effort to keep feelings out of awareness, there is alienation of affect.

Alignment Arrangement in a straight line, bringing line into order.

Alignment of fractured bone In fracture bone cortex, periosteum and the surroudning musculature are disrupted. Alignment of fractured bone can be maintained by three point pressure.

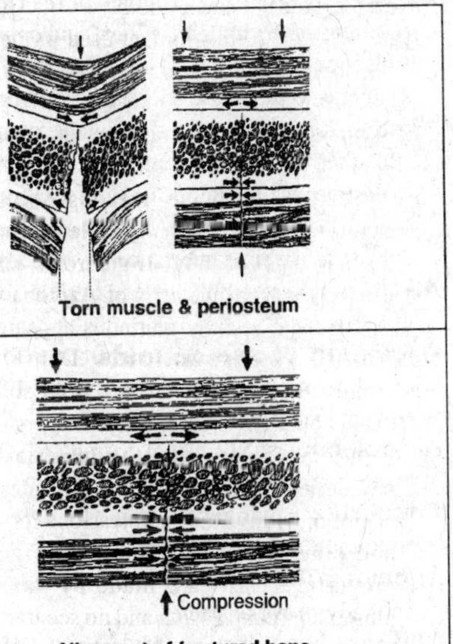

Alignment of fractured bone

Alimentary canal The digestive tract comprising mouth, oeso-phagus, stomach, duodenum, small and large intestines.

Alimentation The entire process of nourshing the body which includes mastication, swallowing, digestion, absorption and assimilation.

Alimentology The science of nutrition.

Aliphatic When the carbon-carbon bonds in a hydrocarbon are all single bonds i.e., the compound is saturated, the compound is referred to as an aliphatic compound.

Alkalemia Arterial pH>7.45 or H+ ion. concentration < 35 mmol/L.

Alkali reserve The amount of alkali that is available for neutralizing the acid produced such as hydrochloric acid.

Alkaline encrusting cystitis Alkaline urine may lead to deposition of phosphate crystals on the bladder mucosa. Synchronous lacerations, ulceration or necrosis of bladder mucosa are necessary for full mani-festations of disease.

Alkaline fermentation Fermentation in which the pH level rises to 7.5 or higher, allowing growth of the essential microorganisms but inhibiting growth of organisms that might otherwise spoil food.

Alkaline tide The slight change in blood pH toward the alkaline side following a meal.

Alkaliphilic Growing optimally in an alkaline setting.

Alkaloids Nitrogen-containing organic compounds of plant origin; often basic, and having intense biological activity.

Alkalosis There are two types of alkalosis, metabolic and respiratory. Metabolic alkalosis may be due to too much consumption of antacids or losing too much acid in vomiting. Respiratory alkalosis is caused by a reduction in the level of carbon dioxide in blood and may result due to deep and fast breathing.

Alkalotic Referring to the condition of alkalosis.

Alkannet Colouring obtained from root of Anchusa tinctoria.

All or none When stimulated, a muscle fiber will contract fully or not at all; whether a contraction occurs depends on whether the stimulus reaches the required threshold.

Allantois A tubular diverticulum of the posterior part of the yolk sac of the embryo. It passes into the body stalk through which it is accompanied by the allantoic (umbilical) blood vessel, thus taking part in the formation of the umbilical cord; later, it fuses with the chorion and helps to form the placenta. A small, vascularized membrane between the chorion and amnion of the fetus that serves as an early site for blood formation.

Allatotropin A neuropeptide that stimulates the synthesis of juvenile hormone by the corpus allatum.

Allele One of two or more alternate genes that occur at a particular locus of a chromosome which decide alternate inherited characteristics.

Allen's test It is used to assess the potency of radial and ulnar arteries at wrist. Pressure is applied over

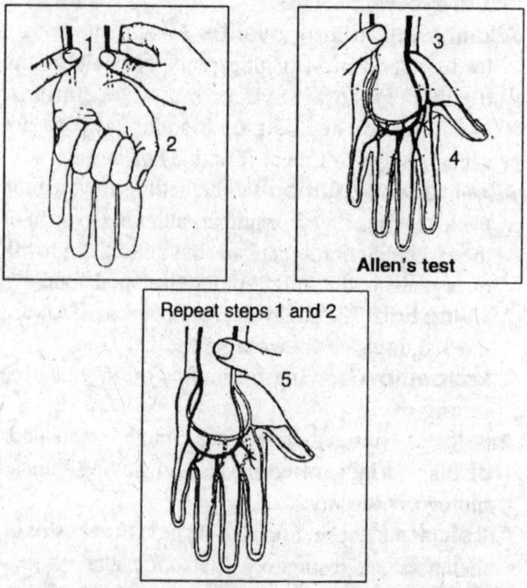

Allen's test

the radial and ulnar arteries at wrist. The patient is asked to open and close the hand and then hold. The colour of the palm changes. The pressure is released from the radial side and normally palm should return to normal colouring. This is repeated for ulnar artery. A similar test is used for digital vessels.

Allergen An antigenic substance that produces hypersensitivity, which may be inhaled, ingested, or injected, or may produce a reaction upon contact with the skin.

Allergic angiitis An inflammation of the small (dermal) blood vessels with polymorphonuclear infiltrate; cutaneous vasculitis.

Allergic blood transfusion reaction Blood contains various antigens and antibodies when transfusion starts. The donor blood may cause allergic reactions in form of skin rash or itching, shivering or severe reaction like difficulty in breathing and laryngeal oedema. Transfusion is to be discontinued. In mild cases anti-histamines are given. Adrenaline may be required in severe reaction.

Allergic gingivitis It is also known as plasma cell gingivitis. It is a lesion of marginal and attached gingiva. Most cases are allergic response to chewing gums. Lesion abruptly ends at the mucogingival junction. However, it may not involve the mucosa of palate, lip and tongue. The involved mucosa is red, swollen and sometimes granular. Patients may complain of burning sensation or pain. The discomfort is far less than clinical appearance will show. In some cases it is restricted to a few isolated areas of gingiva and ulceration is rare.

Allergic sialadenitis These may be accompanied by angioedema, skin rash and other signs of allergy. Diagnosis should be made cautiously. It is a self-limiting disease although secondary bacterial infection has been reported.

Allergy Allergy is inappropriate or the exaggerated reactions of the immune system and only occur on subsequent exposure. The function of immune system is to recognise antigens of microorganisms and to form antibodies. It sensitises white blood cells that will interact with these antigens leading to destruction. In allergies a similar process occurs except that the immune system forms antibodies against a harmless substance, by mistake.

Allicin Sulphur compound responsible for flavour of garlic.

Allocation of scarce resources Process of deciding how to distribute limited life-saving equipment or procedures.

Allochthonous Not native, rising from outside a given system or habitat.

Allocortex Phylogenetically old, three-layered cortex in the temporal lobe.

Allodynia Pain due to a stimulus that does not normally provoke pain.

Allogeneic Refers to the genetic differences between individuals of the same species.

Allogenic Graft Grafting material harvested from the same species as the recipient, but of a different genotype e.g., a graft taken from one human and transplanted into another.

Allograft Tissue or organ graft between allogeneic individuals.

Allometry The study or measurement of body size and its consequences.

Allopathy A theory and philosophy to treat diseases based on clinical and research evidence.

Alloplast A graft of an inert metal or plastic material.

Alloplastic Graft Biotolerant grafting material that is synthetic, derived from a nonliving source.

Allostasis The ability to achieve stability or homeostasis through change. Through allostasis the autonomic nervous system the hypothalamic pituitary-adrenal axis and cardiovascular, metabolic and immune systems protect the body by responding to internal and external challanges.

Allostatic load The ongoing level of demand for adaptation in an individual. An elevated level may be an important contributor to many chronic diseases.

Allosteric enzyme A regulatory enzyme, with catalytic activity modulated by the noncovalent binding of a specific metabolite at a site other than the active site.

Allosteric site The specific site on the surface of an allosteric enzyme molecule to which the modulator or effector molecule is bound.

Allotype An ellelic varient of an antigen which because it is not present in all individuals, may be immunogenic in members of the same species which have a different version of the allele.

Alloy Material that exhibits metallic properties and is composed of more elements, at least one of them is a metal.

Aloe vera Its moisturizing ability is its most widely recognised characteristic. It penetrates the skin. It regulates moisture and absorb UV light. Cleopatra is said to have attributed her beauty to it. It helps in healing the burns. Verapab lotion is available in Indian maket.

Alogia A decrease in speech fluency caused by a mental deficiency or an episode of dementia.

Alopecia Loss or absence of hair noticeable on scalp. Male pattern baldness is the commonest. This pattern is inherited. Normal hair is lost initially from the temples or crown. The affected area gradually becomes wider as the line of normal hair recedes. In generalised alopecia hair falls in large amounts.

All the hair fall in resting phase and then fall out at one go. Causes include mental trauma, chemotherapy, typhoid fever, etc. Localised alopecia may be caused by burns or radiation therapy. Excessive pulling of hair style may also be the cause. Fungal infection, weakness of hair shafts may also result it. Alopecia areata is a disorder of hair loss of localised circular areas of coin size. Sudden shock may be the cause. Recovery is practically assured.

Alpha A cell in the pancreatic islets that secretes glucagon.

Alpha cell Pancreatic cell that secretes glucagon.

Alpha fetoprotein Plasma protein produced by fetus.

Alpha motor neuron The motor neurin that innervates extrafusal fibers of skeletal muscle.

Alpha rhythm A thythimioc electroencephalographic waveform with a frequency ranging from 7 to 11 hertz that can be recorded from the scalp of a subject who is resting with closed eyes.

Alpha sympatholytic A drug that inhibits alpha adrenergic receptors of the autonomic nervous system.

Alpha1 (a1) receptor Alpha-adrenergic neuroreceptors that are located primarily in the vascular and intestinal smooth muscle, where they elicit contraction or relaxation, respectively.

Alpha1-acid glycoprotein A subgroup of the alphaglobulin fraction of blood; one of the most common plasma proteins.

Alpha1-antitrypsin deficiency A genetically determined autosomal recessive disorder in which the glycoprotein alpha1-antitrypsin the major protease inhibitor of human serum is deficient; persons with the disorder are predisposed to juvenile hepatic cirrhosis and pulmonary emphysema

Alpha-adrenergic receptor A subclass of neuroreceptors located at the norepinephrine synapses of the sympathetic (adrenergic) division of the autonomic nervous system; further divided into $alpha_1$ and $alpha_2$ categories.

Alpha-laval centrifuge Continuous bowl centrifuge for separating liquids of different densities, widely used for cream separation.

Alphatoxin of Staphylococcus This toxin is most important in producing pathogenicity. In cultures it is produced only under aerobic conditions. It is haemolytic, leucocidal and cytotoxic.

By its action on smooth muscles toxin causes constriction of small vessels, ischaemia and necrosis of affected tissue. It acts on cell membrane and may cause septicaemia. The toxin is antigenic and toxoid is prepared by treating with formalin.

Alport's syndrome It is of an autosomal dominant inheritance. Males die in early age. There will be haemorrhagic nephritis and progressive nerve deafness. Eyes will develop anterior lenticonus, subcapsular cataracts, thinning of lens capsule, fundus albi punctata and retinopathy.

ALT Alanine amino transferase, an enzyme liberated into the blood stream when hepatocytes are destroyed or damaged; serum levels are determined for evidence of hepatitis.

Altered states of awareness Conditions of consciousness which include sleep and dreams, the hypnotic and drug induced state, and meditation. The comparison is with the normal waking state. On this basis there is some criticism that sleep and dreams do not constitute altered states of awareness, for they occur regularly in daily life.

Alternate birth centre (ABC) An organisation of a hospital or a free-standing labour and delivery area that provides a home-like atmosphere. It has liberal policies regarding the presence of family and friends, labour practices, no separation of parents and infant, and early discharge.

Alternate host One of two possible hosts that a microbe may infect.

Alternate therapy Different diagnostic and and therapy systems that differ from and in some cases oppose conventional medicine practice.

Alternating Pulse Fluctuation between a weak and a strong beat.

Alternative medical therapy Treatment outside the mainstream of traditional medicine.

Alternative medicine Known as complementary medicine, methods of therapy that use techniques which are not normally part of standard or orthodox medicine such as osteopathy and acupuncture. Every culture has its folk medicine and traditional healers who use methods and beliefs handed down through generations. These range from physical and manipulative methods such as acupuncture, osteopathy, acupressure, homeopathy, naturopathy, faith healing, reiki, and herbal treatment. Many alternatives take a holistic approach to medicine.

Alternative sweeteners Nonnutritive sweeteners (or artificial sweeteners) synthetically produced to be sweet-tasting but which provide no nutrients and few, if any, calories; include aspartame, saccharin, and acesulfame K.

Alu repeates A DNA System that is used to trace ancestral heritage. This DNA consists a family of exact repretitive sequences scattered throughout the human genome.

Aluminium crown Temporary metal crown designed to be placed on a tooth to provide function, protect the tooth from thermal changes, and eliminate mesial drift and trauma.

Aluminium hydroxide It reacts with HCl to form aluminium chloride which reacts with intestinal secretions to produce insoluble salts, especially phosphate. It acts as antacids. It does not alter systemic acid-base balance.

aluminous porcelain A strong dental porcelain that is 40 to 50% by weight alumina, a crystalline material made of aluminum oxide (Al_2O_3).

ALV Available lysine value.

Alveolar Relating to or involving the alveoli.

Alveolar bone The bone that encases and supports the teeth; appears radiopaque.

Alveolar bone loss A loss of bone that surrounds and supports the teeth in the maxilla or mandible.

Alveolar crest The most coronal portion of alveolar bone found between the teeth; it is composed of dense cortical bone and appears radiopaque.

Alveolar duct Part of the respiratory passages beyond a respiratory bronchiole; from it arises alveolar sacs and alveoli.

Alveolar macrophage Highly phagocytic cell found in alveolar walls of the lungs. Also called a dust cell. Scavenging host-defense cells that reside in the alveoli englufing inhaled particles, including microorganisms. They destroy some engulfed organisms directly, while others replicate within them, triggering the release of mediators of cellular immunity.

Alveolar mucosa Covering of bony process of maxilla and mandible loosely attached to bone.

Alveolar oxygen concentration Other factors remaining constant PaO_2 is directly proportional to barometric pressure. As ventilation increases PaO_2 rises towards PO_2 at the inspired gases. Rising oxygen consumption of 500 ml/minute may result in hypoxia. Fall in cardiac output means that less oxygen is removed from alveolar gas.

Alveolar pressure Air pressure within the limgs.

Alveolar process It is a part of the maxilla and mandible forming and supporting the teeth. Alveolar process has two parts, alveolar bone proper and supporting bone. Alveolar bone proper consists of a thin lamella of bone surrounding the root. Fibres of periodontal ligament are attached to it. While supporting bone surrounds the alveolar bone proper and acts as a support in its function. Supporting bone consists of compact cortical plates of vestibular and oral surfaces of alveolar process and spongy bone found between cortical plates and alveolar bone.

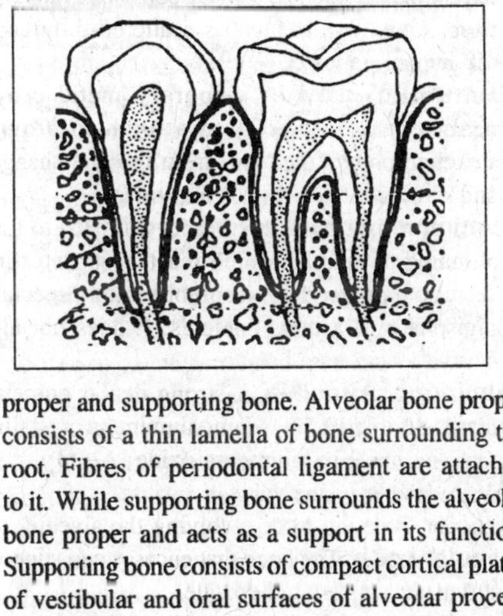

Alveolar proteinosis It is a chronic progressive disease of unknown aetiology. It is characterised by progressive dyspnoea, pulmonary infiltration and pulmonary insufficiency. Chemically material is phospholipids. Treatment is most unsatisfactory.

Alveolar ridge Bony ridge (alveolar process) of the maxillae or mandible, which contains the alveoli (sockets of the teeth).

Alveolar sac A collection or cluster of alveoli that share a common opening. Each alveolar duct ends in several sacs that resemble a cluster of grapes. A cluster of alveoli that share a common chamber or central atrium.

Alveolar surfaces The combined area of the alveoli.

Alveolar-arterial defects An imperfection or absence of the alveolar/arterial blood supply.

Alveolectomy Excision of portion of alveolar process to aid restoration of tooth.

Alveolitis It is the inflammation of alveoli in the lungs with thickening of walls which reduces the efficiency and elasticity of lungs. Most common cause is allergy to wheat pollens. Fibrosing alveolitis is an autoimmune disorder. X-ray shows alveolitis as mottled areas across the lungs. Lung capacity or lung function test is reduced. Treatment includes corticosteroids.

Alveolus Terminal part of respiratory tree, the site of gas exchange. About 3 x 10^8 exist in both lungs. Total surface area 70-80 m^2.

Alveoplasty Reshaping of endululous ridge.

Alveus Refers to the thin layer of white matter on the surface of the hippocampus.

Alzheimer's disease It is a progressive disease in which nerve cells degenerate in the brain and brain substance shrinks. It causes dementia known

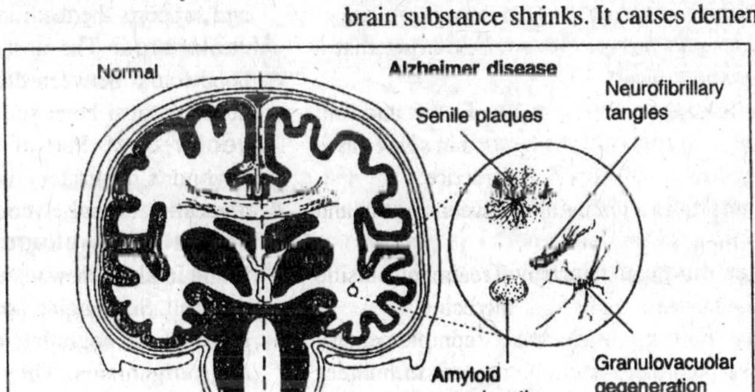

as presenile dementia. It is generally seen after the age of 65. Fifteen per cent cases are having family history. Exact cause is not known. Person becomes forgetful, anxious and depressed. In later stage there may be severe memory loss. Person remembers long ago events of childhood but fails to recall what happened yesterday. They become disoriented. Mood changes are sudden and unpredictable. In last stage they may develop hallucinations and delusions. Keeping the victim well nourished, exercised and occupied helps to alleviate anxiety.

Amalgam Alloy, one of the constituents being mercury; dental amalgam is a combination of

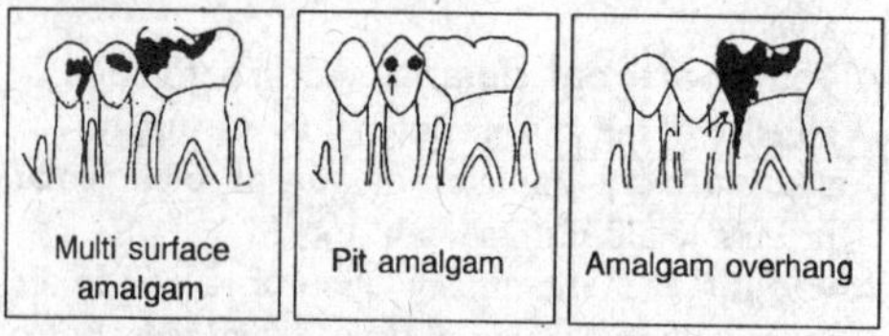

alloys commonly including silver, tin, and optionally copper or zinc mixed with mercury.

Amalgam matrix A thin metal form, usually stainless steel, adapted to a prepared cavity to supply the missing wall so the amalgam will be confined when condensed into the cavity preparation.

Amalgam tatoo Fragments of amalgam frequently become embedded in the oral mucosa and form the pigmented patches resembling melanomas. Dense tatoos may be radio opaque.

Amalgamator A mechanical device used to triturate the ingredients of dental amulgum to a mass.

Amastigote The aflagelleted stage of parasites such as Leishmania. Amastigotes are obligate intracellular parasites of mononuclear phagocytes of the vertebrate host.

Amaurosis fugax syndrome There will be malignant hypertension, atherosclerosis, expanding lesions of frontal or temporal lobe and vascular insufficiency. Ocular features may include partial blindness in short attacks to permanent complete blindness. There may be signs of arteriolar sclerosis.

Ambiguity Having more than one meaning. Simultaneous conflicting emotions, attitudes, ideas or wishes.

Ambiguous genitalia A form of physical development resulting from virilization of external genitalia in females or inadequate virilization of genitalia in males. In the case of the virilized female infant, the clitoris is enlarged with varying degrees of labial fusion which may resemble a scrotum.

Ambisexuality The normal occurrence of male and female function in one and the same individual, either as simultaneous or as sequential hermaphroditism.

Ambivalence The coexistence of contradictory emotions, attitudes, ideas, or desires with respect to a particular person, object, or situation. Ordinarily, it is not fully conscious and suggests psychopathology only when present in an extreme form.

Amblyopia It embraces all the condition of optic nerve damage due to ingestion of exogenous poisons, drugs and tobacco. Most common of these are tobacco, ethyl alcohol, quinine, ethambutol and oral contraceptives. Some of these affect ganglion cells of retina. Earliest complaint is of fogginess of vision more in day light rather than dull light. On ophthalmoscope there is normal fundus or slight temporal pallor of optic disc. There is central field defects. Loss of vision is due to degeneration of ganglion cells of retina at the macular area.

Ambubag Portable resuscitation device that provides manual inflation of the lungs. An Ambubag is usually used with supplemental oxygen.

Ambulatory blood pressure monitoring A technique for measuring blood pressure over prolonged periods of time in free living subjects. Practically every half an hour for 24 hours B.P. is checked.

Ambulatory electrocardiogram Continuous recording of heart rate and rhythm during normal activity.

Amelia Congenital absence of a limb or limbs.

Ameloblast Epithelial cell of the enamel organ; functions in the formation of enamel.

Ameloblastic fibroma It is an odontogenic tumour composed of both epithelial and mesenchymal elements. It constitutes 2.5 per cent of all odontogenic tumours of jaws and affects younger age group specially males. The premolar and molar area is preferred site of it and tumour is often associated with an impacted tooth. Lesion is slow growing and may be asymptomatic. It produces enlargement of jaw and migration of tooth. It appears as multilocular areas of radiolucency with expansion of cortex of jaw. The tumour has calcified tissue component. It is not encapsulated like the odontogenic adenomatoid tumour and does not diffusely infiltrate the surrounding marrow spaces like ordinary ameloblastoma. It has great potential for recurrence and can undergo malignant transformation to ameloblastic fibrosarcoma. Treatment includes wider excision and careful follow up.

Ameloblactic fibro-odontoma Lesions consist of calcified dental tissues as well as actively proliferating odontogenic epithelium and mesenchyme. It occurs more in childhood. Tumours are more common in mandible and 80% occur in posterior part of jaw. It is asymptomatic but may enlarge and deform the involved bone. On X-ray it shows irregular radiopacity surrounded by or associated with a radiolucent zone. Microscopic sections show areas of calcified and uncalcified hard dental tissue. It is not an aggressive lesion. Local conservative removal and curettage is curative.

Ameloblat Epithelial cell of the enamel organ which functions in the formation of enamel.

Amelogenesis imperfecta A severe hypoplasia or agenesis of enamel that is inherited as a dominant characteristic.

Amenorrhoea It is an absence of menstrual periods. If menstruation does not start till the age of 16 it is called primary amenorrhoea and after it permanent or temporary cessation of menstruation is called secondary amenorrhoea. Main aim of primary amenorrhoea is delayed puberty which may be due to disorder of endocrine system. It may be due to pituitary tumour, hypothyroidism or adrenal tumour. The commonest cause of secondary amenorrhoea is pregnancy. On family planning pills also menstrual cycle may cease.

Ames test A quick ban frequently used test to estimate the mutagenic potential of a chemical substance.

Ametropia It is a condition in which the incipient parallel rays of light from a distance of more than 6 metres do not come to focus upon the retina when the eye is at rest. Axial ametropia is due to abnormal length of eyeball. An eyeball longer than normal results in myopia and eyeball shorter than normal results in hypermetropia. Curvature ametropia is due to abnormal curvature of refractive media of eyeball, cornea and lens. More curvature of cornea or lens results in myopia and less curvature of cornea or lens results in hypermetropia. Index ametropia is due to change in the refractive index of lens. A high refractive index of lens nucleus results in myopia. This is seen in aged with sclerosis of lens nucleus.

Amicus Curiae "A friend of the court." A person who has not right to appear in a suit (no standing), but is allowed, at the court's discretion, to present legal arguments or evidence to the judge.

Amimia A disorder of language characterised by an inability to gesticulate or to understand the significance of gestures.

Amination An addition of amino group to an organic compound to produce an amine.

Amino acid pool The assortment of amino acids available to cells.

Amino acid profile Amino acid composition of protein.

Amino acids These make basic structural units of proteins. Individual amino acid molecules are linked together by chemical bonds. Quality of protein depends on composition of amino acids. There are 20 amino acids out of which 12 can be synthesized by body and rest 8 are known as essential amino acids.

Amino sugars Sugars that contain an amino group.

Aminoaciduria An excess of amino acids in the urine.

Aminocyclitol A cyclitol with one or more hydroxyls substitued by amino groups.

Aminoglycoside A low-molecular-weight saccharidic substance based mainly on aminated sugars. Aminoglycosides are a class of antimicrobial agents that inhibit protein synthesis; used widely against gram-negative bacteria. These are bactericidal. They act inside the cell by binding in the ribosomes.

These are water soluble and do not readily cross cell membrane. Half-life is 2 to 5 hours and are eliminated unchanged mainly by glomerular filtration so dose reduction may be needed. These are effective against staphylococci and aerobic gram-negative organisms. It is effective against septicaemia, pelvic and abdominal sepsis. Gentamicin is very effective against bacterial endocarditis.

Aminoglycoside drugs Antibacteria drugs that are active against gram-negative, some gram-positive and anaerobic bacteria.

Aminogram Diagramatic representation of amino acid composition of protein.

Aminopeptidase An intestinal peptidase that releases free amino acids from the amino end of short, chain peptides.

Aminophylline A mixture of theophylline and ethylenediamine used to treat bronchial asthma. It dilates the bronchi. It increases blood pressure and increases urine flow. Side effects include vomiting, headache and dizziness.

Aminopterin Aminopteroy-laglutamic acid specific antagonist to folic acid.

Amiodarone A coronary vasodilator used in the treatment of symptomatic supraventricular and ventricular arrythmias.

Ammeter An instrument for measuring the strength of current in amperes.

Ammonia Colourless, pungent smelling gas, highly soluble in water and toxic to all human cell.

Amnesia It is a loss of memorising information stored in memory. In such people short-term memory is retained for seconds only. Usually long-term memory is more affected in head injury, degenerative diseases and Alzheimer's disease.

Amnesic syndrome A profound deficit in learning and memory usually associated with bilateral damage to the diencephalon.

Amnestic aphasia Fluent speech with circuminocution and vague expressivity conveying little precise information, difficulty in finding words particularly nouns, slight impairment of understanding of sppech. Occurs with lesions in temporoparietal lobe.

Amniocentesis It is a diagnostic procedure in which a small amount of amniotic fluid is withdrawn from amniotic sac, a membrane surrounding the fetus in uterus It is done to detect fetal defects such as Down's syndrome and other sex-linked disorders. It can diagnose haemolytic anaemia of newborn and respiratory distress syndrome. Genetic amniocentesis is done between 16th and 18th weak of gestation.

Amnioinfusion Infusion of lactated Ringer's solution or isotonic solution into uterine cavity to reduce umbilical cord compression.

Amnion The amniotic cavity enlarges more than the growing embryo. The amnion is attached to the chorion and fetal surface of placenta in a loose manner and can be easily separated from above. Exchange of amniotic fluid between fetal and maternal compartments takes place.

Amnioscope An instrument for examination of the fetus and amniotic fluid by passage through the maternal abdominal wall into the amniotic cavity, thus permitting direct visualisation.

Amnioscopy It is direct visualization of amniotic fluid by means of an illuminated cone shaped hollow tube introduced through dilated cervix.

Amniotic cavity Fluid-filled cavity surrounding and protecting the developing embryo.

Amniotic cell division This is equal to fragmentation. Nucleus divides by a process of fission and resulting daughter nuclei may not be equal in size. The chromosomes are not equally ensured between the daughter cells. This type of cell division results in formation of binucleated or multinucleated cells.

Amniotic fluid It is a clear fluid which surrounds the fetus in uterus throughout pregnancy. Fluid is contained in amniotic sac. Child moves freely being attached to placenta by umbilical cord. The fluid is produced by the cells lining the membrane

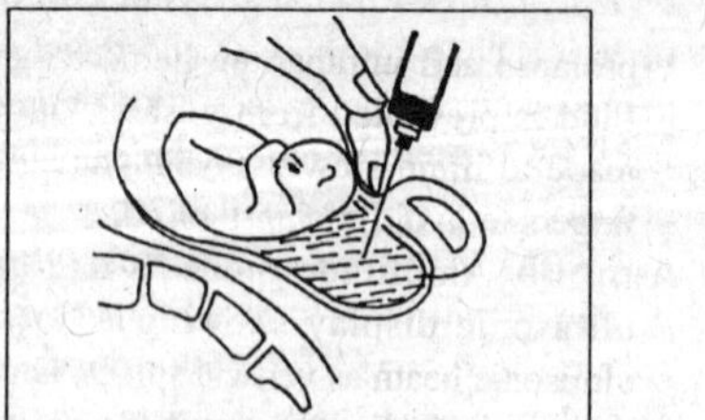

Amniotic fluid

and is constantly circulated. It is swallowed by fetus, absorbed into the blood stream and again passed as urine. Amniotic fluid is 90 per cent of water. Remaining part consists of substances found in plasma. By 35 weeks the amount of fluid is 2 pint. Amniotic fluid appears after first week of conception.

Amniotic fluid embolism An embolism in which amniotic fluid with its particulate matter is drawn into pregnant woman's circulation, lodging her lungs.

Amniotic fluid index (AFI) A measurement of the largest amniotic fluid pocket in each of the four abdominal quadrants. The AFI normally ranges between 8 and 26 cm. An AFI <8 represent reduced amniotic fluid volume; values <5 cm are associated with significantly increased perinatal morbidity.

Amniotic membrane The tiny crescentic line that constitutes the amniotic membrane can be seen within the gestational sac in the first trimester with high quality ultrasound system. It encloses the amniotic cavity. The yolk sac lies the extracelomic cavity outside the amniotic membrane. At about 4 weeks the amniotic sac is about the same size as the yolk sac. Both lie within chorion.

Amniotomy It is a method of induction of labor used in combination with oxytocin drip. For it cervix must be effaced and 2 cm. dilated with head deeply engazed. Complications of it are cord

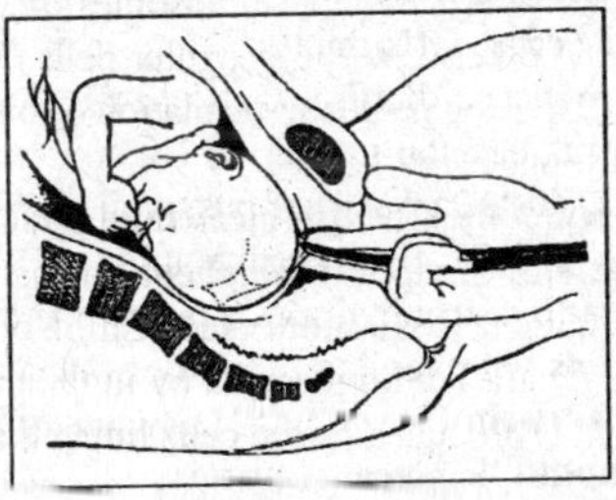

prolapse and intrapartum hemorrhage. Amniotic fluid is prevented from gushing out rapidly and made to drain slowly by tamponing cervix with fingers to avoid prolapse of cord.

A-mode Amplitude mode, a one-dimensional ultrasonic display showing echoes along the ultrasonic beam as vertical spikes. On a horizontal time axis indicates depth or reflectors. The amplitude of spikes reflects the echo strength.

Amoebiasis It is very common and is caused by *Entamoeba histolytica*. It happens where public hygiene is poor. *Entamoeba* is single-celled organism that multiplies by simple division and moves around in intestine. Many people carry it in their intestines and excrete amoebic cysts without any symptoms. Some strains may invade intestinal wall and cause bleeding. Ulcers are formed in intestinal walls. Stools may be loose with rumbling pain in stomach. Some may develop full-blown dysentery. If liver abscess develops then person may develop shaking chills, fever, loss of weight and painful enlargement of liver. Chloroquine and metronidazole destroy it.

Amoebic liver Clinical manifestations include fever with loss of appetite and right upper abdominal pain. Liver is enlarged and tender. Jaundice is minimal. Metronidazole is effective if given for 7 days.

Amoebic liver abscess This is a common type of metastatic amoebiasis occurring in 2 to 5% cases. During the course of formation of ulcer in large gut vegetative forms of *Entamoeba* enters inside the portal venous radicals in submucous coat and as emboli enter the liver. Fever comes with chill and rigor and goes away with sweating. Hectic type of fever is seen. Pain is in right hypochondric region.

Sometimes haemoptysis with typical chocolate-coloured sputum is seen. Tongue is dry and oedema may be present. Right lower chest will be restricted in movements, will show diminished vocal fremitus and impaired note on percussion. On auscultation breath sounds and vocal resonance are diminshed. Sometimes frank signs of effusion may be obtained. Liver abscess may burst at various sites. Metronidazole and chloroquine are helpful.

Amorphine Lacking specific form or shape; unorganised.

Amorphous 1. Having no definite form; shapeless 2. Having random arrangement of atoms 3. In pharmacy, not crystallized.

Amphetamines These are psychostimulants. It acts by releasing noradrenaline stored in nerve endings in both the CNS and periphery. Subject becomes euphoric and fatigue is delayed. Physical and mental performance may improve. While large doses may result in anxiety and feeling of nervous and physical tension. Person in heavy doses may develop confusion. Mild dependence on prescribed amphetamines may develop in unstable personalities, depressives and tired. Students consume it to keep awake for continuing studies during examination time. Its use in sport is abuse. It suppresses appetite too.

Amphiarthrosis Slightly movable joint such as the joint joining the two pubic bones.

Amphid A small depression or pit located anteriorly on the body surface of most nematodes and believed to be a chemoreceptor.

Amphimixis Sexual reproduction; the mixing of the genes from two distinct individuals, involving the recombinational effects of meiotic reduction and fusion of gametes.

Amphoteric Capable of donating and accepting protons, thus able to serve as an acid or a base. Referring to or describing a type of monogonont female capable of producing both AMICTIC and MICTIC eggs.

Amplification of transmission The increased spread of infectious disease, occuring naturally or because of facilitating factors such as nonsterilized needles and syringes.

Amplifying host A host that serves to increase the natural pool of an invading pathogenic agent.

Amplitude The intensity of a stimulus; in audition, amplitude is roughly equivalent to loudness.

Ampoule Ampoule has a narrow upper portion—the stem, wider lower portion—the body with neck which may be constricted or smoothly curved. For filling in syringe the content to be injected apply spirit to neck, tap gently the upper portion. Then cut the neck with file. Aspirate the fluid in syringe without pushing the air into the ampoule.

Ampule Small, sterile all-glass or plastic container used for medication.

Ampulla A saclike enlargement of a duct or tube.

Ampulla of vater Heparorpancreatic ampulla.

Amputation It is a surgical removal of a limb or part of limb usually following a crush injury, destruction of tissue by frostbite or gangrene. This operation is done in such a way that artificial limb may be fitted. It requires skilled dressing.

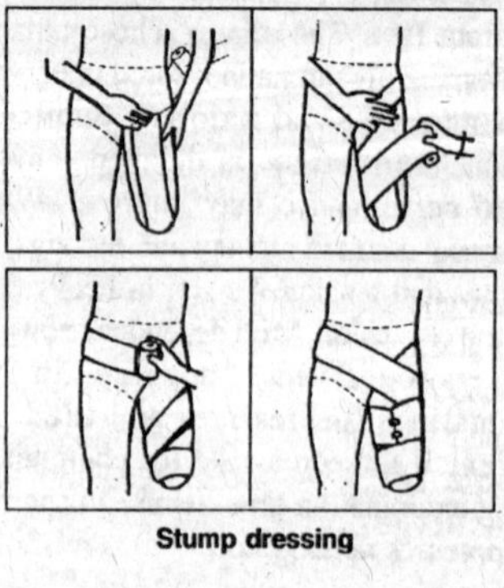

Stump dressing

Amulgum retrograde Silver amalgam filling placed in apex of tooth after an apicoectomy.

Amygalin Glucoside in almonds, apricot and cherry stones hydrolysed by enzyme emulsion to glucose.

Amygdala Small wallnut shaped brain area in the center of brain involved in fear response.

Amygdalo A combining from denoting relationship to an almond-shaped structure or to the tonsil.

Amylase One of a group of starch-splitting enzymes that cleave starch, glycogen, and related polysaccharides.

Amylasuria The presence of amylase in the urine.

Amylodyspepsia Inability to starch dyspepsia.

Amyloid A type of age pigment which accumulates in nerve cells. It inhibits metabolic process in nervous system.

Amyloidosis In it substance known as amyloid is deposited in tissues of body. It contains protein and starch. It may be caused by rheumatoid arthritis, multiple myeloma and tuberculosis. Amyloid may deposit in any organ, liver, kidney, tongue, spleen etc. If it is deposited in heart then it may cause arrhythmias. If intestines are affected it may cause diarrhoea. In primary amyloidosis deposits develop in skin, as slightly raised, waxy spots, clusted around armpits, groin, face and neck. There is basically no teatment.

Amyloins Carbohydrates that are complexes of dextrins with varying proportions of maltose.

Amylophagia Pica of corn and laundry starch.

Amylopsin Pancreatic amylase.

Amyotrophic lateral sclerosis Motor neuron disease of unknown aetiology characterised by progressive degeneration of cortico-spinal tracts and anterior horn cells or bulbar efferent neurons. Commonly known as "Lou Gehrig's disease."

Anabiosis Return to life; the restoration of life processes in a dormant organism that did not have the external appearance of life.

Anabiotic Apparently lifeless, but still capable of living.

Anabolic steroids Androgens are protein anabolic agents but their clinical use for this purpose is limited by the virilisation. These have little use in male osteoporosis. The use of androgens in general wasting is justifiable in extreme debilitating disease such as after major surgery, long illnesses and severe ulcerative colitis. Itching of biliary obstruction is relieved. They should be given in intermittent course of 3 to 12 weeks with similar intervals to reduce unwanted effects specially liver injury.

Anabolism A phase of metrabolism involving chemical reactions within cells that result in the production of larger molecules from smaller ones; specifically, the synthesis of protein, glycogen, and fat.

Anabolite A product of anabolism.

Anaclitic Literally, leaning on. In psychoanalytic terminology, dependence of the infant on the mother or mother substitute for a sense of well being (e.g. gratification through nursing). Normal behaviour in childhood, pathologic in later years if excessive.

Anaclitic depression A severe form of depression identified by Spitz in infants who experienced prolonged separations from their mothers.

Anacrotic pulse It is represented by a small slow rising pulse with a notch or an extra wave. It is of no special clinical significance but may be seen in aortic stenosis.

Anadromy A type of life cycle in which fish migrate from freshwater to seawater and then return to freshwater to spawn.

Anaemia In it haemoglobin level falls below normal. Haemoglobin molecules are carried inside RBCs and function to carry oxygen from lungs to tissues. It is maintained by strict balance between RBC production in bone marrow and RBC destruction in spleen. Normal blood haemoglobin is 14 to 16 gm/100 ml in male and 12 to 14 gm/100 ml in females. Concentration below 10 gm causes headache, tiredness and lethargy. Below 8 gm/100 ml may cause difficulty in breathing and palpitation.

Anaemia, aplastic In it RBCs, WBCs and platelets are reduced in number. It is caused by production failure of stem cells in bone marrow. It may be caused by anticancer drugs or by radiation therapy. Long-term exposure to fumes of benzene may cause this. It is most common around the age of 30. Feeling of tiredness is the most common symptom. WBC deficiency increases susceptibility to infections while deficiency of platelets may lead bruising and bleeding gums. Sometimes bone marrow transplantation is needed

Anaemia, haemolytic It is caused by premature destruction of red cells in blood due to haemolysis. Bone marrow has the capacity to increase RBC production six times. Destruction may result due to abnormal rigidity of cell membrane which may be an inherited defect. Symptoms may be pallor, headache, fatigue and shortness of breath on exertion. There may be jaundice too. Blood smear under microscope will show abnormally large number of immature cells. These RBCs may be abnormal in shape.

Anaemia, iron deficiency It is caused by deficiency of iron if insufficient iron is available to the bone marrow. It occurs when iron loss with any extra demand is more than supply from diet. It may be caused during disease, heavy menstrual period, peptic ulcer or cancer. Prolonged treatment with anti-inflammatory drugs and hookworm infestation of intestine may lead to it. There may be poor absorption of iron from digestive tract. There may be diet which may not be providing sufficient iron. Along with fatigue there may be sore tongue, sore mouth, brittle nails, breathlessness and pain in chest.

Anaemia, megaloblastic It is caused by deficiency of Vitamin B_{12} or folic acid. These interfere with the production of red blood cells in bone marrow. RBCs formed are enlarged and deformed known as macrocytes. Vitamin B_{12} is found only in non-vegetarian and dairy foods. Excess of vitamin B_{12} is absorbed in liver. In pernicious anaemia stomach lining is not able to produce intrinsic factor which helps in absorption of vitamin B_{12}.

Requirement of vitamin B_{12} is so less that even pure vegetarians do not develop its deficiency. Folic acid deficiency may also cause anaemia but plenty of folic acid is available from green leafy vegetables. Deficiency may be found in young children and old people. Symptoms include sore mouth and tongue.

Anaerobic Able to live and grow only when oxygen is absent.

Anaerobic bacteria Microorganisms that exist without oxygen.

Anaerobic glycolysis The conversion of glucose to lactic acid to provide energy in the absence of oxygen.

Anaerobic pathway A form of energy production that does not require oxygen.

Anaerobic respiration The use of ions or molecules, usually inorganic other than molecular oxygen to accept electrons derived from energy-conserving oxidation reactions by cells.

Anaerobic threshold The limit of the ability of the blood to buffer the by-products of anaerobiosis e.g. lactic acid ; the onset of plasma lactate accumulation; an indirect measure of an individual's endurance.

Anaerobic treatment A biological treament process in which no oxygen is available. Electron acceptors may be organic substrates sulfate, nitrate, or carbon dioxide. The last is more common for treatment of high-strength industrial wastewaters with conversion of a large portion of the organic carbon to methane.

Anaesthesia There is absence of all sensations. It may happen if all nerve tissues are damaged by injury or disease. Anaesthesia is induced artificially to abolish pain during surgical procedures and child birth. Two types of anaesthesia are there. Under local anaesthesia person remains conscious and sensation is abolished only in localised area temporarily. It can be given as eyedrops, sprays, creams. In general anaesthesia, whole of body is anaesthetised.

Anaesthesia dolorsoa Pain in anaesthetic area, typically following destructive treatment of trigeminal neuralgia. It may develop after many months and is not responding even to further surgery.

Anaesthesia general Application of anaesthesia which makes a patient unconcious.

Anaesthesia stages

Stage one of analgesia.

- Normal reflexes
- Ends with loss of eyelash reflex and unconsciousness.

Stage two of excitement

- Irregular breathing
- Dilated pupils
- Vomiting, laryngospasm
- Loss of eye lid reflex

Stage three

Surgical anaesthesia

Anaesthesia, dental A loss of sensation induced in a patient to prevent pain during dental manipulations. Mostly local anaesthesia is given. For dental filling surgeons do not use anaesthesia. For other purposes lidocaine or procaine is injected into gums. Sometimes if gum is inflamed and bleeding then injection is not given directly but around the affected part and is known as peripheral nerve block. Sometimes additional sedation is given. In periodontal surgery general anaesthesia is given.

Anaesthesia, general In it patient is rendered unconscious and remains in this state for long. Loss of sensation and consciousness is induced in a patient by anaesthetist who gives combination of drugs by injection and inhalations. The primary aim of anaesthesia is to abolish pain, awareness, muscle tone and cardiovascular reflexes. Complications of general anaesthesia may be low blood pressure, myocardial infarction and respiratory failure.

Anaesthesia, local There is loss of sensation induced in a limited region of a person's body to prevent pain. For minor stitching, etc. injection is given directly at the location. In severe cases nerve block may be done. Nerves can also be blocked as they branch off from the spinal cord known as epidural anaesthesia. It is generally used in child birth and surgery of lower limbs. Throat, larynx and respiratory passages can be sprayed locally before bronchoscopy.

Anagen One of three main stages in the hair growth cycle, anagen is the phase of active growth. In a healthy human scalp approximately 85-95% of the follicles are in anagen. In human scalp hairs, the duration of the anagen phase ranges from 2 years and 2 months to 6 years and 6 months.

Anal canal The terminal tubular portion of the large interstine that opens through the anus of the G.I. tract.

Anal character Qualities such as stubbornness and excessive orderliness, presumably relating, in the Freudian view, to early toilet training.

Anal fissures These are longitudinal breaches in anal mucosa which occur at the anterior and more commonly the posterior aspect of anal canal as far as the pectinate line. Cause is unknown but a few may have inflammatory bowel disease. Chronic fissures contain fibrous tissue and are marked superiorly by a hypertrophied anal papilla and inferiorly by a sentinel tag. Spasm of sphincter causes pain and relief of spasm allows healing of fissure.

Anal glands Enlarged and modified sweat glands that empty into the anal opening.

Anal intercourse It is the coitus in which male organ is inserted into the partner's anus, usually after lubrication and stretching with fingers. Anal intercourse is practised by homosexuals and is termed as sodomy.

Anal sphincters Ring-shaped banks of muscles in the anus.

Anal stage The second stage in the psychosexual stages postulated in psychoanalysis, concerning chiefly toilet training and the development of related habits, such as cleanliness, neatness, obedience, and so forth.

Anal triangle The subdivision of the female or male perineum that contains the anus.

Analeptic drugs These are the drugs which stimulate breathing and are used in the treatment of apnoea in a newborn. These work by stimulating the respiratory centre.

Analgesia A mild to moderate lessening or dulling of central nervous system function, thereby rendering the client conscious, but sedated, and experiencing a decreased level of pain.

Analgesic Drug that relieves pain without causing loss of consciousness.

Analgesic drugs These are the drugs which relieve pain. Narcotic analgesics are codeine, morphine, pethidine while non-narcotic drugs are acetaminophen, aspirin and sodium salicylates. Non- narcotics drugs are used in mild pain, headache and backache.

When these fail narcotic drugs are used. When any infection is developed they produce prostaglandins which trigger transmission of pain signals to the brain. Non-narcotic work by preventing prostaglandin production. etaminophen blocks the pain impulses in the brain itself thereby preventing the perception of pain. Narcotic analgesics block pain impulses at specific sites known as opiate receptors in the brain and spinal cord. Side effects of aspirin include nausea, vomiting due to irritation of stomach mucosa. Narcotics may produce constipation and euphoria.

Analog Something that has very similar properties to another, but also is different in some fundamental way; for example; 1. a gene that is structurally or functionally similar to another, but not related by descent. 2. a naturally occurring or synthetic compound with structural similarity to natural nucleobases or nucleosides.

Analogy The fact of being an analog.

Analysis Critical review of collected data to identify and remedy gaps and inconsistencies and compilation of that data in an organized manner, so as to determine those concerns or problems with which the client need assistance or guidance. The analysis phase ends with the identification of the pertinent nursing diagnosis.

Analysis of covariance (ANCOVA) A form of analysis of variance in which the effect of an intervening variable is mathematically removed from the analysis.

Analysis of variance (ANOVA) A widely used statistical procedure for determining the significance of differences obtained on an experimental variable studies under two or more conditions. Differences are commonly assigned to three aspects; the individual differences among the subjects or patients studies, group differences, however, classified (e.g. by sex) and differences according to the various treatments to which they have been assigned. The method can assess both the main effects of a variable and its interaction with other variables that have been studied simultaneously.

Analyst The person, usually with medical training, who conducts psychoanalytic sessions—a psychoanalytic therapist.

Analyte The analyte of a sample is a substance searched for and identified by chemical analytical means.

Analytic psychology The approach to psychoanalysis presented by Carl Gustav Jung—a significant concept in this approach is the collective unconscious.

Anamorph A sexual stages of a fungus.

Anaphase The third stage of mitosis in which the chromatids that have separated at the centromeres move to opposite poles of the cell.

Anaphylactic shock It is severe and may even be life threatening. Bites and stings may cause it. Injection of penicillin, antitetanus serum and local anaesthetic may result it. Entry of allergen into blood provokes the release of massive amount of histamine and other chemicals. Blood vessels dilate lowering the BP. There may be itching, bronchospasm, swelling of tongue and throat. In emergency, epinephrine IV may be given immediately. Intramuscular (IM) hydrocortisone and oxygen inhalation are necessary. Antihistaminic drugs should be given.

Anaphylactoid purpura It develops in children between the age 4 and 16 years. Headache, loss of appetite and abdominal pain are early symptoms. Joint involvement manifests as periarticular pain, tenderness and minimal swelling. Colicky abdominal pain, malaena or haematemesis develop. Kidneys may be involved. Usual course of illness is 4 weeks.

Anaphylactoid reaction Clinically it is similar to anaphylactic reaction except that it dont involves immunoglobulin cross linkage.

Anaphylaxis An acute, severe, allergic reaction characterised by sudden collapse, shock, or respiratory and circulatory failure following the injection of an allergen; increased susceptibility to an allergen resulting from previous exposure to it.

Anaphylaxis mechanism As a result of original sensitisation with antigen, specialised cytotropic antibody is formed which binds to mast cells and basophils, respiratory tract and vascular endothelium. In man anaphylaxis is entirely due to IgE antibodies when same antigen is again absorbed. The histamine released as a result of anaphylaxis leads to vasodilatation, increased capillary permeability and smooth muscle contraction.

Anarthria Unintelligible speech resulting from a brain lesion, particularly in the brain stem, causing severe impairment of the motor-speech system.

Anastomosis It is the connection between two vessels or tubes in body. It may occur naturally or be created surgically as is done in by-pass surgery in intestine and heart ailment.

Anatomic barriers Anatomic structures determined by the shape and fit of the bones at the joint.

Anatomic crown Portion of dentin covered by enamel.

Anatomic dead space Spaces of the nose, pharynx, larynx, traceha, bronchi, and bronchioles that contain 150 mL of tidal volume; the air does not reach the alveoli to participate in gas exchange.

Anatomic dead space volume The volume of gas that occupies the nonrespiratory conducting airways.

Anatomic position Body position is vertical, facing forward with hands to the sides and the palms facing forward to assist in body part identification.

Anatomical classification of placenta previa Type I- Minor portion of placenta lies below the lower uterine segment. Type II Most of placenta lies below uterine segment. Type III Placenta covers the internal OS when OS is closed. Type IV Placenta completely covers the internal OS when it is dilated.

Anatomical position A position of the body universally used in anatomical descriptions in which the body is erect, facing the observer, the upper limbs are at the sides, the palms are facing forward, and the feet are flat on the floor.

Anatomy The branch of science concerned with the structure of the body and the relationship of its organs.

Anchorage The supporting base for orthodontic forces that are applied to stimulate tooth movement.

Anchovy A fish

Anderson-Warburg syndrome It has sex-linked inheritance. Mental retardation ranges from imbecility to idiocity. There will be microphthalmos with extensive destruction of all ocular structures, blindness at birth, iris atrophy, iritis, corneal opacification and lenticular destruction.

Androgen drugs These are group of drugs having similar actions as androgen hormones. Testosterone is the most common example. Androgens are used in male hypogonadism to stimulate the development of sexual characters, growth of pubic and facial hair and enlargement of genitals. These are commonly used by athletes and body builders to increase muscle bulk and strength. Adverse effects include fluid retention, weight gain, increased cholesterol level and may even damage liver. If taken by females it may deepen their voice and develop male characters. During pregnancy and breastfeeding these should not be given.

Androgen hormones These are produced by specialised cells of testes in males and adrenal glands in both sexes. Ovaries are also secreting very small amount of androgens. The production of androgens by testes is controlled by certain pituitary hormones. It affects growth of penis, facial and body hair. These increase bulk of shoulders. It promotes aggressiveness. Excess androgen in males causes premature development of sex feelings. Initially these increase bone growth but later on height is decreased because androgens cause long bones to stop growing.

Androgen inhibitor A substance that decreases androgen production or expression.

Androgenesis A phenomenon in which chromosomes are completely of paternal origin.

Androgogy Principles of teaching adult learners.

Androgyny The expression of both traditionally feminine and traditionally masculine attributes.

Android Pelvis The brim is heart shaped. The widest transverse diameter intersects the AP of the brim nearer to the sacrum. AP diameter is 10.2 cm and the widest transverse diameter is 12.9 cm. The side walls are convergent and the ischial spines are prominent.

Anecdotal procedure Includes categories and classifications of procedures, technologies, or euipment that have not received the benefit of the experimental method. Items included in this definition originate and depend upon experience and observation only.

Anecdotal records Personal, handwritten account of an incident.

Anechoic Normal urine and bile are anechogenic, i.e. they have no internal echoes.

Anemia Low red blood cell count.

Anencephaly There is absence of brain, cranial vault and spinal cord. Most affected children are stillborn and survive for a few hours. On ultrasound it is easily seen. This happens due to failure of development of neural tube.

Anergy panel A panel containing several pravalent antigens that are injected to assess immuno-competence. At least one of the antigens should elicit a reaction if the immune system is not impaired.

Anesthesia The loss of sensory perception.

Anesthesiologist Physician who administers chemical agents that temporarily eliminate sensation and pain.

Anesthetist Specialists who administers anesthesia.

Anesthetization The production of insensibility to pain.

Anesthetize To put under the influence of anesthetics.

Aneuploidy A condition of numeric chromosome errors, which result in major developmental defects of the fetus.

Aneurysm This is ballooning of an artery due to the pressure of blood flowing through a weakened area. Weakening may be due to disease, injury or congenital defect in the artery wall. Aorta may have dissecting aneurysm.

There is usually severe pain and vessel may rupture. It may be due to congenital weakness of middle layer of artery.

In Marfan's disease middle layer of wall of aorta is defective leading to aneurysm. Due to atherosclerosis aneurysm develops in lower part of vessel. Aneurysm may rupture causing fatal loss of blood and severe damage to brain. MR angiography is a better tool to diagnose aneurysm.

Aneurysm of aorta It is a permanent localised dilatation of aorta due to destruction of its wall. It may be congenital or inflammatory. Aneurysm of ascending aorta may produce dull chest pain due to erosion of rib and a local bulging on right side of sternum. If right bronchus is compressed there may be cough, collapse of lung and secondary infection. Aneurysm of arch of aorta will compress mediastinal structures. There will be cough and tracheal tug. There will be inequality of pus on two sides. Clinical features will include bloated face, non-pulsatile engorgement of jugular veins, hoarseness of voice and deep boring pain over sternum.

Angathia A congenital condition characterized by total or partial absence of a jaw.

Anger A negatively toned emotion, subjectively experienced as an aroused state of antagonism toward someone or something percieved to be the source of an aversive event. An unpleasant emotion ranging in intensity from irritation or annoyance to fury or rage that is emotional side of hostility.

Angiitis It is the inflammation of blood vessel. Symptoms vary widely. These may include arthritis, rashes and even kidney failure. Corticosteroids are helpful.

Angina innocens Functional type of angina is known as pseudoangina. Evidence of functional angina is increase of pain after exertion, not during it. Presence of palpitation, giddiness and fainting attacks, presence of precordial hyperaesthesia, evidence of unstable nervous system or history of nervous breakdown will be there. Still organic angina has to be ruled out. Safest criterion is pain in relation to exercise and only during exertion then it is true angina.

Angina pectoris It is pain in chest, arms and jaw due to lack of oxygen to the heart muscle mostly during activity and exercise when demand of oxygen is more. Atherosclerosis and coronary artery spasm are the main cause. It is common in men after the age of 50. Patient feels sensation of pressure over chest.

It usually starts in the centre of the chest and can spread to throat, upper jaw, back and arms. Pain comes on when heart is working harder and requires more oxygen and is relieved by a short rest. There may be nausea, sweating and giddiness. A prolonged and more serious attack of angina may be due to myocardial infarction. Attacks of angina may be relieved by nitroglycerine which increases flow of blood through heart. If nitroglycerine is not effective and is causing severe headache, beta-blockers and calcium channel blockers may be given.

Angio catheter Indications of putting catheter are hemodyanmic monitoring arterial blood sampling and frequent blood draw requirement.

Placement of arterial lines is generally done in ICU settings.

Angioataxia Irregular tension of a blood vessel.

Angioblastic tissue The primordial mesenchymal tissue that develops into embryonic blood cells and vascular endothelium.

Angiocarditis Any inflammatory disease of the heart and blood vessels.

Angioedema Allergic reaction is known as angioneurotic oedema. It is similar to urticaria. There is large, well-defined swelling of sudden onset in skin, larynx, etc. This swelling may last for several hours. Common cause is sudden allergic reaction to eggs or sea food in general. The symptoms include sudden difficulty in breathing, speaking and swallowing, accompanied by swelling of lips, face and neck. Angioedema of throat and larynx may be life threatening because it can block airway causing suffocation. Treatment includes injection epinephrine, tracheostomy in severe difficulty of breathing and injection of corticosteroid.

Angiogenesis The formation of blood vessels.

Angiogram Image of blood vessels obtained by intra-arterial injection of radioopaque fluid.

Angiography It is a procedure that enables blood vessels to be seen on film generally after giving radiopaque dye. But with the availability of MRI now dye is not needed for angiography. Carotid angiography is performed on patients suffering from angina and ischaemic attacks to see whether there is blockage or narrowing in one of carotid arteries supplying blood to brain. Cerebral angiography is done for showing aneurysm. Contrast medium is usually injected into the vessel to be examined through a fine catheter. Catheter is inflexible plastic tube inserted into the femoral artery or just over elbow or the carotid arteries. A needle is inserted into the artery.

A long wire with a soft tip is inserted through the needle, needle is removed and catheter is then threaded over the wire into blood vessels. Under X-ray control the tip of catheter is introduced into the vessel under study and contrast medium is injected and X-ray pictures are taken. In digital subtraction angiography (DSA) computer is used to process and subtract or remove unwanted background leaving the vessel well seen to be studied. Very little contrast is needed. With the help of MRI, angiography can be done with or without contrast just within 5 minutes with the help of 1.5 Tesla unit.

Angiolipsis Pressure on an artery, direct or indirect; e.g., in the intervertebral foramen I.V.F. through pressure generated by a discopathy, in the foramina transversarii through osteogenic reactions.

Angiomas These are true vascular neoplasms, conspicuous causing function impairment. It presents as flat or slightly prominent painless tumour area generally with assoicated discolouration and irregularity of overlying skin. Angiomas in mucosa usually produce a deep red and purple discolouration.

Tumour may be soft, tense and easily compressible. On straining tumour may produce prominent swelling. Multifocal occurrence is possible.

Angioneurotic oedema There is allergic reaction resulting in itching and swelling of skin. The allergen may be a drug or certain foods. Extreme cold or heat may also result it

Angiopathy Any disease of the vessels.

Angioplasty It is a technique of treating stenosis or occlusion of a blood vessel or a heart valve by introducing a balloon into constricted area.

It is also done in the treatment of coronary arteries There is always a slight risk of damaging the artery. It is a very effective method, successful for 2 to 3 years but after it stenosis may develop again.

Angiostrangiloidiasis *Angiostronglus cantonensis* is a parasitic roundworm. Its larva develops in giant land snail. When larvae are ingested they migrate to CNS where they cause radiculoencephalomyelitis.

Angiotensin Either of two forms of a protein associated with regulation of blood pressure. Angiotensin I is produced by the action of renin on angiotensinogen and is converted by the action of ACE (angiotensin-converting enzyme) into angiotensin II, which stimulates, aldosterone secretion by the adrenal cortex, stimulates the sensation of thirst, and causes vasoconstriction with resulting increase in systemic vascular resistance.

Angiotensinogen A protein found in the blood which gives rise to angiotensin I after renin, an enzyme secreted from the kidney, acts on it.

Angiotonic Increasing the vascular tension.

Angle line Any place where two tooth surfaces meet.

Angle of impact The acute angle formed between the direction of a blood drop and the plane of the surface its strikes.

Angle of Laurin With the knee 20° of flexion the lateral patellofemoral angle is measured Normally angle will open laterally when the angle of Laurin is positive.

In case of abnormal patellar tilt the angle of Laurin is negative and suggests an abnormal medial opening.

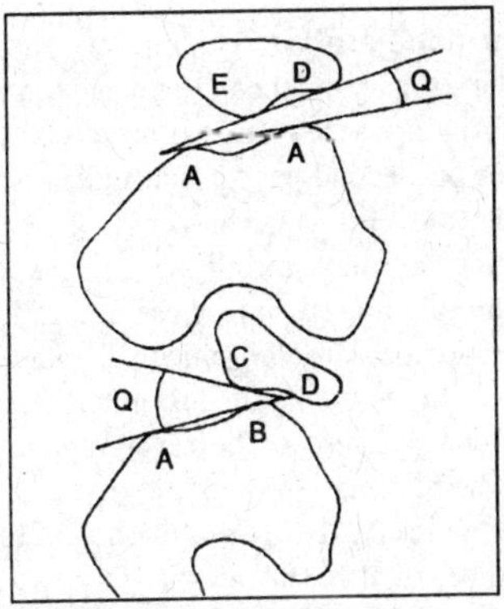

Angle point Any point where three tooth surfaces meet.

Angle's classification of malocclussion Classification of the different forms of malocclusion set up by Edward Angle, an orthodontist (1855-1930). Class I normal anteroposterid relationship of mandible to maxilla. The mesiobuccal cusp of the maxillary first permanent molar occludes with the buccal groove of the mandibular first permanent molar. Class II the posterior relationship of the mandible to the maxilla.

The mesiobuccal cusp of the maxillary first permanent molar occludes mesial to the buccal groove of the mandibular first permanent molar. Division of this classification may exist. Class III : the anterior relationship of the mandible to the maxilla. The mesiobuccal cusp of the maxillary first permanent molar occludes distal to the buccal groove of the mandibular first permanent molar, subdivision may occur.

Angle-angle diagrams Diagrams in which angular displacements of adjacent joints in the sagittal plane are plotted against each other.

Angstrom A linear unit of measure equivalent to 1/100,000,000 of of a centimeter. Angstrom was a Swedish physicist. Unit of length equivalent to 0.000000001 m (1/10,000,000,000 of a meter or about 1/250,000,000 of an inch). (A) A unit of length (10^{-8} cm) used to indicate molecular dimensions.

Angstrom unit One ten millionth part of a millimeter.

Angular Having corners or angles.

Angular acceleration The rate of change of the angular velocity of a body segment with respect to time. Angular acceleration is usually measured in radians per second per second (radians/s^2).

Angular cheilitis It is characterised by fissuring, cracking, burning and dryness at the angles of mouth. Saliva seeps into these cracks leading to maceration of skin. The patients lick the corner of the mouth. Riboflavin deficiency and fungal injection may cause it. The use of nystatin ointment helps the patients.

Angular velocity The rate of motion in rotation of a body segment around an axis.

Angulation of teeth Each tooth has been placed at the angle that best withstands the line of forces

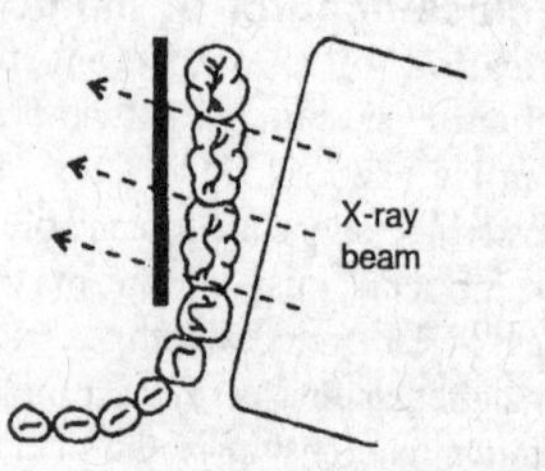

Incorrect angulation resulting overlapped contacts

brought against it during function. If angle is not correct tooth is placed at disadvantage. The teeth are placed so that their axes on either right or left are placed at acute angle to median line.

Anhidrosis Inability to produce or secrete sweat.

Anhydrite The natural anhydrous form of calcium sulfate.

Anhydrous Containing no water.

Anima In Jungian psychology, a person's inner being as opposed to the character or persona presented to the world. Further, the anima may be the more feminine "soul" or inner self of a man; the animus the more masculine soul of a woman.

Animal protein factor Vitamin B_{12} which is not found in vegetarians.

Animal reservoir A source in nature in whcih an infectious agent can be maintained for occasional or usual transmission to human beings by a vector.

Animalcules A historic term used for the microscopic organisms first described by Leeuwenhock.

Animus That part of the collective unconsciousness which, according to Jung, includes the masculine side of the female. Women show male traits through the animus.

Anion Negatively charged particle.

Anion gap Difference between measured cation and anion concentration.

Anion-exchange resin A polymeric resin with fixed cationic groups; used in the chromatographic separation of anions.

Anionic detergents A detergent in which the cleansing action resides in anion. Soaps are anionic.

Anions Ions that are negatively charged, such as chloride, bicarbonate, and phosphate.

Aniridia It is a rare condition in which iris is extremely rudimentary. It has the following features. The pupil appears very large. On focal illumination and slit-lamp examination the margin of lens, the zonules and even ciliary process can be seen. Diminution of vision along with marked photophobia is seen. Person may develop nystagmus and is likely to develop granuloma.

Aniseikonia A difference in the refractive power of two eyes is the most frequent cause of an aniseikonia. In these cases the retinal image differs in size. A functional aniseikonia may be caused by anomalous distribution of the visual receptor cells in retina. Patching one eye should immediately relieve the difficulties.

Anisometropia It is a dioptric condition of the refraction wherein refraction of two eyes is unequal in its degree or kind. It is found in every possible variety. One eye is emmetropic and the other eye may be myopic or astigmatic. Binocular vision is a rule of low degree of anisometropia. The vision may be unilocular. It is seen in cases where one eye is low ametropic and the other is having a very high refractive error.

Anisotropic An object or substance that exhibits different behavior when exposed to polarized light propagated in different directions.

Ankle It is the joint between talus which articulates with lower end of tibia and fibula. This joint is commonly sprained. The resultant swelling is best treated by cold compression for several hours and strapping the joint with crepe bandage.

Ankle foot orthoses Plastic leaf spring (PLS) dorsiflexion assist orthoses are perhaps the most

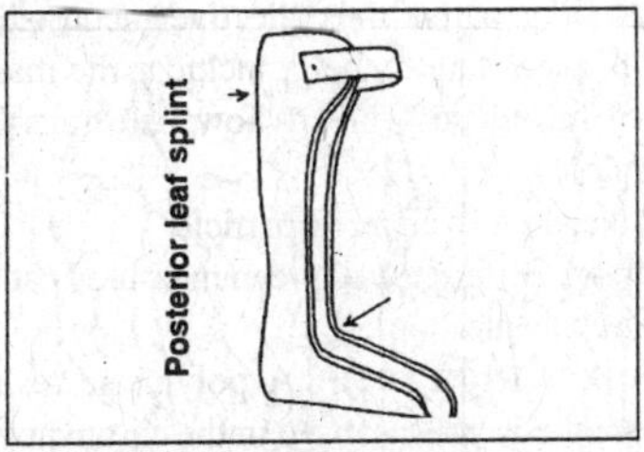

used device. The unobstructive braces slip into most patient's shoes easily and provide support in footdrop.

Ankle tapping It is done to prevent ankle sprain. More the external support ankle has smaller the chance of sprain. Excellent method of preventing

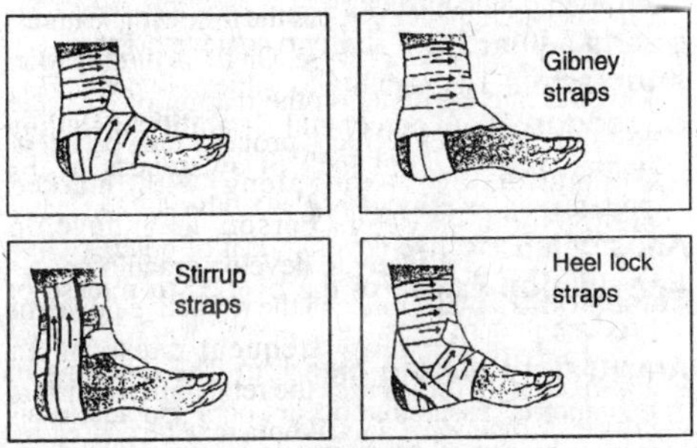

sprain is to tape your ankle before competition. There are different styles of tapping.

Ankyglossia Abnormally short lingual frenum that limits movements of tongue.

Ankyloblepharon It is a condition in which there is an adhesion of margins of two lids. It may be congenital or acquired, partial or complete. In congenital there may be one or more tags of skin In acquired ankyloblepharon adhesion may be at places or along the whole lid margin. Most common cause is symblepharon and ulceration of lid margin.

Ankyloglossia In this condition ventral surface of the tongue is partially or completely attached to the oral floor. The fixation results from the fact that the lingual frenum is attached too forward toward the tip of the tongue. Treatment is surgical only.

Ankylosing spondylitis It is an inflammatory disease affecting joints between vertebrae and sacroiliac joints. Cause is unknown. It is more common in men between the age of 20-40 years. It may run in families. It starts from discomfort in lower back with pain and stiffness which becomes worse while resting. Exercise helps in reducing pain. Loss of appetite, tiredness and occasionally redness of eyes due to iritis is seen. There is no curative treatment.

Ankylosis In it there is complete loss of joint movement. This may result due to injury, infection or fusion done surgically.

Ankylostomiasis It is a disorder resulting from infestation with the hookworm Ankylostoma, common in tropical region with poor sanitation. The live larvae remain in soil and penetrate the skin of humans. They travel in the blood stream to lungs through stomach to small intestine. Symptoms include pain in abdomen, diarrhoea and weakness and anaemia.

Anlage An embryonic precursor; the earliest discernible development of an organ or part.

Annatto A yellowish red vegetable dye made from pulp around the seeds of a small tropical tree, used in colouring cheese.

Annealing Heating of a material, such as metal or glass, followed by controlled cooling to remove internal stresses and created a desire of strength, toughness, temper, or softness within a material.

Anniversary reaction An emotional response to a previous event occurring at the same time of year. Often the event involved a loss and the reaction involves a depressed state. The reaction can range from mild to severe and may occur at any time after the event.

Annular detachment of cervix It detaches spontaneously during labour and is delivered on top of child's head. The detached part of cervix may be circular or flat disc like It may occur in primigravida getting oxytocin. Bleeding is minimal.

Annular pancreas It is the second part of duodenum and is surrounded by a ring of normal pancreatic tissue. It may be one inch thick to cause even duodenum obstruction below the opening of common bile duct. Annular pancreas develops due to faulty migration of anterior pancreatic bud. Mostly it is asymptomatic but may cause fullness and discomfort after meals. Pancreatitis and duodenal ulceration are complications. When obstruction is severe, division of contricting ring is required.

Annulment A ruling that marriage was never properly formed.

Annulus fibrosis Concentric layers of fibrous tissue surrounding the nucleus pulposus of the intervertebral disc.

Anode Positive terminal of an x-ray tube. The anode consists of a tungsten target embedded in a copper stem and set at an angle to the cathode. The anode is the location where x-rays originate in the tube, thus it is often called the target or focal spot.

Anodyne Any agent that neutralizes or relieves pain.

Anomally An organ that is malformed or in some way abnormal with reference to form, structure or position.

Anomalous speech representation A condition in which a person's speech zones are located in the right hemisphere or in both hemispheres.

Anomaly An organ or structure that is malformed or in some way abnormal with reference to form, structure, or position.

Anomia 'Without names'. Inability to name common objects.

Anomie Apathy, alienation, and personal distress resulting from the loss of goals previously valued. Durkheim popularised this term when he listed it as a principal reason for suicide.

Anopsla 'Without vision'.

Anorchia The absence of both testicles.

Anorectal abscess *Escherichia coli* is the most common causative factor. In 20% cases *Staphylococcus aureus* is causative factor. In 90% cases the abscess commences as an infection of an anal gland. Other causes are penetration of rectal wall. Patient of diabetes and AIDS may cause anorectal abscess. These are of 4 types, perianal, ischiorectal, submucous and pelvirectal.

Anorectal syndrome This syndrome is characterised by itching, irritation, soreness and burning of rectum, redness about the anus, diarrhoea, are other systemic manifestations.

Anorexia Lack or loss of the desire to eat, aversion to food.

Anorexia nervosa It is a condition of self-imposed starvation resulting in emaciation. Disease is most common amongst young girls. Patients have an intense preoccupation with staying slim.

Fear of obesity may be associated with distorsion of body image. Evidence of depressive or schizophrenic psychosis is unusual but obsession and hysterical features are common. There is

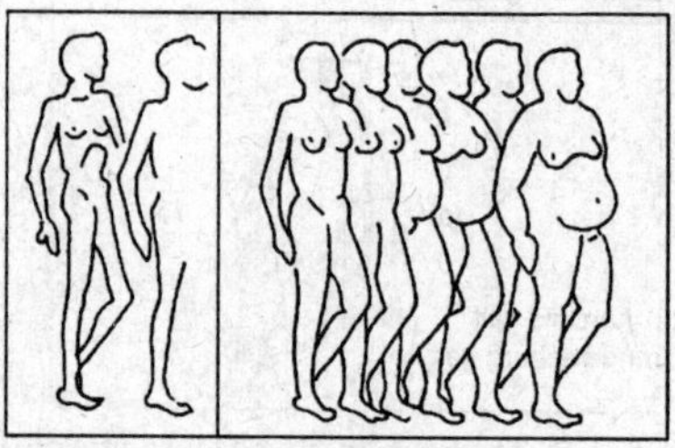

progressive weight loss and condition mav be complicated by vomiting and diarrhoea. There may be emaciation due to loss of muscle bulk, bradycardia, cyanosis and cold extremities. There will be normal secondary sexual development but invariable amenorrhoea.

Anorgansmia The inabilityto achieve orgasm.

Anorgasmia The inability to achieve orgasm.

Anosognosia A perceptual disability including denial, neglect, and lack of awareness of the presence or severity of one's paralysis.

Anostosis Defective development of bone.

Anovulation Failure of the ovaries to release or produce mature eggs.

Anovulatory uterine bleeding The shedding of endometrial tissue that occurs on a sporadic basis in the absence of ovulatory cycles.

Anoxia Absence of oxygen to the body tissues, to be differentiated from hypoxia.

Anoxybiosis A condition of life in the absence of oxygen.

Ansa hypoglossi Ansa cervicalis.

Antacids These contain compounds of magnesium or aluminium which have a long lasting effect. Sodium bicarbonate produces rapid but short-lived life. Antacid drugs neutralise stomach acid. It gives sufficient time to mucous membrane of stomach to heal. Side effects include constipation.

Antagonist A chemical compound that counteracts or blocks the actions of another chemical.

Antagonist muscle Those having opposing actions; for example, muscles that flex the upper arm are antagonists to muscles that extend it.

Antalgic gait It is very typical of unilateral pain. There is lateral displacement of head and neck, trunk towards the involved weight bearing side. Patient subconsciously tries to decrease the forces through the joint by shifting his weight over the affected joint. Trendelenburg gait typically shows

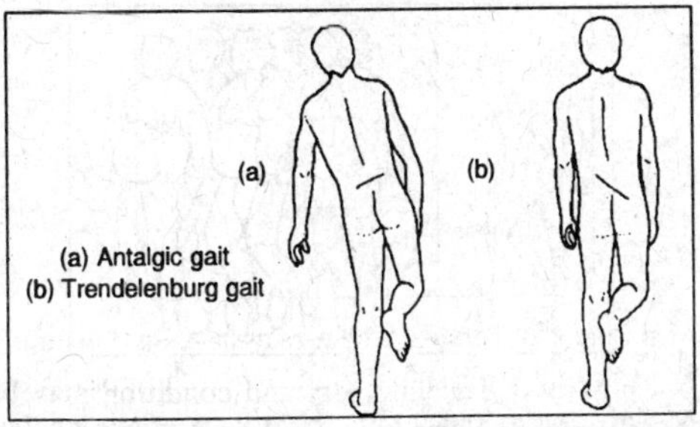

(a) Antalgic gait
(b) Trendelenburg gait

excessive pelvic tilt on the side opposite the involved stance limb. When standing on one leg the centre of gravity of body is brought over the weight bearing leg by action of gluteal muscles on that side tilting the pelvis. Thus the pelvis is raised on the swing phase leg. Trendelenburg positive test shows that buttock on the weight bearing leg fails to rise.

Antebrachial Refers to the forearm

Antebrachium The forearm.

Antecedents Events that immediately precede behavior and influence its frequency.

Antecubital Refers to the elbow.

Antecubital fossa Triangular fossa anterior to elbow joint. It contains median nerve, branchial artery, radial nerve and biceps tendon.

Antefebrile Before the onset of fever.

Anteflexion A uterus that is bent forward just above the cervix.

Antemortem During the life of an organism.

Antenatal Occurring before birth.

Antenatal care As soon as woman misses her one or two periods, she should get her antenatal check up to establish diagnosis and to have necessary advice. Antenatal care includes training for motherhood.

Antenatal medicine Prenatal medicine.

Antepartal The period from conception to the onset of labor; prenatal.

Antepartum A term referring to the time interval prior to the birth process.

Antepartum haemorrhage There is vaginal bleeding after the onset of third trimester. Antepartum haemorrhage is due to defective placenta. Placenta may be low lying close to birth canal. Bleeding can also be caused by cervical erosion or lesions of vagina. Bleeding is painless. When placenta is partly separated from uterus there may be more bleeding with abdominal pain. Ultrasound is the best diagnostic tool. When bleeding is severe baby may not get oxygen hence caesarean section may have to be done.

Anterioposterior (AP) View describes the direction of the roentgen ray beam through the patient from anterior to posterior.

Anterior That which goes first; in humans, towards the belly or front.

Anterior beaking of vertebra Central beaking is found in Morquio's syndrome while lower end beaking is found in achondroplasia, cretinism, Down's syndrome, Hurler's syndrome and neuro muscular diseases.

Anterior cardiac veins Three or four small veins receiving blood from the right ventricle

Anterior chamber It is a space bounded in front by the cornea and behind by a strip of anterior surface of ciliary body, the iris and lens in the pupillary area. The diameter of anterior chamber varies from 12.4 to 13.3 mm. It is about 3 mm deep in centre and becomes shallower at periphery. Anterior chamber is deep in myopia, total posterior synechia and in aphakia. The anterior chamber becomes shallow in glaucoma and hypermetropia.

Anterior chamber cannula This cannula is attached to a syringe with saline or an irrigation fluid bottle and used to wash out the cortical matter in an extracapsular cataract surgery. It can be used

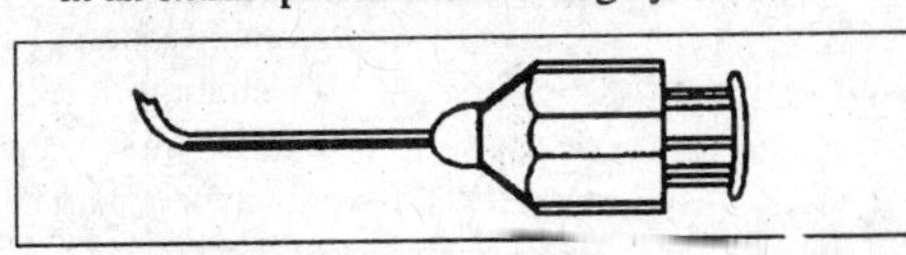

to push in the vision or pilocarpine in the anterior chamber. An irrigation-aspiration unit is better to clear the cortical matter, than this conventional method.

Anterior cord syndrome Incomplete spinal cord lesion with primary damage in the anterior cord; loss of motor function, and sense of pain and temperature; perseveration of proprioception, kinesthesia, and vibration below the level of the lesion.

Anterior cruciate ligament (ACL) It is located on anterior surface of tibia. It is composed of two bands, a small anteromedial bank. It is 50% weaker than that of posterior cruciate ligament. Avascular structure gets its supply from genicular arteries.

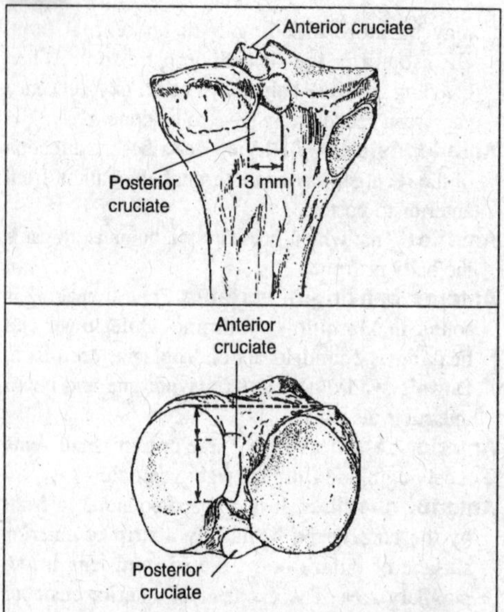

Attachment anterior and posterior cruciate ligament on the tibia.

Internal rotation of tibia is limited by ACL. Excessive rotation occurs after an injury to ACL. There may be an associated injury to meniscus.

Anterior drawer test The anterior drawer test may indicate the severity of ankle injury. It is performed by stabilising the tibia and grasping the calcaneus

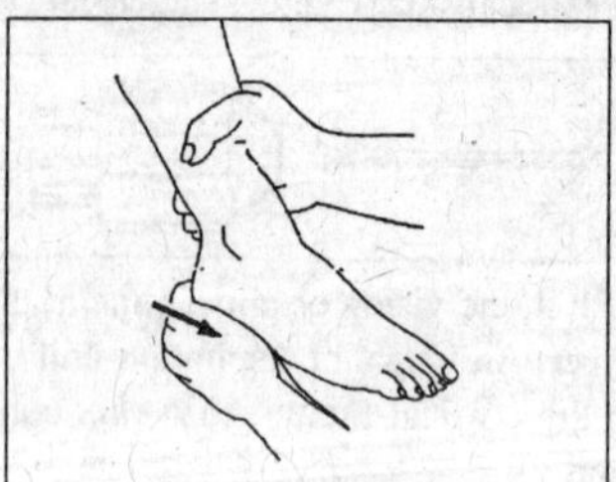

Anterior drawer test

while exerting a gentle anterior force. Increased forward translation of talus in the ankle indicates damage to the anterior talofibular ligament.

Anterior horn The part of the spinal cord grey matter containing motor neurons; also called the ventral horn or motor horn.

Anterior interosseous nerve syndrome Syndrome is characterised by weakness of the flexor pollicis longus, flexor digitorum profundus and

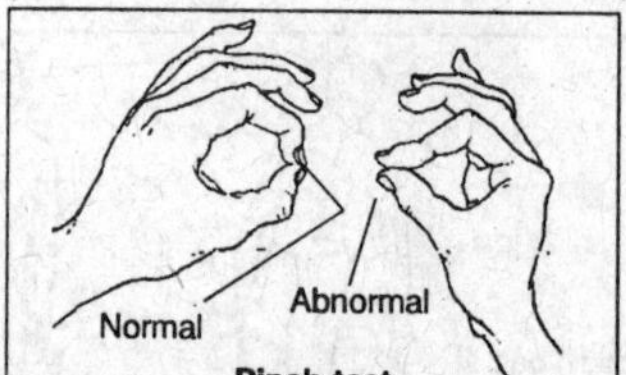

Pinch test

pronator quadratus. There may be a mild ache in proximal forearm. Patient loses the ability to perform the 'pinch test'. There may be variability in the degree of muscles. Surgical decompression is the treatment.

Anterior interventricular artery The anterior interventricular branch of the left coronary artery; left anterior descending artery.

Anterior interventricular sulcus A groove on the anteriosuperior surface of the heart that marks the location of the interventricular septum.

Anterior leaflet of the mitral valve The larger of the two cusps of the mitral valve; it has no basal zone; also called the anteriomedial, aortic, or septal leaflet.

Anterior metatarsalgia It is defined as pain with direct palpation of the plantar aspect of metatarsal head. It is due to increased pressure there. It may

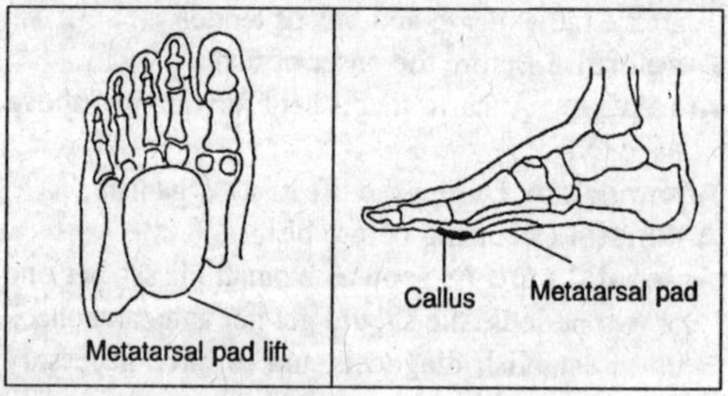

be caused by depressed metatarsal, elongated metatarsal, decreased plantar fat pad and accessory sesamoid bones. Treatment includes by decreasing pressure under the affected metatarsal head. Metatarsal pads can be used to unload one of the lesser metatarsals.

Anterior Nasal Spine A median bony process, adjacent to the inferior margin of the anterior aperture of the nose, formed by a forward prolongation of the two maxillae. An important anatomic landmark and subperiosteal implantology.

Anterior open bite The deficit in overbite will produce the condition of an anterior edge to edge bite or an anterior open bite. A cross bite occurs if the buccal cusps of maxillary tooth are in a position lingual to that of mandibular tooth. In deep overbite mandibular incisors impinge on palate.

Anterior papillary muscles Arise from the interior border of the moderator band in the right ventricle and from the sternocostal wall of the left ventricle.

Anterior pituitary Portion of the pituitary derived from the oral epithelium.

Anterior pulmonary plexus A network of nerves formed by branches of the vagus nerves and the deep cardiac plexus supplying anterior branches of the bronchi and the pulmonary and bronchial vessels.

Anterior root The bundle of axons of efferent (motor) fibres that emerge from the anterior (ventral) sides of the spinal cord.

Anterior segmental bronchus The portion of the tracheobronchial tree arising from the right or left upper lobe bronchus that is distributed to the anterior segment.

Anterior spinal artery syndrome There is impaired blood supply to anterior two-third of spinal cord which includes the corticospinal lateral spinothalamic tracts and anterior horns of grey matter caused by thrombosis. Person may develop quadriplegia with loss of sense of position. Arms may be impaired. Sense of pain and temperature will be disturbed. Nystagmus may develop.

Anterior vaginal wall retractor It has oval fenestrated ends. These fenestrations have transverse serrations. These oval loops are set at a particular angle. To visualise cervix and anterior fornix it is used with Sim's speculum.

Anteroclusion Malocclusion of the teeth in which the mandibular teeth are in a position anterior to their normal position relative to the teeth in maxillary arch.

Anterograde Moving or extending forward.

Anterograde amnesia A form of forgetting, in which the individual has no memory for events which happened after a traumatic incident or surgery. The individual can remember prior experiences, even those dating from childhood, but cannot recall events subsequent to some brain trauma.

Anterograde transport Axonal transport from soma to nerve terminals.

Anterolateral Situated in front and to one side.

Anterolateral pathway Sensory pathway that conveys information related to pain, temperature, crude touch, pressure, tickle, and itch.

Anterolateral thoracotomy An incision into the anteriolateral aspect of the chest wall.

Anteromedial basal segmental bronchus The portion of the tracheobronchila tree arising from the left lower lobe bronchus that is distributed to the anteriomedial basal segment.

Anteromedian Situated in front and toward the median plane.

Anteroposterior Extending from the front backward.

Anterosuperior Situated in front and above.

Anteroventral Situated in front and toward the ventral surface.

Anteversion A uterus which is tipped abnormally forward.

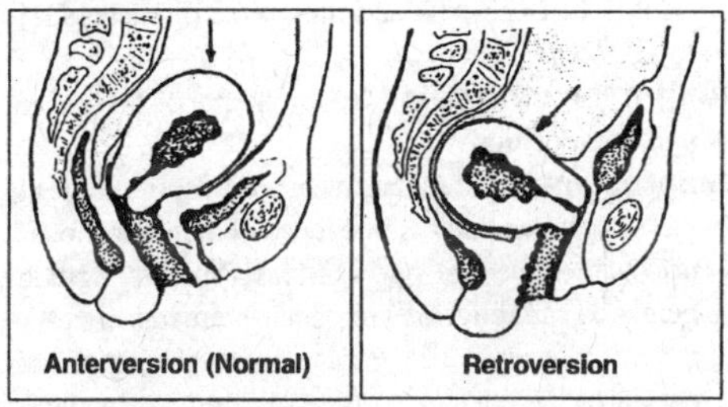

Anterversion (Normal) Retroversion

Anteverted uterus Uterus is usually 8 to 9 cm long from the cervix to the fundus and is normally found in an anteverted position with the cervix pointing downwards backwards.

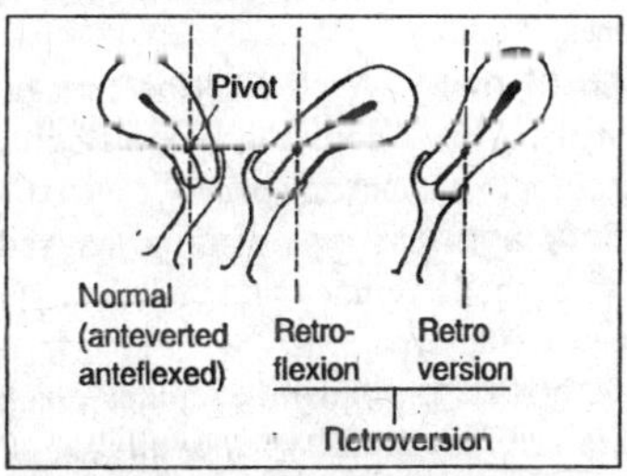

Anthelmintic enema It is given to destroy worms. For removal of worms second cleansing enema may be given, if not evacuated fully. Solution of Quassia 150 to 246 CC sodium chloride 8 gm per 500 CC of water is given. Hypertonic solution after Quassia solution may be repeated till all worms come out.

Anthracycline An antineoplastic agent; a glycoside antibiotic used in the treatment of solid tumors e.g., breast, ovarian, small cell bronchogenic cancers.

Anthrax It is a necrotic ulcer of skin or of mucous membrane, produced by gram-positive spore forming *Bacillus anthracis*. Source of infection is wool, shaving brushes and infected animals. It gives rise to a small, erythematous macule which appears on exposed part of skin, Macule enlarges and becomes oedematous so as to create a papule and lastly necrotic ulcer covered with slough. Lesion is necrotic but not very tender. Regional lymph glands enlarge and suppurate frequently. There may be fever and fulminating septicaemia.

Anthropoid pelvis The anterio-posterior diameter of the brim is longer than transverse diameter. Anterior segment of brim is less oval compared to the posterior segment. Pubic arch is narrow but well shaped and measures 70 degrees. AP diameter of inlet is 12 to 13 cms and transverse diameter 11.5 to 12.5 cm.

Anthropometric data Measurements of body size and composition.

Anthropometry It means measurement of different parts of human body. Some measurements are noted down after the age of 21. Measurements include height on standing, different measurements of head, ear, middle and little finger, outstretching arms, colour of iris, etc.

Anti-actinic lens Lens absorbs ultraviolet radiation to a much greater extent than a white spectacle lens.

Antiandrogen A substance capable of antagonizing and reducing the biological effects of androgenic hormones.

Antianginal drug A medication that dilates coronary arteries, improving blood flow to the myocardium to prevent angina.

Antianxiety agent A type of drug that reduces anxiety; benzodiazepines and sedativehypnotic agents are of this type.

Antianxiety drugs Benzodiazepines and beta-blockers are two main types available. These provide temporary relief from anxiety. These are sometimes used to calm a person before surgery. Benzodiazepines promote mental and physical relaxation by reducing nerve activity while beta-blockers reduce the physical symptoms of tremors and palpitation.

Antibacterial drugs Drugs to kill bacteria or inhibit bacterial replication.

Antibiotic A chemical substance derived from fungi or microorganisms which, in dilute solutions, can destroy or inhibit the growth of bacteria and other microorganisms; used in the treatment of infectious diseases of man, animals, and plants. These are drugs used to treat infection caused by bacteria. Previously these were derived from moulds and fungi, but now these are made synthetically. Some antibiotics are effective against only specific bacteria.

While broad-spectrum antibiotics are effective against a wide range of bacteria. Sometimes more than one antibiotics are used to increase efficiency. These also prevent infection where immune system has become weaker. Resistance develops if a person fails to take full course. Side effects that may develop are oral thrush, vaginal candidiasis and itching.

Antibiotic resistance The ability of bacterials to withstand the killing effect of antimicrobial agents.

Antibody Antibody is serum protein which is formed in the blood, lymph and various secretions of the body in response to antigenic stimuli and reacts specifically with that antigen in some observable manner *in vivo* or *vitro*. Antibody is usually obtained from serum although all the body fluids contain some antibody.

Antibody-mediated immunity That component of immunity in which lymphocytes (B cells) develop into plasma cells that produce antibodies that destroy antigens.

Anticaking agent A substance that keeps salts and powders free flowing used in table salts.

Anticancer drugs These are used to treat cancer specially lymphomas, leukaemias. Most anticancer drugs are cytotoxic, i.e. chlorambucil, cyclophosphamide, fluorouracil and methotrexate. Others are synthetic sex hormone drugs, i.e. androgen, oestrogen and progesterone drugs. Choice of drugs depends on type of cancer. All anticancer drugs kill cancer cells by preventing them from growing and dividing. Side effects include loss of hair, depression of bone marrow, anaemia and abnormal bleeding.

Anticarcinogenic Inhibiting or preventing the development of cancer.

Anticariogenic Suppressing the development of caries

Anticarious anticariogenic.

Anticholinergic drugs It is a group of drugs that blocks the effects of acetylcholine, a chemical released from nerve endings. Choline triggers activity of muscle contraction, increases secretions in mouth and lungs and slows the heart beat. Anticholinergic drugs are used in irritable bowel syndrome, Parkinson's disease and asthma.

Anticipatory grieving Grieving that beings before a loss actually occurs.

Anticipatory stress Stress experienced as one waits and or prepares for a stressful event.

Anticoagulant These are substances which prevent or slows the clotting of blood. Commonly used anticoagulants are coumarin, heparin and warfarin. These are sometimes used to treat circulatory disorders associated with arteriosclerosis or to break up blood clots.

Anticoagulant drugs A group of drugs used to treat and prevent abnormal blood clotting hence are used to treat thrombosis, stroke or transient ischaemic attack. Heparin, warfarin and dicoumerol are common drugs. Heparin blocks the activity of coagulation factors. These do not dissolve thrombus.

Anticodon A base triplet provided by three nucleotides within a loop of transfer RNA that is complementary in its base pairing properties to a triplet (the codon) in mRNA. The matching of codon to anticodon provides the mechanism for translating the genetic code into a specific sequence of amino acids.

Anticomplement A substance that inactivates. Opposes, or counteracts the action of complement.

Anticonvulsant drugs It is a group of drugs including clonazepam, diazepam, phenytoin, valproic acid used in treatment of seizures. These drugs are to be taken on a regular basis to reduce frequency and severity of seizures. After brain surgery and head injury these are also given to prevent seizures. In long-term treatment more than one anticonvulsants are given. Seizures are caused by abnormally high level of electrical activity in the brain. Anticonvulsant drugs have an inhibitory effect that neutralises electrical activity. Side effects include reduced concentration, impaired memory, poor coordination and fatigue.

Antidepressant drugs These drugs are used in treatment of depression. These include tricyclics, amitryptyline, lithium, etc. Antidepressant drugs are given when depression lasts more than a few days. Symptoms of depression may be lethargy, loss of appetite or sex drive with a feeling of despair. Some antidepressant drugs trigger the release of chemicals in the brain that activates nerve activity. These take at least 10 days to start its beneficial effects. Most antidepressant drugs cause dryness of mouth, blurred vision, dizziness and drowsiness. Overdose may even cause death.

Antidiarrhoeal drugs These should be given if diarrhoea persists more than 24 hours. Bulking agents which contain fibre in diet absorb water from faeces making it more solid while narcotic antidiarrhoeal drugs affect the muscles in the wall of intestine. This slows the passage of faeces and allows more time to absorb water.

Antidiuretic Suppressing the secretion of urine.

Antidiuretic hormone ADH is released from posterior part of pituitary gland. It causes reduction of water lost in urine. It helps in maintaining the optimum amount of water in body. Production of ADH depends on hypothalamus. Synthetic ADH is given via the nose or by injection to treat diabetes insipidus.

Antidote Remedy for counteracting a toxin, poison, or harmful effect.

Antidotes These reduce or abolish the effects of poisons through a variety of mechanisms. There may be receptors which may be activated, blocked or bypassed. Certain enzymes may be inhibited or reactivated. These may displace poison from tissue binding sites.

Antidromic Usually refers to nerve impulses which, travelling proximally along one branch of a Y-shaped sensory nerve fiber, arrive at the junction and travel distally along the other branch.

Antidromic conduction A nerve impulse that moves in the opposite direction than normal.

Antiembolism stockings Elastic stockings.

Antiemetic drugs These are the drugs used to treat nausea and vomiting caused by motion sickness, vertigo, radiation therapy, etc. In morning sickness of pregnancy they can be used also. Some antiemetic drugs reduce nerve activity at the base of brain, suppressing vomiting reflex while other antiemetics prevent vomiting by relaxing the muscles in lower part of stomach.

Antienzymes If certain enzyme is repeatedly injected, a substance is produced in serum which prevents the normal action of enzyme injected. The substance is called antienzyme. Known ones are antipepsin, antirenin, antitrypsin and antiurease.

Antiflux A substance that inhibits the action of flux, thereby reducing the flow of a solder, used to confine the flow of the molten solder.

Antigen An antigen is a substance which when introduced parenterally into the tissues, stimulates the production of an antibody or immune cell and which can combine specifically. To be antigen the substance must have inherent ability to induce the formation of antibodies. Antigen has to be foreign and molecular weight should be more than 5000.

Antigen-antibody reaction The combination of an antibody with the antigen of the type that initially stimulated the formation of the antibody, causing the agglutination, precipitation, fixation, or phagocytosis of the antigen.

Antigen-binding receptor Molecule on the surface of lymphocytes that specifically binds antigens.

Antigenic determinant A cluster of epitopes.

Antigenic determinant site The region of an antigen molecule that specifically reacts with particular antibodies. A large antigen molecule may have a number of such sites.

Antigenic drift Change of antigenic structure caused by amino-acid substitutions, which themselves result from the accumulation of random point mutations in the gene.

Antigenic shift Major change in the surface antigens of a viral influenza strain, with the potential to create worldwide epidemics (pandemics).

Antigenic site The portion of a molecule that stimulates production of an antibody or to which an antibody binds.

Antigenic variation Change of antigenic structure due to active specific mechanisms hapening at higher frequencies than random mutation rates.

Antigenicity The capacity to act as an antigen.

Antigen-presenting cell Special class of migratory cells that process and present antigens to T cells during an immune response; APCs include macrophages, B cells, and dendritic cells, which are present in the skin and in mucous membranes.

Antihistamine A drug that inhibits the action of histamine.

Antihistamine drugs These block the effects of histamine. Histamine is released during allergic reaction. These drugs are used in the treatment of urticaria and itching with redness. Such drugs may be used in common cold and allergic rhinitis. These suppress vomiting reflex also. These drugs block the effect of histamine on skin, eyes and nose. These prevent histamine to irritate nerve fibres. Side effects include drowsiness and dizziness.

Anti-infective drug resistance The ability of a virus, bacterium, or parasite to defend itself against a drug which was previously effective. Drug resistance is currently occuring for bacterial infections such as tuberculosis and gonorrhoea, for parasitic infection such as malaria, and for the human immunodeficiency virus (HIV).

Antilymphatic serum It is the preparation containing antibodies that reduces the action of leucocytes. Such cells are part of body's immune system. Their action has to be suppressed to prevent rejection following transplant surgery.

Antilymphocyte globulin (ALG) An immunosuppressant; used to suppress the cell-mediated immune response to transplanted tissue e.g., liver, heart.

Antilytic Inhibiting or suppressing lysis.

Antimetabolite A chemical compound that resembles a substance occuring naturally and prevents its metabolism.

Antimicrobial A substance that destroys or prevents the development or action of microbes.

Antimicrobial agents Chemicals that limit the number of infectious microorganisms by destroying them or suppressing their growth.

Antimitotic Inhibiting or preventing mitosis.

Antimonial Pertaining to or containing antimony.

Antimyosin imaging Trials with indium-III labelled antibodies to cardiac myosin have been preferred. Images are taken 24 to 48 hours after injection to allow clearance of blood pool activity. Antimyosin is a more specific indicator of acute infarction than ^{99m}Tc bone agents and there is no rib or sternal take up to obscure cardiac image. It is more useful in assessment of patients with acute MI to distinguish between infarcted and severely ischaemic tissue. It also has a role in the evaluation of cardiac transplants by detecting patchy areas of necrosis associated with rejection.

Antinatriuresis Inhibiting the excretion of sodium in the urine.

Antineoplastic drugs Medications used to destroy or slow the growth of malignant cells.

Antineoplastic therapy A substance, procedure, or measure that prevents the pfoliferationof maligant cells; usually chemotherapy, radiation therapy, surgery, biological response modifiers, or bone marrow transplantation.

Antineuralgic Alleviating or counteracting neuralgia.

Antineuritic Preventing or relieving inflammation of a nerve. It counteracts neuritis such as thiamine.

Antiodontalgic Relieving toothache.

Antioxidant A substance that prevents or delays oxidatioin. These are most common groups of food additivies used to prevent change in colour or flavoured caused by oxygen in air. Antioxidants prevent rancid taste and odour from developing in fats and oils during storage.

Antiporter A membrane transporter protein catalyzing coupled, simultaneous counter transport across the membrane of two solutes in opposite directions.

Antipsychotic Favourable modifying psychotic behavior and symptoms.

Antipsychotic drug Sometimes called major tranquillisers, these drugs are administered in cases of extreme emotional disorders, including depression and the manic depressive state. They also may be used to reduce delusions and hallucinations

Antipyretic drugs These are the drugs which reduce fever. Most common is paracetamol. Paracetamol is deethylated active metabolite of phenacetin and is in use since 1950. It is good and promptly acting antipyretic. It raises pain threshold but is having weak anti-inflammatory component. In contrast to aspirin paracetamol does not stimulate respiration or affect acid-base balance. It does not cause gastric irritation. Paracetamol is safe and well absorbed orally, only one-third is protein bound in plasma and uniformly distributed in body.

Antipyretics Drugs that reduce fever.

Antiretroviral agent Any drug used in treating patients with human immunodeficiency virus HIV infection.

Antiscorbutic Preventive or curative of rickets.

Antisense A region of DNA or RNA sequence that is complementary, is of opposite polarity, and hybridizes to a naturally functional target sequence, resulting in decreased function.

Antisepsis Prevention of infection of a body surface usually skin or oral mucosa, through the application of an antimicrobial agent.

Antiseptic It is a substance that will inhibit the growth and development of microorganisms without necessarily destroying them. This term refers to nontoxic and nonirritant antimicrobial agent that may be applied superficially to body surface.

Antiserum These are the preparations obtained from blood of animals that contain antibodies against a specific disease such as tetanus. Antisera are used in certain blood tests also.

Antisialagogue A drug that reduces, slows, or prevents the flow of saliva.

Antisialic Checking salivary secretions.

Antisocial personality Pattern of recurrent antisocial, deliquent and criminal behavior that begins in childhood and is manifested by disturbances in many areas of life, family relations, service, school and marriage.

Antisocial personality disorder The behaviour disorder shown by an individual who is hostile to the laws and norms of his or her culture. The person fails to observe rules which govern conduct in his or her society.

Antispasmodic drugs These are the drugs which relieves the spasm of involuntary smooth muscles. These are used in irritable bowel syndrome and irritable bladder. These may have an anticholinergic effect, blocking the action of acetylcholine which stimulates muscle contraction.

Antispastic Antispasmodic with specific reference to skeletal muscle.

Antitermination A process in which RNA polymerase is modified by cellular factors so that it makes transcripts at an increased elongation rate and it becomes resistant to transcription terminators.

Antithermic Reducing temperature.

Antithrombin A substance capable of neutralizaing the action of thrombin and thus limiting or restricting blood coagulation.

Antitrismus A spasm that prevents closure of the mouth.

Antitussive These drugs act on coughing centre in brain to suppress cough. Codeine is also antitussive.

Antivenom It is the most effective therapeutic agent available for a snake bite. Before giving it wait for clinical evidence of poisoning. Besides helping in reducing systemic toxicity antivenom prevents or lessens local effects of necrosis. Each ml of antivenom will neutralise following amount of dried venom, cobra—0.6 mg, common krait—0.45 mg, Russel viper—0.6 mg and echis—0.45 mg. Antivenom dose for children is same as for adults.

Antiviral drugs Drugs that kill virus are difficult to develop because viruses live only within body cells and there is danger that antiviral drugs will damage the host cell as well as the virus. But a few drugs have been found effective against herpes virus. Antiviral drugs reduce the severity of disease. Some antiviral drugs disrupt chemical processes necessary for viruses to grow and multiply within cells. Side effects include anaemia due to bone marrow damage.

Antiviral resistance The developed resistance of a virus to a specific drug.

Antivitamin Substances that interfere with function of vitamins. Thiaminase of raw fish destroys thiamine, methotrexate inhibits folate. An antimetabolite against a vitamin which it replaces or competes metabolically.

Vitamin	*Antivitamin*
Biotin	Avidin
Folacin	Methotrexate
Niacin	Pyridine 3sulfonic acid
Pyridoxine	INH
Riboflavin	Galactoflavin
Vitamin K	Dicumrol

Antral trocar and cannula It is used in case of sinusitis not responding well to medical treatment. Puncture is both for therapeutic and diagnostic purposes. Site of puncture is through the inferior meatus. The trocar is then removed leaving cannula in place. The patient is made to sit leaning forward with a bowl below his or her chin to collect the washings. Washing is performed using syringe and warm saline at 37°C. Be careful not to puncture orbital floor.

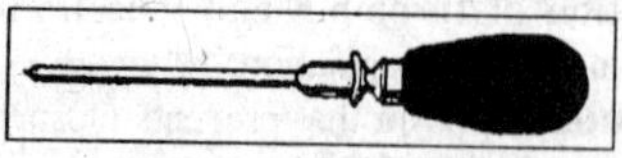

Antritis Inflammation of an antrum, chiefly after the maxilgical excision of an antrum.

Antrobuccal Pertaining to or communicating the maxillary antrum and buccal cavity, as an antrobuccal fistula.

Antrolith It is a relatively rare lesion similar to rhinolith. It is produced by the calcification of a nidus which may be a blood clot or pus. Antroliths may be true and false. Antroliths are usually greyish-black in colour. These may be small and asymptomatic. Some may be round while others may be irregular. Treatment includes removal.

Antrophine Nalorphine.

Antroscopy Examination of an antrum with the antroscope.

Antrum The fluid-filled compartment of the mature follicle.

ANUG Abbreviation for acute necrotizing ulcerative ginvitis, a recurrent periodontal disease primary involving the interdental papillae, which undergo necrosis and ulceration.

Anuria In it there is complete cessation of urine production by kidneys. It shows kidney damage because even in severe dehydration some of urine is produced.

Common causes are reduced blood flow in shock or severe kidney damage resulting in acute renal failure or tubercular necrosis.

Anus This is the end of alimentary tract through which faeces are expelled from body. It is 4 mm long and is extension of rectum as it passes backwards and downwards. There are two rows of sphincters, internal and external on which man has voluntary control. Rarely there may be imperforate anus.

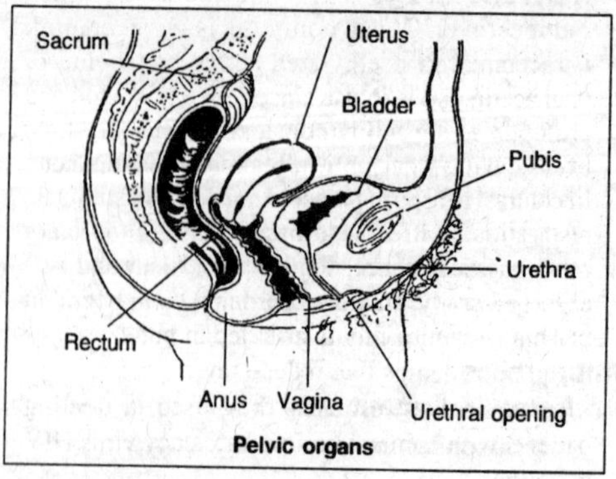

Pelvic organs

Anxiety It is an unpleasant emotional state ranging from mild unease to intense fear. Certain level of anxiety is needed to keep up better performance but it becomes a symptom when it starts to inhibit thoughts and disrupts normal day today activities. Person may develop palpitation and feeling of tight chest. There may be headache, spasm in back and inability to relax.

Anxiety disorder A form of mala-djustment characterised by widespread anxiety without an obvious source and with no obvious defensive reaction.

Anxiety, neurosis It is the most common form of psychoneurosis. It may create all kinds of visceral symptoms. Fears of mental illness, suicide or death are common. Acute panics lasting for hours with emotional distress occur. He or she fears to meet people, fears to walk in crowd and may remain sitting in house. During sleep nightmares are often present. Visceral symptoms are almost present. Seminal emissions persist. Patient cannot explain why he or she dreads these things but realises their absurdity.

Anxiolytic Anxiety or stress reducing.

Anxiolytic drugs Antianxiety drugs; usually act as GABA (gama-aminobutyric acid) angonists.

Aorta Large elastic artery that is the main trunk of the systemic arterial system which carries blood from the left ventricle of the heart and passes through the thorax and abdomen.

Aortic arch syndrome It is a pulseless disease, non-specific aorto-arteritis. It is more common in Japan.

Predominantly it affects young females. There is narrowing of branches of aorta. The arterial pulse is diminished or absent in upper extremity. Headache, syncope and visual disturbance may develop. Person will have muscular wasting and paraesthesia. There will be hypoplastic aortic knuckle.

Aortic area The region of the chest, second intercostal space along the right sternal border, where the normal and pathologic sounds made by the aortic valve are traditionally said to the best appreciated.

Aortic bodies Peripheral chemoreceptors near aortic arch similar in function and structure to carotid bodies.

Aortic body Cluster of receptors on or near the arch of the aorta that respond to alterations in blood levels of oxygen, carbon dioxide, and hydrogen ions (H^+).

Aortic dissection Passage of blood into aortic wall involving media of vessels. Atherosclerosis usually occurs in ascending aorta while due to hypertension it involves branch of aorta.

Aortic insufficiency There is leakage of blood through the aortic valve resulting in backflow of blood into left ventricle. It may be congenital or may be inflammatory. It can occur in intravenous drug users. Rheumatic fever may cause it. It may or may not cause any symptom. Doppler echocardiography will show the blood flow across the valve.

Aortic reflex A reflex concerned with maintaining normal systemic blood pressure.

Aortic regurgitation There is retrograde flow of blood through the aortic valve during diastole. It cause left ventricular hypertrophy and dilatation with increased stroke volume.

Aortic semilunar valve The semilunar valve consisting of three cusps of tissue is located at the base of the aorta where it arises from the left ventricle; the cusps overlap during ventricular diastole to prevent leakage of blood from the aorta into the left ventricle.

Aortic sinuses Three dilations above the attached margins of the cusps of the aortic valve at the root of the aorta.

Aortic stenosis Narrowing of aortic valve opening causes obstruction of blood flow. Walls of left ventricles become thickened. The most common causes are atherosclerosis, cardiomyopathy and rheumatic fever. It may be diagnosed on routine examination. But person may develop fainting attacks and lack of energy, chest pain or exertion and difficulty in breathing. Heart valve surgery may be done.

Aortic vestibule The portion of the left ventricle immediately below the aortic orifice.

Aorticopulmonary septum The spiral septum formed from the bulbar and truncal ridges that separates he bulbus cordis and the truncus arteriosus into a ventral pulmonary trunk and dorsal aorta.

Aortocaval compression Compression of great vessels against vertebral bodies by the gravid uterus.

It may result in hypotension, bradycardia or syncope.

APACHE scoring system Acute physiology and chronic health evaluation was described in 1981 for assessing the severity of illness of individual patients and predicting the risk of hospital mortality.

Apathic Without sensation and feeling.

Apathy There is general lack of interest in oneself or one's surrounding. Sometimes it develops in normal person also otherwise it is a symptom of depression.

Apatite Inorganic compound with a complex formula containing calcium and phosphate; makes up the inorganic portion of bones and teeth.

Apert's syndrome It is inherited as recessive form. Severe form is described as carpenter's syndrome. There will be oxycephaly, syndactyly, synostoses and synarthroses of shoulder and elbows. Orbit may be shallow, exophthalmos, ptosis, strabismus, nystagmus and optic atrophy.

Apex Extremity of a conical or pyramidal structure; the apex of the heart is the rounded tip directed anteriorly and slightly inferiorly.

Apex beat It results from the impact of left ventricle against chest wall. It is located at midclavicular line in the 4th and 5th intercostal space localised to a point not more than 2 to 3 cm. It is shifted downwards and laterally in left ventricular enlargement and aortic regurgitation.

Hyperdynamic apical impulse is noted in ventricular septal defect (VSD), patent ductus arteriosus (PDA), thyrotoxicosis and severe anaemia. Mitral and aortic regurgitation will also produce it. In it there is an increase in amplitude but is of brief duration.

Heaving apex is well sustained with swift exaggerated upstroke seen in aortic stenosis and systemic hypertension. In mitral stenosis apical tap is brief but prominent due to accentuated first heart sound.

Apex of the heart The conical extremity of the heart formed by the left ventricle.

Apexification A method of inducing apical closure or the continued apical development of the root of an incompletely formed tooth in which the pulp is no longer vital.

Apexigraph A device for determining the position of the apex of a tooth root.

Apexogenesis Treatment of a vital pulp by a pulp capping or pulpotomy to permit continued closure of the open apex and growth of the root.

Apexograph A delicate, flexible braoch used for exploring the apical portion of the root canal of a tooth.

Apgar scoring system A system for appraising the condition of a newborn on the basis of heart rate, respiratory effort, muscle tone, reflex irritability, and colour. The maximum score is 10. The evaluation is done at 60 seconds after birth, then again at 5 minutes and at 10 minutes if the neonate is unstable.

Aphagia Failure to eat; may be due to an unwillingness to eat or to motor difficulties, especially with swallowing.

Aphakia It is a condition of eye in which lens has been removed, either removed surgically or dislocated by trauma. There may be hypermetropia of about 10 dioptres. There is complete loss of accommodation. The retinal image is about one-quarter larger than the emmetropic retinal image. This enlarged image also causes diplopia if the opposite eye has a normal vision. The diplopia is due to disparity of retinal images of two eyes, the normal and aphakic eye.

Aphasia It affects the ability to speak and write due to cerebral dysfunction. A stroke or head injury is the most important cause. Damage to Broca's area causes difficulty of language. Speech is non-fluent and laboured and is known as expressive aphasia. While in global aphasia there is total inability to speak, write or understand spoken or written words. Some recovery after speech therapy is possible.

Aphonia There is total loss of voice. It may be due to sudden emotional stress. Vocal cords fail to meet as normal when patient tries to speak. There is no treatment except reassurance and psychotherapy.

Aphrodisiacs These are most wanted substances to increase sex desire and sex performance. Ginseng, rhinoceros horn, oysters are among many others. Person after consuming these develop confidence and some of them perform better too. Alcohol can encourage sexual desire. Best known aphrodisiacs is *shilajeet.* Marijuana, yohimbine and amyl nitrate help in sex desire. In men who have a testosterone deficiency the hormone may restore both libido and potency.

Aphthous major This condition occurs exclusively on the salivary glands. It begins as small, smooth, painful red nodules or plaques that soon ulcerate. The crater like, painful ulcers are much larger and deeper and heal much more slowly than do aphthous ulcers. Healed ulcers leave scar. Microscopic features are those of non-specific ulcer over a salivary gland bearing mucosa.

Apical Pertaining to or situated at the apex, as a tooth root.

Apical complex A combination of structures found in the apical region of sporozoites and merozoites of members of the phylum Api-complexa.

Apical curettage Curettage of diseased periapical tissue without excision of root tip.

Apical foramen Channel located at the conical tip of the root or roots of each tooth through which the pulp receives its vascular and neural supply.

Apical heart rate Number of ventricular contractions per minute.

Apical pulse Measurement of the heartbeat as taken with the stethoscope placed over the apex of the heart.

Apical segmental bronchus The portion of the tracheobronchial tree arising from the right upper lobe bronchus that is distributed to the apical segment.

Apical-radial rate Number of sounds heard at the heart's apex and the rate of the radial pulse during the same period.

Apicoectomy Surgical procedure whereby the apical portion of the root is removed, usually after the root canal filing has been completed.

Apicomplexa pneumocystitis carnll Belongs to phyllum Apicomplexa. The taxonamic group was established to accomodate profojoans structures known as atypical complex.

Aplasia Abnormal development or congenital absence of an organ or tissue.

Apnea Absence of respirations, usually temporary in duration.

Apneic spells Cessation of breathing for more than 15 seconds accompanied by cyanosis or bradycardia.

Apneusitc area Portion of the respiratory center in the pons the sends stimulatory here impulses to the inspiratory area that activate and prolong inspiration and inhibit expiration.

Apneustic center A collection of nuclei (nerve cell bodies) in the brain stem that participates in the rhythmic control of breathing.

Apnoeic oxygenation Method of delivering oxygen to the lungs by insufflation during apnoea.

Apocrine A type of secretion in which the secretory products accumulate at the apical end of the cell; the entire free end of the cell is then pinched off leaving the remainder of the cell to repeat the process. Glands whose cells contribute cytoplasm to its secretion; sweat glands that produce organic secretions traditionally are called apocrine. The sweat glands now are known, however, to be merocrine glands.

Apocrine gland A type of sweat gland that functions in evaporative cooling. It may respond during periods of emotional stress.

Apocrine sweat gland Secretory glands located in the axillae and genital regions that become active at puberty. It responds to emotional and sexual stimulation.

Apocrinic Referring to a multi-cellular gland, such as the mammary or axillary sweat gland, that extrudes some cytoplasm as it secretes its product.

Apoenzyme The protein portion of an enzyme to which the prosthetic group or coenzyme is attached.

Apoferritin The protein part of ferritin, the iron storage complex in the intestinal mucosal cells.

Apolipoprotein The protein component of a lipoprotein.

Apolysis The release of gravid, or egg-filled, proglottids from tapeworm strobila.

Apomixis Asexual reproduction without chromosome reduction or fusion of gametes.

Aponeuroses Aponeuroses are collagenous sheets or ribbons that resemble flat, broad tendons. Aponeuroses may cover the surface of a muscle and assist in attaching superficial muscle or separate structure.

Apoptosis A normal type of cell death that removes unwanted cells during embryological development, regulates the number of cells in tissues, and eliminates many potentially dangerous cells such as cancer cells. During apoptosis, the DNA fragments and the cytoplasm shrinks, but the plasma membrane remains intact. Phagocytes engulf and digest the apoptotic cells, and an inflammatory response does not occur.

Aporeceptor A steroid receptor not bound by a hormone.

Aposia Absence of feeling of thirst.

Apothecia Cup-shaped or saucer-shaped sexual reporductive structures formed by certain fungi.

Apparent leg length discrepancy This is measurable difference in the two legs from the umbilicus or xiphisternum to the medial malleolus.

Apparent shortening of limb Adduction contracture of one hip joint results in aparent shortening while real shrotening results from damage to bones.

Appeal A complain to a superior court to reverse or correct an alleged error committed by a lower court.

Appellant The party who appeals the decision of a lower court to a higher, appellate court.

Appellate Court A court which has the power to review the actions and decisions of a lower court. Supreme Court has final appellate jurisdiction over all the courts in the States.

Appellee The part against who an appeal to a higher court is taken.

Appendage Something that is attached.

Appendicectomy Appendix is a blind-ended sac leading off to caecum. The inflammation of it results in pain abdomen in right iliac fossa, fever, and vomiting. The preferred treatment is surgical removal of appendix known as appendicectomy.

Appendicitis It is an acute inflammation of appendix. Appendix is narrow, finger-shaped tube branching off the large intestine. It is 3.5 inches long. Sometimes it becomes inflamed and obstructed due to faeces or pinworm. It becomes swollen and inflamed. To start pain is around naval and within hours this develops into a sharper more localised pain in right iliac fossa. There may be a slight fever, loss of appetite, nausea and vomiting. In severe case if delayed may perforate causing peritonitis. Surgical removal is the choice on repeated appendicitis.

Appendicitis and pregnancy Appendicitis is more often seen in first two trimesters. Gravid uterus causes confusion in diagnosis. Pain in appendicitis is constant; intestinal obstruction causes intermittent pain. Pain in appendicitis is usually gradual in onset as opposed to sudden pain in hollow viscous lesions. While in pregnancy appendicitis results in diffuse pain in later part of pregnancy. Sickness and vomiting is more frequent. The mortality of appendicitis in pregnancy is high due to delay in diagnosis.

Appendicular Refers to the upper and lower extremities of the body.

Appendicular skeleton The bones of the upper and lower extremities of the body.

Appendix Smaller structure usually attached by one end to a larger structure; a small blind extension of the colon attached to the caecum.

Apperception Perception as modified and enhanced by one's own emotions, memories, and biases.

Appetite The desire for food.

Appetitive stimulus A stimulus that induces an exploratory response.

Appliance Dental device used to position or maintain the position of teeth, such as space maintainers in orthodontics and pediatrics.

Application objective In education, a learning objective which requires the student to make some application, using previously learned principles and facts in a new situation. The learner must apply knowledge to a new problem.

Applied psychology Psychologists who attempt to utilise or apply scientific discoveries for some practical purpose. The emphasis is upon using currently existing knowledge for the benefit of humanity rather than upon the discovery process.

Applied research Research intended to solve existing problems, as opposed to basic "research," which seeks knowledge for its own sake.

Appointment schedule list Printed list denoting patient appointments in chronologic order for each day. This posting of activities is placed in treatment rooms and other frequently used areas.

Appositional growth To place one layer of bone, cartilage, or other connective tissue against an existing layer; increases the width or diameter of bones.

Appraisal A congnitive analysis of an imaginative event.

Appressorium In certain parasitic fungi, a flattened, but swollen, hyphal structure from which the infection emerges to penetrate the host.

Approach-avoidance conflict A situation of indecision involving a single object or event which has both attractive and aversive features. When two or more such objects or events are involved, the situation is called double approach-avoidance.

Appropriateness of medical care The proedures being performed are properly selected and carried out by trained personnel in the proper setting.

Approximal Situated close together.

Approximate To come together, as in the edges of a wound.

Approximation The technique of pushing muscle fibers together in the belly of the muscle.

Approximations, method of A procedure in operant conditioning by which an organism learns a certain behaviour in a step-by-step fashion, each step involving a response slightly more complex than the one preceding it. The correct behaviour at each step is reinforced until that step is mastered. Then, the next step, which is still closer to the final criterion, is reinforced, and so forth.

Apraxia A disorder of voluntary learned movement that is charactrized by an inability to perform purposeful movements and which cannot be accounted for by inadequate strength, loss of coordination, impaired sensation, attentional deficits, or lack of comprehension.

Apraxia 'without movement' Inability to carry out voluntary movements in the absence of paralysis.

Apron A piece of clothing worn as a protection for the body in front.

Apterous Lacking wings.

Aptha A small ulcer on the oral mucosa.

Aptitude The capacity to learn readily and attain a high level of accomplishment in a given area, such as music, mathematics, or mechanics. It refers to potential, rather than actual accomplishment.

Aptitude test A measure of the capacity to learn readily and to achieve a high level of skill in a specific area, such as music, mathematics, or mechanics. It refers to potential rather than actual accomplishment.

Apyrene sperm A type of sperm unique to Lepidoptera in which there is no nucleus, and the sperm do not fertilize the oocytes

Aquathermia pad Electrical heating or cooling device.

Aqueous Watery or waterlike; referring to a medication prepared with water.

Aqueous humor Watery fluid that fills the anterior chamber of the eye, in front of the lens.

Arachin One of the globulin protein in peanut.

Arachnodactyly A hereditary metabolic disorder characterised by abnormally long and slender fingers and toes. Also called Marfan's syndrome.

Arachnoid matter The weblike middle covering of the central nervous system.

Arachnoiditis It is a chronic inflammation and thickening of arachnoid matter, the middle of three meninges. It may develop even after several years of meningitis or subarachoid haemorrhage. It may cause headache, epileptic seizures, loss of vision and slowly progressive spastic paralysis.

Arantius's nodules Nodular, fibrous thickenings at the midpoints of the free edges of the semilunar cusps of the aortic valve.

Arbitration A private, nonjudicial proceeding in which two or more parties agree to allow one or more arbitrators to decide disputed issues.

Arbor vitae The branching arrangement of white matter within the cerebellum.

Arbovirus It is one that multiplies in a blood-sucking arthropod and is transmitted by bite to a vertebrate. The great majority of those that infect man are either Toga viruses or Bunya viruses although few others also cause human disease. These are susceptible to other and to sodium deoxycholate, the presence of RNA in the virus and antigenic relationship with an established arbovirus.

Arbuscule A structure produced by a fungus, responsible for nutrient and carbon exchange between plant and fungus.

Arbutamine A new pharmacologic agent used for stress testing; this medication increases cardiac contractility as well as the rate of contraction acting as a catecholamine.

Arch palatoglossal Extension from soft palate to the base of tongue.

Archaea A group of prokaryotes that constititue a phylogenetically separate domain of organisms distinct from the other two domains, the Bacteria Eubacteria and Eukarya. Archaea are often found living in extreme terrestrial or aquatic environments such as hot springs, under-sea thermal events, or under conditions of high alkalinity.

Archebiosis A term coined by Bastian in 1870 to describe life arising from strictly inorganic starting materials.

Arches Ridges are stacked, one above the other, entering the pattern area from one side, gently rising, falling and existing on the other side.

Arches, lumbocostal Arcuate ligaments.

Archimedes' principle Archimedes principle states that when a body is immersed in a fluid, it experiences a buoyant force equal to the weight of fluid that the body has displaced.

Architomy A form of asexual reproduction in which simple subdivision of the worm is followed by regeneration of the missing parts.

Archival data Records or documents of the activities of individuals, institutions, or governments found in sources such as medical records, voter registration rosters, newspapers and magazines, and meeting minutes.

Archwire Wire applied to two or more teeth through fixed attachments to cause or guide tooth movement orthodontically. Full archwire extends from the molar region on one side of the arch to the opposite side; sectional archwire extends to include only a few teeth on one side or an anterior segment.

Arciform Having a shape like an arc or bow.

Arcuate Shaped like an arc or bow.

Arcus senilis It is a grey white ring in cornea developing in old age. It overlies the outer rim of iris. It is encircled by a narrow zone of unaffected cornea. Arcus senilis is caused by degeneration of fatty material within cornea. It starts in lower part of cornea. It does not affect visual acuity.

Ardee Denture reliner probably prepared from ethyl alcohol plasticizers and acrylic resins.

ARDS Adult Respiratory Distress Syndrome.

Area postrema A nucleus in the brainstem that is sensitive to blood-borne toxins and causes vomiting.

Area sample A sample which includes subgroups of people or items from certain geographic areas in the same proportion as they appear in the population. In a given region, if two-third of the population lives in Orange County, one-sixth in Brown County, and one-sixth in White County, then the sample is composed of people from these same counties in these same ratios.

Within each county, however, the sample is selected on a random basis.

Areola of breast It is the pigmented area that surrounds the nipple. Colour varies from pink to brown or black.

After pregnancy areola deepens and when lactation starts, pigmentation diminishes. It is sexually very sensitive part.

Areolar A type of connective tissue consisting of fibers and a variety of cells embedded in a loose matrix of soft, sticky gel.

Argentaffin Having affinity for or staining readily with silver and chromium salts.

Argentic Containing silver.

Argillaceous Made up of clay.

Argol Crust of crude cream of tartar.

Argyll Robertson pupil Argyll Robertson pupil is small, unequal and irregular pupil which responds to convergence accommodation but not to light or shade and responds poorly to mydriatics. It is generally seen in neurosyphilis but may also be occasionally seen in encephalitis, vascular and traumatic lesions, cerebral tumours, diabetes and chronic alcoholism.

Argyremia The presence of silver or silver salts in the blood.

Argyrophil Staining or easily impregnated with silver.

Arhrophyma The swelling of a joint.

Arhtrosis A joint or articulation.

Ariboflavinosis A disese resulting from the deficiency of riboflavin.

Arkansas stone Natural abrasive stone used to sharpen instruments.

Arm The portion of the upper extremity from the shoulder to the elbow.

Arm ergometry A loss of rhythm; an irregularity of the heart beat.

Armamentarium The materials and tools available to dental personnel for ally types of dental procedures.

Arnold-Chiari malformation This disorder is characterised by hydrocephalus and hindbrain anomalies. There is frequent associated spina bifida cystica. Cerebellar tonsils are displaced through the foramen magnum and ventral displacement and caudal kinking of lower pons. Fourth ventricle is elongated and angulated. Hydrocephalus may develop due to obstruction of aqueduct stenosis.

Aroinatase An enzyme belonging to the P450 family of enzymes. It is primarily responsible for the metabolism of testosterone to oestrogen.

Aroma Aromas are volatile compounds which stimulate odor receptors of olfactory organs of nose. Taste is the result of non volatile substances which stimulate gustatory sense organs of tongue.

Aromatase A cytochrome P-450 steroidogenic enzyme that converts androgens to estrogens.

Aromatherapy It is the systemic use of essential oils in holistic treatments to improve physical and emotional wellbeing. Essential oils are extracted from plants, leaves, flowers and roots, from woods, resins of trees and from zest of citrus fruits. These oils can be used in many ways, i.e. lotions, soaps, oil bath. Most effective way is introducing the oil to the body by massage.

Aromatic When a hydrocarbon has a benzene ring incorporated into its structure.

Arousal A state of activation, surprise and intensity.

Arousal level The degree of emotional response in an individual. The term refers more to the behavioural than to the feeling or physiological components of emotion.

Arousal techniques These are the activities that tend to be sexually stimulating, including mouth-to-mouth deep kissing, kissing and biting ear-lobes, neck, thighs and buttocks, etc.

Arrector pili Smooth muscles of the skin, which are attached to hair follicles; when contraction occurs, the hair stands up, resulting in "goose flesh".

Arrest of descent Failure of the fetal head to descent for more than 1 hour in a nullipara and more than 5 hours for a multipara.

Arrest of placenta due to constriction ring Constriction ring is usually at the junction of upper and lower segment. Uterus is globular and there is not much of bleeding.

Arrest of placenta in lower segment It happens due to poor expulsive power of the uterus or of the abdominal muscles. Usual signs are vaginal bleeding, globular shape of fundus and permanent lengthening of cord. Lower pole of uterus is broadened. Immediate bimanual removal of placenta is a must.

Arrested caries Caries may cease to progress in which instance it is referred as arrested caries. This usually occurs on the occlusal surfaces where because of breakage of enamel walls, a large carious lesion becomes exposed to the cleansing action of tooth-brushing, saliva and mastication. The soft dentin is then worn off, leaving a hard, eburnated layer of black or brown dentin.

Arrhenotoky The development of males from unfertilized eggs.

Arrhythmia It is an irregular heart beat due to malfunctioning of sinoatrial node. Usual symptoms are chest pain, breathlessness and palpitation. It may lead to heart block.

Arrhythmia, cardiac It is an abnormality of the rhythm or rate of heart beat. Heart beat is 100 per minute in tachycardia and 60 per minute in bradycardia. The beat may originate at the sinus node or some other area of heart. In tachycardia (pulse between 100-160 per minute) the rhythm may be regular originating in sinoatrial node. In supraventricular tachycardia rate is faster 120-200 beats per minute. Beat may arise anywhere in the conducting tissue above the ventricles. When rapid irregular beat arises it is called ventricular tachycardia. In atrial flutter atria beat regularly about 200-400 beats per minute. In atrial fibrillation there are completely irregular ventricular beats. A slow regular beat is called sinus bradycardia. In coronary heart disease arrhythmia develops. Any sudden arrhythmia can cause faintness or dizziness due to reduction of blood flow to brain. Drugs are available and lastly pacemaker can be fitted.

Arrhythmogenic Capable of producing cardiac arrhythmias.

Arsenic It is an element and its poisonous form is trioxide. In trace amount it is present in water. It is being used for homicidal poisoning being colourless and tasteless. Acute poisoning primarily affects the lining of intestine producing painful symptoms. There will be nausea, vomiting, diarrhoea, and burning of throat if not treated well. Chronic poisoning develops weakness, tiredness, scaly skin and swelling of lining of mouth. There may be tingling and numbness in hands and feet. Gastric lavage, replacement of fluid and dimercaprol is the line of management.

Arsenic poisoning The average daily arsenic intake in adults is 0.5 to 10 mg. Environmental arsenic exists mainly as sulphur complex. Acute intoxication features develop within 30 minutes of exposure. There is usually a metallic taste in mouth and a slight odour of garlic in breath along with a dry mouth and dysphagia. Severe nausea, vomiting and colicky abdominal pain and profuse diarrhoea develop. Capillary damage leads to generalised vasodilatation, cyanosis, hypoxic encephalopathy, seizures, acute renal failure and death can occur.

Cardiac manifestations include acute cardiac myopathy. After 2 to 4 weeks of acute ingestation patients may develop hair loss and Maes's line over nail plates. A sensorimotor peripheral neuropathy may develop within 2 to 8 weeks. In severe cases the patient may develop flaccid quadriplegia.

Art Ability to perform an act skillfully.

Art and science Certain artists like Leonardo-Da-Vinci and others have drawn line sketches showing coitus, delivery, etc. which are perfect examples of correct anatomy of human figure.

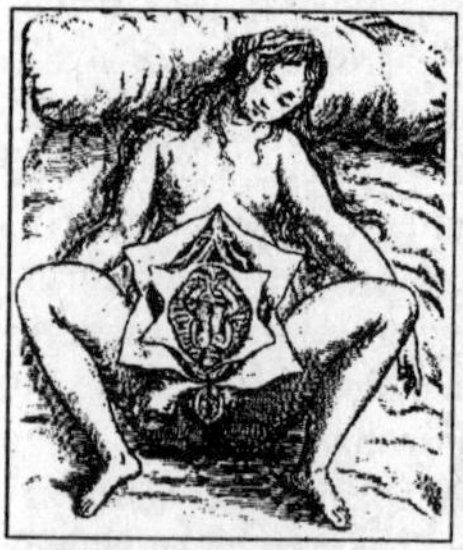

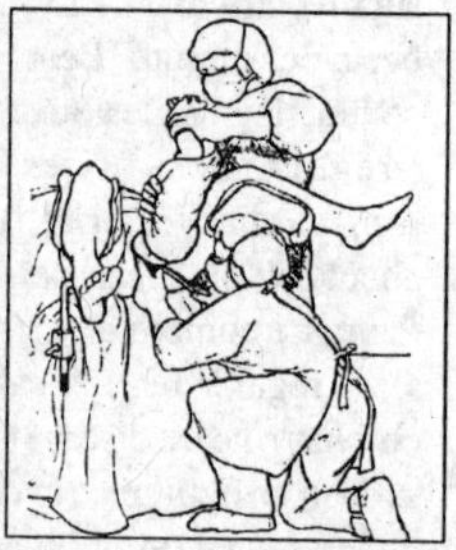

Artefact In radiography, a substance or structure not naturally present in living tissues, but of which an authentic image appears in a radiograph; a blemish or an unintended radiographic image that may result from the faulty manufacture, manipulation, exposure, or processing of an X-ray film.

Arterial blood gas Laboratory test using blood from an artery.

Arterial blood pressure The blood pressure is the pressure of blood on the arterial walls, the systolic pressure normally is 120 mm Hg. It is the pressure during contraction, the diastolic pressure is 80 mm Hg at the end of diastole. The difference between them is pulse pressure. It depends on cardiac output and peripheral resistance. Mean arterial pressure is diastolic plus roughly one-third of pulse pressure.

Arterial blood sample Arterial blood is taken out for blood gas estimation. Collect 3 to 5 ml of arterial blood for gas analyser. Sample has to be sent for immediate analysis.

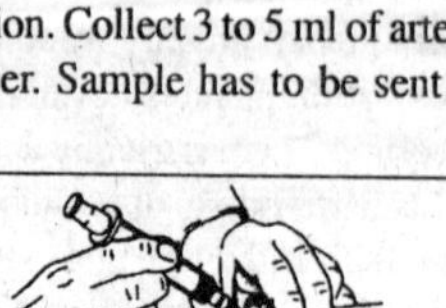

Collection of arterial sample

Arterial catheterisation This is the introduction of fine flexible, polythene catheter into a big artery to introduce radiopaque dyes to study the size of artery, constriction, obstruction or dilatation of artery. The common femoral artery is used to study arterial condition of aortic, mesenteric, iliac and popliteal artery.

Arterial circulation Movement of oxygenated blood under pressure from the heart to the body through the arteries.

Arterial injuries It is generally a complication of fracture. There may be transection of artery, contusion of artery with endothelial rupture and thrombosis. There may be arterial spasm.

Arterial pulse Radial pulse is the most commonly examined arterial pulse. Its examination is facilitated by slight flexion. It should be counted for one complete minute. The heart rate is increased in fever, anxiety, exercise, thyrotoxicosis and anaemia. Heart rate is decreased in athletes, myxoedema, hyperbilirubinaemia, raised intracranial pressure and complete heart block.

Arterial puncture It is a simple and repeatable method for obtaining arterial blood sample. The analysis of arterial PO_2, PCO_2 and pH level provides valued information about respiratory and cardiovascular system (CVS) function and acid-base status. It is useful in respiratory failure, cardiovascular arrest and for research work.

Arterial ulcer of leg This is known as ischaemic ulcer. Mostly these occur on toes, dorsum of foot or heel. There is history of intermittent claudication and rest pain particularly in a person who is chronic smoker. Arterial ulcers are very painful. Peripheral arterial pulses are absent or poor. The arterial ulcer varies in size and shape. The edge is punched out because healing by surrounding tissues is poor or absent. The skin at the edge may be greyish blue in dry pale skin, loss of hair, fissuring of nails. Surrounding tissues are usually cold.

Arterila catheter A hollow, tubular device placed intra-arterially to allow the passage of fluid into or out of the artery.

Arteriography Opacification of arterial system by means of percutaneous arterial needle puncture or placement of percutaneous intra-arterial catheter. According to puncture site of organ to be visualised different terminologies such as femoral, hepatic and transfemoral arteriography are used.

Arteriole A small arterial blood vessel just proximal to the capillaries containing a large proportion of smooth muscle relative to its size.

Arteriosclerosis It causes thickening and loss of elasticity of artery walls. Atherosclerosis is the most common amongst arterioscleroses. While inflammation of arteries is known as arteritis and will cause narrowing.

Arteriosclerotic lesion A lesion or growth in arteries that narrows the lumen, or passage, and makes the walls of the arteries less elastic; commonly called hardening of the arteries.

Arteriosclerotic retinopathy Arteriosclerotic changes in vessels are related to the duration of hypertension. Arterios clerotic changes are due to thickening of walls of retinal arteries. In grade I : there is broadening of light streak from retinal vessels. The vein at crossing is not visible due to thickening of arterial wall.

In grade II there is deflection of vein at arteriovenous crossing. In grade III there will be copper wire arteries. There will be tapering off vein on either of arteriovenous crossing and deflection of vein at right angle to artery. In grade IV there will be silver wire arterioles. There may be degenerative changes at the macula and optic disc appears pale and atrophic. Some cases present with branch vein occlusion.

Arteriovenous fistula This is a condition in which an abnormal communication between an artery and a vein established. It may be a congenital malformation or acquired due to trauma of a penetrating wound. As arterial blood directly drains into the adjacent vein, the vein becomes dilated gradually, tortuous and thick walled. The collaterals increase in size and become tortuous. Operation becomes difficult and hazardous. There becomes marked fall of diastolic pressure with rise in pulse pressure. In superficial communication there is pulsatile swelling in limb. There will be presence of distended superficial veins. Locally extremity becomes warmer.

Arteritis Inflammation of an artery.

Artery Blood vessel that carries blood away from the heart. It is a blood vessel that transports blood away from heart. All arteries except pulmonary artery carry blood that has been oxygenated in the lungs. Walls of arteries are elastic and consist of 3 layers. There may develop aneurysm, arteriosclerosis or atheroma.

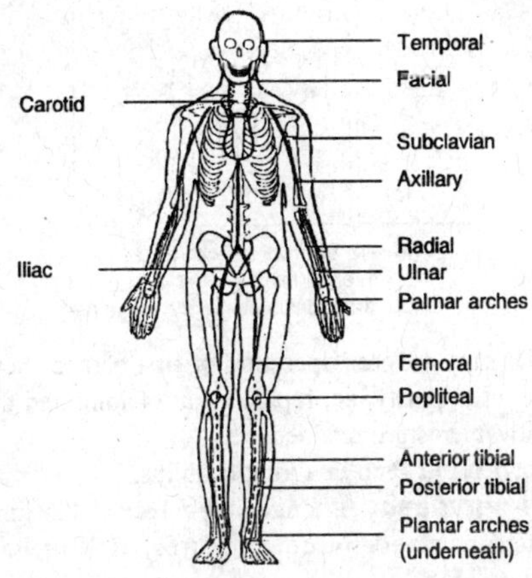

Arterial system

Artherosclerosis A form of arteriosclerosis. The inner layers of artery walls are made thick and irregular by deposits of a fatty substance. The internal channel of the arteries becomes narrowed and blood supply is reduced.

Arthralgia It means pain in joints. Arthritis is inflammation of joint characterised by pain, swelling, stiffness and redness.

Infective arthritis is due to invasion of bacteria into joint. It may also develop from infection elsewhere as in mumps, gonorrhoea and rheumatic arthritis. In osteoarthritis there is wear and tear of joint after the age of 50. In rheumatoid arthritis there is an autoimmune disorder. Many joints are involved and become stiff and deformed.

Arthrectomy Excision of a joint.

Arthrempyesis Suppuration in a joint.

Arthrocele A swelling of a joint.

Arthrocentesis Surgical puncture or aspiration of a joint.

Arthrochalasis Abnormal relaxation or flaccidity of a joint.

Arthrochondritis Inflammation of the cartilage of a joint.

Arthrodesis It is a surgical procedure in which two bones in a diseased joint are fused and movements are restricted.

Sometimes it is done because the pain and deformity

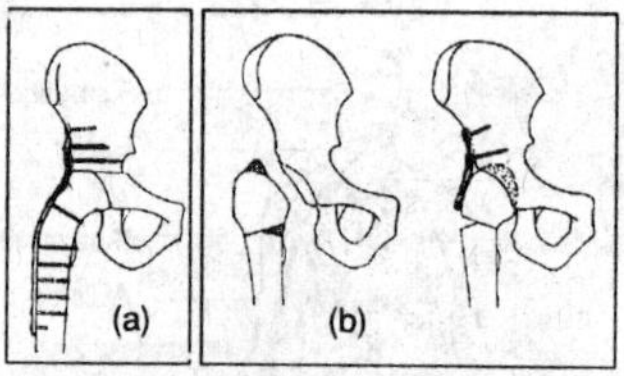

(a) Hip arthrodesis with rigid internal fixation
(b) Arthrodesis of a girdle stone hip

was very severe. Operation of first choice should be arthroplasty, i.e. replacement of joint and thus movements are retained.

Arthrodynia Pain in a joint or joints.

Arthrogryposis A congenital defect of the limbs characterized by contractures, flexion, and extension.

Arthrology The scientific study of the structure and function of joints.

Arthroplasty Any surgical reconstruction of a joint; may or may not involve prosthetic replacement.

Arthropods Invertebrate animals such as insects, mites, spiders and ticks, relevant as carries of infectious diseases between humans or between other animals and humans.

Arthropysosis The formation of pus in a joint cavity.

Arthrosclerosis Stiffening or hardening of the joints.

Arthroscopic portals Careful attention should be paid to portal placement so as to minimise the potential for injury to superficial structures.

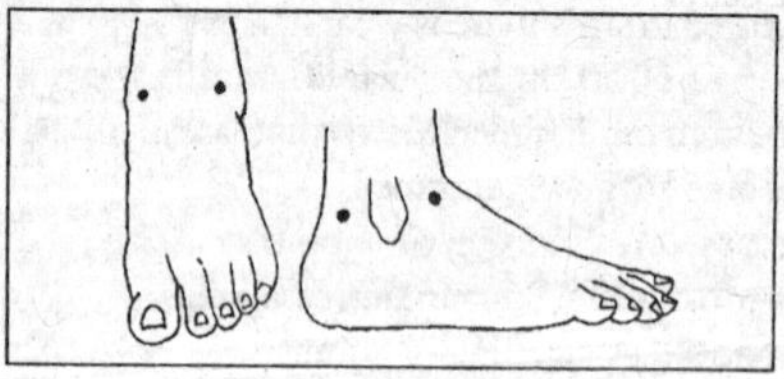

Arthrosteitis Inflammation of the body structures of a joint.

Arthrosynovitis Inflammation of the synovial membrane of a joint.

Arthrotomy Surgical incision of a joint.

Articular cartilage Cartilage covering the joint ends of bones.

Articular eminence A rounded projection of the temporal bone located anterior to the glenoid fossa; appears radiopaque.

Articular meniscus Fibrous cartilage found in the articular capsule.

Articulation Contact relationship of the maxillary and mandibular teeth when moving into and away from centric occlusion.

Articulation disorder Omission or incorrect production of speech sounds due to faulty placement, timing, direction, pressure, speed of response, and neural integration of all events.

Articulator A device that reproduces the hinge motion of the jaw ; used in the production of dental restorations and devices to ensure correct occlusion.

Artifact A voltage signal generated by a source other than the one of interest.

Artificial active immunisation This is the resistance induced by vaccine, preparations of live or killed organisms or their products.

Artificial airway Use of an oral or nasal endotracheal tube for short-term artificial ventilation or tracheostomy for long-term artificial ventilation. •

Artificial airways These are used to relieve an obstruction, to protect the airway, to facilitate suctioning and to give artificial ventilation. These can be : nasal airways which cannot breath at their own, and oral airway is used to keep the tongue from falling back into the throat required for postoperative patients until they recover from anaesthesia.

Artificial blood Artificial solutions capable of gas transport and 0_2 delivery to the tissues. There is no need of blood cross matching.

Artificial heart A mechanical pump used to replace a diseased heart.

Artificial insemination The introduction of semen into the cervix by means of an instrument instead of coitus is known as artificial insemination for purpose of pregnancy. In first type husband's semen is introduced because intercourse is not feasible due to physical injury and deformity or impotency. There may be severe acidity of vagina which is hostile for sperms. Second type is when semen of unknown person is used if man is infertile. It can also be used by a woman who wants children but has no male partner. It is always better to use fresh semen. Although semen can be frozen in liquid nitrogen for years.

Artificial intelligence The capacity of computers to solve problems—the use of machines for purposes which, in the human being, would be called artificial thinking.

Artificial kidney It is known as a kidney machine which fulfils the action of kidney in case of a kidney failure. Technique of renal dialysis or haemodialysis is used. Blood from arm or leg of a patient is pumped through a dialyser in which a semipermeable membrane separates the blood from dialysing fluid. Waste products in the blood pass through minute holes in membrane which are too small to allow passage of blood cells. The filtered blood is pumped back into patient's circulation.

Artificial menopause The cessation of menstruation by artificial means such as irradiation or surgery

Artificial pacemaker An electronic device implanted beneath the skin with an electrode that extends to the heart; provides periodic electrical stimuli to the heart and substitutes for a faulty SA node.

Artificial respiration It is a forced introduction of air into the lungs of a person who has stopped breathing. It may be given mouth to mouth or mouth to nose. Once respiration is fully stopped it should be started within six minutes otherwise it can cause death. When there is no breathing, chances are there that heart has stopped beating. When breathing is weak and shallow and movements of chest are minimal and hardly any breath can be felt, mouth to mouth respiration is easy and most effective. You should exhale with the victim's inhalations. If mouth is injured then mouth to nose respiration will help. For that take a deep breath and seal your mouth around the victim's nose.

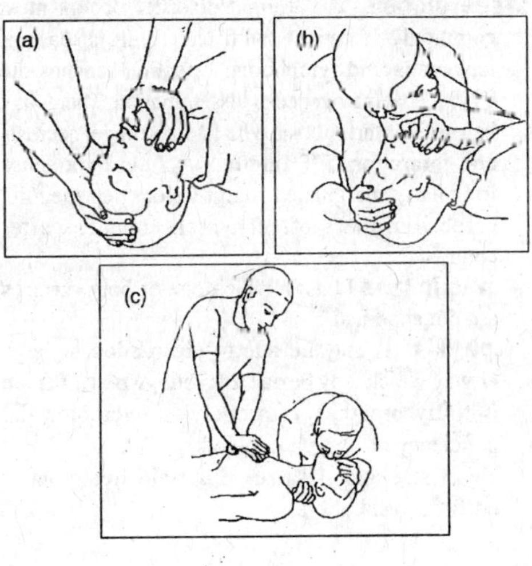

Artificial RNA RNA molecules expressed from genes that have been introduced into cells, or RNA molecules synthesized in cell-free systems.

Artificial rupture of membrane For this it is necessary that cervix is soft and effaced and admits the index finger easily. This is called 'ripe' cervix. Amniotomy performed on unripe cervix fails to induce labour.

Artificial sweetners These are synthetic substances, substitutes of sugar used by people on reducing diets, by diabetics and by food industry. Saccharin is 500 times sweeter than sugar and has no calories. But on long run it may cause cancer bladder. Aspartame is 200 times sweeter than sugar although its sweetness is destroyed on heating and is virtually calorie free. It may cause some neurological disorders after prolonged use. Sorbitol is present naturally in certain fruits.

Artrial natriuretic hormone (ANH) Hormone secreted by the heart cells that regulates fluid and electrolyte homeostasis.

Aryepiglottic folds The posterior boundary of the larygeal inlet formed by the ligamentous and muscular fibers between the epiglottis and arytenoid apex.

Arytenoid Shaped like a jug or pitcher, as the arytenoid cartilage.

Arytenoid cartilages A pair of small cartilages located on the superior aspect of the larynx.

Asbestosis Pulmonary compromise resulting from an accumulation of asbestos fibers in the lungs and from the associated inflammatory response, ultimately leading to pulmonary fibrosis.

Ascariasis It is a roundworm between 6 and 15 inches in length and lives in small intestine. Many worms be there at a time. Mild infestation may cause nausea, abdominal pain and irregular bowel movements. Worm may be passed via rectum or be vomited out. Heavy worm infestation may result in anaemia.

Ascending activating system A group of neurons, each of which contains a common neurotransmitter, that have their cell bodies located in a nucleus in the basal forebrain or brainstem and their axons distributed to a wide region of the brain.

Ascending aorta The first part of the aorta between its origin from the heart and the arch of the aorta.

Ascending colon The portion of the large intestine between the cecum and the hepatic flexure.

Ascending reticular activating system (ARAS) A polysynaptic chain of reticular formation neurons involved in maintaining the conscious state.

Ascending urinary tract infection Causes include uretheritis, cystitis, ureteritis and pyelonephritis.

Ascentidng reticular activating system A polysynaptic chain of reticular formation neruons involved in maintaining the conscious state.

Ascher's syndrome It is of rare occurrence and is related to thyroid gland. Symptoms start at puberty. There may develop goitre and reduplication of upper lip. Eye symptoms include bulging of orbital fat, protrusion of lacrimal gland and blepharochalasis.

Aschheim-Zondek test It is the earliest test of pregnancy as the reaction develops as early as 13 to 14 days after conception and within 2 days after the first missed period. It gives positive reaction through out the pregnancy and till a period of 7 days after termination of pregnancy. This test is based on the fact that in a pregnant women an abnormal amount of anterior pituitary like hormone of chorionic villi are excreted in the urine and shortly after puerperium this stops. But this test is positive in hydatidiform mole, chorion epithelioma and during first week of puerperium.

Aschoff bodies These are small, oval-shaped perivascular granulomas in the myocardium with central areas of necrosis, lymphocytes, occasional plasma cells, and large multinuclear histiocytes, and are often seen in rheumatic carditis.

Ascigerous Describing tissues in which asci are produced, or fungi having such tissue; generally refers to the sexual stage in Ascomycetes.

Ascites It is the collection of fluid in peritoneal cavity between two layers and commonest causes are heart failure, nephrotic syndrome, liver cirrhosis and malignancy. There may be abdominal discomfort, with difficulty in breathing. Treatment depends on the cause.

Ascoli test Extract of infected tissues of animal when carefully layered over immune serum produces a ring of precipitate. This test is used for confirmation of diagnosis of anthrax.

Ascorbic acid It is the chemical name of Vitamin C. It is important for growth and maintenance of bones, teeth and gums. It is present in fresh fruits and vegetables. Mild deficiency may cause weakness, general aches and pains. Severe deficiency leads to scurvy and anaemia. Daily requirement of Vitamin C is 50 mg.

Asepsis Practices that decrease or eliminate infectious agents, their reservoirs, and vehicles for transmission.

Aseptic In medicine, referring to the absence of infectious organisms. In fermentation, referring to the absence of contaminating microorganisms.

Aseptic technique It develops a germ-free environment to protect a person from infection. This technique is needed for any procedure in which there is danger of introducing infection into the body. All persons who come in contact of patient must scrub their hands and wear gowns and disposable gloves. Instruments have to be autoclaved. The area under operation is to be cleaned with antiseptic solutions of iodine and surrounding skin is covered with sterile dressings.

Asexual reproduction Reproduction without the union of gametes having taken place.

Ash Residue left behind after all the organic matter has been burned off.

Asparate An acidic amino acid with excitatory or neurotransmitter activity, released from presynatptic nerve terminals within the brain.

Asparatic acid The non essential amino acid.

Aspergillosis This fungal disorder occurs most commonly in patients with underlying disease of leukaemia and lymphoma. Infection reaches the CNS by haematogeneous dissemination. There may be vascular thrombosis with haemorrhage, necrosis and infarction. CT findings include hypodense irregularly marginated round lesions representing cerebritis, mass effect which enhances after contrast.

Aspheric lens Lens in which one or both surfaces are not spherical.

Asphyxia It may be due to obstruction of large airway which may be due to a foreign body. Person initially breathes vigorously to overcome the deficiency of oxygen in blood.

Heart rate and BP rises. First aid treatment is artificial respiration.

Asphyxia neonatorum Failure to establish spontaneous respiration even although the fetus is born alive. If breathing does not occur within a minute of delivery asphyxia is labelled.

Asphyxiant A substance capable of producing asphyxia.

Asphyxiation Inability to breathe.

Aspirant Fluid or particulate that is aspirated.

Aspiration It is a withdrawal of fluid or tissue from the body by suction. Aspiration biopsy is the removal of tissue or fluid for examination of suction through a needle attached to a syringe. Cells obtained are examined for cancer. Aspiration pneumonia is inflammation of lungs that results from inhalation of foreign material.

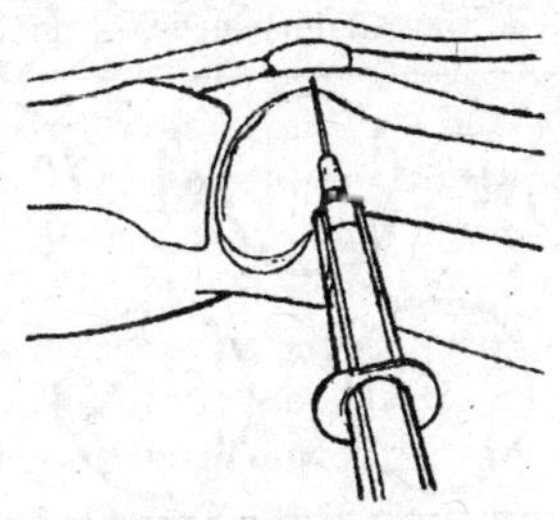

Aspiration of the knee joint

Aspiration pneumonia Inflammation of the lung parenchyma resulting from the entrance of oral or gastric contents into the bronchi.

Aspirator An apparatus employing suction.

Aspirin It is a painkiller used in headache and bodyache. 100 mg tablet is used for heart patients because it reduces the stickiness. It reduces the production of certain prostaglandins responsible for inflammation, pain and fever. It may cause irritation of stomach lining resulting in nausea. Prolonged use may cause bleeding and peptic ulcer.

Assault Intentional, unlawful act of bodily injury to another by force or unlawfully directing force toward another person so as to create a reasonable fear of imminent danger, coupled with the apparent present ability to do the harm threatened if not prevented. A completed assault is battery. In a dental setting, the unconsented touching of the body would be assault and battery.

Assay Determining the amount or purity of a chemical substance in alloys, mixtures, living tissues, or any other system, by means or biological methods.

Assertiveness training A procedure in which subjects are taught appropriate interpersonal responses involving frank, honest, and direct expression of their feelings, both positive and negative.

Assessability of medical care Care can be readily evaluated.

Assessment (1) A continuously evolving process of data collection in which the nurse, drawing on the past and the present, is able to predict or plan the future. Typically it is the initial phase of the nursing process that progresses into diagnosis, planning, intervention, and evaluation; (2) The first step of the medical care process, which involves the gathering of data through reviewing the human situation and the physical, emotional, and social status of the patient to obtain complete the accurate data for the purpose of determining needs for care.

Assignment The transfer of rights or property to another. This is commonly done by physicians when assigning their delinquent accounts to a collection agency.

Assimilate To take a new concept and incorportate into existing knowledge.

Assimilation In this context, the incorporation of inorganic compounds, such as ammonia or sulfate, into organic intermediates of cellular metabolism.

Assimilationist To assimilate means to lose individual identity cultural, racial, sexual traits to align more closely with social norms. A common example of assimilation is the experience of immigrants who do not pass their native language to their children.

Assimilatory reduction The reduction of a compound for the purpose of introducing its building elements into cellular material.

Assistance reflex During voluntary movement, positive feedback from actively stretched neuromuscular spindles reflex.

Assisted suicide Suicidal act in which the individual is assisted

Associated cortex Neocortex that is outside the primary sensory or motor cortex; it functions to produce cognition.

Associated reactions Automatic responses of the limbs as a result of action occurring in some other part of the body, either by voluntary or reflex stimulation. In hemiplegia, these reactions are stereotyped and abnormal.

Association area A portion of the cerebral cortex connected by many motor and sensory fibers to other parts of the cortex. The association areas are concerned with motor patterns, memory, concepts of word hearing and word seeing, reasoning, will, judgment, and personality traits.

Association cortex Area of cortex receiving afferents from one or more primary sensory areas.

Associations Relationships or among events—a form of learning in which the basic elements are stimulus-response connections. The strength of the association is influenced by the frequency with which the events are presented together.

Associative Nitrogen fixation by free-living bacteria in the rhizosphere.

Associative learning A form of learning in which two or more unrelated stimuli become associated with each other so that either can elicit the same behavioral response.

Associative play Group play without group goals.

Assoication cortex Area of cortex receiveing afferents from one or more primary sensory areas.

Assumptions Taken for granted without examination.

Astaxanthin A carotenoid pigment, the pink colour of salmon muscle.

Astereognosis Literally, "without tactile knowledge of space." A disability associated with lesions in the parietal lobe, characterised by inability to recognise objects or geometric forms by touch.

Asterognosis Refers to inability to identify common objects by touch alone.

Asteroid hyalosis It is characterised by appearance of small white dot-like bodies in the vitreous. These asteroid bodies are attached to interlacing fibres of vitreous, therefore these bodies move only on movement of eyeball, otherwise these remain suspended in vitreous. These are asymptomatic and do not interfere in vision. These are easily seen by torchlight on routine examination.

Asthenozoospermia poor motility of sperm within the ejeacualate.

Asthma There are recurrent attacks of breathlessness accompanied by wheezing. Asthma may be due to inhaled allergy from pollens which often cause allergic rhinitis. Other common allergens are hous[e] dust, animal fur or feathers. Emotional factors ma[y] precipitate the factor. Attacks are most frequent i[n] early morning. Main symptoms are breathlessness dry cough and a feeling of tightness in the chest During severe attack breathing becomes difficul[t] causing sweating, rapid heart beat and anxiety Person may develop cyanosis. Broncho-dilator ma[y] be used.

Astigmatism It is a dioptric condition of refractio[n] wherein a point of focus of light cannot be formec upon retina. The astigmatism can occur due to erro[r]

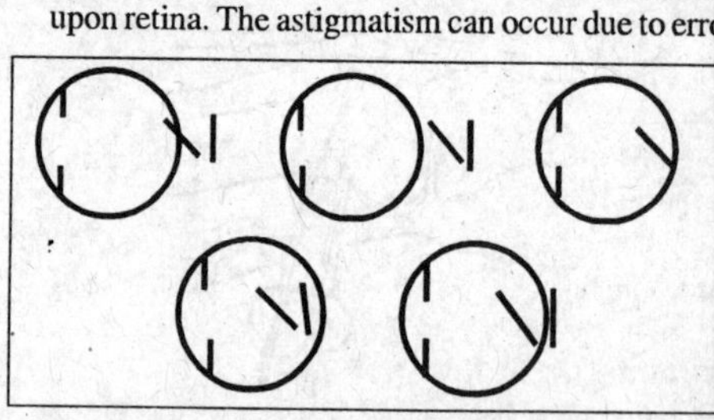

of curvature of centring or of refractive index. Curvature astigmatism is due to change in curvature of cornea. It is usually a congenital anomaly. Acquired astigmatism may be due to trauma and operative scar at limbus.

Astrand exercise protocol A graded exercise test protocol for treadmill or bicycle ergometers; treadmill; constant 5 mph speed; after 3 minutes at 0% grade, the grade is increased 2.5% every 2 minutes; bicycle; constant 50 or 60 rpm, after 3 minutes at 0 W resistance, the resistance is increased by 25 W every 2 minutes.

Astringent A topical substance that causes constriction of tissues ypon application; commonly used for cleansing the skin.

Astringent enema This is used in case of colitis or dysentery to remove spasm of inflamed and irritated mucosa. The solution used is a mixture of tannic acid 2 gm in 500 cc of water of silver nitrate 2 % in 500 cc of water. Temperature is maintained at 105°F.

Astrobiology The stud of life in the universe; the chemistry, physics and adaptations that influcence the origins, evolution, and destiny of life. A term used to describe a new field that will expand upon the limited studies embraced within the field of exobiology.

Astrocyte A neuroglial cell having a star shape that participates in brain development and the metabolism of neurotransmitters, maintains the proper balance of K^+ for generation of nerve impulses, and provides a link between neurons and blood vessels.

Astrocytoma These are most common type of glioma, a tumour arising from glial cells within the nervous system and are composed of astrocytes. These develop mostly in cerebrum. There are four grades. Grade I is slow growing and grade IV are fastest growing and in grade four life expectancy is only 12 to 15 months. MRI is the best tool to diagnose it.

Asymmetric growth retardation Growth of head and long bones is asymmetrically spared relative to abdomen and viscera. This is reflective of fetal nutritional status with decreased subcutaneous fat, brown fat and liver glycogen stores.

Asymmetric tonic neck reflex (ATNR) Head rotation to the left causes extension of the left arm and leg with flexion of the right arm and leg; head rotation to the right causes the reverse pattern.

Asymmetrical pelvis Oblique deformity results from subluxation or tuberculosis of hip joint. Pelvis on diseased side is small. Patient throws all weight on the healthy side.

Asymmetry Lack or absence of symmetry of position or motion. Dissimilarity in corresponding parts or organs on opposite sides of the body which are normally alike.

Asymptomatic It means without symptoms. Blood pressure and diabetes are mostly accidentally diagnosed from a routine blood and urine test. In dental cases person may be having cavity without pain because pulp has not been exposed so far. Similarly early cancer cases may not be producing pain or loss of weight.

Asymptomatic bacteriuria There is presence of significant numbers more than 100,000 organisms in urine without any associated symptoms.

Asymptomatic carrier A person harboring an infectious microbe without symptoms of the disease but with the capacity to transmit to other persons.

Asymptomatic infection The presence of a virus, bacteria, or protozoa in the mother and/or fetus, without causing symptoms of manifestations of clinical disease.

Asynclitism An oblique presentation of fetal head in labour.

Asynergia Loss of ability to associate muscles together for complex movements.

Asynergy Lack of muscular coordination in special function.

At water factor Factors used to calculate energy available from food stuffs after allowing for the losses of digestion and incomplete combustion of nitrogen part of proteins.

Ataraxia A state of complete serenity without impairment of mental or physical functions.

Ataxia There is incoordination of gait and balance and is caused due to damage of cerebellum and spinal cord. Alcoholism may also result in such imbalance. Multiple sclerosis and brain tumour may also result it. The typical ataxia is when gait is lurching and unsteady and walking person has tendency to fall on the affected side. He or she may overshoot while picking up the fallen objects.

Ataxia-telangiectasia It is a genetic, multisystem disorder inherited in an autosomal recessive manner. The disorder is genetically heterogeneous. Clinical features include telangiectasia, cerebellar ataxia, ocular motor apraxia and high incidence of neoplasia. Cerebellar ataxia is noted towards the end of second year of life. Such patients have higher incidence of lymphomas and T-cell leukaemia and primary carcinoma of breast, salivary glands and stomach.

Atelectasis Collapse of a part of lung caused by obstruction of bronchus. After collapse lung loses its elasticity and cannot take air. Blood passing through cannot absorb oxygen or dispose of carbon

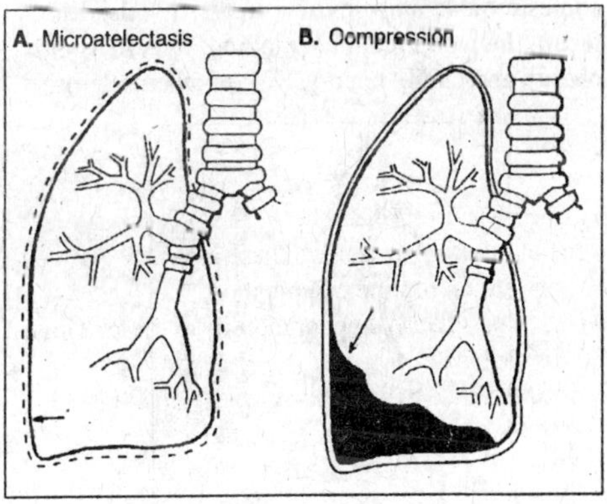

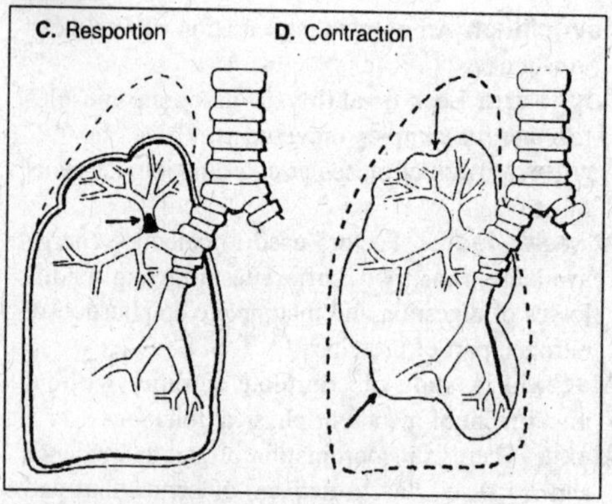

dioxide. In newborn it may prove fatal. It becomes difficult to breath for a man. There may be cough and chest pain. Once obstruction is released due to postural drainage or antibiotics, lungs may reinflate. Antibiotics may be helpful.

Atenolog (Tenormin) A beta-adrenergic blocking agent.

Atherogenesis The development and accumulation of atherosclerotic plaque in arteries.

Atheroma Well-circumscribed, rounded, subcutaneous mass of variable size which moves with the skin. Mass is painless and common sites to be involved are mastoid and posterior auricular surface.

Atherosclerosis In it inner wall of blood vessel thickens causing narrowing of lumen and obstructing blood flow. The plaques consist of lipoproteins, decaying muscle cells, fibrous tissue and clumps of blood platelets. It may take place in persons with high concentrations of blood cholesterol. It may involve heart vessels. Risk factors include cigarette smoking, hypertension, obesity and family history. Risk of atherosclerosis

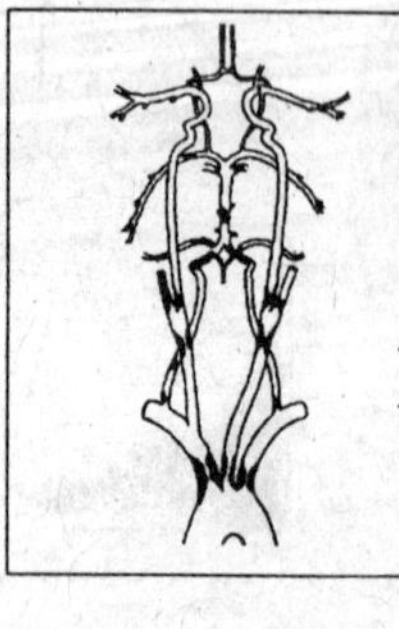

Circle of Willis. Shades show site of atheromatous plaques

increases with age above 50. It causes no symptoms unless the disease is severe. Later on it may cause symptoms of angina pectoris. Restriction of blood flow to legs causes intermittent claudication. Narrowing of arteries to brain causes transient ischaemia. Medication is unnecessary. Anti-coagulants have been tried to check secondary clotting and embolus formation.

Atherosclerotic occlusive disease The blockage of blood vessels as the result of atherosclerotic plaque formation.

Atherosis Lipid deposits in the initma of arteries that produce a yellow swelling on the endothelial surface.

Athetoid Purposeless weaving motions of the body or extremities.

Athetosis This is a slow, irregular, sinus movement seen in limbs specially after perinatal brain injury involving striatum. Pseudoathetosis is a quiet different disorder in which there is abnormal posturing of the outstretched hands due to disturbed sense of finger position.

Athlete A person who participates in sports as an amateur or a professional. Athletes require precise use of their bodies.

Athlete's foot It is a common illness where skin between the toes becomes itchy and sore. It cracks and peel away and occasionally blisters may be formed. It is a fungal infection caused by Tinea pedis. Sometimes it clears up without medication. Careful drying up of part and putting antifungal powder or applying antifungal tube helps the person.

Atmospheric pressure Pressure exerted by the atmosphere. Atmospheric pressure at sea level is 760 mm Hg.

Atom The small particle of an element that is composed of protons, neutrons, and electrons.

Atonia The absence or lack of normal muscle tone.

Atonia No tone Even resting muscles have a certain level of activity, or tone, that can be blocked by inhibiting motor neurons to produce a condition of atonia.

Atonic Lacking the tone or strength that is normally present.

Atonic seizures It begins in childhood and is associated with diffuse brain lesion. The child's head may drop for few seconds or loss of tone may be generalised with sudden falling to the ground. These may occur many times a day.

Atony It is a complete loss of tone in muscle. Muscle becomes flaccid. It may be caused after injury to nerves. Muscles of arm become atonic after injury to brachial plexus.

Atony of uterus It accounts for about 80% of PPH. Violent mass aging, squeezing and pushing of uterus downward cause irregular contraction of uterus and partial separation of placenta.

Atopic Atopic eczema is an allergic eczema.

Atopic dermatitis An allergic skin reaction to agents such as poison ivy and poison oak; a type of delayed hypersensitivity.

Atopy It is a predisposition to various allergic reactions. Such patients suffer from one or more allergic based disorders such as asthma, eczema and allergic rhinitis. It may be caused by absorption of abnormally high levels of allergens in first few weeks of life. There is also a distinct genetic or inherited basis to atopy.

ATP Adenosine Triphosphate, the energy-rich molecule synthesized in energy-yielding reactions and consumed in biosynthetic processes.

Atraial natriuretic Peptide hormone, produced by the atria of the heart in response to stretching, that inhibits aldosterone production and thus lowers blood pressure.

Atretic Without an opening. Atretic ovarian follicles are those that fail to ovulate.

Atria A chamber or cavity to which are connected several chambers or passageways.

Atrial ectopic beats Impulses arising from abnormal pace maker sites with in the atria.

Atrial fibrillations These are lack of coordinated atrial contractions resulting from impulses from many different parts of atria reaching the AV node in quick succession, only some of which are transmitted.

Atrial flutter Arrhythmia resulting from rapid atrial discharge.

Atrial gallop The triple cadence of heart sounds heard by auscultation and characterized by an audible sound (fourth heart sound) occurring in late diastole in addition to the normal first and second heart sounds; presystolic gallop.

Atrial gland An elaboration of the secretory epithelium that secretes several peptides.

Atrial kick The increased ventricular stroke volume resulting from the priming force of atrial contraction immediately before ventricular contraction.

Atrial natriuretic Hormone released from cells in the atrial wall of the heart when atrial blood pressure is increased; acts to lower blood pressure by increasing the rate of urine production.

Atrial septal defect (ASD) It is the most common congenital heart disease. It is in two forms, ostium primum defect or ostium secundum defect. A degree of left to right shunt depends on size of defect. Person loses weight and develops respiratory infections.

There will be palpable left parasternal heave. Pulmonary component of second sound is loud. Middiastolic murmur across tricuspid valve and right sided S_3 are heard in left lower sternal region due to increased blood flow especially when shunt is 2%. Central cyanosis may be present. ECG will show right axis deviation, right ventricular hypertrophy with persistent deep S-waves in V5-V6.

P wave may be inverted in lead III. X-ray will show right ventricular enlargement, prominent pulmonary arteries and increased pulmonary vascular markings. Ascending aorta is small. Osteum secundum type is due to defective formation of septum secundum. It may be due to defective formation of septum. It will cause shunting of blood from left to right atrium and then to right ventricle and pulmonary trunk causing hypertrophy and dilation of these.

It develops slowly and symptoms appear in 3rd and 4th decade. Symptoms include dyspnoea, palpitation and rarely cardiac failure. ECG may show incomplete right bundle branch block.

Atrial tachycardia Depolarization of the atria at a rate in excess of 100 per minute.

Atrioventricular (AV) bundle Bundle of modified cardiac muscle fibres that projects from the AV node through the interventricular septum; conducts action potentials from the AV node rapidly through the interventricular septum; also called the bundle of His.

Atrioventricular (AV) node The portion of the conduction system of the heart made up of a compact mass of conducting cells located in the septum between the two atria.

Atrioventricular bundle The portion of the conduction system of the heart that begins at the atrioventricular (AV) node, passes through the cardiac skeleton separating the atria and the ventricles, then extends a short distance down the interventricular septum before splitting into the right and left bundle branches. Also called the bundle of His (HISS).

Atrioventricular canals The left and right halves of the atrioventricular canal of the heart tube, formed by the union of the dorsal and ventral endocardial cushions.

Atrioventricular dissociation Electrically unrelated ventricular and atrial activity.

Atrioventricular node A microscopic aggregation of specialized cardiac fibers located in the interatrial septum of the heart that are a part of the conduction system of the heart; AV node.

Atrioventricular valve Valve located between the atrium and the ventricle of the heart, the tricuspid valve between the right atrium and right ventricle and the bicuspid or mitral valve between the left atrium and left ventricle.

Atrium One of the two chambers of the heart that collects blood during ventricular contraction and pumps blood into the ventricles to complete ventricular filling at the end of ventricular relaxation; the right atrium receives blood from the inferior and superior venae cavae and from the coronary sinus, and delivers blood to the right ventricle; the left atrium receives blood to the left ventricle.

Atrophic non reactive union Bone ends are atrophic having tapered appearance. There is lack of surrounding callus.

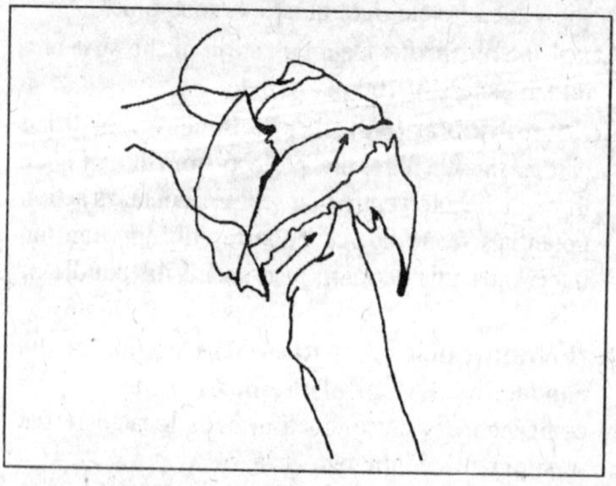

Atrophy It is a shrinkage in the size of cell due to loss of cell substance. It may be caused by decreased workload, loss of innervation, inadequate nutrition and aging. Atrophic cells have diminished function but are not dead. There is a shrinkage or wasting away of tissue or organ due to reduction in size and number of its cells. Atrophy is generally caused by its disuse of parts or by poor nutrition or poor circulation.

Atrophy of pulp Reticular atrophy is really an artefact but at one time it was believed to be a regressive change of pulp. Microscopic sections show numerous spaces and interweaving bundles of fibres in the pulp.

Atropine It is the drug used in inflammation of iris and corneal ulcer. It is put to dilate the eye pupil before it is being examined. It's action is utilised in premedication before general anaesthesia. Along with antibacterial drug it is being utilised for antispasmodic effect.

Atropine sulphate It is the racemic mixture of dextro and laevo-hydroscyamine. It reduces secretion of saliva. It can be used to depress the cardiac vagus especially in patients on digitalis. It counteracts bradycardia in high spinal block and so raise blood pressure. It can be used as a cycloplegic and to depress the oculocardiac reflex in ophthalmic operations. It competes with acetylcholine at the site of muscarine activity. It stimulates the medulla and higher centres and directly stimulates the respiratory centre to counter effect of morphine. It results in paralysis of sphincter of iris resulting in dilated pupils. Sweat, bronchial and salivary glands are paralysed. It acts as a bronchodilator. The tone of peristalsis, gut and kidney are decreased. It crosses the placenta rapidly. Usual dose is 0.5 to 1 mg intramuscularly. Milk secretion is not affected.

Attached gingiva The portion of the gingiva that is firm, dense, stippled, resilient, and tightly bound to the underlying connective tissue, periosteum, bone, and the underlying cementum if present, thus being relatively immovable.

Attachment An enduring emotional tie between persons that develops and grows overtime and that is not transient or easily abandoned. Attachment is specific and unique to the involved individuals and implies love, tenderness, and affection. Involved individuals seek proximity to each other and yearn to be in each other's presence. Attachment relationships can withstand anger, frustration, and periods of separation.

Attachment of cranial nerves The olfactory nerve (1) in bundles enters the olfactory bulb, and the optic nerves (2) lead back to the optic chiasma. The oculomotor nerves (3) emerge from interpeduncular fossa behind the mamillary bodies. The trochlear nerves (4) emerge dorsally below the caudal colliculus and wind around the cerebral peduncles. The trigeminal nerves (5) are attached to the later surface of the pons where motor and sensory roots may be distinguished. The abducent nerves (6) emerge between the pyramids and pons, the facial (7) and vestibulocochlear (8) nerves emerge in the cerebelloponto-medullary angle. The glosso-pharyngeal (9) vagus (10) and cranial accessory (11) nerves emerge between the olives and the inferior cerbellar peduncles, the hypoglossal nerves (12) emerge between the olives and pyramids.

Attachment site A site on a phage (attP) or chromosome (attB or Att Y, phi 80, etc.) at which a site-specific integrase can join circular phage DNA and host chromosome.

Attachment width Distance in millimeters from the base of the pocket to the mucogingival line. Indicates width of attched gingiva.

Attack rate The proportion of exposed persons who become ill. Ths is the customary measure used to establish the severity of a disease outbreak.

Attar Any essential or volatile oil of vegetable origin.

Attempted suicide A suicide act in which an individual survives.

Attention span The length of time that a person is able to concentrate on a given task.

Attenuate To weaken.

Attenuated vaccine Vaccine derived from microorganism or virus whose virulence has been weakened because of passage through another host.

Attenuation Reducing, thinning, or weakening; reduction of the virulence of a virus or pathogenic microorganisms, as by successive culture or repeated inoculation; in radiography, the process by which a beam of radiation is reduced in energy when passing through some material.

Attenuator An RNA sequence involved in regulating the expression of certain genes; functions as a transcription terminator.

Attestation Signing a written statement that a document is correct or that you have witnessed the document being signed.

The witnesses to a living will may attest that the patient making the will was of sound mind and made the will of his or her own volition.

Atticitis Inflammation of the attic.

Attitude A posture or position of the body. The relation of fetal parts to each other in the uterus. The basic attitude is either flexion or extension.

Attitude of fetus It is the relation of fetal head and limbs to its trunk. Normal attitude is flexion. The fetus forms a compact ovoid mass fitting the uterine cavity.

Attitudes States of mind, feelings.

Attractant A chemical that causes a positive chemotaxis response.

Attraction The tendency of teeth or other maxillary or mandibular structures to become superior to their normal structure.

Attributable risk The rate of the disorder in exposed subjects that can be attributed to the exposure derived from subtracting the rate (usually incidence or mortality) of the disorder of the non-exposed population from the corresponding rate of the exposed population.

Attributable risk percent The percentage of overall risk of disease outcome within a exposed person.

Attributable risk percent in the exposed Answers the following question: Among those with the risk factor, what percentage of the total risk for the disease is due to the risk factor?

Attribution theory Study of the process by which people attribute characteristics to other individuals —the attempt to identify the ideas or procedures that people use in making inferences about other people's personality and behaviour.

Attrition Normal loss of tooth substance due to frictioin caused by physiologic forces.

Atypical antidepressants Includes compounds that act similarly to tricyclic antidepressant but have a different chemical structures.

Atypical chest pain Angina that does conform to the typical or normal form.

Auctorsion The twisting of an artery with a needle to control hemorrhage.

Audioanesthesia Multifrequency sound played to patients through head phones in order to reduce pain.

Audiogram It is a graph produced by result of certain hearing tests which shows that at what level of intensity an individual can hear sounds of different frequencies. Audiologists conduct hearing tests and may not be qualified doctors. While in audiometry, machine produces sounds of defined intensity and frequency and hearing of each ear is measured.

Audiologist A sepecialist in evaluation and rehabilitation of those whose communication disorders centre in whole or in part in the hearing function.

Audiometry Measurement of hearing acuity at various sound frequencies.

Audiopsychic area (area 22) It occupies the whole of superior temporal gyrus except in upper part. Its pyramidal layer is deeper and granular layers are shallower than audiosensory cortex. A special part of superior and middle temporal gyri on the left side is concerned with the understanding of spoken speech words. Stimulation of this area 22 may also cause adversive movements of head and eyes.

Audiosensory area (areas 41 and 42) It is largely hidden in Sylvian fissure and a limited part of it extends for a short distance at the superior lip of temporal lobe. Area is rich in cell and fibres. In this area the auditory impressions reach consciousness as sounds and their pitch, quality and loudness are differentiated.

Auditors Inspectors who examine patient records.

Auditory Pertaining to the ability to hear and interpret sounds, localize sounds, and discriminate foreground from background sounds.

Auditory coding The use of microelectrodes for recording responses from single nerve cells in the temporal lobes.

The aim is to determine transmission of auditory information from one neural site to another.

Auditory localisation Naming or pointing to positions from which sounds emanate.

Auditory ossicles Bones of the middle ear; the malleus, incus, and stapes.

Auditory tube A narrow canal that connects the middle ear chamber of the pharyns; also called the eustachian canal.

Auer bodies These are rod-shaped structures in the cytoplasm of the immature myeloid cells, and are seen in acute myeloblastic leukaemia.

Auerbach's plexus and ganglia Mysenteric portion of the nerve plexus.

Auger spectroscopy A Technique used to study the surface composition of substances, specially of low atomic weight elements. This is done by detecting the characteristic energies of electrons emitted from a surface targeted with high energy electrons.

Augmentation A procedure performed to create an increase in size or volume, In alveolar ridge augmentation, various grafting materials alone in combination are used to increase the size of atrophic areas.

Augmentation of labor Artificial stimulation of uterine contractions that have become ineffective.

Augmentative communication Communication through the use of mechanical devices that expand the individual's ability to communicate.

Aura It is a peculiar warning sensation which precedes before epilepsy, migraine and certain other diseases. A migraine attack may be preceded by a feeling of elation, unusual wellbeing and drowsiness. There may be flashing lights before the attack. While an epileptic aura may be of a distorted perception, hallucinatory sound or smell. These symptoms subside the moment real illness starts.

Aural Pertaining to the ear.

Aural speculum It is a cone-shaped, tubular made of metal and is available in various sizes. It is used to examine auditory meatus with proper size speculum. The light is focussed through the speculum to visualise the outer ear canal. It is used in myringotomy operation and to assess damage.

Aural syringe It is a metallic syringe with a long metallic cannula. Piston is having ring attached and there are 2 more rings attached to the syringe. It gives a good grip during syringing. It is used to remove foreign body and wax from ear canal. It also helps in removing dried discharge of chronic suppurative otitis media. To avoid injury to

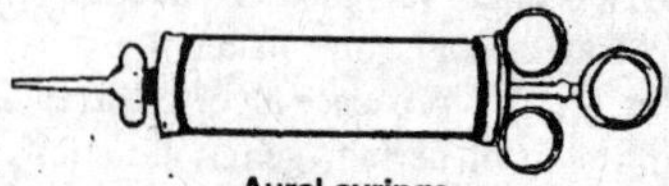

Aural syringe

tympanic membrane jet of fluid should not be very forceful and nozzle should not be introduced inside ear canal. Jet of fluid should always be towards roof of the canal.

Aural-perceptual approach First of the two analyses realized by phoneticians in a speaker recognition procedure. It consists in a detailed auditory analysis.

Auricle Part of the ear attached to the side of the head; earlike appendage of each atrium of the heart.

Auricular acupuncture This is an acupuncture to the outer ear where particular areas can be used to treat conditions of particular parts of body.

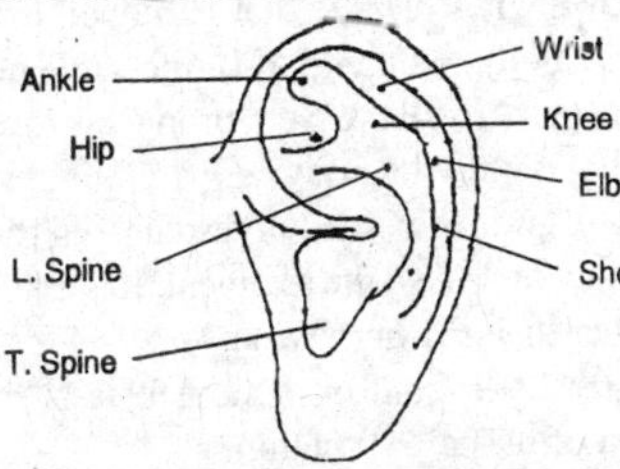

Auricular acupuncture points

Connection between ear and sciatic nerve was mentioned by Hippocrates. Various parts of body are represented in ear. Needles placed in these areas can result in pain relief of the affected part. One area represented in ear is of 0.2 mm.

Auricular erysipelas Swelling, tension and redness of the auricular skin. Erythematous redness area is sharply demarcated and skin appears glossy. Earlobe is mostly involved. There is moderate pain or only a sensation of fullness and heat.

Auricular fibrillation It is essentially an auricular disturbance due to multiple ectopic foci causing irregular ventricular response affecting the pulse in its rate/rhythm and volume so that no beats are equal. These may be caused by rheumatic heart disease, thyrotoxicosis and acute febrile disease. There will be palpitation, and effort dyspnoea. Pulse is absolutely irregular and average rate is 100 to 120/minute.

Volume of pulse differs from beat to beat. There is gross cardiac irregularity which increases after slight exercise and may vary from 100 to 180/minute. ECG shows characteristic 'F' or fibrillary waves and absence of 'P' waves.

Auricular flutter Auricular impulse formation occurs at the rate of 250 to 350 per minute. Since AV node cannot transmit more than 220 impulses there is physiological AV block. Symtoms include palpitation, breathlessness and pain in chest. Flutter should be suspected when pulse is regular at the rate of 120 to 170 per minute and is not influenced by change of posture, exercise and emotional upset. Sometimes flutter waves may be seen in jugular veins. Pulse rate may vary from time to time depending on degree of AV block. ECG may show rapid regular F waves giving rise to saw tooth well seen in V_1.

Auricular perichondritis There develop extreme tenderness on pressure of affected cartilage area, circumscribed redness and doughy thickening of overlying skin. There will be pad-like swelling chiefly affecting anterior side of auricle.

Auriculotemporal syndrome It follows the injury to the fibres of temporal auricular nerve during operation of parotid abscess or suppurative parotitis. Characteristic features include that cheek becomes red, hot and painful with appearance of beads over perspiration. Sometimes during shaving there is cutaneous hyperaesthesia in front and above ear. Usually the symptoms passes off within a few years. Otherwise avulsion of auriculo-temporal nerve will result in effective treatment.

Auscultable fetal heart sound It is the most convincing sign of pregnancy. It can be heard at 24 the week of pregnancy. Uterine souffle is also heard over fibroid.

Auscultate To listen/heart/lung sounds.

Auscultation The examination procedure of listening for sounds produced by the body to detect or judge an abnormal condition.

Auscultatory gap The fading away and the reappearance at a lower pint, of the sounds that indicate systolic blood pressure; in hypertensive patients this may lead to the recording of falsely low as much as 25 mm Hg systolic blood pressure values (it maybe avoided by pumping the sphygmomanometer 30 mm Hg beyond palpable systolic pressure).

Austin-Flint murmur An early, soft, low-pitched, rumbling, mid diastolic murmur heard at the apex. It is found in aortic regurgitation and also in left ventricular dilatation.

Australopithecus (southern ape) The earliest known humanlike animals, one species of which gave rise to the lineage that led to modern humans.

Authenticity and integrity analysis The ability to detect falsificatons on audio recordings presented as evidence.

Authoritarian personality A cluster of personality traits reflecting a desire for security. These traits might include a rigid, highly conventional outlook, extreme obedience, scapegoating of minority group members, and a desire for structured lines of authority. The pattern is assumed to develop from the child's interaction with a domineering parent.

Autism This is a condition in which children fail to form relationship with others. It is rare in girls and boys suffer more. From the very beginning child does not like being cuddled or picked up. He or she avoids eye to eye contact and prefers playing alone. He does not observe social conventions and remains aloof to the feelings of others. He does not like to be disturbed. In such children delay in speaking is very common. There is no specific treatment for it.

Auto tolerance Ability to accept an antigen in the body without raising a pathogenic inflammatory response.

Autoantibody response The formation of antibodies in response to antigenic constituents of one's own tissue.

Autoclave These are routinely used for sterilisation of surgical liners, gloves, gauze, cotton, glass items and rubber items. Twenty-two pound pressure is employed for 30 minutes. At 15 pounds there is red mark for caution. Keep required items to be sterilised in drum having perforated windows. Pour water to the body of autoclave up to 3 to 4 inches till metallic base or stand inside body just touches water. Now put the sterilising drum inside and close the lid. Now put the autoclave to heat. When the required pressure of 22 pounds is reached steam passes pushing through safety valve in whistling manner. Now by releasing steam from adjustment mechanism, pressure is maintained at desired level and within desired time.

Autocrine Relating to or acting upon itself; e.g., an autocrine product affect the same cell that produces it.

Autoeroticism Sensual self-gratification. Characteristic of, but not limited to, an early stage of emotional development. Includes satisfactions derived from genital play, masturbation, fantasy, and from oral, anal, and visual sources.

Autogamous Capable of or involving autogamy.

Autogamy Sexual reproduction by fusion of gametes from a single parent organism, resulting in self-fertilization.

Autogenetic inhibition Negative feedback from Golgi tendon organs causing a muscle to relax.

Autogenic relaxation Self directed lessening of tension.

Autogenous graft Tissue that is moved from one part of the body to other part of the same person.

Autogenous infection Self-produced infection; originating within the body.

Autograft A graft of tissue harvested from the same individual who is also the recipient. It is taken from a site other than the burn wound.

Autogregulation Control of homeostasis through alteration of tissue or function.

Autoimmune disorder There are many diseases such as rheumatoid arthritis, systemic lupus erythematosus (SLE), insulin-dependent diabetes caused by a reaction against the organs or tissues of his own body.

There develops a hypersensitivity disorder in some cases. Auto immune process can have various results, i.e. slow destruction of a particular type of cell or tissue, stimulation of an organ into specific growth or interference in its function. Endocrines are mostly affected.

Autoimmunization The induction in an individual of an immune response to its tissue constituents, which may lead to pathological sequelae, Autoinfection Infection by an agent already present in the body or transferred from one part of the body to another.

Autoinfection Reinfection by a parasitic organism without its leaving the host.

Autointoxication Intoxication by some poison generated within the body.

Autokinetic effect The apparent drifting of a small fixed spot of light in an otherwise completely dark room.

Autolet A small instrument with a lancet used to obtain a capillary blood specimen.

Autologous transfusion Self-donated blood.

Autologus blood transfusion Transfusion of blood into a patient having been donated by same patient.

Autolysin Endogenous murein hydrolases that cleave bonds in the peptidoglycan sacculus, that are critical for, the mechanical strength of the structure and thus cause lysis of the bacterium.

Autolysis Self-destruction of cells by their own lysosomal digestive enzymes after death or in a pathological process.

Automated external defibrillator Device that delivers an electrical charge to the heart.

Automated fingerprint Identification systems. All computer systems that perform fingerprint searching.

Automated monitoring devices Equipment that allows the simultaneous collection of multiple vital sign data.

Automatic movement Movments performed without conscious effort that align body parts, restore balance, or maintain balance.

Automatic postural synergies Discreate patterns of leg and trunk muscle contractions characterized by consistency in muscle combinations, timing, and intensity; they are used to preserve standing balance.

Automatic speaker recognition ASR relies on computer methods, based on information theory pattern recognition and artificial intelligence.

Automatic temperature regulation Regulation of body temperature by involuntary thermo effector responses to heat and cold that modify the heat production and heat loss.

Automatic thoughts Thoughts that are involuntary and difficult to inhibit.

Automaticity A cell's ability to initiate its own depolarization.

Automixis Asexual reproduction with chromosomal reduction but without fusion of gametes.

Autonphagous Capable of or carrying out a process of autophagy.

Autonome A cutaneous area innervated by autonomic nerves originating from a particular segmental level.

Such an area can often be visualized with thermographic methods.

Autonomic A division of the nervous system that supplies the sensory innervation for the smooth muscles, heart and glands. It is divided into the parasympathetic (craniosacral) and the sympathetic (thoracolumbar) systems.

Autonomic (involuntary) nervous system A division of the nervous system that supplies the sensory innervation for the smooth muscles, heart, and glands. It is divided into the parasympathetic (craniosacral) and the sympathetic (thoracolumbar) systems. Sympathetic nervous system heightens activity in the heart increasing beating and breathing rate.

It has two chains of nerves that pass from spinal cord throughout the body. Into these tissues the nerve endings release the neurotransmitter chemicals, epinephrine and norepinephrine. This system decreases the activity of digestive system, increases contractions of urethra while ejaculation and dilating the pupils. The parasympathetic nervous system is composed of one chain of nerves that passes from brain and another that leaves the lower spinal cord. This system releases acetylcholine which has opposite effects of epinephrine.

Autonomic dysreflexia (hyperreflexia) Exaggerated autonomic nervous system responses.

Autonomic effector Tissues to which autonomic neurons conduct impulses.

Autonomic ganglion A cluster of sympathetic or parasympathetic cell bodes located outside the central nervous system.

Autonomic hyperflexia There is an increased sensitivity of sympathetic reflexes in patients with spinal cord injury above thoracic 5/6 vertebra.

Autonomic nervous system System which regulates non voluntary body functions by means of reflex path ways.

Autonomic neuron Motor neurons that make up the autonomic nervous system.

Autonomy The moral principle that indivuduals should be permitted to be self-determining.

Autonomy versus doubt In Erikson's psychosocial stages, the second crisis in which the issue is the amount of freedom to be allowed to the developing child.

An appropriate amount leads to autonomy: too much or too little freedom may prompt the child to become fearful in one way or another, leading of doubt, rather than autonomy.

Auto-oxidation Oxidation which takes place spontaneously and which leads to rancidification.

Autopagnosia Impairment of body scheme.

Autophagy A process of self-digestion by cells that are starved of amino acids in which portions of the cytoplasm are circumscribed by endoplasmic reticulum and then catabolized as an internal supply of nutrients.

Autophosphorylation reaction The catalysis of the phosphorylation of a residue found on itself by an enzyme.

Autopsy Examination of the deceased's body performed after a person's death to confirm or determine the cause of death.

Autoradiography It is a method by which biologically active tissue, often live animals are given a radiolabelled compound typically labelled as beta-emitter.

After metabolic processing of substance the tissue is sliced and put adjacent to a photosensitive film or increasingly to a digital device. Thus a spatial distribution of the radiotracer in the slice can be identified.

Autoreceptor A presynaptic receptor acted upon by the transmitter released at the same nerve ending.

Autoreceptors Sites on the nerve axon terminal which respond to the neuron's own neurotransmitter.

Autoregulation A local, automatic adjustment of blood flow in a given region of the body in response to tissue needs.

Autorelese The spontaneous tearing of tissue. It is usually caused by an outside applied force.

Autortroph An organims that can synthesize its own complex molecules from very simple carbon and nitrogen sources, such as carbon dioxide and ammonia.

Autoshaping A process in operant conditioning in which the response is acquired despite the absence of any obvious reinforcement. The individual seems to develop this behaviour apart from regular reinforcement.

Autosoma Pertaining to an autosome.

Autosomal dominant inheritance A disorder expressed when only one abnormal autosomal allele is present and the corresponding gene on the homologous chromosome is normal.

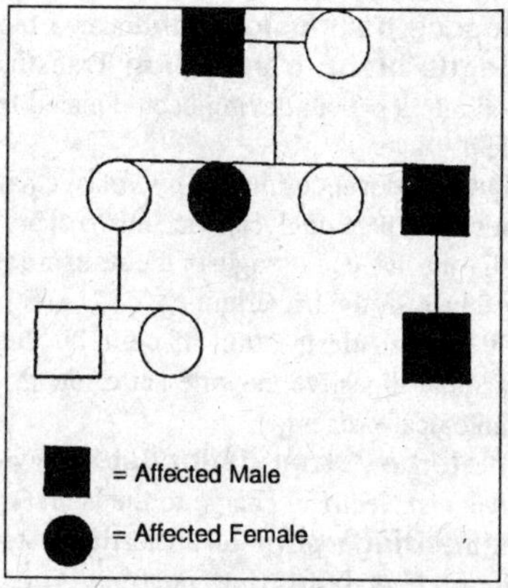

Autosomal recessive disorder A condition in which both members of a gene pair are abnormal.

Autosome Any chromosome other than a sex chromosome; normally occur in pairs in somatic cells and singly in gametes. The 22 human chromosomes that do not express triats related to sex.

Autotraction It is a multiplane automatic traction with a force determined by the patient.

Autotrophy The fact of being an autotroph; using Co_2 as a sole source of carbon.

Auvard's speculum It is a self-retaining type of speculum provided with a lead weight and suitable curvature to retract the posterior vaginal wall. It is used in lithotomy position. It is used in major vaginal operations.

Auxiliary Giving support; helping; aiding; assisting.

Auxillary personnel Non professional aids who assist the responsible professional in the provision of professional services.

Auxins Plant hormones produced in growing buds.

Auxostat A continuous culture system in which a growth-dependent parameter is held constant and all other parameters, including the specific growth rate, vary accordingly.

Auxotrophy The inability of a mutant organism to produce an essential component or growth requirement.

AV bundle Fibers in the heart that relay a nerve impulse from the AV node to the ventricles; also known as the bundle of His.

Availability of medical care The provision of care during the hours and days when people need it.

Avascular not supplied with blood vessels.

Avenin The glutelin protein present in oats.

Aversion therapy The use of classical conditioning procedures to remove unwanted positive emotional responses, such as the desire for alcohol, smoking, and sexual relations with persons of the same sex. For example, an electric shock, nauseous drug, or some other negative stimulus is paired with alcohol on numerous trials, thereby creating an aversive reaction towards the alcohol consumption.

Aversive stimulus A stimulus that includes avoidance and escape response.

Aviation medicine It is the speciality concerned with the physiological effects of flight and its treatment in air. Increasing altitude causes a fall in pressure of oxygen and resulting in hypoxia. Hypoxia and anxiety can lead to hyperventilation. The changes in cabin pressure affect the body's gas containing cavities specially middle ears, facial sinuses, lungs and intestines. During descent of aeroplane if preventive measures are not taken it may cause pain in ears.

Avidin A basic protein in chicken egg white, which binds biotin, rendering it inactive. A diet consisting of large amounts of raw egg white may produce biotin deficiency.

Avirulen Not virulent; unable to cause disease due to resistance of the potential host.

Avirulence A lack of virulence; the inability of a pathogen race or strain to cause disease on a particular strain.

Avitaminosis A disease or condition resulting from a deficiency of one or more vitamins in the diet.

Avogadros' hypothesis At constant temperature and pressure, equal volumes of all ideal gases contain same number of molecules.

Avoidance A cluster of symptoms including behavioral and psychic avoidance such as avoidane of thoughts, feeling and reminders of trauma, emotional numbing and loss of interest in activities.

Avulsed tooth Tooth that has been abnormally luxated from its alveolar support, commonly as a sequele to trauma; also "evulsed".

Avulsion Pulling or tearing of a piece of bone away from the main bone.

Aw Attachment width.

Award The amount of money a court orders a party in a legal proceeding to pay.

Axes Lines, real or imaginary, about which movement take place. There are three basic types of axes at right angles to each other.

Axial Line of plane running parallel to the long axis of an object.

Axial line A line of reference in the hand or foot. In the hand, the axial line extends in line with the third metacarpal and the third digit. In the foot, the axial line extends in line with the second metatarsal and the second digit.

Axial loading of vertebrae Axial compressional loading has been implicated as the loading mechanism of injury for severe vertebral injuries.

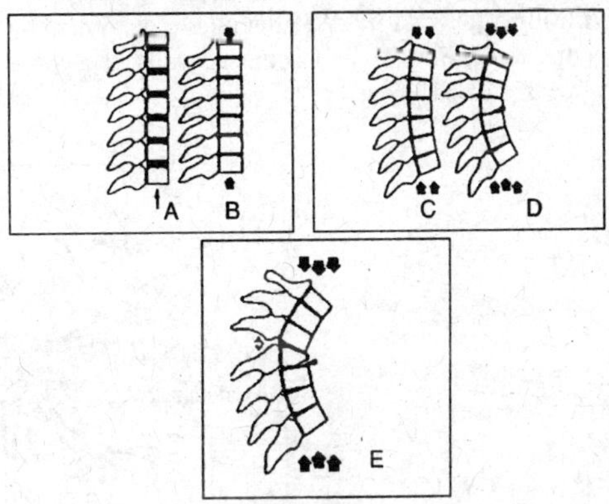

Axial loading

With the head in flexion cervical vertebrae are aligned in a segmental column. Impact causes loading along the longitudinal axis of cervical vertebra leading to compression fracture. Initially the disc absorbs the energy. Later on deformation and buckling occur. It may result in subluxation and disc herniation.

Axial skeleton The bones of the head, neck, and torso.

Axilla The depressed hollow commonly called the armpit.

Axillary tail Wedge of tissue extending from the breast into the axilla.

Axillary thoracotomy An incision into the chest wall in the region of the axilla.

Axillary-femoral bypass A surgical procedure that circumvents flow-limiting occlusions of the infrarenal aorta and iliac arteries by creating a tunnel from the axillary artery, beneath the pectoralis major, into the subcutaneous tissue of the lateral chest wall, passing medial to the anterior superior iliac spine to reach the ipsilateral femoral artery.

Axiobuccogingival pertaining to or formed by the axial, buccal, and gingival walls of a tooth cavity preparation.

Axiobuccolingual Pertaining to the long axis of the buccal and lingual surfaces of a posterior tooth.

Axiogingival Pertaining to or formed by the axial and gingival walls of a tooth cavity preparation. Also called as axiocervical.

Axioincisal Pertaining to or formed by the axial and labial walls of a tooth cavity preparation.

Axiolionguo-occlusal Pertaining to or formed by the axial, lingual, and occlusal walls of a tooth cavity preparation.

Axis Axis are lines, real or imaginary, about which movement takes place.

Axis (prosthetic) Component of the prosthetic knee unit; creates the connection between the thigh piece (socket) and shank; may be either a single axis hinge or polycentric linkage.

Axlla The depressed hollow commonly called the armpit.

Axoaxonic synapse A synapse between two axons.

Axodendritic synapse A synapse between an axon and a muscle.

Axolemma 'Husk' covering the central part or 'axis' of a nerve fiber.

Axon The part of the neuron which carries the nerve impulse away from the cell body and into another nerve fibre or neural structure. The axon of a motor neuron carries the nerve impulse into the muscle fibre—the axon of a sensory neuron carries

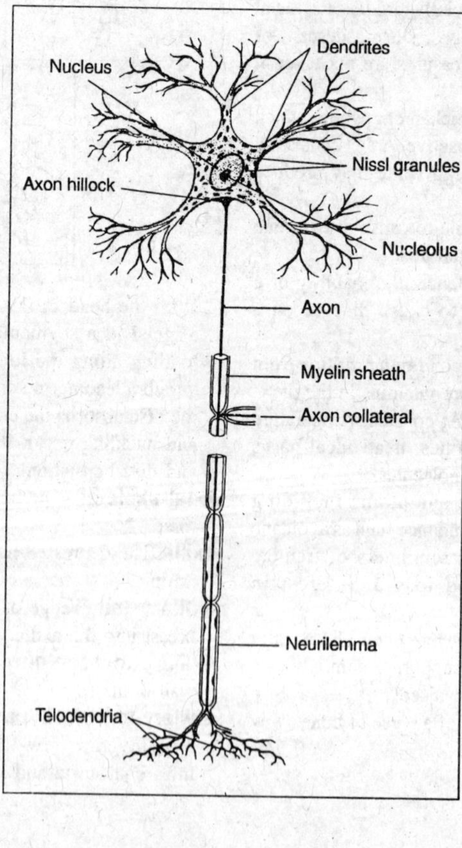

impulses into synaptic connections with the dendrites of a motor or an association neuron.

Axon collateral A branch of an axon.

Axon hillock The part of the axon that is adjacent to the cell body and is the location where the action potential begins.

Axoplasmic flow Flow of neuroplasm along the axon between synapses and toward and away from end organs.

Axosomatic synapse A synapse between an axon and the cell body of a neuron.

Axostyle A tube-shaped sheath of microtubules observed in many flagellates, that usually extends from a basal body to the posterior end.

Axosynaptic synapse A synapse between an axon and another synapse.

Azathioprine (Imuran) An immunosuppressive agent used in organ transplantation; a cytotoxic agent used in the treatment of autoimmune hemolytic anemias, systemic lupus erythematosus, and rheumatoid arthritis.

Azeotrope Mixture of two or more liquids whose components cannot be separated by distillation.

Azoospermia There is an absence of sperms from semen causing infertility in males. Congenital azoospermia may be due to chromosomal abnormality, failure of testes to descend into the scrotum and absence of vas deferens.

In some males pituitary gland produces insufficient amount of hormone to produce sperms. The most common cause of azoospermia is vasectomy. Azoospermia can be produced by temporary or permanent failure to produce sperm. Diagnosis is made by analysing at least two samples of semen collected a month apart.

Blood samples are analysed for FSH levels. If biopsy of testes is normal it means blockage is somewhere else. Injection of FSH may cause puberty to develop. Artificial insemination may help in becoming father.

B

B cells A lymphocyte; activated B cells develop into plasma cells, which secrete antibodies into the blood.

Babbling Sometimes considered the second stage in language acquisition, after unpatterned cooing. Occurring around the fifth month, it is the regular repetition of certain sounds, such as "wa-wa-wa-wa."

Babinski sign In Babinski sign when the lateral aspect of the sole of the foot is stroked with a pointed needle from the heel towards the toes, the plantar reflexes show dorsiflexion of great toe and fanning of other toes. It indicates lesion in the corticospinal tract, but may also be present in normal infants. This sign is seen in spinal paralytic poliomyelitis, Friedreich's ataxia, parkinsonism, cerebral haemorrhage, and bacterial meningitis.

Babinski-Nageotte syndrome There will be contralateral hemiparesis and disturbance of sensibility. Person will have ipsilateral cerebellar hemiataxia. Eye symptoms include enophthalmos, ptosis and miosis.

Baby massage oil The importance of tradiational baby massage for its caring and soothing effects and its role in tactile communication is well established. Massage tones up and relaxes the soft tissues and improves the baby's coordinated physical skills and activities. Baby Olemessa massage oil contains vitamin E. It contains no synthetics and perfumes. Olemessa baby soap contains olive oil besides rose extract and glycerine. It contains mild antibiotic chamamile. Olemessa bath oil is also available.

Baby blues An information term for a self-limited episode of unexplained sadness experienced by as many as 60% of women in the postpartum period, usually beginning three days to a week after delivery.

Bach flower remedies In 1930 Edward Bach a prominent homeopath and bacteriologist, developed 38 flower remedies to treat various emotional problems. Flower extracts are taken by mouth and a few drops are placed under tongue four times a day. Bach remedies are included in homeopathic pharmacopoea. Infusion of flower in water is known as 'mother stock' which is diluted by brandy and is ready for use.

Bachmann's bundle The portion of the specialized conduction system of the heart that is a continuation of the right arterial anterior internodal tract into the left atrium.

Bacillus Calmette-Guerin(BCG) vaccine A live bacterial antigen vaccine that gives partial immunity against Mycobacterium tugerculosis infection.

Bacitracin It is an antibacterial drug used for skin and eye infections. It is generally mixed with neomycin and polymyxin B. It is usually applied to the skin as a powder or ointment to the skin and ointment to the eye. It is not absorbed orally hence is given in injection form. Prolonged use can cause damage to the kidney. It is a polypeptide antibiotic that is bactericidal for many gram-positive species. Except *Neisseria* it has little effect on gram-negative organisms. Resistance to drug rarely develops. It resembles penicillin in its mode of action.

Back bone Vertebral or spinal column.

Back The posterior part of the body; the dorsum.

Back fire fracture A fracture of radial styloid.

Back ground radiation The sum total of radioactivity measured in given area.

Back knee It is a hypertension of knee.

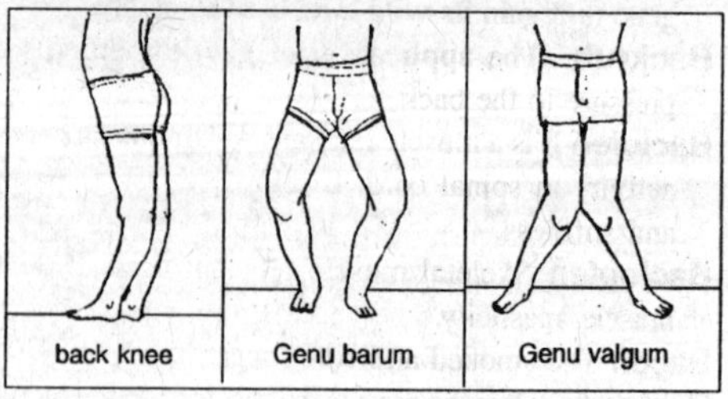

Back labour It occurs in 20-25% cases of delivery. Position of fetus is such that the back of head is directed to the mother's back or turned toward her sacrum. It is most uncomfortable to mother.

Back of infant Infant's back should be slightly flexed, freely movable and free of defects. Infants should kick both legs.

Back pain People most likely to suffer back pain are those whose job involves much heavy lifting and carrying or those who spends long periods

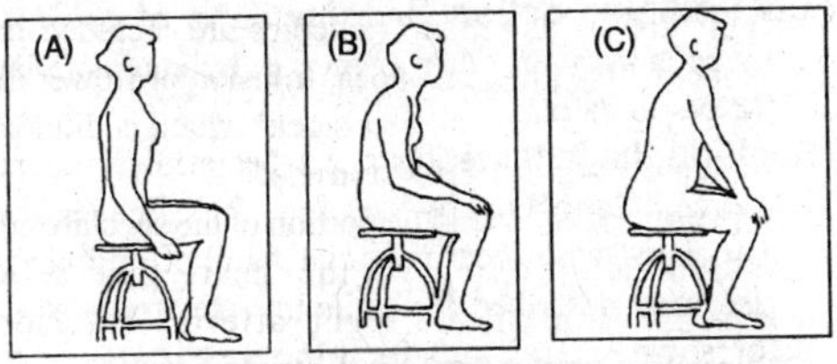

(A) Correct sitting posture (B), and (C) Incorrect posture

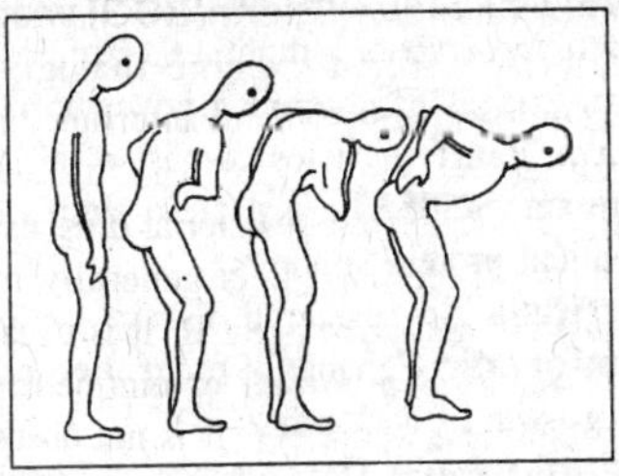

sitting in one position or bending awkwardly. Obesity, slipped disc may result in back pain. Osteoarthritis can cause persistent back pain, ankylosing spondylitis, stiffness and loss of back mobility. Fibrositis results in pain and tenderness in muscles of back pain. Rest and sleep on a firm mattress with non-steroidal anti-inflammatory drugs (NSAIDs) relieve pain. In severe cases surgery may be required.

Back seam In shoe terminology a posterior seam joining the quarters of uppers.

Back-mutation A mutation that causes a mutant gene to regain its wild-type base sequence.

Backrub The application of gentle methodical pressure to the back.

Baclofen It is a muscle relaxant which blocks nerve activity in spinal cord. It relieves muscle spasm and stiffness.

Baclopfen Skeletal muscle relaxant used to treat muscle spasticity.

Bacon The smoked and cured meat from pig.

Bacteremia It is the presence of bacteria in the blood stream and may result after tonsillitis or minor operation. Bacteraemia may lead to septicaemia.

Bacteria It may cause disease. Abundant in air, soil and water contains most bacteria which are harmless to humans. Some cause disease and are known as pathogens. These are classified on the basis of shape, cocci (spherical) bacilli (rod shaped) and spirilla (spiral shaped). Cocci cause pneumonia, tonsillitis, meningitis and skin infections. Bacilli produce leprosy, tuberculosis, dysentery, typhoid and whooping cough. Spirilla causes yaws, syphilis and leptospirosis. Bacteria reproduce by dividing into two cells which in turn divide and so on. This division can take place every 20 minutes. It produces poisons which are harmful to human body. Main form of treatment is antibiotic. Diphtheria, tetanus and botulism are treated by injection of antiserum. These are the smallest, unicellular, free living organisms which do not contain chlorophyll. These do not show branching except higher bacteria such as actinomycetales. There are about 1600 species. Bacterial size is measured and expressed in micrometre. These measure 0.5 to 1.2 micromillimetre in diameter. These have four types, coccal or spherical, bacillary or cylindrical, the vibrio and spirillar form or spirochetes.

Bacterial Relating to, caused by, or involving bacteria.

Bacterial artificial chromosomes (BACs) Vectors based on plasmid F origin of replication. Such vectors, which can carry 24 to 100 kbp, are stable in E. coli.

Bacterial capsule Capsular substance is usually antigenic which plays an important role in determining immunological specificity of bacteria. Most of the substances forming bacterial capsule are polysaccharide such as pneumococci. Capsular substance is antigenic. Capsulated bacteria more or less form mucoid colonies.

Bacterial mastitis It commences acutely. It is associated with lactation. Affected breast will show signs of inflammation, later on abscess will form. Appropriate antibiotics should be used and infected breast should be emptied by breast pump.

Bacterial meningitis It presents with fever, general malaise, headache and vomiting. Patient remains drowsy and confused. If not treated person may undergo stupor and unconsciousness. There will be signs of meningeal irritation, i.e. stiff neck and unconsciousness. Patient with meningeal fever may have a petechial rash first visible on conjunctivae but later becoming widespread over trunk and limbs. There may be profound hypotension and child may develop seizures. Papilloedema may be present due to diffuse cerebritis and generalised cerebral oedema.

Bacterial resistance Ability of bacteria to servive in the presence of antibacterial drugs.

Bacterial sialadenitis The term sialadenitis means inflammation of salivary glands. Bacterial sialadenitis occurs in children or the aged and produces recurrent, acute, painful enlargement of the involved gland. The overlying skin may be red and milking or compressing the gland will give a purulent discharge at the duct orifice. Pain and swelling are not related to eating. *Streptococcus viridans* causes lesion in children while *Staphylococcus aureus* in geriatric patients. Treatment includes heat application, pain relieving drugs and antibiotics. Microscopic section shows oedema and infiltration of the ducts and lobules by polymorphonuclear leucocytes.

Bacterial spore A resistant form of bacteria encapsulated by a thick cell wall that enables the cell to survive in environment unfavorable to immediate growth and division; not a reproductive mechanism.

Bacterial translocation Passage of bacteria across the bowel wall via lymphatics into hepatic portal circulation and then to systemic circulation.

Bactericidal Capable of killing bacteria.

Bacteriemia Presence of bacteria in blood.

Bacteriochlorophyll Forms of chlorophyll present in photosynethetic bacteria.

Bacteriocyte An insect cell harboring symbiotic microorganisms.

Bacteriology It is the study of bacteria that causes disease. Louis Pasteur started it followed by Robert Koch. To identify bacteria it must be isolated. A throat swab, specimen of urine, faeces, blood sputum or pus is taken from an infected person and examined by one of these methods : Staining makes it possible to look and differentiate bacteria under microscope—Generally Gram's staining is used; To culture sample material is used into a nutrient where bacteria multiply, then different antibiotics are introduced and their effect is studied; antibody testing is done by extracting serum from the blood of an infected person and sample of suspected bacteria is added. If doubt is correct there will occur clump formation.

Bacteriolytic Pertaining to or causing destruction of bacteria.

Bacteriolytic action Breaking down of bacteria by an enzyme or other agent e.g. by antibacterial factors in saliva.

Bacteriophage Bacteriophage as becteriolytic agent was first discovered by Twod in 1915. Phages are associated with most bacterial families and have also been described for actinomycetes for yeasts, for spirochaetes and for blue green algae. A coliphage for instance will not lyse a *Staphylococcus* or a diphtheria bacillus. However some phages have a much wider host range than others. Phage particles consist of a nucleic acid core surrounded by a protein shell made up of identical protein subunits.

Bacteriosis Any bacterial disease.

Bacteriostatic Capable of preventing or inhibiting the growth of bacteria.

Bacteriotoxemia The presence of bacterial toxins in the blood.

Bacteriotoxic Toxic to bacteria.

Bacterium A prokaryotic microorganism which is typically unicellular.

Bacteriuria Bacteria in the urine.

Bacteroides A genus of anaerobic non spore forming gram negative rods. They are found in oropharynx.

Bactofugation Belgian process for removing bacteria from milk by high speed centrifuging.

Bag bath Technique for bathing that involves the use of 8 to 10 premoistened, warmed, disposable cloths contained in a plastic bag.

Bag of bones Descriptive term applied to severely comminuted and displaced intercondylar fractures of distal humerus.

Bag of waters When cervix opens the lower pole of fetal membranes these tend to bulge into cervical canal. It contains a little liquor amnii which passes below the presenting part and known as bag of waters. When the finger is passed into cervix during path this bag will be found to be convex.

Bagging A resuscitative procedure in which oxygen is administered by bag and mask ventilation at a rate of 40 to 60 breaths per minutes to deliver oxygen into the newborn's bronchi.

Bainbridge's reflex An atrial stretch reflex that causes changes in heart rate; it is elicited when the right atrial pressure rises sufficiently to distend the right atrium.

Bait Plant and animal materials placed in a hunting area in such a manner as to draw the target animal to the hunter.

Baker's cyst Cystic swelling behind the knee in the popliteal fossa.

Baker's yeast A micro organism, one of the fungi. Baker's yeast has replaced brewer's yeast in baking.

Baking powder Mixture that liberates carbon dioxide when moistened or heated.

Balance The stability produced on each side of a vertical axis. The center of gravity is maintained over the base of support.

Balance theory A theory of attitude formation and change which stresses the tendency to seek equilibrium in our attitudes, in which all important elements are harmonious.

Balanced anesthesia Combinations of drug and technique to provide adequate analgesia, anesthesia and muscle relaxants.

Balanced traction A type of traction produced by balancing the extremity in a traction apparatus against counter force other than patients body weight.

Balanitis It is the inflammation of glans penis. It gives rise to painful or itchy penis. Entire area may be red or moist. Uncircumscised man is more prone. Washing, caring and one course of antibiotic will help.

Balanoposthitis It is an inflammatory condition of glans penis. The condition presents with soreness and irritation. Glans penis appears red with painful erosions. Retraction of foreskin may reveal accumulation of thick, yellow, subpreputial discharge with offensive smell. Inguinal lymph glands may be enlarged and painful. In severe cases there may be severe tissue damage and deformity. Inflammation of the prepuce is known as posthitis, inflammation of glans is balanitis. Lichen planus and psoriasis affect the penis. Drug hypersensitivity can affect the skin of penis. In mild case symptom is only itching and more discharge. In severe cases glans and foreskin are red, raw and pus exudes. Monilial infection may be present.

Balans chair It was designed with the 'wedge' concept in mind. Person requiring a loss of lumbar

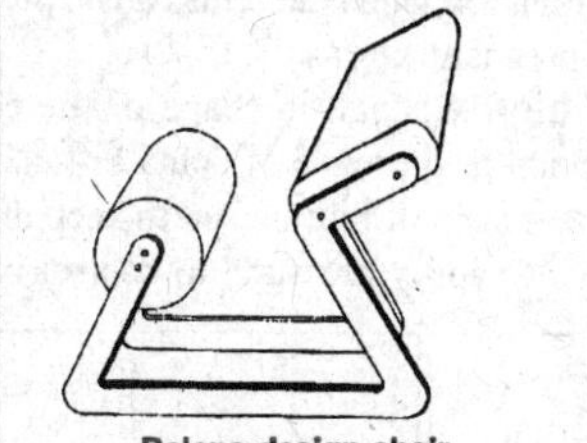

Balans design chair

lordosis may need to add a wedge to this chair. It blocks the pelvis into an anterior tilt. These allow only one sitting pattern.

Baldwin aeroplane splint A shoulder abduction orthosis.

Balint's syndrome It is a bilateral lesion of parietooccipital region. Affected patients are unaware of objects otherwise familiar to them. There will be tonic and motor phenomenon of upper limbs and loss of body coordination and optic ataxia.

Balke's exercise protocol A graded treadmill exercise test protocol consisting of stages of variable duration with incremental speed and grade change at each stage.

Ball and socket joint The articular surfaces are reciprocal segments of a hypothetical sphere i.e., hip and shoulder joint.

Ballism With reference to the flailing movements that follow damage to the subthalamic nucleus.

Ballismus and hemiballismus There is wide ranging throwing, lightening-like movements appearing in several limb segments. Patient may suffer collision, trauma and muscle tears. The rare hereditary degenerative ballismus is bilateral.

Ballistocardiography Detection of body motion resulting from movement of blood within the body.

Balloon catheter It is a type of catheter with one or more balloons which when inflated keep the catheter in place or apply pressure on vessel and organ. Simplest type is Foley's catheter used to drain the bladder. Catheter is passed into the bladder and water is pushed while urine flows out of bladder from second outlet. Another type of balloon catheter is used to expand narrow arteries. This technique is known as angioplasty.

Ballottable Capable of exhibiting ballottement.

Ballottement Literally means tossing. A term used in examination when the fetus can be pushed about in the pregnant uterus.

Banana sign Change in shape of the cerebellum that occurs in presence of spina bifida.

Bandage A strip of fabric used to keep dressings in position, to apply pressure, to control bleeding or

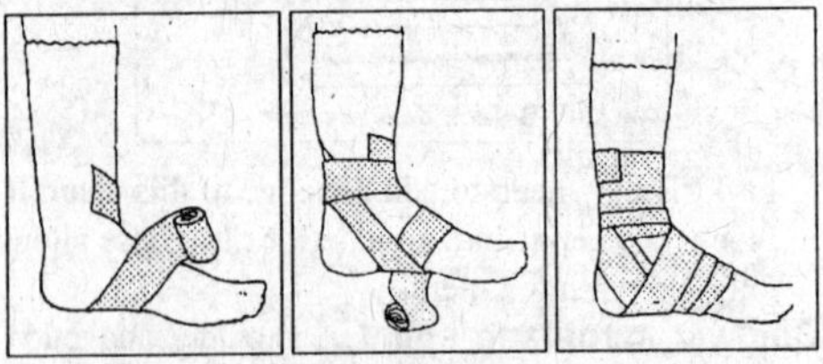

Bandaging of ankle

to support a sprain. Roller bandages are commonly used. While triangular bandages are made for slings.

Bandl's ring A groove on the uterus at the upper level of the fully developed lower uterine segment; visible on the abdomen after hard labour as a transverse or slightly slanting depression between the umbilicus and the pubis. Shows overstretching of lower uterine segment. Resembles a full bladder.

Band-shaped keratopathy It is a degenerative condition of cornea associated with varied ocular conditions such as chronic glaucoma, chronic uveitis, keratitis, phthisis bulbi and hypercalcaemia. It manifests in interpalpebral area. The opacification begins just below and inside of limbus. There is deposition of calcium salts in the subepithelial space and Bowman's membrane and superficial stroma. The overlying epithelium is intact. It is irregular. The opacity is grey or white and is dotted with small round dots. Keratoplasty is effective in providing good vision.

Bang's disease The disease is transmitted to man from animals or animal products containing bacteria of genus *Brucella.* Infection results from ingestion of infected animal tissue, milk products or through skin wounds. Person will develop fever, icterus, weakness, sweats and general malaise. Ocular symptoms include conjunctivitis, optic neuritis, papilloedema, vitreous opacities and raised intraocular pressure.

Bankart lesion A traumatic detachement of fibrocartilaginous labrum from anterior rim of glenoid.

Bar Metal segment of greater length than width that serves to connect two or more parts of a removable partial denture.

Barbiturate poisoning These are used as sedatives and anticonvulsants. Sodium salts of barbiturates are more rapidly absorbed from the gut as compared to free acids. Potentially fatal dose of phenobarbital is 6 to 10 gm, as in 2 to 3 gm of amobarbital or petobarbital short-acting barbiturates, particularly those with short half-lives are more toxic than long-acting compounds such as phenobarbital and barbital. It produces depression of CNS producing stupor and coma and depression of cardiovascular system producing bradycardia and hypotension. Pupils are initially constricted and react to light but in course of barbiturate poisoning pupillary dilation occurs due to hypoxia. Respiratory depression is an early feature. Early deaths are due to cardiorespiratory arrest.

Barbiturates These depress activity of brain. These are habbit forming. Overdose can be fatal. Phenobarbital is still used in treatment of epilepsy and thiopental remains a drug of choice for anaesthesia. Barbiturates reduce the sensitivity of brain cells to abnormal electrical activity as seen in epilepsy. Adverse effects include drowsiness, staggering gait and excitability in a few cases.

Barefoot doctor It is a popular term for a minimally equipped, indigenous rural medical worker in a poor country. These are trained to give first aid treatment in minor injuries and handling common day today diseases.

Barefoot impression The impression left by the planter area of the bare foot. This would include the contour and placement of the toe pads, the contour of the ridge that separates the ball of the foot from the toe pads, the contour and width of the arch and heel, and the overall length of the foot.

Bargaining Psychological mechanism for delaying the inevitable.

Barium enema This is given for diagnostic purpose of lower large gut and X-ray is taken after giving barium solution. The amount of barium depends on the area to be visualised. In certain colonic conditions it is used as activation of colon. Substance known as varipaque on phial in 2000 cc of water is given. It is a radiographic examination of colon using barium sulphate suspension as contrast medium. General contraindications for all barium enema studies are peritonitis, free intraperitoneal air, allergy to barium suspension and risk or perforation.

Barium meal A meal containing barium sulphate.

Barlow splint Immobilization used in the treatment of congenital hip dislocation. Lower end of splint is molded around thighs.

Barodontalgia The sudden acute pain response in a tooth under reduced atmospheric pressure, notably during high-altitude flying.

Barophile Literally, pressure lover; an organism that lives optimally at a pressure greater than atmospheric pressure; e.g., certain deep-sea bacteria. Thus, barophilic.

Baroreceptor Sensory nerve endings in the walls of the atria of the heart, aortic arch, and carotid sinuses; sensitive to stretching of the wall caused by increased blood pressure; also called a pressoreceptor.

Baroreceptor reflex Process in which baroreceptors detect changes in blood pressures and produce changes in heart rate, force of heart contraction, and blood vessel diameter that return blood pressure toward normal levels.

Baroreceptors Stretch receptors in the walls of blood vessels and heart.

Barosymapathetic reflex Reflex reduction of sympathetic tone in response to a rise of arterial blood pressure.

Barotrauma There develop acute hearing impairment, unilateral or bilateral with vertigo and otalgia. There may be tinnitus and middle ear effusion.

Barovagal reflex Reflex reduction of heart rate in response to a rise of arterial blood pressure.

Barr body The persistent mass of the material of the inactivated X chromosome in cells of normal females. Also called sex chromosome.

Barr's Triad Decrease in height of inter-vertebral space, lumbar scoliosis and absence of lumbar lordosis.

Barre Lieous syndrome resulting from europathogenic reflexes caused by pathomechanics of the cervical spine.

Barrel Part of a syringe that holds the medication.

Barrett's syndrome The syndrome is characterised by columnar transposition of squamous epithelium of lower oesophagus or formation of peptic ulceration due to chronic reflux oesophagitis. There is an association of hiatus hernia. Ulcer progresses to strictures. There is strong predisposition of malignancy. Person develops heart burn due to gastrooesophageal reflux, epigastric discomfort and pain during swallowing.

Barrier An obstacle which impedes achievement of a goal. It may be internal, within the individual, or external, imposed by the environment, which includes other individuals.

Barrier membrane A device used to help confine a grafted area, help prevent overexpression and movement of the grafting material, and control the growth of undesirable tissue into the healing site.

Bartholin's glands Glands situated one on each side of the vaginal canal opening into the groove between the hymen and the labia minora.

Barto'n fracture This is due to a fall on the outstretched hand. The intra-articular oblique fracture involves the dorsal margin of distal radius. There may be dislocation of wrist joint.

Barton's forceps It is applied for delivery of head of occipito transverse position as this forceps can be applied more easily. It consist of hinged anterior blade and a posterior blade with exaggerated cephalic curve.

Barton's Tongs A metallic clamp that attaches to the parietal bone of skull used in injuries of neck.

Bartter syndrome It develops due to excessive chloride, potassium and sodium wasting in thick ascending limb of loop of Henle.

Clinical features include failure to thrive, polyuria, polydypsia and recurrent source of dehydration. Treatment with potassium chloride supplement is necessary.

Basal body temperature (BBT) The resting temperature taken in the morning before arising or performing any activity. Characteristic changes in BBT that usually occur in fertile women are used to identify the time ovulation has occurred.

Basal cell carcinoma Generally it develops on face and neck. Basal cell carcinoma is the most common skin cancer. Direct skin damage from ultraviolet radiation is the cause. It starts as a small, flat nodule and grows slowly breaking down at the centre forming an ulcer. It never metastasise. Treatment includes surgical removal followed by radiation therapy.

Basal cell epithelioma It is slow growing, gradually assuming a nodular shape and often covered by a small, recurring crusts of blood. The lesion matures in months or years to a firm, painless nodule of a waxy colour with telangiectasia, often with central umbilication and a pearly border. These tumours do not tend to metastasise and transformation to squamous cell carcinoma is rare.

Basal cell naevus syndrome It is also known as Goltz syndrome. The syndrome is autosomal inherited dominant type. It consists of a widespread skeletal and dental anomalies and jaw lesions. Clinical features include temporoparietal bossing, prominent supraorbital ridge, broad nasal root, mental retardation and nerve deafness.

Basal cells Undifferentiated cells in parts of the airways lined by pseudostratified epithelium; basal cells mature to replace other epithelial types.

Basal chordae Chordae tendlneae that arise directly from the ventricular wall to attach to the basal regions of the leaflets of the valves of the heart.

Basal Energy expenditure Energy requirements for patients suffering from diesese or injury are increased and are often expressed as a percentage above the estimated basal energy expenditure. BEE is an important part of energy requirement for any non active person.

Basal ganglia Nuclei at the base of the cerebrum, diencephalon, and midbrain involved in controlling motor normal functions.

Basal nucleus A mass of nerve cell bodies located deep within a cerebral hemisphere of the brain; also called basal ganglion.

Base Any substance that is a proton acceptor; or any substance that binds to hydrogen ions; lower part or bottom of a structure; the base of the heart is the flat portion directed posteriorly and superiorly; veins and arteries project into and out of the base, respectively.

A chemical substance that in solution yields hydroxyl ions and reacts with an acid to form a salt and water. A base turns red litmus paper blue and has a pH higher than 7.0.

Base ball elbow Arthritic changes in base ball pitchers. Changes include olecranon and distal humeral hypertrophy, joint space narrowing, loose bodies and calcification at the flexor muscle origin.

Base excess (BE) A measure of the metabolic acid-base status; if a positive value, a measure of metabolic alkalosis; if a negative value a measure of metabolic acidosis; the amount of acid or alkali that would have to be added per unit volume of whole blood at 37°C and at a PCO_2 of 40 mm Hg to achieve a pH of 7.40.

Base metal A non-noble metal, such as steel or nickel - chromium alloy, used to make dental instruments and restorations.

Base of support Area on which an object rests.

Base of the heart That portion of the heart bounded by the bifurcation of the pulmonary trunk superiorly, the coronary sulcus inferiorly, the sulcus terminalis on the right, and the oblique vein of the left atrium on the left.

Base resistance The ability of a microbial strain to exist for an extended period at pH values too alkaline for growth, retaining the ability to be cultured after alkali is neutralized.

Base, Intramucosal Insert The portion of the intramucosal insert that seats within the acrylic receptor site on the denture's mucosal surface.

Baseball finger An avulsion of the common extensor tendon with a fragment of a bone from its insertion at the base of distal phalanx of finger. It is caused by baseball striking the finger tip.

Basedow's syndrome There is diffuse goitre, inherited as a simple autosomal recessive disorder. There will be tachycardia, anxiety, insomnia, loss of weight, hyperhidrosis, myocarditis and atrial fibrillation. Eye symptoms include exophthalmos, swelling of eyelids, papilloedema and increased intraocular pressure.

Baseline data Information that describes the status of the client before treatment.

Baseline film X-Ray taken prior to treatment for comparison purpose.

Basement membrane The structure that attaches most epithelia (exceptions include lymph vessels and the liver sinusoids) to underlying tissue; consists of carbohydrates and proteins secreted by the epithelia and the underlying connective tissue.

Baseplate A temporary from representing the base of a denture and used for making maxillo-mandibular relation records, arranging artificial teeth.

Bases These are applied in thicker layers protection to the pulp. Bases must be strong enough to support a restorative material during its placement.

Basiar membrane A membrane in the cochlea of the internal ear that separates the cochlear duct from the scale tympani and on which the spiral organ (organ of Corti) rests.

Basic cardiac life support (BCLS) The emergency procedures of establishing an airway, providing breathing, and performing cardiac compressions as needed; cardiopulmonary resuscitation (CPR).

Basic care facility Agency that provides extended custodial care.

Basic dye A dye consisting of a cations as the actively staining material.

Basic research Scientific studies aimed at the acquisition of further knowledge. There is no practical purpose, the goal is to obtain and disseminate information, regardless of its potential value. Compare with applied psychology.

Basic rest-activity cycle (BRAC) A cycle in humans that has a period of about 90 minutes in which the level of arousal waxes and wanes.

Basic solution Solution with less hydrogen ions than hydroxide ions; has a pH greater than 7.

Basidium An enlarged club-like cell that bears basidiospores usuallly four in number formed after nuclear fusion and meiosis.

Basifacial Pertaining to the lower part of face.

Basihyal Body of hyoid bone.

Basilar membrane In the cochlea, the receptor surface that transduces sound waves not neural activity.

Basinasial Pertaining to the basion and the nasion.

Basipetal Descending or developing in the direction of the base.

Basitemporal Pertaining to the lower part of the temporal bone.

Basket ball foot It is a medial subtalar dislocation caused due to fall on a basket ball court.

Basket forceps Surgical instrument used in arthroscopic surgery. These may be straight or angled.

Basophil A white blood cell (leucocyte) that stains with basic dyes; characterised by coarse granules in the cytoplasm. Also a type of cell found in the anterior pituitary.

Bass technique Toothbrushing technique used in periodontal disease the bristles are positioned in the sulcus, in contact with the gingiva and tooth simultaneously, and with gentle vibration the brush is moved in short back and forth strokes. The brush is advanced around the mouth, on the cheek and tongue surfaces, until all areas have been thoroughly brushed.

Bassen-Kornzweig syndrome A congenital disorder characterised by steatorrhoea, malabsorption of fat, acanthocytosis, retinitis pigmentosa, ataxia, mental retardation, and often retarded growth.

Bastede's sign This sign is considered to be positive when the colon is inflated with air through a rectal tube. Pain and tenderness occur in the right iliac fossa, and is seen in cases of appendicitis.

Batcheolar plasters Casts applied to hold the hips in abduction and medial rotation.

Bateman prosthesis It is a bipolar femoral head prosthesis.

Batozon's plexus Valveless extradural venous plexus composed of anterior and posterior longitudinal veins communicating at each vertebral level.

Batson's plexus A complex network of nonvalvular veins in and around the vertebral column.

Battered baby syndrome It is a form of child abuse by frustrated parents. Signs on children are bruises, cigarette burns, bites and malformed fractures. Whole family needs treatment.

Battery An unconsented, harmful, or offensive touching.

Battle dore placenta When the cord iserts at the placental margin rather than at centre.

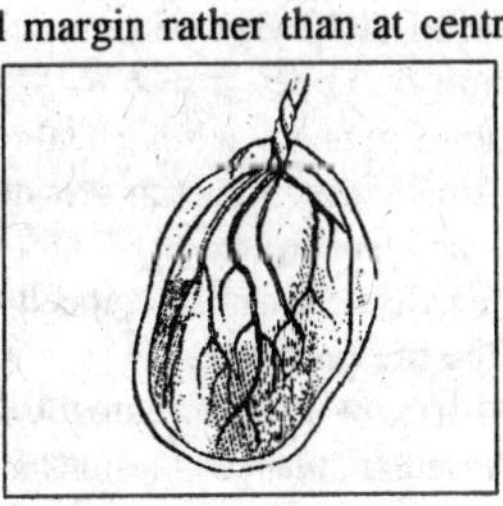

Battle's sign Clinical sign indicating basilar skull fracture.

Battledore placenta When the cord is inserted at the margin of placenta instead of centrally. This has no clinical significance.

Baues' theorem Answers the two important questions that remain unanswered by sensitivity and specificity: (1) If the test results are positive, what is the probability that the patient has the disease? (2) If the test results are negative, what is the probability that the patient does not have the disease?

Bayonetted Descriptive term used for fracture fragments that are opposed and overlapped.

Bazzana's syndrome It is a rare disorder. There is progressive deafness caused by otosclerosis. Visual fields are contracted concentrically and retinal vessels will be tortuous.

BBT Chart Special thermometer for recording BBT marked in tenths to enable patient to read more easily is used.

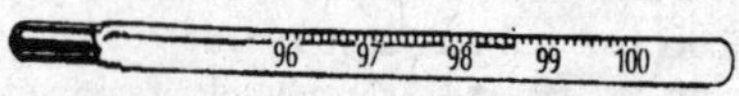

Special thermometer for recording BBT

B-cell A specialized lymphocyte that produces humoral, or circulatory, antibodies.

BCG vaccination Bacille Calmette-Guerin is a vaccine giving immunity against tuberculosis. It is prepared from weakened strain of bovine

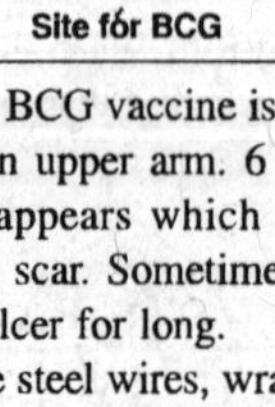

Site for BCG

tubercle bacilli. BCG vaccine is usually given to a child at birth on upper arm. 6 to 12 weeks later small pustule appears which heals completely leaving a small scar. Sometimes it does not heal and leaves an ulcer for long.

Bead High tensile steel wires, wrapped with rubber, that hold the tire on the rim.

Bean's syndrome It is an autosomal dominant disorder. Vascular cutaneous lesions may be found anywhere on the body. There may develop profuse sweating and visceral lesions are common. There may be subconjunctival haemangioma with overlying fibrosis and AV malformations.

Beans Seeds of wide variety of leguminous plants.

Bearing down Reflex effort by the mother to help with the uterine contraction.

Beating Beating is a single or tow handed stroke in which the loosely clenched fist strike the part so that the dorsal aspect of the middle and distal phalanges of the fingers and the heel of the hand makes contact with the tissues.

Beau's lines Transverse furrows that occur on the finger nails and toe nails following wasting disease.

Beaver's knife Brand name for thin, disposable, flexible knife used in meniscal surgery.

Bechterew's test It is a method to detect sciatica. If sciatica is present, patient sitting will be able to straighten each knee by turn but not both at a time.

Beck Depression Inventory (BDI): A brief questionnaire used to measure the severity of depression; developed by Aaron Beck.

Becker muscular dystrophy This is a milder variant of Duchenne dystrophy. Onset of weakness is at about the age of 10 and patients are able to walk till mid twenties. It shows low amount of dystrophin or of low molecular weight.

Beclomethasone It is a corti-costeroid drug prescribed as a nasal spray to relieve allergic rhinitis. It helps in reducing inflammation and mucous production. In asthma it reduces wheezing and coughing. It reduces frequency of attacks of asthma too. It is given when bronchodilators alone are not helpful. It takes several hours to have its effect. Side effects include hoarseness and throat irritation.

Bed bath Washing with a basin of water at the bedside.

Bed board Rigid structure placed under a mattress.

Bed count The number of beds regularly maintained by a hospital.

Bed rest Prescribed or self imposed restriction to bed for therapeutic benefit.

Bed side X-Ray X-Ray examination conducted while patient remains in bed.

Bed sores These are known as pressure sores also. These develop in bed-ridden patients mostly unconscious and immobile specially in cases of spinal cord injuries who are having loss of sensation. Constantly wet skin due to incontinence of urine may also cause it. These start as red, painful areas that become purple before the skin gives way. Once broken they enlarge, deepens and are very slow to heal. Antibiotics, keeping the part dry, changing the position off and on helps the sufferer.

Bedpan Seat-like container for elimination.

BEE Abbreviation for basal energy expenditure.

Beeswax A low melting wax that is an ingreident of many dental waxes.

Beet sugar Sucrose extracted from sugar beet.

Beeturia Production of red pigmented urine after eating beet root.

Beevor's sign When lower part of the rectus abdominis muscles are paralysed the umbilicus moves upward on raising the hand. This sign is seen in the nerve lesions between 8th and 11th thoracic segments.

Behavior modification The use of one or more number of techniques based on learning theory to effect specific changes in behaviour.

Behavior specialists A member of a multidisciplinary cardiac or pulmonary rehabilitation team; a mental health professional.

Behavioral analysis The detailed analysis of behaviour which is considered essential before treatement is taken.

Behaviour In its broadest sense, anything an organism does; any response made by an organism. Some psychologists prefer to limit usage of this term to responses that can be observed or measured.

Behaviour therapy A mode of treatment that focuses on modifying observable and, at least in principle, quantifiable behaviour by means of systematic manipulation of the environment and behavioural variables thought to be functionally related to the behaviour. Some behaviour therapy techniques are operant conditioning, shaping, token economy, systematic desensitisation, aversion therapy, and flooding.

Behavioural information In the structure-of-intellect model of intelligence, a content dimension which concerns knowledge about the significance of human actions. This information is sometimes called "body language". People who use behavioural information are allegedly adept at understanding the feelings and thoughts behind overt actions.

Behaviourism An approach to psychology first developed by John B. Watson which rejected the notion of mental states and reduced all psychologic phenomena to neural, muscular, and glandular responses. Contemporary behaviourism emphasises the study of observable responses but is directed toward general behaviour rather than discrete acts. It includes private events such as feelings and fantasies to the extent that these can be directly observed and measured.

Behcet's syndrome There develops recurrent genital and oral ulceration associated with iritis. Retinal vessels and cerebral vessels develop vasculitis. Cerebral venous circulation is occluded by inflammatory process. Syndrome includes episodes of sudden dysfunction of cerebral hemispheres. Course of disorder is similar to multiple sclerosis.

Beikost Supplemental or weaning foods.

Belching It is a noisy return of air from the stomach through mouth. It may be due to swallowing air, eating and drinking too much and too quickly. Each act of belching further swallows air. In dyspepsia belching may give relief.

Beliefs Concepts that a person holds to be true.

Bell stage Third stage of formation of the enamel organ.

Bell stethoscope Stethoscope is of 2 types : one is diaphragm type used better to listen lung sounds, another is bell type. Bell type is used better to listen heart sounds.

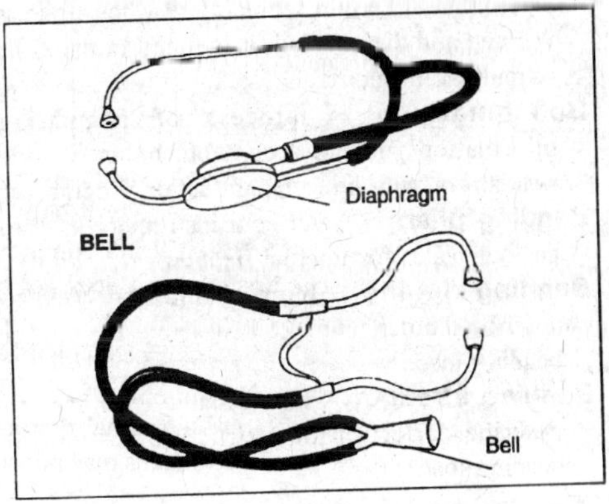

Bell's law The law describing nerve function. Anterior roots of spinal nerves are motor and posterior roots are sensory nerves.

Bell's muscle Lateral edges of the trigonal muscle of the urinary bladder.

Bell's palsy It results due to the paralysis of muscles supplied by the seventh cranial nerve. The cause may be unknown or there may be malignant tumour of parotid or may be after surgery of parotid. Some cases may be due to herpes simplex type I virus. Paralysis is always unilateral On the affected side eyes cannot be closed, the mouth droops and saliva escapes from the corner of mouth. Due to paralysis of facial muscles person becomes expressionless and has difficulty in mastication and speech.

Bell's phenomenon Bell's phenomenon represents that in case of peripheral facial paralysis any attempt of closure of the eyelid of the affected side requires outward and upward movement of the eyeball.

Belly The abdomen. The gaster or prominent, fleshy part of a skeletal muscle.

Belly of muscle The prominent, fleshy, central portion of muscle.

Belts Rubber layers, filled with cord or steel, located beneath the tread surface. They provide the tire an additional stability. Rubber layers, filled with cord or steel, located beneath the tread surface. They provide the tire an additional stability.

Bemyelination Destruction or removal of the myelin shealth of nerve tissue by a disease process.

Bence Jones protein Bence Jones protein, if present in the urine, can only be found as precipitate at certain temperature when urine is warmed and then cooled. It is found in the urine of multiple myeloma.

Benchmarking A process of comparing information with an acceptable industry-wide standard or with other rehabilitation programs.

Bending pliers A hand held instrument used to contour plates for internal fixation.

Bending rigidity A biomechanic term used to describe the deflection of a structure per unit of bending load.

Bending strength A biomechanic term used to describe deflection of a structure per unit of bending load.

Benedikt's syndrome There is lesion of inferior nucleus rubber with obstruction of third nerve. Arteriosclerotic occlusion of branches of basilar artery, trauma, haemorrhage in mid brain and neoplasms are the most common cause. There will be contralateral hemiparesis, coarse tremor of upper extremity, absent deep sensibility and ipsilateral ataxia.

Beneficence The moral principle that people should act to promote the welfare of others.

Benign Mild in character or nonmalignant; does not spread to distant sites. Not malignant; not recurrent; favourable for recovery.

Benign cementoblastoma It is rare and reaches a much larger size than cementoma and may lead to jaw expansion. It is attached to the root of an erupted permanent tooth and is seen in mandibular molar region. Patients are young and it appears as a radiopacity with a peripheral radiolucent border on X-ray.

Benign essential tremor a tremulous disorder commonly.

Benign essential tremor A tremulous disorder commonly attributed to parkinson's disease.

Benign hyperkeratosis It is the most common white lesion of oral cavity and constitute about 70% cases of all white lesions. It is more common in males. Mandibular mucosa, cheek, lip, palate are commonly involved. Lesion may be elevated or flat. Habitual cheek biting may result in it. On microscope it is characterised by a thickened layer of keratin. There may be thickening of epithelial ridges and stratum malpighii. If the cause is removed it disappears spontaneously in 2 to 3 weeks. Lesions do occur after excision.

Benign nephrosclerosis It includes abnormalities of kidney induced by benign hypertension, with associated hyaline arteriosclerosis. There develops narrowing of arterioles caused by thickening of walls. Large arteries may show fibroelastic hyperplasia. It rarely causes renal failure but mild proteinuria can happen.

Benign paroxysmal positional vertigo This syndrome is characterised by violent attacks of paroxysmal vertigo provoked by certain positions of head. There are no auditory symptoms. Provoking lesion lies in labyrinth. There is history of violent vertigo provoked by turning into a particular direction—say to remove book from high shelf or on bed. Nystagmus is rotatory.

Benign prostatic hypertrophy A noncancerous enlargement of the prostate in older men.

Benign tumor A relatively harmless neoplasm.

Benjmin-Allen syndrome It is a brachial arch syndrome. Clinical features include lymphadenopathy, cutaneous naevoid lesions, incomplete alopecia and marked mental retardation. There may be bilateral dermoids of conjunctiva, and follicular hyperplasia of conjunctiva.

Bennett's fracture It is an intra articular fracture subluxation at the base of the first metacarpal.

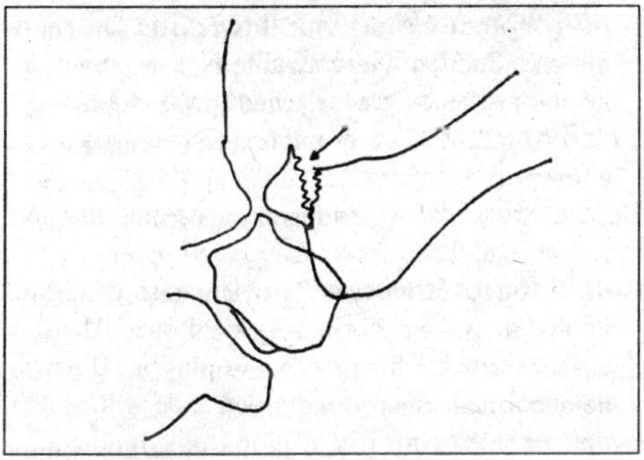

Benthic Relating to or found in the benthos, the region at the bottom of an ocean or at the soil-water interface of an ocean.

Benzene intoxication It is obtained by fractional distillation of coaltar naphtha. It is a colourless, volatile liquid which is highly inflammable. Inhalation of benzene at a concentration of 20,000 ppm is fatal. Ingestion of 30 ml is lethal. It is a narcotic poison and produces dizziness, tinnitus, dyspnoea, cyanosis, delirium and seizures. It is irritant to eyes and may develop local erythema. On ingestion it develops pain in mouth and epigastrium, vomiting, dizziness, flushed face and delirium. Later respiratory failure and coma may result.

Benzidine test Very sensitive test for presence of blood.

Benzoate A salt of benzoic acid.

Benzodiazepine toxicity These are used as sedatives, hypnotics, anxiolytics, muscle relaxants and anticonvulsants. These effects are produced by binding of the drug to the specific receptors in the central nervous system. These are completely safer and 25 to 30 times drugs can be consumed without any significant CNS depression. Deaths attributable to benzodiazepines taken alone are extremely rare. Patient will be drowsy, stuporous and ataxic or may present with a low-grade coma. Most overdosed patients will become easily arousable or awaken within 12 to 36 hours, secondary to drug distribution. Absent brain stem reflexes, unilateral plantar extensor reflexes and skin blisters are rare. After recovery patient may remain dizzy, depressed and apathetic for longer period.

Benzodiazepines These have hypnotic, sedative, anxiolytic, anticonvulsant and muscle relaxant actions. They attach to a specific GABA receptor. They may act chiefly on brain reticular activating system. These shorten the time taken to go to sleep, decrease intermittent awakening and increase total sleep duration. Slow absorption and long half-life give smooth action. Diazepam have half-life of 30 hours. The more slowly absorbed oxazepam may be preferred. It is used to treat anxiety, panic attacks and insomnia. Tolerance occurs with chronic use and there is cross-tolerance within group.

Benzylpenicillin (penicillin G) It is used when high plasma concentration is required. It is highly effective against *Streptococcus pneumoniae*, Lancefield group A and B haemolytic streptococci. *Enterococcus faecalis* is less susceptible. It is the drug of choice for meningococcal meningitis, tetanus, syphilis and diphtheria. The main hazard is allergic reaction. Angioneurotic oedema is a serious hazard.

Bereavement Loss through death crisis. A self limited response to hazardous events and experienced as a painful state. It can last from a few hours to few weeks.

Beriberi This develops due to deficiency of vitamin B_1 in the diet. It may be common in alcoholics and who are starving for long. Thiamine is found in whole grain, cereals, meat, green vegetables, potatoes and nuts and is essential for metabolism of carbohydrates. In dry beriberi person develops numbness, burning sensation of legs and wasting of muscles. In severe cases child may become emaciated, virtually bed-ridden and paralysed. In wet beriberi main problem is heart failure. There may be congestion in legs and oedema. Child will have poor appetite. Thiamine tablets may be given after a course of injections.

Berry aneurysm Congenital weakness in the vascular wall of circle of Willis are common. The weakened walls allow the artery to bubble out like a small balloon. These aneurysms are often seen as small bumps or berries known as Berry aneurysm. The weakened wall may rupture, producing cerebral hemorrhages specially in hypertensive cases. Vascular walls may also be weakened by the invasion of an atherosclerotic plaque.

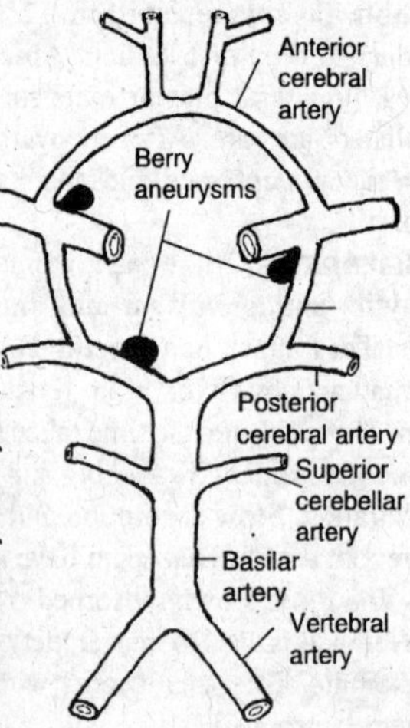

Sites of Berry aneurysm

Berylliosis Poisoning by fumes or dust of the metal beryllium, usually resulting in pneumonitis.

Best estimate Estimate achieved with the statistical model that produces the smallest sum of the squared error terms.

Beta cell Pancreatic islet cell that secretes insulin. Insulin-producing cells situated in the islets of langerhans of the pancreas.

Beta rhythm A thythmic electroencephalographic waveform with a frequency ranging from 15 to 30 hertz that can be recorded from the scalp of an alter subject or a subject in REM (rapid eye movement) sleep; also called an active or desynchronized pattern.

Beta-adrenergic blocker Any substance that results in the selective inhibition of the responses of effector cells to beta-adrenergic stimuli.

Beta-adrenergic blocking agent Drug that binds to and prevents adrenergic receptors from responding to adrenergic compounds that normally bind to beta-adrenergic receptors and cause them to function; beta-adrenergic blocking agents are used to treat certain arrhythmias in the heart and to treat tachycardia.

Beta-blocker drugs These are given to treat heart disorders specially angina pectoris, hypertension and cardiac arrhythmias. Sometimes these are prescribed after myocardial infarction also. These may be prescribed to prevent migraine attacks. These may be occasionally used as eyedrops in cases of glaucoma. Side effects include worsening of symptoms of asthma, bronchitis and lung disease. Sudden withdrawal may exaggerate the symptoms hence gradual withdrawal is advised.

Betadine Solution of providone-iodine used as an antiseptic

Beta-endorphin An endogenous peptide that has actions similar to those of ingested opium.

Beta-lipoproteinaemia This is a rare condition known as Bassen-Kornzweig syndrome. There is absence of beta lipoproteins in plasma. But will be abnormally shaped red blood cells with spikes on surface, retinitis pigmentosa leading to blindness, progressive ataxia, fatty infiltration of enterocytes. Plasma vitamin E levels are very low. There is now good evidence that early intensive and continued repletion with vitamin E prevents neurological deterioration.

Betamethasone It is used in the treatment of inflammation specially eczema and psoriasis and to reduce severity of asthma and arthritis. It is occasionally used to treat cerebral oedema. As side effect it may cause thinning of skin.

Betatron A machine that produces high speed electron through magnetic induction.

Betel Leaf of creeper piper betel which is chewed for its stimulating effect due to presence of alkaloids coline and gavacoline. Leaves are chewed with lime and nuts and Areca catechu.

Between-groups mean square Same as Between-groups variance.

Between-groups variance Measurement of the variation between the means of more than one group, based on the independent variables under study.

Bevel The inclination that one surface makes with an another when not at right angles. In cavity preparation a cut that produces an angle or more than 90 degrees with a cavity wall.

Bevelling (of bone) The process of smoothing the cut ends of bone to prevent rough edges that could cause skin irritations from pressure against the prosthetic socket.

Bevelling Making an angle in which one surface meets another at other than 90°.

Bezoar In it a ball of food and mucus, vegetable, fibre, hair or other indigestible material is found in stomach. These are rare in adults. These can cause loss of appetite, constipation, nausea and vomiting. If these pushes down to intestine then may result in obstruction. Barium meal X-ray is diagnostic.

Bezoars Physical obstacles created by tangles of fibrous material in the gastronitestinal tract that may cause dangerous gastrointestinal obstructions.

Biangled Having two angles or bends.

Bias The introducitonof error that produces deviations or distortions of data that are predominantly in one directoin, as opposed to random error. Same as differential error.

Bias angle The angle of the cords in a bias or bias belted tire, with respect to its centerline.

Biattenuation The nonengineered, natural decomposition of organic contaminants in soil and ground water system.

Biceps brachii Muscle in the anterior arm with two heads or origins on the scapula and an insertion onto the radius; flexes and supinates the forearm.

Biceps femoris Powerful flexor of the lower leg.

Bicipital Having two heads.

Bicipital syndrome Symptom complex produced by a dislocation of long head of biceps brachii from inter tubercular or biceps groove.

Bicipital tendinitis A painful affliction of tendon of long head of biceps muscle.

Bicipital tuberosity The prominence of neck of radius for attachment of biceps tendon.

Biconcave lens Lens which has two concave surfaces.

Bicornuate uterus Having two horns that, in the embryo, failed to attain complete fusion.

Bicuspid A tooth with two cusps.

Bicuspid valve Valve closing the opening between the left atrium and left ventricle of the heart; has two cusps; also called the mitral valve.

Bicycle spoke injury Injury of lower spoke seen in children when a foot is caught between the spokes of cycle.

BID Latin meaning twice a day.

Biemond's syndrome There is simple recessive, hypophyseal infantilism. Person will have mental retardation, polydactyly, genital dystrophy and absence of secondary sex characteristics.

Bier Block A method of intravenous regional anesthesia.

Bifacet dislocation of vertebrae It is due to flexion and rotation mechanism. It may cause tetraplegia.

Bifid Divided into 2 parts.

Biforate Having two foramina or openings.

Bifurcation Division into two parts or branches, as any two roots of a tooth.

Bigelow 'Y' ligament The iliofemoral ligament.

Bigeminal Paired Especially, the occurrence of heart beats in pairs.

Bigeminal Pulse Two regular pulse beats followed by a long pause.

Bihormonal Containing two hormones; specifically, in the case of gonadotropes, a cell that contains both LH and FSH.

Bilateral On both sides of the body and bilateral integration The ability to coordinate both sides of the body during activity.

Bilateral stance time The length of time up to 30 seconds that a subject can stand upright in the parallel bars bearing weight on both lower extremities.

Bilateral symmetry Refers to organs or parts that are present on both sides of the body and very similar in appearance on each side. For example, the hands are bilaterally symmetrical, whereas the heart is not .

Bile It is a liquid secreted by liver. It carries away waste products formed in the liver and helps in breaking down fats and its absorption. These are stored in gall bladder and reaches there through bile ducts. From gall bladder it reaches to duodenum. Any blockage in duct will result in accumulation of bile in liver and development of jaundice due to accumulation of bilirubin. It may be caused by gall stones, tumour of pancreas compressing lower end of common bile duct and cholangiocarcinoma. Obstructive jaundice results in pale coloured faeces and dark urine as well as yellow colour of sclera and skin. Ultrasound is a helpful diagnostic tool.

Bile duct Ducts that collect bile from the liver join as one large duct underneath the hepatic duct. From this the cystic duct leads to gall bladder. In gall bladder bile is stored, when bile is needed it turns down to the cystic duct to common bile duct and into the duodenum.

Bile salt Organic salt secreted by the liver that functions to emulsify lipids.

Bilharziasis Endemic haematuria occurs mostly in Middle East. Adult female worm *Schistosoma hematobium* lives in portal system. Symptoms include urticarial eruptions, terminal haematuria, frequency, perineal, penile and suprapubic pain and aching in lumbar area. The blood is bright

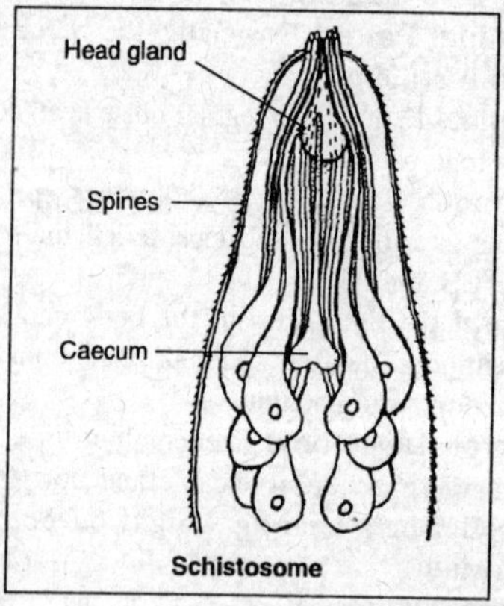

Schistosome

red, occurs at the end of micturition and increased by exercise. Cystoscopic examination reveals round yellowish white, pseudo tubercles and ulcers. Later on papillomata and sandy patches may be seen. Secondary bacterial infection is possible.

Biliary atresia A congential condition in which the mahor bile duct is blocked, limiting the availability of bile for fat digestion.

Biliary cirrhosis It is an uncommon liver cirrhosis resulting from disease or defects of bile ducts. In primary cirrhosis duct within liver becomes inflamed and destroyed. Symptoms include itching followed by jaundice and enlargement of liver. There may be abdominal pain and fatty diarrhoea. Liver function test gives clue to the diagnosis. Secondary cirrhosis develops due to prolonged bile duct obstruction or biliary atresia. There will be abdominal pain, tenderness, liver enlargement, fever with chill.

Biliary colic There is severe pain in right upper quadrant. Pain is severe and mimic like that of heart attack, often lasts upto an hour and may radiate to right shoulder. Injection Fortwin gives relief. Ultrasound scanning is helpful in diagnosing it.

Biliary obstruction Causes includes primary sclelrosing cholangitis, gall stones, carcinoma of common bile duct and head of pancreas. There will be jaundice, conjugated hyperbilirubinemia and clay coloured stools.

Bilingual A person who has enough control of two languages to function well with both languages in a number of different contexts.

Bilirubin Bile contains bilirubin and biliverdin. Bilirubin represents the breakdown of haemoglobin. It is orange yellow coloured and becomes visible through sclera in case of jaundice. Normal bilirubin level in blood is 0.8 mg per cent.

Bilirubin encephalopathy Brain damage resulting from deposits of unconjugated bilirubin in brain tissue.

Biliverdin A greenish pigment in bile formed by oxidation of bilirubin.

Bimalleolar Ankle fracture A fracture of the ankle in which both the distal fibula and medial malleolus are broken.

Bimanual palpation uterus Uterus can be palpated bimanually. Finger of one hand through vaginally and another hand externally.

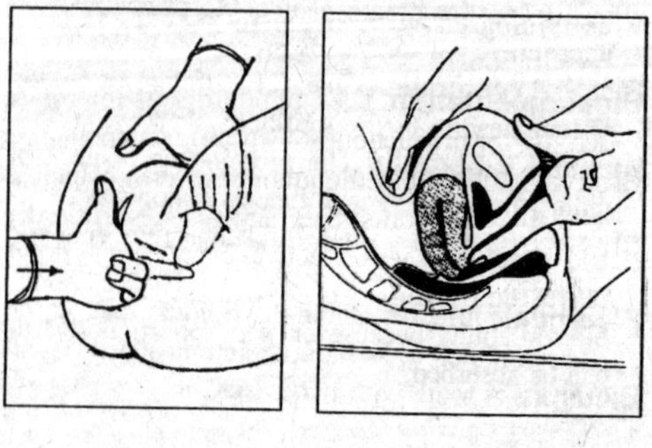

Bimanual removal of placenta If within 30 minutes placenta does not come out and manual compression fails bimanual removal of placenta may be practiced. If there is free flow of blood after delivery placenta is to be removed manually.

Binangle A dental instrument having two angulations in the shank connecting the handle, or shaft, with the working portion of the instrument, known as the blade, or nib.

Binary variables Same as Dichotomous variables.

Binaural cues Pertaining to both ears.

Binder Bandage made of a large piece of material to fit and support a specific body part. A substance, generally sticky that holds the solid particles in a mixture together preserving physical form of mixture.

Binders Substances occurring in plant foods that combine with minerals to form undigestible compounds that cannot be absorbed.

Binding site The specific area of an enzyme molecule to which other molecules can attach in a chemical reaction.

Binocular cues Visual cues that require the use of both eyes working together.

Binocular perception Perception attained through simultaneous use of both eyes.

Binocular visual field The visual field common to both eyes.

Binuclear family Divorced families with coparenting arrangements.

Bioactive Having an effect on or eliciting a response from living tissue.

Bioaerosol An aerosol of living matter; i.e., an air-bone suspension of microorganisms, microbial byproducts and/or pollen.

Bioassay Determination of the active power of a sample of a drug by noting its effect on animals, as compared with the effect of a standard preparation.

Bioaugmentation The stimulation of microbial activity for production of a specific compound.

Bioavailability It is the amount of drug which is available to blood stream and reaches to tissues and organs. This way effectiveness of various drugs is tested. Drugs given orally have lesser bioavailability because only a proportion of drug can be absorbed.

Biocatalyst A biochemical compound particularly an enzyme that catalyzes chemical reactions.

Biochemical marker In biotechnology, an indicator of biodegradation or biotransformation.

Biochemicla oxygen demand The quantity of oxygen that aerobic bacteria in sewage will deplete form the water.

Biochemistry It is the science which studies the chemistry of living organisms including human beings. The chemical process providing energy, eliminating their waste, damage and repair, normal growth and abnormal cell division are all studied in biochemistry. Studies of hormones, gases and chemical constituents all are studied and blood tests, liver and kidney functions tests all are done under it.

Biocidal Capable of killling living organisms.

Biocide Any agent that kills living organisms. Specifically, a chemical susbstance or composition used to kill microorganisms considered to be undesirable; i.e., pest organisms.

Biocompatible The ability of the material to perform with an appropriate host response in a particular situation; does not cause harm to the body; nontoxic (note that even biocompatible materials may cause allergic reactions in some people)

Bioconversion The process by which drugs are converted into other substances in a biological environment.

Biocytin The conjugate amino acid residue arising from covalent attachment of biotin, through an amide linkage.

Biodevelopmental Pertaining to both the biological and the developmental processes.

Bioelectric Current The electrical or electrochemical phenomenon that appears in living tissues, as may be generated by muscle, nerve tissue, and bone during function.

Bioelectric impedance analysis A method using a very mild electric charge to estimate lean body mass in order to determine body fat composition.

Bioelectric Signal A bioelectric potential or current that triggers a biologic response that may enhance or retard physiological activity.

Bioengineer A person who has knowledge of both engineering and biology and functions as a scientist or inventor in health care fields in which engineering principles and components are used.

Bioenrichment Enrichment of the protein, essential amino acid, or vitamin content of food through growth and synthetic activities of microorganisms overgrowing the substrate.

Bioethanol Ethyl alcohol produced by yeast fermentation for use as a fuel or industrial commodity.

Bioethics Rules or principles that govern right conduct, specially those relating to heath care.

Biofeedback A condition in which an electroencephalograph, electrocardiograph, or comparable device is used to present information to an individual about his or her bodily functioning, such as type of brain waves being emitted or rate of heart beat. Studies have indicated that with this information some persons are able to alter the relevant bodily processes. The use of instrumentation to provide information (feedback) about variations in one or more of the subject's own physiologic processes not ordinarily perceived, e.g. brainwave activity, muscle tension, or blood pressure. Such feedback over a period of time can help the subject learn to control certain physiologic processes even though he or she is unable to articulate how the learning was achieved.

Biofilm A biologically active layer on a surface or interface, consisting of a complex association of microorganisms, microbial products, water, and suspended dissolved solids.

Bioflavin It is known as vitamin 'P' also. It is found mainly in pulp and connective tissue of citrous fruits. It builds resistance to infection.

Biofouling Damage caused to a surface by microorganisms attached to the surface.

Biofunctionability The quality of being both compatible and functional with the biologic environment in implant dentistry, with regard to force transfer within physiological limits of health.

Biogenic Produced or formed by organisms, such as the formation of some metal sulfide deposits.

Biogenic amine hypothesis The concept that abnormalities in the physiology and metabolism of biogenic amines, particularly catecholamines (norepinephrine and dopamine) and an indole amine (serotonin), are involved in the pathogenesis of certain psychiatric illness. The concept was derived originally from a serendipitous discovery that monoamine oxidase (MOA) inhibitors and certain tricyclic durgs had moodelevating properties, and that these agents exerted dramatic effect on brain-monoamine functions. The findings that phenothiazines inhibit dopamine activity in the brain further support this theory and suggest that a disorder of dopamine metabolism may be implicated in the aetiology of schizophrenia. Disorders in norepinephrine and serotonin activity have been implicated in the aetiology of depression and mania.

Biogenic amines Organic substances of interest because of their possible role in brain functioning. Subdivided into catecholamines (e.g. epinephrine, dopamine, norepinephrine) and indoles (e.g. tryptophan, serotonin).

Bioinert Having minimal effect and eliciting a minimal response from living tissue.

Bioleaching The solubilization of metal values from an ore by microbially mediated oxidation of the minerals.

Biologic defense mechanisms Methods that prevent microorganisms from causing an infectious disorder.

Biologic dressing Biologic tissue used to cover a burn wound.

Biologic rhythms Cyclical variations in physiologic and biochemical function, level of activity, and emotional state. Circadian rhythms have a cycle of about 24 hours; ultradian rhythms are shorter than one day; and infradian rhythms may be weeks or months.

Biological clock Data which the DNA the cell has inherited and which determine the life span of cells. It determines the life span of person, time of menopause and balding. A regular time schedule of biological activities. Examples are menses, the time regulated release of hormones and periods of sleep and wakefulness.

Biological dressings The use of homologus or heterologus skin for coverage.

Biological family Family relationships defined by genetic connection.

Biological filtration Process in which cells alter the contents of the filtered fluid.

Biological value It is the efficiency with which protein furnishes the proper proportion and amounts of essential or indispensable aminoacids needed for synthesis fo proteins in human. Egg protein has the highest biological value. The BV is defined as Nitrogen obtained Nitrogen absorbed

Biological vector An arthropod used by a disease-producing organism for transmission and as a vehicle for reproduction and/or development.

Bioluminescene The emssion of visible light by living organisms.

Biomagnetometry Like EEG, biomagnetometry is a non-invasive procedure to record eletrical activity of brain. Minute electrical currents that flow through neurons generate a magnetic flux which is detected by complex antenna coils and is converted as electrical signals. It has better diagnostic value in seizures. It is useful in study of auditory and visual function.

Bio-markers Biochemical structures that may be characteristic or indicative of a particular plant or animals family, genus, species or subspecies.

Biomaterial Any substance other than a drug, synthetic or natural, that can be used as a system or part of a system that treats.

Biome A region of the earth having a distinct form of vegetation; e.g., a tropical forest.

Biomechanical cleansing Process of flushing a root canal with sodium hypochlorite to clean and remove debris from the canal.

Biomechanical engineering It is the use of engineering expertise to create and apply devices and machines towards assistance for or within the human body. It is mostly useful in making artificial joints. This is a branch which applies engineering principles and methods to human body to explain how it functions and to treat them. This branch has made artificial joints, pacemakers, renal dialysis machines and artificial heart valves

Biomechanics Application of mechanical laws to living structures. The study and knowledge of biological function from an application of mechanical principles.

Biometrics The use of physical features and characteristics, i.e. face, fingerprints, handwriting, retina patterns, etc. to identify a person because those features and characteristics are unique to that individual.

Biomolecule An organic compound normally present as an essential component of living organisms.

Biooxidation pretreatment The microbial oxidation of minerals in order to release a metal value contained within the mineral.

Biopesticide A living microbial pathogen that selectively infects and kills its insect or weed host, or that is a microbial antagonist of a plant pathogen.

Biopsy It is a diagnostic method in which tissues are removed from the body for examination under microscope. Most of these procedures are minor and do not require any anaesthesia. Microscopic examination of tissue gives a correct diagnosis. One can confidently diagnose whether tissue is benign or malignant and if malignant, gland biopsy may show its extent.

Biopterin An enzymatic cofactor derived from pterin and involved in certain oxidation-reduction reactions.

Bloreactor A closed vessel or system used for fermentation or enzyme reaction.

Biosensor An instrument that combines a biological recognition unit with a physical transducer.

Bioslurry treatment Accelerated biodegradation of contaminants by the suspension of contaminated soil or sediment in water through mixing energy.

Biosphere All the living matter on or in the earth, the seas, and the atmosphere.

Biostatic Describing an agent that inhibits or halts growth and multiplication of organisms.

Biosterol Obsolete name for vitamin A.

Biosurfactant A biodegradable surfactant produced by micro-organisms or enzymes.

Biosynthesis The chemical synthesis of materials in living plants/materials.

Biot's respiration It is a kind of respiration which is completely irregular in rhythm, depth and rate, and may sometimes be noisy and stertorous. It is encountered in meningitis and bulbar poliomyelitis.

Biotic pertaining to life

Biotin A vitamin, an enzymatic cofactor involved in carboxylaction reactions.

Biotope A specific, defined site or environment containing a biological community.

Biotoprotein A soluble biotin protein complex that occurs naturally.

Biotransformation The alteration of the structure of a compound by an organism, especially a microorganis.

Biotroph Literally, eater of life; an organism that requires nutrients from a living host in order to grow and reproduce, thus, biotrophic.

Biotrophy The fact or process of feeding by extracting nutrients from living host tissues.

Biovar An infrasubspecific grouping of isolates of a species differing in biochemical or physiological properties.

Biparietal diameter It is 9.5 cm, distance between the two parietal eminences.

Bipartite patella A congenital anomaly of patella in which an accessary ossification center gives the patella the appearance of being in two pieces.

Bipennate Denoting muscles that have a fibre architecture coursing obliquely on both sides of a tendon.

Biphysical profile Five fetal parameters are used as biophysical assessment of fetal well being. These are fetal breathing movements, gross body movements, fetal tone, reactive fetal heart rate and amniotic fluid volume.

Bipolar affective disorder Alternating periods of depression and mania.

Bipolar disorder An emotional disorder in which the feelings vary from extremely positive to extremely negative. The former is called a manic state—the latter is the depressive state. Previously, this condition was known as a manicdepressive disorder.

Bipolar illness Synonm for manic depressive illness.

Bipolar neuron A neuron with one axon and one dendrite.

Birefringent The property of a substance of doubly refracting a beam of light.

Birth The act or process of being born.

Birth defects These are abnormalities obvious at birth or detectable early in infancy. Congenital defects are birthmarks and spina bifida. Some children are born with more or less than 23 pairs of chromosomes as in Down's syndrome. Genetic defects are inherited from one or both parents. Example of genetic defects at birth are achondroplasia and albinism. Accidental irradiation damages unborn child and exposes to develop leukaemia in later life. If mother suffers from German measles in first three months of pregnancy then chances are there that child may suffer from eye, ear or heart abnormalities. If child has too less of amniotic fluid child may develop clubfoot.

Birth fathers Men who are biologically generative through procreation and they provide care to infant.

Birth injuries These are damages sustained during birth. In normal vaginal delivery all babies suffer some sort of injuries but during forceps delivery cephalhaematoma may be formed. In breech deliveries nerves of shoulder region are sometimes injured causing temporary paralysis. Broken clavicle may result in difficult delivery. Many cases of cerebral palsy and mental retardation may be due to birth injury.

Birth marks These are areas of discoloured skin present from birth. Most common are moles. Strawberry marks are hemangiomas. Strawberry disappears gradually after 6 months but portwine stains seldom fades, laser treatment may prove helpful. Sometimes mole may change into malignant melanoma. If a mole rapidly becomes irregular and suddenly increases and changes its shape then it requires careful watch.

Birth plan Planning of couple for giving birth to their children.

Birth trauma The physical injury that occurs during labor and delivery.

Birth-room A room with home like decor in which the patient labours, delivers and recovers.

Biscodyl suppository This is a popular 10 mg suppository. This procedure is based on peristalsis in large bowel by reflex action by contact with mucosal nervous plexus. A combination of biscodyl two tablets of 10 mg each orally at bed time followed by suppository in the morning is routinely followed in many hospitals in case of preoperatory enema.

Biscuit Essentially a bakery confectionary dried down to low moisture content.

Biscupid valve One of the two AV valves, it is located between the left atrium and ventricle and is sometimes called the mitral valve.

Biscuspid Premolar.

Biscuspidization Surgical procedure used in endodontic treatment when severe bone loss is confined to the furcation area. The process creates two biscuspids (premolars) from a mandibular molar.

Bisecting technique Intraoral radiographic technique in which the x-ray beam is directed perpendicular to a line bisecting the long axis of the tooth and the film plane.

Bisexual This term is often used to describe people whose sexual objects of choice include both men and women.

Bisexuality It is the sexual attraction to both sexes, not merely in fantasy but also in performance. These people can achieve orgasm with either sex through at times they may be preponderantly active with males and at other time with females.

Bishops hand A low ulnar nerve palsy causing clawing of ring and small fingers.

Bismuth poisoning The oral manifestations consist of metallic taste, burning sensations of oral mucosa and a bismuth line. Some cases show pigmented patches in other areas also. Microscopically granular deposits of a black pigment bismuth sulphide are seen in submucosa. Sulphide is produced from food debris of mouth to produce bismuth sulphide which in turn deposits as an insoluble precipitate.

Bismuthia Discolouration of mucus membrane and skin from bismuth poisoning.

Bite open Condition in which the anterior teeth of two arches dont meet when posterior teeth are in centric occlusion.

Bite registration An impression of the occlusal surfaces of the teeth, taken with the upper and lower teeth in contact; used to orient casts accurately on an articulator.

Bite splint Removal clear acrylic appliance used to relax T.M. joint muscles.

Bitemporal diameter It is 8 cm and is the greatest distance between two halves of coronal sutures.

Biteplane A removable appliance that covers the occlusal surfaces of teeth to prevent their articulation.

Bitewing Intraoral radiograph depicting the crowns of maxillary and mandibular teeth and interdental bone crests. A bitweing radiograph is made using a film positioned by special tabs on which the teeth are closed.

Bitewing intraoral radiograph Intraoral radiograph records on a single film the outline Position, and mesiodistal exent of crown, neck and coronal third of roots.

Bite-wing radiograph A dental radiograph that reveals the crowns of both the maxillary and mandibular teeth on the same film; the primary use of a bite-wing radiograph is to detect interproximal caries.

Bitot's spots These are small, circumscribed, lustreless, greyish white, foamy, greesy, triangular deposits on bulbar conjunctiva of both eye, and are seen in vitamin A deficiency.

Biuret test For proteins. Violet colour is developed when a drop of copper sulphate is added to a solution of protein in caustic soda.

Bivalved cast Cast that is cut in two lengthwise pieces.

BK Mole syndrome It is an autosomal dominant disorder. There will be many large, irregular, variable naevi occurring mainly on upper part of trunk and extremities.

BKA Below knee amputation.

Black eye Sometimes eye injury is followed by bruised appearance of skin around eye. Any direct blow damages capillaries below skin causing blood to leak and collect there and the skin around eye is thin and loose, bruise looks darker in colour.

Black hairy tongue White hairy tongue may accumulate foreign pigment and appear as black hairy tongue. Pigmentation of the attached gingiva has been seen in postmenopausal state and after the use of tranquillisers, oral contraceptives and antimalarial drugs.

Black head It is a type of acne and is semisolid black capped plug of greasy material blocking the sebaceous gland. These generally develop in chest, face and shoulder.

Black lung disease Same as Coal worker's pneumoconiosis.

Black out It is brief and momentary. There is loss of consciousness similar to fainting.

Black powder Also known as gunpowder; a mixture of potassium nitrate, carbon and sulfur.

Black widow spider venom A poison, produced by the black widow spider, that promotes the release of acetylcholine from the synapse.

Blackfan-Diamond syndrome A rare congenital disorder associated with red cell aplasia producing profound anaemia in the infants.

Blackhead When sebum accumulates, darkens, and enlarge some of the ducts of the sebaceous glands; also known as a comedo.

Blackout A condition characterized by failure of vision and momentary unconsciousness, due to diminished circulation to the brain.

Blackwater fever Massive lysis of vertebrate erythrocytes that, at times, accomapnies falciparum malaria.

Bladder A sac, usually referring to the urinary bladder.

Bladder calculi Bladder calculi may be the result of stones passed down the ureter which have lodged and enlarged in the bladder. There will be sudden cessation of urinary stream during voiding with severe penile or perirenal pain and passage of small amount of blood. Pain is relieved when patient lies down and stone falls back away from trigone.

Bladder injury Obstetric traumatic injury to bladder may be due to pressure necrosis of bladder base due to prolonged compression of the bladder wall between the fetal head and mother's pubis.

Bladder irrigation It is done in severe and recurrent infection of bladder to reduce infection. It helps in cleaning bladder from blood and mucus and to relieve pain. For irrigation one can use normal saline solution, KMnO 1:1000 or 4 gm of boric acid in 500 cc of water. At one time you can introduce 30 cc of solution.

Bladder neck The smooth muscle at the base of the bladder. When contracted, it blocks the flow of urine into the urethra or prevents the flow of semen into the bladder.

Bladder neck descent It is due to poor pelvic floor support. It may be due to raised intraabdominal

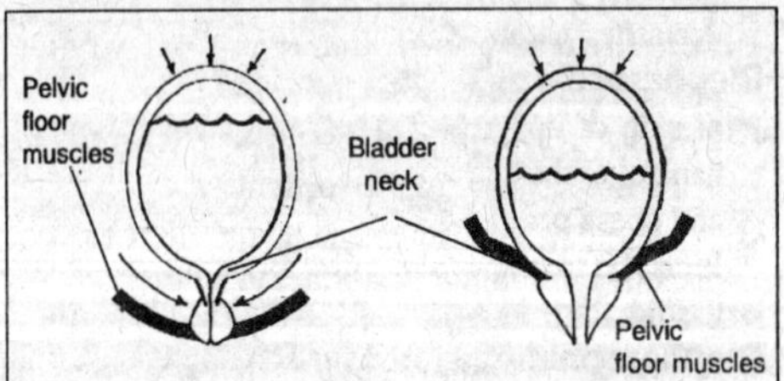

No bladder neck descent   Bladder neck descent

pressure which normally occludes the bladder neck. Prolapse may also occur where there is disruption of pubourethral ligament.

Bladder sound It is a metallic rod, 10" long. It is gradually curved at distal end and is not graduated. It is used to determine the limits of bladder during operation and to diagnose a calculus in bladder.

Bladder tumours Many bladder tumours are benign papillomas. These are small wart-like growths but have potential to change into malignancy. Haematuria is the main symptom.

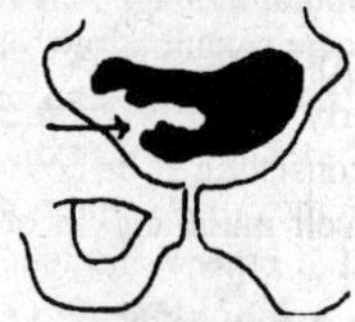

Bladder tumour

Passing of urine becomes painful. If growth blocks urethral opening it may develop back pressure in kidney and hydronephrosis may develop.

Blade The flat, cutting part of a knife. 2. the end portion of a dental instrument designed for cutting, probing, or scraping, connected by a shank to the handle.

Blade holding forceps Nowadays, this is the most common method practised by the sugeons to make an incision for cataract surgery fixed in the forceps. The razor blade is for incision.

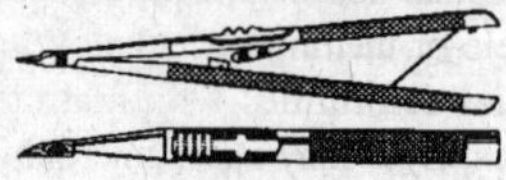

Blade holding forceps

Blair fusion A technique of ankle repair intended for patients with a vascular necrosis of talar body.

Blanch A white spot seen in the skin when pressure is applied. This is an indication of the presence of viable capillary beds; the blanced area will become pink when pressure is released if the capillary bed is perfused.

Bland Mild or soothing.

Bland diet It means a diet without spices or excess ghee/oil, residue and not to cause irritation to gastric mucosa. Vegetables containing excess cellulose do not come under bland diet. Bland diet includes, *kheer, khichdi*, custard, milk, curds, jellies, ice creams, etc.

Blast trauma to hearing There is first a short positive pressure wave reaching very high pressure levels of thousands of pounds per square inch lasting about 5 ms followed by a longer lasting

negative phase below atmospheric pressure as long as 30 ms.
The cochlear damage caused by blast is usually severe hearing loss with tinnitus. Recovery after a shortwhile is common but some high tone loss often persists. Tympanic membrane may even perforate. Vestibular damage may result in vertigo.

Blastocele Cavity in the blastocyst.

Blastocyst Early stage of mammalian embryo development consisting of a hollow ball of cells with an inner cell mass and an outer trophoblast layer.

Blastocyst hatching The process in which the blastocyst emerges from the zona pellucida prior to implantation.

Blastocyte An embryonic cell that has not yet become differentiated.

Blastoderm The outer layer of cells of a fertilized ovum in the blastula stage.

Blastomere A cell in the early preimplantation embryo.

Blastula An earlystage of prental developing between the morula and embryonic period.

Blatt's syndrome Distichiasis is usually inherited as an autosomal dominant disorder. There will be meningocele or meningoencephalocele. One may have cranial deformities with malformations of facial bones. Eyes may show microphthalmos.

Bleacher A chemical agent that removes stains or color skin.

Bleaching The act or process of removing discolorations from the crowns of pulpless teeth through the use of chemical agents, usually but not necessarily in combination with heat. Oxidizing agents, such as 30 percent hydrogen peroxide solution, are generally used.

Bleaching agent Agent used in modification or removal of discolouration.

Bleb A sac containing fluid or gas; refers to the coalescent alveolar sacs formed from the destruction of alveolar septa as the result of pulmonary disease e.g., emphysema.

Bleeding Temporarily it can be controlled by putting firm pressure over a pad on the bleeding site. Maintain this pressure until bleeding is controlled and then apply a firm bandaged dressing. If wound is in upper limb place a sling. Treat for a shock.

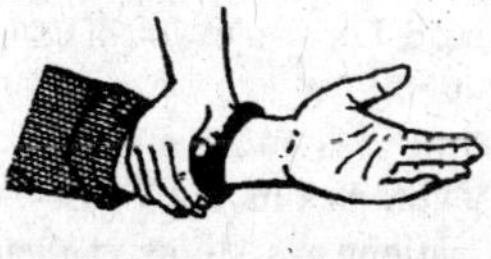

Control of bleeding by direct pressure

Bleeding disorder Haemophilia and Christmas diseases are disorders resulting from deficiencies of two coagulation factors called factor VIII and factor IX. Individuals with any of these disorders can bleed internally without warning. Such deficiency may develop due to liver disorder, vitamin K deficiency or the use of anticoagulant drug. Coagulation defects are investigated by blood clotting tests. Too less of blood platelets may also be the reason.

Blennadenitis Inflammation of mucous glands.

Blennorrhea Excessive discharge of mucus;

Blepharitis Inflammation of eyelids with redness, irritation and scaly skin of lid margin may result in burning and discomfort of eyes. In some cases roots of eyelashes may become infected. Dandruff or eczema of scalp may be an associated finding. Swabbing with warm water may remove scales. Marginal blepharitis generally recur. It is chronic inflammation of lid margins. Ulcerative blepharitis is due to infection. It usually follows chronic conjunctivitis due to staphylococci. Squamous blepharitis is due to metabolic factor. The patient complains of mild lacrimation, itching and photophobia. Some may complain of crusts at the lid margin. There may be complaint of falling of eyelashes with swollen and thick lids.

Blepharochalasis It is a condition of redundancy of skin of upper eyelid forming a fold of skin to hang over the upper lid margin. It is seen in elderly and obese people. It does not interfere with vision. It can be treated by excision of the excess skin of the lid.

Blepharophimosis Abnormal narrowness of the palpebral fissures.

Blepharoptosis Drooping of the upper eyelid.

Blepharospasm This is a focal dystonia affecting the orbicularis oculi and neighbouring facial muscles. By blepharospasm is meant an involuntary sustained and forced closure of eyelids. Bright light may precipitate it. There may be shaking of head. Local injection of botulinum toxin may prove useful.

Blighted ovum It is an anembryonic pregnancy. The sac develops but the embryo does not. Clinically patient has slight vaginal bleeding. Pregnancy test may be positive even though no embryo is present. The growth of the sac will not increase as it would have in normal pregnancy. Although eventually a blighted ovum will abort.

Blind lithopaxy It is now rarely utilized. There are two basic ways to hold the lithotrite and grasp the stone. The funnel and sugar tongs technique.

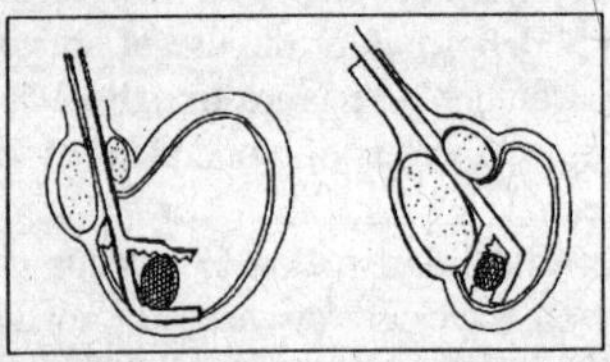

Blind spot It is a small, oval shaped area on the retina where the optic nerve joins the eyeball. This area is not sensitive to light because there is no light receptor.

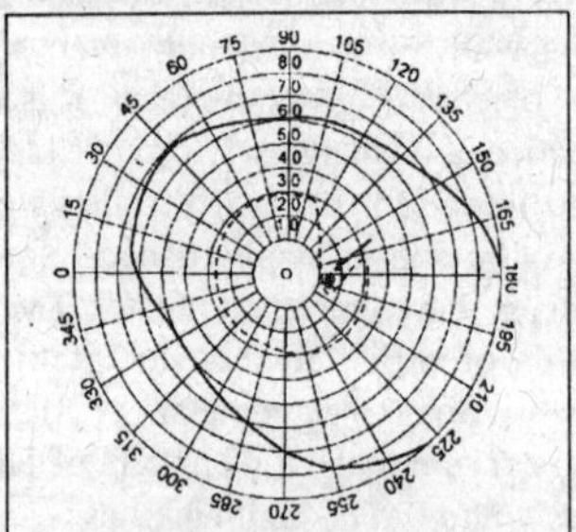

Baring of the blind spot

Blindness There is severe loss of vision which cannot be corrected by glasses. Vision markedly hampers day to day working. It is usually defined as corrected visual acuity of 20/200 or less in better eye or a visual field of no more than 20 degrees in better eye. It may result from injury, disease or degeneration of optic nerve. Cataract is a common cause of blindness. In glaucoma pressure in the eyeball causes degeneration of the nerve fibres of optic nerve disc.

Blindsight Patients with cortical blindness ay perceive movement in the peripheral field without being ale to see anything there.

Blinking-to-light reflex Reflex blinking in response to a flash of bright light.

Blinking-to-noise reflex Acousticofacial reflex causing the orbicularis oculi to twitch in response to a loud sound.

Blister There is collection of fluid beneath the outer layer of skin. It forms a raised area usually oval or circular. The fluid in it is serum that has leaked from blood vessels in underlying skin due to damage. Burns and friction are the common causes. Certain diseases as impetigo, erythema multiforme may also cause it. Small blisters develop in herpes zoster. Blister should be left to heal at its own, i.e. it should not be burst.

Blob A region in the visual cortex that contains color-sensitive neurons, as revealed by staining for cytochrome oxidase.

Block anesthesia Anesthesia which acts on larger terminal branches of nerves.

Blockage The process of blocking or obstruction; the condition of being blocked or obstructed.

Blocking A sudden obstruction or interruption in spontaneous flow of thinking or speaking, perceived as an absence or deprivation of thought.

Blood It is a red coloured fluid that circulates in our arteries and veins. It transports oxygen and has a vital role in body's defence mechanism. It seals damaged blood vessels, protects the injury with a clot and helps to repair a damage. Average human being is having about 5 litres of blood in body. At rest 5 litres of blood is pumped by the heart via arteries and returns back by veins. During exercise pumping capacity increases 3 to 4 times. Half of the volume is RBC and WBCs. Remainder is a fluid called plasma which contains dissolved proteins, sugars, fats and minerals. Plasma is a straw coloured fluid consisting mainly of water with a salt content.

Blood clotting Blood begins to clot within seconds once skin is cut. Clot helps to seal damaged blood vessels. But thrombi formed inside major blood vessels are cause of many heart attacks. Blood coagulation is triggered by chemicals released either by activated platelets or by tissue. Fibrin formation is the end product.

Blood products Blood may be stored either as a whole or separated into various components. Each product has a specific utility. *Whole blood* is used to restore blood volume after severe bleeding, whole blood can be kept well for 3 to 4 weeks after donation. *Packed red cells* is prepared after removing plasma. It is used to treat some form of anaemia. It raises haemoglobin without overloading fluid to the patient. In chronic anaemia it is fruitful. *Frozen red cells* can be preserved for longer period at very low temperatures. Generally RBCs of rare blood group are preserved this way. *Platelets* are extracted from whole blood in concentrated form. These are useful in dysfunctions of blood clotting. *White blood cells* can be separated from normal blood and can be used in life threatening infections. *Frozen fresh plasma* is prepared by separating and freezing the plasma as soon as possible after blood collection. Being rich in clotting factors it is used to correct many types of bleeding disorders. *Plasma protein solution* is liquid part of any blood and not used within 3 weeks of collection then it is converted into concentrated solution of protein. It can be used in patients of shock. Purified albumin preparations are used to treat nephrotic syndrome. *Clotting factors VIII and IX* can be prepared for treatment of haemophilia.

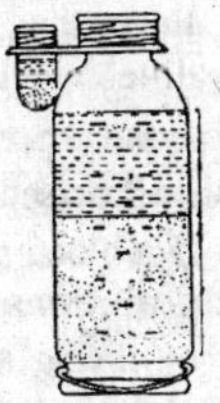

Bottle of blood

Blood bank In this blood is stored, categorised according to blood group. In latest blood banks test of HIV is done before it is issued to be given to needy patient.

Blood brain barrier Number of subrtances in the blood that transfer into brain cells is limited. Major source of energy to brain is glucose which can pass the barrier, other sugars cannot. Since the brain depends on glucose hypoglycemic states cannot bring on convulsions as in insulin shock.

Blood cells There are mainly two types of cells, RBCs and WBCs. *RBCs* form about 40 per cent by volume. These are formed in bone marrow by a series of divisions. These carry oxygen from lungs to tissues. Cells released from bone marrow are called reticulocytes, over 2 to 4 days these develop into mature cells. One cubic millilitre of blood contains about 5 million RBCs, each of which is doughnut shaped, about 7.5 thousandanth of a millimetre in diameter and much thicker round the edge than centre. It helps the cells to squeeze through narrow vessels. Cell is packed with haemoglobin. Oxyhaemoglobin formed when oxygen combines with haemoglobin is responsible for bright red colour. Each RBC also contains enzymes, minerals and sugars which give energy to maintain shape, structure and elasticity. Lifespan of RBCs is 120 days. As cells age, their internal chemical machinery wears out, they loose elasticity and are trapped in small vessels. These are then destroyed by a type of WBCs. Lack of RBCs results in anaemia. *White blood cells*. These are called WBCs and their role is to protect the body against infection and to fight infection. These are bigger than RBCs and about 5500 to 11000 per cubic millilitre of blood. *Platelets* are smallest type of blood cells and are more numerous than WBC about 250,000 per cubic ml of blood. These have role in blood clotting.

Blood citrated Blood that has been prevented from clotting by addition of citrate which combines with calcium.

Blood colour index A figure gained by dividing the hemoglobin percentage by the red cell percentage. In most anemias the result is below 1, but in pernicious anemia it is significantly above 1.

Blood culture A laboratory test on serum to determine presence of infection in the blood. It is done to detect circulating microorganism.

Blood disruption When a child is deprived of their main attachment object, whether for short or long term.

Blood doping A practice used to improve athletic performance by removing red blood cells weeks before an event and then reinfusing them just before competition to increase the oxygen-carrying capacity of the blood.

Blood filters Devices for removing microaggregaties during blood transfusions.

Blood function Blood transports O_2 from the tissues to the lungs. It transports substances absorbed from the intestines to the tissues. It transports metabolic waste products to the organs of excretion. It transports hormones and vitamins which are chemical regulators of metabolic process. It maintains acid-base equilibrium of body. It contains agglutinins, precipitins and antitoxins which combat toxic agents.

Blood groups Landsteiner found 4 groups of blood A, B, AB and O. The most common of the ABO group is 'O' followed by A, then B and finally AB. 'O' group is a universal donor and AB is a universal recipient. Another blood group system, i.e. Rh factor was discovered in 1940 during experiments in Rhesus monkeys. This factor is found in 85 per cent people and is known as Rh positive and rest are Rh negative. Transfusion of Rh-positive blood into an Rh-negative patient causes serious reaction. With the help of ABO group it can be established that a particular man is not the father of the child. But it cannot be shown positively that a particular man is the father by blood grouping.

Blood incompatibility This is due to mismatched blood transfusion. The incompatibility reaction produces immediate symptoms. There will develop shivering of body, rise in body temperature, pain in lumbar region, nausea and vomiting. Late symptoms are jaundice and oliguria.

Blood islands Clusters of mesodermal cells on the outer surface of the yolk sac that differentiate into the first blood cells.

Blood plasma The liquid portion of the blood, free of its formed elements and particles.

Blood pressure It is the pressure within the artery and is measured by sphygmomanometer in millimetres of mercury. It is recorded as systolic when ventricular contraction sends more blood into arteries and diastolic the lowest when the heart is in the phase of relaxation. The normal range of BP is 110 to 130 systolic and 70 to 90 mm Hg as diastolic. The readings are affected by emotions, age, posture and disease. In women BP is little lower than man. As age advances BP rises. The difference between systolic and diastolic readings is pulse pressure and is 30 to 50 mm Hg.

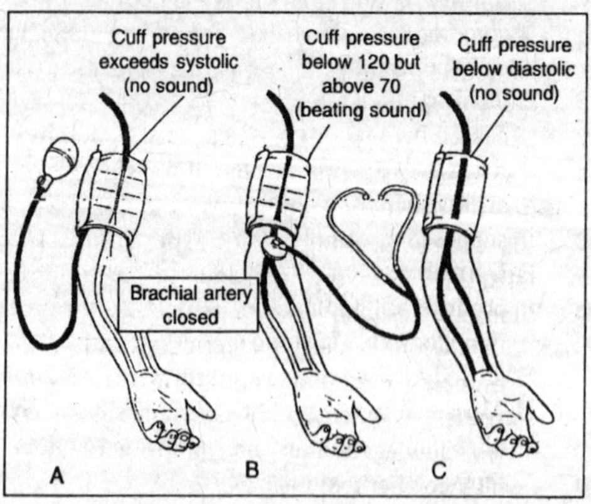

Blood pressure gradient The difference between two blood pressures in the body.

Blood smear A thin blood smear can be prepared by taking a drop of blood on a grease free slide

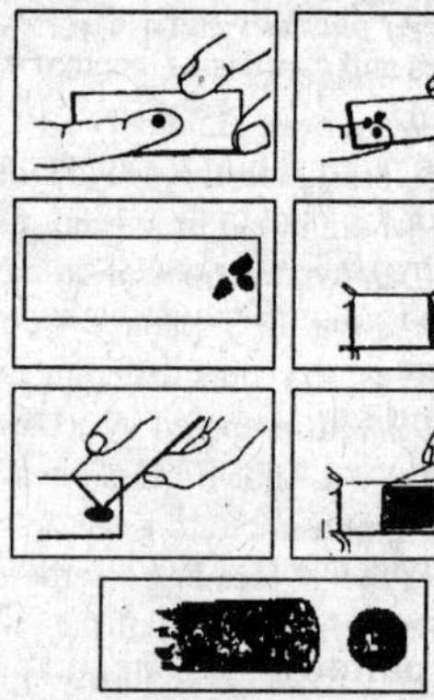

Preparation of thick and thin smear

and spreading it evenly across the slide by means of a smooth edged spreader. For RBC morphology or differential count a thin smear is required.

Blood storage Viability of red cells is defined as at least 70% survival 24 hours after transfusion. During storage following occurs. Lactic acid increases and pH is reduced as low as 6.7-7.0. Increased potassium ion concentration up to 30 mmoL/Liter can be seen. Reduced ATP and glucose consumption occurs.

Blood transfusion Blood transfusion is done to compensate the loss of blood or to correct anaemia. It may also be required after internal bleeding. Thalassaemia requires frequent transfusion. In an exchange transfusion nearly whole of recipient blood is replaced by blood of donor. Before transfusion blood must be crossmatched to ensure compatibility. In it recipient's blood is taken, blood group is identified and is matched with suitable donor's blood. It can be done in less than one hour. Blood is transfused in arm vein. Usually 300 ml blood is transfused between 2 and 3 hours. If blood is not properly matched it may result in shock and kidney failure. In elderly people it can overload the system.

Blood type Blood groups indentified by genetically determined antigens on the surface of red blood cells. The different types of blood that are identified by certain antigens in red blood cells (A,B, AB, O, and Rh-negative or Rh-positive).

Blood typing Identification of genetically detrermined antigens on the surface of the red blood cell, used to determine a person's blood group.

Blood vessels These include arteries, arterioles, veins, venules and capillaries through which blood is transported.

Blood volume Normal blood volume may be taken as 85 ml/kg or 7.7 % of body weight. These values are lowered by 10 % in elderly patient. About half of total blood volume is contained by systemic venous system.

Blood warming coil Device constructed of coiled plastic tubing used to warm reserve blood before massive transfusion.

Bloodstain Evidence that liquid blood has come into contact with a surface.

Bloodstain pattern The categorization of an observed distribution of blood and bloodstains at a crime scene into characteristic patterns. The patterns then can be assigned to probable causes, time sequences, number of events and approximate points of origin to assist reconstruction of events.

Blood-testis barrier (BTB) A barrier formed by Sertoli cells that prevents an immune response against antigens produced by spermatogenic cells by isolating the cells from the blood.

Bloody show Mixture of cervical mucus and blood from ruptured capillaries in the cervix. Bloody show often preceedes labor and increased with cervical dilation.

Bloom's syndrome An autosomal recessive disorder associated with telangiectatic butterfly erythematous areas on face and sometimes on forearm and hand, and primordial dwarfism.

Bluck's fascia The fasical support structure of the deep structures of the penis.

Blue baby Due to lack of O_2 new-born can be cyanotic, or looking blue may be due to congenital mitral stenosis. Surgery can correct such defects.

Blue dot cataract It is also known as punctate cataract. The spots are multiple and scattered all over the lens. Under slit-lamp beam these appear as tiny blue dots. Sometimes these dots get crowded in the Y-sutures. These do not disturb the vision and are of no significance.

Blue naevus It is a special type of intradermal naevus. It is flat, or slightly raised, hairless lesion. Surface is smooth and shiny colour is uniform and varies from blue to bluish black. These are commonly seen over face, dorsum of hand and foot and buttocks. Microscopically the cells are elongated, star shaped having dendrites. The cells are melanin containing and situated deep in dermis in strap-like manner or in whorls. Epidermis itself is normal. It is a benign lesion but may undergo malignant change in its intradermal portion.

Blue sclera Normal sclera is white and opaque. Thinning of sclera allows the underlying uveal tissue to be seen therefore sclera appears blue in colour. In normal infants sclera may be seen as blue. It may be noted in keratoconus and keratoglobus. Blue sclera is seen in osteogenesis inperfecta and Marfan's syndrome. Treatment is not required.

Blue value It is an index of free soluble starch.

Blunt affect Lack of emotional expression, affective flattening.

Blunted heart rate response A less than anticipated heart rate for the amount of work being performed; Flat heart rate response.

Blurred vision Vision may be diminished or distorted. It is not double vision. Sometimes part of vision is only affected. After the age of 40 it may be seen that person starts blurring of words while reading and after the age of 45 most people require glasses. Refractive error is the most common cause of blurring vision. It may be myopia or hypermetropia.

Blushing There is reddening of face temporarily caused by dilation of vessels. Some women blush when they see or talk about their boy-friends. It is an involuntary function to embarrassment. It is supposed to be a good quality of girls.

B-Lymphocytes White blood corpuscles which produce antibodies according to directives of T lymphocytes. These are produced in bone marrow.

BMI Body mass index

B-Mode Brightness mode, a two-dimensional ultrasound image display composed of bright dots representing the ultrasound echoes. The brightness of each dot is determined by each amplitude. B-mode image is produced by sweeping a narrow ultrasound beam.

BMR Basal metabolic rate

Board of nursing Regulatory agency that manages the provisions of a state's nurse practice act.

Bobath The main features of bobath technique are :

Reflex inhibitory patterns :- to inhibit abnormal tone assocaited with abnormal movement patterns and abnormal posture.

Sensory motor experience

Facilitation techniques for mature postural reflexes.

Key points of control - for inhibition or facilitation.

Development sequence is followed and adapted to each child.

Bobath method Therapeutic exercises for patients with lesions of CNS.

Bochdalek's gap Lumbocostal trigone.

BOD Biological oxygen demand.

Body Unified and complex assembly of structurally and functionally interactive components.

Body alignment Refers to the condition of joints, tendons, ligaments, and muscles in various body positions.

Body cast Form of a cylinder cast that encircles the trunk of the body instead of an extremity.

Body cavity A space within the body that contains various internal organs.

Body composition Assessment to identify the percentage of the body that is lean tissue and the percentage that is fat.

Body exploration In this act various parts of the partner's body are touched, stroked and manipulated, specially erogenous areas.

Body fat It may be white and brown fat. White fat is most of the fat while brown fat is only in neck and upper part of back. White fat is stored in adipose cells and serves as energy store. Brown fat produces heat instead of chemical energy. Brown fat decreases with age and increases with increased exposure to cold environment. Skin fold thickness can be translated into terms of body fat. Normal fat content is 15% for a male and 19% for female by weight.

Body fluid Body water and its dissolved substances; constitutes about 60% of total body weight.

Body heat balance The steady state relation in which the heat produced by the body equals that lost to environment.

Body image A visual and mental image of one's body that includes feelings about one's body, especially in relation to health and disease.

Body implant That portion of an endosteal implant that is placed within bone.

Body language Nonverbal communication behaviours that are accomplished by the movement of body, by presentation of ourselves to the world and by use of our personal space.

Body mass index Weights in kilogram (Height in meters)^2 Normal values in men range from 20 to 25 and in women 19 to 24. A BMI over 25 is distinct in obesity.

Body mechanics Proper balance of the skeleton by muscular alignment which favours function with the least amount of expended energy; refers to a dynamic position as opposed to posture, which is alignment in a rigid position.

Body mechanisms Study of the static and dynamic human body to note the mechanical integration of the parts, and to endeavor to restore and maintain the body as nearly as possible in normal mechanical condition.

Body odour This is caused by sweat. Sweat itself has no odour but when left over armpit, bacteria ferment and give typical odour. Sweat may also smell after consumption of onion and garlic. Apocrine glands are present in armpits and groin which contains proteins and fatty materials favourable to growth of bacteria. Proper washing and putting dusting powder helps the person.

Body of the sternum The middle segment of the sternum.

Body plethysmograph It is a airtight box which can enclose a human being studied for lung volumes and pressure.

Body plethysmography The measurement and recording of changes in volume usually lung volumes obtained by placing the body in a chamber that surrounds it completely.

Body powered prosthetic device One that is manipulated by the patients remaining group of muscles and not by power.

Body scheme Consciousness of the relative position of body parts; a function of area 40 (inferior parietal lobe). The awareness of the body and the relationship of body parts to one another.

Body segment The area of the body between joints that provides movement during walking and balance.

Body substance barrier Material such as gloves, mask, and isolation gown, that prevent exposure to infected body substances.

Body supports Pillows, folded blankets, foam forms, or commercial products that help contour the flat surface of a massage table or mat.

Body systems approach Collection of data according to the functional systems of the body.

Body temperature The normal temperature by mouth is 36.9°C or 98.4°F ranging from 97.4 to 99°F. In rectum it is one degree higher than mouth. In axilla or groin it is one degree lower than by mouth 97.6°F. Hyperpyrexia is over 40.6°C or 105°F. Moderate fever is 38.3°C-39.4°C or 101-103°F. Low fever is regarded between 37.2-38.3°C or 99-101°F. Subnormal temperature is 35-36°C or 95°-97°F.

Bodymass index Numeric data used to compare a person's size in relation to norms for the adult population.

Bodywork A term that encompasses all the various forms of massage, movement, and other touch therapies.

Boggy Inadequately contracted and having a spongy rather than firm feeling, descriptive of the postdelivery uterus.

Bohler splint A hand splint used for immobilisation of phalangeal fractures.

Bohler's angle In case of calcaneum Bohler's angle help in evaluating depression.

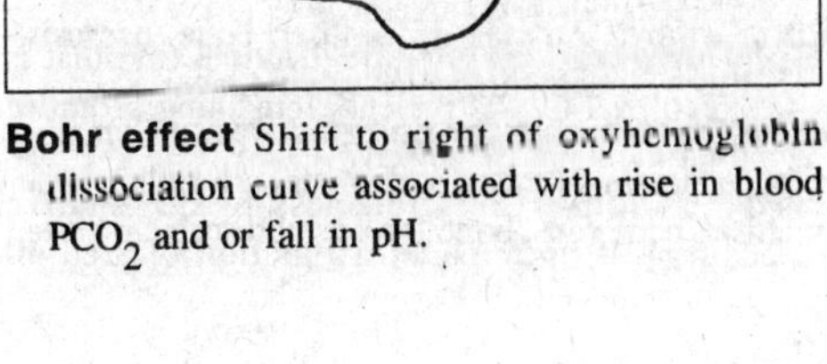

Bohr effect Shift to right of oxyhemoglobin dissociation curve associated with rise in blood PCO_2 and or fall in pH.

Bohr equation It is an equation to derive physiological dead space. Expired CO_2 = inspired CO_2 + CO_2 given out by lungs.

Boil It is an inflamed, pus filled area of skin usually a hair follicle. Armpits, groin and back are the most common sites. Usual cause of boil is infection with *Staphylococcus aureus*. Boil generally starts as a red, painful lump. As time passes it fills with pus and becomes rounded with a yellowish tip. In case of diabetes these generally do not heal automatically. Antibiotics are effective otherwise surgically, it can be drained easily. It is an acute staphylococcal infection of a hair follicle with suppuration and central necrosis. There develops a painful and indurated swelling. It gradually extends. After 2 days centre softens discharging pus. A blind boil is one which subsides without suppurations. Boil may result in a sinus or fistula.

Bologna cast Plaster cast application in which generous amounts of cotton padding are applied to the limb and then compressed to achieve appropriate tension.

Bolognini's symptom It represents a feeling of crepitation occurring from gradual increasing pressure on the abdomen, and is seen in cases of measles.

Bolt A metallic device used in internal fixation.

Bolus A moistend mass of food that is swallowed from the oral cavity into the pharynx.

Bolus administration Undiluted medication given fairly quickly in a vein.

Bolus dose Larger dose of drug administered initially or when pain is intense.

Bolus feeding Instillation of liquid nourishment four to six times a day in less than 30 minutes.

Bomb calorimeter It is an apparatus measuring calories stored in food or any organic material. The apparatus is insulated throughly against loss of heat and the amount of heat produced by the change in temperature of a measured amount of water on electrical charge.

Bonafide In good faith; openly, honestly, or innocently; without knowledge of fraud; without fraudulent intent.

Bond energy The energy required to break a bond.

Bonding 1. Adhesion of orthodonitic attachments to the teeth without use of an interposed band or the adhesion of a restorative, such as composite material, to the tooth. The etched enamle provides a slightly porous surface for the bonding material to adhere. The composite resin material then adheres to the bonded resin.

Bonding Forming a relationship The term is sometimes used synonymously with 'attachment' but in this book has been reserved to refer to the early relationship between very young infants and their caregivers, as well as the relationship between some non-human young and their caregivers.

Bone It forms the skeleton of body. Bone is composed of calcium and phosphorus making it hard. The surface of bone is covered with periosteum. Periosteum contains a network of blood and nerves. Beneath the periosteum is hard, dense shell of compact or ivory bone. Inside this is cancellous and spongy part. The growth of bones is a balance between the activity of its two constitutents, osteoblasts and osteoclasts. Osteoblasts encourage the deposit of the mineral calcium phosphate on the protein framework of the bone. Osteoclasts remove minerals from bone. Actions of these are controlled by growth hormone secreted by pituitary gland, oestrogen and testosterone. Most bones develop in fifth or sixth week of pregnancy. This cartilage begins to be replaced by hard bone. At birth many bones consist mainly of cartilage which will ossify later on. There are 206 bones in body. It represents a form of connective tissue comprising a matrix of strands of collagen permeated by calcium salts. Outer portion of bone is hardest known as periosteum. Growth of bones is controlled by growth hormone.

Bone age The age of patient based on the degree of skeletal maturation.

Bone bank A place in which homogenous bone is preserved and stored for use as allograft.

Bone block A segment of bone that is surgically transposed to create bony impingement and thus block motion at a joint.

Bone broth Prepared by prolonged boiling of chopped bones.

Bone chips Small pieces of cancellous bone generally used to fill in bony defects and to precipitate recalcification.

Bone cyst It is a cavity of bone usually filled with fluid. It typically develops at one end of a long bone and is diagnosed accidentally being

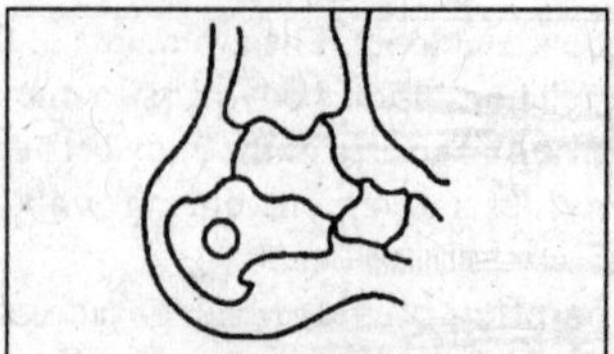

Bone cyst

asymptomatic. Generally when pathological fracture develops it comes to notice on X-ray. Minor operation of scrapping the cyst and filling with bone chips is helpful.

Bone Enhancement Any procedure that increases the volume of available bone, including grafting, nerve respositioning, ridge expansion, and distraction osteogenesis.

Bone graft It is an operation in which a small piece of bone is taken from one part of the body to repair bone damage in other part. Bone graft is attached to the defective bone and provides bone growth stimulating hormone/protein. Bone graft ultimately dies but it acts as scaffold upon which new bone can grow. A bone graft has four main uses, to encourage a fracture to heal, to restore bone lost through injury, to replace bone removed surgically because of disease and to provide a peg to join the bones of a diseased or unstable joint. It may be used for cosmetic purpose too. The most common source of bone is iliac crest because it contains a large amount of cancellous bone which helps graft to be 'taken'. Other sources are ribs and ulna. The wound heals within a week or two.

Bone grafting Transplanting bone tissue from one part of the body to another.

Bone holding forceps A device for holding a bone.

Bone imaging X-ray shows bone structures clearly. So it is best for diagnosing fractures and tumours. CT is still better. MRI is better for lumbar spine and disc pathology. Radionuclide scanning is able to reveal bone function, the rate of blood flow to the bone and of cell activity within it. It helps in diagnosing the spread of cancer to bone.

Bone infarct An area of localised bone necrosis. X-Ray will show irregular calcification.

Bone instruments for dental surgery Common bone instruments used in dentistry are mallet, bone chisel, bone files, bone forceps and surgical burrs.

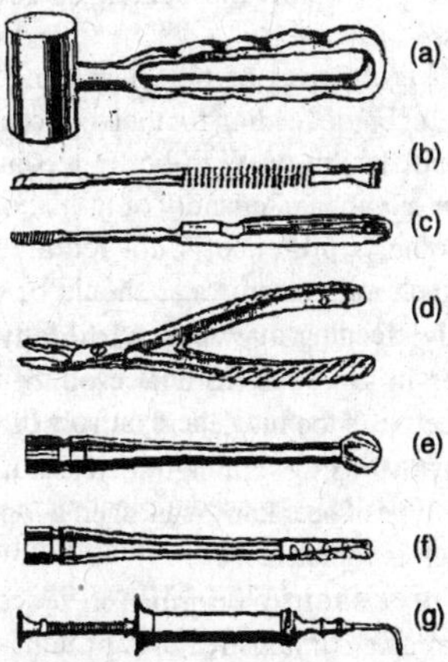

Bone instruments :
(a) Mallet (b) Bone chisel
(c) Bone file (d) Bone forceps
(e) Surgical burrs (f) Hunt syringe

Bone islands An asymptomatic bone lesion noted as sclerotic density.

Bone lamella Bone having the appearance of layers of thin leaves or plates produces by the lines that represent periods of inactivity of bone formation.

Bone loss Dental X-ray shows the dental professional to view the amount of bone remaining rather than the bone lost. The amount of bone loss can be estimated a difference between physiological bone level and height of remaining bone.

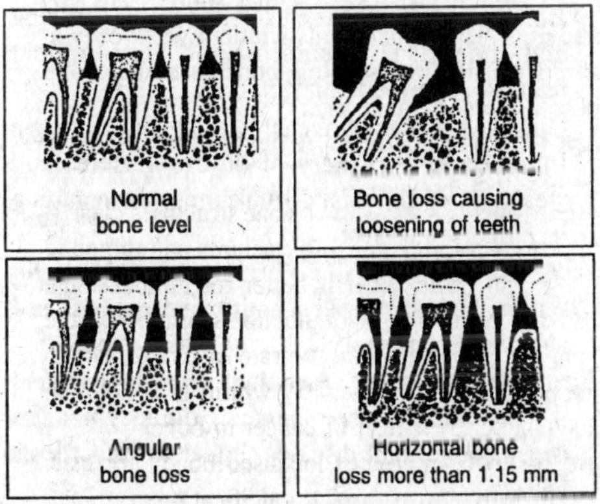

Bone marrow It may be red or yellow. Red bone marrow is blood producing tissue present in all bones. During teens, it is gradually replaced in some bones by less active yellow marrow. In the adult, red marrow is confined chiefly to spine, sternum, ribs, clavicle, scapulae and skull bones. Red bone marrow produces red blood cells. The blood cells go through various stages of maturation in red bone marrow before being relieved in circulation. Yellow marrow produces the white cells but is composed mainly of fat and connective tissue. In aplastic anaemia marrow fails to produce normal amount of blood cells. It may overproduce certain blood cells in polycythaemia and leukaemia.

Bone marrow aspiration It is a technique of obtaining semisolid bone marrow tissue for histologic and histochemical examination. Marrow aspirations can also be cultured for bacteria and fungi and used for chromosome studies. Preferred site for marrow aspirations is posterior iliac crest. Sternal marrow aspiration bears risk. It is done to define mechanism of anaemia, thrombocytopenia, dysproteinaemia, and leukaemia. It can be done in Hodgkin's lymphoma.

Bone marrow biopsy It is a way to obtain sample of cells from the bone marrow. It is useful in the diagnosis of many blood disorders, including anaemia, leukaemia, bone marrow failure and certain infections. Trephine biopsy requires a long, thick needle for removal of bone core. Bone marrow biopsy may be performed repeatedly to monitor the response of a disease to treatment.

Bone marrow harvest Taking of bone marrow for transplantation.

Bone marrow transplant In this, bone marrow replaces malignant or defective marrow in patient. Healthy bone marrow is taken from donor who has similar tissue, usually brother or sister. Being risky it is done only in fetal blood and immune disorders, i.e. severe aplastic anaemia, leukaemia, etc. Infection is a common complication.

Bone marrow transplantation Procedure to replace diseased marrow or to reconstitute marrow following high-dose chemoradiotherapy to eradicate malignancies.

Bone meal Prepared from degreased animal bones and used as supplement of calcium and phosphate.

Bone mineral densitometry A variety of non-invasive techniques are available to measure bone mass. Current equipment in nuclear medicine uses a dual energy X-ray absorptiometer. The patient lies compfortably on the scanning couch and machine is able to offer a choice of skeletal site for assessment. Osteoporosis is the main indication, since reduced bone mineral density is an important factor in the consideration of fracture risk.

Bone palantine Forms the hard palate.

Bone punch It is used to cut the bone during dacryocystorhinostomy operation.

Bone swaging Lateral displacement of alveolar bone into an adjacent vertical bony defect.

Bone wax A refined bee's wax used to stop bleeding.

Bony labyrinth A series of chambers within the pertous part of the temporal bone associated with

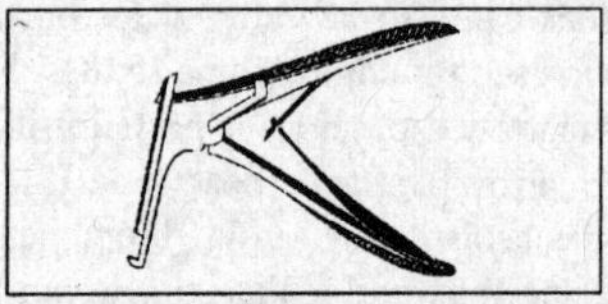

the vestibular organs and the cochlea. The bony labyrinth contains a fluid called perilymph.

Boot A high quarter shoe in which the quarters covers the malleoli to any point up to hip.

Boot top fracture A transverse fracture of the distal 1/3 of the tibia.

Booth test The clinical examination to assess the inegrity of the transverse humeral ligament.

Borax Sodium salt of boric acid.

Borborygmus Audible abdominal sound produced by hyperactive intestinal peristalsis.

Border molding Shaping of an impression material by the manipulation or action of the tissues adjacent to the borders of an impression.

Borg scale A numerial scale of 1 to 10 (or sometimes 6 to 20) for the rating of perceived exertion of exercise.

Borrowed Servant An employee temporarily under the control of another.

Boss A rounded or knoblike protuberance from the surface of bone.

Bosworth fracture Fracture and dislocation of ankle with entrapment of fibula behind the tibia.

Bosworth screw A screw designed for the internal fixation of the clavicle to the base of coracoid.

Botallo's duct and ligament Ductus arteriosus and ligamentum arteriosum.

Bothrium A groove on the scolex of some of tapeworms.

Bottle feeding Instead of breast feeding some females prefer bottle feeding for their convenience, certainty and flexibility. With bottle feeding one can monitor quality and quantity of milk. For such feeding mother's presence is not required. For preparing such milk clean water should be boiled properly. Overfeeding may make child fatty.

Bottom filler In shoe, the material used for filling the cavity between the insole and outsole of shoes.

Bottom-fermenting Describing the yeasts used to produce the type of beer known as lager, as opposed to ale which is topfermented.

Bottom-up processing Information processing guided by simple stimulus features of units rather than by a person's general knowledge, beliefs or expectations.

Botulin toxin A toxin, associated with food poisoning, that blocks the release of acetylcholine from the synapse. Clinically it is used to block unwanted activity in muscles.

Botulism The paralytic illness is due to toxin producing organism which may be consumed along with food. It is the most lethal toxin. It readily crosses the gut mucosa, is taken up by synaptosomes and is then transmitted to neurons. Muscle fibres are easily denervated and toxin binding is irreversible. Recovery takes a longer time.

Botulism in adults presents with nausea, vomiting and abdominal discomfort and neurological features soon predominate.

Cranial nerves are affected with ophthalmoplegia followed by weakness of bulbar muscles and weakness of limbs and trunk muscles including respiratory muscles.

Mental state remains normal and there is no sensory signs. Polyvalent antitoxin should be used alongwith respiratory and circulatory support.

Bouchard's nodes Osteophyte formation around the proximal interphalangeal joints typical of degenerative joint disease; similar to Heberden's nodes.

Boundary Personal space that exists within an arms's length perimeter. Personal emotional space is designated by morals, values, and experience.

Bounding Pulse A pulse that is difficult to obliterate; usually owing to high blood volume within a vessel; artery has a feeling of tension on palpation.

Boutonniere deformity Finger deformity with flexion of the proximal interphalangeal joint and hyperestension of the distal interphalangeal joint. Rupture, avulsion or laceration of the central extensor slip results in a boutonniere deformity. Finger adopts the posture of flexion of the PIP joint and hyperextension of DIP joint. Loss of continuity of central slip allows stretching of the triangular ligament. There will be pain and swelling. Conservative treatment is used for closed injuries to the tendon and small avulsion fractures.

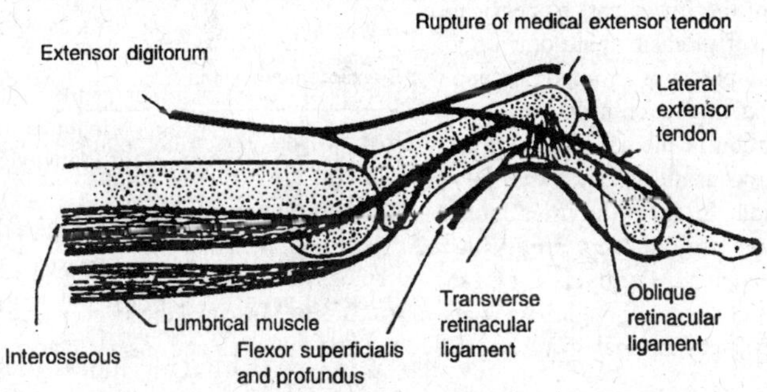

Boutonniere deformity

Bow legs It is known as genu varum in which lower legs bow inward resulting in the knees being separated when ankles are touching. Bowing is most common in tibia. One or both legs can be affected. It is corrected naturally by the age of three. If no braces have to be used, this structural deformity is frequently accompanied by compensatory deformities in feet.

Bow sign X-Ray indicative of severe spondylolisthesis, usually of L5—S1. In AP view of density that gives the appearance of a bow with its convex surface downwards.

Bow string sign A sign elicited on examining for radiculopathy.

Bowel incontinence Inability to voluntarily control the passage of feces and gas.

Bower's disease It may occur in genital region above the age of 35. In males it is seen as a thickened, grey white plaques over the shaft of the penis. Microscopic features include marked epithelial atypia with complete loss of normal surface maturation.

Bowing fracture A traumatic injury seen in growing bones in which bone is deformed beyond full elastic recoil.

Bowleg Genu varum.

Bowler's thumb A perineural fibrosis of the ulnar digital nerve of the thumb caused by repetitive compression which occurs while grasping of bowling ball.

There will be tingling and hyperesthesia around pulp space of thumb.

Bowman's capsule The enlarged end of the nephron; Bowman's capsule and the glomerulus make up the renal corpuscle.

Box toe A tip of shoe. A stiffener is used to maintain the shape of a shoe toe.

Boxer fracture These are common fractures which occur after striking a closed fist. The head of metacarpal is forced into flexion. Crape bandage is to be applied. Fracture of the neck of the fifth metacarpal associated with volar displacemnet of metacarpal head.

Boxing The building of vertical walls, usually of wax, around an impression to produce the desired size and form of the base of cast.

Boxing (an impression) Enclosure of an impression by the building up of vertical walls to produce the desired size and form of the base of the cast. It also preserve certain details of the impression.

Boyd & Anderson technique It is a method used to attach distal rupture of biceps tendon.

Boyd sisk procedure A surgical technique for the repair of recurrent posterior shoulder dislocation.

BPH Benign prostatic hyperplasia.

Brace Is an orthopaedic appliance or apparatus used to support, align or hold parts of the body in a correct position.

Brachalgia Nerve rood pain in upper limb.

Brachial Pertaining to the arm.

Brachial plexus It is a collection of large nerve trunks that pass from the lower part of cervical spine and upper part of thoracic spine down the arm. Injury to brachial plexus is an important and common cause of partial or complete loss of movement and sensation in the arm. Damage of brachial plexus may occur during birth specially in breech presentation. In severe injuries, both upper and lower roots are damaged producing complete paralysis of arm. Paralysis may be temporary if tear is not severe enough. Brachial plexus can also be affected by cervical rib infections or tumours.

Brachial artery It is the continuation of axillary artery from lower border of teres minor to antecubital fossa where it divides into radial and ulnar artery.

Brachial palsy during delivery This injury is usually unilateral. When it is bilateral cord injury should be suspected. Erb's palsy is commonest type. Hands hangs passively.

Brachial plexus A network of nerve axons of the anterior rami of spinal nerves C5, C6, C7, C8 and T1. The nerves that emerge from the brachial plexus supply the upper limb.

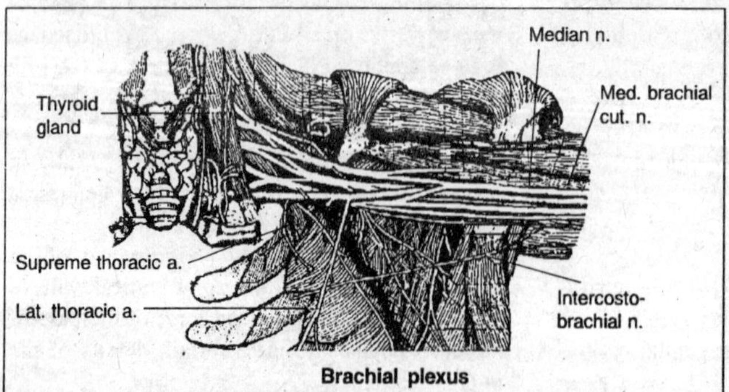

Brachial plexus

Brachial plexus block Regional anesthesia of arm, fore arm and hand given as supraclavicular or axillary injection.

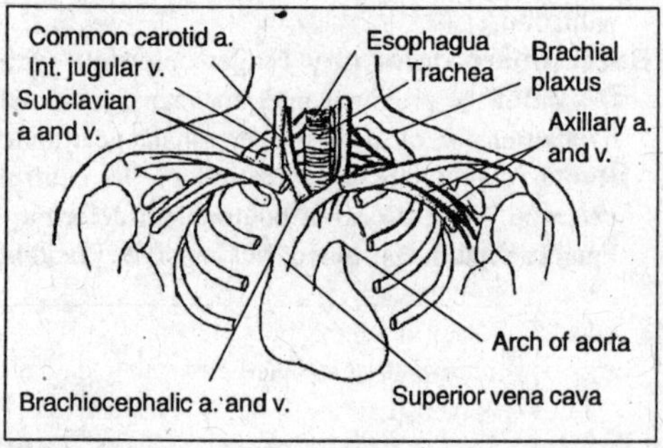

Brachialgia Person complains of pain or stiffness in arm. It is often accompanied by pain, tingling or numbness of hands and finger. There is weakness of hand grip. Underlying disease may be of frozen shoulder or cervical osteoarthritis.

Brachialis Muscle of the anterior arm that originates on the humerus and inserts onto the ulna; flexes the forearm.

Brachy pelvis Oval type of pelvis.

Brachygnathia Marked underdevelopment of mandible.

Bracket Small metal attachment fixed to a band for the purpose of fastening the archwire to the orthodontic band.

Bradform frame A canvas bed suspended from rectangular poles that have an opening for the buttocks. It allows bed pan placement.

Bradycardia In this condition heart rate is below 60 beats per minute, Many people who exercise regularly and vigorously and in athletes pulse rate is lowered. Although person is normal while in myxoedema or heart block or betablockers may also result in bradycardia. Sudden lowering of pulse may cause fatigue.

Bradykinesia Abnormal slowness of movement; sluggishness of physical and mental responses.

Bradykinins Short polypeptides that stimulate vasodilation and other cardiovascular changes.

Bradyphagia Eating very slowly.

Bradypnea Breathing that is normal in rate but abnormally slow (less than 12 breaths per minute).

Bradyzoite In Toxoplasma, the slowly dividing, infectious, asexual stage found within tissue cysts in the intermediate host.

Bragard's sign Test for presence of lumbosacral radiculopathy.

Braille It is embossed dots that enables blind people to read and write. It was developed in France by Louis Braille. It is based on six raised dots which can be arranged in different combinations to form 68 symbols. There are two grades. In grade I each symbol represents individual letter or punctuation while in grade II symbol represents words.

Brain It controls body's functions and is organ of speech, thought and emotions. Brain and spinal cord constitute central nervous system and controls basic functions such as heart beat, breathing, temperature, etc. Brain interprets sensations from nerves extending from CNS to different parts of body. The nerve pathways that control internal body functions such as heart rate, sweating, temperature, digestion are called autonomic nervous system. In somatic nervous system nerve pathway carries sensations to brain from sense organs and message from brain to muscle to act. *Brainstem* and *cerebellum* are concerned with control of vital functions, i.e. breathing, maintenance of blood pressure and cerebellum with muscular coordination and posture.

Cerebrum consists of two hemispheres and constitutes 70 per cent of weight of total nervous system. Certain of sulci and gyri are noticeable and divide into distinct occipital, parietal, temporal and frontal lobes. It consists of grey matter with nerve cells arranged in 6 layers. It has centres for thought, movement and sensations. Beneath the cortex there is white matter of nerve fibres. Deeper within hemispheres are basal ganglia. Some higher centres of speech and writing are controlled from one dominant cerebral hemisphere. In right handed people this is left hemisphere. The whole of brain and spinal cord is encased in three layers of meninges. CSF flows between two of these layers. Brain supply is from circle of Willis supplied by carotid arteries.

Brain abscess Abscess may arise through direct extension of infection in middle ear or mastoid cavity or in paranasal sinuses. Haematogeneous infection occurs as a result of metastatic infection from elsewhere in body. Clinical features include seizures, altered consciousness and focal neurological signs depending on location. Abscesses are easily seen on CT and MRI. Surgical excision or resection/aspiration are the methods available. Abscesses secondary to sinus infection respond very well to penicillin.

Brain attack Stroke.

Bain bridge reflex Reflex tachycardia following rapid infusion of fluid and increasing venous return.

Brain contusions It may develop directly at the impact point or countercoup to the injury. These are mostly found under the depressed fracture. Cerebral gyral crests are bruised by jagged-edged bones in the skull base. Bilateral contusions are asymmetrical. Patient with small cerebral contusions may present with focal deficit with normal consciousness. It develops immediately following injury. On CT haemorrhagic contusions appear as heterogeneous hyperdense lesions. These are surrounded by irregular hypodense mass.

Brain electrical activity mapping (BEAM) Computer-enhanced analysis and display of electroencephalographic and evoked response studies. In evoked response studies, a stimulus (e.g. flashing light) is presented to the patient and the responses are recorded electrically from scalp electrodes. Computers translate the information into a topographic, coloured display of electrical activity over the surface of the brain. Useful in diagnosing seizure disorders and seems to be helpful in looking at atypical psychiatric presentations.

Brain haemorrhage It is bleeding within or around the brain caused due to trauma or spontaneous rupture of blood vessels. These are of 4 types : subdural haemorrhage, extradural haemorrhage, subarachnoid haemorrhage and intracerebral haemorrhage. *Extradual* and *subdural haemorrhages* generally result from a blow to head. It may result in headache, drowsiness, confusion and even paralysis of one side. *Subarachnoid* and *intracerebral* haemorrhages occur spontaneously and generally results due to rupture of aneurysm or due to hypertension.

Brain imaging Conventional X-ray is not of much use. It gives information about skull erosion, fracture and calcification due to disease. CT introduced in 1971 gives clear picture of the ventricles and can reveal tumours, blood clots well. Contrast studies are also possible. MRI is latest and does not give radiation and gives clearcut and detailed information. Radionuclide scanning uses radioactive isotopes to detect tumours but is not very informative in comparison to MRI. Ultrasound is used in pregnancy or in very young babies. Any technique that permits the *invivo* visualisation of the substance of the central nervous system. The best known of such techniques is computerised axial tomography (CAT), commonly called the CAT scan. However, two newer methods of brain imaging, positron-emission tomography (PET) and magnetic resonance imaging (MRI), are based on different physical principles but also yield a series of two-dimensional images (or slices) of brain regions of interest. A number of other related techniques, such as ultrasound, angiography in its various forms, radionuclide scans, regional cerebral blood flow (RCBF) measurements, brain electrical activity mapping (BEAM) and its variants, and even the older pneumoen-cephalogram (PEG) also provide images of some aspects of the central nervous system, but are generally more limited in the structures visualised or degree of resolution, or some other parameter, than CT, PET, and MRI.

Brain localisation The effort to identify mental and behavioural functions related to certain areas of the brain, such as mapping the sensory and motor areas adjacent to the central fissure.

Brain plasticity The ability of the brain to change its structure in response to experience, drugs, hormones, or injury.

Brain syndrome There is a disturbance of consciousness, intellect or mental functioning of organic origin and not psychological. Cause is degenerative, metabolic or infection, trauma or stroke. Symptoms include from confusion to coma, restlessness and disorientation. Hallucinations and delusion can also be seen.

Brain topography Surface of brain is generally divided into four lobes, termed frontal, temporal, parietal and occipital. Each surface is folded and convoluted and each ridge is called a gyrus and each groove is called a sulcus. Central sulcus divides frontal and parietal lobes.

Fissure of Sylvius divides temporal and frontal or parietal lobes.

Brain tumour Brain tumours may be primary arising from tissue or metastasis from lung and breast.

About 60 per cent are gliomas. Symptoms include muscle weakness, loss of vision or other sensory disturbances, speech difficulties and epileptic fits. MRI is a better tool for diagnosis.

Brain wave in orgasm During orgasm brain waves are unique and dont occur with other types of activities. People find orgasmic experience difficult

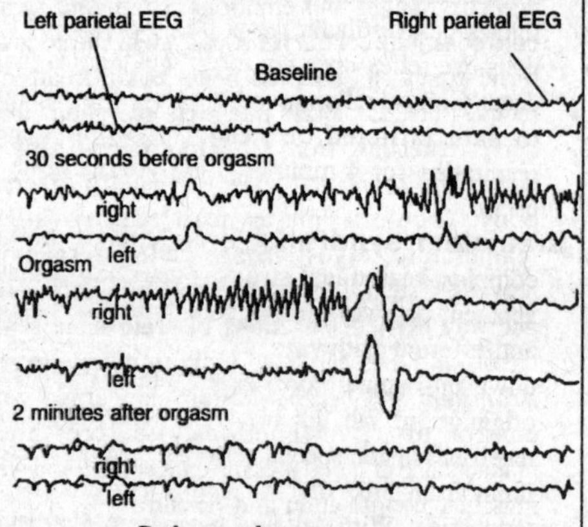

Brain wave in orgasm

to describe. The slowing of brain wave cycles and increased in amplitude indicates its emotional intutive character.

Brain waves Electrical activity produced as a result of action potentials of brain neurons.

Brain-derived neurotrophic factor (BDNF) A 'nourishing' factor that promotes survival and normal functioning of cortical neurons.

Brainstem The brainstem consists of three main parts, called medulla, pons and mid brain. *Medulla* resembles a thick extension of spinal cord. It contains 9th to 12th cranial nerves and thus relays taste sensations from tongue. It also contains nerve cells involved in heart beat, breathing, blood pressure. *Pons* contains thick bundles of nerve fibres connecting with cerebellum. Pons contains nuclei of fifth to eighth nerves and relays sensory information from ear, face and teeth. It is responsible for facial expression. *Mid brain* is the smallest section of brainstem. It contains nucleus of 3rd and 4th cranial nerves which control eye movements and size of pupil of eye. It also coordinates limb movements. Damage to medulla may cause immediate death while damage to reticular system may cause coma. Degeneration to mid brain causes parkinsonism. Damage to specific cranial nerve can have specific effect, i.e. facial palsy in 7th cranial nerve, tongue wasting in 12th cranial nerve.

Brainstem death It was clinically described in 1959. For this diagnosis all signs should be present for at least 12 hours. Pupils have no response to light. Oculovestibular reflex becomes absent. The dolls-eye reflex does not mean that there is brain death. Corneal reflex becomes absent. No response to pain inflicted on head. No spontaneous respiration for 4 minutes. EEG confirmation is useful.

Brainstem syndrome Brainstem is highly complex anatomical structure carrying somatic apparent pathways from spinal cord to thalamus and efferent pathways from cerebral peduncle down into spinal cord. Brainstem is the site of origin of 3rd, 7th, 9th and 12th cranial nerves and receives somatic special sense or visceral afferent input from 5th, 7th, 8th and 9th cranial nerve territories. With all this brainstem syndrome produces complex neurological symptoms.

Brainstem tumour Sign of increased cranial tension are present. Reflexes in lower limbs are exaggerated. Pontine tumours affect the 6th and 7th cranial nerves. Cerebellar dysfunction is often present. Surgical excision is very difficult.

Brainwashing A pattern of interrogation and indoctrination. It is a persuation which allegedly radically alters beliefs against the will of the individual.

Bran Outer layer of cereal bran.

Branched-chain amino acids (BCAA) Leucine, isoleucine, and valine.

Branchial cyst It is circumscribed movable swelling on the lateral side of neck. 10 to 20 per cent may be at the angle of mandible between the age of 20-40 years of age. It arises from epithelial inclusions within the cervical lymph nodes. Under microscope study shows that branchial cysts are usually lined by stratified squamous epithelium and are surrounded by lymphoid tissue. If aspirated or drained, branchial cysts recur. Excision is the treatment of choice.

Branching programme An approach to programming in education which includes detours for the purposes of remediation. The learner who misses a series of frames takes a branch or detour, involving extra frames, to gain the necessary knowledge or skill to complete the rest of the programme.

Branchiofaciolingual Pertaining to or affecting the arm, the face, and the tongue.

Brand slipper sock test A method for semiquantitative dyanamic pressure assessment inside a shoe.

Brandy A spirit distilled from wine.

Braxton Hicks contractions Uterine contractions, occurring periodically during pregnancy, thereby enlarging the uterus to accommodate the growing fetus. During the third trimester, they are felt as a painless hardening or tightening of the uterus. They can become painful and are often difficult to differentiate from labour. Also called BH sign. This sign appears at about 28th week of pregnancy or earlier as painless, irregular, brief uterine contractions and pressure which disappear on walking or exercises. It is a normal phenomenon of pregnancy.

Breach of contract Failing to comply with the terms of a contract. A branch can occur through failing to comply at all, through incomplete compliance, or through untimely compliance.

Bread Usually refers to a loaf made from wheat or mixture of many cereals.

Bread lactein Loaf with added milk usually 6% milk.

Break To interrupt the continuity, or an interruption in the continuity of a structure, especially bone.

Break through pain Intermittent episodes of pain despite continued use of analgesics.

Breakbone fever An arbovirus-caused disease.

Breast Female breast produces milk for child and has secondary sexual characteristic too. Female breast contains 15 to 20 lobes of milk secreting glands. These have outlet in nipple. The breast

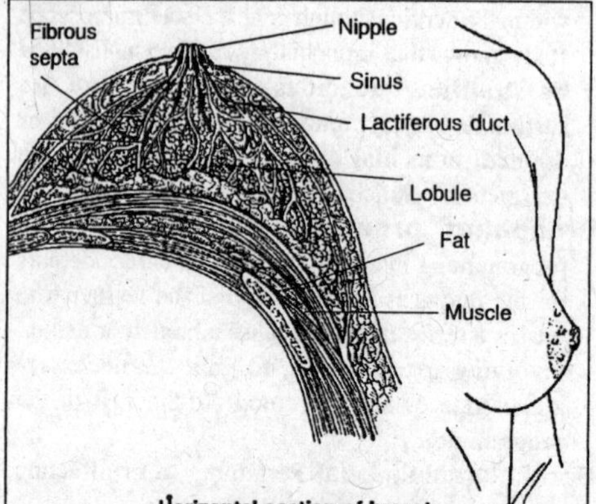

Horizontal section of breast

contains no muscles. Actually these are modified sweat glands. At birth there is a nipple with rudimentary milk ducts. At puberty due to hormonal effect it starts developing. Areola swells and nipple enlarges.

Breast bone The sternum

Breast cancer The incidence of breast cancer is known to be raised who started menses at an early age. No definite cause has been proved. The most common site is upper and outer part of breast. Lump is felt than seen. In some nipples may be retracted. Ladies should examine their breast while taking bath, as soon as they feel lump they should consult doctor. Now this cancer is having better prognosis. Excision of lump, breast, lymph glands + radiotherapy and chemotherapy help.

Breast changes during pregnancy Increased vascularity, sensation of heaviness and pain appear as early as six weeks. By 8 weeks nipple and areola becomes dark. Secondary areola develops after 16 weeks. Montgomery's tubercles due to enlarged sebaceous glands becomes prominent at 8th week. Clear fluid can be expressed during 20 weeks.

In first pregnancy whole gland increases in size and undergoes a true hypertrophy. It affects not only glandular acini but also the connective tissue. When hypertrophy is well marked clear pale yellow secretion can usually be expressed. Nipple and primary areola become more deeply pigmented. Areola becomes more prominent. An increased vascular supply is indicated by dilated veins under the skin. The breasts can become engorged with blood and secretion makes them swollen and painful.

Breast duct A mainframe tubular structure of the glandular component of the breast tissue.

Breast feeding This is the natural way of feeding the child. It contains well-balanced food having protective quality. It has antibodies against gastroenteritis. After delivery child may be put on breast immediately. It gives physical closeness and strengthen the bond. Once child has started sucking, mother should give whole of areola in his or her mouth. This helps to stimulate flow and child will not bite the nipple causing cracks. Baby should be allowed to suck for a few minutes at a time. Engorged breasts may be uncomfortable to mother on occasions. Manual expression of breast milk is advised. Proper care should be taken of cracked nipples.

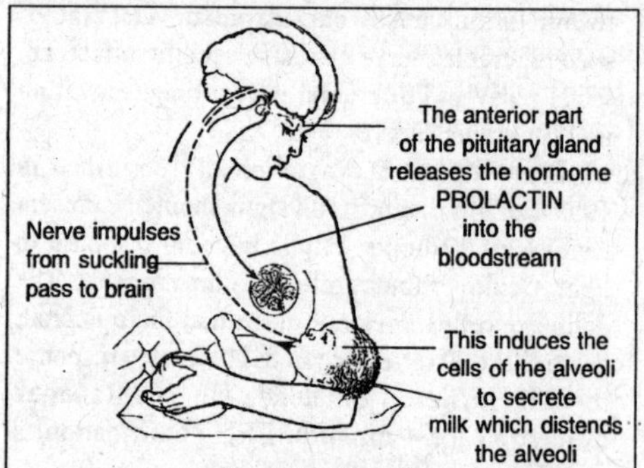

The prolactin reflex

Breast lump This is a mass which can be felt in breast. About 80 per cent lumps are benign. Most common is fibrocystic disease or fibroadenosis. In it one or more cysts and thickening of milk glands develop. In young women common lump is mostly fibroadenoma. It is a benign growth and is usually round, firm and rubbery. It is painless and is not attached to skin. It moves freely. A lipoma is a benign, painless tumour, made of fatty tissue changing the size and shape of breast. Intraductal papilloma is a wart-like growth and there is discharge.

Breast milk It is the ideal food for babies. It is fresh & almost bacteria free. Fat globules of human milk make very fine emulsion and makes digestion easier. Protein content of cows milk is twice of that of mother's milk Human milk contains more of sugar making it more palatable.

Breast milk jaundice Exact cause is not known though pregnandriol and unsaturated fatty acids in milk have been implicated in causation. If reductase in breast milk breaks down conjugated bilirubin in the gut it increases bilirubin load via enteropeptic circulation.

Breath Normally it should be free from any kind of odour. In ketosis breath is sweet, while in alcoholism it is alcoholic. Large cavity in lungs in bronchiectasis produces putrid breath. The sickly odour of bronchiectasis may be intermittent, lasting a few days and disappearing.

Breath holding spasm These generally occur between the ages of 6 months and five years. Child starts crying after he or she is hurt, admonished, frustrated or frightened. After a bout of crying most of air in lungs is exhaled and breath is held in expiration for a few seconds and child becomes blue and limp. If the hypoxia continues for 10 to 15 seconds convulsions may occur.

Breathing It is the process by which air passes into and out of lungs. It allows blood to take up oxygen and disposal of carbon dioxide. It is controlled by respiratory centre which is present in mid brain. Respiratory rate varies from 13 to 18 breaths per minute. When air is inhaled the diaphragm is relaxed, flattens and ribs contract and pull the cage upwards and outwards. Lungs expand when air is exhaled and chest muscles and diaphragm relax. When lungs contract these squeeze out the air. Lungs hold about 1.5 gallons, i.e. 6 litres of air at one time.

Breathing difficulty There is a change in rate and depth of breathing and breathing is effortful. Accompanied features may be pain in chest, coughing and wheezing Overweight people often experience difficulty in breathing during exertion. Severe anxiety during times of stress and tension can bring an attack of hyperventilation. Damage to brainstem due to transient ischaemic attack or a head injury can alter the breathing activity. On high altitude due to lack of oxygen lungs have to work hard to meet the requirement. In severe anaemia, lack of RBCs results in insufficient oxygen to lungs and one has to breath fast. Any block in airway will cause distress in breathing pattern. Pneumonia, pneumothorax, pleural effusion, pulmonary oedema will increase the rate of respiration. Any pain due to fracture of ribs or during rib movement will make normal breathing difficult.

Breathing exercise Breathing exercises are often recommended in chronic chest diseases and after operation. In yoga deep rhythmic breathing is used to achieve a state of relaxation. Even during child birth breathing exercises relax the mother and help in reducing pain.

Breathlessness Laboured breathing is a sign of disorder of respiration and may be caused by emphysema, lung cancer, pleurisy, pneumonia and tuberculosis. At high altitude person develops laboured breathing due to O_2 thinning.

Breech delivery Generally baby projects his or her head first during delivery but in some cases bottom may be a presenting feature. By around 32 weeks most babies assume a head down position in uterus but 1 to 3 per cent may have head on the top of uterus. By 34 weeks obstetricians try to turn a baby with breech presentation into head down position. If it fails and mother's pelvis is short, caesarean section has to be done to deliver the child.

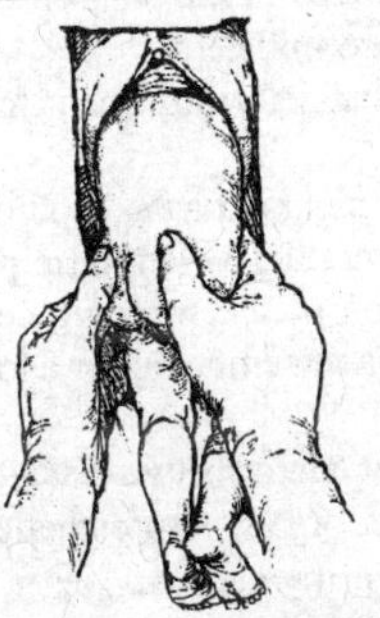

Breech presentation extraction of the body

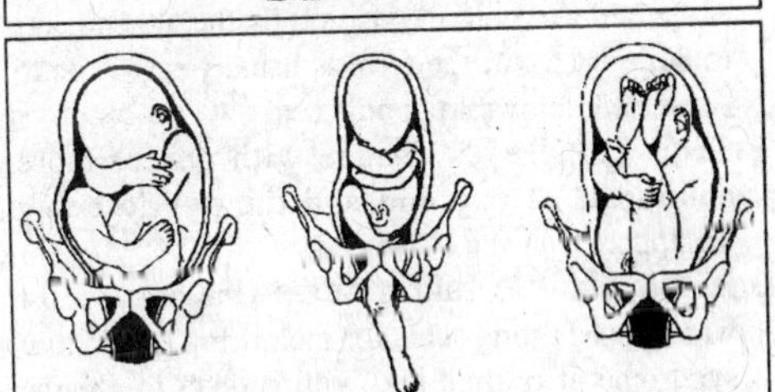

Complete breech

Footling breech

Frank breech

Breech extraction In breech extraction entire body of the fetus is extracted by obstetrician. For it cervix must be fully dilated.

Breech-classification (i) Complete-Buttocks present with feet and legs flexed on the thighs and thighs flexed on the abdomen (ii) Frank-The buttocks present with hips flexed and the legs extended against the abdomen and chest. It is a most common type. (iii) Incomplete-One of both feet or the knees extend below the buttocks. It is also known as single or double footling breech.

Bregma It is the large diamond shaped membranous space of the junction of sagittal, coronal and frontal sutures. It measures 3 cm in length and 2 cm in breadth at widest part. It closes when child is about 18 months.

Brenner's tumour These usually small, solid tumours are characterised by dense fibrous stroma and nests of transitional cells. These are occasionally encountered in the wall of mucinous cystadenomas and are unilateral.

Brevicollis A congenital deformity characterised by shortness of knee.

Bridal night The first night a married couple spend together after the wedding when anticipation is high and the euphoria of the wedding ceremany still has its effect. It is remembered for a long time by both the partners.

Bridge A structure that connects two distant points, including parts of an organ. A prosthetic dental appliance which replaces lost teeth, being supported and held in position by the attachments to adjacent teeth; the term is usually restricted to fixed nonremovable appliances.

Bridge cantilever Bridge with one or more abutments at one end and the pontic being unsupported at the other end.

Brief psychiatric rating scale One of the most widely used rating scale for measuring psychiatric syndrome at basline and with respect to change overtime. It allows the rapid assessment of symptoms such as depression, anxiety, delusion and hallucination.

Briefs Written arguments on questions of law or fats to assist the judge in making a decision. Maybe filed by the parties to the lawsuit or by amicus curiae.

Brightness The intensity aspect of light—the visual dimension represented by the black-white continuum. Also, a high level of intelligence, in contrast to dullness.

Brightness gain It is a measure of ability of an image intensifier to convert arriving X-rays into the brightest possible image on the output screen. This is often measured using the conventional factor Gx.

Brim Inlet of pelvis.

Brim sign A thickening of pelvic brim.

Brime (Brief Isometric Exercise) Gerber and Hicks devised this program of increasing muscle strength without raising blood pressure significantly. the regime is, one to six isometric contractions, held for 3-6 seconds, with 20 seconds rest between contractions.

Brine A strong salt solution used in preservation of fish, meat & vegetables.

Brisement A closed manipulation of stiff shoulder.

Bristle polishing A polishing brush with natural or synthetic bristle.

Bristow procedure A technique for the repair of anterior shoulder dislocation.

Brittain arthrodesis A technique of extra articular hip fusion.

Brittle The property of being easily broken or shattered; fragile or crisp. Prone to fracture or failure when the proportional limit of a material is exceeded.

Brittle bones Pathological affections of bone in which ductiblity is lost.

Broach An instrument with numerous protruding barbs from a metal shaft. It is generally used to engage the dental pulp for extirpation.

Broad ligament A double fold of parietal peritoneum attaching the uterus to the side of the pelvic cavity. Fibrous sheath covered by peritoneum extending from each side of the uterus to the lateral wall of the pelvis.

Broad ligament of uterus It is a triangular shaped double fold of peritoneum which lies on either side of the uterus.

Broca's aphasia The lesion in this case is in posterior part of left third frontal convolution, inferior motor cortex and adjacent insula. Spontaneous language production is slow with very few words per minute and much effort is expended on initiation. Retrieved words are noun. Few or no conjunctions are used and verb tenses are incorrect. The normal rhythm of speech is lost.

Broca's area Pars triangularis (area 44) and pars anterior (area 45) of the frontal operculum, involved in generating speech.

Broca's convolution Posterior end of left inferior frontal gyrus.

Brodmann number Broadman divided the brain cortex according to their functions and each area was give a specific number.

Brodmann's areas Brodmann has divided brain into different areas which perform special function. *Occipital lobe* : Area 17—Visual cortex, Area 18-19—visual associa-tion areas; *Parietal lobe* : Area 3.1.2—principal sensory area, Area 5.7—sensory association area, Area 41—primary auditory cortex, Area 42—associative auditory cortex, Area 38, 40, 21, 20, 22—association areas; *Frontal lobe* : Area 4—principal motor area, Area 6—Part of extrapyramidal circuit, Area 44—motor speech area, Area 8—conjugate eye movement, Areas 38, 40, 20, 21, 22—association area. The most well known name associated with mapping functional areas of cortex is Broadmann who in 1909 described 52 fields. Later scientists divided as many as 200 fields and more are likely to be identified. Broadmann's area 4 (motor strip) or areas 1,2,3 (primary sensory areas) Broca's areas 44 and 45 are familiar as the motor speech areas. Most areas have complex functions. Speech function occurs at least in seven areas. Some are concerned with perception of auditory impulses whereas others are essential for the interpretation and appreciation of intricate sounds. Still other synthesise data into a sensory language pattern. Some connections are responsible for turning the head following sound.

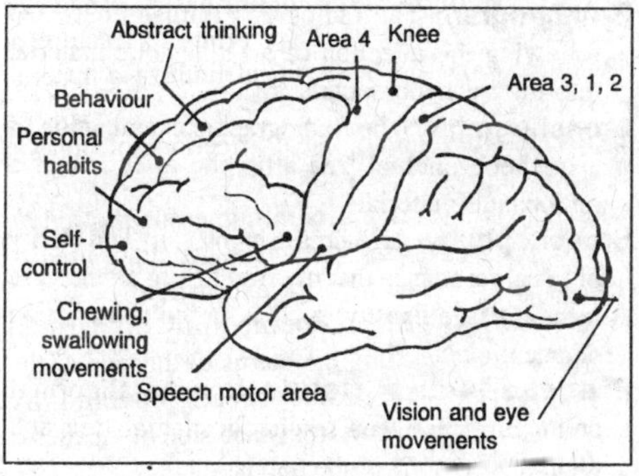

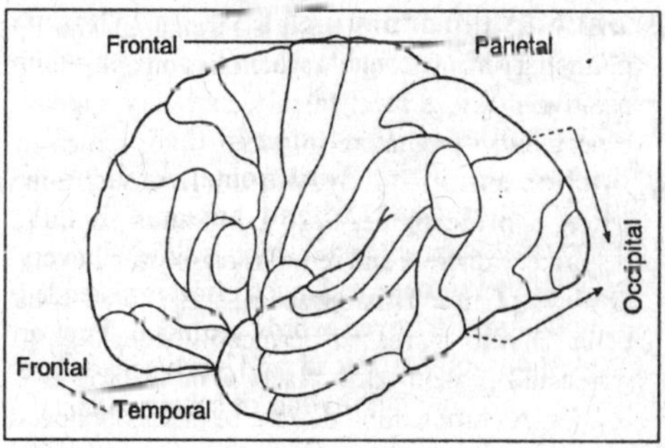

Bromelin A proteolytic enzyme from pine apple that digest protein.

Brominated vegetable oil Chemically vegetable oils i.e. olive, sesame, corn or cotton seed whose density has been increased to that of water combining with bromine. Lighter than water oils are dispersed through out the drink. Otherwise they will float on the surface.

Brominism A condition of poisoning produced by excessive use of bromine or a bromine compound; the symptoms produced are an eruption of acne upon the face and body, toms products are an eruption of acne upon the face and body, headache, coldness of the extremities, fector oris, sleepiness, weakness, and impotence.

Bromosulphthalein retention test A known amount of dye is injected and the amount of dye remaining in the serum is measured usually after 45 minutes so as to determine the amount cleared by the liver and excreted in the bile. From this liver function test, hepatic cell damage and biliary obstruction can be established if the amount of retention of bromosulphthalein exceeds to more than 4 per cent.

Bronchi The branches of the trachea.

Bronchial asthma and pregnancy There is no evidence that bronchial asthma improves with pregnancy because of increased plasma cortisol level and higher plasma histaminase which neutralises bronchial spasm. There is no particular indication of therapeutic abortion.

Bronchial breath sounds The sounds normally heard over the large bronchi on auscultation of the chest; the inspiration to expiration ratio is typically 1 to 1; and abnormal sound when heard over the peripheral lung tissue.

Bronchial breathing These are of three types, high pitched, or tubular breathing, medium pitched or true bronchial breathing, low pitched or cavernous breathing. This sound is a variety normally heard over trachea and other areas. It is heard when the sound produced in a dilated bronchus or cavity is conveyed to the surface.

Bronchial buds Outgrowth of the primordial bronchus of the fetus from which the bronchi and lungs eventually form.

Bronchial drainage The removal of secretions from the bronchi; postural drainage.

Bronchial glands Mucous and seromucous glands, the secretory units of which lie outside the muscular layer of the bronchi.

Bronchial tree The trachea, bronchi, and their branching structures up to an including the terminal bronchioles.

Bronchiectasis There is dilatation of bronchi specially terminal part at the bases of lung due to infection. In this condition there is green foul smelling sputum early morning. Person is trained to be in definite position while lying down to drain sputum. A course of antibiotic helps in chest infection. Even if severe symptoms persist then surgery may be needed.

Bronchiole Branch of a tertiary bronchus further dividing into terminal bronchioles (distributed tolobules of the lung), which divide into respiratory bronchioles (distributed to alveolar sacs).

Bronchiolitis It is an acute infection of the lungs mainly affecting babies and young children in which bronchioles become inflamed. Adult bronchiolitis may follow bronchitis due to influenza virus. It can pass on from one person to another. Symptoms include cough, shortness of breath, and in severe cases child may become blue due to cyanosis. There will be crepitations throughout lung. Antibiotics and in some cases even cortisone and artificial ventilator may be needed.

Bronchitis, chronic Bronchitis is regarded as chronic when sputum is coughed up on most of days during at least three consecutive months in at least two consecutive years. It results due to widespread narrowing and obstruction of airways in lungs. Cigarette smoking and atmospheric pollution may be the cause. Symptoms include cough, breathlessness, pain but no fever. In old age person may develop emphysema also.

Bronchoconstriction A reduction in the luminal caliber of a bronchus or bronchi.

Bronchodilation The act or process of increasing the calibe of bronchi.

Bronchodilators These drugs widen airways in lungs. Narrowing of bronchioles obstructs the flow of air into and out of lung and results in difficulty in breathing. Bronchodilators increase the flow of air and improves breathing. These are of three principal types : sympathomimetic drugs, anticholinergic drugs, and xanthine drugs. Drugs can be given by inhaler or in tablet form.

Bronchogenic carcinoma There will be persistent cough. Pain is pleuritic type or behind the sternum. The unexplained haemoptysis in a middle-aged is common. Shortness of breath appears early, when bronchus is occluded by growth. Infection arises distal to block. Recurrent pleural effusion takes place. When apex is involved pain may be radiated to neck and shoulder. Dysphagia may develop. Pulmonary osteoarthropathy and clubbing are noted.

Bronchogram The radiographic image obtained following the injection of a radiopaque material into the tracheobronchila tree.

Bronchography The Radiographic examination of a tracheobronchial tree after the injection of a radiopaque material.

Bronchophony An increase in intensity and clarity of vocal resonance that my result from an increase in lung tissue density, such as in the consolitaion of pneumonia.

Broncho-pleural fistula It is an abnormal connection between tracheobronchial tree and pleura.

Bronchopulmonary dysplasia Chronic pulmonary insufficiency associated with long-term positive-pressure mechanical ventilatory support, especially in premature infants.

Bronchopulmonary dysplasia It is suspected when a preterm neonate continues to have respiratory distress and remains on oxygen beyond 28 days of life. This causes damage to alveolar cells. Due to increased permeability leakage of water and protein takes place. Overall prognosis is poor. A chronic lung disease in infants believed to be associated with oxygen toxicity. It is often preceded by severe respiratory distress syndrome and treatment in a high oxygen environment.

Bronchopulmonary lavage It is performed in pulmonary alveolar proteinosis to remove accumulated lipoproteinaceous material. It may be done in asthma and cystic fibrosis.

Bronchopulmonary segments The largest subdivisions of a lobe of the lung; each is fed by direct branch from a lobar bronchus.

Bronchospasm Abnormal contractio of the smooth muscles of the bronchi.

Bronchus One of several large air passages in the lungs through which pass in spired air and exhaled gases.

Broomstick cast A cast used to maintain abduction of hips.

Brow It is the area bounded by orbital ridges and coronal sutures.

Brow presentation Fetal position in which the largest diameter of the fetal head, the occipitomental, presents at the pelvic inlet.

Brown dermatome Electrically powered instrument used for cutting skin grafts.

Brown fat Highly vascular specialised fat found in new born that provides more heat than other fat when metabolised.

Brown tumor Localized lytic lesion seen in bones of patients with hyperparathroidism.

Brown-Marie syndrome Cause is unknown and is due to simple recessive inheritance. There will be hereditary ataxia, choreiform movements, athetosis, phyramidal tract paresis and speech difficulties. Eyes may show nystagmus, strabismus, ophthalmoplegia, Argyll Robertson pupil, retinitis pigmentosa, optic nerve atrophy and retrobulbar neuritis.

Brown Sequard syndrome It is caused due to lesion of spinal cord. There will be homolateral spastic paralysis with loss of contralateral pain and temperature sensations and sphincteral disturbances. There will be loss of ipsilateral deep joint tendon and vibratory sensations below the level of lesion. There will be sluggish pupillary reaction to light with nystagmus. There is hemisection of cord. There will be ipsilateral lower motor neuron paralysis of muscles supplied by segment of cord. There will be ipsilateral anaesthesia of skin supplied by the segment of cord which is involved and contralateral loss of pain and temperature sense below the level of cord lesion. One will have ipsilateral loss of two-point discriminatory sense below the cord lesion.

Bruce effect The termination of pregnancy prior to implantation when a female is exposed to the odors of an unfamiliar, reproductively active male.

Bruce exercise test protocol A graded treadmill exercise test protocol consisting of stages of 3 minutes' duration with incremental speed (1.7, 2.5, 3.4, 4.3, 5.0, 5.5, 6.0, 6.5 mph) and a grade (2%) change at each stage.

Brudzinski's sign It is considered to be positive when abrupt flexion of neck of patient lying supine with legs extended results in an involuntary flexion of thighs. It is seen in meningeal irritation.

Brufen Half-life is 2 hours. It is well absorbed after an oral dose and is inactivated by metabolism. Fenbrufen has half-life of 10 hours. Naproxen's half-life is 14 hours. So Naproxen and Fenbrufen can be given twice daily. Main advantage over aspirin is lower incidence of adverse effects on GIT. Gastric bleeding may occur.

Bruit Abnormal sound or murmur created by turbulent blood blood flow heard while auscultating an organ, gland, or artery.

Brushfield's spot White spots on iris.

Brushing It is a device useful in reducing dental plaque at gingival margin. Interproximal brushes are useful in cleansing interdental areas. Some patients prefer these brushes to floss since less dexterity is required. Brushing is as important for massage as it is for cleansing. Brushing once or twice daily is needed to remove all plaques and debris. The handle of the brush should be suitably shaped for a firm, comfortable grip. The head of the brush should be small enough to insert into all areas of mouth yet large enough to cover several teeth at a time. Bristles should be of equal length.

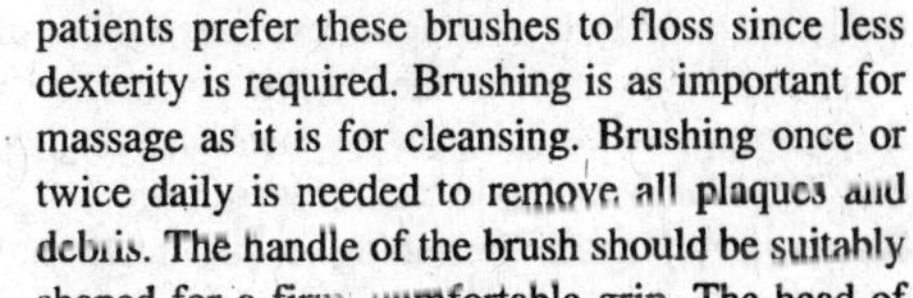

Different stages of occlusal brushing

If they are soft then should be arranged closely in two or more rows. If they are hard then should be widely spaced. 3 to 5 minutes brushing is sufficient. No single method of toothbrushing has been demonstrated to be totally adequate for all patients.

Bruxing Excessive chewing or grinding of the teeth.

Bruxism The involuntary grinding or clenching of teeth. It is usually unconcious. It is associated with fatigue, anxiety, emotional stress of fear.

Bruxomania Day time grinding or clenching of teeth.

Bryant's traction A technique for application of vertical skin traction for infants and young children with femur fractures. .

Bubble rings Rings in blood that result when blood containing air bubbles dries and retains the bubble's circular configuration as a dried outline.

Bubo A lymphnode that is enlarged secondary to an infection. It may suppurate seen in syphilis, plague, malaria etc.

Buccal Pertaining to or adjacent to the cheek.

Buccal application Drug placement against the mucous membranes of the inner cheek.

Buccal bar An orthodontic appliance auxillary consisting of a rigid metal wire extending from the buccal side of the molar band anteriorly.

Buccal cavity The mouth, or oral cavity.

Buccal object rule A localisation technique that allows the practitioner to determine the position of superimposed dental structures or foreign objects viewed on a dental radiograph.

Buccinator Muscle making up the lateral sides of the oral cavity; flattens the cheeks.

Buccogingival Pertaiing to the cheek and gingiva.

Buccolabial pertaiing to the cheek and lip.

Buccopharyngeal Pertaining to the mouth and pharynx.

Buck's fascia the fascial support structure of the deep structures of the penis.

Bucket-handle rib motion Movement of the lower ribs during respiration such that with inhalation the lateral aspect of the rib elevates, increasing the transverse diameter of the thorax.

Bud scar The chitinrich, convex ringed protrusions that remain on the mother cell surface of budding yeasts following birth of daughter cells.

Bud stage First stage of formation of the enamel organ that has developed from the lamina dura.

Budding A mode of vegetative reproduction in many yeast species whereby a small outgrowth, the daughter bud, appears and grows from the surface of a mother cell and eventually separates to form a new cell at cell division.

Buddy taping Technique for dyanamic splinting of a digit.

Buerger's disease It is also known as thromboangitis obliterans. It is a slow growing ulcer characterised by episodic, segmental inflammation of small and medium sized arteries and veins of lower extremity. There is subsequent occlusion by thrombosis in young smokers. There is arteritis, periarteritis, phlebitis and periphlebitis. The thrombus may become organised and converted into fibrous tissue obliterating the lumen which may get partially canalised. New vascular channels lined by endothelium may be formed in fibrous mass.

Buerger's Exercises This is a pattern of positions designed to encourage the development of a collateral circulation in the legs. The procedure is as follows :- 1. The patient lies supine with the legs supported in elevation (at an angle of 45 to the horizontal) until the skin blanches - about 2 minutes. 2. The patient sits up with the legs dependent until the leg colouris brigh red - about 2 mts. 3. The patient lies with the legs horizontal until the skin colour return to normal - about 5 mts.

Buffer Chemical that resists changes in pH when either an acid or base is added to a solution containing the buffer. Any substance in a fluid that tends to lessen the change in hydrogen ion concentration (reaction), which otherwise would be produced by adding acids or alkalies. A system capable of resisting changes in pH, consisting of a conjugate acid-base pair in which the ratio of portion acceptor to proton donor is near unity.

Buffer pairs Two kinds of chemical substances that prevent a sharp change in the pH of a fluid; for example, sodium bicarbonate ($NaHCO_3$) and carbonic acid (H_2CO_3).

Buffer solutions The power of blood to absorb acid or base without appreciable, change in pH is due to its content of substances which act as buffer.

Buffers Substances which resist a change in pH by absorbing or releasing hydrogen ions when acid or base is added to the solution.

Bular A discredited term usually meaning the calcarine sulcus in the medial wall of the atrium of the lateral ventricle.

Bulbar 'Bulb' of the brain A discredited term usually meaning medulla oblongata.

Bulbar palsy Whatever may be the cause, clinical picture is one of difficulty in swallowing often with nasal regurgitation due to palatal paralysis, dysarthria and often dysphagia. In advanced cases tongue will be wasted. Bulbar palsies due to extrinsic brainstem lesions such as carcinomatous meningitis may have associated sensory signs in distribution of trigeminal nerve.

Bulbourethral Small glands located just below the prostate gland whose mucuslike secretons lubricate the terminal portion of the urethra and contribute less than 5% of the seminal fluid volume; also known as Cowper's glands.

Bulbourethral glands A pair of gland that secrete a viscous fluid into the male uethra during sexual excitement; also called Cowper's glands.

Bulbous cordis The division of the heart tube between the truncus arteriosus and the ventricle.

Bulimia Episodic eating binges or excessive intake of food or fluid, generally beyond voluntary control. Characteristics are self-induced vomiting and purging following eating, which is of the binge eating variety. The resulting loss of body fluids and electrolytes may lead to severe disturbances such as EKG abnormalities and tetany. Sometimes seen as a symptom in anorexia nervosa.

Bulimia nervosa This is considered as a variant of chronic anorexia nervosa syndrome where bouts of pathological overeating occurs. There is a lasting preoccupation with obtaining and defavouring food. A sense of lack of control over eating during episode. One cannot stop or control what or how much one is eating.

Bulk flow The movement of large numbers of ions, molecules, or particles in the same direction as a result of pressure differences (osmotic, hydrostatic, or air pressure).

Bullet A projectile normally made out of lead or lead covered in a thin copper jacket. The bullet only refers to the projectile and not the entire cartridge.

Bullet-Shaped Crown A replacement tooth, usually posteriorly located in a fixed prosthesis because of esthetic considerations, tapered towards the gingiva from every aspect.

Bullous concha Main symptoms include unilateral impediment of nasal respiration. Rhinoscopy shows markedly expanded head of middle turbinate obstructing nasal lumen. Large pneumatised ethmoid cell in the head of middle turbinate are the causative factors.

Bullous emphysema The destruction of alveolar septa and the reduction in the number of alveoli, creating thin-walled cavities (bullae).

Bullous lichen planus These are rare. In this characteristic white line or papule of lichen planus are seen on the peripheral area of vesicle, in the erosion area and in the area of atrophy. It is generally seen on the lateral border of tongue. Microscopic lesions may have several formation of a subepithelial vesicle.

Bumper fracture Compressure fracture of lateral tibial plateau.

Bundle of His A bundle of specialised cardiac muscle fibres that conduct action potentials from the AV node to the Purkinje fibres in the heart. It is composed of spindle shaped cells which intercommunicate and have got scanty striations. Bundles contain many elastic fibres. Its vascular supply is poor.

Bunion Hallux valgus with a painful bursitis over the medial aspect of the first metatarsophalangeal joint.

Bunnel stitched A technique for the end to end sutures of tendon. Criss crossing stitch.

Bunsen burner Small laboratory burner consisting of a vertical metal tube connected to a gas source, which produces a very hot flame from a mixture of gas and air let in through adjustable holes at the base.

Buoyancy The upward pressure exerted by the fluid in which an object is immersed.

Buphthalmic eye Most obvious feature is an enlargement of whole globe, usually into an oval shape giving an appearance of proptosis. Horizontal diameter of cornea is more than 12 mm. Cornea becomes hazy due to striae or oedema. Anterior chamber becomes deep and corneal sensation is diminished. Intraocular pressure is raised. Fundus examination shows cupping of disc. There is triad of symptoms : photophobia, blepharospasm and epiphora.

Buphthalmos There is raised intraocular pressure due to congenital abnormality at the angle of anterior chamber, thereby offering an obstruction to the drainage of intraocular fluid resulting in congenital glaucoma. Simple buphthalmos is caused by primary developmental anomaly at the angle of anterior chamber. It is transmitted as a recessive character.

Bupivacaine hydrochloride This local anesthetic agent was introduced in 1963. It is of slow onset but of longer duration than lingocaine. Effect lasts 3-4 hours for extradural block and up to 12 hours for nerve block.

Bur A rotary dental instrument made of steel or tungsten carbide, held and reloved in a handpiece, deriving power from the dental electric motor or air power. It consists of the shank, which may be tapered, notched, or elongated and smooth to fit into a handpiece.

Bureau-Barriere syndrome This usually occurs in men. Chronic alcoholism and protein deficiency are the principal contributory factors. The pathogenesis is due to degeneration of sensory nerves and dorsal root ganglion. Clinical features include ulceration in foot, tactile anaesthesia and analgesia.

Burkitt's lymphoma It is a small cell lymphoma containing scattered pale macrophages which give the darksheets of cells giving starry sky appearance 95% responds clinically to single dose of chemotherapy.

Burn A lesion caused by contact of heat, radiation, chemical etc. with tissue.

Burn out A state characterized by emotional exhaustion that occurs often after exposure to prolonged stress.

Burn's space Suprasternal fascial space.

Burning feet syndrome This condition is characterised by peripheral neuritis and burning sensation on the soles of feet. It is due to deficiency of B_6 deficiency.

Burning mouth syndrome It is an intraoral pain disorder unaccompanied by clinical signs. It is a diagnosis by exclusion and probably encompasses a fairly heterogeneous group of patients. Some patients may develop burning painful tongue or other oral mucosal surface, dry mouth, taste abnormality or other oral dysaesthesia. Tongue temperature is decreased. Responses to a battery of local sensory stimuli applied to the tongue, lip and other mucosal sites show decreased pain tolerance. Some relief from symptoms is obtained from the use of topical analgesics as 0.5 per cent aqueous diphenhydramine alone or mixed with 0.5 per cent dyclone.

Burnish To condense and polish under the sliding pressure of a smooth hand instrument, as in finishing the surface of a gold restoration.

Burnisher An instrument shape with rounded edges used to burnish, polish metallic surfaces.

Burnishing A process related to polishing and abrading.

Burnout A stress reaction developing in persons working in an area of unrelenting occupational demands. Symptoms include impaired work performance, fatigue, insomnia, depression, increased susceptibility to physical illness, and reliance on alcohol or other drugs of abuse for temporary relief.

Burns-Marshal manoeuvre Baby must be allowed to hang down until the hair at the nape of neck.

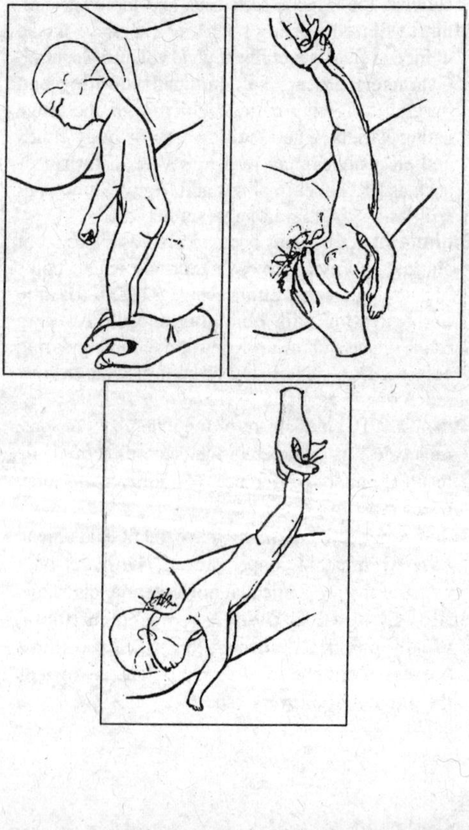

Traction to keep the body taut is exerted while legs are lifted steadily upwards towards the mothers abdomen. Fetus should not be allowed to hang for long otherwise hypoxia may develop.

Burr High speed surgical instrument useful in drilling and enlarging holes in bones or teeth.

Bursa A Saclike structure filled with synovial fluid. Bursae are located at friction points, as around joints, over which tendons can slide without contacting bone.

Bursa of Fabricus A primary lymphoid organ in avian species, located at the cloacalhind gut junction; it is the site of B cell maturation.

Bursae Small, cushion like sacs found between moving body parts making movements easier.

Bursitis There is inflammation of bursa and it becomes swollen. It is the result of pressure friction. Patellar bursitis happens due to prolonged kneeling on hard surface and olecranon bursitis from prolonged pressure of elbow joint against a table. Deltoid bursitis if remain untreated may result in frozen shoulder. Treatment is generally rest. Applying an ice pack may relieve pain. Infection may be treated with antibiotic and drainage. Local injection of corticosteroid may help.

Burst A term for the abrupt release of many progeny viruses upon the disintegration of the infected cell in which the virus has been growing.

Burst fracture vertebra It is a failure of spine under compression of the anterior and middle column involving mostly lower thoracic or thoracolumbar junction. There may be spinal or neurological instability. CT scan will help in knowing spinal canal compression. If fracture is greater than 60% an anterior surgical procedure with buttress grafting is indicated.

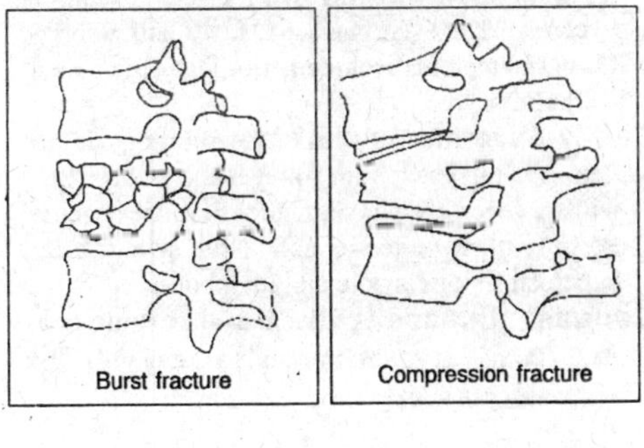

Burst fracture — Compression fracture

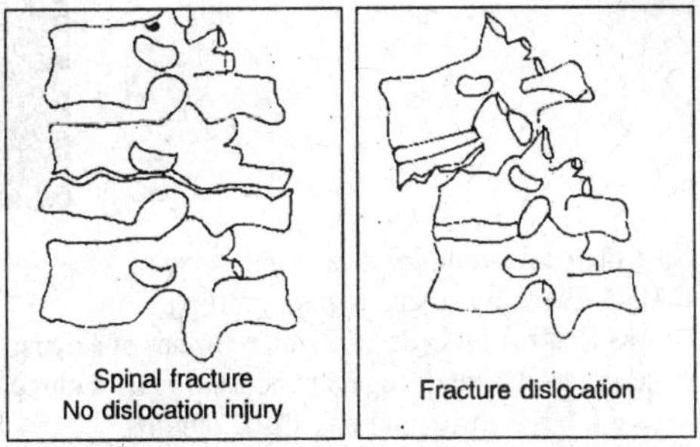

Spinal fracture No dislocation injury — Fracture dislocation

Butt To place directly against the tissues covering the residual alveolar ridge.

Butter An edible animal fat, obtained from milk and cream made solid by churning. Butter can be made from fresh or slightly acid milk. It can be sweet or salted with moderate amount of vitamin A.

Butter fat It can be separated into high and low melting fractions. Repeated separation of solidified portion will result in a lower melting solid fraction. Higher melting butter fat is suitable for icecreams and chocolates while low melting is used as table butter.

Butter milk Sour fluid is obtained by separating the butter fat from cream or milk which has been churned.

Butterfly fragment Comminuted wedge shaped fracture that has split off from the main fragment.

Butterfly vertebrae Biconcave vertebrae with notching of end plates by nucleus pulposus.

Buttock The lump or fleshy mass on the posterior aspect of the lower trunk, formed primarily by the gluteal muscles.

Butyric acid It is a saturated fatty acid that occurs as a glyceride to the extent of about 5 to 6 % butter. It is a mobile liquid mixing in all proportions with water, alcohol and ether.

Bypass operation It is the procedure to bypass the blockage or narrowing of an artery or vein or any part of digestive system. Arteries can become blocked or narrowed by atheroma. These blocks can be bypassed using section of artery, vein or synthetic tubing. Veins are bypassed most commonly with diseases of liver such as portal hypertension or oesophageal varices.

Byssinosis An asthma-like pulmonary syndrome resulting from inhalation of textile dust (e.g., cotton dust).

Bystander effect The tendency for an individual to be less likely to help as the number of other people present increases.

C

Ca Chemical symbol for calcium.

CABG Coronary artery bypass grafting.

Cable graft A procedure in which strands of a donar nerve are bundled together and the ends sutured to the larger proximal and distal stumps.

Cachectic Relating to cachexia.

Cachexia This is an appearance of profound illness. There is massive loss of weight either due to lack of food or due to starvation. Chronic diseases such as tuberculosis and cancer may result it.

Cacolalia Expression of absence situations.

Cacosmia Persistent experience of bad odour.

Cadaveric muscle changes Immediately after death all muscles of body become flaccid. Lower jaw falls while limbs remain mobile. Gradually molecular death takes place and is manifested by stiffening or rigidity.

Cadaveric spasm It is the continuation of contraction of muscles even after death. It is not rigor mortis because muscles still have not undergone any change. They still possess molecular life. Rigor will supervene later fixing the muscles rigidity in their contracted position. The suicider who shoots himself in the head will be found with the pistol firmly gripped in his hand.

Cadence Number of steps per unit of time; may be measured in centimeters as the number of steps per second (cadence=number of steps/time). A simple method of measuring cadence is by counting the number of steps taken by the patient in a given amount of time.

Cadmium tungstate It is a scintillation crystal used in many CT scanners. It has a fast speed of response and little afterglow. It is not hygroscopic.

Caecum A blind sac forming the beginning of the large intestine.

Caesarean section Child is delivered through caesarean section. Indications include extreme degree of pelvic contraction, large fibromyoma, big ovarian cysts, tumours of pelvic bones, undilatable and indivisible structures of cervix and vagina. Non-selective indications include failed trial labour and fetal distress. All cases of failed forceps are to be delivered through caesarean section.

Caesarean section in multiple pregnancy Indications include prolapse of cord if first fetus is breech, toxemia of pregnancy, placenta praevia, abruptio placenta locking of twins and big size fetus.

Caesarian section It is defined as delivery of the child through an incision of the abdominal wall and uterus after 28th week of pregnancy. Hysterotomy is the essence of the operation.

Cafe au lait spots Light brown birth marks.

Caffeine It is a stimulant present in caffeine seeds, tea leaves and kola nuts. Certain popular drinks contain coffee. Persons who consume more than 6 cups of coffee, may suffer withdrawal symptoms such as tiredness, headache and irritability due to physical dependence. It may help in relieving migraine along with ergotamine.

Caffeinism The official diagnostic category for excessive caffeine consumption to a point of intoxication.

Caffey's disease There is an enlargement of affected bones and patients are below 6 months of age. Child develops fever, total WBC count and increased ESR rate. Alkaline phosphate level is increased. In majority of cases mandible is involved. X-ray shows thickening of cortex. Lower border of mandible is bulged. Corticosteroids help the patients.

Caffey's syndrome It is also known as infantile cortical hyperostosis and cause is unknown. There will be cortical swelling over regions of cortical hyperostosis, severe anaemia, fever and pleurisy. Ocular symptoms include periorbital oedema and tenderness.

Caffey-Silverman syndrome Aetiology is not known but it develops in younger age group. There will be fever, dysphagia and periorbital oedema. Person will have tender soft tissue swelling and hyperostosis of clavicle and long bones.

Cahgas' disease A disease also known as American trypanosomiasis, caused by Trypanosoma cruzi.

Calabar swelling Calabar swelling is slightly inflamed, oe̊dematous, swelling of hen's egg size occurring in any area but mostly on the wrist and forearm which persists for a few days and then subsides. It is seen in loaiasis.

Calamine It is a pink substance consisting of zinc oxide and is used in skin powders and ointments. It relieves irritation of skin and has cooling effect. It is used in dermatitis, insect bite and sun burn.

Calamitous death A premature or unexpected death.

Calcaneal Pertaining to calcaneus.

Calcaneal frontal plane motion The bisection of calcaneum should show 10° of eversion measured from the reference line of distal one third by leg. Inversion should measure 20°.

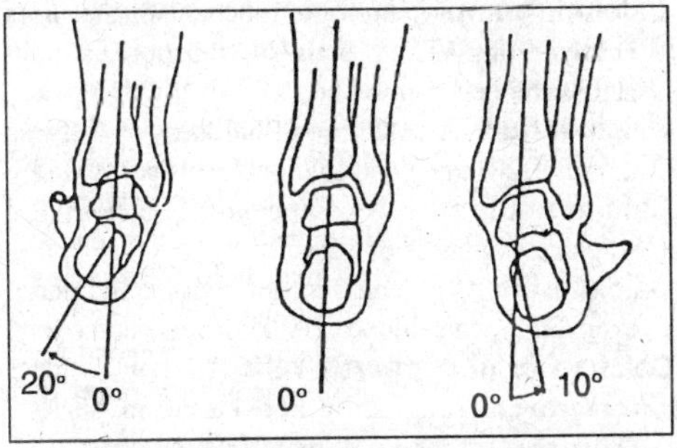

Calcaneal index Method used in diagnosis and grading of osteoporosis based on trabecular pattern of calcaneus.

Calcaneocuboid joint The articulation between calcaneous and cuboid bone in foot.

Calcaneous Heel bone; largest tarsal in the foot.

Calcaneous gait Typical walk of patient with paralysed gastronemius soleus muscles.

Calcaneovalgus A foot deformity in which there is increased dorsiflexion of ankle and lateral deviation of foot. Usually seen with paralytic disorder.

Calcaneum It is a thick, stout heel bone but can be fractured if person falls directly impacting the bone. Multiple fractures of this bone may cause permanent damage to the joint inturning the foot in and out. In case of fracture plaster is to be applied. Inflammation around the fascitis causes pain and tenderness under the heel when standing or walking.

Calcaneus secundarium An accessory bone of the foot. It projects from the dorsal and distal end of calcaneus.

Calcar avis Elevation produced by the calcraine sulcus in teh medial wall of the atrium of the lateral ventricle.

Calciferol Synthetically produced Vit. D.

Calcific metamorphosis of pulp Frequently observed phenomenon seen as reaction to trauma.

Calcific tendinitis Inflmmatory involvement of a tendon associated with calacium deposits; commonly affects the supraspinatus and biceps tendons in the shoulder.

Calcification It is the deposition of calcium salts in body tissues. It is normal in bone and teeth formation and is necessary for healing of fractures. In injured muscle calcification is possible. It is common in arteries affected by atherosclerosis. In parathyroid disorder calcium level in blood is raised.

Calcified cartilage Hyaline cartilage in which mineral salts have been deposited. Normally found in growth plate.

Calcination A process of removing water by heat.

Calcinosis Deposition of calcium salt in various tissues due to hypercalcemia.

Calcitonin It is a hormone produced by thyroid gland. It controls the level of calcium in the blood. It slows down the loss of calcium from bone. It is used in the treatment of Paget's disease. In Paget's disease bones become deformed and multiple fractures develop. Calcitonin is used to treat hypercalcaemia. It relieves nausea and vomiting.

Calcitonin generelated peptide (CGRP) A peptide released by chollnergic end feet that synapse with muscles; the corelease of CGRP increases the force with which a muscle contracts.

Calcitriol Active vitamin D hormone that raises blood calcium levels.

Calcium A chemical element with atomic number 20, atomic weight 40.08. Serum calcium level ranges from 8.5 to 10.5 mg/ml. Body contains about 1.1 kg of calcium. It is essential for the functioning of cells. It helps in contractions of muscles and transmission of nerve impulses from nerve endings to muscle fibres and in clotting of blood too. It is an important constituent of teeth and bones. Vitamin D and some hormones control the level of calcium by regulating absorption and excretion of calcium by kidneys. Parathyroid hormone and calcitonin control the regulation of calcium. Milk, green leafy vegetables, drumsticks are good source of calcium. In mild cases of hypocalcaemia there may not be any symptoms. In severe cases tetany may develop. There may be cramp-like symptoms of hand, feet and face. It may also lead to softening of bones. Children may develop rickets and adults may result in osteomalacia. Hypercalcaemia results in depression and kidney stones.

Calcium antagonist These drugs cause blockade of slow calcium ion influx into the contractile and conducting myocardial cells resulting in slow conduction, prolonged refractory period and depression of contractility. Verapamil, nifedipine and diltiazem are common drugs of this group.

Calcium carbonate Crystalline compound $CaCo_3$ occuring naturally in bone and shells.

Calcium channel blockers It is used in angina pectoris and high blood pressure. It works with interfering of muscle contractions. It causes prevention of movement of calcium across the membrane and as a result muscle relaxes and dilates. It slows the passage of nerve impulses through heart muscle helping certain types of arrhythmias. Side effects include increased headache, flushing and dizziness.

Calcium chloride A calcium salt $CaCl_2$ used in solution to restore electrolyte imbalance.

Calcium hydroxide An astringent compound used topically in solutions.

Calcium hydroxide base The base paste contains calcium tungstate, tribasic calcium phosphate and zinc oxide in glycol salicylate. Fillers such as calcium tungstate or barium sulphate provide radiopacity. Although setting times vary between 2.5 and 5.5 minutes, compressive strengths of these elements continue to increase over 24 hours period. The calcium hydroxide base may provide some thermal insulation to the pulp if used in thick layer. A thickness greater than 0.5 mm is not suggested. Some solubility of calcium hydroxide is necessary to achieve its therapeutic properties. Calcium hydroxide bases have low values of tensile strength.

Calcium hydroxide-liner It is a basic compound with pH 11. It is mildly irritating to vital pulp tissue and has and has bacteriostatic properties. It may be a liquid containing compound calcium hydroxide suspended in solvent. As a past calcium hydroxide is suspended in methylcellulose.

Calcium lactate A preparation of calcium used for dietary supplement.

Calcium oxalate A compound occuring naturally in urine as a crystal sediment and abnormally in renal calculi.

Calcium oxide Quick lime.

Calcium phosphate It contains calcium and phosphate radicle.

Calcium propionate The calcium salt of propionic acid is a chemical used to prevent growth of mold and certain bacteria in bread and rolls and also prodcue a calcium supplement to diet.

Calcium pump A biologic mechanism that uses energy from ATP to actively transport calcium across the cell membrane.

Calcium rigor A condition of hardness or stiffness of muscles when blood calcium levels get too high.

Calcium sulphate A compound of calcium and sulphate as plaster of Paris.

Calcium tetany A condition of spasms and nerve excitability when blood calcium levels get too low.

Calcium to phosphorus ratio 1:1 ratio is ideal for growth, pregnancy and lactation period. Otherwise 1:1.5 ratio is required.

Calcium tungstate screen An intensifying screen containing calcium tungstate as the X-ray luminescent material. Calcium tungstate screens emit light in the blue range with an emission maximum of about 420 nm.

Calculus It is a calcified deposit on teeth. But generally these may be small, hard crystalline mass precipitated from bile or urine. Gall bladder and bile duct stones are prone for it. Stones may be symptomless or may develop severe radiating pain.

Calculus, dental These are hard, crust-like deposits found on crowns as well as roots of teeth. This is also known as tartar. Actually mineral salts of saliva are deposited in existing plaques. These are of two types : (*i*) general place of deposition are inside surfaces of lower incisors and outer surfaces of upper molars; and (*ii*) supragingival calculi are white or yellow while sublingual calculi are black or brown. Both types of stones are hard and it is not very easy to remove them. These become continuously covered by plaque. These cause inflammation and destruction of gums. By professional scaling these can be removed.

Calculus, subgingival Calculus found below the gingiva; appears radiopaque.

Calculus, supragingival Calculus found above the gingiva; appears radiopaque.

Calcur The thickened plate of cortical bone at the medial inferior edge of femoral neck.

Calf Popular name for the prominent muscle mass in the back of leg below knee.

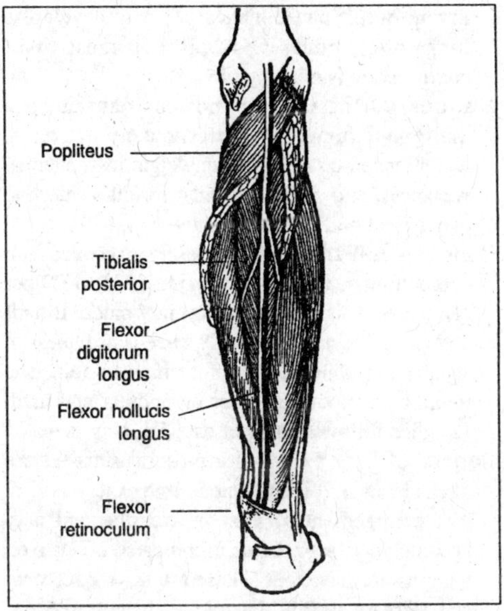

Caliber The diameter of a gun barrel and a term frequently used to describe the type of ammunition a particular weapon can fire.

Calipers An instrument having two adjustable curved legs or jaws, used for measuring the thickness or diameter of an object.

Caliper and rule It is used to measure the length of the muscle to be resected or the distance to which the muscle is to be recessed during squint surgery. It is also used during surgery on levator muscle for ptosis.

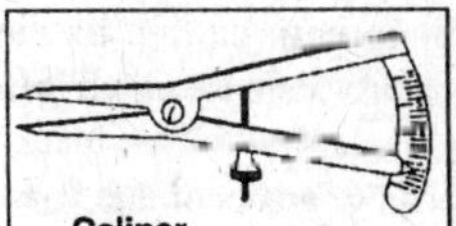

Caliper

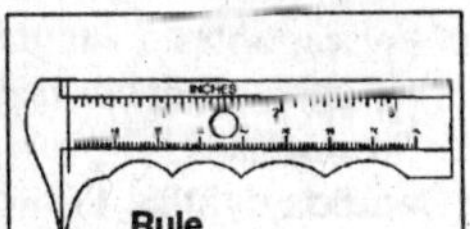

Rule

Caliper rib movement Movement of lower ribs during respiration such that the ribs move anteriorly with inhalation.

Call girls A call girl does not work on street or in hotel but out of posh apartments and her pimp is often a business manager. All males are not welcome and her charges are higher. These girls may be used by some rich influential people to get their work done from bureaucrats and diplomats. Solicitation is by telephone.

Call-Exner bodies The fluid-filled spaces between follicular granulosa cells that coalesce to form the antrum.

Callosity Callus

Callus It is a benign condition of cellular proliferation of epidermis produced by repeated pressure or friction. Calluses develop due to certain occupation or habit. Histopathologically condition produces localised hyperkeratosis and marked thickening of stratum corneum. It presents with firm, raised, superficial, less demarcated, flattened, plaque of hyperkeratosis with localised area of compact scales. These are usually painless and can cause irritation.

Callus skin It is an area of thickened skin. It is caused by regular or prolonged friction. Manual labourers are prone to develop on their palms and hands. Runners and joggers on their soles and instrumental musicians on their tip of fingers. If scaled it will recur again.

Calmodulin A receptor protein for Ca^{2+} located within the cytoplasm of target cells. It appears to mediate the effects of this ion on cellular activities.

Calor A localized increase in body temperature, being a cardinal sign of inflammation.

Calorie It is a measure of energy. It is the energy required to raise the temperature of 1 kg of water by 1°C from 14.5 to 15.5. Each gram of fat gives 9.1 calories while carbohydrate and proteins give 4.1 calories. If you consume calories more than your requirement you are bound to gain weight. To deposit one pound of weight you have to consume 3500 extra calories. Direct calorimetry is the usual method of calculating the calorie value of small amount of food. The amount of energy required to raise the temperature of 1 kg of water 1°C from 14.5° C to 15.5°C.

Calorie equivalent The number of calories produced per liter of oxygen for each oxidizing food stuff is the calorie equivalent.

Calorie requirement The amount of energy required to maintain life is the sum of total calories needed to satisfy requirement for basal metabolism.

Fat	*weight Kg*	*K cal avilable*
Adipose tissuee	15	141,000
Glycogen		
Muscle	12	48000
Liver	0.7	280
Glucose		
Extracellular	0.04	80
Protein		
Muscles	6	24,000
Total energy available 205840		

Calot, triangle Cystophepatic triangle.

Calvin cycle The cyclic pathway used to fix carbon dioxide and produce triose phosphates.

Calyx The small containers into which urine flows as it leaves the collecting ducts at the tip of the renal pyramids; the calyces come together to form the renal pelvis.

Camper's fascia Fatty part os superficial fasica on lower abdomen.

Camperwell life events An interview based procedure for evaluating the presence, severity and origins of stressful events.

Canal A tube-like passageway through bone that houses nerves and blood vessels; appears radiolucent.

Canal pulp Part of pulp cavity located in root.

Canaliculi An extremely narrow tubular passage or channel in compact bone.

Canaliculus Tiny canal in bone between osteocytes containing osteocyte cell processes; a cleft-like lumen between the cells of each hepatic cord. A microscopic channel in bone tissue that connects lacunae.

Canalis opticus syndrome There is loss of vision after blunt injury to head. There may be spontaneous unior bilateral reversible or irreversible amaurosis. In case of complete blindness there may be absence of pupil reaction.

Canal-root Space inside the root which holds the pulp tissue.

Cancellous bone Refers to a lattice-like structure; also known as spongy or trabecular bone; appears radiolucent.

Cancellous bone graft Any bone graft analogus or otherwise in which cancellous bone is used in blocks and stripes.

Cancer It is a rapid and abnormal growth of cells. Skin, breast, lungs and pancreas are the most common part of body to develop it. It can also develop in bone marrow, lymphatic system and bones. The growth of a cancer begins when the oncogens in a cell or cells are transformed by agents known as carcinogens. Years may pass before the growth of cells cause symptoms. Even during occult phase metastases may develop in lung, liver, bones and brain. In most cases confirmation is done by biopsy.

Cancer cachexia A syndrome caused by a malignant tumor characterized by anoresia, alterations in taste sensation, weight loss, anemia, weakness, and emaciation that results in decline of physical and mental functions;

Cancer of gall bladder It is closely associated with cholelithiasis. Calculi are found in 70 to 90 per cent cases. It is more common in women. Biliary colic may occur but normally there is heaviness in right upper abdomen. Tumour may be felt. It is round and smooth but later on nodular and hard. Jaundice follows. Surgical excision may help.

Cancer of liver Pain is an almost constant feature of cancer liver. It is continuous with exacerbations. The enlargement of liver is irregular and may become very large. Often umbilicated nodules on margins are made out. These are hard, consistent and increase rapidly. Jaundice is usually present. Deep jaundice for 5 to 7 weeks in old age always leads to suspect cancer. Ascites usually develops. Spleen is not enlarged. General condition of patient is bad. Fever may occur at intervals. It is usually fatal in 6 to 12 months.

Cancericidal Destructive to cancer or malignant cells.

Candida albicans A yeast-like fungus that causes infections in the human being, commonly involving the mucous membranes of the mouth and vagina. During pregnancy, women are more susceptible to candidal infections due to the changed pH of the vagina and increased glycogen in vaginal cells.

Candida cystitis Predisposing factors of this yeast cystitis are antibiotics, diabetes mellitus, permanent indwelling catheter, steroid treatment, chemotherapy of urogenital tract anomalies. *Candida albicans* is the usual causative agents.

Candida oesophagitis It is most common in patients with metabolic abnormalities or other lower resistance. It also occurs in setting of HIV infection, reflux oesophagitis, achalasia and broad-spectrum antibiotic therapy.

Candidosis Infection with Candida albicans also known as candidiasis and thrush.

Cane A type of walking aid.

Canidae An animal family of the order carnivora, composed of wolves, foxes and dogs.

Canine tooth The tooth with the longest crown and the longest root, which is located lateal to the second incisor.

Cannabis Mild hallucinogenic drug obtained from cannabis sativa plant. It is a mixture of 60 chemicals.

Cannibalism The eating of members of the same species; e.g., an adult bird killing and eating eggs or young birds.

Cannula A tube for insertion into a duct or cavity; during insertion into a duct or cavity; during insertion its lumen is usually occupied by a trocar.

Canthal Pertaining to a canthus.

Canthi The palpebral commissures, or angles at which the eyelids meet.

Cantle A piece or fragment.

Canula A hollow tube designed for insertion into a body cavity either to aspirate or to introduce medication.

Canulated nail A general class of nail having a lumen in center.

Cap stage Second stage of formation of the enamel organ.

Capacitance vessels The large venules and veins that from a large, variable-volume, and low-pressure reservoir.

Capacitation The process by which a spermatozoon is conditioned to fertilise an ovum after it is exposed to the female reproductive tract.

Capacity for growth One of three fundamental characteristics of human uniqueness postulated in the humanistic approach to personality. It emphasises that human beings have high level goals and values and seek to achieve satisfaction in these ways, as opposed to such basic goals as seeking food, safety, and the capacity for development in psychological direction.

CAPD Continuous ambulatory peritoneal dialysis.

Capener's method A method of measuring degree of spondylolisthesis.

Capillary Minute blood vessel consisting only a simple squamous epithelium and a basement membrane, major site for the exchange of substances between the blood and tissues.

Capillary action Movement of a liquid at the point of contact with a solid.

Capillary bleeding It is caused by damage to the smallest blood vessels generally in the skin or mucous membrane. Blood oozes for some time over the whole surface of the wound but soon clots and bleeding stops spontaneously.

Capillary blood pressure The blood pressure found in the capillary vessels.

Capillary circulation It contains 5% of circulating blood volume which passes from arterioles to venules via capillaries with in 2 seconds.

Capillary closing pressure The amount of external pressure required to close off the blood flow to the capillaries.

Capillary electropherograph Instrument for capillary electrophoresis.

Capillary enzyme immunoassay Immunoassay carried out in a capillary electrophoresis sysstem in which electrophoresis produces the separation of free antigen from the antigen bound to the antibody.

Capillary fragility test Sphygmomanometer cuff is applied below the elbow and a pressure midway between the systolic and the diastolic is maintained for 15 minutes. When the test is positive there appears large number of petechiae, and is seen in cases of vitamin C deficiency.

Capillary refill time Amount of time taken by blood to resume flowing in the base of the nail beds.

Capillary stasis Stagnation of blood in the capillaries.

Capitaiton basis for payment Payment of primary care physicians on a "per head" basis. Although patients vary in their need for and use of medical services, the physician receives the same amount of money per patient per year.

Capital epiphysis The proximal epiphysis of femur. It ossifies in 4-5 months. It fuses at about 16-18 years.

Capitate One of the bones of carpus.

Capitation Strategy for controlling health care costs by paying a fixed amount per member.

Capitellum The rounded bony prominence of lateral aspect of distal humerus that articulates with humerus.

Capitulum A small, anterior projection of acarines that bears the mouth parts.

Caplan syndrome This is characterised by pneumoconiosis and rheumatoid arthritis. It is usually seen in coal miners, pottery workers. There will be cough with expectoration due to bronchitis. Sputum may be black in coal miners. Right ventricular failure supervenes as terminal event. Fibrotic nodules of 0.5 to 3 cm diameter peripheral parts of lungs are seen.

Capnography It is a continuous measurement and pictorial display of CO_2 concentration.

Capping An active process whereby cross-linking of cell surface molecules e.g. by antibody leads to aggregation and subsequent migration of the molecules to one pole of the cell.

Capreomycin It is a cyclic polypeptide antibacterial drug. It is used in TB resist to other therapy.

Caproic acid A standard fatty acid occuring in cow and goat butter and coconut fat.

Capsid The protein coat or shell that contains the nucleic acid genome of the virus particle.

Capsomere Represents the individual morphological units on the surface of capcid.

Capsule Found in diarthrotic joints, holds the bones of joints together while allowing movement and is made of fibrous connective tissue lined with a smooth, slippery synovial membrane.

Capsulectomy Any surgical procedure for excision of whole or part of capsule.

Capsulitis Inflammation of shoulder capsule is more common in shoulder joint and complains of pain in shoulder and develops stiffness soon after.
For about 3 months pain and stiffness increase and thereafter remain static. During next 3 months pain reduces and range of movements increases gradually. Manipulation under anaesthesia is helpful.

Capsulotome or cystitome The purpose of this instrument is to rupture the anterior capsule of the lens. Many surgeons use a injection needle 22 gauge, shaped according to their own requirements and needs. It works very well and can be disposed off.

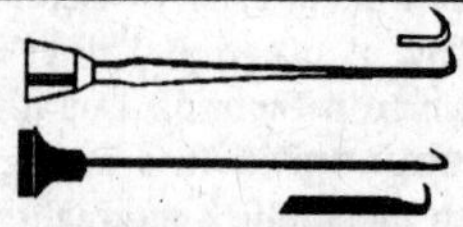

Capsulotome or cystitome

Capsulotomy Incision into a joint space.

Captopril An antihypertensive agent; an angiotension-converting enzyme inhibitor.

Caput index X-Ray technique used to determine femoral head sphericity using arthrographic measurement.

Caput succedaneum In it presenting part is edematous. The presenting part is surrounded and compressed by cervix except in the region of cervical opening. The part underlying orifice is under less pressure and results in exudation of fluid and extravasation of blood into the subcutaneous tissues. So caput succedaneum may be over vertex, face or buttocks. It disappears within 48 hours.

Caput ulnal syndrome Affection of radio ulnar joint in rheumatoid hand. Pain develops at ulnar head.

Carat 1. A measure of fineness of gold; pure gold being 24 carats or having 24 parts of gold and 18-carat gold having only 18 parts of gold and 6 parts of another metal.

Carbamazepine It is an anticonvulsant drug chemically related to tricyclic drugs. It reduces seizures caused by abnormal nerve signals in the brain. It is also given to relieve neuralgia. It may be helpful in certain psychological or behavioural disorders.

Carbamazepine intoxication It is used as anticonvulsant drug and also in treatment of painful neuropathies. Acute ingestions of over 10 mg/kg of carbamazepine are likely to produce toxicity. Intoxication results in nystagmus, dysarthria, vertigo, dilated pupils and confusion. In severe intoxication coma, myoclonus, respiratory depression, and apnoea occurs. Patients may develop hypertension, gastric emptying may be delayed.

Carbaminohemoglobin The compound formed for the union of carbon dioxide with hemoglobin.

Carbanion A negatively charged carbon atom.

Carbenoxolone This aids mucosal protection perhaps by increasing mucus secretion, reducing diffusion of H^+ ions and reducing cell loss, and it also has mild anti-inflammatory actions. It is effective in healing gastric ulcer some 40 to 70 % in 6 weeks and also in duodenal ulcer. Given in doses of 300 mg/day for 2 weeks, then 150 mg for 4 weeks leads to substantial mineralocorticoid effects in many patients.

Carbicarb It is a buffer composed of 0.3 M sodium carbonate and 0.3 M sodium bicarbonate used to treat acidosis.

Carbocation A positively charged carbon atom; also called a carbonium ion.

Carbohydrate Sugar and starch are well known carbohydrates. Before they are used by the body complex, carbohydrates are to be broken into simple monosaccharide sugars, glucose, galactose and fructose. The enzymes of saliva starts breaking down. Cellulose remains unaffected by saliva. The monosaccharides are then absorbed through the intestinal wall. Brain cells and RBCs require glucose to survive. When blood sugar is high after meals, carbohydrate metabolism is controlled by insulin.

Carbohydrate loading The method used by athletes to increase the stores of muscle glycogen, allowing more sustained aerobic exercise.

Carbohydrate oxidation The process in which O_2 unites with carbohydrate to form CO_2, water and heat and chemical energy through the terminal respiratory chain. Heat represents the energy available for maintenance of body temperature. Chemical energy mainly in the form of ATP is used for and physical work.

Carbohydrate storage It is stored in the liver and other cells as the polysaccharide glycogen. Glycogen has protective action too.

Carbohydrates Nutrients that contain molecules of carbon, hydrogen, and oxygen.

Carbon dioxide It is a colourless gas with pungent odour in high concentration. Molecular weight is 44. Critical temperature is 31°C. Critical pressure is 73.8 atmosphere. Cylinders of CO_2 are painted grey. Carbon dioxide oxygen premixed cylinders are available in various combinations. Cylinders are filled at 137 atmosphere. More than five per cent concentration of CO_2 may cause distress, dyspnoea, and headache. At 30 per cent person will develop coma, Normally inspired air contains 0.03 per cent while expired air contains 4%. Alveolar air contains 5 to 6 per cent. It is useful in increasing depth of anaesthesia rapidly when volatile agents are in use. The addition of a little CO_2 for no longer than 5 minutes stimulates depth of respiration. It is useful to widen the glottis and facilitate blind intubation. It has been given during anaesthesia to increase cerebral blood flow in arteriosclerotic patients undergoing surgery.

Carbon dioxide narcosis Loss of consciousness caused by severe hypercapnia. Arterial PCO_2 exceeds 200 m.m. Hg.

Carbon dioxide withdrawal Sudden fall of PCO_2 may result in hypotension. There may develop hyperkalaemia and dysrhythmia. Shift of oxygen-haemoglobin dissociation curve impedes oxygen exchange at tissue level. Rapid following of chronic hypercapnia in respiratory failure can lead to convulsions and death unless the alkalaemia produced is corrected.

Carbon disulphide It is a colourless, transparent fluid with sweetish aromatic odour. It is soluble in fat. Acute exposure is not common. In acute form neurological features predominate. After ingestion patient develops spasmodic tremors. There develops cyanosis, large pupils, pallor, hypothermia, confusion, delirium and finally coma. Less serious manifestations include hemiplegia, unsteadiness in arms and legs. Late features are of parkinsonism.

Carbon fixation reactions In photosynthetic cells, the light-independent enzymatic reactions involved in the synthesis of glucose from CO_2, ATP, and NADPH, also known as the dark reactions.

Carbon markings Carbon paper is put in between teeth articulation to find out high points.

Carbon monoxide (CO) A gas that acts as chemical neurotransmitter.

Carbonaceous Containing or composed of carbon.

Carbonic anhydrase Zinc containing enzyme catalysing the reaction of CO_2 and water to form carbonic acid. It readily dissociates to bicarbonate and hydrogen ions and is not found in plasma.

Carboxyhemoglobin The result of the union of carbon monoxide with hemoglobin.

Carboxypenicillins Antibacterial spectrum is that of ampicillin but have the additional capacity to destroy *Pseudomonas aeruginosa.* It is given parentrally. It inactivate aminoglycosides if both drugs are given in same syringe.

Carboxypeptidase A pancreatic protease that hydrolyzes polypeptides into amino acids.

Carbuncle This is a cluster of boils caused by *Staphylococcus aureus.* Common sites are the back of neck and the buttocks. These mostly develop in diabetics. If diabetes is present then blood sugar is to be controlled by antidiabetic drugs first and then antibiotics will be helpful.

Carcinogen Any agent capable of resulting in cancer is known as carcinogen. Amongst them common are polycyclic aromatic hydrocarbons. Exposure of ultraviolet rays over years may result in skin cancer. Asbestos fibres are another known physical cause of cancer. Certain viruses are believed to be responsible for cancer of cervix, the hepatitis B has been identified to cause liver cancer.

Carcinogenesis The process of cancer production.

Carcinoid syndrome The syndrome occurs commonly with tumours arising from the embryological midgut. 10% of such tumours give rise to the carcinoid syndrome. Syndrome occurs when the primary tumour is clinically silent. At this time liver may be large, hard and irregular. Symptoms are episodic. There are attacks of flushing of skin mostly confined to upper half of body and associated with cyanosis. There may be associated salivation, lacrimation, conjunctival oedema, palpitations and hypotension, emotional stress. Alcholol and trytophan containing foods may precipitate it. In 30% cases bronchospasm may worry the patients.

Carcinoid tumour These are APUD tumours usually of G.I.T., sometimes in the respiratory tract and elsewhere. These are multiple, slow growing but malignant. Microscopically these are localised within gut wall with considerable fibrosis around. Rarely they may ulcerate. There may be massive enlargement of draining lymph nodes even while the primary growth is small. Hepatic spread is late. Microscopically carcinoid tumours consist of nonencapsulated collections of uniform polygonal cells with speckled chromatin cells occurring in cluster. Local tumour is usually asymptomatic. Local extension may lead to colicky pain, intestinal obstruction, perforation and haemorrhage.

Carcinoma A malignant tumour derived from epithelial tissue.

Carcinoma of vulva 2 to 3 % of all malignancies of genital tract are vulval carcinoma. Mostly are squamous type. It is not related to parity. Pruritus is the most common symptom. There may be vulval swelling, or ulcer. Lesions bleed on touch and there may be an offensive discharge. Pain is a late feature of carcinoma. Advanced lesions may lead to stenosis of urethra. Inguinal lymph nodes are enlarged.

Carcinoma endometrium It may be diffuse or localised. Pain is a late symptom. Diagnosis is made by examining tissue obtained by endometrial biopsy or by curettage.

Carcinoma in situ These are mucosal lesions resembling leukoplakia in all respects except that dyskeratosis involving epithelial strata. It appears as a white plaque or an ulcer, erosions or reddened area. Lesions of floor of mouth, tongue and lips are most aggressive.

Carcinoma in situ in pregnancy The peak incidence of carcinoma in situ coincides with the most active child bearing years. Pregnancy by itself produces a completely benign reversible change by way of basal cell hyperactivity. With carcinoma in situ normal vaginal delivery is possible.

Carcinoma of pancreas About 80% cases arise from epithelium. Most patients are middle-aged. Weight loss is an early manifestation. Epigastric discomfort or pain with a bloating feeling occurs in majority. Pain radiates to back and may be relieved by leaning forward. Jaundice is common with carcinoma of head. Diabetes mellitus found in non in elderly obese should raise suspicion. There may be palpable mass in epigastrium. Ascites indicates metastasis. Ultrasound and endoscopic retrograde cholangiopancreatography (ERCP) helps in diagnosis.

Carcinoma penis It mostly occurs in middle-aged and elderly people. In 95% cases, it is squamous cell carcinoma and is more common in poor class having poor hygiene. Lesion usually occurs on glans penis and the inner surface of prepuce near reflection from the corona. Growth commonly starts as a wart or an ulcer. Growth is slowly growing and remains localised for many months. Spread to the body of penis is restricted by Buck's fascia. Urethra remains spared even in long standing cases. Distant metastasis by blood is rare. Patient presents with a lump or an ulcer. If infected lesion may be painful. Inguinal glands will be enlarged. Anaemia, loss of appetite and loss of weight are rare.

Carcinomatosis Presence of one or more enlarging carcinoma in different sites due to metastasis forms an original malignant tumour. X-ray and radioisotope imaging is helpful. Chemotherapy or radiation therapy may be given. Metastasis from testis, prostate and thyroid may be treated with prolonged abetment of symptoms.

Carcinophobia Fear of carcinoma.

Cardia output Volume of blood pumped by heart per minute. It is equal to stroke volume X heart rate.

Cardiac Each complete heartbeat, including contraction and relaxation of the ateria and ventricles.

Cardiac muscle dysfunction (CMD) A term that has gained popularity in describing an apparently common finding in patients with heart and lung disease.

Cardiac anomalies Anomalies that result from congenital heart defects. These include transposition of the great vessels, atrial septal defect, patent ductus arteriosus, ventricular septal defect, coarctation of the aorta, the tetralogy of Fallot, and others.

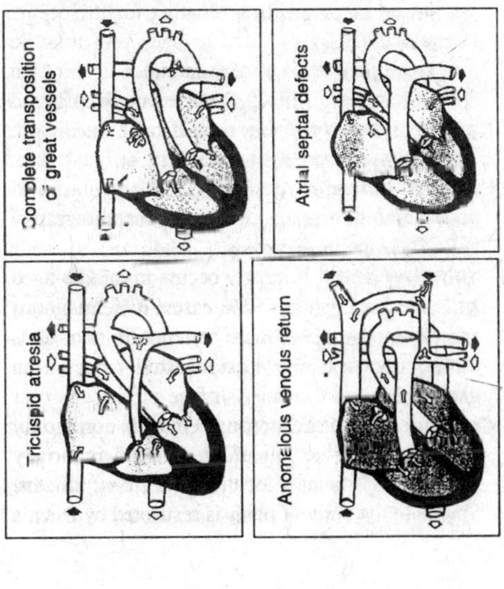

Cardiac arrest The most common cause is myocardial infarction. Other causes include respiratory arrest, electrical injury, hypothermia, loss of blood, drug overdose and injection anaphylactic shock. Patient collapses suddenly with loss of consciousness. Pulse is not felt and neither respiratory movements are seen. If a person is breathing normally then he or she has not suffered cardiac arrest. Cardiac arrest may respond to IV infusion of epinephrine + calcium. In extreme cases direct injection of epinephrine into heart may help. Electrical pacemaker may help.

Cardiac asthma Acute pulmonary oedema resembling asthma.

Cardiac catheterisation Diagnostic indication includes assessment of congenital and acquired malformation of coronary arteries and valves. It is used for endomyocardial biopsy for transplant rejection and measurement of blood gases and shunt quantification. It is useful in recording of bundle of His and transcoronary ultrasound. Therapeutic uses include percutaneous transluminal cutaneous angioplasty, balloon dilatation of mitral, pulmonary and aortic valves. Coronary stenting, coil placement, ablation of AV node can be helped by cardiac catheterisation.

Cardiac cirrhosis The fibrotic reaction that occurs within the liver as the result of prolonged congestive heart failure.

Cardiac cycle It is the operation of heart from one heart beat to another. It comprises events of one systole and one diastole.

Cardiac decompensation Impaired cardiac output for which the reasons are not entirely understood.

Cardiac dilatation It happens when heart is failing to keep pace with demand. Slight dilatation is immediate physiological response of heart to increased work. If increased work continues hypertrophy follows. Cardiac dyspnoea is always accompanied to cardiac enlargement. Hypertensive heart disease, syphilis, coronary arteriosclerosis, emphysema may cause it. Usually left side is first affected and its failure later causes right ventricle to fall.

Cardiac dysrhythmias It includes all conditions where cardiac rate and rhythm will be altered or there is defect in conductive system. It may have its origin in SA node, atrium, AV junction or in ventricle.

Cardiac failure Usually defined as inability to produce sufficient output for the body's requirement and venous return.

Cardiac glycoside Drugs to treat supraventricular arrhythmias and cardiac failure.

Cardiac hypertrophy It is an increase of muscular substance of heart and its weight which is normally 250 gm in women and 300 gm in men. There will be increase in precordial dullness in downward and outward direction in left ventricle hypertrophy. In right ventricle there will be outward enlargement. Impulse of apex is undue forcible, heaving or thrusting, and thrust is being generally felt in epigastric notch. On auscultation first sound is loud and prolonged. Hypertrophy is caused by increase in work.

Cardiac impression The indentations on the inner surfaces of the lungs that outline the contact areas of the heart.

Cardiac index A relative measure of cardiac output based on body side; expressed in terms of volume (L) Per area (m^2) per unit of time (minute).

Cardiac ischemia Impaired blood flow to the heart.

Cardiac jelly The noncellular material between the endothelial lining and the myocardial layer of the early embryonic heart.

Cardiac massage Periodic compression of heart and chest in order to maintain cardiac output.

Cardiac muscle Muscle of the heart, consisting of striated muscle cells. These cells are interconnected into a mass called the myocardium.

Cardiac neurosis It is an excessive anxiety about heart condition. It generally develops after myocardial infarction. Person experiences chest pain, lethargy, palpitation and breathlessness but on examination cardiologist will not find any organic cause. It simply requires psychotherapy.

Cardiac notch A roughly V-shaped depression in the anterior border of the left lung at the level of the fourth costal cartilage.

Cardiac oedema It is due to diminished cardiac output and fall in filtration pressure in renal glomeruli and leads to sodium retention. Oedema develops in most dependent part. Dyspnoea precedes dropsy. Heart failure with congestive heart failure is known as congestive cardiac failure. Oedema in absence of dyspnoea and cardiac enlargement is not due to heart disease.

Cardiac output Volume of blood pumped by either ventricle of the heart per minute; about 5 litres/min for the heart of a healthy adult at rest.

Cardiac pacing Repetitive electrical stimulation of cardiac activity used to treat brady or tachy arrhythmias.

Cardiac plexus The anastomosing network of sympathetic and parasympathetic (vagus) nerves that surround the arch of the aorta and the pulmonary artery before continuing to the atria, ventricles, and coronary vessels.

Cardiac psychosis A disorganization of thought process associated with fear and anxiety following heart attack.

Cardiac rehabilitation A multidisciplinary program designed to assist patients with cardiac disease to achieve their optimal physiologic, psychological, and functional status through the use of education and exercise to decrease the risk of a secondary event.

Cardiac rehabilitation center A facility in which cardiac rehabilitation is conducted.

Cardiac risk index Goldman cardiac risk index was derived in 1977. Nine risk factors were identified.

- MI within 6 months — 10 points
- Elevated JVP — 11 points
- Ventricular ectopic beat>5 min — 7 points
- Age > 70 years — 5 points
- Emergency operations — 4 points
- Severe aortic stenosis — 3 points
- Poor condition — 3 points
- Abdominal/thoracic operation — 3 points

Patients scoring above 25 are having higher risk.

Cardiac silhouette The outline of the heart seen on a radiographic image of the chest.

Cardiac sphincter A ring of muscle between the stomach and esophagus that prevents food from reentering the esophagus when the stomach contracts.

Cardiac tamponade Compression of heart by fluid within in the pericardium, restricting ventricular filling and reducing stroke volume and cardiac output.

Cardiac transplantation Cardiac transplantation is the last hope for those patients who are resistant to medical and surgical therapy of heart ailment. Recipient should be otherwise healthy with lungs and normal healthy kidneys. With availability of cyclosporin A, graft rejection rate has declined and one year survival rate can be predicted to be around 80% with 3% decrease for every year.

Cardiac vein Any vein that carries blood from the myocardial capillary beds to the coronary sinus.

Cardiacplegia Intentional cardiac arrest caused by coronary perfusion with cold electrolyte solution to allow cardiac surgery.

Cardinal movements Positional changes that help the fetus meet minimal resistance as it passes through the birth canal. These movements include descent, flexion, internal rotation, extension, external rotation, and expulsion.

Cardinal number A number that represents quantity.

Cardinal symptoms Most characteristic symptoms of any disease.

Cardinal trait According to Allport's theory of personality, a single outstanding characteristic that dominates a person's life; few individuals are characterized by a cardinal disposition.

Cardiogenic Of cardiac origin.

Cardiogenic cords Strands of mesenchymal cells that develop in the cardiogenic area of the presomite embryo.

Cardiogenic shock A condition arising when the blood supplying to the body tissues in insufficient because of inadequate cardiac output.

Cardiokinetic Stimulating the action of the heart.

Cardiologist A physician who specializes in the diagnosis and treatment of disease of the heart.

Cardiology The study of the heart and diseases associated with it.

Cardiomegaly There is enlargement of heart and there is hypertrophy of heart muscle. Hypertension causes the wall of left ventricle to thicken. In pulmonary hypertension both ventricles may be thickened. Dilatation of a heart chamber may be due to heart valve incompetency. Certain types of cardiomyopathy can also lead to swelling of a chamber. Heart failure will result causing breathlessness and swelling of the legs and hands.

Cardiomyopathy The disease may be infectious, metabolic or nutritional. It may be toxic or degenerative. *Hypertrophic* type is usually familial. *Dilated cardiomyopathy*, muscle cell metabolism is abnormal and walls of heart tends to dilate.

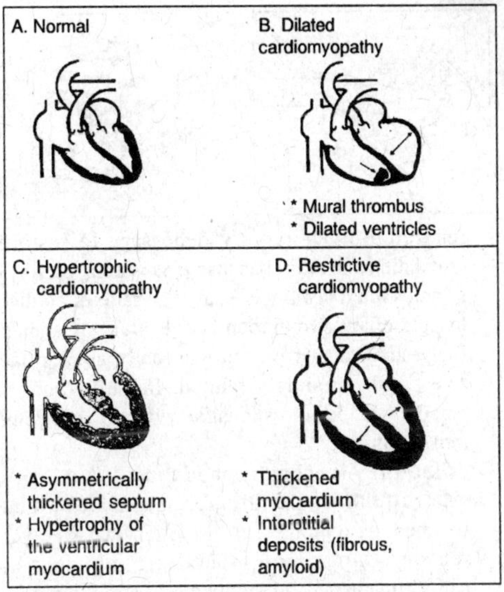

Restrictive cardiomyopathy is caused by scarring of endocardium. Heart muscle disorder may be due to poisoning. Person may develop fatigue, chest pain and palpitation. Heart failure may cause difficulty in breathing and oedema. ECG shows enlarged electrical impulses on the tracing due to heart muscle hypertrophy.

Cardiomyoplasty An alternative to heart transplantation, this surgical procedure takes a transformed, fatigueresistant skeletal muscle often the latissimus and wraps it around the patient's heart; this muscle is then electrically stimulated to contract with systole.

Cardionihibitory Restraining or inhibiting the movements of the heart.

Cardiopathy Any disease of the heart.

Cardiopulmonary arrest Sudden cessation of respirations, pulse, and circulation.

Cardiopulmonary resuscitation It is a life-saving cardiac massage and mouth to mouth

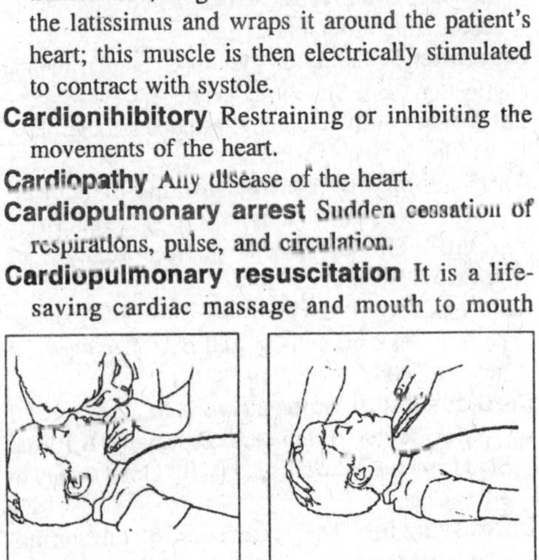

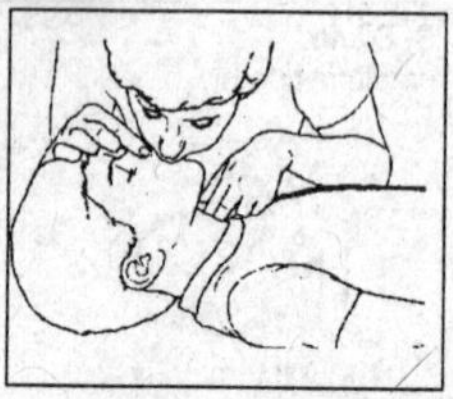

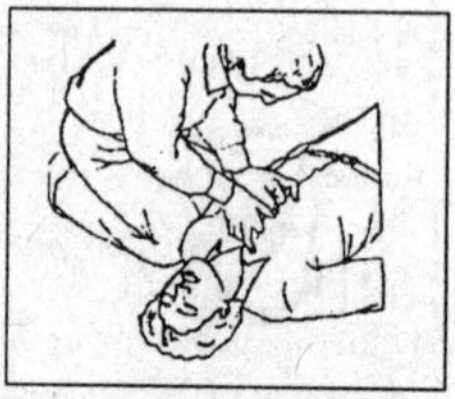

resuscitation. It is very necessary to restore circulation for brain because if it is delayed for 3 minutes brain death will start. The ratio of cardiac to pulmonary stimulation is 5:1. But one should first establish that person has really got cardiac arrest and not simply fainted. In cardiac arrest person will be unresponsive with no breathing movements.

Cardioquin An antiarrhythmic drug.

Cardioregulatory centre Specialised area within the medulla oblongata of the brain that receives sensory input and functions to control parasympathetic and sympathetic stimulation of the heart.

Cardiothymic silhouette The line of demarcation between the thymus gland and the heart in the superior mediastinum; sometimes visible in radiographic images of the chest.

Cardiotocography This involves a continuous recording of fetal heart rate. The machine calculates the rate. A normal trace shows a short-term variation of greater than 5 beats, a rate between 120 and 160 beats per minute spontaneous acceleration of fetal heart rate is a good sign.

Cardiotoxic Having a deleterious or detrimental effect on the action of the heart.

Cardiovascular Pertaining to the heart and blood vessels.

Cardiovascular center Groups of neurons scattered within the medulla oblongata that regulate heart rate, force of contraction, and blood vessel diameter.

Cardiovascular endurance The ability of the body to take in, deliver, and obtain oxygen for physical work.

Cardiovascular homeostasis Maintenance of cardiovascular parameters, especially B.P. and blood volume at levels optimal for blood supply to all organs.

Cardioversion The restoration of the normal rhythm of the heart by electrical countershock.

Care of umbilical cord The umblical cord should be doubly clamped and cut in between two clamps and ligated doubly. The first ligature should be 2.5 cm from the umbilicus. A separate pair of scissors should be used for cutting. Cut end of cord should be touched with savlon and be left without dressing.

Carebaria A form of headache with distressing sensation of pressure/heaviness.

Career A chosen pursuit; a life's work.

Caregiver Any person involved in the identification or prevention of illness or in the treatment or rehabilitation of the patient; includes the psychiatrist and other members of the traditional treatment team as well as community workers and other non-professionals.

Caretaker-child interaction The mutual responsiveness between a child and the adults responsible for that child's care.

Caridac vein Any vein that carries blood from the myocardial capillary beds to the coronary sinus.

Caries These are most common diseases of man. It is decalcification and disintegration of hard dental tissue. Diet rich in fermentable carbohydrate promotes caries. Bacteria destroy the protein

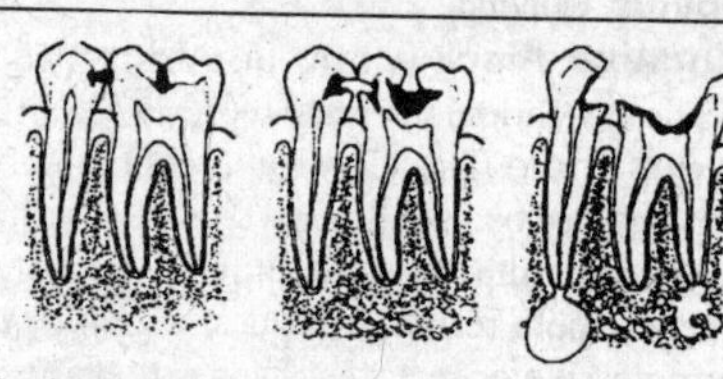

A. Proximal caries reaching to dentin
B. Severe proximal and occlusal caries nearing pulp chamber
C. Caries invading pulp chamber

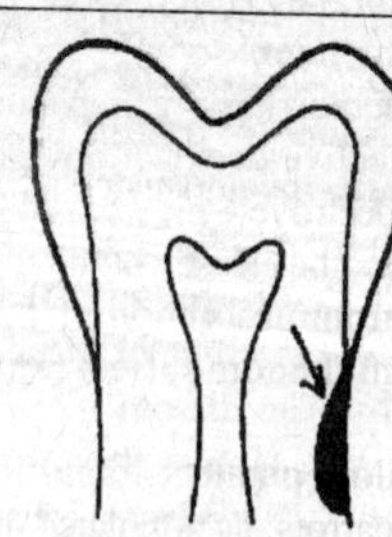

Root caries, Enamel is not involved

content of teeth. The bacteria primarily responsible for dental decay in man are *Streptococcus mutans*. These organisms proliferate in the supragingival dental plaque. Rate of caries initiation and extension depends on the susceptibility of enamel. Under low magnification, a smooth surface carious lesion appears triangular with the apex of cone pointed toward the dentin. Section through a carious lesion in dentin shows four zones. Deepest zone is that of fatty degeneration of dentinal tubules. Next is zone of sclerosis. Coronal to zone of sclerosis is a zone that shows decalcification and invasion of tubules by microorganism. Most superficial zone of lesion consists of completely necrotic dentin.

Caries ceremental Decay found on tooth root.

Caries removal The Process of arresting the decay through mechanical removal.

Carina The ridge separating the openings of the right and left main bronchi at their junction with the trachea.

Caring skills Nursing interventions that restore or maintain a person's health.

Cariogenesis Development of caries.

Cariogenic Conducive to caries.

Carminative A solution to provide relief from gaseous distention.

Carneous mole The term mole is applied to an ovum blighted by pathological conditions affecting its coverings during early months of gestation. Carneous mole results from destruction of ovum by progressive or recurrent haemorrhages usually but not invariably before the formation of placenta, i.e. during the first 3 months of pregnancy. It is completely enveloped in the thick, very vascular decidual membrane. Blood mole is formed by repeated slight haemorrhage or by a slowly progressive haemorrhage which does not cause rupture of protective decidual covering of ovum. An ovum thus destroyed, may be retained in uterus for many weeks. The effused blood then undergoes consolidation from absorption of fluid, and wall of dead ovum become firm and fleshy in consistency.

Carotene A yellow pigment found in plants such as squash and carrots; accumulates in the lipids of the stratum corneum and in the fat cells of the dermis and hypodermis and used as a source of vitamin A.

Carotenoids Fat extracted from any tissue is always more or less yellow. It is due to fat soluble pigments called lipochrome or carotenoids. These may be easily obtained from carrots and plant leaves. 1000 kg of carrots contains 25 gm of carotene. Carotene can be broken down to vitamin 'A' in liver. Carotenes are present in human fat, milk, serum and nervous tissue.

Carotid body tumour Carotid body is situated at the bifurcation of carotid artery and is the most important moiety of the chemoreceptor system. The cells of this system are sensitive to changes in pH and temperature. It is usually unilateral. There develops a lump at bifurcation. This lump does not move vertically but only side to side. Arteriography shows carotid fork to be splayed and a blush outlining the abnormal tumour vessels.

Carotid arteries Either one of the two main right and left arteries of the neck.

Carotid artery surgery It is done in patients with carotid stenosis. It reduces a risk of CVA by more than 50 percent.

Carotid artery syndrome Causes include microemboli, atherosclerotic plaques, arteritis between the age of 50 and 70 years. There will be transient cerebral ischaemia with contralateral weakness of arm and leg. Hemisensory disturbance and mental confusion will take place. Person may develop lacrimation, homolateral transient painless visual loss, photopsia, retinal infarcts and cataract.

Carotid body Chemoreceptor located in the carotid artery that detects changes in the oxygen, carbon dioxide, and blood acid levels.

Carotid duplex ultrasonography A diagnostic procedure to identify plaque, stenoses, and occlusions of internal, common, and external carotid arteries and flow direction in vertebral arteries.

Carotid endarterectomy The excision of occluding material e.g., thrombus from the carotid artery.

Carotid insufficiency The sudden occlusion of common carotid artery causes permanent central nervous deficits while slowly growing occlusion may not develop it. Carotid stenosis not caused by trauma or neoplasia may be asymptomatic. Symptoms depend on degree of stenosis. A sudden bilateral occlusion of external carotid may lead to severe necrosis of various sites in head and neck.

Carotid massage The manual rhythmic compression of the carotid sinuses at the bifurcation of the common into the internal and external carotid arteries in an effort to slow the heart rate.

Carotid pulse It is a smooth, relatively rapid upstroke and a smooth more gradual downstroke, interrupted only briefly at the pulse peak.

Carotid sinus Enlargement of the internal carotid artery near the point where the internal carotid artery branches from the common carotid artery; contains baroreceptors.

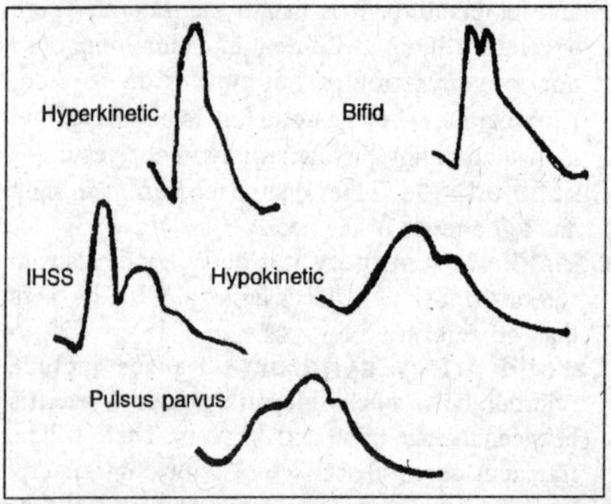

Carotid sinus reflex A reflex concerned with maintaining normal blood pressure in the brain.

Carotidynia There develops throbbing pain along one side of neck from lower jaw to clavicle, lasting from minutes to several hours. Tenderness over carotid artery shows increased pulsation.

Carpal Pertaining to the wrist.

Carpal bones The eight small bones of wrist.

Carpal height The distance between the distal cortex of capitate and prominent proximal lunate, as measured along the long axis of third metacarpal.

Carpal tunnel The space between the flexor retinaculum of wrist and carpal bones through which flexor tendons of fingers, pollicis longus and median nerve passes.

Carpal tunnel syndrome It is the compression of the median nerve in the carpal tunnel with paraesthesia and pain on the palmar aspect of the thumb, index, middle and ring fingers radiating to forearm.

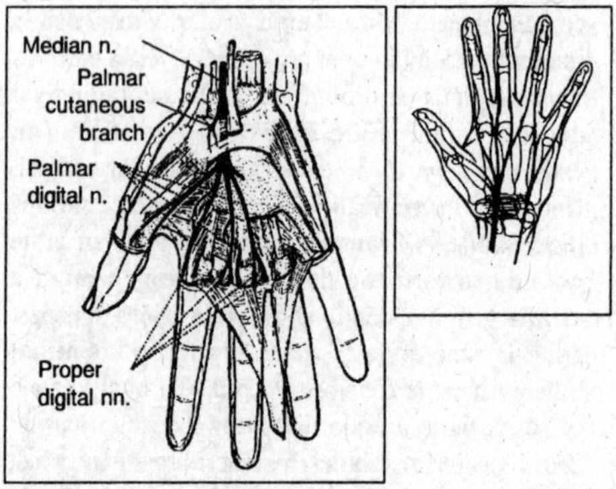

Carpectomy A surgical procedure to excise carpal bone.

Carpule Cylindrical device that holds medication before and during administration.

Carpus The proximal prodion of the hand that contains the eight carpal bones.

Carr splint A splint used for the first aid treatment of distal upper extremity injuries.

Carrier An infected person who harbours a specific infectius agent in the absence of discernible clinical disease and serves as a potential source of infection.

Carrier molecule Protein that extends from one side of the cell membrane to the other; binds to molecules to be transported and moves them from one side of the membrane to the other.

Carrying angle A normal carrying angle is present at the elbow along the longitudinal axis in anatomic position with arm extended. The angle normally is 5 degrees in men and 10 to 15 degrees in women. An increased carrying angle can be caused by lateral epicondylar fracture that damages the epiphysis which may also lead to delayed ulnar nerve palsy. Carrying angle should be bilaterally symmetric.

Carter-Robbins test In this test intravenous infusion of hypertonic saline does not cause any decrease in urinary flow in diabetes insipidus. In psychogenic diabetes insipidus, however, the urinary flow decreases and the urinary specific gravity increases during or immediately after the infusion.

Cartilage It is a variety of connective tissue, firm yet elastic and is associated with bony framework of body. In is non-vascular and its nutrition is maintained by imbition of tissue fluid through matrix. It covers articular ends of bones, costal or rib cartilage, nasal cartilage, cartilages of larynx and trachea. These are of 3 types : *fibrocartilage* makes up much of the tendons and intervertebral disc, *elastic cartilage* forms the outer ear flap, and third one *hyaline cartilage*, the rigid tissue which forms the larynx and upper respiratory tract.

Cartilaginous Consisting of or of the nature of cartilage.

Cartilaginous joint A joint without a synovial (joint) cavity where the articulating bones are held tightly together by cartilage, allowing little or no movement.

calcifications. These tend to grow in lobules and is identified by lobulated growth.

Cartridge The unit of ammunition that consists of a case containing primer and propellant.

Cartridge case A cartridge case contains all the components of modern ammunition in an easy to handle weatherproof package. It also seals gas, the breech of the gun on firing.

Cartwheel fracture Fracture of distal femoral epiphysis.

Caruncle A convex connective tissue structure of the endometrium that is covered by a layer of luminal epithelium; characteristic of the uterus of ruminants and developing into the maternal half of the placentome.

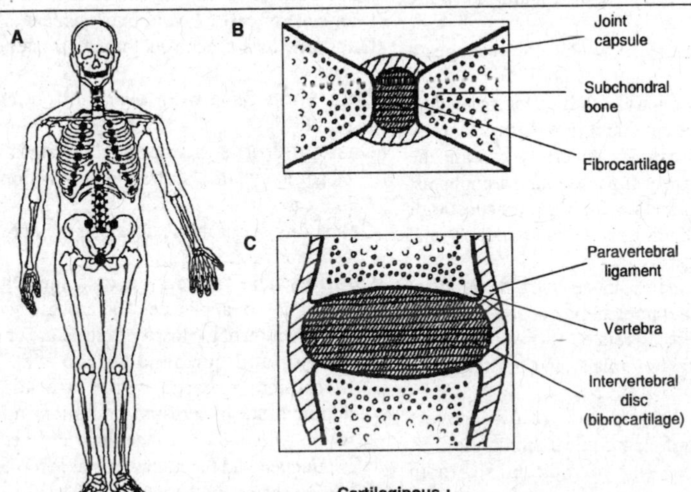

Cartilaginous :
(A) Distribution (B) Symphis pubis (C) Intervertebral joint.

Cartilaginous tumor These can be recognised by popcorn like punctate, annular or comma shaped

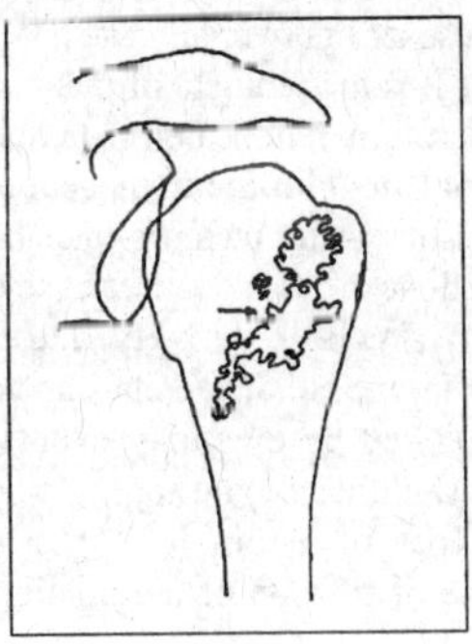

Carver A knife or any other instrument used for carving or fashioning an object by cutting, such as one used for shaping artificial teeth and dental wax or amalgam.

CASA Computer-assisted semen analysis, the automated analysis of sperm swimming patterns, used to help identify treatment effects on sperm. Poor CASA values may correlate with reduced fertility.

Case A person who has a disease of interest.

Case brace Combination of a brace within a cast at a joint.

Case definition Characterizes the clinical manifestations of the condition under investigation. The case definition provides the inclusion and exclusoin creteria that are used to determine which subjects are cases and which are not cases in an outbreak investigation.

Case fatality The proportion of persons with a particular disease with in a specified period of time.

Case fatality ratio The proportion of clinically ill persons who die of the condition under study. this is a marker of virulence.

Case finding The process of searching for asymptomatic diseases or risk factors among people while they are in a clinical setting.

Case history Assembled data which reconstruct an individual's past with the aim of understanding his or her present problems and aiding in future adjustment.

Case method Pattern in which one manages a patient's care for a designated period.

Case report A descriptive study of an individual patient presented in narrative form. Details included in such a study generally contain the patient's health history and presenting complaints, any relevant examination findings, diagnostic or analytical conclusions, intervention protocols, and outcomes assessment.

Case sequencing In implant dentistry, the protocol followed for a dental implant procedure, including timing of treatment as related to healing, tissue integration around the implant, and prosthodontic restoration.

Case series A descriptive study of two or more patient's with significant clinical similarities.

Case stabilization Use of rods, pins, broom handles, or sticks to lend stability to a particular cast.

Caseation The breakdown and necrosis of a diseased tissue into a dry, amorphous, cheese like mass.

Casein A white amorphous, colloidal aggregate, soluble in acids, that is found in milk and that is composed of several proteins together with calcium and phosphorus.

CASH Cortical androgen stimulating hormone, a human pituitary factor proposed as the primary regulator of adrenal androgens due to its ability to stimulate adrenal androgen secretion in vitro.

Casoni reaction Even though not so specific Casoni reaction is used for the diagnosis of *Echinococcus* infection in which case intradermal administration of inactivated hydatid fluid produces both immediate and delayed reaction.

Cassette Light-tight container in which X-ray films are placed for exposure to X-radiation; usually backed with lead to eliminate the effect of backscatter radiation.

Cast A small mass of hardened material formed within a cavity in the body and then discharged from the body; can originate in different areas and can be composed of various materials.

Cast (kast) An accurate reproduction or a replica of an object or part produced in a plastic material which has taken form in an impression or mould. A positive reproduction of a maxillary or mandibular arch or a portion thereof made from an impression of that arch.

Cast bender A heaving forcep used to bend a part of edge of cast to avoid impingement.

Cast saw Saw used to cut through plaster to remove cast.

Cast shoe Shoe worn over the foot encased in plaster.

Cast syndrome A series of client signs indicative of an untoward claustrophobic reaction to being in a cast.

Caste Any set of individuals that are specialized in behavior, as in social insects.

Casting The fabrication of a metallic dental restoration or appliance. The process involves the reproduction of the lost tooth structure or appliance in wax and surrounding the wax with an investment material which is a mixure of a hemihydrate of gypsum and silica mixed with water. After the investment has hardened, the wax is removed and the molten metal is forced into the space vacated by the wax.

Casting machine Mechanical device used for throwing or forcing a molten metal into a refractory mold.

Casting tape Rolls of adhesive or resinimpregnated tape for use as lightweight casts.

Castration It is the removal of man's testes with or without scrotum. If done before puberty it prevents the normal development of secondary sexual characteristics. After puberty voice becomes deep. It may be done in case of cancer or severe infection.

Castration anxiety Anxiety due to fantasised danger or injuries to the genitals and/or body. May be precipitated by everyday events which have symbolic significance and appear to be threatening, such as loss of a job, loss of a tooth, or an experience of ridicule or humiliation.

CAT Abbreviation for computerized axial tomography.

Cat eye syndrome Causative factor is one extra chromosome, a G-chromosome which may be from 13-15 or 21-22 chromosome.

There may be anal atresia, preauricular fistulae and heart anomalies. Eye features include microphthalmos, strabismus, choroidal coloboma and epicanthal folds.

Cat gut It is a chemically toughened fibre made from intestine of a sheep. It is used for sutures because it is readily biodegradable and can held two edges of a wound together long enough for healing.

Catabasis The stage of decline of a disease.

Catabolism The portion of metabolism associated with the breakdown of organic molecules, in contrast to anabolism, which is associated with chemical synthesis.

Catalase Enzyme which breaks down hydrogen peroxide. it is an antioxidant and is found in all tissues which use oxygen.

Catalepsy Diminished responsiveness as in trance; the limbs remain immobile.

Catalyst A substance that induces an increased rate of chemical reaction without taking active part in the reaction.

Cataplexy Sudden loss of muscle tone, triggered by an emotional change such as laughing or anger.

Cataract In cataract there becomes loss of transparency of the lens of eye.

It never causes complete blindness because howsoever lens may become densely opalescent it will transmit some of light. It is caused by attrition in the protein component of the lens. Cataract develops in both eyes but one may be severely affected. Old age may be the predisposing factor. It may be caused by direct injury. Cataract is entirely painless and causes visual symptoms only. Progress of symptoms is very slow. Treatment includes lens transplantation.

Cataract knife The purpose of cataract knife is to give an incision during cataract surgery. Introducing infection from outside is the risk.

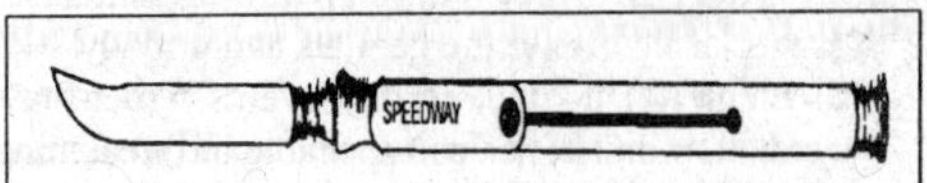

Catarrhal tracheobronchitis Viral infection that usually begins in the nasopharyngeal area and ascends within several days to include trachea. Retrosternal, dry cough and moderate fever develop. There is significant malaise. It is of highly contagious viral aetiology.

Catatonia Immobility with muscular rigidity or inflexibility and at times excitability.

Catatonic type A form of schizophrenia characterised by such symptoms as extreme negativism, physical rigidity, and holding bizarre postures.

Catch trials A research procedure designed to minimise or eliminate faking or dishonesty among subjects. In a test of auditory ability, for example, during one trial the tone might not be presented at all, yet the subject would be asked to describe what he or she had heard.

Catchment area A geographic area for which a mental health programme or facility has responsibility for its residents.

Catecholamines A term for the three neurotransmitter agents (norepinephrine, epinephrine, and dopamine) which are formed from the amino acid tyrosine and are structurally related to the substance catechol.

Categorical theory Descriptive theory in which the characteristics that describe a phenomenon are exhaustive.

Catgut Sheep's intestine prepared as a suture and used for ligating vessels and closing soft tissue wounds.

Catharsis A release of tensions by expressing pent up emotions and by reliving early traumatic events, an aspect of psychotherapy often encouraged by the therapist. The expression of ideas, thoughts and expressed material that is accompanied by an emotional response and that produces a state of relief to the individual.

Catharsis hypothesis The conjecture that the expression of anger and other emotional reactions leads to decrease of these feelings. The hypothesis is not well supported.

Cathartic An agent that causes evacuation of the bowels.

Cathechol-o-methyl transferase (COMT) The enzyme that catalyzes the degradation of the catecholamines norepinephrine and epinephrine at the synaptic junction.

Catheter care Hygiene measures used to keep the meatus and adjacent area of the catheter clean.

Catheter hub Plastic threaded connection at end of an intravenous catheter.

Catheter irrigation Flushing the lumen of a catheter.

Catheterisation It means introduction of a catheter into a hollow or tubular organ. Usually in nursing catheterisation implies introduction of a catheter

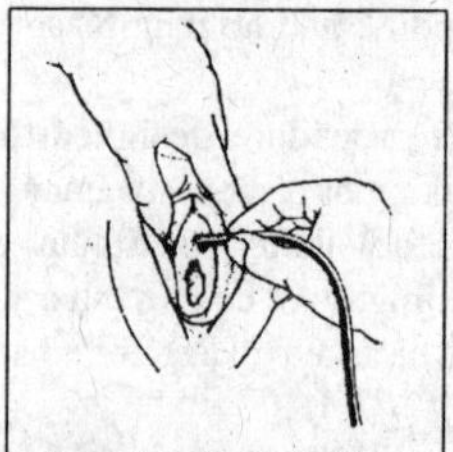

Female catheterisation

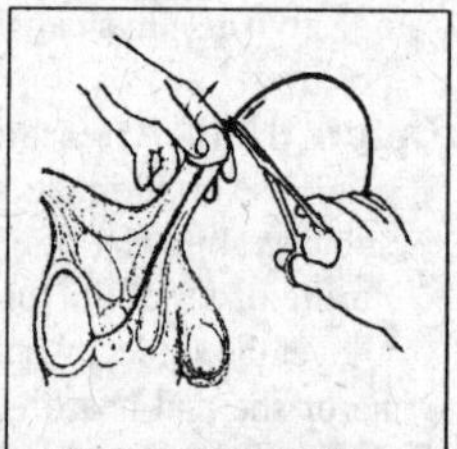

Male catheterisation

into urinary bladder to empty urine. These may be made up of rubber, polythene, hard rubber and metal catheters.

Cathexis Attachment, conscious or unconscious, of emotional feeling and significance to an idea, an object or most commonly a person.

Cathode Negative terminal of an x-ray tube. The cathode consists of a helical tungsten filament within a molybdenum reflector cup. The function of the cathode is to produce a cloud of electrons.

Cations Positively charged ions, such as sodium , potassium, calcium and magnesium.

Caton index It is the ratio between the patellar articular length and distance between distal pole of patella and tibial tubercle. The ratio is 0.8 in normal knees with 30 degrees of fexion.

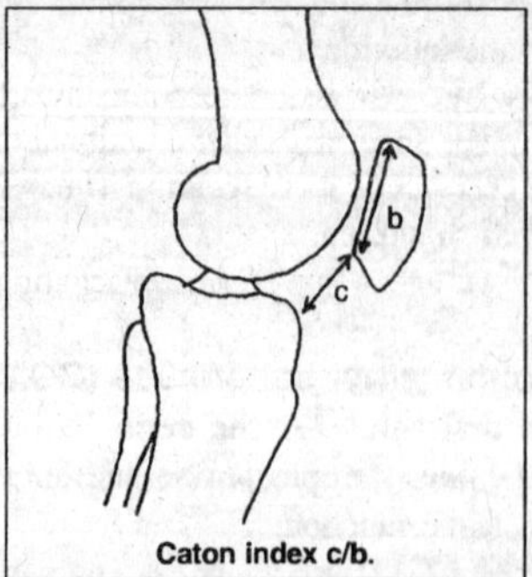

Caton index c/b.

Cauda equina The nerve roots progresses longer to make their exit at the spinal level below their respective vertebra. In the lumbar region these elongated roots form cauda equina which traverses the lower lumbar vertebral spinal canal.

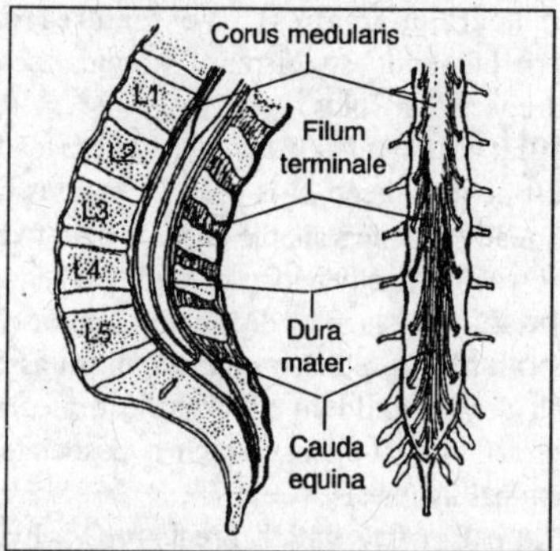

Cauda equina lesion Damage to peripheral nerve roots below the first lumbar vertebra; some regeneration is possible.

Cauda equina syndrome Usually spinal cord terminates at the lower borders of the body L_2. Large central disc protrusion at L_4/L_5 may result in compression not only on L_5 roots bilaterally but also on all sacral roots as they stream caudally.

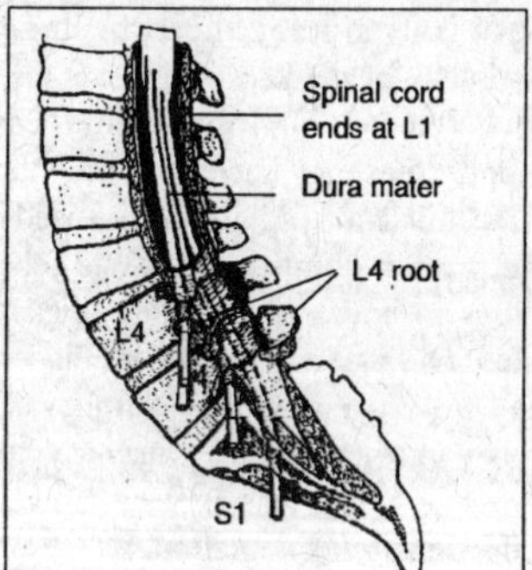

Patient will loose control of his sphincters and will feel numbness of the buttocks and backs of his thighs. It is sometimes difficult to distinguish lesion of cauda equina from an acute plaque of demyelination in conus medullaris. In both cases, there will be loss of sphincter control and weakness and sensory loss. In acute conus lesion all tendon reflexes of legs will be lost.

Caudal Toward the tail or inferiorly.

Caudal anesthesia The term applied to analgesia or anaesthesia resulting from the introduction of the suitable analgesic or anaesthetic solution into the caudal canal (non-closure of the laminae of the last sacral vertebra). Pelvic/perineal anesthesia produced by injection of local anesthetic through the sacral hiatus into the epidural space.

Caudal regressive syndrome Severe malformation that results in failure of development of sacrum, lumbar spine and lower extremity.

Caudate Having a tail.

Causalgia It refers to burning pain in the area of previous injury or surgical procedure. In the oral region it occurs following tooth extraction. After a few days of extraction the socket is the site of intense burning pain though the wound is completely healed. Pain is transitory.

Cause of action A set of facts or legal circumstances that can support a claim for relief in the courts.

Caustic An agent that burns or corrodes; destroys living tissue; having a burning taste.

Cautaneous sense Relating to the skin sense, as in responses to touch or temperature.

Cauterization Destruction of a tissue with cautery.

Cavernous sinus It lies on each side of sella turcica where each surrounds the internal carotid artery and traversed by nerves going to orbit. Cavernous sinuses of two sides communicate with each other through an intercavernous sinus.

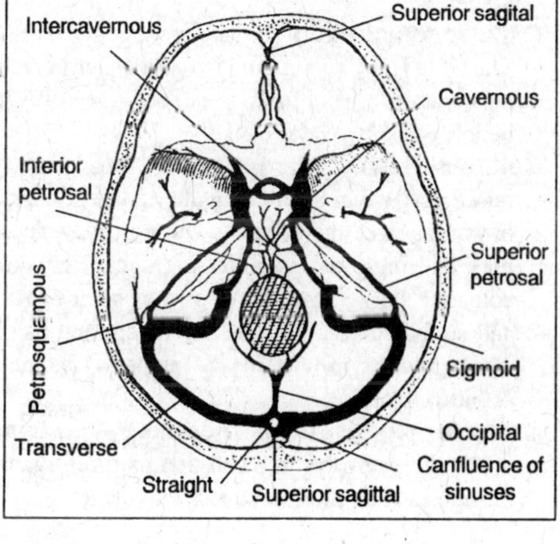

Cavitation The development process that forms spaces among cells of a tissue and by which these developing spaces coalesce to form a cavity.

Cavity A hollow or space or a potential space within the body or a body organ.

Cavity classification Carious lesions are classified according to the surfaces of a tooth on which they occur (labial, buccal, occlusal, etc.) type of surface (pit and fissure or smooth surface). and numerical grouping.

Cavity lining Material applied to the prepared cavity before the restoration is inserted to seal the dentinal tubules.

Cavity preparation Tooth prepared by a dentist to recieve restoration.

Cavity pulp Pulp chamber and pulp canal.

Cavity wall One of the enclosing sides of a prepared cavity. Walls take the name of the surface of the tooth adjoining the involved surface toward which it is placed.

Cavity-Tooth Hollow place or space in a tooth; dental caries.

Cavus Increase in the height of the longitudinal arch of the foot.

CBC Complete blood count.

CBCA Criteria-based content analysis.

CCD Charged coupled device.

CD antigen Cluster of differentiation designation assigned to leukoctye cell surface molecules which are identified by a given group of monoclonal antibodies.

CD-4 Cell A specialised cell of T portion of the immune system also known as helper T lymphocyte. This cell is responsible for maintaining immune competence and is one of the cells infected selectively with HIV virus and destroyed.

CD-8 cells These are cytotoxic activated by CD 4 cells to kill target cells.

CDA Certified Dental Assistant a person who has met specific criteria and who has successfully completed a credentialing examination.

CDC Centers for Disease Control and Prevention.

CDH Congenital dysplasia of hip.

CE Capillary electrophoresis.

Cecum The pouchlike portion of the large intestine to which the ileum of the small intestine is attached.

Celibacy It is the condition of total abstinence from sexual activity involving the partner. Although in celibacy some religious groups demand total abstinence from any sexual activity, some self-professed celibates admit to masturbation.

Cell It is the elementary structural and functional unit composed of a mass of living substance protoplasm and cytoplasm containing a specialised plasmatic body nucleus and enclosed by a semipermeable membrane. Membrane is a film of lipoprotein molecules.

Cell body The principal portion of a cell such as a neuron, which contains genetic material and most of the cell cytoplasm.

Cell cycle The sequence of events that ocurs during the growth and division of tissue cells.

Cell differentiation The process by which pluripotential cells differentiate into specialized cells such as osteoblasts, osteoclasts, fibroblasts, and erythroblasts.

Cell division Process by which a cell reproduces itself that consists of a nuclear division (mitosis) and a cytoplasmic division (cytokinesis); types include somatic and reproductive cell division.

Cell membrane Two layer of phospholipid molecules that surround the cell, separating its contents from the extracellular fluid; membranes that surround components inside the cell also are bilayer.

Cell nests In it epithelial cells of epidermis proliferate into the dermis in column separated from one another by the connective tissue. In course of time the central cells being the oldest undergo some degenerative changes as found in normal surface epithelium and are finally converted into a hyaline structureless mass of keratin. This process is known as keratinisation or cornification. Cells nests are relatively slow growing tumour and have high degree of cell differentiation. It has poor sensitivity to radiotherapy. Radiotherapy is the choice of treatment.

Cell nucleus It is a specialised plasmatic body, denser than ordinary mass of cytoplasm and bounded by a viscid membrane. It contains a thin network of fibres supporting a special particle called nucleolus. It contains nucleo proteins, lipids and large amount of calcium. Its action is concerned with cell division and multiplication. It is the seat of intracellular oxidation and takes an active part on active part in metabolic process.

Cell sorter An instrument that uses optical or mechanical technologies to allow the separation of cells on the basis of size of cellular properties.

Cell wall One of the outer layers of the bacterial cell that protects the cell from osmotic perturbations and provides mechanical protection to the fragile cellular membrane.

Cell-adhesion molecule (CAM) A chemical to which specific cell can adhere, thus aiding in migration.

Cell-generated signal A physical, mechanical, chemical, or electrical signs that originates from a cell to influence a physiologic process of tissue growth or repair.

Cell-mediated immune response Specific immune response mediated by T cells and activated macrophages, rather than by antibody.

Cell-mediated immunity A tissue-based cellular response to foregine antigens. The response involves mobilization of killer T cells.

Immunological defense provided by T cell lymphocytes that come within close proimity of their victim cells.

Cellular ageing A number of functional and morphologic alterations occur in ageing cells. There develops reduced oxidative phosphorylation by mitochondria, diminished DNA and RNA synthesis of structural and enzymatic proteins. There will be irregular and abnormally lobed nuclei.

Cellular dehydration The lack of water in the cells. The body is dry due to fluid loss through urination, perspiration, and so forth. This condition needs to be alleviated by water intake.

Cellular naevus It presents with flat, slilghtly raised, soft, circumscribed papule, nodule or plaque of varying sizes. It may be anywhere on body. These may be single or multiple, pigmented or skin coloured. Larger ones are known as giant naevus and surface of naevus may be smooth and hairy. The pigmented naevus may be single as slate blue or bluish black.

Cellular respiration The energy-releasing metabolic pathways in a cell that oxidize organic molecules such as glucose and fatty acids.

Cellular tolerance A change that takes place in a cell in which the activity of the cell adjusts to the excitatory or inhibitory effects of a drug.

Cellulase A family of enzymes that hydrolyzc B-14, glucosidic bonds in native cellulose and derived substrates.

Cellulitis 1. Any inflammation of cellular tissue 2. A spreading, diffuse, edematous, sometimes suppurative, hot, inflammatory lesion, associated with infection with invasive bacteria, principally streptococci, capable or producing hyaluronidase and fibrinolysins. Unlike in an abscess, which is well defined and localized, in cellulitis infection tends to spread through tissue spaces and cleavage planes owing to breaking down of hyaluronic acid.

Cellulittis It is a skin infection resulting in local inflammation, warmth, erythema and pain with fever and leucocytosis. Lymphangitis and lymphadenitis may be present.

Cellulose It is a very stable insoluble compound and is the main constituent of the supporting tissues of plants. It forms a considerable part of our vegetable food. Herbivorous animals with the help of bacteria can utilise a considerable proportion of cellulose while man is unable to do so. It adds bulk to the intestinal contents, thereby stimulating peristalsis and elimination of food residues.

Cement base A cement, a layer of insulated, sometimes medicated dental cement placed in a deep portion of a cavity preparation to protect the pulp. It reduces the bulk of the metabolic restorations or eliminate even undercuts in a tapered preparations.

Cement retention The use of cement for the retention of an abatement or prosthesis.

Cement sealer It is a compound used in filling of a root canal. It is inserted in plastic form which solidifies after placement. It fills the irregularities of canals too.

Cement zinc oxide It is a least irritating cement. It is a powder of zinc oxide with strengtheners and acceleractors.

Cementicle It is a calcified body sometimes found in peridontal ligament specially in older person Degenerated epithelial cells from the nidus.

Cementoblasts Cells that form the cementum.

Cementoenamel junction (CEJ) The junction between the cementum and enamel of a tooth.

Cementoid It is the most recent layer covering the surface of cementum that is uncalcified.

Cementum It is a specialised, calcified connective tissue covering the anatomic root of a tooth. It gives attachment to a periodontal ligament.

Center of gravity Point at which the mass of an object is centered.

Center of mass Point in the body or body part at which all mass seems to be concentrated.

Center of ossification An area in the cartilage cells hypertrophy and then secrete enzymes that result in the calcification of their matrix, resulting in the death of the cartilage cells, followed by the invasion of the area by osteoblasts that then lay down bone.

Center of pressure It is a way of visualising the force against the ground. The movement of center of pressure along the bottom of the foot in a normal person follows a consistent pattern.

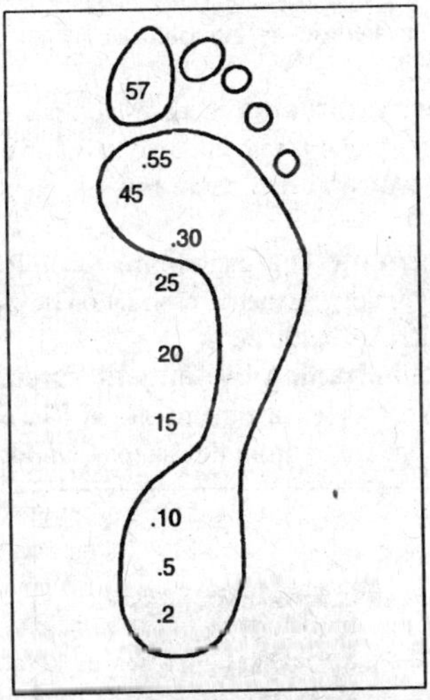

Centering The ability to focus the mind by screening out sensation.

Center-surround receptive field A visual receptive field having a center surrounded by a ring of opposite sign.

Centigrade Body temperature is measured in centigrade.

Centigrade scale Scale that uses 0°C as the temperature at which water freezes and 100°C as the point at which it boils.

Centimeter 1/100 of a meter; approximately 2.5 cm equal 1 inch.

Central anticholinergic syndrome It is the syndrome following use of anticholinergic drugs specially hyoscine. Person may develop, confusions, agitation, hallucination, muscle incoordination and convulsions.

Central canal A microscopic tube running the length of the spinal cord in the gray commissure. A circular channel running longitudinally in the center of an osteon (Haversian system) of mature compact bone, containing blood and lymphatic vessels and nerves. Also called a Haversian.

Central cord syndrome Incomplete spinal cord lesion producing greater neurologic involvement in upper extremities.

Central core disease It is a mild usually non-progressive myopathy presenting in infancy with hypertonia and proximal muscle weakness. The "cores" are central zone seen in type I muscle fibres. The disorder is inherited as an autosomal dominant.

Central disc protrusion It causes compression of the cauda equina. It may involve two nerve roots or may involve all the nerve roots in the cauda equina.

Central dogma The organizing principle of molecular biology : genetic information flows from DNA to RNA to protein.

Central field charting by tangent screen For this a tangent screen of 1 metre is used. The patient is seated one metre from the screen, comfortably,

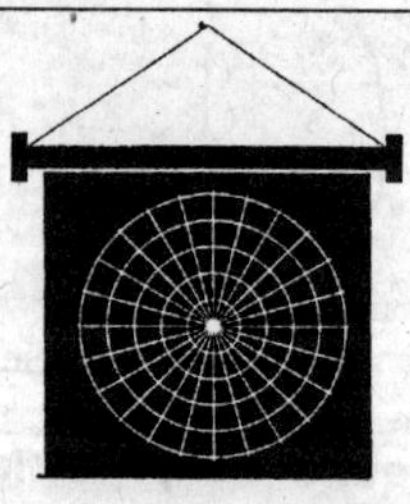

Tangent screen

fixing the eye to be examined and adjusting the chair, so that the eye under examination is in line with the fixation spot in the centre of screen, the other eye being covered. A white test object 5 mm, is brought in from the side at 15° intervals, by a black thin test rod on which the test object is attached, the patient giving a signal, on seeing the test object.

The response is to be charted on the chart by the surgeon or he or she can put pins with black heads at the point on the screen where the patient made a signal, and later chart it out in one sitting. The blind spot is charted out with this tangent screen. The normal blind spot is located, about 13 to 18° temporal to central fixation and just inferior to fixation point. An abnormally large blind spot can be due to papilloedema.

Central frenum Fold of membrane connecting the lip of the tissue.

Central giant cell granuloma It is a tumour-like growth located within the central jaw. Peripheral gingiva may be involved. It is seen below the age of 20. Mandible is more commonly involved. Lesion is generally asymptomatic but is usually expansile. Regional tooth may migrate. X-ray shows a single cystic area or a soap bubble-like deformity.

Under microscope it consists of numerous multinucleated giant cells dispersed throughout the lesion. Soap bubble-like appearance is not diagnostic because aneurysmal bone cyst, myxoma and ameloblastoma also have soap bubble lesions. Local curettage is the treatment of choice.

Central incisors Cutting teeth; the first of the four anterior teeth of either jaw.

Central limit theorem For reasonably large samples, the distribution of the means of many samples is normal.

Central nervous system Portion of the nervous system consisting of the brain and spinal cord.

Central occlusion Contact that is made when maxillary and mandibular jaws are closed in most stable position.

Central pain Any pain associated with a lesion in CNS.

Central pain syndrome It develops as an injury to CNS. Spontaneous pain and pain evoked by innocuous stimuli are most prevalent symptoms of CPS.

Central pattern generator A neural circuit giving rise to rhythmic motor activity.

Central prolapse disc Central prolapse of disc at L4-L5 is capable of damaging all roots below L5.

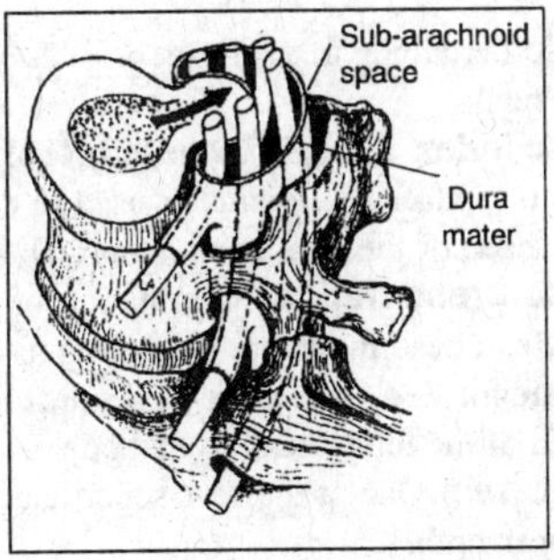

The most anterior roots L5-S2 are the most vulnerable.

Central ray A hypothetical X-ray whose direction of travel corresponds to the geometric centre of a useful beam of X-radiation.

Central retinal artery occlusion Occlusion of the central retinal artery can occur due to emboli, vaso-obliteration and raised intraocular pressure. Emboli is the most common cause. Emboli material from the heart or carotid artery reaches the eye directly through the ophthalmic artery, a branch of internal carotid. The common cause for vaso-obliteration is arteritis. There is sudden loss of vision. Patient realises that vision is fading and finally goes. Vision is reduced to perception of light. Retinal veins are of normal calibre. If not treated well optic disc becomes atrophic.

Central retinal vein occlusion Vein is compressed by thick and arteriosclerotic artery. It is more common in primary open angle glaucoma. Periphlebitis has a role. The symptoms depend upon the location of occlusion and involvement of macula. There is complaint of loss of vision. Patient may complain of metamorphopsia. Under ophthalmoscopy veins are dilated and tortuous. Haemorrhages may be flamme-shaped or dot and blot type covering entire fundus oedema of retina with cotton-wool spots. There will be macular oedema. Macula may show pigmentation and degenerative changes. Neovascularisation leads to vitreous haemorrhage.

Central serous chorioretinopathy It is a common disorder of macula of unknown aetiology between the age of 20 and 40 years. The patient presents with complaints of blurred vision associated with positive scotoma, microscopsia and metamorphopsia. On ophthalmoscopy there is an oval or round elevation at the posterior pole with a glistening reflex at a border. On slitlamp biomicroscopy there is an elevation of posterior pole with a fluid which is clear and transparent. Fluorescein angiography shows a hyperfluorescent spot at the site of leakage. Recurrence is common and prognosis is favourable.

Central tinnitus Diffuse head tinnitus without laterality. The masking level well above threshold and equal in both ears combined with sensorineural hearing loss. Central vestibular dysfunction is common.

Central trait A trait which is at the core of the personality, a trait which influences our judgement of an individual in a global way. For example, the warm-cold dimension influences our judgement about other characteristics of an individual, such as whether that person is honest, outgoing, and even artistic.

Central venous catheter A hollow, tubular instrument passed through a peripheral vein into

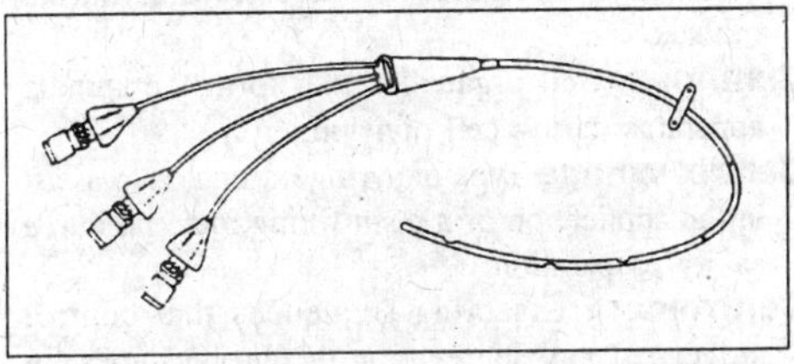

the vena cava immediately proximal to the right atrium; used for the measurement of right atrial pressure or the infusion of fluids and medications.

Central venous pressure A measurement of ventricular end diastolic presure with the help of central venous catheter transducer system normally it measures 5 to 12 cms.

Centration The tendency of a child in Piaget's second stage of intellectual development, the preoperational stage, to focus attention on the dominant stimulation. The child's attention is so fixed on the height of a beaker, for example, that he or she ignores the operations which have been performed on the contents of the beaker.

Centreline The middle of the tire tread, as divided around the circumference.

Centriacinar emphysema A condition resulting from the destruction of the septal walls of the alveoli surrounding the central terminal bronchioles; centrilobular emphysema.

Centric occlusion Relationship of opposing occlusal surfaces that provides the maximum planned contact and/or intercuspation. It should exist when the mandible is in centric relation to the maxilla.

Centric relation Most retruded physiologic relation of the mandible to the maxillae, a position that can exist at various degrees of jaw separation and that occurs on the terminal hinge axis.

Centrifugal Moving away from a centre; efferent or exodic.

Centrifugation The process of separating the lighter portions of a solution, mixture, or suspension from the heavier portions by centrifugal forces.

Centrifuge An apparatus that use centrifugal force to separate or remove particulate matter suspended in a liquid.

Centriole Small organelle that divides and migrates to each pole of the nucleus; spindle fibres extend from the centromeres to the centrioles during mitosis.

Centrioles Cell organelles that form the spindle apparatus during cell division.

Centrix syringe Type of syringe designed to assist in the application of a resin filling material into a cavity preparation.

Centromere Cisacting sequences that control movement and segregation of chromosomes. In eukaryotic microbes, centreomeres are attached to microtubules of the mitotic spindle apparatus. In prokaryotic microbes, the centromere and its attachment structure are less well defined.

Cephal hematoma This is a common form of birth injury but is seldom seen before second day of life. This is a localised subperiosteal collection of blood usually over parietal region. Swelling is fluctuant. It may be unilateral or bilateral. Cephal hematoma is harmless and disappears spontaneously

Cephalad Toward the head.

Cephalhaematoma This is due to subperiosteal haemorrhage over one or more of bones of skull. It is due to slow ooze of blood following minor trauma to the head during delivery. A few days after birth baby develops a soft, fluctuant, painless swelling confined to the area of skull bone. A hard rim around periphery gives an alarming impression of depressed fracture.

Cephalic pertaining to the head, or to the head end of the body.

Cephalic index The ratio of the biparietal diameter to the occipitofrontal diameter used to determine if the shape of the fetal head is normal.

Cephalic presentation Presentation of any part of the fetal head in labour. Cephalic presentations are categorized into groups according to the relation of the fetus' head to its body.

Cephalic vein One of the four superficial veins of the upper limb.

Cephalocaudal Progression from head to toe.

Cephalocaudal development A gradient of growth particularly in the embryonic stage, proceeding for head to tail. In a fetus, the head is likely to be more fully developed than the trunk and lower body parts.

Cephalogram Extraoral radiographic examination of the head.It is most frequently used in orthodontics to measures and study maxillofacial growth or relationshops of maxilla and mandible. A cephalogram is made by placing the patient's head in a special positioner that maintains precise alignment of head to film.

Cephalometer An orienting device for positioning the head for radiographic examination and measurement.

Cephalometrics Scienctific study of measurements of head.

Cephalometry Measurement of the bony structure of the head using reproducible lateral and anteroposterior radiographs.

Cephalopelvic disproportion (CPD) A condition in which the fetal head is diproportionately large for passage through the maternal pelvis.

Cephalosporins They were first obtained from fungus cephalosporium. Their molecule is closely related to that of penicillin. These impair bacterial cell wall synthesis and hence are bactericidal. This is excreted in urine unchanged. These have half-life from 1 to 4 hours. Wide distribution in body allows treatment of infection in bone, soft tissue and muscle. Most usual allergic reactions are of penicillin type.

Cer regulon The set of genes directly regulated by the complex of cylic adenosine monophosphate and its receptor, the CAP protein.

Ceramic A class of materials composed of metallic oxides and minerals, having the characteristics of high stiffness and compressive strength, low thermal and electrical conductivity, brittleness, and low chemical reactivity.

Ceramide A class of lipids which dont contain glycerol.

Cercaria It is equipped with a tail that enables it to swim. Human lung fluke have minute tails, limiting the cercaria to crawl on a substrate rather than swim.

Cerclage Encircling a part with a ring or loop of wire to affix the adjacent ends of a fractured bone. Encircling of the cervix with suture to prevent recurrent spontaneous abortion caused by early cervical dilatation.

Cercomer The posterior extension of procercoid and cysticercoid larvae, usually retaining the oncospheral hooks.

Cerea flexibilitas The waxy flexibility often presents in catatonic schizophrenia in which the patient's arm or leg remains in the position in which it is placed.

Cerebellar rigidity Increased tone of extensor muscles caused by an injury to cerebellum.

Cerebellar ataxia Ataxia of cerebellar origin.

Cerebellar cognitive affective syndrome Constellation of symptoms associated with cerebellar pathology.

Cerebellar gait An uncordinated gait due to cerebellar degeneration. Unsteady gait is wavering and lurching in character.

Cerebellar peduncle An aggregation of nerve fibres connecting the cerebellum with the brain stem.

Cerebellar signs Ataxia/intention tremor (in particular) associated with cerebellar pathology.

Cerebellar tumours Medullo-blastoma is very common causing truncal ataxia. These are fast growing and death may occur in one year. Usual tumour in cerebellar hemi-sphere is an astro cytoma. There is ataxia and incoordination on the side of lesion. Nystagmus is observed on lateral gage.

Cerebellum It is the part of the hind brain which is responsible for maintenance of posture, balance and coordination of movement. It is located behind the brain stem. Disease of cerebellum can result in abnormalities of posture or movement. It may cause jerky, staggering gait and slurred speech. There may be jerky eye movement, i.e. nystagmus. Alcohol intoxication impairs function of cerebellum.

Cerebellum, Functions It rearranges, synthesises and redistributes afferent impulses. It also serves as a discharging centre to the musculature of body. It modifies muscle tone by influencing the brain stem nuclei. It influences the postural activity mainly on its side of body.

Cerebral Pertaining to the two hemispheres of the brain.

Cerebral irritation It develops 3 days after injury and is caused by cerebral oedema. Patient is not concious but takes no interest in surroundings. He or she usually prefers to lie curled up in bed and turned away from light with the eyes closed and resist to open them.

He or she does not want to be aroused. Recovery may be apparently complete but in some cases headache, irritability, depression or lack of concentration persist.

Cerebral palsy It is a non-progressive disorder of movement and posture which results due to damage of brain generally during early childhood.

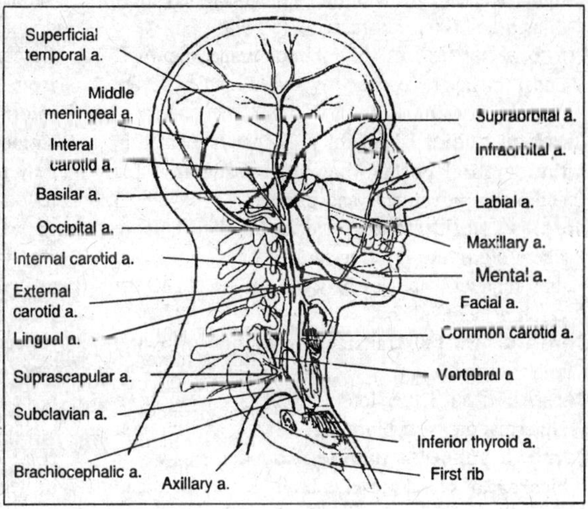

Child suffers from spastic paralysis, i.e. abnormal stiffness and contractions of muscles. There may be ataxia and involvement of writing movements. In 90 per cent cases damage occurs before birth. During first year, cerebral palsy is not recognised and muscles become hypotonic. There may be feeding difficulty. Child may have delayed development. Mental retardation in 75 per cent children develops with lower IQ level of below 70. It is incurable. Physical therapy is required to teach the child to control balance. Inadequate speech can be helped by speech therapy.

Cerebral aqueduct A channel through the midbrain connecting the third and fourth ventricles and containing cerebrospinal fluid. Also termed the aqueduct of Sylvius.

Cerebral arterial circle A ring or arteries forming an anastomosis at the base of the brain between the internal carotid and basilar arteries and arteries supplying the brain. Also called the circle of Willis.

Cerebral blood flow About 700 ml/minute. Hypercapnia increases cerebral blood flow.

Cerebral compression After head injury patient becomes restless and passes then into profound unconsciousness. His face becomes flushed and pulse becomes slow and bounding. Respiration is slow and deep frequently stertorous. The temperature may be unequal, being higher on paralysed side. Pupil on the side of lesion dilates after initial contraction, having poor reaction to light. In last stages both the pupils become widely dilated and fixed not reactive to light.

Cerebral herniation Shift of brain tissue side ways, under the falx cerebri or downward causing severe neuralgic dysfunction.

Cerebral nuclei Islands of gray matter located in the cerebral cortex that are responsible for automatic movements and postures.

Cerebral peduncles A paired bundle of nerve fibers along the inferior surface of the midbrain that conduct impulses between the pons and the cerebral hemispheres.

Cerebral shock Transient hypotonia following injury to the brain.

Cerebral steal Diversion of blood flow away from abnormal areas of brain e.g. infarcts and tumors.

Cerebral vascular accident Sudden rupture or blockage of blood vessel in brain. It may be due to bleeding, thrombosis or embolism. There may be intracerebral haemorrhage or subarachnoid haemorrhage.

Cerebral venous thrombosis Causes of CVT include pyogeni meningitis, systemic lupus erythematosus (SLE), head trauma, dehydration and severe heart failure. It should be suspected when there is papilloedema, extensive bilateral haemorrhagic infarction not confined to vascular territory, persistent seizures and prominent headache prior to stroke. Diagnosis is best established by MRI that shows absence of blood flow in involved venous sinus.

Cerebroside A fatty acid glycolipid compound present in myelin sheath of nerve fibres identified as white matter.

Cerebrospinal fluid About 500 ml is secreted in 24 hours from choroid plexuses of third, fourth and lateral ventricles, i.e about 0.5 ml/minute. It contains protein derived partly by filtration of serum, partly from brain interstitial fluid and brain cells and partly from cells of theca. It is clear and colourless with slight opalescence due to globulin. Specific gravity is 1003 to 1009 at 37°C. The viscosity averages 1.006 centipoise similar to normal saline. Density is more dependent on temperature and on the contained sodium.

Cerebrospinal otorrhoea Fracture of temporal bone is the most common cause of cerebrospinal otorrhoea since bone is widely related to subarachnoid spaces of middle and posterior cranial fossa.

Cerebrospinal fluid (CSF) leakage may also arise from congenital fistula between lateral end of internal acoustic meatus and vestibule due to surgical trauma or cholesteatoma. Bleeding which may mask the cavity usually ceases within first few days after injury. Flow is often profuse. CSF appearing in discharge from ear is a serious warning of possible meningitis.

Cerebrotonia Temperament characterised by such features as restraint, shyness, hypersensitivity, and reflection.

Cerebrovascular accident (CVA) A hemorrhage or cessation of blood flow through cerebral blood vessel resulting in destruction of neurons; commonly called a stroke. Thrombosis, embolism or hemorrhage in or arount the brain.

Cerebrum It is the most developed part of the brain. It has two cerebral hemispheres. Cerebrum consists of billions of inter-connected nerve cells called nuclei. It has grey and white matter. Much of the sensory information from eyes and ears and skin reach its final destination in cerebral cortex. In cerebrum these are analysed. For different sensations different centres are located in cortex. For example, visual perception is located in occipital lobe, touch and pressure sensations are in postcentral gyrus. Hearing and smell are located

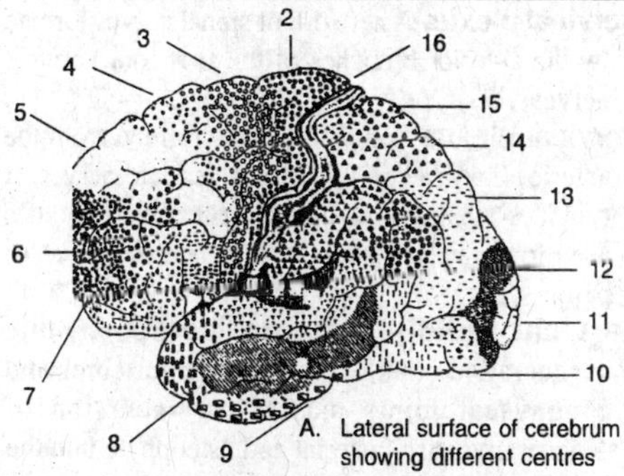

A. Lateral surface of cerebrum showing different centres

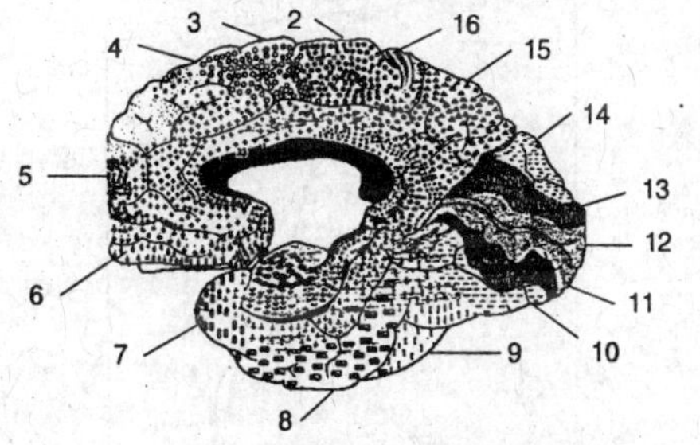

B. Medial surface of cerebrum

in temporal lobe. Damage to particular region may cause specific syndromes. If frontal lobe is damaged there may develop mental apathy and self-neglect while with parietal lobe injury there may be loss of sensory discrimination. Loss of memory may be the result of temporal lobe insult. Cerebral disease causes nonspecific symptoms such as headache and epilepsy.

Ceremic It is a compound formed by union of a metallic and non metallic element. Most of these materials are oxide formed by union of oxygen with metals such as silicon, aluminium, calcium and magnésium glass. Fine crystal and gypsum are ceremics.

Cericodorsal Pertaining to the neck and the back.

Certification A designation by a private or governmental body that a person or entity has satisfied a preetablished set of standards or requirements. In medicine, it is common for governmental agencies to defer to certifications by private, voluntary organizations such as the Joint Commission.

Certiorari A legal order directing a lower court to transmit the record of a proceeding to an appellate court for review.

Certitude The highest degree of belief.

Cerumen The waxy secretion produced by the ceruminous glands in the external ear canal.

Cerumen impaction Abrupt unilateral or bilateral hearing loss sometimes with associated tinnitus. Pain occurs only if the plug is very large and hard. Pain increases with chewing.

Ceruminous gland A modified sudoriferous (sweat) gland in the external auditory meatus that secretes cerumen (ear wax).

Cervial halter Support for the head, made of cotton material, used for traction.

Cervical Pertaining to the neck or a necklike portion of an organ.

Cervical angina A pseudoangina resulting from referred pain from cervical dysfunction. Costly and hazardous cardiologic workups are often fruitlessly endured by patient's with this disorder.

Cervical burnout A radiolucent artefact seen on a dental radiograph resulting from the differences in densities of adjacent tissues.

Cervical cap A small cup like device placed over the cervix to prevent sperms to enter.

Cervical cellulitis It is a diffuse, usually fulminating bacterial soft tissue infection of neck dissecting along the planes of cervical fascia and great blood vessels. It develops as a severe systemic illness with septic temperatures, dysphagia and stridor. There may develop possible symptoms of thrombophlebitis.

Cervical changes during pregnancy Softening of cervix usually begins during second missed menstrual period. It feels likelips or lobe of ear. It is due to increased blood supply. The glands of cervical mucosa undergo marked proliferation and

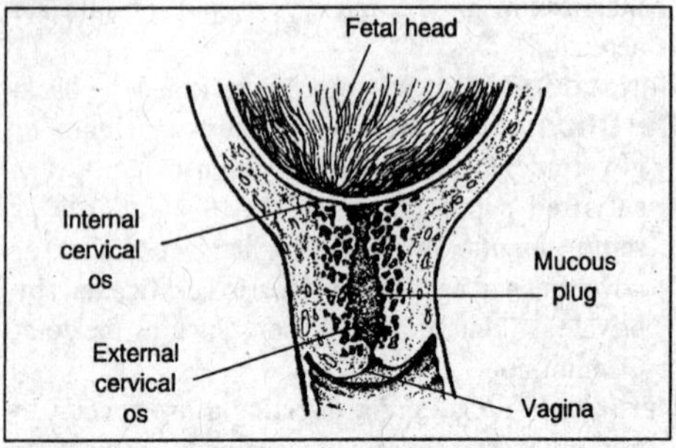

distend with mucous. This creates a mucus plug that seals the uterus from contamination by bacteria in vagina.

Cervical collar Foam or rigid splint around the neck.

Cervical curve Spinal curvature with an apex from C_1 to C_6 vertebra.

Cervical dilatation Enlargement of the cervical os from an orifice of a few millimeters in size to an aperture large enough to permit the passage of the fetus (ie, a diameter of about 10 cm)

Cervical dilators Hegar's cervical dilators are available of different sizes and diameters. These dilators are not tapering and are of same thickness. These are made of gradually increasing sizes. These are used in dilatation and curettage, MTP, insufflation tests and for relieve of spasmodic dysmenorrhoea.

Cervical dystocia Cervical dilatation occurs very slowly although uterine action is normal in primigravida. In multipara cervical dystocia occurs due to cervical scarring following cauterization, radium burn etc. Pain and uterine contraction are normal to begin with. Cervix is rigidly firm.

Cervical effacement The process in which the uterine cervix changes from a 3-4 cm fibrous cylinder to a lumen in continuity with the lower pole of the uterus.

Cervical erosion It is the bacterial invasion and destruction of an area of tissues on the surface of neck of uterus. It is prompted usually by infection in the vagina or due to hormonal imbalance. In this area healing is problematic and may result in vaginal discharge or bleeding.

Cervical ganglion A cluster of postganglionic sympathetic nerve cell bodies located in the neck, near the cervical vertebrae.

Cervical migraine A syndrome characterized by headache, neck pain, vertigo, and loss of cervical range of motion at the gross and segmental levels, particularly in rotation.

Cervical mucus The secretion of mucous membrane of the cervix.

Cervical orthoses A device prescribed to neck intended to control and restrict head and neck motions.

Cervical pleura The serous membrane that covers the uppermost aspect of the lunging the neck.

Cervical plexus A network of spinal nerves formed by the anterior branches of the first four cervical nerves.

Cervical plexus block Plexus is formed from the anterior branches of upper four cervical nerves. It provides analgesia of upper cervical dermatomes used for head and neck surgery and treatment of pain.

Cervical radicular syndrome Spondylotic degenerative changes in the intervertebral and apophyseal joints may allow incursion of degenerative disc material and osteophyte into the

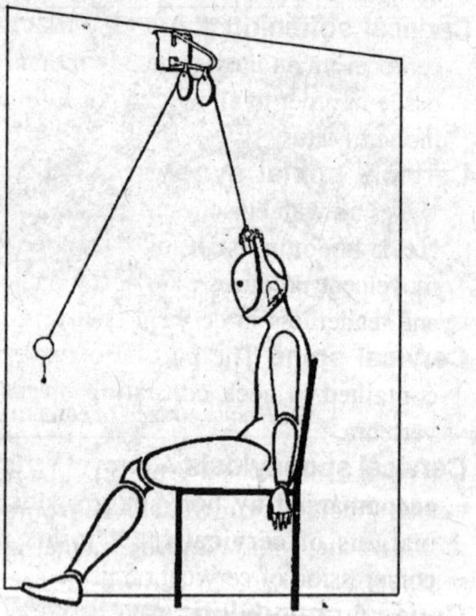

foramina through which spinal roots exit from the canal. The sixth and seventh cervical roots are commonly involved. There will be deep boring pain referred to shoulder. There may be tingling pain in little finger and thumb. Biceps tendons are depressed. In 7th nerve root syndrome pain is referred to arm and to chest wall. Triceps reflex is depressed. Cervical collar helps the patient.

Cervical rib It is a congenital disorder. Lowest cervical vertebra is overdeveloped to form a rib. It may be partially or fully developed rib. It may be asymptomatic or may have pain and tingling in the forearm.

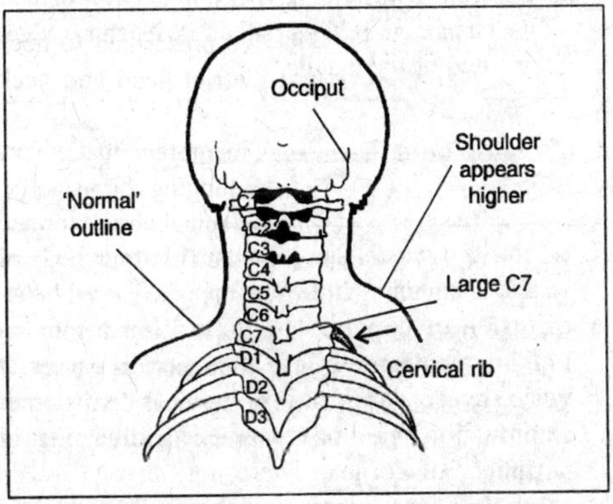

Cervical ripening The maturational process of softening and effacement of the cervix.

Cervical scoliosis Scoliosis having its apex between C_1 and C_6.

Cervical softening A process that transforms the cervix from an inextensible to a highly complaint tissue in order to allow dilation for the passage of the term fetus.

Cervical spinal syndrome Sometimes person wakes up with episodes of cervical muscle spasm. Neck becomes stiff or a sudden unguarded movement produces pain accompanied by spasm and tenderness in cervical spinal muscles.

Cervical spine The portion of vertebral column contained in neck consisting of seven cervical vertebra.

Cervical spondylosis A rorm of vertebral arthritis accompanied by bony outgrowths around the margins of cervical facet joints resulting in compression of cervical nerve roots.

Cervical spondylotic myelopathy There may be clumsiness of one or both hands. The cause of myelopathy is compression of spinal cord. Postmortem studies show loss of myelin around cord, compression results in secondary ischaemic effects. Cervical collar is of much use.

Cervical tear Some degree of cervical laceration in primipara is unavoidable. Deep cervical tears may occur in spontaneous labours specially in breech

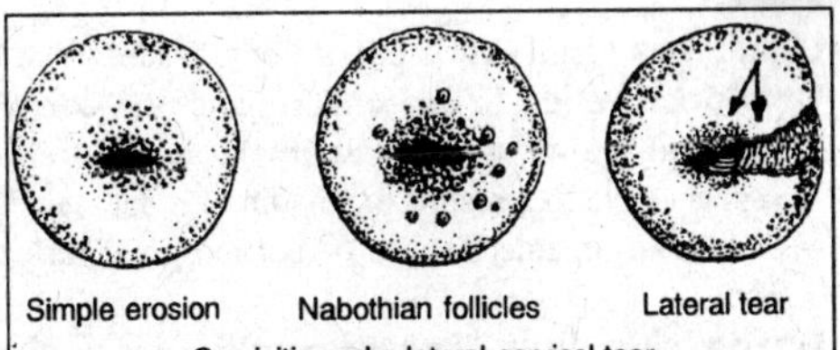

Cervicitis and a lateral cervical tear

presentation. Tear usually occurs at lateral wall and may even involve uterine artery. Deep cervical tear is suspected even though the uterus is firmly retracted.

Cervical tinnitus It is usually unilateral and seldom bilateral. It is constant and very rarely pulsatile. Sound tends to be more noticeable early in the morning than in the evening. Tinnitus changes pitch and loudness frequently with changes in head position. Tinnitus is combined with fluctuating, usually low frequency sensorineural hearing loss with direction changing provoked nystagmus.

Cervicitis It is due to vaginal infection or injury during child birth. It may be symptomless. Chronic

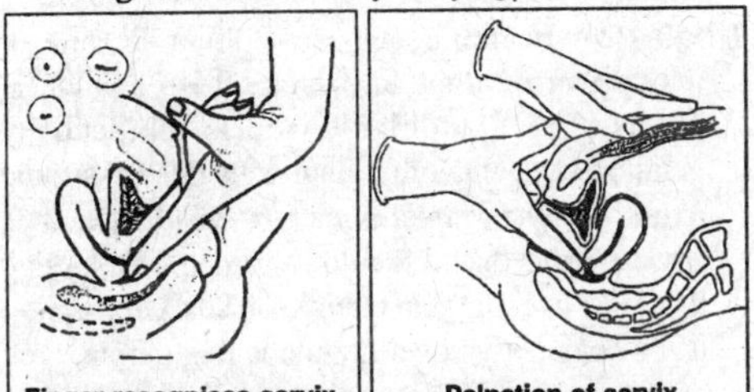
Finger recognises cervix
Palpation of cervix

cervicitis may produce a vaginal discharge, bleeding from vagina specially after coitus. Untreated cervicitis can cause endometritis or salpingitis. If child is to be delivered it may cause neonatal ophthalmia.

Cervicodorsal Pertaining to the neck or a necklike structure.

Cervicodynia Pain in the neck.

Cervicogenic headache A headache with the site of origin in the cervical spine.

Cervicothoracic curve Spinal curvature with an apex at C_7 or T_1.

Cervix Lower part of the uterus extending to the vagina.

Cestode Any tapeworm or platyhelminth of the class Cestoidea.

Chachexia General wasting of body tissue.

Chaddock reflex In this stroking over the skin of external malleolus and along the dorsolateral aspect of the foot results extension of great toes. It is seen in organic disease of corticospinal reflex paths.

Chadwick's sign The blue-purple color on the mucous membrane ot the vagina just below the urethral orifice, caused by increased vascularity.

Chain of infection Sequence that enables the spread of disease-producing microorganisms.

Chain, sympathetic Sympathetic trunk.

Chaining Learning related behaviours in a series, in which each response serves as a stimulus for the next response, as when a child learns to write his or her name letter by letter. When the child writes the name quickly and as a single unit, the chaining is complete.

Chairside assistant Dental health care workers whose primary responsibility is to assist the dentist or independently perform clinical treatment for the patient.

Chalazion It may occur as a solitary nodule or multiple or in crops in eyelids. It is common in adults. The glandular tissue is replaced by granulations containing giant cells due to chronic irritation by organisms of low virulence. It is advisable that the lid should be palpated by passing the finger over the skin of both the lids. On eversion of lid conjunctiva over nodule is red, purple, grey or even yellow. Grey colour indicates that the granular mass has been converted into a jelly-like mass. A yellow point indicates that it has been infected. Some cases may show a granular mass sprouting through conjunctiva. Large nodule in upper lid may give rise to dropping of lid because of weight.

Chalazion clamp It is used to fix the chalazion during its incision and curettage. It has a plate and a ring. The plate side is kept on the skin and ring towards the conjunctiva. Trap the nodule between the ring and press, evert and tighten the screw. The ring demarcates the border and plate protects the underlying structures from damage.

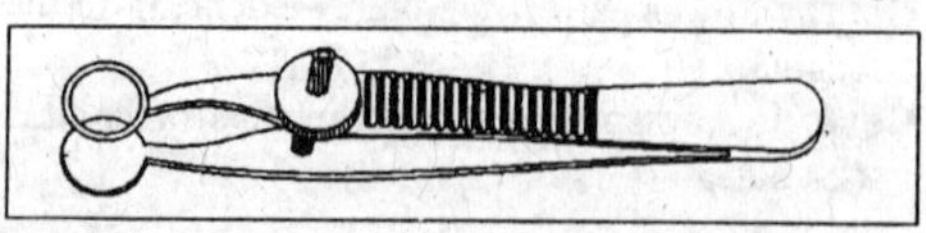

The clamp also acts as a haemostat. Incision should be vertical and deep enough to cut the capsule of the gland. The contents are scooped out by a chalazion scoop.

Chalazion scoop It helps to scoop out the contents of the chalazion. It has small cup with sharp edges at one end of the handle.

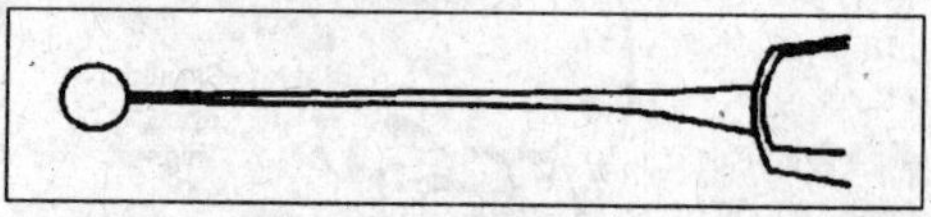

Chalcosis It occurs due to retained foreign body of an alloy containing little pure copper. There is slow diffusion of copper. The deposition occurs in limiting membrane of eye. Reaction to copper is very severe suppurative type. On slit-lamp examination one notices greenish blue ring in periphery of cornea. There may be sunflower cataract of lens. Many particles may be seen in aqueous humour. Iris shows greenish colour. There are refractile deposits in retina.

Chalk Used as polishing agent in dentistry and frequently as an ingredient in dentifices.

Chamberien forcep Each branch is about 12 inches long and had a fenestrated blade with a cephalic curve. Branches can be separated and can

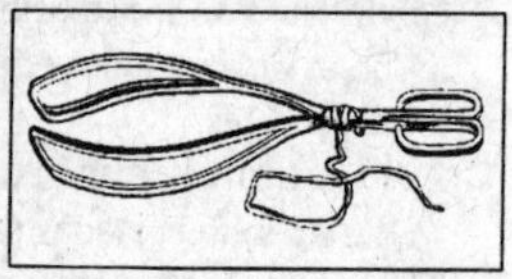

be inserted individually. The forceps then function as a first class lever.

Chamberlains line A line used to assess basilar impression.

Chance fracture These occur in car passenger after road accident. Lumbar fractures are unstable. Fracture in the horizontal plane of neural arch and vertebral body produced by acute spinal flexion.

Chance node An element in a decision analysis that represents a point at which specified outcomes are determined on the basis of probability.

Chancre Primary lesion of chancre is usually in the genital area. It appears after 3 weeks of exposure and starts as a macule. Then it becomes papule and later on ulcer. The ulcer has indurated borders. The lips are the most common site for primary syphilis. The chancre disappears within 1 to 4 weeks. Under microscope it shows an ulcer with oedema and dense infiltration by plasma cells, macrophages and lymphocytes. PAM is the line of treatment.

Chandler disease Idiopathic asceptic necrosis of femoral head.

Change of shift report Discussion between a nurse from the shift that is ending and personnel coming on duty.

Channel An opening in a protein that is imbedded in a cell membrane and allows the passage of ions through the cell membrane.

Chaperone Proteins that function to support another proteins or growing polypeptides in a particular conformation. Proteins that are required for the correct folding of newly synthesized proteins. They also prevent protein denaturation during stresses, and can renature damaged proteins.

Chaperone proteins Protein required to proper folding and assembly of another protein.

Chapman's reflexes Tender zones at various locations on the body surface, correlated by Frank Chapman, D.O., with lymphatic stasis in various internal organs, and more recently correlated by George Goodheart, D.C., with lymphatic stasis in various skeletal muscles. A synonym is neurolymphatic reflexes.

Chapple test A method of evaluating congenital dislocation of new born hip.

Character Personality viewed from the standpoint of what is ethical or moral, such as a person's honesty— ordinarily it has reference to relatively fixed traits.

Character defence Any character or personality trait which serves an unconscious defensive purpose.

Characteristic Pertaining to a character.

Charas Hashish.

Charcoat Joint It is a rapidly progressive degeneration of a joint characterized by degeneration of cartilage with spur formation and debris, bone fragmentation, dislocation and swelling. A neurogenic arthropathy producing chronic progressive degeneration of one or more joints which are relatively painless with pronounced swelling, and characterised by formation of synovial effusion of osteophyte, relaxation of ligaments, and hypermobility of the joint, leading to sensory disturbances. It is seen in tabes dorsalis, diabetic neuropathy, leprosy, syringomyelia, and tumour or injury to the spinal cord of peripheral nerve, and subacute combined degeneration of pernicious anaemia.

Charcot's triad Cardinal symptoms of multiple sclerosis—intentional tremor, scanning speech, and nystagmus.

Charisma The ability to arouse or inspire others via skilled, emotional communication.

Charle's law At constant pressure, the volume of a fixed mass of gas is proportional to its temperature.

Charley Horse A colloquial term referring to a soreness, cramping and stiffness of a muscle.

Charnley arthodesis It is a technique for intra articular fusion of a joint using a temporary external fixation apparatus.

Chart Binder or folder that enables the orderly collection, storage, and safekeeping of a patient's medical records.

Charter's technique Method of toothbrushing in which the brush is held horizontally, with the bristles lying against the teeth and gingivae and pointed in a coronal direction at 45 degreees so that the bristles lie half on the teeth and half on the gingivae. A vibratory cycle of a very constricted diameter is negotiated so that the brush head moves circularly but the brush bristles remain fairly stationary while being agitated. The circular vibration loosens debris and pumps the bristles into interproximal areas to massage the tissues.

Charting Process of writing information.

Charting by exception Documentation method in which only abnormal assessment findings or care that deviates from the standard is charted.

Chassaignac's tubercle The anterior tubercle on the transverse process of sixth cervical vertebra.

Chauffeur's fracture Fracture of radial styloid.

Cheatle forceps It is a heavy stainless steel forceps without locking system. It is used to hold sterilised

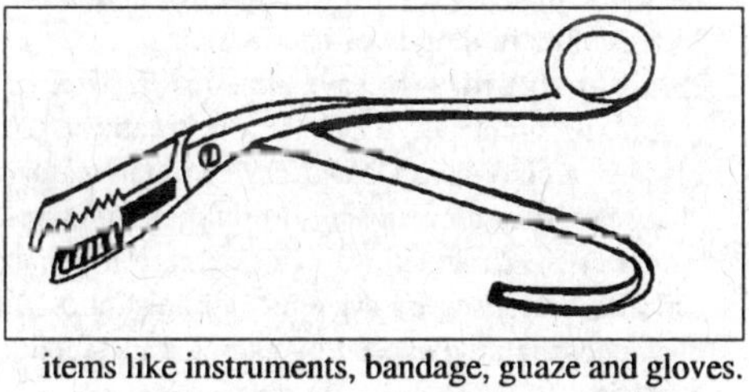

items like instruments, bandage, guaze and gloves. It is kept in bottle dipped in Savlon solution.

Checkboard pattern A square set of equal size black and white squares placed adjacent to each other is used to check visual acuity.

Checklist Form of documentation in which the nurse indicates with a check mark or initials that routine care has been performed.

Chediak-Steinbrinck-Higashi syndrome An autosomal recessive disorder characterised by anaemia, lymphadenopathy, hepatosplenomegaly, thrombocytopenia, structural abnormalities of leucocytes with cytoplasmic inclusions and Dohle's bodies, and increased susceptibility to cold.

Cheek biting Chewing of ones buccal mucosa. It may result due to malocclusion, or due to lack of coordination in the chewing cycle.

Cheilectomy The surgical excision of bony protruberances from edges of an articular surface which interfere with joint motion.

Cheilitis Inflammation of the lips.

Cheiloangioscopy Observation of the circulation in the blood vessels of the lip.

Cheilocarcinoma Carcinoma of the lip.

Cheilorraphy It is the corrective surgery of restoration of lips.

Cheilotomy Incision into, or removal of part of lip.

Chelation Binding of a metallic ion with a structure so that the ion is inactivated.

Chellion The corner of the mouth.

Chemical Relating to chemistry, especially to the characteristics of atoms and molecules and to their interactions.

Chemical bond Force of attraction in a molecule or compound that holds its atoms together. Examples include ionic and covalent bonds.

Chemical burn Chemical burn of the oral mucosa presents as a white lesion. This leads to a white irregular patch of tissue coagulation. After the necrotic surface sloughs off leaving a raw red, bleeding area.

Microscopic finding is of necrosis.

Chemical cystitis Intravesical instillation of cytotoxic agents or BCG for the treatment of bladder carcinoma can lead to severe inflammatory changes of bladder wall and surrounding structures which cause irregular wall thickening on CT. It can also be caused by systemic administration of cyclophosphamide caused by excreted metabolite acrolein.

Chemical degestion The chemical altering effects of digestive secretions, gastric juices, and enzymes on food substance composition.

Chemical element Unit of matter that cannot be decomposed into a simpler substance by ordinary chemical reactions. Examples include hydrogen (H), carbon (C), and oxygen (O).

Chemical formula Symbols of atoms used to indicate the composition of a molecule.

Chemical messengers Substances produced by endocrine or non-endocrine cells that bind to a receptor on or in a target cell to elicit control or function of the cell.

Chemical neurotransmitter A chemical that binds to a receipts site of a membrane protein.

Chemical reaction The combination or separation of atoms in which chemical bonds are formed or broken and new products with different properties are produced.

Chemical score of proteins Chemical score of protein is determined as the ratio between the concentration of a limiting essential amino acid in a test protein with its concentration in the reference protein.

Chemical shift imaging It is a type of MR spectroscopy in which spatially localised spectra are obtained using technique in which spectroscopic data are acquired simultaneously from a large volume of sample and then decoded into a number of spatially resolved spectra.

Chemical substance abuse Both physical dependence and psychologic dependence on the use of chemical such as alcohol or illega drugs to modify mood and performance and to escape from anxiety.

Cigarette smoking is also a form of chemical dependence or substance abuse.

Chemical synapse When stimulated by an action potential, a synapse that releases a chemical into the synaptic cleft.

Chemistry Science dealing with the atomic composition of substances and the reactions they undergo.

Chemoarchitecture The relationship between cellular topography and the cellular machinery used in signal detection and processing.

Chemoattractant A hormone or chemical agent that attracts other cells.

Chemoheterotroph An organism that uses organic carbon both as a source of carbon and as a source of energy, thus, chemoheterotrophic.

Chemoheterotrophy A type of metabolism in which cellular carbon is derived from organic carbon compounds, with energy derived form its oxidation.

Chemonucleolysis Injaction of chymopapain to reduce disc herniation.

Chemoreceptor A neuroreceptor that is stimulated by the presence of the chemical molecules .

Chemoreceptor reflex Process in which chemoreceptors detect changes in oxygen levels, carbon dioxide levels, and pH in the blood and produce changes in heart rate, force of heart contraction, and blood vessel diameter that return these values toward their normal levels.

Chemoreceptors A receptor that detects substances according to their chemical structures. This includes smell and taste receptors.

Chemosignal A chemical released externally by one individual that can induce physiological or behavioral change in another individual; pheromone.

Chemosis Oedema of conjunctiva is termed as chemosis. On the inflammation of conjunctiva, there is exudation from conjunctival capillaries. The conjunctiva becomes swollen and gelatinous in appearance. The chemosis affects mostly the loose bulbar conjunctiva and the fornices. In case with severe chemosis, swollen bulbar con-junctiva forms a wall around the cornea overhanging the corneal margin affecting the nutrition of cornea from the perilimbal capillaries.

Chemotactic Relating to or able to produce chemotaxis.

Chemotaxin A factor that induces a process of chemotaxis.

Chemotaxis Movement of a cell or organism towards or away from a chemical substance. Specifically, the directed migration of cells towards an inflammatory site.

Chemotherapeutic agent It is a chemical agent which is used to kill or inhibit the growth that are used to kill or inhibit the growth of microorganism already established in the tissues of the body. The object is to kill microorganisms without significant harmful effects on host. Chemotherapeutic agents need to act at a concentration that can be tolerated by the tissues of the host and therefore they must have a selective toxicity for the microorganism compared with the host.

$$\text{Index} = \frac{\text{Maximum tolerant dose}}{\text{Minimum curative dose}}$$

Chemotroph An organism that obtains energy by metabolizing organic compounds derived from other organisms.

Cherry red spot Cherry red spot at macula is the most striking fundus picture seen in a rare group of diseases such as Tay-Sachs' disease, Neimann-Pick disease, Sandhoff disease and sialidosis type I and II. All these diseases are characterised by intracellular deposition of certain glycolipids in various tissues of body. In retina lipids are stored in ganglion cell layer giving it a white appearance.

Cherry red spot myoclonus syndrome There may be development of a slowly progressive neurological illness where most crippling symptom is myoclonus, seizures, decreased muscle tone, speech disorder and hyperactive reflexes. There will be cherry red spot of macula, horizontal nystagmus and white dot and flake lens changes with decreased visual acvity.

Chest Thorax.

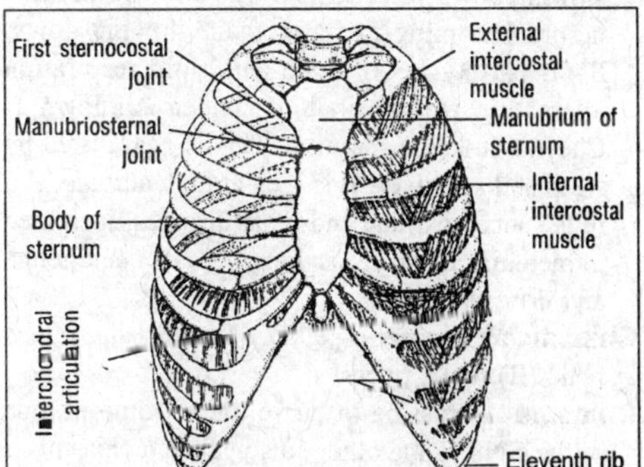

Chest pain Most common cause is strained chest wall, i.e. fibrositis. Pressure on a nerve root attached to spinal cord may result in sharp chest pain. Disc prolapse although not very common in dorsal spine may cause pain. Chest pain may be caused by pleurisy. Bronchitis, pneumonia may also result in pain. Malignant tumour of lung may cause pain as they grow. Acid reflux is a cause of heartburn. Most important is the pain of angina or myocardial infarction. Stable angina may be present for months. Myocardial pain may be referred to arms and is of cruciating nature. Pain of pericarditis is also felt in centre of chest. Valvular defect pain is sharp on the left side. Chest pain may be result of anxiety and stress.

Chest physical therapy A multifaceted area of practice that includes many evaluation and treatment techniques with the goals to improve airway clearance, ventilation, and exercise tolerance; reduce work of breathing; and restore patient to fullest potential.

Chest physiotherapy Techniques for mobilizing pulmonary secretions.

Chevron osteotomy Any V shaped osteotomy.

Chew-in technique The method by which the dentist records a patient's occlusal paths in wax patterns to be used in making restorations.

Chewing gum Partially evaporated milky juice of latex of sapodilla tree, plus sugar, balsum of Tolu and flavour.

Cheyne-Stokes breathing There is impairment of suppression of respiratory centre in the brain as may occur in coma or under sedation. There is slowing down of or temporary halt of respiration before becoming fast and again slowing down. Short paroxysms of deep and rapid respiration alternating with periods of apnoea is known as Cheyne-Stokes respiration. This is aggravated by sleep and sedatives. It is seen at high altitude, and in advanced cardiac and renal diseases, increased intracranial pressure, asthma, severe pneumonia, and drug poisoning.

Chiasm A crossing; especially the crossing of the optic (II) nerve fibers.

Chiasma A crossing of nerve tracts from one side of the CNS to the other , also called a chiasm.

Chiasma 'Crossing' Refers mainly to the optic chiasma.

Chicago test A clinical test used in differentiation of disc disease and back strain.

Chicken pox Portal of entry of virus is the respiratory tract. Incubation period is 2 weeks. It may start with fever followed within a day by sudden eruption of crops of skin lesions. Lesions are distributed centripetally on trunk.Successive crops of vesicles appear at a rapid rate and various stages macule, papule, vesicle, pustule and scab formation lesions are seen at one point of time. Itching develops. Lesions are superficial and do not not leave marks. Varicella pneumonitis is more common and may prove serious. Fatal cases may be associated with hepatitis.

Chief cells Cells in the lining of the stomach that secrete digestive enzymes.

Chiene's line A line used in evaluation of a femoral neck fracture. The level of greater trochanter on one side may be compared with that of other side by drawing lines.

Chigger A mite of the family Trombiculiadae.

Chignon New born scalp oedema created by a vacuum extractor.

Child care Supplemental care for children provided by persons other than parents.

Child molestation It is the sexual abuse of children by such acts as fondling, stroking the child's genitals, exhibitionism and intercourse. It is of brief contact and is different from rape or other violent sexual acts.

Childbearing cycle The period to time, beginning with the preconceptual period and prenatal period of pregnancy, the labor and birth, and the postpartum period, during which the woman's body returns to the normal prepregnancy physiological state and family adapts to a new member.

Childbed fever An older term for puerperal fever.

Childhood From infancy to puberty.

Childhood stressor These include parental loss, neglect and physical and sexual abuse in addition to poverty and parental conflict.

Chill It is a sudden feeling of cold that may or may not be associated with shivering. Fever may be accompanied by chills because the blood heat is inappropriate to the environmental temperature. Persistent chill is an indication of infection or of strong anxiety.

Chilled shot Lead shot containing more than 0.5% alloying metal to increse its hardness.

Chinese clock Chinese have a concept that energy flows through particular organs and meridians in a specific order and at a specific time of day or night. Energy is said to commence in lungs at 3 AM and remains at high level until 5 AM when it flows into the colon for 2 hours, then to stomach,

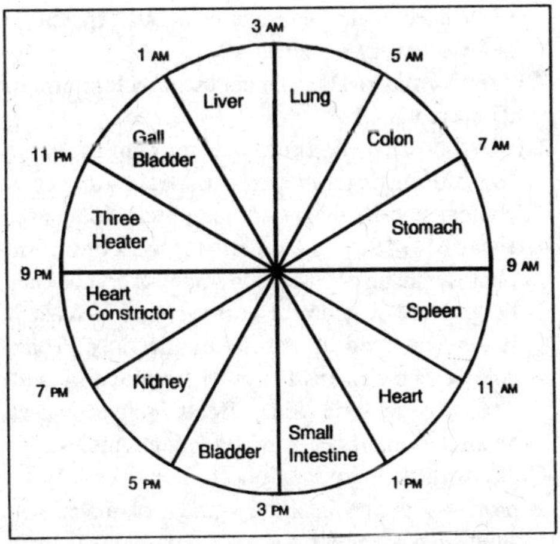

spleen, heart and throughout body In the lung meridian is at its peak energy at between 3 AM and 5 AM and lowest energy level at 3 PM and 5 PM. Treatment for a diseased organ or meridian is most beneficial if it can be done during peak energy time.

Chip fracture A small avulsion fracture in which only a fragment or a piece of cortex has been separated from main body.

Chiral Having the property of chirality; describing a moecule that cannot be superimposed on its mirror image.

Chirality The property of a molecule with carbon atoms to which four different ligands are bonded tetrahedrally. This gives a pair of steroisomers per chiral carbon atom that exhibit mirror symmetry, but cannot be superimposed on each other.

Chiropractic analysis The clinical assessment of a patient's state of biomechanical and neurologic integrity, primarily for the purpose of characterizing subluxation.

Chiropractic Biophysics Technique (CBP) A full-spine technique in which postural analysis and other physical examination findings are correlated with x-ray signs. The patient is positioned in the mirror image of the postural distortion during adjustment.

Chiropractic philosophy A conceptual framework in health care characterized by a profound respect for the organism's adaptive vitality and by an emphasis on removing interference to the organism's ability to sense its internal and external environment.

Chiropractice It is concerned with treatment of mechanical disorders of joints specially spinal joints and their effect on nervous system. It was known to Hippocrates some 2500 years ago and it was the work of Canadian born Daniel Palmer known as chiropractice therapy. The term subluxation is used by chiropractors to describe the condition of bones which are out of alignment and thus interrupts the flow of energy.

Chisel A dental instrument, the cutting edge of which is in line with the center of the handle; used for planing or smoothing a surface, as during cavity preparation.

Chisel and hammer It is used to cut the bone during dacryocystorhinostomy. Many surgeons use an electric drill instead of this.

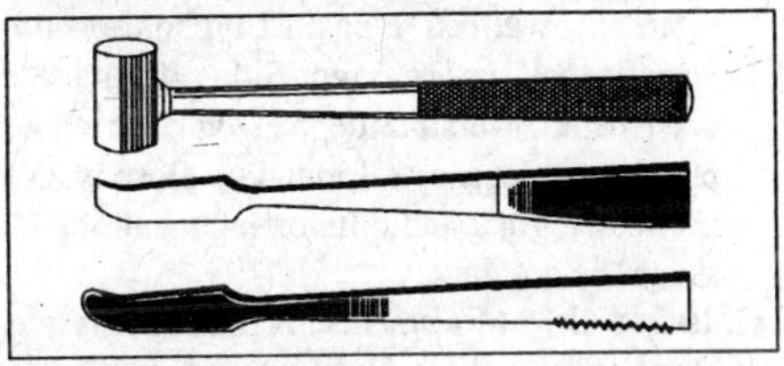

Chisel fracture Incomplete fracture of medial portion of radial head.

Chisel Instrument designed after the carpenter's chisel 1. As a hand cutting instrument the device is used for cutting or cleaving hard tissue; the instrument is beveled with a cutting edge on one side only It can have a straight or angled shank. 2. As a scaler the instrument has a single blade perpendicular to the long axis of the instrument shank and handle and is used in pulling action to remove calculus.

Chlamydia Most prevalent sexually transmitted disease, characterized by frequent, painful, or burning urination and low back pain.

Chlamydia trachomatis An organism responsible for a spectrum of diseases including cervicitis, urethritis, acute salpingitis, and ednometritis.

Chloasma It is the hyperpigmentation of skin specially cheeks. It may occur due to oestrogen taking as oral contraceptives. Exposure to sunlight may accentuate the pigmentation. The condition presents with superficial, non-elevated, smooth, often poorly, defined brownish patchy pigmentation. Lesions are distributed symmetrically over bridge of nose, upper lip, cheeks and forehead. Disease is asymptomatic. Local application of hydrogen peroxide may be beneficial. Salicylic acid 3 to 5% ointment is also useful. In women chloasma gravidarum produces mask-like darkening of face during pregnancy involving cheeks, temples and forehead. Lesion generally disappears after delivery.

Chloral hydrate It is a sedative introduced in 1869 and has a half life of 8-10 hours. It causes minimal cardiovascular or respiratory depression.

Chloramphenicol It is primarily a bacteriostatic but may be bactericidal against *Haemophilus influenzae, Neisseria meningitidis* and *Streptococcus pneumoniae*. Chloramphenicol penetrates well into tissues including the CSF and brain. It is effective against typhoid bacilli but ciprofloxacin is preferred. Side effects are dose dependent, reversible depression of erythrocyte, platelet and leucocyte formation. Dose is 250 mg six hourly. Total and differential count of patients should be got done.

Chloride shift Movements of chloride ions into red blood cells as 0_2 is given up and exchanged for $C0_2$ in tissues.

Chloroazodin An antibacterial substance that slowly liberates chlorine.

Chloroform It is a colourless liquid. It produces a vapour that if inhaled acts as a general anaesthesia. Its use as anaesthetic has been abandoned because of its low margin of safety, cardiac and liver toxicity. It was first prepared by Justus Von Leibig in 1831, and was used in humans in 1847. Prolonged inhalation of 2% vapour may produce respiratory arrest. Nowadays it is not used due to tissue toxicity and action on heart and may result in death. Cardiac depression increases with depth of anaesthesia. It has gone into disrepute how due to hepatic toxicity.

Chloroform intoxicity It has a narrow margin of safety as it causes cardiac and respiratory failure simultaneously. Fatal dose of ingested chloroform is 10 ml. Inhalation of chloroform at 10 ppm may be fatal. Chloroform results in varying degree of anaesthesia and cardiac dysfunction. Jaundice can occur within 2 to 3 days due to hepatotoxicity. 5ml of IV injection can cause drowsiness, hypotension and pulmonary oedema.

Chloroformism The habitual use of chloroform for its nacrcotic effect.

Chlorophylls A family of green pigments functioning as receptors of light energy in photosynthesis; magnesiumporphyrin complexes.

Chloroplasts Chlorophyllcontaining photosynthetic organelles in some eukaryotic cells.

Chloroquine It is useful in prevention of malaria. It may be used as antirheumatic drug. Today chloroquine remains the main treatment of acute attacks of malaria. Side effects include nausea, headache, diarrhoea and abdominal cramps.

Chloroquine intoxication It is used both in the prophylaxis and in the treatment of malaria. In adults ingestion of 1.5 gm of chloroquine is toxic. The lethal dose for adults and children is 2.0 gm and 35 to 50 mg/kg respectively. Toxic symptoms develop within 1 to 3 hours of ingestion. Drowsiness is often the earliest feature and may appear within 10 to 30 minutes of an overdose, other features are headache, phobia, diplopia, seizures and circulatory arrest. Blurring of vision is common clinical feature including vomiting, nausea and epigastric distress. Chloroquine produces vasodilatation and hypotension. Sudden fall of BP is characteristic Ventricular tachycardia and fibrillation are noted. Hypokalaemia is always present. Auditory disturbances are always noted in chronic cases.

Chlorpromazine It is an antipsychotic drug used to depress abnormal behaviour. It is used in the treatment of mania, schizophrenia and dementia. It is not curative but gives symptomatic relief. It is used in nausea and vomiting. Side effects include slowed reaction and blurred vision. Alcohol should not be consumed with this drug.

Choanal atresia Symptoms include complete unilateral or bilateral nasal obstruction. Persistent purulent coryza on the obstructed side develops with inability to blow the nose. It is transmitted as a dominant trait.

Choane The two posterior openings from the nasal cavity into the nasal pharynx; also called the internal nares.

Chocking It is an obstruction of airway. In the unconscious supine patient airway obstruction may occur when a relaxed tongue falls against a posterior larynx. Trauma may cause it and laryngeal oedema and tumours may result it. Manual abdominal thrusts are indicated in the conscious patient. Intrathoracic pressure is increased to blow the obstruction out of the airway. Abdominal thrust is given by pressing fist four times into victim's abdomen with quick inward and upward thrust. There is partial or complete inability to breathe due to obstruction of the airway due to food, fish bone or another swallowed foreign body. If obstruction is partial person may still breath. Airway may be blocked at pharynx, larynx and trachea. If food and drink go to trachea it may be choked. Emergency treatment in the term of cricothyrotomy or tracheostomy may have to be performed.

Choke Interior constriction at or near the muzzle end of a shotgun barrel bore for the purpose of controlling the spread of the shot. The tighter the degree of choke, the smaller the pattern of shot at the target.

Cholagogue A substance that stimulates emptying of gall bladder and flow of bile.

Cholangitis It is the inflammation of common bile duct (CBD) due to bacterial infection or blockage by gall stone. There will be recurrent bouts of jaundice. Person will have pain in abdomen and symptoms may be mild or life threatening. Ultrasound and liver function test help in diagnosis. Antibiotics and higher amount of fluid intake will be able to control fever and infection. Some cases may require surgery.

Cholecystectomy The surgical removal of the gallbladder.

Cholecystitis It is an inflammation of gall bladder causing severe abdominal pain. *Acute cholecystitis* is mostly caused by gall stones. The trapped bile gives an opportunity to develop infection. Repeated acute attacks of acute cholecystitis will lead to *chronic cholecystitis*. In it gall bladder wall thickens. Ultrasound helps in diagnosis. Most cases subside without the need of urgent surgery.

Cholecystokinin It is much more widely distributed than secretin found in CNS, thyroid, pituitary and colonic nerve as the I cells of duodenum and jejunum. It is released by gastric acid and by fats and amino acids in the duodenum. It helps in production of pancreatic enzyme. It results in gall bladder contractions and increase in hepatic bile flow. It stimulates calcitonin release. No clearly defined clinical syndrome of excess production of secretin or CCK are known.

Cholecystokinin-pencreozymin (CCK) A hormone that initiattes pancreaticexocrine secretions, acts against gastrin, and activates the gallbladder to release bile; secreted by the small intestine.

Choledochal cyst There is partial and intermittent obstruction to the flow of bile through the ampulla of Vater. The CBD is dilated into a cystic enlargement. Patients have history of abdominal pain and jaundice intermittently. Cystic swelling is felt in right upper quadrant.

Cholera It is an infection of small intestine caused by *Vibrio cholerae*. It results in watery diarrhoea. If not treated properly person dies due to dehydration. It starts in epidemic form of sudden vomiting and diarrrhoea. About 500 ml of fluid is lost every hour and may result in death in a few hours. Toxin increases the passage of fluid from the blood stream into the large and small intestine. So, treatment includes replacing the lost fluid with glucose saline drips. Tetracycline will help in checking diarrhoea. To prevent cholera, vaccine is available.

Cholestasis Elevated bilirubin is mostly conjugated and alkaline phosphatase and other bile duct enzymes are elevated. Serum cholesterol concentration is raised. Asparate transaminase are normal. Cholestatic jaundice may arise from either extrahepatic or intrahepatic causes. One of earliest symptoms is pruritus which is severe during night. Right upper quadrant pain suggests a gall stone within duct. Painless obstructive jaundice is due to carcinoma head of pancreas. The light coloured stools are due to failure of bile pigments to enter the intestinal tract. Intrahepatic cholestasis is caused by viral hepatitis and drugs like phenothiazines. It may recur.

Cholesteatoma It accounts for less than one per cent of all peria pical pathological radiolucencies. There is formation of few localised cholesterol crystals which form due to fatty degeneration in dental granuloma. It may develop in the wall of radicular cyst also.

Cholesterol It is an important constituent of blood. It is also involved in formation of hormones and bile salts. It is made in liver and helps in transportation of fats. High level of cholesterol results in atherosclerosis and ultimately heart attack and stroke.

HDL is protective cholesterol while LDL increases the risk of cardiac diseases. Ratio of HDL and LDL should not be more than 1:4. Low consumption of saturated fats and exercise helps keeping in control of LDL. Accepted level of total cholesterol should be between 150 and 200 mg per cent.

Choline A natural substance obtained from food and converted into the neurotransmitter acetylcholine.

Cholinergic Denoting nerve endings that liberate acetylcholine as a neurotransmitter, such as those of the parasympathetic system.

Cholinergic fiber Axons whose terminals release acetylcholine.

Cholinergic neuron A neuron that contains acetylcholine in its synapses.

Cholinergic syndrome Muscarinic poisoning syndrome comprises salivation, lacrimation, abdominal cramps, urinary incontinence, vomiting, sweating, pulmonary oedema and confusion. Common causes include organophosphorus and neostigmine and mushrooms.

Chondral Pertaining to cartilage

Chondroclasis The resorption or crushing of cartilage.

Chondroclast A giant cell implicated in the resorption of cartilage.

Chondrocostal Pertaining to rib and costal cartilage.

Chondrocytes Cartilage- forming cells.

Chondrodysplasia An hereditary disorder of cartilage formation.

Chondrodystrophy Heterogeneous group of disorders due to defective cartilage formation. There will be disproportionately short stature.

Chondroepiphysitis Inflammation of epiphyseal cartilage.

Chondrogenesis Formation of cartilage.

Chondroitin sulfate An amorphous matrix material found outside connective tissue cells.

Chondrolysis Degeneration of cartilage cells resulting in cell death.

Chondromalacia A pathologic state of softening with subsequent fibrillation, fissuring and erosion of articular cartilage.

Chondromalacia patella Pathological changes in articular cartilage of undersurface of patella resulting in anterior knee pain.

Chondromas A benign tumor of cartilage.

Chondromucoprotein Constituent of ground substance of cartilage.

Chondromyoma A benign tumor with myxomatous and cartilaginous elements.

Chondromyxoid fibroma There may be pain and swelling of long duration. Under microscope one is able to see chondroid material mixed with myxomatous and giant cells. On X-ray lesion is destructive, eccentric in position in the metaphysis of long bones specially tibia. It is smooth outlined and sclerosis is usually present.

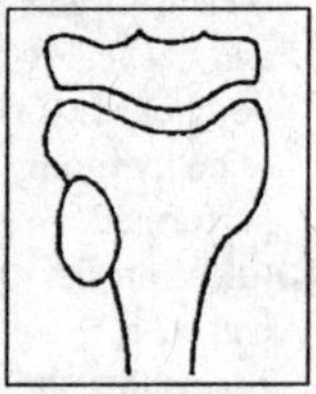

Choparts amputation An amputation of foot through the mid tarsal joint.

Choparts joint The mid tarsal joint of foot consisting of talonavicular and calcaneocuboid joint. Transverse tarsal joint.

Chordae tendineae Tendinous strands running from the papillary muscles to the free margin of the cusps that make up the tricuspid and bicuspid valves; prevent the cusps of these valves from extending up into the atria during ventricular contraction.

Chordates members of the phylum of animals having a notochord; includes the fishes, amphibians, reptiles, birds, and mammals.

Chordee An abnormal bending of the penis during erection. Significant bends may effect the ability to have normal intercourse.

Chordomas These are congenital neoplasms originating from notochord remnants. They are located within clivus. They may also originate within the sella or middle fossa. Early symptoms include ophthalmoplegias and lower cranial nerve dysfunction. Skull X-ray usually shows bone erosion of the clivus and posterior sella region.

Chorea It is the name given to rapid, irregular, involuntary, jerky movements which flow randomly from muscle to muscle. Movements are never co-ordinated, although may be followed by a voluntary movement involving the same part of body.

Chorea 'dance' Involunatary movements representing fragments of motor programs.

Choreoathetosis Movement disorder with features of both chorea and athetosis; frequently seen in cerebral palsy.

Chorin Develops into an important fetal membrane in the placenta.

Chorioamnionitis An intrauterine infection involving mononuclear and polymorphonuclear leucocytic infiltration of the fetal membranes and amniotic fluid.

Choriocarcinoma It develops from placenta in the uterus and is trophoblastic type. It follows an abortion. If remain untreated it invades and destroys the walls of uterus. It may spread to vagina and vulva. There may be persistent bleeding after childbirth or after an abortion. There may be difficulty in breathing, fatigue and tiredness. If any lady has hydatidiform mole should be kept in watch. Ultrasound is a good tool to diagnose. Treatment with anticancer drugs and hysterectomy will help.

Chorion The outermost extraembryonic membrane that becomes the principal embryonic portion of the placenta; serves a protective and nutritive function.

Chorion epithelioma It is a highly malignant neoplasm of fetal tissue. It is very proliferative, invades blood vessel and is highly vascular. Clinical features include uterine hemorrhage, foul stained vaginal discharge. Manifestation of secondary metastases includes dysponea and hematuria.

Chorion leave The smooth part of chorion.

Chorionic Relating to or involving the chorion.

Chorionic gonadotropins Hormones that are secreted as the uterus develops during pregnancy.

Chorionic villi Connected with the blood vessels of the chorion to the placenta.

Chorionic villus One of the fingerlike projections growing in tufts on the external surface of the chorion.

Chorionic villus sampling A method of fetal cell analysis during the first trimester, in which placental and chorionic tissue are collected, processed and reviewed.

Choroid It is a vascular layer between the sclera and retina and extends from the ora serrata to aperture of optic nerve in the sclera. It is loosely attached with sclera so that there is potential space between the two, the epichoroidal space. Choroid provides nutrition to the retina. The choroid is drained by the veins. As the choroid is loosely attached to the overlying sclera, detachment of choroid can occur. Choroid is supplied with sensory nerve fibres from trigeminal nerve. Portion of the vascular tunic associated with the sclera of the eye, functions to prevent scattering of light.

Choroid detachment After an intraocular operation there may occur detachment of choroid. Clinically anterior chamber is very shallow or absent. On ophthalmoscopy a dark mass is visible in upper quadrant.

Choroid plexus 'Membranous network' of capillaries invested with choroidal epithelium, within the ventricles of the brain.

Choroideraemia It is a condition where choroid and pigment epithelium of retina are completely absent except in a region around macula. Nights blindness is the common presenting symptom. There develops extreme concentric contraction of visual fields. Visual acuity is usually diminished and blindness is a rule after the age of 60. On ophthalmoscope fundus shows pepper and salt appearance in the periphery of fundus.

Chose family Family relationships defined by anything besides genetics, e.g., love, sex, affection, money, housing.

Chrioangioma It is the commonest placental tumor. It is likely that groups of blood vessels and stroma in a single vellus proliferate.

chroma The term used in the munsell color system to describe the intensity or extent of saturation of a certain color.

Chromatid One of a pair of identical connected nucleoprotein strands that are joined at the centromere and separate during cell division, each becoming a chromosome of one of the two daughter cells.

Chromatids Duplicated chromosomes, joined together at the centromere, that separate during cell division.

Chromatin Threadlike structures in the cell nucleus consisting primarily of DNA and protein. They represent the extended form of chromosomes during interphase.

Chromatolysis It is the process of disintegration and disappearance of chromatin brought about by various agencies, fatigue, certain poisons and decreased blood supply is called chromatolysis.

Chromatophilic substance Rough endoplasmic reticulum in the cell bodies of neurons that functions in protein in the nucleus of a nondividing or interphase cell.

Chromoatography Process of separating chemical substances by their differential absorption to an insoluble matrix.

Chromogen To produce any substance that may give origin to a coloring matter.

Chromograinins A class of acidic proteins present in large secretory granules in neuro endocrine tissue.

Chromomycosis It is a slowly progressing granulomatous infection of skin. The fungi is *Cladosporium* which is dark brown, thick walled with round cell, usually arranged in clusters. Infection develops on exposed parts. Lesion is dull red sharply demarcated patch with an indurated base containing small, itching papules at the site of inoculation. New crops of lesion may appear over path of lymphatic drainage. Slowly hard, greyish or dull red, cauliflower-like warty growths occur along lymphatics of the affected area. Secondary bacterial infection is common. Regional lymph glands enlarge. Antifungal treatment helps.

Chromosome It is a gene containing filamentous structure in a cell nucleus. the number of chromosomes per cell nucleus is constant for each species like 46 chromosomes in human cell.

Chromosome disorder Abnormality of the chromosome number or structure.

Chromosomes These are the thread-like structures present in nuclei of cells. Chromosome carries the inherited, genetic information, growth and functioning of entire body. Each and every cell of body contains similar type of chromosomes because each is derived from one cell only after repeated divisions. Chromosomes determine the shape of eyes, nose, colour of hair, skin and pupils. Each chromosome contains up to several thousand genes arranged in single line. Chemically a chromosome consists of extremely long chain of hereditary substance DNA alongwith a coating of protein. Total unit is known as chromatin. The sequence of chemical units in DNA provides the coded instructions for cellular activities. Out of 23 pairs of chromosomes 22 are the same in both sexes known as autosomal chromosomes. One member of each is derived from mother and another from father. The other two chromosomes are called sex chromosomes. In women they are known as 'X' chromosome while in men one is 'X' chromosome and another very small 'Y' chromosome. 'Y' chromosome is responsible for male characteristics. In its absence female pattern is developed.

Chronaxie It is the minimal time required for excitation of a tissue by an electric current which has double the threshold intensity of a stedy current. Chronaxie of a motor nerve is always the same as that of muscle it supplies. Long chronaxie indicates a less excitable tissue hence it measures the excitability of a tissue. Different muscles have different chronaxies.

Chronic Characterised by a long, slow course, as compared with acute.

Chronic gastritis It is a chronic form of dyspepsia. There will be pain or distress in epigastrium specially after fried food. Pain may be in back or to shoulder. It may be relieved by eructation. Appetite is diminished. There is a bad taste in mouth. The tongue is dry, flabby and indented by teeth. There are languor, headache, depression, disturbed sleep, fatigue, discomfort and drowsiness after meals. In first stage of congestion hydrochloric acid is diminished. Second stage is mucous catarrh in which there is large secretion of mucus and hydrochloric acid is completely absent. In third stage there is atrophy of mucous membrane. Macrocytic anaemia may be associated, affected and its failure later causes right ventricle to fall.

Chronic progressive chorea It is a hereditary disease characterised by choreiform movement and progressive dementia. It is caused by degeneration of corpus striatum and the ganglion cells of forebrain. Heredity plays an important part. There is an atrophy of cerebral cortex and corpus striatum. Acetylcholine and gammaaminobutyric acid (GABA) is seen in corpus striatum. First symptom is jerky involuntary movement of face and upper extremity. Gradually dysarthria and ataxia develop and patient becomes dementiated.

Chronic adhesive pericarditis This occurs following an attack of fibrinous pericarditis leading to adhesion between two layers of pericardium. There is indrawing of posterior or lateral aspect of chest wall during systole. Apex beat is fixed and does not change with change of posture.

Chronic brain syndrome Permanent and generalized loss of cerebral function that may include disorientation, memory loss, confusion, and stereotyped behavior.

Chronic carriers It is one who harbours pathogens for long period, a year or so and is able to transmit the disease to others.

Chronic catarrhal laryngitis Causative factor is inadequate voice rest in acute laryngitis. Inhalation of dirty environment and smoking may result it. Hoarseness becomes more severe in morning than evening. Patient develops habit of throat clearing. Dryness of throat and foreign body sensation develop.

Chronic constrictive pericarditis It usually results from tuberculous pericarditis. It is the result of healing of tuberculous pericarditis. Heart cannot dilate during diastole. Renal retention of sodium and water takes place. Symptoms include dyspnoea on exertion, precordial pain and discomfort. Gradual swelling of abdomen and feet is seen. On bending person may become faint. Neck veins are markedly engorged. Pulse shows increased rate with low volume. Limbs become cold. Cyanosis is present. Later oedema may appear. Apex beat is feeble.

Chronic dieting syndrome A lifestyle inhibited or controlled by a constant concern about food intake, body shape and/or weight that affects an individual's physical and mental health status.

Chronic exercise Exercise usually performed for 6-8 weeks or longer.

Chronic fatigue syndrome A muscle may fatigue due to disordered neuromuscular transmission. On exercise, intracellular acidosis may occur out of proportion. Rise in high energy phosphate and changes in muscle metabolism have been reported in studies of NMR spectroscopy in patients with postviral fatigue syndrome. Malaise and fatigue are common in those given interferons in trials of treatment of multiple sclerosis.

Chronic hunger A continual experience of undernutrition.

Chronic hypertension A hypertensive vascular disorder that is unrelated to pregnancy and is evident prior to gestation or persists postpartum.

Chronic hypertrophic gastritis There is gross rugal thickening sometimes throughout the body and fundus of stomach or sometimes on the lesser curvature. There may be marked elongation of gastric pits and hyperplasia of mucous secreting cells. Gastric acid secretion is markedly depressed or absent. Hypoalbuminaemia may develop. Person complains of pain, nausea, vomiting or hypoproteinaemic oedema. No drug is of much help.

Chronic illness One that comes on slowly and lasts a long time.

Chronic illness pattern The "long haul" in which families permanently reorganize their daily routines to accommodate long-term diseases and conditions.

Chronic inflammatory demyelinating neuropathy It develops over months and years. There is no family history of disease. Protein in CSF is increased but there are no or a few lymphocytes. Segmental demyelination and remyelination develops, nerve may become thickened and palpable. Nerve conduction velocities are slow. Steroids are helpful.

Chronic intestinal ischaemia Many patients with multiple occlusions involving arteries supplying small bowel may not develop any symptoms. Symptoms may be precipitated by the fall of BP. In severe ischaemia the bowel wall shows pathological effects and eventually ulcer and stricture formation. The symptoms are abdominal pain or discomfort specially after food when more blood is required at the site.
There will be epigastric bruit and weight loss. Diarrhoea or constipation may occur. Malabsorption is a common feature.

Chronic laryngitis Repeated acute attacks, excessive speaking, singing, teaching, overuse with faulty production of voice, nasal obstruction and mouth breathing may result it. These usually go on and ulcerate. Nasal sinusitis is very common.

Chronic leukaemia Course may extend up to many years. There is insidious beginning with enlargement of spleen, lymph nodes and weakness. Chronic myelocytic leukaemia is characterised by great increase in leucocytes in blood. Many immature cells, myelocytes and myeloblasts are present and total blood count may reach to 500,000 per cubic millimetre. Platelet count increases. Chronic lymphocytic leukaemia is having lower white cell count usually less than 100,000 cubic millimetre of which 90 per cent or more are lymphocytes. Oral symptoms are always present and consist of gingival hyperplasia. These are constant in monocytic form. In majority of cases gingival infiltrates are found. Under microscope lesions show dense infiltration of connective tissue by immature cells of lymphoid and monocytic series.

Chronic obstructive pulmonary disease (COPD) A progressive and irreversible condition identified by obstruction of air flow, chronic bronchitis, asthma, and emphysema.

Chronic pain Continuous or recurrent pain lasting longer than 3 months.

Chronic pancreatitis It is characterised by destruction of exocrine tissue in pancreas by inflammation with fibrosis. The pathology is patchy at first causing early enlargement later may be atrophy. The main duct may become dilated, generally or focally and smaller ducts become irregularly involved. Histologically there is inflammation and later on fibrosis. Protein plugs are developed in ducts followed by calculi. True and pseudocysts follow. Calcification may occur. Nerves within pancreas are infiltrated. The pain may be episodic and may be exacerbated by food. There may be intervals of freedom. Pain is epigastric, radiates to back and may be to right or left or upwards or downwards and may be exacerbated by alcohol. Pain may be severe in particular posture often involving flexion of trunk, vomiting may give relief. Mild jaundice occurs. Majority of cases are due to high alcohol consumption. There develops deposition of protein plugs in pancreatic ducts. It leads to ductular dilatation followed by acinar atrophy. It is not a reversible process. Nonalcoholic pancreatitis may be due to malnutrition. In younger patient it presents with pancreatic calcification and diabetes mellitus. It can be due to autoimmune disease and coeliac disease. Symptoms include persistent upper abdominal pain. Pain radiates to back. Pain is deep seated and may be relieved by antacids. Protein plugs calcify.

Chronic poisoning, arsenic It is much insidious in nature and skin toxicity begins with a persistent erythematous flush leading to hyperkeratotic skin. Pigmentation is patchy. Hyperkeratosis is more prominent in distal parts of body. Anaemia and leucopenia are almost universal. Peripheral neuropathy usually a symmetrical sensorimotor polyneuropathy is the hallmark of the arsenic poisoning. Other features include nausea, vomiting, headache and irritability.

Chronic pyelonephritis One or both kidneys may be affected. There may be scarring of varying degree with reduction in size of kidney. Patchy fibrosis with lymphocytic infiltration, tubular atrophy, periglomerular fibrosis and disappearance of nephron are the microscopic findings. In majority of cases there may be tiredness, lassitude, ill health, repeated attacks of fever with pain in lumbar region, dysuria and frequency of urine. Hypertension is not a usual presenting feature. Urine shows albumin and a few pus cells. WBC casts are pathognomonic. Culture may show *E. coli*. Blood urea level is high. Urinary enzymes specially LDH and GOT are reduced.

Chronic rhinopathy Chronic runny nose with a viscous, mucoid, usually colourless discharge. Initially intermittent and alternating nasal obstruction, later becoming constant and usually bilateral. Rhinoscopy shows dark red or pale livid, swollen turbinates. Occasionally polyp formation may develop. Secondary dacrocystitis, epiphosa and pharyngitis may develop.

Chronic sclerosing' osteomyelitis It is known as diffuse sclerosing osteomyelitis, develops specially in females in third decade. Mandible is commonly involved; premolar and molar areas are the usual sites. Teeth may or may not be present in area. Affected area may be enlarged. There may be repeated jolts of pain around jaws. There is swelling and trismus. Some persons may remain asymptomatic. Jaw develops cotton wool or pagetoid appearance. Disease is extensive but is self-limiting. Antibiotic and cortisone therapy is helpful.

Chronic septic lymphadenitis Nodes become moderately enlarged, slightly tender, elastic with or without matting. In the cervical group sepsis of mouth and scalp are the cause while any infection in leg will result in enlargement of inguinal glands.

Chronic ulcerative colitis An inflammatory process confined to the mucosa of any or all of the large intestine.

Chronic venous insufficiency Abnormal circulatory condition characterzied by decreased return of the venous bloood from the legs to the trunk of the body.

Chronobiology The science or study of temporal factors in life and disorders, such as the sleep-waking cycle, biologic clocks and rhythms, etc.

Chronological age Age in years.

Chronotropism The rate of cardiac muscle contraction.

Chuck Device, commonly made of metal, inside the heard of high speed handpieces that is used as a retentive mechanism to hold a bur or stone in place.

Chunking The grouping of items for facilitating memory. A dozen household items, perhaps too much for a child to remember in a series, are grouped into four chunks, those concerning food, furniture, transportation, and play. The child's task is to remember the four chunks and then the two, three, or four items in each chunk.

Churg-Strauss syndrome Aetiology is not known. There is allergic granulomatous angitis involving muscular arteritis and neigbouring veins. Clinical features include fever and arthritic attack, pulmonary infiltration and eosinophilia. Peripheral nerves are involved. There is glomerulosclerosis leading to renal failure. There will be GIT bleeding, perforation and infarction.

Chvostek's sign In this sign a light tapping on the course of facial nerve produces facial contraction or twitching. It is present in hypoparathyroidism and in condition associated with hypocalcaemia. A clinical sign of tetany. All the facial muscles supplied by facial nerve will contract on tapping of nerve anterior to ear.

Chyle Milk coloured lymph with a high fat content.

Chylomicron Protein-coated spherical structure that contains triglycerides, phospholipids, and cholesterol and is absorbed into the lacteal of a villus in the small intestine. The first liprproteins formed after absorption of lipids from food.

Chylous ascites The ascitic fluid is milky white and on microscopy shows chylomicrons—small particles of triglycerides which clear on adding ether or other fat solvents. It can occur hereditary lymphangiectasia or filariasis and destruction of the cisterna chyli. Turbidity is due to presence of many endothelial and inflammatory cells secondary to chronic irritation.

Chyme The mass of partially digested food that passes from the pylorus of the stomach into the duodenum of the small intestine.

Chymopapain An enzyme used for chemonucleolysis.

Chymotrypsin A pancreatic protease that hydrolyzes peptides into dipeptides.

Cicatricial entropion It occurs due to trachoma in its fourth stage. There are various grades of cicatrisation of tarsal plate from thickening of lid margin. During the whole process of cicatrisation there are symptoms of irritation, congestion, mild discharge, vascularisation and watering of eye. On eversion of upper lid, signs of different grades of trachoma are seen in form of follicles.

Cicatrix Scar is characterised by excessive collagenation of granulation tissue.

Cigarette smoker's lip It is a localised, usually well-defined flat or slightly elevated lesion of lip. Lesion begins as a reddened area but becomes more white with time. Person may have burns over fingers also. It is a diagnostic clue. It generally does not transform into malignancy.

Cilia Hair-like projections found on epithelial cell surfaces, capable of whip-like beating motions, propelling the extracellular fluid past the cell surface.

Cilial Microscopic hairlike process that move in a wavelike manner on the exposed surfaces of certain epithelial cells.

Ciliary body It forms a ring which is about 59 mm on the nasal side and 6.7 mm on temporal side . The ciliary body starts from the ora serrata. It is easily recognised by its black colour in comparison to choroid which is brown in colour. The part of ciliary body just beyond ora serrata is smooth and therfore is known as pars plana. Region of ciliary processes is known as pars plica. The ciliary body consists of six layers.

Ciliary ganglion It is a minute body of 2 m.m. diameter lying on the lateral side of optic nerve between the nerve and lateral rectus.

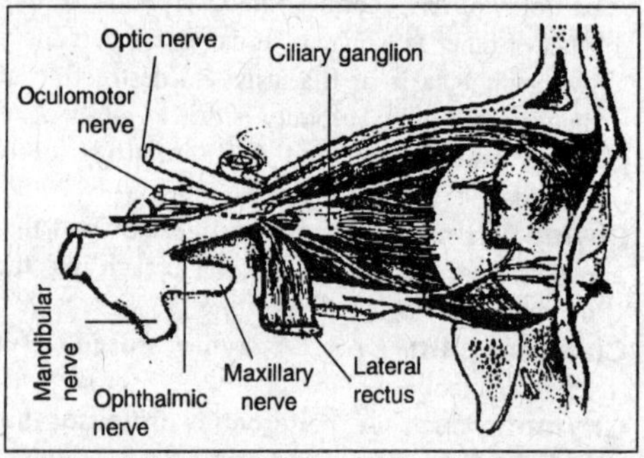

Ciliary injection Blue red, lie in the deep tissue, the individual blood vessel not recognisable, more marked towards the limbus and fading out away to limbus seen in keratitis, scleritis, iritis, iridocyclitis and acute glaucomatous attack.

Ciliated epithelium It lines whole of air passages except the uppermost nostrils, tympanic cavity and auditory tubes, testis and uterine tubes. Ventricles of brain and central canal of spinal cord is also lined by it. It helps in moving out an irritant particles from the respiratory passage and help in their expulsion. It sets up a current in stagnant cerebrospinal fluid for its circulation.

Cilium A hair or hairlike process projecting from a cell that may be used to move the entire cell or to move substances along the surface of the cell. Plural is cilia.

Cilium placenta cilia One of the hair-like projections of a structure such as the fallopian tube. The cilia of the fallopian tube beat in such a manner as to direct any overlying fluid in the direction of the uterine cavity. Thus, the cilia are partially responsible for the transportation of an ovum along the tube.

Cingulotomy Section/excision of anterior cingulate cortex, usually for relief of pain.

Cingulum Portion of incisor teeth and canines, occurring on the lingual or palatal aspects, that forms a convex protuberance at the cervical third of the anatomic crown. Represents the lingual or palatal developmental lobe of these teeth.

Ciprofloxacin Half-life is three hours. It is effective against a range of bacterial but particularly the gram-negative organisms. Chlamydia and mycoplasma are sensitive but most anaerobes are not. It is indicated against urinary tract, respiratory and GIT infection. Dose is 250 to 500 mg twice a day. It impairs the metabolism of theophylline.

Circadian Rhythm with a period of about 24 hours.

Circadian clock An internal timing device that regulates the expression of circadian rhythms. In mammals, a master circadian clock is located in the hypothalamic suprachiasmatic nucleus.

Circadian oscillator A theortical pacemaker with an output that repeat once per day.

Circadian rhythms Physiological changes that repeat at about 24 hours intervals. These are often synchronized with changes in the external environment, such as the day-night cycles.

Circuit training An exercise program in which an individual performs a series of activities one after another.

Circular folds Permanent, deep, transverse folds in the mucosa and submucosa of the small intestine that increase the surface area for absorption.

Circular friction In this, the fingers are closed together or slightly apart. Pressure is applied with fingertips and maintained as the fingers describe a series of small circles. The tissues are rolled over the underlying structures.

Circulation time Time required for blood to pass from the right atrium, through pulmonary circulation, back to the left ventricle, through systemic circulation to the foot, and back again to the right atrium; normally about 1 min.

Circulatory overload Severely compromised heart function.

Circulatory overloading During rapid transfusion a low arterial and raised venous pressure are evidence of cardiac overloading. The rate of drip should be 1 to 3 ml/kg per hour. Signs of overloading are tightness in chest, cough, dyspnoea, cyanosis, tachycardia and basal crepitations. Pulmonary oedema may develop.

Circulatory system This system includes heart and blood vessels. The systemic circulation begins at the left side of the heart. Left atrium receives oxygenated blood from pulmonary circulation. This blood is ejected to left ventricle. Left ventricle

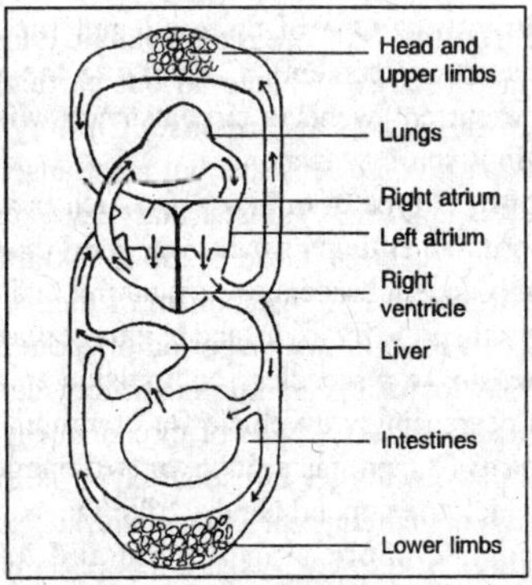

acts as a pumping station and sends blood to aorta. Other branches of aorta carry this blood to different parts of body. From these arteries to arterioles and then to capillaries. Capillaries have very thin walls to pass nutrients from blood to tissues in one direction and carbon dioxide and other wastes in other direction. Capillaries deliver deoxygenated blood to venules which join to form veins. These carrry the blood to veins which return the blood to right atrium. From right atrium the blood will enter the pulmonary circulation. In lungs CO_2 is removed and oxygen enters in. The reoxygenated blood enters the left atrium through left ventricles.

Circumcision Excision of the long preputial skin to expose the glans penis and the corona glandis under general or local anaesthesia. When phimosis is asssociated with narrow external urethral meatus particularly in congenital variety meatotomy is performed. When it is associated with considerable inflammation circumcision at a later date.

Circumduction A circular motion of the swinging leg that includes the hip motions of abduction, external rotation, adduction, and internal rotation. This gait deviation may be used to compensate for inadequate hip or knee flexion and/or insufficient dorsiflexion.

Circumduction gait In this one lower limb is swinging forward in a hemicircular fashion with knee extended.

Circumduction of the trunk Combination of forward flexion, right lateral flexion, extension, and left lateral flexion in succession, which produces a circular movement of the trunk.

Circumflex artery A branch of the left coronary artery that passes to the diaphragmatic surface of the left ventricle.

Circumflex vein The veins that travel circumferentially around the corpora cavernosa, joining the emissary veins to the deep dorsal vein of the penis.

Circumvallate papillae Large V-shaped projections on the dorsal surface of the tongue.

Circumvallate placenta Membranes are folded back on the fetal surface of the placenta, exposing a ring of the fetal surface around the umbilical cord. There is an increased risk of retained placenta leading to postpartum hemorrhage.

Ciribart embolism Blocking of a coronary blood vessel by a clot.

Cirrhosis In it there is chronic damage to liver cells. It results in impaired function of liver. Heavy consumption of alcohol is the main cause of cirrhosis. Women are more susceptible to alcoholic cirrhosis. A special pattern of liver inflammation is present before cirrhosis. To start cirrhosis may be symptomless. Most common symptoms are mild jaundice, oedema, mental confusion and haematemesis. Men may loose body hair. Ascites develops due to low protein level in blood. High pressure in veins results in oesophageal varices. Coma and confusion result from accumulation of toxic material. Hepatoma, a primary cancer of liver may result as a complication. Diagnosis of cirrhosis is confirmed by biopsy.

Cirrhotic peritonitis A low-grade infection of the peritoneal cavity is not uncomon complication of cirrhosis, particularly if there is ascites. Local signs may be restricted to minimal tenderness but patient's condition rapidly deteriorates with increasing ascites, hepatic encephalopathy and rather rarely a fever. Blood culture of fluid is positive in 50 to 60% cases, the most common being *E. coli.* Even local instillation of antibiotics is not very helpful and prognosis is poor.

Cirrus The penis or ejaculatory duct of a flatworm.

Cis-fatty acids Cis indicates the configuration of the duble bond in a natural oil.

Cisplatinum intoxication It is an alkylating agent which is extensively used in treatment of small cell carcinoma of lung, bladder and cervical carcinoma. Two to three times of maximum therapeutic dose of 100 mg/sq metre over 3 to 4 days may produce toxicity but taken as single dose may prove fatal. Myelosuppression resulting in pancytopenia is a common toxic feature. Nephrotoxicity may occur around sixth day. Neurotoxicity is characterised by loss of hearing. There develops altered speech, impairment of taste, numbness of hands and feet. There will be decreased or absent distal reflexes.

Cisterna chyli An enlarged pouch on the thoracic duct that serves as a storage area for lymph moving toward its point of entry into the venous system.

Cisterna magna Cerebellomedullary cistern.

Cisternal puncture This is an alternate procedure for removal of CSF from spinal canal. Spinal canal is entered through a point between occiput and first cervical vertebra. Needle is short one not to pierce medulla oblongata of brain. It is used to introduce radiopaque dye and to drain out or flush out infected material. Procedure is similar to lumbar puncture.

Cistric acid cycle The second series of chemical reactions in the process of glucose metabolism; it is an aerobic process.

Cistron The basic unit of genetic function. The term usually refers to a gene or coding region for a protein. A unit of DNA or RNA corresponding to one gene.

Citric acid cycle Series of chemical reactions in which citric acid (six-carbon molecule) is converted into a four-carbon molecule, carbon dioxide is formed, and energy is released; the released energy is used to form ATP; the four-carbon to form citric acid and start the cycle again.

Civil law Statutory law as opposed to common law or judge-made law. Statutes that protect the personal freedoms and rights of individuals.

Claim A demand for compensation, benefits or relief.

Claim form Statement listing services rendered, the date of the services, and itemization of fees. The completed and signed form serves the carrier as the basis for payment of benefits.

Clavicle The collar bone.

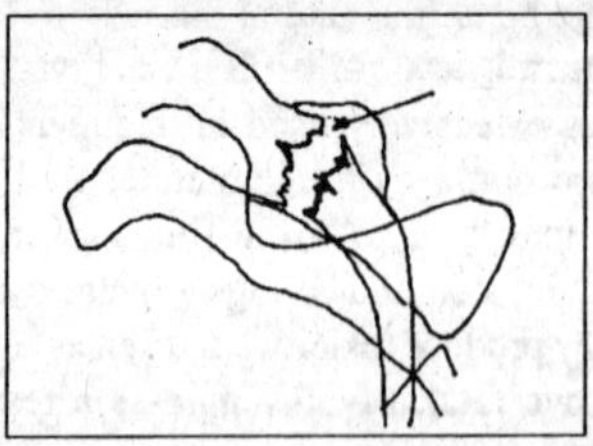

Clairvoyance One of three alleged capacities of extrasensory perception, involving the ability to know current events or circumstances without any obvious sensory awareness.

Clanging A type of thinking in which the sound of a word, rather than its meaning, gives the direction to subsequent associations; punning and rhyming may substitute for logic, and language may become increasingly a senseless compulsion to associate and decreasingly a vehicle for communication.

Clapping Clapping is a single or two-handed stroke in which the cupped hands strike the skin surface rapidly, compressing the air and causing a vibration wave to penetrate the tissues.

Clara's cells Nonciliated epithelial cells that are most prevalent in the terminal airways; Clara's cells are believed to play a secondary role in the production of surfactant.

Clarification of feelings An approach in personal-centred counselling in which the counsellor attempts to express the other person's feelings in a clearer form. The counsellor, by his or her manner or choice of words, attempts to reveal more precisely what has been said or what the interviewee is feeling.

Clasp Part of a removable partial denture that acts as a direct retainer and/or stabilizer for the denture by partially encircling or contracting an abutment tooth.

Claspknife rigidity Initial resistance to passive movement followed by collapse of resistance; a sign of upper motor neuron disease.

Class A group of items or substances which have common properties.

Class switching The process by which a B cell changes the class but not specifity of a given antibody it produces, e.g., switching from an IgM to an IgG antibody.

Classical conditioning A form of learning, as in the experiments of Pavlov, in which a previously neutral stimulus becomes a conditioned stimulus—capable of eliciting a given response— after being repeatedly presented with an unconditioned stimulus. The process is sometimes called stimulus substitution because a new stimulus evokes the response in question, such as salivation.

Classification The orderly arrangement of individuals into units on the basis of similarity;

each unit should be homogenous and different from all others.

Classification of fingerprints The systematic arrangement of fingerprints in pattern groups according to established criteria. Classification is made possible by the search of one fingerprint against a collection of many, and the rapid elimination of most of them, based solely on pattern information. No information about the fingerprint other than the classification detail was required to conduct a search.

Claudication Roman emperor Claudius suffered from this disease. There is cramp-like pain in limbs which increases on walking. It occurs due to blockage of arteries by atherosclerosis. Patient develops pain while working and often has to take rest in between in order to work again. This is known as intermittent claudication.

Claustrophobia It is an abnormal terror of being confined to or contained is an enclosed, windowless room. On occasion psychotherapy helps.

Claustrum The 'barrier' of gray matter between insula and lentiform nucleus.

Clavicle Collar bone, connects the upper extremity to the axial skeleton.

Claw hand In this deformity proximal phalanges are hyper-extended while the other phalanges are flexed. Paralysis of interossei and lumbricalis is commonly the cause of the condition. Muscles are supplied by ulnar and median nerves so the injury of these nerves will also result in it.

Claw toe The proximal and distal interphalangeal joints are hyper-flexed and metatarsophalangeal joint is dorsally subluxated.

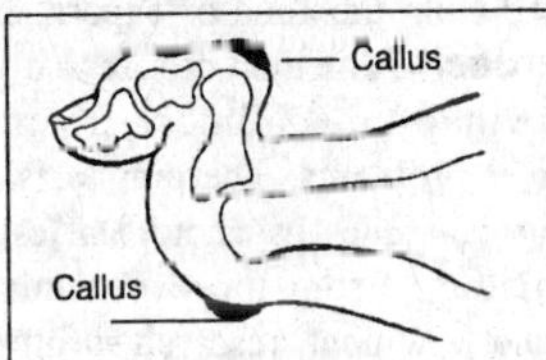

Claw toe

Clay shoveler's fracture Avulsion fracture of spinal process of C_7

Clean Freedom from or removal of all matter in which microorganisms may find favourable conditions for continued life and growth.

Clean-catch specimen Voided sample of urine that is considered sterile.

Cleaning of gloves These should be washed with soap and water, then with cold water. It should be checked for any hole or tear. For oridinary ward use these should be wrapped in cloth and boiled for 3 minutes. For surgical use, they should be dried in shade, and powdered and packed in glove wrapper. Then these should be autoclaved. Gloves should never be cleaned with any antiseptic or disinfecting fluid.

Cleaning of sinks Sinks should be cleaned daily or at definite intervals to avoid contamination and blockage in drainage channels. Detergent powders can be sprinkled and rubbed vigorously with damp cloth and then rinse with plain water and dried with dry cloth.

Cleaning window doors All doors and windows should be washed with soap water properly. Then it should be rinsed with plain water and dry swabbing is to be done. Glasspan should be cleaned by soap and rinsed with plain water. Soda and other detergent powder should not be used for wooden surface as it may spoil the polish of wood.

Cleaning, general rules Dry cleaning is never advisable. It spreads disease easily. Dusting should be done after sweeping only. Use a damp duster for collecting dust. Every time dust with clean duster only. Collect dust at one place to avoid flying from place to place. Dusting is to be done preferably without disturbing or removing the patient from bed. It should be done from top to bottom, i.e. from upward to downward direction.

Cleansing enema This is carried out to ensure that lower colon and rectum are free from faecal matter. This is given prior to rectal operation or before giving a retention enema. Enema solution used may be normal saline; 600 to 1000 cc. It is necessary to measure the washout fluid before it is given and also measure the returned fluid to make sure that no fluid has been left in bowel.

Clearance Condition in which bodies may pass each other without hindrance; also, the distance between bodies.

Clearance angle The angle formed between the clearance face and the circumference of the bur.

Clearance dynamics The temporal pattern of disappearance of substance from circulation, a body part or the body.

Clearance face The surface of the blade that follows behind the cutting edge as the bur rotates.

Cleavage The process of rapid miotic cell division during the development of a fertilized ovum, in which male and female chromosomes mingle and split forming two sets of 46 chromosomes.

Cleavage furrow Appears at the end of anaphase and begins to divide the cell into two daughter cells.

Cleft Vertical soft tissue defect in which the gingival margin dips sharply and abruptly in an apical direction, then moves back up again.

Cleft lip Congenital incomplete closure of the lip.

Cleft palate Congenital fissure of the palate and roof of the mouth.

Cleistothecium The closed, fruiting body of an Ascomycete fungus which contains sexually produced ascospores.

Clelands ligament A fibrous tissue band on the lateral side of fingers that help stabilise the skin during movement.

Clenching It is the non functional forceful intermittent application of mandibular teeth against the maxillary teeth.

Clergyman's hand Tendon ruputure in rheumatoid arthritis especially of the lateral extensor tendons of hand, gives rise to a clergyman's hand.

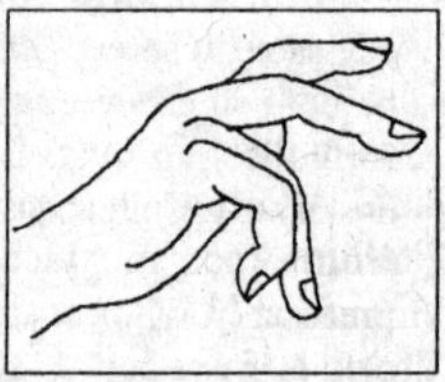

Clerical aptitude The abilities required of office workers; usually perceptual speed, language and numerical facility, and also finger and manual dexterity. For example, using and maintaining a file efficiently requires all of these capacities.

Clever Hans phenomenon The unconscious tendency of an individual to signal his or her thoughts to another individual. For example, the head, eyes, or upper body are moved upward or downward, indicating agreement or disagreement. The term takes its origin from the famous horse in Berlin, Clever Hans, which seemingly could follow all sorts of difficult commands verbal. His success was based on his ability to note small movements of his master's head, which indicated when to begin and stop tapping.

Client outcome The results desired from the massage and the massage therapist.

Client-centered therapy Rogerian concept of humanistic psychology that places the client at the center of all decision making.

Climacteric Menopause is defined the time at which menstruation ceases whereas climactaric is the phase of waning ovarian activity. It may start two or three years before the menopause and can continue for 2 to 5 years after it. So it is a phase of adjustment between active and inactive ovarian function. Initially ovulation fails, no corpus luteum is formed and no progesterone is secreted by ovary. Thus menstrual cycles are anovulatory and may be irregular. Later oestrogenic activity also diminishes and atrophic endometrium leads to menopause.

Climate control Mechanisms for maintaining temperature, humidity, and ventilation.

Climatic bubo It is an acute and chronic contagious disorder produced by serotypes L_1 and L_2. Its incubation period is 3 to 12 days for genital lesions and 10 to 30 days for inguinal bubo. Lymph glands are enlarged, usually matted and show local areas of softening with abscess cavities and formation of granulation tissue. The bubos may shrink and form fibrous mass or burst discharging a purulent fluid and leave chronic ulcer with sinuses. Blocking of lymphatics may occur resulting in elephantiasis.

Clinic An establishment where patients are admitted for study and treatment by a group of practitioners.

Clinical Pertaining to a clinic or to the actual observation and treatment of patients, as distinguished from theoretic or experimental.

Clinical approach A method of research which is an outgrowth of the clinical treatment of psychological problems. The emphasis is upon interviewing techniques, psychological testing, and the case history. From these procedures for diagnosis and treatment, research information is gained.

Clinical chart Legal record of all existing dental conditions and treatment performed for a specific patient.

Clinical crown That portion of enamel visibly present in the cavity; the portion of a tooth that is occlusal to the deepest part of the gingival crevice.

Clinical death Absence of peripheral pulse, heart beat and effective circulation with dilated pupils non responsive to light and absence of breathing.

Clinical diagnosis Determination of disease by examining the patient.

Clinical evaluation Collection of data by a physician for the purpose of determining the health status of an individual. The data include information obtained by history; clinical findings obtained from a physical examination; laboratory tests including radiographs, electrocardiograms, blood tests, and other special tests and diagnostic procedures; and measurements of anthropometric attributes and physiologic and psychophysiologic functions.

Clinical examination Visual and tactile scrutiny of the tissues of and surrounding the oral cavity.

Clinical family health model Examined from this perspective, a family is healthy if its members are free of physical, mental, and social dysfunction.

Clinical hypothyroidism A disorder characterised by decreased production of T4, T3, by the thyroid gland.

Clinical pathways Standardized multidisciplinary plans for a specific diagnosis or procedure that identify specific aspects of care to be performed during a designated length of stay.

Clinical psychologist A person with a Ph.D. in psychology, specially trained to assess and treat mental disorders and behavior problems.

Clinical psychology Concerned with diagnosis and treatment of mental and behavioural disorders. Many clinical psychologists work in collaboration with psychiatrists.

Clinical responsibility A defendent's state of mind at the time of the alleged crime. A person cannot be convicted of a crime if it can be proved that he lacked the ability to formulate a criminal intent at the time of the alleged crime because of "criminal insanity".

Clinical resume Summary of previous care.

Clinical scenario One or two or more alternative paths of management available in a decision analysis.

Clinical thermometer It is used for knowing the body temperature. Temperature is usually taken in mouth but can be taken in rectum, axilla, groin and popliteal space. The temperature is recorded in a temperature chart at 4-hourly interval or twice a day in ward. Before and after taking the temperature the thermometer is shaken to bring mercury to 36.6° C. It should be shaken down with quick twist of wrist. Thermometer should be washed in cold tap water and not in hot water. Then put it in 1% Savlon.

Clinical trials These are done to determine whether a treatment is useful, how it is as compares with other treatments, how it affects different group of people in different doses, side effects felt etc.

Clinitest A test that measures the amount of glucose and acetone in a urine specimen.

Clinitron bed A special bed containing an airfluidization mattress that conforms to the shape of a person's body to reduce pressure exerted against skin and soft tissues.

Clinodale The most superior point on the contour of anterior clinoid.

Clip Any device that grips or holds something tightly.

Clipping injury fracture A fracture involving the distal femoral or proximal tibial epiphysis specially in foot ball players.

Clique Subgroup composed of a few members who are part of a large group. A few boys or girls may form exclusive friendships, shunning other members of their class, thus becoming a clique within the classroom of 30 students.

Clisis Attraction or inclination.

Clitellum The glandular girdle involved in cocoon formation in oligochaetes and leeches.

Clitoris It is an erectile organ of the female external genitalia that is homologous with the penis in males. It is partly concealed by the labia minora but a free extremity appears as a rounded tubercle.

Cloacate Having a cloaca; involving or trasported by the cloaca.

Clockwise rotation Used in describing rotation of the thorax or pelvis. With the transverse plane as a reference and 12 o'clock at midpoint anteriorly, rotation forward on the left is clockwise rotation.

Clonal animal A clone ; i.e., an animal in which the genetic entity is composed of multiple "bodies" that are physiologically separated

Clonal selection The selection and activation by antigen of a lymphocyte bearing a complementary receptor, which then proliferates to form an expanded clone.

Clone It means the true copy. Clones of cells are descended from one original cell. Clones of genes are duplicate of single gene. Clones of organisms can be produced by removing the nucleus from a cell of one individual and transplanting it into the egg cell of another individual.

Clones The descendants of a single cell.

Clonial deletion A process by which contact with antigen at an early stage of lymphocyte differentiation leads to cell death by apoptosis.

Cloning A reproductive technique that involves the insertion of nuclei from an embryo, embryo cell line, fetal cell line, or adult somatic cell line into the cytoplasm of a mature egg that has had its own chromatin removed. These embryos may develop to term in some animal species.

Cloning vector A DNA molecule suitable for transporting new genetic material into host bacteria.

Clonus A pyramidal lesion may also be accompanied by clonus. This is easily elicited at the ankle but may also be found at knee and wrist. At ankle a brisk passive dorsiflexion of foot results in reflex plantar flexion. As long as pressure in the direction of dorsiflexion is maintained by examiner's hand, rhythmic clonic plantar flexion occurs.

Cloquet's septum node Femoral septum; lymph node at the femoral ring.

Closed drainage system Device used to collect urine from a catheter.

Closed panel In a prepayment plan, a group of dentists sharing office facilities who provide stipulated services to an eligible group for a set premium. For beneficiaries of plans using closed panels, choice of dentists is limited to panel members. Dentists must accept any beneficiary as a patient.

Closed reduction Manipulation or setting without open surgical correction of a fracture.

Closed swinging It is an extramarital sex in which the husbands and the wives exchange partners and pair off going to separate sites to have intercourse in privacy. The couples usually agree to return to a particular place after sometime so that they might return home with their own spouses.

Closed system A system that exchanges neither matter nor energy with the surroundings.

Closed wound One in which there is no opening in the skin or mucous membrane.

Closed-head injury A head injury in which there is little or no damage to the skull.

Closed-loop system A movement control process that employs feed-back against a reference for correctness for computation of error and subsequent movement correction.

Closing volume The lung volume at which airway closure begins during expiration; and index of the status of the small airways.

Closing wedge osteotomy It is done mostly for a varus deformity. A wedge of bone based laterally

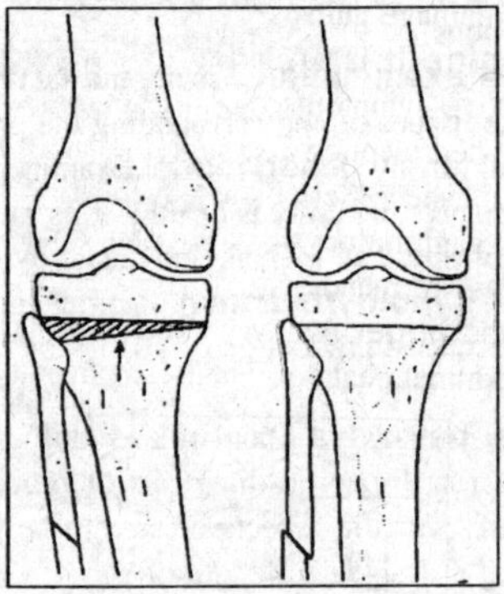

is removed. The fibula is also divided to allow it to shorten slightly.

Clostridium tetani These are gram-positive strict anaerobe, terminal spore giving drumstick appearance, motile, proteolytic and does not ferment common sugars. It produces very powerful exotoxin and produces tetanus. Organism is motile with numerous peritrichate flagella. Spores develop in about 2 to 10 days and are round. It grows on ordinary culture media.

Closure, principle of The principle that when we view fragmentary stimuli forming a nearly complete figure, we tend to ignore the missing parts and perceive the figure as whole.

Clot The semisolid mass of fibrin threads and trapped blood cells that forms when blood coagulates.

Clot retraction The consolidation of a fibrin clot to pull damaged tissue together.

Clotting It is a process of coagulation at a site of wound or otherwise. It is a part of healing. It all happens as a result of chemical reaction involving enzyme thromboplastin which convert soluble fibrinogen in the plasma to insoluble strands of fibrin.

Clotting factor One of many proteins found in the blood in an inactive state; activated in a series of chemical reactions that result in the formation of a blood clot.

Clove oil It is colourless and may be pale yellowish derived from dried flower buds of *Eugenia caryophyllus*. Applied on tooth cavity it is antinfective and acts as analgesic also. So housewives use it as a domestic remedy of toothache. But being strong if used very frequently may damage gums.

Clozapine It is effective in both positive and negative symptoms of schizophrenia resistant to other neuroleptics. Extrapyramidal effects are mild and transient. Serious disadvantage is that it may cause agranulocytosis. Precautionary leucocyte counts are mandatory.

Clubbed finger A finger with bulbous enlargement of terminal phalanx. There is convexity of curved nail.

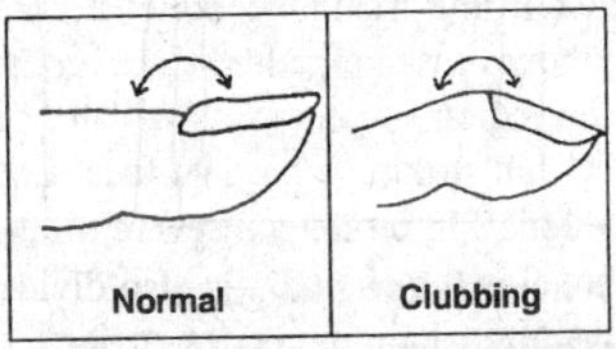

Cluster headache These consist of unilateral supraorbital headaches of deep aching quality which reaches maximal severity with rapidity. These headache frequently awaken the patient. Associated symptoms include lacrimation and conjunctival and facial reddening. Attacks last several hours. These headaches occur in cluster lasting several weeks. It may be caused by abnormal vascular reaction in carotid.

Cluster marriage It is an unconventional lifestyle in which several married couples live together and have sexual access to each other.

Cluster suicides Multiple suicides, usually among adolescents, in a circumscribed period of time and area. Though to have an element of contagion.

Clutch To grip or hold tightly or firmly. A device for gripping the teeth in a dental arch. Also, one to which face-bow or tracing devices may be attached rigidly.

Cluttering Symptoms include hurried muddled speech that has been poorly prepared before utterances and may be difficult to understand due to omission of sounds and words. Speech is often monotonous and non-musical.

Clutton's joints Clutton's joints are painless symmetrical effusion of the large joints with very little impairment of function, and are seen in cases of congenital syphilis.

CMV Cytomegalovirus.

Coactivation (a) Simultaneous activation of alpha and gamma motor neurons; (b) simultaneous activation of motor neurons supplying prime movers and antagonists.

Coagulation Formation of a solid from a liquid, especially in blood where it is known as clotting.

Coagulation factor A group of substances present in blood plasma that result in conversion of blood from a liquid.

Coagulopathy A pathological condition affecting the ability of the blood to coagulate.

Coagulum A clot or curd.

Coal worker's pneumoconiosis A disease that is caused by chronic inhalation of coal dust, is characterized by pulmonary inflammation or fibrosis, and is also known as black lung disease.

Coalescent opacities The blending or fusing together of opaque regions in a radiographic image.

Coalition A group formed for a particular purpose.

Coaptation Proper adaptation or union of parts to each other, such as the ends of a fractured bone or the edges of a wound without overlap.

Coaraction of aorta There is a congenital localised narrowing of aorta. It generally develops after the origin of subclavian artery, so blood supply to lower part of body is reduced. To overcome this deficiency heart works harder and results in hypertension in

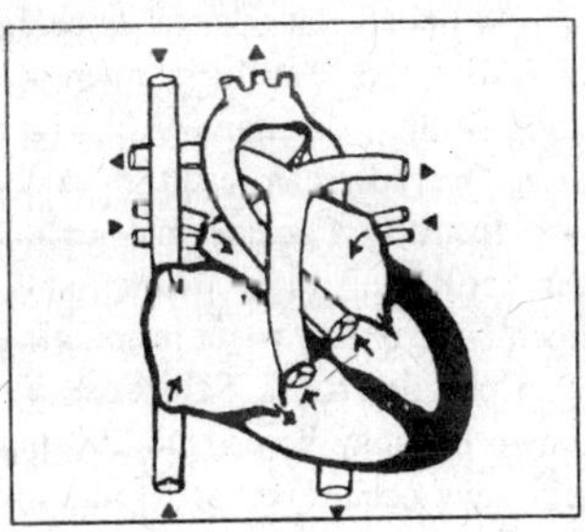

upper part of body. Symptoms develop in early childhood and includes headache, weakness, cold legs and heart failure. There will be weak pulse in groin. Surgery is the only way of treatment.

Coat A membrane or other structure covering or lining a part or organ.

Coating A substance applied to all or a portion of the body of a dental implant with the goal of improving rate and quality of healing.

Cobalamin It is necessary for demethylation of tetrahydrofolate and thus for DNA synthesis. It is formed from cyanocobalamine. Deficiency leads to megaloblastic anaemia, degeneration of brain, spinal cord and peripheral nerves. It results in sore tongue and malabsorption. Daily requirement of cobalamin is 3.0 mg/day. Absorption takes place in terminal ileum. The neurological complications specially spasticity develop only after prolonged severe deficiency but may be permanent.

Cobb elevator It is used for periosteal stripping with flat spoon shaped elevating surface attached to a handle.

Cobb's method A technique for measuring the angle of scoliotic curve on AP X-Ray spine.

Cobra bite Swelling does not usually appear until two or three hours after bite. Necrosis develops more rapidly as a wet gangrene within a few days due to cytotoxic effect. Local symptoms start within 6 to 8 minutes and include a reddish, tender spot at the site of bite along with a mild burning pain. Neurotoxic and cardiovascular features develop within 30 to 60 minutes.

Cardiovascular depression is seen as sweating, cold extremities, hypotension and ECG changes may be more prominent.

Cocaine It was once used as a local anaesthetic for minor surgeries and sprayed in pharynx area before doing endoscopy. Onset of anaesthesia is fast and lasts for 4 hours. But cocaine is being abused by drug addicts for euphoria purposes. Regular inhaling of drug can damage the lining of nasal mucosa. Overdose can result in cardiac arrest.

Cocaine toxicity Cocaine may be obtained as a water soluble crystalline salt, cocaine hydrochloride or as a water in soluble free cocaine base in powder form. Safe dose of cocaine is unknown but may be around 200 mg. Although toxicity may occur even at 20 mg. It can be fatal after ingestion of 1 to 3 gm of cocaine. Toxic symptoms include tachycardia, hypertension, hyperthermia, increased respiratory rate, seizures, respiratory arrest and cardiovascular collapse. CNS stimulation results in behavioural and psychiatric abnormalities such as hyperactivity, irritability, insomnia, mood liability agitation and psychosis. Arrhythmias are common as cocaine leads to sympathetic stimulation and myocardial ischaemia. It can produce myocardial infarction, renal infarction and limb ischaemia. Vasodilatation may lead to shock. Pneumomediastinum and pneumothorax have been reported in patients who smoke or snuff cocaine.

Coccal Resembling or pertaining to cocci.

Coccus A spherical or ovoid bacterium.

Coccygeal Pertaining to the region of the coccys; the caudal termination of the vertebral column.

Coccygeus muscle pain In 20% cases pain may be due to trauma. In 80% coccyx itself is normal and the pain in this region is as a result of spasm developing in levator ani and coccygeus muscles.

Coccyx It is a triangular bone. It consists of four tiny bones fused together. Coccygodynia is a pain in the region of coccyx. It usually begins after a direct fall striking a hard surface. Local heat may give relief. In prolonged severe disability surgical removal is the choice.

Coccyxalgia Pain in coccyx region.

Cochlea The spiral portion of the inner ear that contains the spiral organ i.e. organ of Corti.

Cochlear duct The membranous cochlea consisting of a spirally arranged tube enclosed in the body cochlea and lying along its outer wall. Also called the scala media.

Cochlear implant An electronic device that is implanted surgically into the inner ear so that it stimulates the basilar membrane to transduce sound waves into neural activity and allow deaf people to hear.

Cochlear nerve A branch of the auditory nerve that sends auditory information from the cochlea to the brain.

Cockayne syndrome It is an autosomal dominant disorder. Clinical features include photosensitivity, dwarfism, loss of fat, mental retardation and atrophic hyperpigmented skin with decreased sweating. Person will develop premature greying of hair. Eyes show cataract, exophthalmos, retinal pigmentation and optic atrophy. Gait is unsteady with limited joint mobility.

Cock-up toe Deformity with dorsiflexion of the metatarsophalangeal joint and flexion of the interphalangeal/distal interphalangeal joint.

Cock-up toe Deformity with hyperextension of the metatarsophalangeal joint and flexion of the proximal and distal interphalangeal joints.

Cocoa butter The fat removed from coca beans during their conversion into chocolate and cocoa. It is used in making candy and sustained relense tablets. It is whitish yellow and smells of cocoa.

Cocogeusia A bad taste even when there is nothing in the mouth.

Co-contraction Simultaneous contraction of prime movers and antagonists.

Cocphoria A generalized feeling of unhappiness.

Cocyxgectomy Surgical excision of coccyx.

Code A collection of the existing laws, rules, or regulations. A system of symbols, such as letters, words, or other marks, to represent something, e.g., a system of symbols for representing information in a computerized data bank or information system.

Code of ethics Statements describing ideal behavior.

Codeine Half-life is 3 hours. It is of low efficacy, 10 per cent is converted to morphine. Dependence occurs but much less than morphine. Its use is for mild or moderate pain and cough. It controls diarrhoea too resulting in constipation.

Codman exercise Shoulder mobilization exercise.

Codman's sign Clinical sign of rotator cuff injury. When deltoid contracts suddenly without support, pain develops.

Codon The sequence of three bases in mRNA that specifies a given amino acid, and determines the position of that amino acid in a polypeptide chain through complementary base pairing.

Coefficient A weighing factor use in an equation, with the weight based on the relative importance of the factor in predicting the outcome.

Coeliac disease This is a gluten enteropathy characterised by deformity of the normal villous pattern of mainly jejunum resulting in impaired absorption. The real sensitivity occurs with gluten present in wheat. It produces shortened and blunted villi, hyperplasia and crypts. Onset is gradual. Diarrhoea is most important symptom. Flatulence is marked resulting in doughy feel. Pallor and anaemia gradually develops. Clubbing of fingers takes place. There will be low-grade pyrexia.

Coeloblastual A simple blastula-like larva.

Coelom The abdominal cavity.

Coelome The general cavity of coelomate animals, vertebrates and invertebrates.

Coenurus A larval tapeworm of certain cyclophyllideans in which numerous scolices bud from an internal germinal epithelium.

Coenzyme A nonprotein organic molecule that activates an enzyme; many are derived from vitamins. An example is nicotinamide adenine dinucleotide (NAD), derived from the B vitamin niacin. It is an organic substance superficially associated with enzyme. Enzyme is a conjugated protein in which co-enzyme forms prosthetic group. Several co-enzymes of enzymes are concerned with oxidation and reduction containing phosphoric acid.

Cofactor A substance needed for the catalytic action of an enzyme; generally used in reference to inorganic ions such as Ca++ and Mg++.

Cognition Mental processes involved in the acquisition and use of knowledge, such as attention, thinking, problem solving, and perception; cognitive learning emphasizes these processes in the acquisition of new behaviors.

Cognitive appraisal An assessment of the meaningfulness of an event to an individual; events that are appraised as harmful or potentially harmful elicit stress.

Cognitive approach to therapy An approach to therapy which emphasises human thought processes. A most important premise is that irrational thinking underlies emotional or inappropriate behaviour. The aim is to alter the person's thinking and thereby to alleviate maladjustment.

Cognitive awareness The knowledge that one has a deficit.

Cognitive behavior therapy Therapy that integrates principles of learning theory with cognitive strategies to treat disorders such as depression, anxiety, and other behavioral problems such as smoking or obesity.

Cognitive development Beginning in infancy, the acquisition of intelligence, conscious thought, and problem-solving abilities. An orderly sequence in the increase in knowledge derived from sensorimotor activity, has been empirically demonstrated by Piaget.

Cognitive disorders Habitual errors in logic.

Cognitive dissonance theory A theory of attitude formation and change which indicates that persons try to achieve consistency and avoid dissonance: when dissonance arises, it may be handled by changing one's attitude, rationalising, selective perception, and other means.

Cognitive domain In the learning process, emphasis upon the development of knowledge and understanding. These learning objectives concern primarily mental activities.

Cognitive dysfunction The impairement or biasing of information processes such as perceptual, attentional and memorial function caused by temporary physiological and mood states.

Cognitive egocentrism Part of Piaget's second stage of intellectual development, the preoperational stage. The child does not understand that other people do not have his or her thoughts. The child apparently thinks that everyone has the same thoughts of knowing everyone else's thoughts.

Cognitive map A mental representation of an external area that is used to guide one's behavior.

Cognitive neuroscience The study of the neural basis of congnition.

Cognitive processes A general term emphasising knowledge, understanding, and awareness on the part of the organism—it includes the processes of perceiving, remembering, and reasoning. In this approach to learning, the contribution of the organism is emphasised.

Cognitive psychology An area of psychology which focuses upon mental activities, especially perceiving, thinking, remembering, reasoning, and other forms of problem solving.

Cognitive reappraisal A form of coping that focuses on changing one's attitude toward a stressful situation.

Cognitive specificity Thoughts and images that are specific to diagnostic categories.

Cognitive style Subtle differences in left vs right cerebral function.

Cognitive therapy A treatment method particularly for depressive disorders, that emphasises the rearrangement of a person's maladaptive processes of thinking, perceptions, and attitudes.

Cognitive-physiological theory The view that physiological arousal and an interpretation of the stimulating circumstances are the chief elements in determining the effective component of emotional experience.

Cogwheel rigidity A rachet like response to passive movement characterized by an alternate giving and increased resistance to movement.

Cohesion Cohesion in a liquid is the attractive force exerted by each molecule on those surrounding it, which results in a resistance to any object passing through the liquid.

Cohort An important form of epidemiologic investigation to test hypotheses regarding the causation of disease. The distinguishing factors are : (*i*) the group or groups of persons to be studied (the cohorts) are defined in terms of characteristics evident prior to appearance of the disorder being investigated; (*ii*) the study groups so defined are observed over a period of time to determine the frequency of the disorder among them.

Cohort design An epidemiological research design that works forward from cause of effect; contrast with *casecontrol design*, which works from effect to cause.

Cohort study An observational study in which subjects are sampled based on the presence or absence of a risk factor of interest. These subjects are followed over time for the development of a disease outcome of interest.

Coining The process of applying controlled pressure, stress, and heat in shaping a metal in a mold or die. In implant dentistry, the coining process permits formation of desired implant configurations and alteration of physical properties to enhance function.

Coitus Sexual union between a female and male involving insertion of the penis into the vagina.

Coitus interruptus It involves the withdrawal of man's erect penis from the woman's vagina before ejaculation. It may be frustrating and inefficient method of contraception and woman also does not enjoy sex. Risks of getting pregnant are very high (25%).

Coitus reservatus It is the deliberate suppression of orgasm in the male, achieved through practice in approaching ejaculation without reaching an orgasm. Some people apply an opium paste over penis to reduce its sensitivity.

Colchicine Half-life is one hour. It rapidly relieves pain and inflammation most effectively if it is used within 24 hours of onset of attack. Rapid effect confirms the diagnosis of gout. It is absorbed from gut and some is metabolised in liver and excreted unchanged in bile and reabsorbed from gut. In acute gout 1 mg may be given by mouth followed by 0.5 to 1 mg 2 hourly. Benefit is felt within 2 to 3 hours and is marked within 12 hours. Adverse effects may be severe with abdominal pain, vomiting and diarrhoea.

Cold abscess It is a slow forming abscess associated with tuberculosis. It can develop anywhere in the body. Mostly warmth and other signs of inflammation are not there. There is only local tenderness on pressure.

Cold abscess in neck On occasions there is soft swelling. Cold abscess is noted due to accumulation of pus of TB in posterior triangle. There is no sign of inflammation and so the abscess is not hot and red as in pyogenic abscess. Being of low tension it is less painful. It may be due to caseation of tuberculous lymphadenitis in the cervical region commonly found in upper half of anterior angle of neck. Secondary to tuberculosis spine it is commonly found in posterior triangle of neck.

Cold bath Temp. 10°C-21°C. Decreases development of orthostatic hypotension.

Cold forging In implant dentistry, repetitive impact loading in the absence of applied heat.

Cold injury It is a localised tissue damage due to cold, e.g. frost-bite. The frost-bitten area becomes white and hard. It is caused by direct exposure to air or restriction of blood supply to area. People who sit at the bank of river dipping their foot for hours regularly may also develop it. Blood restriction to the area may cause gangrene and then surgical amputation remains the choice of treatment.

Cold intolerance It is a clinical condition usually described as marked sensitivity exposure to cold may be due to neurologic or vascular etiology.

Cold narcosis A state or stupor, unconciousness or arrested activity produced by cooling.

Cold pack It is to reduce to calm an irritable and restless patient. It reduces blood circulation and reduces pulse. It helps in bringing down the body temperature. Take two bedsheets for cold pack, fold one sheet crosswise and another as lengthwise. Put bedsheets in cold water tub. Roll patient and place bedsheet folded crosswise under patient. Cover patient with bath blanket wiring out second sheet and place it over the front of the patient. Place cold compress over head.

Cold shock response A rapid change in gene expression that occurs when there is a temperature shift to a low temperature.

Cold sponging Cold or tepid sponging is a general application of moist cold liquid usually water to cool the skin and reduce body temperature. Temperature of water for tepid sponging is 78°F to 80°F. It is used to reduce body temperature. It stimulates blood circulation and respiratory movement. It is used to stimulate excretion through kidney and skin. It quietens nervous and delirious patient.

Cold spot Area with little or no radionuclide concentration.

Cold sterilization Means of killing some microorganisms by immersion in a cold chemical solution.

Cold therapy Local application of cold decreases metabolism, circulation, pain, muscle spasm and inflammation but increases stiffness. Following

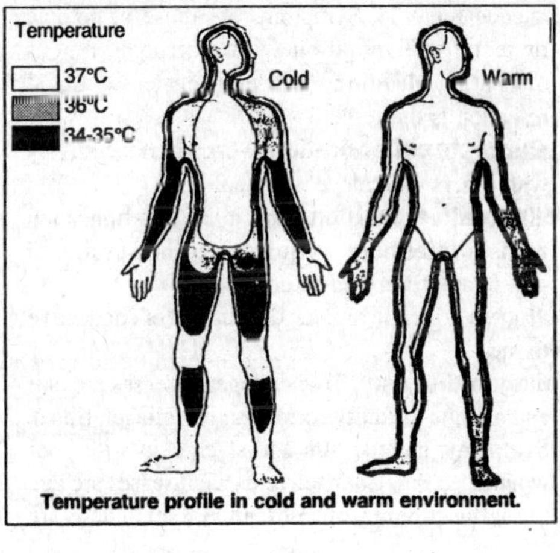

Temperature profile in cold and warm environment.

injury ice is initially applied to reduce the metabolic demands of tissues during the period of hypoxia, to decrease bleeding and minimise oedema. Although ice application is initially painful, within a few minutes pain decreases and part becomes relatively anaesthetised. Compression and rest should be maintained.

Colic It is a severe spasmodic pain. It occurs in waves of increasing capacity. It reaches a peak, abates for sometime and again increases in intensity. Actually when affected part contracts, pain increases. A stone in bile duct or in ureter will cause colic pain while intestinal colic is caused due to obstruction.

Colicin A bacteriocin produced by Escherichia coli or closely related enteric species.

Coliform A membrane of a group of bacteria that has traditionally been used as an indicator of the presence of pathogenic microorganisms in water.

Colitis It is the inflammation of colon causing diarrhoea with blood and mucus. There may be abdominal pain with fever. It may be caused by infection due to bacteria, virus or amoeba. Most infections causing colitis resolve itself without treatment. Amoebic infection can be treated with metronidazole.

Colitis cystica Mucous cysts of no consequences may be seen in the mucosa. In the submucosa and muscularis, the cysts may be surrounded by inflammatory reaction leading to considerable tissue swelling. Cause is not known. The important differential diagnosis is a mucus secreting adenocarcinoma. Symptoms are those of colonic or rectal inflammation with diarrhoea, mucus discharge, bleeding, pain and tenesmus. Local resection is the remedy.

Collaborate collaboration Working cooperatively with others to achieve a mutual goal.

Collaborative problem Physiologic complication whose treatment requires both nurse-and physician-prescribed interventions.

Collagen Principle organic constituent of connective tissue.

Collagen diseases True collagen diseases are rare and are due to faulty formation of collagen fibres. Symptoms include thin and slack skin with poor wound healing. Connective tissue diseases are due to malfunctioning of immune system. These are common and include rheumatoid disease, SLE periarteritis nodosa, scleroderma and dermatomyositis.

Collagen vascular disease Diverse group of systemic diseases characterized by diffuse abnormalities of the vasculature and inflammatory lesions involving the joints, muscles, and connective tissue.

Collagenase An enzyme that hydrolyses peptides containing proline including collagen and gelatin.

Collar cuff Cervical spondylitis is the common cause of neck pain and surgery is not that easy. To restrict the neck movements certain varieties of collar cuffs of foam and elastic material are available to be used.

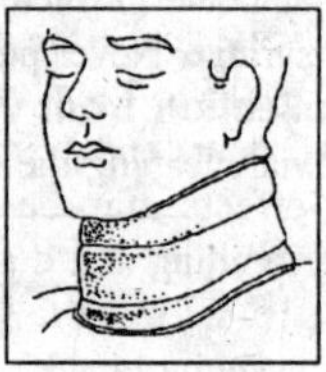

Collar stud abscess In third stage of lymphadenitis, abscess remains deep to the deep cervical fascia. Ultimately the fascia is eroded at one point and the pus tracks into superficial space and now it is known as collar stud abscess. The superficial abscess gradually enlarges and becomes obvious on inspection. In untreated cases the overlying skin becomes ischaemic and reddish blue at the centre of an abscess. Ultimately skin at centre necroses and gives away leading to a chronic discharging sinus papillomatous and darker.

Collar, Nylon The disposable sheath supplied with an intra mucosal insert that protects against cement medium expressing into the retentive area under the head when the insert is affixed into its acrylic receptor site.

Collateral ligament stability The basic strategy is to apply to valgus stress to test the medial collateral ligament and a varus stress to test the lateral collateral ligament. In each case the degree of both angulation and pain produced is compared with the other side.

Collecting duct Straight tubule that extends from the cortex of the kidney to the tip of the renal pyramid; filtrate from the distal convoluted tubules enters the collecting duct and is carried to the calyces.

Collection from ampoule Ampoule has a narrow upper portion the stem, wide lower portion the body with neck which may be smoothly curved.

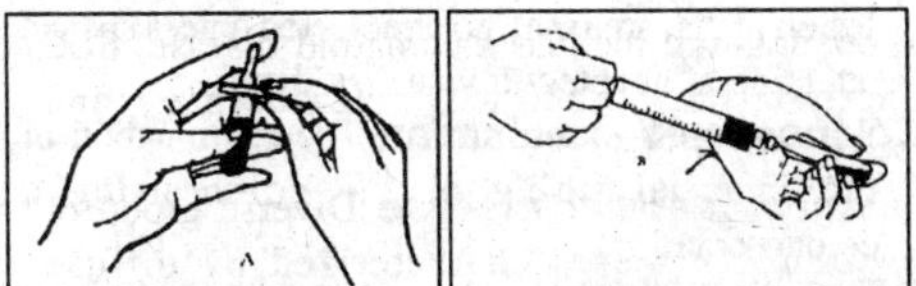

(A) Ampoule holding with file in position

(B) Ampoule held with syringe aspirating contents

After applying spirit break away the stem either by a gentle pressure or by cutting by file. Hold the ampoule in tilted fashion and collect the fluid in syringe. Never push air in ampoule.

Collection from vial Rotate and gently shake the vial cleaning the rubber cap with spirit inject air

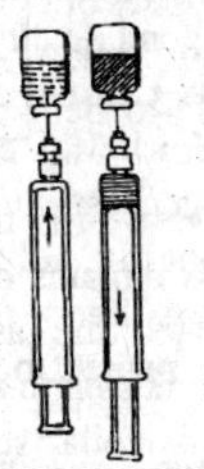

Collection from vial

equivalent to the amount of liquid to the aspirated. Then keeping the needle tip in liquid turn the vial up side down and collect the liquid in syringe.

Collective tubule A straight part of a renal tubule formed by distal tubules of several nephrons joining together.

Collective unconscious In Jungian theory, a portion of the unconsciousness common to all people; also called "racial unconscious."

Collectivistic society A culture where individuals share tasks, belonging and income. The people may live in large family groups and value interdependence, unlike individualistic societies.

Colles' fascia Superficial perineal fascia membranous, deep to the tela subcutanea.

Colliouli Four small elevations (superior and inferior) in the posterior portion of the midbrain concerned with visual and auditory reflexes.

Colliculus One of four small mounds on the dorsal side of the midbrain; the superior two are involved in visual reflexes, and the inferior two are involved in hearing.

Collimation Restricting the side of the x-ray beam by absorbing divergent x-rays with metal tubes or diaphragms interposed in the path of the beam. Rectangular colimators limit. The primary beam to approximate the size of intraoral radiographic film.

Collimator An arrangement of openings or slits that limits a stream of particles to a beam in which all particles move in nearly the same direction.

Colloid A suspension of fine particles (less than 1gum in size) dispersed throughout a liquid, such as water (i.e., hydrocolloid).

Colloid solutions Water and molecules of suspended substances, such as blood cells, and blood products such as albumin.

Colloidal bismuth It forms a protein coagulum on the ulcer surface. It is as effective as cimetidine in both gastric and duodenal ulcer. Its disadvantages are blackening of tongue and stool and foul ammonical odour of liquid preparations. It may lead to bismuth encephalopathy on long-term use.

Colloidal osmotic pressure Force for attracting water.

Colloids Undissolved protein substances.

Coloboma It is a congenital defect of the eye in which the tissues of the uvea and associated retinal tissues are deficient. It is due to defective closure of embryonic cleft. Coloboma occurs in lower part of eye. The typical coloboma of iris is pear shaped runs downwards and slightly inwards and extend from pupil towards ciliary body. While a typical coloboma of fundus is oval in shape with rounded apex towards the optic disc which may or may not be involved. Choroidal vessels are at edges. Vision is affected and there is scotoma in the field of coloboma.

Colon It is 2.5 inches wide and 4.5 feet long M-shaped loop in the abdomen. It is irregular in outline. It has four parts, ascending, transverse, descending and sigmoid colon. Ascending colon starts at caecum and extends upto liver. Point is known as hepatic flexure. Then it passes to spleen below stomach and this bend is known as splenic flexure. From here it turns downwards to the brim of pelvis where it becomes S shaped sigmoid colon. The function of colon is to absorb water and small amount of minerals. When intestinal contents enter the colon digestion is completed.

Colon spasm It is more common in young and middleaged. There is persistent abdominal pain and discomfort of nagging character. Pain is liable to colicky exacerbations which may be more marked after bowel evacuation. There are attacks of constipation during which stools may be hard. During attack mucus may be passed in masses, shreads or casts of several shapes. There may be intestinal flatulence and abdominal distension due to carbohydrate fermentation. *E. coli* may infect the urinary tract. Sigmoidoscopy helps in diagnosis.

Coloniality The behavior of birds or other animals whereby many individuals breed in close proximity, interact with each other, and usually join in group defense against predators.

Colonic function Major functions of colon are absorption of salts and water motility to move intestinal content onwards and storage of luminal contents before defaecation. Colectomy which is very well tolerated may have significant consequences in condition of high sodium losses such as fever, sweating and larger small bowel effluent. Water is also conserved. Of about 1500 ml entering the colon each day only about 100 ml leaves it.

Colonic irrigation It is also known as enterolysis. The process involves introduction of large amount of fluid into large bowel for flushing purpose and allow return of washout fluid. Fluid is introduced in slow and steady stream. It is used to clean the colon of faeces, gas, excess accumulated mucus, microorganism and toxin in dysentery. It helps in relieving pain and discomfort out of distension of large gut. It is used to prepare patient before surgery of large gut.

Colonization Condition in which microorganisms are present but the host manifests no signs or symptoms of infection.

Colonoscopic blind spot Wherever bowel bends at an angle, a colonoscopic blind spot exists. A lesion in that area may go undetected unless speical attention is devoted to visualise them.

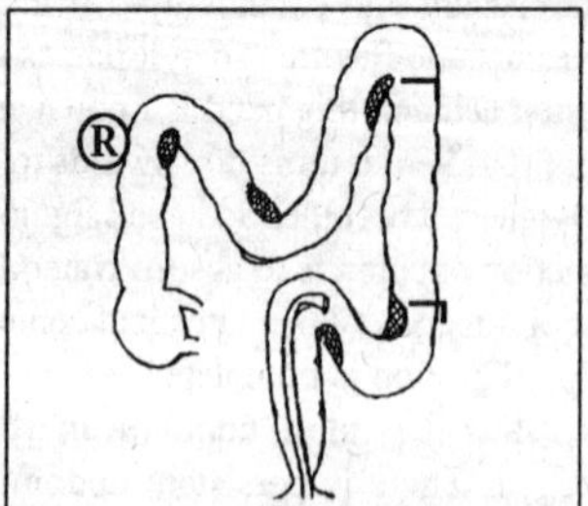

Colonoscopic examination The examination of the mucosal lining of the colon using a colonoscope.

Colony A multiple group of organisms that are physically connected to one another.

Colonyforming unit A colony formed from a group of micro-organisms rather than from one.

Color agnosia An inability to recognize colors.

Color constancy Phenomena whereby the perceived color of an object tends to remain constant, regardless of changes in illumination.

Colostomy Opening to some portion of the colon.

Colostrum It is a yellowish fluid containing more protein, minerals in good quality and quantity but less sugar and fat. Colostrum particles are considered to be epithelial cells which have undergone fatty degeneration. Its high gamma globulin level probably helps for providing antibodies, IgA has been demonstrated in colostrum. It gives protection against enteric infection.

Colour asthenopia It is a condition in which the patient has normal colour vision but after prolonged stimulation the differential threshold for colour increases.

Colour constancy The tendency for an object to be perceived as maintaining its basic colour despite changes in illumination, as when snow is seen to be white even though in shade or at dusk it has a purple cast.

$$\frac{\text{The presence of Hb}}{\text{The presence of RBCs}}$$

is called colour index. Normally it is one and indicates relative haemoglobin content of average corpuscles.

Colour vision The ability to discriminate among different parts of colour spectrum. Different wavelengths produce the sensation of violet, blue, green,

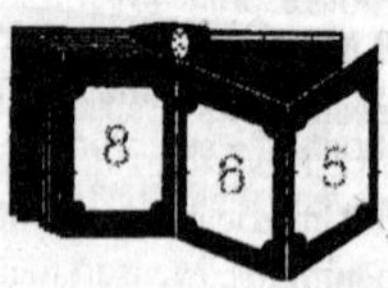

Polychromatic plates of Ishihara

yellow, orange and red (VIBGYOR). White light consists of fairly uniform mixture of all wavelengths of visible spectrum. Eyes have two cells, rods and cones about 4 to 7 million per eye and are more concentrated in macula. Colour vision is more accurate when seen directly instead of seen at periphery. Colour perception requires a minimum level of light for rods to respond. Most cases come to notice when a person is noted making a mistake or when the colour perception is recorded for service. There is practically no treatment of colour vision deficiency.

Colporrhaphy The Operation of suturing the vagina wall for the purpose of narrowing vagina.

Colporrhexis It is rupture of vaginal vault. Vaginal vault rupture without involvement of cervix or corpus is called primary colporrhexis. Secondary colporrhexis is defined as rupture of vaginal value with extension to cervix or lower uterine segment. Complete colporrhexis refers to the injury of vagina penetrating through the entire thickness and overlying peritoneum.

Colposcope An instrument designed for close examination of the cervical tissues, similar to a low-magnification microscope with binocular vision.

Colposcopy The process of evaluating the cervix with magnification to identify abnormal cells.

Colpotomy Any surgical cutting operation upon the vagina.

Column A term used interchangeably for the posterior funiculus of the spinal cord.

Columnar Shape in which cells are higher than they are wide.

Columnar epithelium Height of cells exceeds their other dimensions. It lines whole of interior of stomach and intestines. It lines greater part of male urethra, vas deferens, tubular alveoli of prostate and its function is secretion and absorption.

Coma It is a state of unconsciousness in which person does not respond to stimuli. It results due to damage of limbic system due to head injury or brain tumour, and intracerebral haemorrhage. CT and MRI are best tool to examine it. Other causes include alcohol intoxication, uncontrolled diabetes, hypoxia or meningitis. Measurements of variations in depth of coma are necessary to treat it. In less severe form the person may respond to stimulation by uttering a few words. In severe form person fails to respond to repeated vigorous stimuli. A person may remain in commatose state of deep coma for years with little or no apparent activity in cerebrum.

Coma scale It includes general simple scales

1 = fully awake
2 = conscious but drowsy
3 = unconscious but responsive to pain with flexion
4 = unconscious responds to pain and extension
5 = unconscious with no respond to pain.

Combat stress reaction A term for the acute psychological breakdown experienced by combat soldiers.

Combined transurethral and suprapubic lithoplaxy Under local anesthesia with adequate dilatation of cystostomy track the stones are either

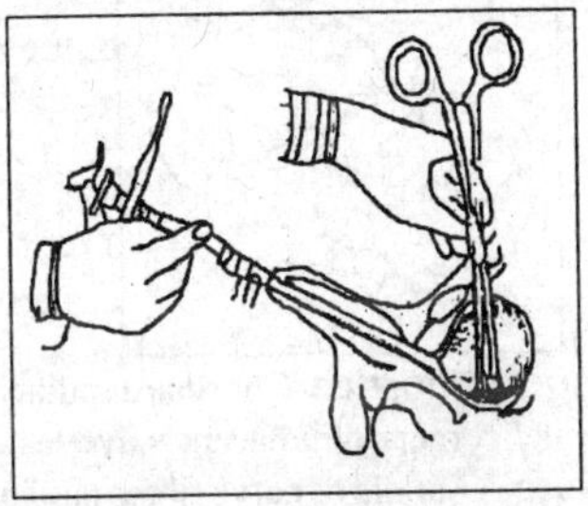

removed intact or piecemeal by same route. With simultaneous cystoscopy through a standard cystoscope the proceedure can be carried out under direct supervision.

Combining sites Antigen-binding sites, antigen receptor regions on antibody molecule; shape of each combining site is complementary to shape of a specific antigen.

Comby's sign It is represented by thin white patches due to degenerated squamous epithelium occurring on buccal mucosae and gums, and is seen in early stage of measles.

Cometabolism The biotrans-formation of a compound by a microoganism that is incapable of utilizing the compound as a source of energy or growth.

Comfort State in which a person is relieved of distress.

Comforting Any action taken to promote comfort of the client, such as a back rub, change in position.

Comforting skills Interventions that provide stability and security during a health crisis.

Coming out The informal process gay people go through in revealing their sexual preference to their family, friends, and coworkers.

Commensal Pertaining to a relationship between to organism in which one organisms benefits and the other is unharmed.

Commensalism A symbiotic relationship between two species in which neither species is physiologically dependent upon the other.

Comminuted calcaneum fracture CT scan precisely show position of bony fragments and extent of depression at the posterior facet of subtalar joint.

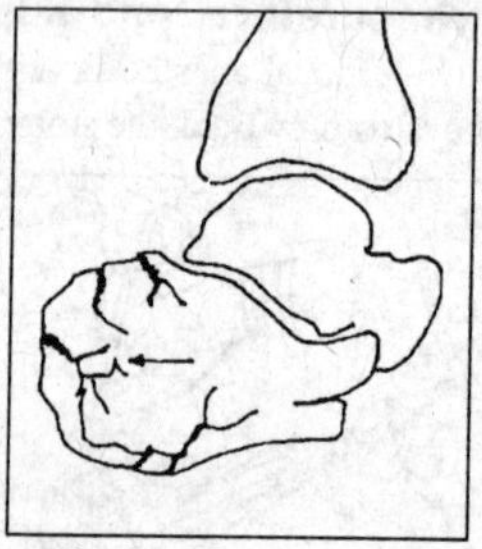

Commissural chordae Chordae tendineae that attach at the corners of adjacent valve leaflets.

Commissure A bundle of nerve fibres passing from one side to the other in the brain or spinal cord.

Commissure labial Lip junction.

Commissurotomy A surgical division of the junction between adjacent cusps of a valve of the heart.

Commitment A legal process for admitting a mentally ill person to a psychiatric treatment programme. The legal definition and procedure vary from state to state although commitment usually requires a court or judicial procedure. Commitment may also be voluntary.

Commode Portable chair used for elimination.

Common ancestor An ancestor from which two or more lineages or family groups arise and so is ancestral to both groups.

Common atrioventricular bundle The collection of specialized myocytes that begins at the atrioventricular node and passes through the annulus of the right atrioventricular valve to the membranous portion of the interventricular septum where it splits into two branches; bundle of His; His-kent bundle.

Common bile duct (CBD) Duct formed by the union of the common hepatic and cystic ducts; it joins the pancreatic duct and empties into the duodenum.

Common descent Refers to individual organ isms or families that descend from the same ancestor.

Common hepatic duct Duct formed by union of the right and left hepatic ducts; it joins the cystic duct to form the CBD.

Common Law Law made by judges in the context of particular cases, and based on decisions made in previous cases involving related facts and laws.

Common mode rejection ratio A ratio expressing an amplifier's ability to reject unwanted noise while amplifying the wanted signal, for example, a ratio of 1000:1 indicates the wanted signal will be amplified 1,000 times more than noise, can also be expressed in decibels (1000:1 equals 60 dB).

Common oviduct In insects, an ectodermal invagination that connects the genital opening with the lateral oviducts.

Common penile artery The continuation of the deep internal pudendal artery after the departure of the perineal artery and the labial scrotal artery.

Commotio retinae It occurs due to contusion injury to the eyeball, i.e. blow. There is a milky area with a promineut red spot in the centre referred as a cherry red spot at macula. This typical appearance is due to oedema at the posterior pole giving a white appearance and macula in centre shines as red spot. Oedema may resolve completely or is followed by degenerative changes at the macula in form of pigmentation or hole at macula. There is marked loss of vision.

Communicable Capable of being transmitted from one person to another.

Communicable disease Infectious diseases that can be transmitted to other people.

Communication Any means by which an individual relates experiences, ideas, knowledge, and feelings to another; includes speech, sign language, body language, gestures, writing; the process by which meanings are exchanged between individuals through a system of symbols.

Community A collection of microbial populations growing together in a defined habitat.

Community as client A broad interpretation of the unit of service that address the entire community's needs.

Community medicine It is the branch of medicine for treating the disorder of entire section of population. It includes preventive and social medicine.

Community-acquired infections Infectious diseases that can be transmitted to other people.

Comolli's sign Clinical sign of scapula fracture.

Comorbidity The association between migraine and another condition that is unlikely to be random or one causing the other.

Compact (dense) bone tissue Bone tissue that contains few spaces between osteons (Haversian systems); forms the external portion of all bones and the bulk of the diaphysis of long bones; is found immediately deep to the periosteum and external to spongy bone.

Compact bone Tightly packed bone that is superficial to spongy bone and covered by the periosteum; also called dense bone.

Companionate love Characterised by deep affection and a realistic outlook. It can be the love among family members or between partners in a couple. It is considered less intense and longer-lasting than passionate love.

Comparative negligence The legal theory that allows the jury to consider the plaintiff's negligence in determining whether the defendant's actions caused the plaintiff's injuries.

Comparative psychology Often used as synonymous with animal psychology. More accurately, the comparison of behaviour at different levels of species development to discover development trends—as in the evolution of intelligence from amoeba to human beings.

Compartment syndrome It is impaired circulation and function of tissues within a fascial compartment with increased pressure within the compartment.

Compatibility It is the degree of matching between two drugs and tissues. It is to be judged carefully in organ transplantation otherwise body will reject the new organ transplanted.

Compatible Capable of existing together in harmony; with medications, suitable for simultaneous administration.

Compensation A defence mechanism, operating unconsciously, by which one attempts to make up for real or fancied deficiencies. Also a conscious process in which one strives to make up for real or imagined defects of physique, performance skills, or psychologic attributes. The two types frequently merge.

Compensation reflex Vestibuloocular reflex compensating for movement of the head; associated with fixation/foveation.

Compensatory acid-base disorder A normal or anticipated attempt to restore the acid-base balance that occurs in response to some disruptive factor.

Compensatory curve In spinal curvature a secondary curve above or below the major curve to maintain normal body alignment.

Compensatory damages Money paid to an injured or wronged plaintiff based on their proven losses.

Compensatory pause The suspension or delay of myocardial electrical activity that may occur following an extrasystole.

Competence The individual's adequacy or capability in given task.

Competent larva A term for a larva that is physiologically and morphologically capable of undergoing metamorphosis.

Competition A form of social interaction in which the goals of group members are incompatible. Any given member can attain his or her own goal only at the expense of depriving another group members are incompatible.

Competitive preference A tendency to choose either a superiority or rivalry resource distribution.

Complainant The individual who claims to be a victim of a crime.

Complaint The written statement in a civil case setting forth the plaintiff's claims and the legal basis for the lawsuit.

Complement A group of a least 20 normally inactive proteins found in plasma that forms a component of nonspecific resistance and immunity by brining about cytolysis, in flammation, and opsonization.

Complement fixation Highly specialized antigen-antibody complexes are formed to destroy a foreign cell.

Complementary medicine The use of therapies traditionally a part of Western health care system but more often an element of Eastern medicine and philosophy.

Complete denture Dental prosthesis replacing the lost natural dentition with associated structures of mandible and maxilla.

Complete inevitable abortion Bleeding is reduced to mere staining, pain ceases and cervix closes. Mistaken diagnosis has often been made. In later months complete abortion resembles a miniature labour. Entire sac with placenta is expelled unruptured. Lochia may persist for some time.

Complete lesion No sensory or motor function below the level of lesion.

Complete protein A protein that contains the essential amino acids in quantities sufficient for maintenance of body and for a normal rate of growth. Egg, milk, cheese and meat are complete foods as proteins. Proteins containing all nine essential amino acids.

Completeness of medical care Adequate attention to all aspects of a medical problem, including prevention, early edtection, diagnosis, treatment, followup measures, and rehabilitation.

Complex A group of associated ideas having a common, strong emotional tone. These are largely unconscious and significantly influence attitudes and associations.

Complex cell Type of visual cortex neuron that responds best to a light stimulus of a particular shape in its receptive field.

Complex regional pain syndrome type 2 It consists of burning pain in distribution of partially damaged peripheral nerve, specially median, ulnar or sciatica. It may develop within month of an injury and may radiate beyond nerve distribution.

Complex regional pain syndrome type I There is continuous pain in part or extremity after trauma but not involving a nerve damage. It becomes worse with movements.

Complex spikes Complex response of purkinje cells to stimulation of olivocerebellar fibers.

Complex tone A sound whose basic wave from although repeated periodical, is more complicated than that of a pure tone; a complex tone contains two or more puretone components.

Complex tone A sound whose basic waveform, although repeated periodically, is more complicated that allows the flow of the substance from an area of high concentration to an area of low concentration.

Complexity In the humanistic view of personality, emphasis upon the extraordinary capacities of human beings, not found in other organisms. Human thinking and problem solving, for example, presumably cannot be fruitfully understood through the study of animals or solely through reductionistic studies, in which the whole is analysed only in terms of its parts.

Compliance A measure of the ease with which a structure such as the lung expands under pressure; a measure of the change in volume as a function of pressure changes.

Complicated myocardial infarction A myocardial infarctions of such severity that there is evidence of continued ischemia, left ventricular failure, shock, serious arrhythmia or other conduction disturbance, or other serious illness persisting beyond the fourth day after the infarction; constitutes a high-risk subset.

Complicating disease A disease forseen or unforeseen occuring in the course of development or treatment of other disease.

Complication An undesired result or misadventure in the medical care of a hospital patient.

Compomelic dysplasia The defect involves a gene encoding a transcription factor related to product of the SRY gene which induces testis development.

Compomer A class of materials having composite and glass ionomer-type characteristics that are mainly used as an anterior restorative; otherwise known as a polyacid modified resin. They are anhydrous.

Composit Tooth coloured restorative material made of a composite or filled resin, used where esthetics are important.

Composite Resinous filling material formed by a reaction of an ether bisphenol A with acrylic resin monomers; initiated by a benzoyl peroxide amine system to which inorganic fillers (glass beads and rods of either aluminum, silicate, quartz, or tricalcium phosphate) are added.

Composite impairment An impairment whose underlying cause includes both direct and indirect effects of the original pathology.

Compound A substance that can be broken down into two or more other substances by chemical means.

Compound naevus It is the combination of both junctional and intradermal components. The intradermal components are inactive and incapable of multiplication or pigment production. But the junctional components are very much prone to malignant change. These appear round and elliptical elevated lesions, the centre being more elevated than periphery. These are light brown to dark in colour. In adolescents compound naevi often grow, become thicker, papillomatous and darker.

Compound presentation Presentation of an extremity that prolapses alongside and enters the pelvis at the same time as the presenting part.

Comprehensive health care Services that meet the total health care needs of a patient.

Comprehensiveness of medical care The extent to which care is provided for all types of health problems, including dental and mental health problems.

Compress Soft pad of gauze or cloth used to apply heat, cold, or medications to the surface fo a body part.

Compresses Moist cloths that may be warm or cool.

Compression A load that pushes the fibers of a material together along its long axis; it results in, or tends to cause, a shortening and widening of the material.

Compression bandage Any dressing meant to apply pressure to prevent or reduce swelling and to check bleeding.

Compression fracture A vertebral fracture resulting from pressure along the long axis of the vertebral column and closely associated with flexion injuries.

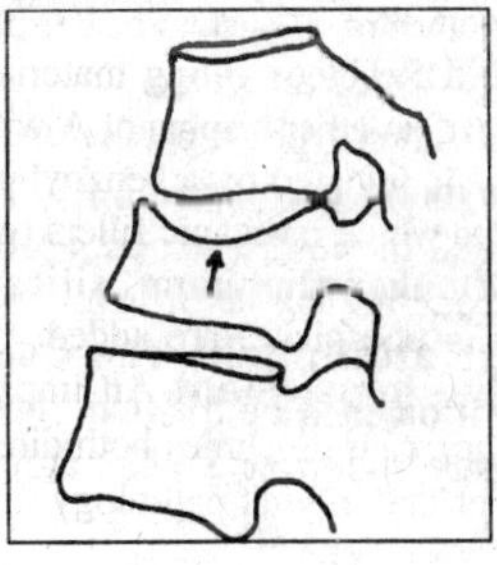

Compression kneading This basic kneading stroke is called 'Palmar' kneading. As its name implies, it involves the entire palmar suface of either or both hands. In this manipulation the tissues are compressed upwards and inwards, in a circular motion against the underlying tissues and then released.

Compression nerve root Sciatica pain is the result of synovitis or periarticular inflammation which irritate and compress the nerve root.

Compression paralysis Partial or complete paralysis caused by pressure on a nerve or spinal cord.

Compression—cervical rib The eighth cervical and first thoracic roots unite to form the lower trunk of brachial plexus lying on the first rib. The lower trunk may be stretched. Patient complains of pain in forearm and weakness in hand. There is wasting of all muscles of hand. Electro-physiological studies show denervation in the wasted muscles. Operative decompression usually relieves pain, once prominent wasting of hand has occurred then recovery of function is possible.

Compressive strength Amount of resistance of a material to fracture under compression or biting forces.

Compules Premeasured units of dental matirials such as single past resin filling material.

Compulsion An insistent, repetitive, intrusive, and unwanted urge to perform an act that is contrary to one's ordinary wishes or standards. Since it serves as a defensive substitute for still more unacceptable unconscious ideas and wishes, failure to perform the compulsive act leads to overt anxiety.

Computed tomography (CT) scan CT image is a display of the anatomy of a thin slice of body developed from multiple developed X-ray

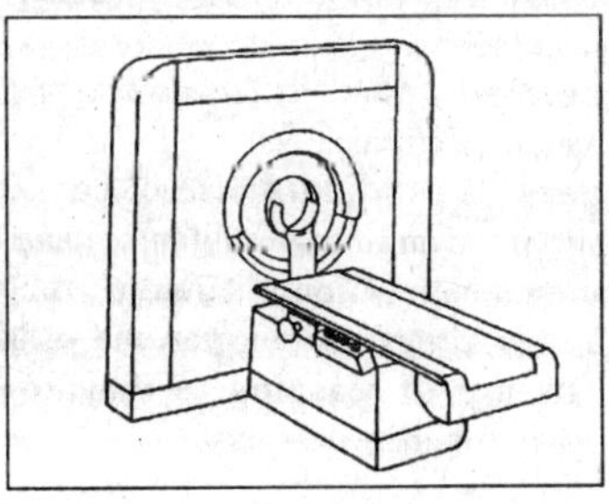

absorption measurements made around the body's periphery. In conventional tomography image of a thin section is created blurring out the information from undesired region. In CT, image is constructed mathemetically using data arising only from section of interest.

Computer graphics The process of generating, creating, visualizing, animating and controlling

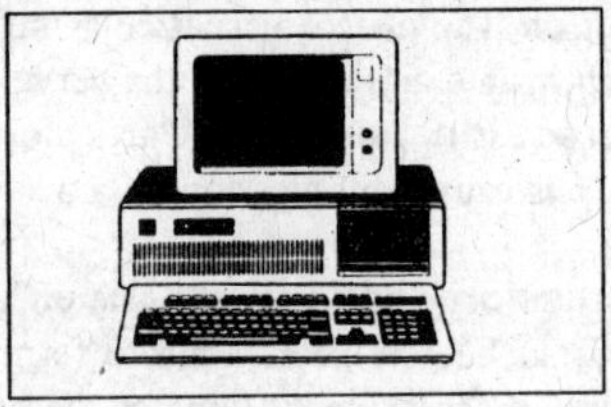

synthetically images by the use of computer methods. Computer graphics are a wide scientific area used. To give some examples for recreation, simulation, illustration and documentation.

Computer model The use of a computer to simulate human thinking. The computer processes are examined to understand the ways in which they represent human thought—they serve as a means for examining symbolic processes.

Computer-assisted instruction Use of a computer to present educational tasks to the student. Often, the tasks are prepared in the form of programmed learning, involving a step-by-step sequence. An important advantage of the computer is that its enormous memory system and immediate recall can be used to present material at the appropriate level for a given individual, in accordance with his or her prior responses.

Computer-Generated Bone Modeling The use of computerized scanning and milling technology to create a replicate model of bone intended to substitute for the stage one surgical process of direct bone impressioning in the subperiosteal implant protocol;.

Computerized charting Documenting patient information electronically.

Computers in medicare Use of computer in medicare is proving very useful in keeping record of patients admission/discharge, record of instruments, drugs, inventories and making of bills. Its use in reaching to diagnosis and investigation is increasing fast.

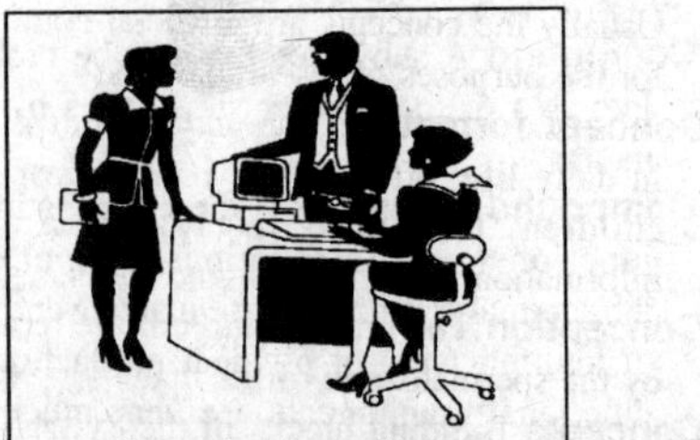

Computers in medicare

Comuting impedance Obstacls or behavioral constraints on movement of goal attainment.

Conative Pertains to one's basic strivings as expressed in behaviour and actions; volitional as contrasted with cognitive.

Concatemer A single molecule of DNA consisting of more than two phage genomes joined head to tail.

Concave A rounded, somewhat depressed surface.

Concavity An area of tooth surface that is depressed into a hollow.

Concentration camp A camp where prisoners of war are confined.

Concentric A shortening contraction; an isotonic contraction.

Concentric lamella Ring of calcified matrix surrounding the Haversian canal.

Concentric muscle contraction Any contraction in which muscle shortens while tension is generated.

Concentric needle electrode Recording electrode consisting of a steel cannula through which is threaded a single platinum wire that is insulated from the needle shaft. The wire and shaft are bared at the tip and the potential difference between them is recorded in the presence of electrical activity.

Concentricity The condition of a circle or circular object having the same center point as another circle or circular object. In drilling, the maintenance of a constant center point of rotation.

Concept An abstract idea or conclusion based on a generalisation from a particular instances, such as "anything burning is hot". A phenomenon expressed in words; sometimes used as a more concrete term than *construct*.

Concept attainment The study of concept acquisition in a controlled setting, often the laboratory, following explicit training procedures.

Usually the concepts are artificial contrived only for the purposes of research.

Concept formation The acquisition of concepts in daily life, often a long process, especially in children. The ability to organize a variety of information into thoughts and ideas.

Conception The impregnation of the female ovum by the spermatozoon of the male.

Concepts Building blocks of theory that represent the main ideas expressed by the theory; sometimes termed variables. They exist on a continuum from empirical, to abstract. Examples of concrete concepts are gender and age; abstract concepts, family and health.

Conceptual model or framework The terms "model" and frame work" are sometimes used interchangeably to mean a set of interrelation concepts that symbolically represent and convey a mental image of a phenomenon. They are less predictive than a theory and only symbolize that there is a relationship among the concepts in the framework. For example, nursing models are not considered stringent enough to be theories because they are not predictive.

Concha Structure resembling a shell in shape; the three bony ridges on the lateral wall of the nasal cavity.

Concomitant Accompanying; accessory; joined with another.

Concrescence The union of two teeth after eruption by the fusion of their cementum surfaces.

Concrete thinking Thinking characterised by immediate experience, rather than abstractions. Seen in persons who have never developed the ability to generalise.

Concurrent disinfection Measures that keep the patient environment clean on a daily basis.

Concussion An impairment of brain function caused by injury to the head. The speed and degree of recovery depend on severity of the brain injury. Symptoms may include headache, disorientation, paralysis, and occasionally unconsciousness.

Condensation A psychologic process often present in dreams in which two or more concepts are fused so that a single symbol represents the multiple components.

Condenser Hand instrument used for placing a restorative material into prepared cavity.

Condensing osteitis It is also known as sclerosing osteomyelitis. It is associated with bone formation rather than bone destruction. Mandible is mostly affected. It is symptom free and is associated with a tooth having pulp or periapical pathology. There are localised radiopacities and under microscope one can see dense bone trabeculae and mild infiltration of plasma cells and lymphocytes. There is no need of treatment in case of nonvital tooth endotonic therapy helps.

Conditioned response In classical conditioning, a response aroused by some stimuli other than that which naturally produces it, such as salivation in response to a tone. In operant conditioning, a response that has become more frequent after being reinforced.

Conditioned stimulus A previously neutral stimulus which acquires the property of eliciting a particular response; it acquires this capacity through pairing with an unconditioned stimulus.

Conditioned response (CR) In Pavlovian conditioning, the learned response to a formerly neutral conditioned stimulus (CS).

Conditioned taste aversion An avoidance of a food or drink that has been followed by illness when consumed in the past.

Conditioning It is the modification by adopting new responses to stimuli. Classical conditioning involves the establishing of conditioned reflex. It is a stimulus that produces a specific response. Operant conditioning relies on reinforcement.

Condom It is made of a thin layer of elastic rubber. It fits over the erect penis and acts as barrier to the transmission of semen into vagina. Condom is 19 cm long and 2.5 cm wide. Certain condoms are lubricated while a few varieties come in ribbed or patterned forms in various attractive colours. It is safe self-explanatory, not bulky and easily available. Disadvantage is that it becomes barrier

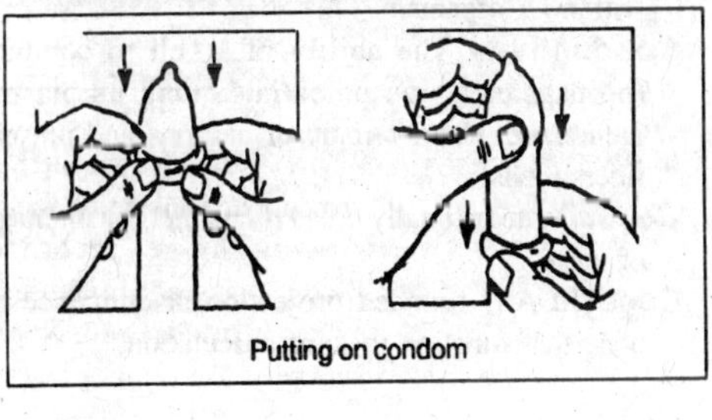

Putting on condom

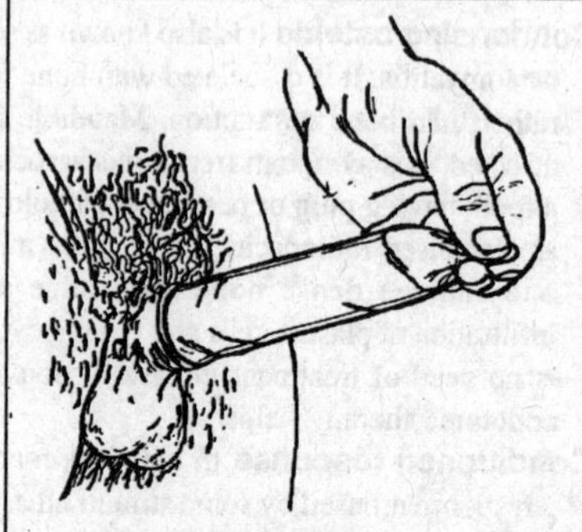

Condom

in skin contact, reduces sensitivity and can be torn or semen may slip while getting it off.

Conduct disorder A behaviour disorder of childhood and adolescence characterised by stealing, running away, frequent fighting or other illegal activities.

Conduction Conveyance of energy, as of heat, sound, or electricity.

Conduction aphasia Aphasia caused by damage to the arcuate fasciculus.

Conduction distance Distance measured in centimeters between two points of stimulation along a nerve in a nerve conduction velocity test.

Conduction system A series of autorhythmic cardiac muscle fibers that generate and distribute electrical impulses to stimulate coordinated contraction of the heart chambers; includes the sinoatrial (SA) node, the artioventricular (AV) node, the atrioventricular (AV) bundle, the right and left bundle branches, and the conduction myofibers (Purkinje fibers).

Conductive deafness Deafness caused by disease in the outer ear canal or middle ear.

Conductive heat transfer The net rate of heat transfer by conduction down a thermal gradient within an organism.

Conductivity The ability of a cell to conduct (propagate) action potentials along its plasma membrane; characteristic of neurons and muscle fibers (cells).

Conduit An arificially created channel for drainage of urine.

Condyle Any rounded projection or eminence of bone that function in joint articulation.

Condyloid joint It is a type or synovial joint in which the rounded condyles of one bone articulate with a shallow elliptical cavity of another.

Condyloma A wart-like excrescence near the anus or the vulva; the flat, moist papule of secondary syphilis.

Condyloma acuminatum It rarely occurs before puberty. It is caused by papovirus and is transmitted by sexual contact. These are mostly situated near coronal sulcus and appear as sharp pointed red, papillary excrescences, sessile or pedunculated and usually moist with offensive discharge. These are premalignants.

Cone An accessory device on a dental X-ray machine designed to indicate the direction of the central axis of its X-ray beam and to serve as guide in establishing a desired source-to-film distance. Such cones may be conical or cylindrical in form; provision for beam collimation and/or added filtration may be incorporated in the construction of the cone.

Cone receptor Cell located in the retina that is stimulated by bright light.

Cone-cut An artefact seen on a dental radiograph when a portion of the film has not been exposed to the X-ray beam; appears as a curved, unexposed radiopaque area.

Cones These have two limbs. Outer one is tapering while inner is broader in the centre. These have a nucleus near the external limiting membrane and terminates by branching in the external molecular layer. These are responsible for vision in bright light, colour vision and acquity of vision.

Cone-vision These are responsible to see colours and require more light.

Confidential communication Communications between persons in fiduciary or confidential relationships. The right of confidentiality belongs to the client or patient, not to the fiduciary. A patient can freely discuss his physician's advice, but the physician cannot freely discuss the patient's condition or the advice given the patient.

Confidentiality The ethical principle that a physician may not reveal any information disclosed in the course of medical attendance.

Configuration In implant dentistry, a specific shape and size or implant.

Configurationalists Gestalt psychologists, who emphasised the study of whole of configurations.

Opposed to the reductionistic viewpoint, which examines a complex event by studying its smaller components.

Confinement A term for procedures used to keep genetically-modified organisms within bounds or limits, usually in the environment with the result of preventing widespread dissemination.

Confirmation The process of establishing beyond reasónable doubt the identity of a substance.

Conflict A mental struggle that arises from the simultaneous operation of opposing impulses, drives, external (environmental) or internal demands. Termed intrapsychic when the conflict is between forces within the personality; extrapsychic, when it is between the self and the environment.

Confluence The process of combining two or more activities at the same time. In families, this may promote togetherness.

Confounding Confusion of two supposedly causal bariables, so that part or all of the purported effect of one variable is actually due to the other.

Confrontation A communication that deliberately invites another to self-examine some aspects of behaviour in which there is a discrepancy between saying and doing.

Confusion A mental state in which reaction of environmental and physical conditions is inappropriate.

Confusional insanity It is characterised by unstable attention, poor perception of present reality, disorientation and inability to act coherently. It results from mental, physical exhaustion and fevers.

Congelation Frostibite or freezing.

Congenic Animals which only differ at a single genetic locus.

Congenital Born with a person; existing from or from before birth, as, for example, congenital disease, a disease originating in the fetus before birth.

Congenital abnormality It is the malformation which is present at birth which may be of known or unknown cause. Common examples are cleft lip, congenital heart disease and dislocation of hip, etc. Person should avail the facility of genetic counselling before deciding to have another child.

Congenital anomaly A structural abnormality that may be hereditary, or that may be due to some influence occurring during gestation or in the process of birth.

Congenital disorders Disorders present at birth that result from faulty embryonic development.

Congenital ptosis It is the most common type and has a strong hereditary tendency. There is drooping of lid since birth. It is unilateral. Lid is smooth, unwrinkled thin, without tarsal fold and may cover the pupil. A case of congenital simple ptosis is most amenable to surgery or resection of the levator muscle.

Congenital synostosis A congenital fusion of two or more bones.

Congenital variation of uterus There may be uterus didelphys, uterus bicornis unicollis, uterus subseptate and uterus septate.

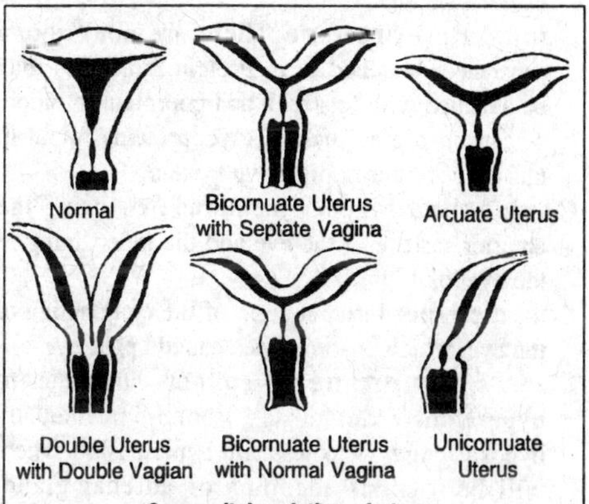

Congenital variation of uterus

Congestive cardiomyopathy Here patients have oedema, breathlessness, engorged neck veins and increased heart rate. Biventricular enlargement is present. Triple rhythm is often present on auscultation over mitral and tricuspid areas. Murmurs of mitral and tricuspid incompetence are present. ECG shows evidence of ventricular enlargement.

Congestive dysmenorrhoea In this patient complains of pain in back and in lower abdomen. It begins a few days before the onset of menstruation and is relieved by bleeding. Although a feeling of heaviness throughout menstruation may continue.

Congnitive control A strategy for thinking about a situation in order to reduce its stressful event.

Congruence In the person-centred approach to personality, the degree to which an individual's experience is compatible with his or her concept of self.

Conidium An asexual fungal spore formed from a generative cell known as a conidiophore.

Conjoined Twins when the division of the germ disc occurs after 13th day of post fertilization. This results in failure in splitting in its entirety and leaves some portions in common.

Conjuctiva The thin membrane covering the anterior surface of the eyeball and lining the eyelids.

Conjugal Involving or taking part in conjugation.

Conjugate movement Movement in parallel, e.g. ocular saccades.

Conjugated proteins These are non protein substances attached to it. Protein molecules may be attached with fats such as lipoprotein in blood, or carbohydrates such as glycoproteins found in mucus. secreted in digestive system.

Conjunctiva Mucous membrane covering the anterior surface of the eye and the inner lining of the eyelids.

Conjunctivitis Inflammation of the conjunctiva of the eye, which is sometimes called "pink eye".

Conn's syndrome Symptoms are due to hyperaldosteronism and is characterised by hypokalaemia, weakness and hypertension. There will be a small adenoma of adrenal gland. Pathologically overactivity of zona glomerulosa is the main cause. Patient feels severe weakness due to potassium deficiency. Polyuria and polydipsia occurs. Tetany type attack may occur. ECG shows prominent 'U' wave and cardiac arrhythmias. BP is high and oedema of dependent parts develops.

Connecting strut A strut on a subperisteal implant the connects and unifies the buccal/labial and lingual main bearing struts.

Connective heat transfer The net rate of heat transfer by convection between an organism and its external environment or the transfer for heat with the blood stream from the thermal core to the heat dissipating surface.

Connective tissue One of the four major tissue types; consists of cells usually surrounded by large amounts of extracellular material; functions to hold other tissues together and provides a supporting framework for the body. It is developed from mesoderm. Cementing substance is markedly developed and all of them give mechanical connection and support.

Connective tissue massage Elibzabeth Dicke, a Germen physiotherapist in 1929 when she herself suffered from pain developed this technique. Later Mackenzie (1909) observed hypertonic alterations

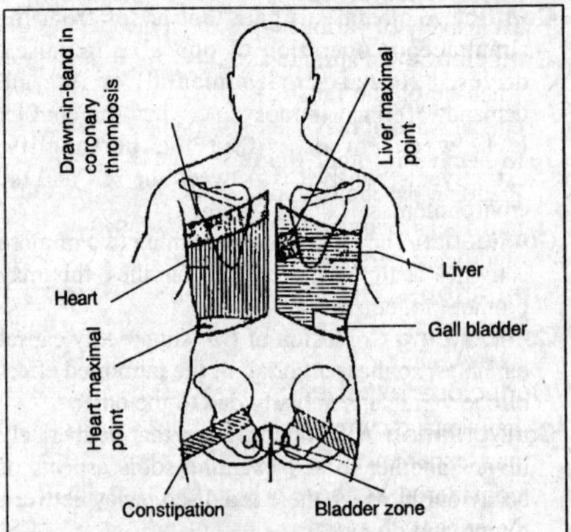

Points for massage

and hypersensitivity in muscles belonging to the same segment as disabled organs. In liver and gall bladder malfunction tension is increased in between the right scapula and vertebral column at the level of T_4T_6.

Connective Tissue Massage or Bindegeweb Massage It is based on peripheral manipulation of the nervous system and produces visceral effects. Specific strokes are applied to reach the connective tissue underlying the skin with the intent of affecting organs whose innervation corresponds to cutaneous dermatomes. It facilitates changes in the autonomic nervous system activity.

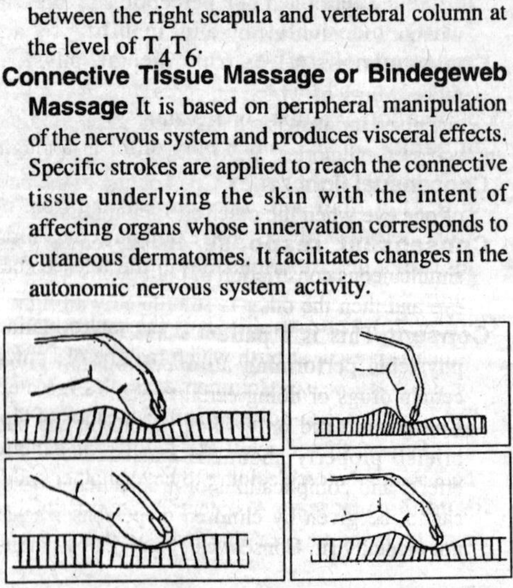

Connective tissue massage stroke The stroke consists of a tangential pull on the skin and subcutaneous tissues away from underlying fascia. It is always a pull on the tissues and never a push or pressure. There are three stages : (*i*) to touch firmly, (*ii*) take up the slack by flexing the distal interphalangeal joints, and (*iii*) one is 'pull'.

Connective tissue membrane One of the two major types of body membranes; composed exclusively of various types of connective tissue.

Conscience An attitude assumed by the individual when he or she fails to conform to the moral or ethical ways of his or her group , or when tempted to behave in other than the approved ways. In Freudian psychology, part of the superego, ideals and ideas acquired from the parents or other significant persons in one's early life.

Conscious The content of mind or mental functioning of which one is aware. In neurology, awake, alert.

Conscious experience Experience of which the individual is currently aware, as distinguished from past experience. Conscious experiences may be considered as those which the individual can describe such as sensory experiences and feelings.

Conscious proprioception Perceived sensations arising within the body, notably from muscle spindles.

Conscious sedation An anesthetic procedure in which analgesia and anesthesia are accomplished without loss of consciousness.

Consciousness A level of awareness that includes those things of which an individual is aware at any given moment, such as current ideas, thoughts, accessed memories, and feelings.

Consensual light reflex Constriction of the pupil of one eye when the other eye is illuminated.

Consensual response Brisk, equal, and simultaneous constriction of both pupils when one eye and then the other is stimulated with light.

Consent This is a patient's agreement with a physician performing an operation and giving certain drugs or doing certain tests.

Consent is valid only when he or she has been briefed properly about the consequences, side effects and complications of procedures. Consent cannot be given by children or persons who are not mentally fit. Consent can be given by parents, sons and relatives who have brought the patient to the clinic.

Consequences Events that follow behavior and influence its frequency.

Conservation withdrawal A parasympathetic survival pattern that is similar to "Playing 'possum" or hibernation.

Conservative focusing A strategy in concept attainment in which each attribute of a concept is examined separately to determine whether it is relevant or irrelevant. Thus, the subject proceeds slowly, step by step, to acquire the concept, rather than guessing or speculating about which characteristics are involved.

Consistency principle The desire of the human being to be consistent, especially with regard to attitudes and beliefs. Theories of attitude formation and change based on the consistency principle include balance theory and congruity theory, which suggest that the individual seeks to avoid imbalance or incongruity in various attitudes.

Consolidation Solidification; the process of becoming or the condition of being solid.

Consolidation theory A view of forgetting which postulates that lack of memory is due to eradication of the trace before it becomes permanent. It is hypothesised that the memory trace needs time in order to become firmly fixed, disruption of the trace during the formative stages can eliminate the possibility of memory.

Constant friction Mechanism that applies uniform resistance throughout swing; may be incorporated in sliding, hydraulic, or pneumatic friction mechanisms.

Constant region Part of an antibody that does not combine with an antigen and is the same in different antibodies; responsible for activation of complement and binding the antibody to cells such as macrophages, basophils, and mast cells.

Constipation Condition in which dry, hard stool is difficult to pass.

Constipation in pregnancy It is physiological with decreased bowel transit time and stool may be hardened.. Dietary modification with increased bulk can help. Laxatives should not be given.

Constitution A person's intrinsic physical and psychologic endowment; sometimes used more narrowly to indicate physical inheritance or intellectual potential.

Constitutional disease It is a systemic disease that involves multiple body systems instead of local involvment.

Constitutional symptoms Any untoward symptoms that beset the body in a generalized manner like fever, malaise.

Constitutional types Constellations of morphologic, physiologic and psychologic traits as earlier poroposed by various scholars. Galen; sanguine, melancholic, choleric, and phlegmatic types; Kieschmer; pyknic (stocky), asthenic (slender), athletic, and dysplastic (disproportioned) types; Sheldon; ectomorphic (thin), mesomorphic (muscular), and endomorphic (fat) types, based on the relative preponderance of outer, middle, or inner layers of embryonic cellular tissue.

Constitutive Relating to or describing continuously expressed or unregulated genes in the absence of an inducer.

Constitutive enzyme An enzyme whose formation is not dependent upon the presence of a specific substrate.

Constitutive expression Gene expression from which RNA synthesis occurs continuously without the requirement of an inducing molecule or complex.

Constitutive gene A gene whose transcription is dependent of RNA polymerase only, and no other regulatory factor.

Constriction Narrowing.

Constriction ring There is localised spastic contraction of a ring of circular muscle at the junction of upper and lower uterine segment around fetal neck in cephalic presentation.

Constrictive cardiomyopathy This is rare and stimulates constrictive pericarditis as the thickened myocardium resists ventricular filling. Clinical features include engorgements of neck veins. Liver is enlarged and on occasion pulsus paradoxus is present. All these features simulate constrictive pericarditis. Heart sounds are normal and there is no ventricular enlargement.

Construct validity A type of validity that assesses the extent to which a test score (variable) correlates with other tests (variables) already established as valid measures of the item.

Consultant He or she is a doctor in private or government job with appropriate qualification and experience. He or she is supposed to be very good in his or her branch and is a senior man or woman.

Consultation A meeting of persons to discuss and decide about treatment etc.

Consumer One who may recieve or is recieving dental service.

Consumer psychology A speciality which focuses upon consumer behaviour of all sorts. The field began with developments in advertising and buying behaviour but has been expanded to include noncommercial purposes, such as campaigns for government projects and opinion surveys for educational and environmental programmes.

contact angle The angle that an adhesive liquid makes with a surface; used as a measure of wetting, where a low-contact angle signifies good wetting and enhances the potential for adhesion.

Contact area Point at which abutment teeth touch each other.

Contact carriers These persons acquire the pathogens from a patient and carry them to infect other person.

Contact interproximal Any point where two teeth touch each other on their side.

Contact lens It is the form of lens used to correct visual defects that is made of plastic or glass and is placed on the front of eyeball in contact with conjunctival membrane. Some lenses may cover sclera. All move with the eyeball giving better peripheral vision than ordinary glasses.

Contact occlusal Any point where two teeth in opposite arches touch.

Contact point Area of the adjustive hand that makes contact with the patient in the delivery of the chiropractic adjustment. There are 12 contact points :

1. Pisiform
2. Hypothenar
3. Metacarpal (knife-edge)
4. Digital
5. Distal interphalangeal (DIP)
6. Proximal interphalangeal (PIP)
7. Metacarpophalangeal (MP or index)
8. Web
9. Thumb
10. Thenar
11. Calcaneal
12. Palmar

Contact precautions Measures used to block the transmission of pathogens by direct or indirect contract.

Contact vulvitis This often results from local reaction to under-garments, chemicals, perfumes, synthetic materials and detergents. It may result in oedema and reddening of vulvar skin and vaginitis. Antihistaminics and steroidal preparations are helpful.

Contagion The transmission of an illnes from one individual to another by contact or by indirect transfer of germs.

Contagionism The principle that disease is transmitted by direct or indirect contact between living organisms, especially humans, in the form of microscopic living entities, e.g. germs.

Contagiosa impetigo It is a superficial infection of skin produced by *Staphylococcus aureus*. It presents with pea sized or larger macular, bullous, pustular or honey coloured, crusted, circinate lesions. Intervening area of skin remains unaffected. Itching is the main symptom. Lesions may heal within 2 to 3 weeks without scarring.

Contagious diseases Infectious diseases that can be transmitted to other people.

Contaminate To render impure by contract or mixture; in sterile technique, to introduce microorganisms.

Contamination The introduction of infectious material on normally clean or sterile sites.

Content analysis A process by which the text of archival records is reduced to quantifiable information.

Contexual threat The level of threat caused or implied by the little event to an average child of the same age, sex and biological characteristics.

Contigs A term for adjacent or partially overlapping clones.

Continence training Process of restoring control of urination.

Continent ostomy Surgically created opening in which liquid stool or urine is removed by siphoning.

Contingency A relationship between a response and its consequence or between two stimuli, sometimes considered a dependency.

Contingency contract A contract with a health professional or other support person that includes the process of setting a goal and identifying costs and rewards of goal attainment. The purpose of the contingency contract is to reinforce behaviors needed to reach a goal.

Contingency table Used to determine whether the distribution of one variable is conditionally dependent upon the other variable.

Continous variables Variables in which data are measured over the range of an uninterrupted numerical scale. Examples are height, weight, and age.

Continuing care Maintenance care; continued periodic reexamination and supervision of periodontal care after completion of treatment procedures.

Continuity of care Uninterrupted patient care despite the change in caregivers.

Continuity of medical care Management of a patient's care over time is coordinated among providers.

Continuous ambulatory peritoneal dialysis (CAPD) An alternative form of treatment for renal failure rather than the more complex and expensive hemodialysis.

Continuous conduction Propagation of an action potential (nerve impulse) in a step-by-step depolarization of each adjacent area of an axon membrane.

Continuous incontinence It occurs in vesico vaginal fistula. Dribbling of urine appearing immediately after instrumentation is traumatic injury during labour. Uretero vaginal fistula following cesarian section also presents with continous incontinence.

Continuous passive motion machine Electrical device that exercises joints.

Continuous positive airway pressure An airway maneuver, in spontaneously breathing patients, in which airway pressure is maintained above atmospheric pressure throughout the respiratory cycle of inspiratory and expiratory phases.

Continuous quality improvement Process of promoting care that reflects established agency standard.

Continuous subcutaneous insulin infusion A method for a controlled introduction of insulin beneath the skin.

Continuous traction It is a way of aligning the bone ends specially if the fracture is comminuted or unstable. It is usually applied by skeletal traction pin because prolonged skin traction may cause blisters. After enough healing has occurred to maintain length and alignment a plaster case is applied.

Continuus irrigation Ongoing instillation of solution.

Contoured seating Custom molded seating surface created by carving foam, building up the surface with pads and blocks, or preforming, based on research about human contours.

Contra-angle Instrument that has two or more offset angles of such a degree that the end of the instrument is kept within 3 mm of the long axis of the shaft; attachment for burs, stones, and disks to provide easy access to all posterior surfaces of the teeth.

Contraception Any device which prevents contraception. Contraception devices tend to represent either a barrier between sperm and ovum or a means of preventing implantation of a fertilised ovum in uterine wall. The most common is condom for males and pills for woman.

Contract A binding agreement between two or more parties.

Contract dentistry Providing dental care under a specific set of guidelines under an accepted agreement.

Contracted pelvis It is one in which one or more diameters are less than minimal normal range by over 1 cm making the delivery of an average sized baby through the natural passage difficult or impossible. It may be classified as contraction of the diameter in any of four major morphologic types and asymmetrical contraction in pelvic deformities.

Contractile unit The sarcomere, the basic functional unit of skeletal muscle.

Contractility The ability of cells or parts of cells to actively generate force to undergo shortening for movements. Muscle fibers (cells) exhibit a high degree of contractility.

Contraction The intermittent shortening of a muscle, especially the uterus during labour in order to expel the contents.

Contraction stress test A method of evaluating FHR in the presence of spontaneous or oxytocininduced contractions. The premise is that oxygenation of a marginally compromised fetus will transiently worsen with uterine contractions.

Contractions Braxton Hicks Uterine contractions, occurring periodically during pregnancy, that enlarge the uterus to accommodate the growing fetus. During the third trimester, they are felt as a painless hardening or tightening of the uterus. They can become painful and are often difficult to differentiate from labor.

Contracture It is a permanent flexing of a muscle because its tissues have shortened or shrunk, cases include thickening and scarring through injury or disease. Surgical remedy is possible.

Contractures-pregnancy Long-lasting, low-amplitude epochs of myometrial activity that occur throughout pregnancy.

Contrafissure A fracture in a part opposite the site of a blow.

Contraindication A circumstance or condition that, because of associated risk, makes the use of a particular intervention inadvisable.

Contraindication to breast feeding In case of open T.B. baby may be at risk of infection. In case of typhoid or septicemia or pneumonia mother may be too weak to feed. Insanity and severe epilepsy is strongly contraindicated.

Contralateral Regers to opposite side of the body compare with ipsilateral, same side.

Contralateral neglect Neglect of a part of the body or world on the side opposite (that is, contralateral) to a brain injury; also called neglect.

Contransport The simultaneous transport, by a single transporter, of two solutes across a membrane.

Contrast medium Substance that adds density to a body organ or cavity, such as barium sulfate or iodine.

Contrast bath Contrast baths are a popular method of treatment following soft tissues and joint injury. The alteration of warmth and cold stimulates blood flow and may assist in reduction of swelling. Recommended procedure is of alternate hot (up to 45° C) and iced water in a ratio of approximately 3:1 minutes. Routine should commence and finish with iced water.

Contrast echocardiography Procedure in which a contrast agent is injected intravenously during an echocardiogram to improve the diagnostic accuracy.

Contrast effect In the study of punishment, the change in the value of an incentive according to another incentive with which it is compared. For example, after regular receipt of a large reward, a small reward appears much smaller than it would otherwise.

Contrast therapy Alternating applications of heat and cold is referred to as 'contrast therapy'. It is directed at improving circulation in injured tissues.

Contributory negligence A legal theory that prevents plaintiffs, from recovering damages if they are even 1% at fault. This has been supplanted in most states by comparative negligence.

Control The term is used in three contexts : (i) the process of keeping the relevant conditions of an experiment constant, (ii) causing an independent variable to vary in a specified and known manner, and (iii) using a spontaneously occurring and discoverable fact as a check or standard of comparison to evaluate the facts obtained after the manipulation of the independent variable.

Control center The component of a feedback system, such as the brain, that determines the point at which a controlled condition, such as body temperature, is maintained.

Control condition Subjects comparable to the experimental group in all respects except for the factor under investigation, usually referred to as the independent variable.

Control group A group of participants in an experiment who receive no 'treatment' so that their behavior can be compared with the participants who do receive 'treatment'; the experimental group. Without a control group we do not know if the experimental treatment did have any effect.

Control recording Audio recording of the voice of a suspected person as representative as possible of her/his intravariability.

Control variable An extraneous factor that might influence the dependent variable, making it difficult to evaluate the effect of the independent variable; in an experiment, attempts are made to isolate or control such effects systematically.

Controlled substances Drugs whose prescription and dispensing are regulating by federal law because they have the potential for abuse.

Conus arteriosus The outflow tract of the right ventricle; infundibulum.

Conus medullaris The inferior, tapering portion of the spinal cord.

Convalescence It is the period of relaxed healing and recovery after an acute illness or surgery. During this period patient may need considerable reassurance and mental support as well as physical assistance.

Convalescent carriers These are persons in whom a limited, localised infection continue for a variable period, weeks or months after clinical recovery from typhoid fever, the organisms may localise in the gall bladder and discharged in faeces.

Convection Transfer of heat energy to air that is flowing away from the skin.

Convenience form Modification's necessary, beyond basis outline form, to facilitate proper instrumentation for the preparation of the cavity or insertion of the restorative material; also, the placing of starting points or slight undercuts to retain the first portions of restorative material while succeeding portions are placed.

Conventional medicine The treatment available in modern system of therapy.

Conventional prosthetic socket It is simply a hard socket with a soft liner in it. The liner is usually made pelite and is essentially a filler to

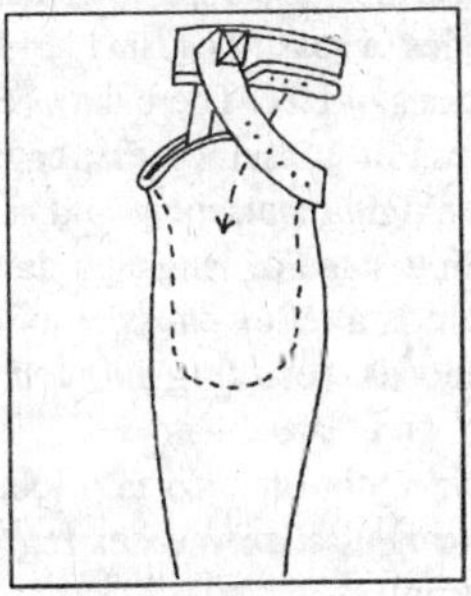

decrease the problems of residue volume fluctuation.

Conventional radiography Use of x-radiation and x-ray film to record an image.

Conventional therapy One or two daily injections of insulin, including mixed intermediate and rapid-acting insulins, daily self-monitoring of urine or blood glucose, and education about diet and exercise.

Convergence The medial movement of the two eyeballs so that both are directed towards a near object being viewed in order to produce a single image.

Convergent strabismus In it deviating eye turns inward. This is very common in children.

Conversation The use of verbal and nonverbal communication to interact with others.

Conversion A defence mechanism, operating unconsciously, by which intrapsychic conflicts that would otherwise give rise to anxiety are, instead, given symbolic external expression.

The repressed ideas or impulses, and the psychologic defences against them, are converted into a variety of somatic symptoms involving the nervous system. These may include such symptoms as paralysis, pain, or loss of sensory function.

Conversion disorder A psychiatric syndrome characterized by disturbances of bodily functions that dont correspond to known patho-physiological mechanism.

Convex Having a surface or boundary that curves or bulges outward, as the exterior of a sphere.

Convexoconcave Convex on one surface and concave on the other.

Convolution An elevation on the surface of a structure and an infolding of the tissue upon itself.

Convulsion It is the muscle spasm of many muscles. There is a series of spasms causing jerking of limbs and contractions of face. There may be fainting or temporary loss of consciousness, causes include epilepsy, meningitis, poisoning and diabetes.

Cooing The first stage of language development , in which there is a reflex emission of air through the vocal chords, resulting in such sounds as "oooohhhh" and "aaaahhhh".

Coolant Air or liquid directed into tooth tissue or restoration to neutralize the heating effect of a rotatory instrument.

Coombs' test Diganostic test using antiimmunoglobulin to agglutinate antibodycoated erythrocytes.

Cooper's ligaments A pectineal ligament, suspensory ligaments of breast.

Cooperative play Organised play with group goals.

Coopernails sign A clinical sign of fracture of pelvis where ecchymosis is present on the perineum, scrotum or labia.

Copal An odorless and tasteless, yellowish to yellowish brown resin obtained from various tropical trees or dug from the ground as a fossil.

Co-parenting Co-operation between divorced parents in the raising of their children.

Copayment Amount or percentage of the total approved amount that the subscriber is obligated to pay. This is not to be confused with deductible amount.

COPD Chronic obstructive pulmonary disease.

Coping The process through which individuals deal with the variety of social and environmental factors encountered in life.

Coping mechanisms Ways of adjusting to environmental stress without altering one's goals or purposes; includes both conscious and unconscious mechanisms.

Coping skills Those abilities that enable an individual to indentify and manage stress and related reactions.

Coping strategies Stress-reduction activities selected on a conscious level.

Coping technique A method for reducing or preventing the onset of negative consequences.

Copoious Present in large quantity.

Copolymer A polymer made from the polymerization of two or more different types of monomers.

Copper Plasma contains 110 mg/100 ml of copper. Copper deficiency results in anemia, hypopigmentation, change in texture of hair, failure of myelination and CNS defects.

Copper dental cement It is a zinc phosphate cement to the powder of which has been added a copper oxide.

Copper-food content

Copper in mg/100 gm of food	
Almonds	1210
Apple	120
Bananas	200
Bread	960
Carrots	80
Cabbage	50
Liver beef	2450
Spinach	197
Sweet potato	184
Walnut	1000
Wheat	787
Mushrooms	1790
Oranges	80
Peas dried	802

Copper-T It is the most common family planning method used by women in India.

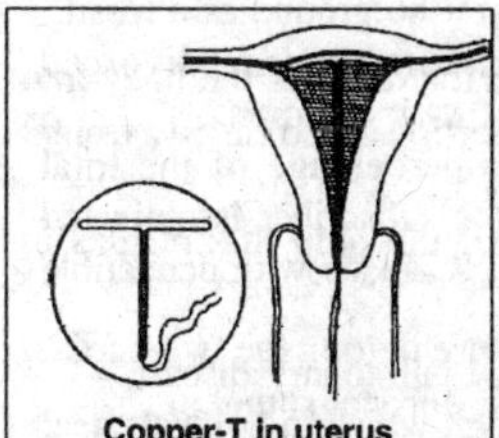

Copper-T in uterus

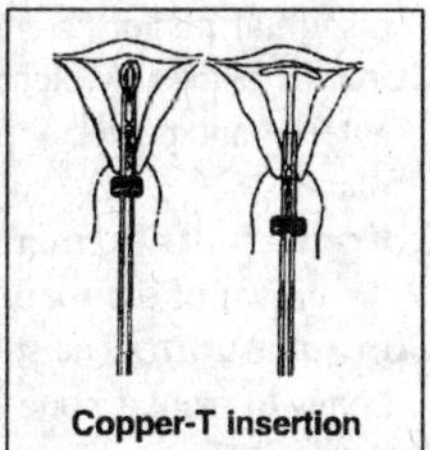

Copper-T insertion

Copping resources The personal and social resources an individual has at his experience of distress.

Copresence The simultaneous participation in perception, experience and activity by two more alters.

Coprotease A protein that acts to stimulate the autoproteolytic activity of another protein.

Copulatory bursa In female insects, a pouch or an expansion of the median oviduct into which sperm are deposited by the male insect during copulation.

Copying mechanisms Unconscious tactics used to protect the psyche.

Coracidium An oncosphere surrounded by a ciliated embryophore.

Coracoacrominal arch The arch like structure located betweeen subacrominal bursa and acromioclavicular joint.

Cord around the neck If cord is found turned round the neck, it is not wise to cut the cord. It will cut off the O_2 immediately. If baby is hypoxic and there is delay in delivery, chances of survival are reduced.

Cord prolapse It is the condition, when membrane rupture allowing a loop of cord of prolapse through the cervical OS. The cord is either in vagina or protruding outside the labia cord compression due to presenting part or due to the spasm of vessels due to change in temperature and may be the end result.

Cordocentesis A technique for obtaining a sample of fetal blood from the umbilical vein for fetal disease diagnosis or therapy.

Cordotomy Surgical interruption of pain pathways in the spinal cord.

Core The central part.

Core temperature The mean temperature of thermal core i.e. interior of body.

Corepressors Adaptor proteins that act as a bridge between nuclear receptors and general transcription factors to inhibit transcription.

Corn It is a benign condition manifested by polished flesh coloured, conical, well-circumscribed, hyperkeratotic nodule occurring in sole due to tight fitting of shoes. It is hard when develop on sole and soft between the toes. It is tender and recurs. Salicylic acid application makes it soft.

Cornea It is the anterior part of the outer coat of eyeball. It is transparent and has more curvature than the rest of the eyeball. It appears elliptical of about 12 mm in horizontal meridian and 11 mm in vertical meridian. The radius of curvature of anterior surface is 7.8 mm and that of posterior surface is 6.5 mm in adults. Cornea is more flat. In the periphery cornea is thicker than at centre cornea is avascular and gets its nutrition for air aqueous humour and diffusion of tissue fluid from perilimbal capillaries. Cornea is very sensitive and is supplied by first condition of ophthalmic division of fifth cranial nerve. The transparency of cornea depends on its hydration and regularity of stromal components. Transparent, anterior part of the fibrous tunic of the eye through which light enters the eye.

Cornea plana It is cogenital sometimes hereditary and occurs in an otherwise normal globe. Peripheral cornea frequently appears like sclera. There is no sharp delineation from the opaque zone to the transparent cornea. Cornea therefore appears extremely small.

Corneal oedema Any inflammatory, traumatic or degenerative lesion of the endoethelium may lead to a more or less pronounced corneal oedema. Cornea is thickened and looks grey. Clinically, cornea loses its normal lustre and appears slightly stippled on slit-lamp examination. Small droplet epithelial elevations are visible.

Corneal reflex Blinking in response to corneal contact.

Corneal scissors, universal These are used to enlarge the incision, for cataract surgery and keratoplasty to cut the corneal button.

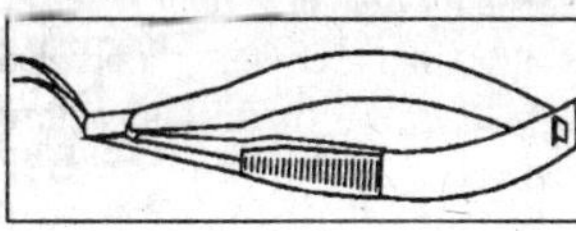

Corneal sensation Cornea is usually sensitive to touch. The sensitivity is reduced in deep herpes simplex, in neuroparalytic keratitis. Hyperaesthesia of cornea may also be observed in zoster ophthalmicus, damage to the trigeminal nerve, after cataract operation.

Corneal trephines These are used for corneal grafting. Available in various sizes. These are calibrated and accordingly one can produce a cut in the cornea depending on the requirement of the surgeon and/or thickness of the cornea.

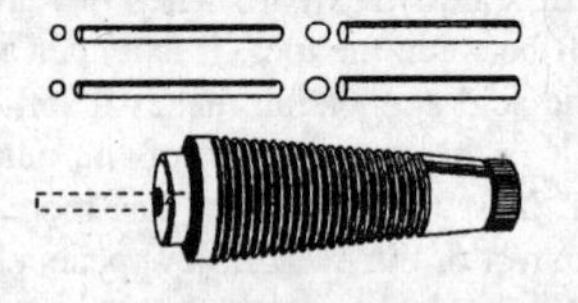

Corneal trephines

Corneal ulcer It is always due to exogenous infection. It develops due to diminished resistance of corneal epithelium and favoured by minute abrasions and corneal oedema. To start, there is localised necrosis involving epithelium and Bowman's membrane. After casting off sequestrum the ulcer appears larger, saucer shaped, the edges projecting above the normal surface of cornea due to oedema. A second zone of infiltration is formed by polymorphs, carrying out their digestive function of macerating and dissolving the necrotic tissue in the base of ulcer. With the regressive stage vascularisation of cornea occurs. If the scar formed on cornea is centrally placed covering pupillary area then it affects the vision. There will be pain associated with blephrospasm, photophobia and lacrimation. There will be intense congestion around cornea and marked loss of vision.

Cornual pregnancy Pregnancy in rudimentary horn is termed cornual pregnancy. Pregnancy has occurred in the cornua when corpus between was present in the ovary on the side of normal uterus suggesting transperitoneal migration of ovum.

Corona radiata The innermost layer of granulosa cells, that is firmly attached to the zona pellucida around a secondary oocyte.

Coronal Literally "like a crown" ; a coronal plane divides the body or an organ into anterior and posterior regions.

Coronal axis It lies in the coronal plane and extends horizontally from side to side. The movements of flexion and extension take place about this axis in a sagittal plane.

Coronal plane A plane that divides the body into anterior and posterior portions; also called a frontal plane.

Coronal pulp Portion of the pulp that resides in the crown of the tooth.

Coronal suture The suture uniting the two parietal bones to frontal bone is coronal suture.

Coronalis Encircling in the manner of a crown; a term applied to vessels, nerves, etc.

Coronaplasty Occlusal equilibration.

Coronary angioplasty It is the treatment of atherosclerotic narrowing and occlusion of coronary arteries by interventional catheter technique. The classic angioplasty procedure is conventional balloon dilatation. The balloon catheter generally is introduced over a guidewire through a guiding catheter. Because of 30 to 45% of restenosis, other angioplasty techniques such as coronary stenting, coronary atherectomy and laser ablation seems to be effective. Limitations of stenting are difficulty of deploying the device, its expense, problem of subacute stent thrombosis and intimal hyperplasia.

Coronary artery bypass It is done in case of myocardial infarction and when coronary arteries are blocked. After coronary angiography if there is sufficient blockage or narrowed lumen, operation is done by grafting an additional vessel to receive blood flow. When disease is localised to one or two segments of artery, it may be possible to relieve blockage by using a technique known, as ballooning angioplasty. The artery is stretched over the narrow segment. Bypass is a lengthy operation done under general anaesthesia with the support of heart lung machine. Hospital stay is about 3 to 5 days.

Coronary artery An artery that carries blood to the muscles of the heart; the left and right coronary arteries arise from the aorta.

Coronary artery spasm An involuntary constriction of the smooth muscle of the coronary arteries.

Coronary atherosclerosis Arteriosclerosis characterized by lipid deposits in the intima; irregularly distributed in large and mediumsized arteries of the heart.

Coronary cataract It manifests at puberty. It is situated in deeper layers of cortex and superficial layer of nucleus. It appears as corona of clubshaped opacities in the periphery of lens. The axial region of the lens and extreme periphery is clear. It is not progressive type of cataract. Slit-lamp under full mydriasis is helpful.

Coronary circulation Normal coronary flow is about 250 ml/per minute or 5% of the resting cardiac output. The volume of oxygen consumed by myocardium at rest is 40 ml/minute or 15% of total body consumption. Blood flow through coronary arteries is continuous throughout the cardiac cycle, about 2/3 occurring at diastole. Coronary sinus drains 90% of blood from left ventricles. Vagal stimulation has no direct effect on coronary circulation. Coronary flow increases if cardiac output increases and as a result of exercise. Angiotensin and vasopressin have a vasoconstrictor action.

Coronary embolism Blocking of a coronary blood vessel by a clot.

Coronary sinus A wide venous channel on the posterior surface of the heart that collects the blood from the coronary circulation and returns it to the right atrium.

Coronary steal Diversion of blood from poorly perfused areas of myocardium to those already adequately perfused.

Coronary thrombosis It is the obstruction or narrowing of one of the coronary vessels by a thrombus, thus depriving the blood supply and oxygen to a specific part of the heart. Then the specific part of heart does not get blood supply of oxygen. It is a major cause of heart disease and death of a patient.

Coronary vein Vein that carries blood from the heart muscle primarily to the right atrium.

Coroner Independent judicial officer of the crown who investigates the circumstances of some death.

Coroner's Jury A special jury called by the coroner to determine whether a person died because of criminal action.

Coronion The tip of the coronoid process of the mandible.

Coronoid fossa The depression in the anterior surface of distal end of humerus into which coronoid process of ulna fits.

Coronoid process Thin triangular rounded eminence originating from the anterosuperior surface of the ramus of the mandible. Provides insertion for the various fiber bundles of the temporal muscle.

Corpora callosum A large tract of white matter within the brain that connects the right and left cerebral hemispheres.

Corpora cavernosa Two columns of erectile tissue found in the shaft of the penis.

Corporate practice of medicine When physicians are employees of nonphysician corporations that are in the business of providing medical services.

Corpus albicans A white fibrous patch in the ovary that forms after the corpus luteum regresses.

Corpus bursa A component of the female reproductive tract where the spermatophore is deposited.

Corpus callosum The connecting structure between the two hemispheres of the brain, currently assumed to be responsible for the development of duplicate memories, one in each of the cerebral hemispheres, it apparently transmits information gained in one hemisphere to the other one.

Corpus cavernosum urethrae Corpus spongiosum penis.

Corpus luteum A hormone-secreting glandular structure transformed after ovulation from a ruptured follicle; it secretes chiefly progresterone, with some estrogen secreted as well. The yellow matter found within the ruptured follicle after the ovum has been discharged.

Corpus spongiosum A spongy body that contains urethral bridge from the prostate to the tip of the glans penis.

Corpus striatum A subcortical mass of gray and white substance in front of and lateral to the thalamus in each cerebral hemisphere.

Corpuscle of touch A touch sensory receptor found in the papillary layer of the dermis of the skin; also called Meissner's corpuscle.

Correct posture Defective posture is the most common cause of backache when sitting, reading, speaking or typing for long periods. One should learn to stand properly and to collect fallen items from gound correctly.

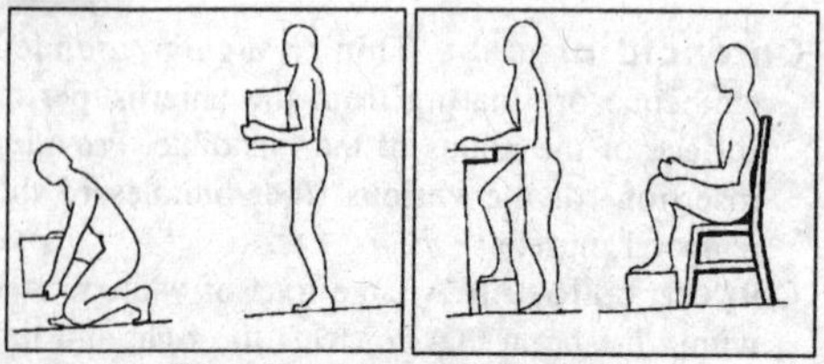

Correct posture to avoid back pain

Corrected gestational age Gestational age that a preterm infant would be if still in utero. May also be called developmental age.

Correlation The degree of relatedness or correspondence between two variables, expressed by a coefficient that can range from +1.00 to -1.00; 0.00 signifies no correspondence.

Corrigan's pulse An extensive form of bounding pulse in which the arterial pulse shows a rapid rise and fall. It is seen in aortic regurgitation but also in patent ductus arteriosus and arteriovenous aneurysm.

Corrode To eat away or wear away, as by rust, causing deterioration of a substance.

Corrosion Tools dental appliances though mode of steel undergo surface and structural deterioration when left unprotected. Deterioration of a metal by chemical or electrochemical reaction is termed corrosion.

Corrosion fatigue Biomechanical term for fatigue failure caused by surface corosion.

Corset It is a device used for backpain and spinal injuries. It is similar to weightlifter's belt. The belt keeps restriction of the movement. Rigid corsets are made of plaster or of lightweight plastic.

Cortex The outer part of an organ such as the brain, kidney, adrenal gland, or hair.

Cortical blindness A total failure to appreciate incoming visual sensory information owing to a lesion in the cortex, rather than injury to the eyes.

Cortical Bone The dense, compact bone that surrounds the medullary cavity.

Cortical bone graft Any autogenous or other bone graft composed of dense, cortical bone.

Cortical column Unit of cortical organization that represents a vertically organized functional unit.

Cortical mosaic Mosaic arrangement created by interdigitation of cortical modules of different kinds.

Cortical type sensory loss Diminution of tactile perception associated with damage to the primary sensory cortex.

Corticated A well-defined outer border of a radiolucent lesion; appears radiopaque.

Corticoids Hormones secreted by three cell layers of the adrenal cortex.

Corticospinal tract A bundle of fibers directly connecting the cerebral cortex to the spinal cord.

Corticosteroid drugs These are the group of drugs similar to the natural corticosteroid hormones produced by adrenal glands. These are used in the treatment of inflammatory intestinal disorders such as Crohn's disease and ulcerative colitis. Asthma, rheumatoid arthritis, eczema and iritis improve with corticosteroids. They are also used to suppress the immune system to prevent rejection of transplanted organ. Side effects include oedema, hypertension, diabetes mellitus, peptic ulcer and development of extra hair on face. They lower the immune system.

Corticosteroid related myopathy Any abnormal condition that affects the muscular tissues, usually proximal muscles.

Corticotrope Cell type in the anterior pituitary that synthesizes and secretes ACTH which in turn stimulates glucocorticoid secretion from adrenal cortex.

Cortin General term for the hormonal secretion of the adrenal cortex.

Cortisol Steroid hormone released by the adrenal cortex; increases blood glucose and inhibits inflammation; it is a glucocorticoid.

Cosmetic dentistry It is the procedure to improve the appearance of teeth. Teeth that are out of alignment can become decayed because such teeth are hard to keep clean. With the help of orthodontic appliance teeth can be moved to correct position. Bonding is used to treat chipped or malformed teeth to close small gaps between front teeth. It may be used to cover stained or coloured teeth. Bleaching is used to treat teeth that have become discoloured because the pulp is dead.

Cosmetic hand An artificial hand in which appearance is emphasized.

Cosmic radiation Cosmic radiation originating outside the atmosphere of earth emanating from galactic or solar sources and consisting of particles capable of producing ionising events. Cosmic rays are primarily charged particles and heavy ions. Secondary cosmic rays may have energies in the hundreds of MeV range.

Cosmid A plasmid cloning vector containing bacteriophage lambda cos sites incorporated into the plasmid DNA.

Costa A striated rod, associated with the basal bodies of many flagellates, that courses along the base of an undulating membrane.

Costal Pertaining to a rib.

Costal angle An angle formed by right and left costal cartilage at the xiphoid process.

Costal cartilage The cartilage that connects the ribs to the sternum.

Costal groove of the rib The groove along the inferior border of the rib dorsally that changes to the internal surface of the rib where it bends.

Costalcartilage Hyaline cartilage that attaches a rib to the sternum.

Cost-benefit analysis Measures and compares the costs and benefits of a proposed course of action in terms of the same units, usually monetary units such as dollars.

Cost-effectiveness analysis Provides a way of comparing the cost of different proposed means to a particualr end in terms of the most appropriate measurement units. Assesses the least costly means of achieving a fixed goal.

Costoclavicular syndrome Symptom is seen in old clavicular fracture with hypertrophied subclavian muscle. When shoulders are moved backwards and downwards, neurovascular compression symptoms occur like pain, paraesthesia, numbness and weakness in arms and hands. On X-ray, fracture of clavicle and anomaly of first rib is seen.

Costophrenic angle The junction of the costal and diaphragmatic pleurae.

Costovertebral angle Angle formed by articulation of ribs with bodies of thoracic vertebra.

Costovertebral pleura The serous membrane that lines the ribs and vertebrae.

Cotransduoible Relating to or involved in contransduction.

Cotransport Active transport process in which two substances are moved together across a cell membrane; for example, sodium and glucose may be transported together across a membrane.

Cotton's fracture An eponym for a trimalleolar fracture of ankle.

Cough It is a reflex action to clear the airways of mucus, foreign body or any other irritant blocking the bronchi. Cough may be a symptom of underlying disease. In case of children, inflammation of upper respiratory tract can narrow airway and result in a barking or whooping cough. In bronchitis, cough contains large amount of infected phlegm.

Sufferer has to cough persistently to bring up phlegm, which may be associated with bleeding. Bronchospasm, as in asthma will cause a dry cough; worse at night. Pneumonia results in painful coughing which may have tinge of blood. Bronchiectasis causes early morning large amount of foul smelling mucopurulent cough. Antibiotics and bronchodilators help the patient.

Cough CPR In it one maintains cerebral perfusion and consciousness during severe arrhythmias by repeated coughing. It has been successful for 1-3 minutes till defibrillator is available.

Cough fracture Bilateral fractures of axillary segments of sixth to 9th ribs. These fractures are non displaced resulting due to violent cough.

Cough impulse test It determines the saphenofemoral incompetency. The fingers are placed over the course of vein just below the saphenous opening and the patient is asked to cough—a palpable fluid thrill and a bruit on auscultation are evident if the valve at the sapheno-femoral junction is incompetent.

Cough syncope During paroxysms of prolonged coughing intrathoracic pressure rises which may cause syncopal attack due to diminished cardiac output, cough-induced peripheral vasodilation and rise in intracranial pressure.

Counseling skills Interventions that include communicating with patients, actively listening to the exchange of information, offering pertinent health teaching, and providing emotional support.

Countebore The slight enlargement at the superior aspect of the osteotomy that allows the next gradual enlargement to take place.

Counter extension Technique consisting of traction on one part of limb while the remainder of limb is held steady.

Counterclockwise rotation Used in describing rotation of the thorax or pelvis. With the transverse plane as a reference and 12 o'clock at midpoint anteriorly, rotation forward on the right is counterclockwise rotation.

Counterconditioning The procedure of classical conditioning, used in therapy to remove some fear or other negative affective state. A positive stimulus is presented in such a fashion that it outweighs the patient's potential negative response to the fear producing stimulus.

Countercurrent heat exchange A process of temperature regulation that occurs within the pampiniform plexus. Cooler venous blood acts as a heat-sink for the warmer arterial blood arriving from the abdomen, thus lowering the temperature of the arterial blood as it reaches the testis.

Counterirritants Counterirritants are substances which are applied to mask the visceral pain by causing irritation at local application over skin. It is used to promote healing to reduce inflammation and to relieve congestion.

Counterirritation Superficial stimulation that relieves a deeper sensation by stimulating different sensory signals.

Counterphobia The desire for seeking out experiences that are consciously or unconsciously feared.

Counterpuncture A second opening made opposite the one.

Counters It is the system used to measure the radioactivity emanating from a sample. There are counters for gamma-emitters and for beta-emitters. In beta-counters, sample is admixed with a scintillation fluid which gives off light when hit by the beta-radiation. The detecter then detects the light emitted which is proportional to beta-radiation present.

Counters are used in nuclear imaging when quantitative data analysis is required as in PET imaging. Gamma-counters detect the emitted gamma-rays using detector system similar to those used in gamma-cameras with light flashes being produced when gamma-rays impinge on scinitillation crystal.

Counterstain A stain applied to render the effects of another stain more discernible.

Countertraction Use of client's body weight or other weights, ropes, and pulleys to counter the pull of the traction weight.

Countertransference The psychiatrist's partly unconscious or conscious emotional reactions to the patient.

Couple A combination of two : a pair.

Coupled reactions Two chemical reactions that have a common intermediate and thus a means of energy transfer from one of the other.

Couplet Two consecutive atrial or ventricular extrasystoles; paired extrasystoles.

Coupling Phenomenon of consistent association of one motion (translation or rotation) about an axis with another motion about a second axis: One motion cannot be produced without the other.

Coupling agent Liquid or gel filling the gap between skin and transducer to avoid intervening air.

Courtship behavior Behaviors exchanged between a male and a female of the same species prior to mating.

Courtship song In songbirds, a type of song given at close range after pairing, influencing mate choice.

Courvoisier's law It is a clinical rule which expresses that the gall bladder is enlarged and often palpable when jaundice appears in biliary obstruction due to neoplasm, but is small and non-palpable in obstruction due to stone.

Couvade Pregnancy related rituals or a cluster of symptoms experienced by some prospective father during pregnancy and child birth.

Couvade syndrome A phenomenon whereby the father or partner manifests pregnancy related symptoms, such as nausea, vomiting, alterations in appetite, weight gain, abdominal pain, backache, leg cramps, elusive toothaches, and other aches and pains in different parts of the body.

Couvelaire uterus It is a rare type of abruptio placentae. The uterus has a purplish coppery colour. The uterine muscle is degenerated and infiltrated with blood. There is dissociation of middle and outer layers. Blood vessel shows acute degenerative arteriolitic changes. Coagulation failure takes place.

Covalent bond Chemical bond that is formed when two atoms share a pair of electrons. A chemical bond that involves sharing of electron pairs.

Cover screw A root form component that closes of the interior receptor area of an implant in the osteointegration healing protocol.

Covert abruptio placentae Abruptio placentae whereby central separation entraps lost blood between the uterine wall and the placenta.

Covert conditioning A procedure in counterconditioning in which the negative stimulus is not actually present but only imagined by the fearful individual. The conditioning procedures are applied to the imagined aspects, at least in the early stages of therapy.

Cow's modified milk One part of cows milk is diluted with three or four parts of water. This reduces the sodium and caseinogen content. Boiling makes caseinogen easily digestible. Addition of a quarter teaspoonful of sugar to each ounce makes up the sugar deficiency.

Cowper's gland One of two glands located at the base of the prostate gland and on either side of the membranous urethra that produce a mucinous substance that lubricates the urethra and coats its surface.

Coxa The bone of the hip.

Coxa plana Flat hip in Perthes disease.

Coxa senilis Degenerative hip disease concomittant with age.

Coxal bone The pelvic bone or hipbone (also known as the os coxae or the innominate bone); formed by fusion of three distinct bones (ilium, ischium, and pubis) during skeletal development.

CPAP mask Device that maintains positive pressure in the airway throughout the respiratory cycle.

CPR Cardiopulmonary resuscitation.

CQT Control Question Technique.

Crack A highly addictive form of cocaine that has been processed to be smoked.

Crack cocaine A class of tests of statistical significance that depend on dividing some parameter (such as a difference between means by the standard error of that parameter.

Cracked nipple This may occur during lactation. It may result in acute infective mastitis. Nipple and areola should be cared well with a lanolin during last 2 months of pregnancy. If nipple is severely cracked during lactation it may be avoided and resumed gradually. When baby vigorously and fruitlessly sucks engorged breasts cracks develop in nipples. These become infected and tender. Cracked nipples may bleed during sucking. In such cases, breast feed may be discontinued for 72 hours and milk may be expressed manually.

Cracking and crackling Damaged articular surfaces produce crepitus when moved. When coarse, it may be appreciated as grating and in badly damaged weight bearing joint; may be clearly audible as creak. But similar sounds arising during shoulder or scapular movements do not indicate of disease. Joint craking, the snapping sound arising from knee during full flexion or from metacarpophalangeal joint during passive hyperextension is due to the cavitation in which a bubble of gas forms within the joint.

Crackle Fine bubbling sound heard on auscultation of the lung.

Crackles Adventitious breath sounds heard on auscultation of the parenchymal tissues of the lungs when fluid has accumulated in the distal airways or when air sac are collapsed and partially reopening during inspiration.

Cradle position A common position for breastfeeding in which the baby is cradled in the mother's arms and brought to the level of her breast for feeding.

Cramp It is a painful spasm of muscle caused by excessive and prolonged contraction of muscle fibres. These occur during or just after exercise due to collection of lactic acid. Profuse sweating, fever, heatwave or prolonged exercise can lead to cramps in resting muscle. Cramps at night may be due to poor circulation of blood into legs but often there may not be any known cause.

Cranial Upward, towards the head.

Cranial mononeuropathies Facial palsies can occur in association with mumps and infectious mononucleosis. Depending upon the extent of the oedematous compression, there will be conduction block with segmental demyelination or infarction of nerve with distal wallerian degeneration. The facial palsy usually becomes nearly complete within a few hours. There may be pain in or behind ear. Face is twisted to the side opposite to the palsy. An early symptom is lacrimation. Weakness usually affects the uper and lower parts of face equally, patient's with Bell's palsy are unable to close eyes on the affected side.

Cranial cavity Space inside the skull that contains the brain.

Cranial nerve One of a set of nerves that controls sensory and motor functions of the head; includes senses of smell, vision, audition, taste, and touch on the face and head. The 12 pairs of nerves that arise from brain and leave the skull through separate apertures.

Cranial vault Eight skull bones that surround and protect the brain.

Craniometaphyseal dysplasia This condition is most common as an autosomal dominant disorder of modelling of metaphysis, sclerosis of skull base and overgrowth of face.

Craniometaphyseal dysplasia syndrome It is different than Pyle's disease. It is inherited in a more severe autosomal recessive form and in a more benign dominant form. Person will develop vomiting, headache, deafness and paralysis of facial muscles. Skull is enlarged with osteosclerosis. Sinuses are obliterated.

Craniosacral Pertaining to parasympathetic nerves.

Craniostenosis Premature closure of cranial sutures resulting in malformation of the skull.

Craniosynostosis There is an early closure of sutures of skull, e.g. Erozon disease or Apert syndrome and rickets. It is to be treated before 6 months of age to avoid damage. Operation is done to separate the skull bones by cutting away fused edges.

Cranium The endochondral bones of the skull that enclose or support the brain and the organs of sight, hearing, and balacne.

Crater formation Formation of interdental depressions in gingival tissue or subjacent bones.

Crawl Reciprocal movement of arms and legs in which the stomach contacts the supporting surface.

Crazing The formation of fine cracks on the surface of a material as a result of stresses built up by dimensional changes within the structure; a common example is crazing of a denture base as a result of stresses produced by alternate drying and soaking.

C-reactive protein An acute-phase reactant to inflammation, recently related to an increased risk for coronary artery disease.

Cream A type of lubricant that is in a semisolid or solid state.

Crease A line or a well-defined depression, usually on the skin, formed in zones of folding, such as those on the palms of the hands.

Creatine An organic compound that combines with phosphate to form creatine phosphate, which serves as a source of energy for anaerobic muscle contraction.

Creatine phosphokinase (CPK) An enzyme that catalyzes the transfer of a high-energy phosphate from phosphocreatine to ADP; creatine kinase.

Creatinine It is formed in the muscles during muscular metabolism. The phosphagen of muscle is broken down during muscular activity into creatine and phosphate. Creatine is dehydrated creatinine.

Creatinine Height index It is an index of skeletal muscle catabolism. It is measured by urinary creatinine excretion for 24 hours divided by expected urinary excretion in normal course.

Creative thinking The ability to produce work that is both novel and appropriate. A novel product is one that is original and not predictable. An appropriate product satisfies problem constraints, fulfills a need, is sensible, and useful.

Crede maneuver Technique for emptying urine from a flaccid bladder; repeated pressure is placed between the umbilicus and symphysis pubis in a downward direction; manual pressure is also placed directly over bladder to further facilitate removal of urine.

Crede's method Manual bladder compression used to stimulate urination.

Credential Letter or certificate given to a person to verify that the person has the right to assume a certain authority or perform an activity.

Creep It is the gradual but permanent change in dimension that occurs in an object exposed to a constant load. Most materials undergo creep at or near of their melting points.

Creeping eruption The irritation and rash caused by hookworm larvae in an unnatural host.

Cremaster muscle Extension of abdominal muscles, in the male it raises the testis.

Crenate Scalloped or notched.

Crenation A notched or scalloped appearance of the red blood cell membrane caused by the osmotic loss of water from these cells.

Crenulations Characteristic ruffles in the outer cell wall layers characteristic of spirochetes of the genus Pillotina.

Crepitus Crackling sound produced by the rubbing together of fragments of fractured bone.

Crescent sign Typical crescent sign in avascular necrosis of femoral head is best visualised in frog position.

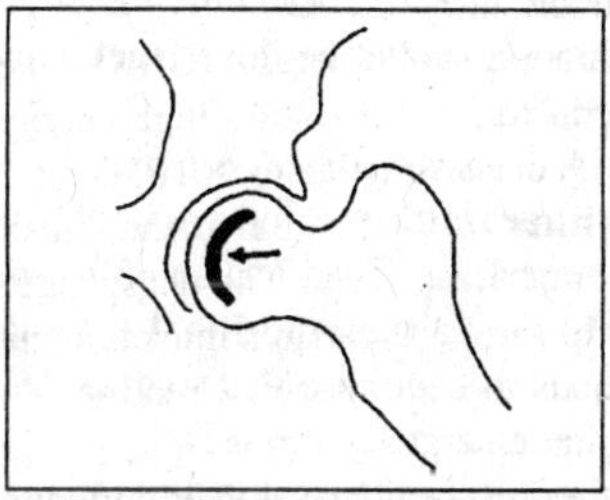

Crescent sublingual It is a crescnet shaped area on the floor of month formed by lingual wall of mandible and the adjacent part of the floor of the mouth.

Crescentic glomerulonephritis It occurs as a consequence of focal necrotizing glomerulonephritis. Inflammatory exudate, along with proliferation of epithelial cells lines the Bowman capsule forming crescent.

Cresol It is used as an antiseptic. Lysol is a mixture of cresol and soap solution. Both cresol and lysol are less toxic than phenol. Local application of 5% solution may produce severe necrosis of local parts which may even need amputation. Inhalation may cause loss of consciousness, shock and cyanosis within a few minutes. Ingestion causes symptoms to develop over 1 to 16 hours. The person may suffer recurrent vomiting and abdominal pain and ulceration in mouth. Late features include chemical alveolitis, myocardial failure, pulmonary oedema and death.

Crest A thickened ridge of bone for the attachment of muscle.

Crest syndrome There develops systemic sclerosis with prominent calcinosis.

Cretinism An abnormality of structure and behaviour which results from insufficient thyroid secretion during early growth. It involves stunted growth, protruding abdomen, and pronounced mental retardation.

Creutzfeldt-Jacob disease It is a rare disorder and older people are generally affected. After a vague prodromal illness of change of mood and general malaise, focal neurological deficits such as dysphagia, ataxia or visual hallucination can occur. Myoclonic jerks are frequent. Later on cortical blindness, rigidity and muscle wasting may occur. Most patients do not survive more than few months. EEG may show stereotyped generalised triphasic complexes occurring once or twice a second. No successful treatment is available.

Crevice A narrow opening due to a fissure or a crack.

Crevice corrosion An accelerated corrosion caused by differences in the concentration of oxygen and pH levels within a groove or crevice compared with sites outside of the crevice; commonly found at the margins of metallic restorations, such as amalgams.

Crevicular fluid Sulcular fluid; characteristic fluid in the gingival sulcus that is similar but not identical to tissue fluid.

Cribriform Perforated.

Cribriform plate Alveolar bone that forms the tooth socket and to which the periodontal ligament is attached.

Cricoarytenoid arthritis Patient complains of pain and feeling of pressure during speech and swallowing. There develops hoarseness or other vocal dysfunction. Laryngoscopy shows redness and oedema with variable fixation of arytenoid cartilage. It may result due to rheumatoid arthritis.

Cricoid cartilage A ring-shaped cartilage that forms the inferior portion of the larynx. Partially ossified, ringlike cartilage that forms the lower part of larynx.

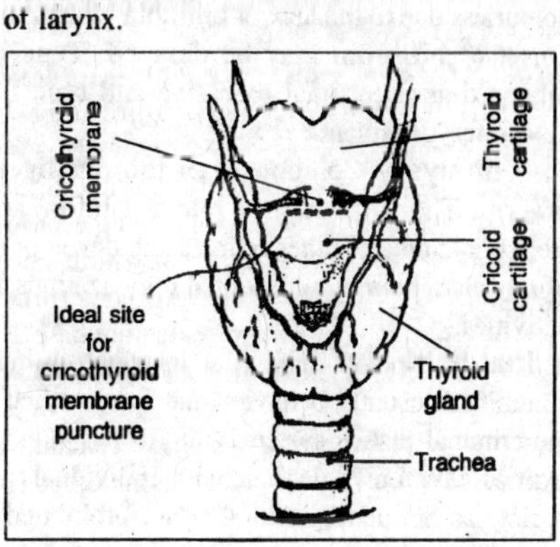

Cricopharyngeal sphincter This lies at the upper end of oesophagus at the level of C_6 and is composed of striated muscle. Its action is voluntary as well as reflex. It acts as a sphincter normally but as a valve when paralysed.

Normally it allows fluids to pass from the pharynx into the oesophagus, but not in reverse direction. When paralysed, it tends to obstruct the passage of fluids from the pharynx to the oesophagus but not in reverse direction. The lower part of oesophagus containing plain muscle is not affected by relaxant while cricopharyngeal sphincter behaves like stripped muscle.

Cricothyroid Pertaining to the cricoid and thyroid cartilages.

Cricothyroid çartilage Less prominent cricothyroid cartilage is located about 1.5 cm inferior to thyroid cartilage. Cricothyroid ligament lies between the criocoid and thyroid cartilages in the neck. It is palpated in most patients with neck extended.

Cricothyroidotomy It is an emergency procedure used for glottic or supraglottic airway obstruction. It is the fastest means of establishing an airway. It can be performed with the percutaneous placement of large bore needle through the cricothyroid membrane.

Cricothyrotomy Formation of an artificial opening in a victim's air passageway through the membrane between the cricoid and thyroid cartilage.

Crigler-Najjar syndrome There is congenital absence of enzyme uridine diphosphate (UDP) glucuronyl transferase. Type I is characterised by the onset of jaundice at birth. Bile secreted is colourless due to the lack of bilirubin glucuronide. Onset of bilirubin may be delayed. Type I is inherited as autosomal recessive and type II as autosomal dominant.

Crime analysis Component of the intelligence process. The revelation of relevant information from crime data or other sources and development of models representing criminal organizations and activities.

Criminal behavior Behaviour in which crime is committed, usually behavior that is identified by the criminal justice system.

Criminal law Laws dealing with individuals and society as defined by acts that are prohibited by stature or regulation and punishable by fine or imprisonment.

Criminal malpractice It happens when a medical man shows gross unskilled or unreasonable carelessness in the course of treatment resulting in serious injury to or death of the patient by acts on omission or commission. When doctor issues false certificate, abort the otherwise healthy female child and does sex detection. Recording of dying declaration should be done legally and carefully by a doctor.

Crisis A decisive moment or point.

Crisis intervention A form of brief psychotherapy that emphasises identification of the specific event precipitating the emotional trauma and uses methods to neutralise that trauma. Often used in hospital emergency rooms.

Crista A crest or ridged structure. A small elevation in the ampulla of each semicircular duct that contains receptors for dynamic equilibrium.

Crista ampullaris A specialized receptor located within the semicircular canals that detects head movements.

Crista galli Projection of the ethmoid bone in the anterior cranial fossa that assists in attaching the dura matter of the brain.

Crista terminalis A muscular ridge that separates the right atrium into two parts.

Criteria Standards upon which a decision can be based; established rules or principles for any given test.

Critical diameter The minimum diameter of an explosive charge that will sustain a detonation shock wave. Strictly this is for an unconfined explosive.

Critical organ It is the organ which during an application of ionising radiation recieves the highest relative dose with respect to its radiosensitivity. In medical imaging, radiation dose given is so slow and low that it is not detrimental to any organ. In nuclear imaging, the critical organ is that which has the highest radiopharmaceutical uptake in relation to its radio uptake.

Critical period A term with special reference to imprinting. It is the period of maximum imprintability, before and after which imprinting is difficult or impossible to obtain. Also, in animals, a period when socialisation is most possible.

Critical period of sex differentiation The period of time when CNS is most sensitive to the organising actions of sex steroids.
Time and length of critical period vary depending on species.

Critical thinking Purposeful, self-regulatory judgement, which results in interpretation, analysis evaluation, and inference, as well as the explanation of the evidential, conceptual, methodological, criteriological, or contextual consideration on which that judgment was based; a statement of expert consensus for purposes of educational assessment and instruction.

Cromoglycate It is used in prophylaxis is of asthma.

Cromolyn sodium (Intal) A prophylactic antiasthmatic agent.

Crop milk A nutritive substance consisting of epithelial cells sloughed from the crop sac wall of incubating and brooding pigeons and doves, regurgitated to the nestings at hatching.

Crop sac An outpocketing of the esophagus that is used as a seed storage organ in many birds and as a source of crop milk in pigeons and doves.

Cross infection Infection contracted by a patient from another patient of staff.

Cross inoculation The ability of bacterial strains from two or more different legumes to each producing nodules on the other's host.

Cross protection The phenomenon in which plant tissues infected with one strain of a virus are protected from infection by other strains of the same virus; protection can thus be conferred by the use of a related mild strain.

Cross sectional study Assessing predictor and outcome variables at same point in time.

Cross talk Activity seen at one electrode site that is generated by a muscle other than the one being monitored.

Crossbite Occlusion that exists when the line of occlusion of the mandibular teeth is anterior and/or buccal to the maxillary teeth.

Cross-contamination Transfer of impurities, infection, or disease from one source to another.

Crosscut A bur with blades slotted perpendicular to its axis.

Crossed & divergent forceps Crossed forceps are with overlapping shanks and 15 cm blades are modifications. Divergent forceps where first

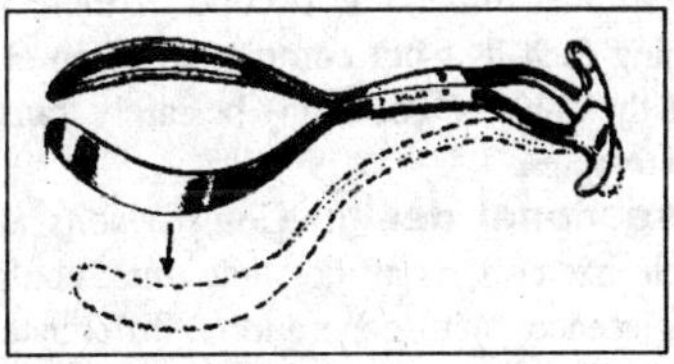

introduced by Thenance in 1781. These are long and unwieldy.

Crossed extensor reflex When limb retracts as a result of the contraction of flexor muscles in response to a stimulus the limb of opposite side extends and is called the crossed extensor reflex. This way person is enable to support himself on the opposite limb when the ipsilateral limb is carried off the ground in response to painful stimulus. Mechanism is also important in walking and running in which there is alteration of flexion and extension of opposite limbs.

Crossed hemiplegia Follows unilateral brainstem lesion affecting one or more motor cranial nerve nuclei (resulting in ipsilateral paralysis) together with corticospinal fibers (resulting in contralateral hemiplegia/hemiparesis).

Crossed leg gait Scissor's gait.

Cross-examination Witnesses who testify in a legal proceeding may be questioned by the opposing counsel to test the truth and credibility of their character and testimony.

Cross-fostering The exchange of offspring between different parents, usually during early development and between different species.

Cross-infections Transfer of infection from one source to another.

Crossing-over The exchange of a portion of one chromatid with another during meiosis. It permits an exchange of genes among chromatids and is one factor that results in genetic variation of progency.

Cross-linking A molecular bridging structure formed by covalent bonds, connecting individual polymer chains to produce a giant polymer network (similar to a spider web).

Crossmatching It is a procedure to match the blood of donor and recipient. In this laboratory procedure red blood cells from donor are mixed with serum of recipient and red blood cells of recipient are mixed with serum of donor. Then both the samples are examined under microscope. If there is any clumping then it is not compatible. If no clotting occurs the donor's blood may be safely transfused to the recipient.

Cross-sectional design Comparisons among multiple age cohorts at the same time; confounds age differences with generational difference.

Cross-sectional ecologic study A study of the frequency with shich some characteristic and some outcome of interrest (e.g., lung cancer) occur in the same geographically defined population at one particular time.

Cross-sectional method A developmental research method involving the comparison of groups of individuals at different age levels. Contrasted with the longitudinal method, where the same individual is observed as he or she grows older.

Cross-sectional study Study documenting the status of a group at a particular point in time.

Cross-sectional survry A survey of a population at a single point in time.

Cross-tolerance A form of tolerance in which the response to a novel drug is reduced because of tolerance developed in response to a related drug.

Cross-validation Assessing the value of a test by using it with a sample of subjects other than the ones employed in its construction; testing with new subjects a set of test items already found to be a value with an earlier group.

Crouch gait Gait with exaggerated flexion of hips and knees seen in spastic paraplegia.

Croup It is a viral function in 90% cases. There develops acute hoarseness of voice, sometimes stridor and nasal discharge. There may be respiratory obstruction due to thick and tenacious secretion of tracheobronchial tree or oedema of laryngeal mucosa. Peripheral circulatory failure may develop.

Crowding The experience of stress in the presence of others. This term has a subjective definition; it is not based on the number of persons per unit of space but upon the individual's reactions to being with other persons.

Crown The part of the tooth that is formed of and covered by enamel.

Crown clinical Portion of tooth exposed beyond the creast of gingiva.

Crown full Cast gold restoration which completely covers the crown of teeth.

Crown gall A tumorous plant disease induced by Agrobacterium tumefaciens.

Crown to rump length The longest demonstrable length of the embryo or fetus, excluding the limbs and yolk sac.

Crowning The phase in the second stage of labour when the largest diameter of the fetal head is visible and circled by the vulva. The anus is open, and the perineum is distended.

Crown-porcelain jacket Full crown usually for anterior teeth made of porcelain.

Crown-Root Ratio The ratio of the height of the crown above the ridge crest to the depth of the root within bone; useful as a prognostic tool.

Crude rates Rates calculated using the entire population at risk; contrast with *specific* and *adjusted rates.*

Cruncle Fleshy protrusion.

Crural Refers to the leg.

Crust injuries The damage or wounds that results from being squeezed between two hard objects.

Crutch gait Gait assumed by a person on crutches by alternately bering weight on one or both legs and on the crutches.

Crutch palsy Temporary or permanent loss of sensation or movement resulting from pressure on axilla from crutch.

Crutches Axillary crutches are prescribed when non-weight bearing gait is required. It is required for patients who require the extra lateral stability. Elbow crutches are indicated for long-term use. These are suitable for both non-and partial weight bearing gaits. These can be easily handled on stairs, for opening doors and getting out of cars. Forearm crutches are particularly useful for them who are

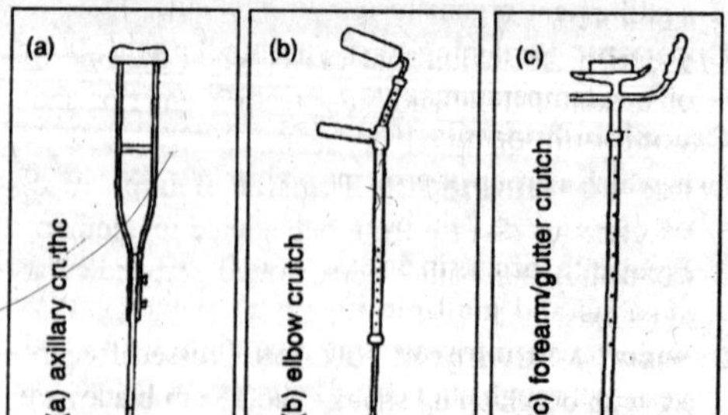

unable to use normal hand grips due to pain or deformity.

Cry genes Genes found in Bacillus thuringiensis and a few other bacteria that encode proteins toxic to insects; the genes are frequently located on large plasmids that maybe transmissible by conjugation between bacteria.

Cryo instruments The present cryosurgical instruments use feron or nitrous oxide or carbon dioxide for cooling effect. The cryoprobes are available in different diameters, 1 mm for intravitreal use, 1.5 mm for cataract extraction,

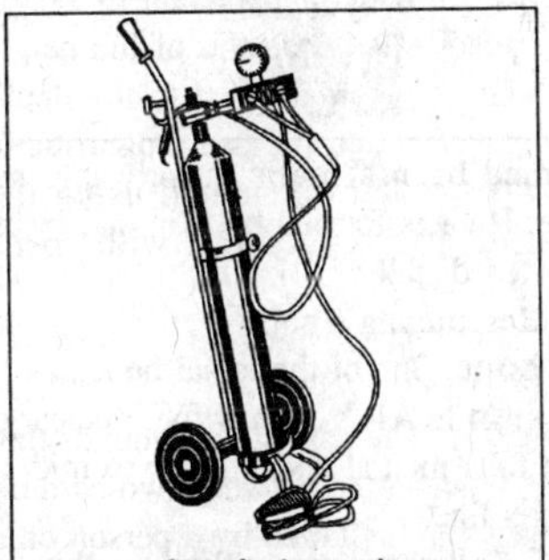

Cryo instrument

2.5 mm for cryopexy of retina and about 4 mm for cyclocryopexy. The cryo units are available with defrosting device also. Disposable cryo units are available for cataract extraction. With feron the temperature at the tip is about –40° to –70°C, with nitrous oxide about –89°C, with carbon dioxide about –78°C.

Cryoanalgesia Use of extreme cold to damage peripheral nerves. It provides relief from pain for several months.

Cryobiosis The existence of life at very low temperatures, the absence of metabolic activity in a still extant organism due to freezing.

Cryogenic Pertaining to or causing the production of low temperatures.

Cryoglobulinaemia It is a haematologic disorder in which a group of proteins precipitate from serum on exposure to cold but redissolve when warmed Frequently occurs in diseases of reticuloendothelial systems and multiple myeloma. There will be widespread intravascular coagulation in small vessels through out body. There may be congestive retinopathy and vitreous haemorrhage.

Cryoprotectant A chemical e.g., glycerol used to protect cells during cryopreservation.

Cryotherapy The cryolesion behaves like a burn but it is almost painless. There are two ways of obtaining a subzero temperature. The open ended spray or using nitrogen in a closed probe the temperature is lowered to –20 degree C. Liquid nitrogen gives a temperature of –180°C and both nitrous oxide and carbon dioxide can be used. Nitrous oxide gives a temperature of –70°C. Usually no anaesthesia is required. It is used in surgery of haemorrhoidectomy and nerve block. Cryoanalgesia produces prolonged but not permanent neural blockade and neuroma formation is rare.

Crypt A pit-like depression.

Cryptobiosis Hidden life; the absence of any evidence of metabolic activity in a dormant organism.

Cryptococcal meningitis This causes chronic basilar granulomatous meningitis, small multiple nodules may also form. These occur in cryptococcal meningitis. Focal neurological deficits, seizures and intracranial hypertension are late findings. There will be elevated cryptococal antigen titre and positive fungal culture.

Cryptococcosis *Cryptococcus neoformans* is usually widely distributed in avian faeces and soil. Cryptococcal meningitis is a frequent opportunistic infection in cases of AIDS. Subacute meningitis may develop. There will be gradually increasing headache. Invasion of subarachnoid space around optic nerve causes early papilloedema. Organism can be found in spinal fluid on repeated examinations. Treatment is amphotericin B, intravenous 0-3 to 0-5 mg/kg day for six weeks.

Cryptogenic Of obscure, doubtful, or underterminable origin.

Cryptogenic fibrosing alveolitis An alveolar inflammatory process of indeterminate etiology that leads to fibrosis of the lungs.

Cryptograph The art of creating and using a method of disguising messages so that only certain people can see through the disguise.

Cryptoorchidism It is the congenital retention of boy's testis in abdominal cavity leaving the scrotum virtually empty at birth. It may require surgical intervention. The possession of only one testis is called monorchidism.

Cryptophthalmus In congenital cryptophthalmus the lids may not be developed at all. There are usually severe anomalies of the globe, sometimes microphthalmos.

Cryptorchidism Failure of one or both testes to descend into the scrotum.

Crystalline Having atoms or molecules arranged in a regular repeating three dimensional patterns. Metals are always crystalline.

Crystalline arthropathy Any joint disease that results from deposition of crystals within the joint.

Crystalloid solution Water and other uniformly dissolved crystals, such as salt and sugar.

C-spine Abbreviation for cervical spine.

CT angiography CTA begins with the acquisition of crosssectional images of an entire volume during arterial phase of enhancement following an IV contrast agent. The stack of slices is then processed to produce a projection image or a 3D rendering of arterial tree.

CT number The attenuation value in the constructed CT image expressed in Hounsfield units. Attenuation number is different for air, blood, bone, etc. and helps in recognising them.

CT scan It is a diagnostic technique in which X-rays are passed through the body at different angles produces clear cross-sectional images. It minimises the amount of radiation. First CT scan came in operation in 1972 for head.

CT-guided interventions Inter-ventional procedures guided by CT. These may be diagnostic and therapeutic. Diagnostic procedures are fine-needle aspirations and core biopsies. Therapeutic interventions include drainage of infected and non-infected fluids, injection of ethanol in lesions like tumours or hydatid cysts, ganglion blockage and intra-articular injections into small joints for pain relief.

Cuban heel A broad high heel.

Cubical epithelium It is distributed in acini of thyroid and mammary glands, tubules of testis and ovary. It lines smallest respiratory ducts. Its function is secretion.

Cubiod Resembling a cube.

Cubital Pertaining to the antebrachium. The cubital fossa is the anterior aspect of the elbow joint.

Cubital fossa It is the triangular space on the anterior aspect of the elbow. Floor of cubital fossa

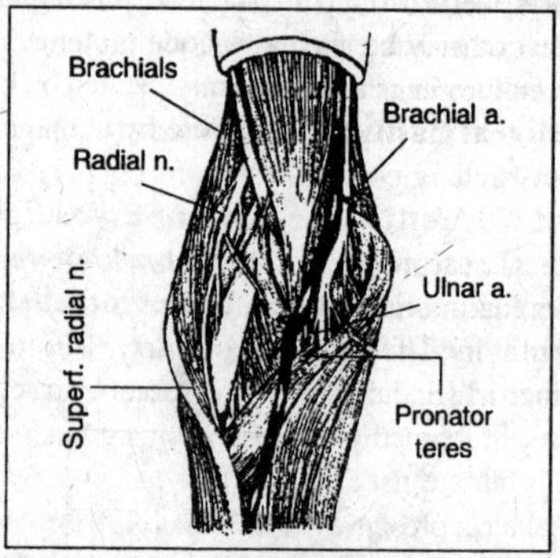

is formed by brachialis muscle and supinator muscle. Roof is formed by skin and fascia. Apex is directed distally.

Cuboid Resembling a cube.

Cuboid bone One of the tarsal bone.

Cuboid sign In AP X-Ray of foot nuclear center of cuboid falls medial and inferior to mid calcaneal long axis line.

Cuboidal Cell shape resembling a cube.

Cuff tear arthropathy Degenerative changes of shoulder joint resulting from massive untreated rotator cuff tear.

Cuing strategies Methods of offering a patient cues to help him or her to perform a given task.

Cuirass A type of negative pressure mechanical ventilator that covers the anterior surface of the thorax.

Culdocentesis It provides a way to sample free fluid seen in cul-de-sac on ultrasonography. This test can differentiate hemorrhage from fluid from a ruptured corpus luteum cyst.

Cullen's sign According to this sign the umbilicus may become bluish due to ecchymoses in cases of intraperitoneal haemorrhage. It is seen in acute pancreatitis and abortion of rupture of tubal pregnancy.

Cult A new religious movement specially that which is secretive, socially isolated, often faddish with unfamiliar rules and rituals and coercive or manipulative or deceptive techniques used to win or keep new converts.

Cultural deprivation The absence of normal learning opportunities for children; an environment which does to offer adequate stimulation for normal intellectual development.

Cultural relativism The value of a behavior or attitude can only be understood within the context of the culture in which it occurs,

Culturally sensitive nursing care Care that respects and is compatible with each patient's culture.

Culture It is a process of growth of bacteria or microorganims or tissue cultivated artificially in the laboratory. The specimen is collected in a sterile container and incubated at body temperature in a chosen culture medium. Generally agar gel or meat based broth are used.

Any bacteria present will multiply to form visible colonies. The type of bacteria can be identified by noting the appearance of the colony. Bacterial cultures can be tested with various antibiotics to determine which antibiotic may be most effective against particular infection.

Culture shock Feelings of isolation, rejection and alienation experienced by an individual or group when transplanted from a familiar to an unfamiliar culture, e.g. from one country to another.

Culture-fair test A test of general intelligence allegedly of the same difficulty for persons from different cultures; the items are presumed to be no more difficult for persons from one culture or another. Attempts to construct a test of this sort have not been notably successful.

Culture-free test A test of general intelligence in which the influence of culture presumably has been eliminated; the items do not pertain to any particular culture. Attempts to construct a test of this type have been unsuccessful.

Cumulativ incidence The total number of incident cases over a specified period of time. Incident cases resulting is death would be included in the cumulative incidence measure but not in the prevelence.

Cumulative dose Term used in radiation medicine to describe the total dose resulting from repeated exposure of same region.

Cumulus oophorus Loosely arranged mass of cells surrounding the ovum in the ovarian follicle. The several layers of granulosa cells surrounding an occyte and supporting the antrum of a Graffian follicle.

Cuneonavicular joint The joint between cuneiform bones and navicular bone.

Cupping The type of *tapotement* that involves the use of a cupped hand; it is often used over the thorax.

Cupula A mass of gelatinous material covering the hair cells of a crista; a receptor in the ampulla of a semicircular canal stimulated when the head moves.

Cupyrene sperm The nucleate sperm of Lepidoptera, used to fertilize the oocytes.

Curare A chemical derived from plant sources that causes flaccid paralysis by blocking A ch receptor proteins in muscle cell membranes.

Curative medicine The effort at treatment in health-care systems.

Curet An instrument with a fine blade, used in curettage. In periodontics, curets are used for cutting the soft tissue wall of periodontal pockets, to remove the inner lining and epithelial attachment, and for removing periodontal fibers from the walls of osseous defects associated with intrabony pockets. Curets are also used to remove calculus fragments and to smooth root surfaces.

Curettage The removal of substances from the wall of a cavity, especially the uterine cavity, with a spoon-shaped instrument called a curette.

Curette These are spoon shaped. The curette has two cutting edges. It removes the soft-tissue wall of the pocket and serves as a root planner. These

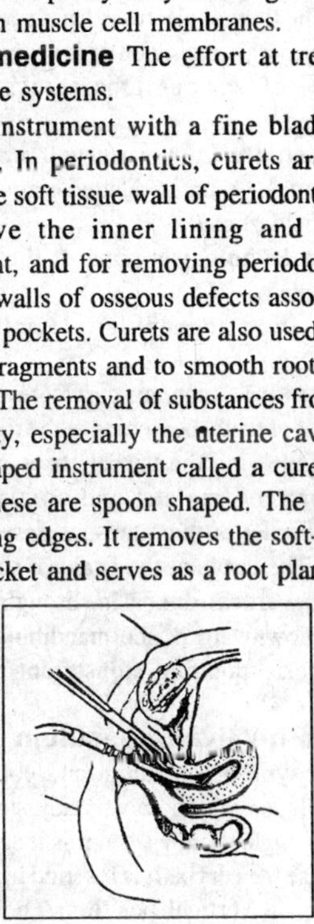

are designed as pull and push instrument. The pull curette is applied to the tooth so that its face makes 80 to 85° angle. The push curette is applied to tooth to make a 15 to 25° angle. It is a instrument for root planning.

Curetting Use of current scalers to remove subgingivual calculus from the root surface of the tooth.

Curie A unit measure of radioactivity. One curie is defined as the amount of radioactivity emitted by 1 gm of radium.

Curing The process by which the denture base material is hardened in a denture mold to form a mold.

Curing light Visible light source used to activate the polymerization of resin restorative materials.

Curli A class of thin, irregular, and highly aggregated adhesive surface fibers expressed by E. Coli and Salmonella enteritidis.

Curling ulcers Peptic ulcers occurring after severe burns.

Current The flow of electrons from a rergion of high negative charge to a regon of low negative charge; the flow of various ions across the neuron membrane.

Current density Current per unit area.

Curriculum A group of relatled courses, often in a special field of study.

Curvature Pathological bend of the spine in the coronal plane.

Curve It is a nonangular deviation from a straightline.

Curve of spee 1. Anatomic curvature of the occlusai alignment of teeth, beginning at the tip of the lower canine, following the buccal cusps of the natural premolars and molars, and continuing to the anterior border of the ramus, as described by von Spee. 2. The curve of the occlusal surfaces of the arches in vertical dimensin, brought about by a dipping downward of the mandibular premolars, with a corresponding adjustment of the upper premolars.

Cuscow's bivalved speculum It is a self-retaining type of speculum and consists of two hinged blades which can be adjusted at desired level and angle. Screw system is there. It is useful to visualise the cervix. It is inserted in vagina being closed up in vertical position. Then blades are rotated by 90° and made horizontal and opened and locked in position. It is very easy to use.

Cushing reflex Hypertension with compensatory bradycardia occurring with acutely raised ICP.

Cushing's syndrome It is a hor-monal disorder caused by an abnormally high circulating level of corticosteroid hormones produced by adrenal glands. In it face appearance is round and red like a moon. The trunk tends to become obese. Purple scratch marks may be seen over abdomen, thighs and breasts. Women may become more hairy. Person may develop mania and depression. Skin becomes thin and is easily bruised.

Cushing's ulcer These are acute ulcers which are usually multiple, superficial and do not penetrate muscularis mucosae. These are located in oesophagus, stomach and duodenum. Steroids, analgesics and alcohol may cause it. Pain is absent, haematemesis and maelena are dominant features. Ulcerated area is visualised on gastroscopy. Antacids in high doses and H_2 blockers are useful. Surgery is to be avoided.

Cushioning effect The shock absorbing quality that directly results from the compression of the periimplant ligament around an osteopreserved dental implant.

Cusp Notably pointed or rounded eminence on or near the masticating surface of a tooth.

Cuspid Canine tooth, serves to pierce or tear food being eaten.

Cuspidor Small sinklike device located near the dental chair into which the patient expectorates.

Cuspids Canines; the four pointed teeth in humans, situated one on each side of each jaw, distal to the lateral incisor; form the keystone of the arch.

Custodial care Provision of board or other non medical assistance to a physically and mentally incapacitated individual on a long term basis.

Custom A practice followed by a particular group or region.

Custom-made tray Acrylic tray customized for an individual patient arch; used in taking final impressions.

Cut off point A value on an ordinary or distinguish categories.

Cutaneous Pertaining to the skin.

Cutaneous amyloidosis It is a rare, chronic and benign conditon arising from deposition of amyloid in skin. Histologically, skin reveals deposition of amyloid in papillae and destruction of elastic tissue. The primary condition gives rise to shiny, smooth, firm, flat topped, waxy or translucent papules over eyelids. Often purpura develops from amyloidosis of small cutaneous vessels. Condition is asymptomatic. Secondary condition presents with extremely itchy, small, normal skin coloured, waxy or translucent papule. No effective treatment of condition is available but spontaneous regression of lesions may occur.

Cutaneous application Drug administration by rubbing medication into or placing it in contact with the skin.

Cutaneous diphtheria It is an infection of skin caused by gram-positive bacteria *Carynebacterium diphtheriae*. It is caused by direct contact of organism secondary to wound. There may be no systemic involvement. It presents with acutely spreading lesions or punched-out ulcers showing formation of adherent dirty grey pseudo-membrane. Edges of ulcers are swollen, rolled and elevated. Ulcers may become chronic. It is treated with subcutaneous administration of diphtheria antitoxin 10,000 to 20,000 units.

Cutaneous larval migrans A condition caused by the migration of nematode larvae in the skin of an unnatural host.

Cutaneous leishmaniasis It is a chronic infection of skin caused by *Leishmania tropica*. Infection is transmitted through bite of sandflies. Following inoculation of the organism, infiltration of corium with plasma cells, large endothelial macrophages produce a nodule. Overlying epidermis becomes thin and atrophic. It presents with chronic, single or multiple slowly growing papule on the exposed part such as cheeks, lips, nose, ears, hands and arms. Papule may ulcerate and become covered by a crust that exudates a sticky secretions. Removal of the crust reveals moist, freely bleeding area. Healing of lesion occurs by granulation leaving a depressed fibrous scar following treatment otherwise also it spontaneously heal after 2 to 18 months.

Cutaneous membrane Primary organ of the integumentary system; the skin.

Cutaneous pain Discomfort that originates at the skin level.

Cutaneous sensitivity The various skin senses; chiefly the experiences of pressure, temperature, and pain through the skin.

Cutaneous sensory receptors Sensory nerves in the skin.

Cutaneous stimulation Stimulation of the skin.

Cutaneous triggering The act of lightly massaging or tapping the skin above the public area to stimulate urination.

Cuticle A thin layer, principally composed of wax and cutin, external to the wall of plant epidermal cells.

Cuticle, primary A delicate membrane covering the crown of a newly erupted tooth; produced by the ameloblasts after they produce the enamel rods. Also called Nasmyth's membrane.

Cuticles Thin edge of skin at the base of the nail.

Cuticular scales Overlapping, transparent cells that make up the cuticle of the hair. They are irregular in shape in human hair.

Cutter A device used for cutting.

Cutting Edge The functional point of intersection of the rake face and clearance face that is directly involved in the cutting action of the bur.

Cuvier, duct of Common cardinal vein.

CVA Warning signs of impendng CVA are drowsiness, dizziness, headache and frequent transient ischaemic attacks. There may be a

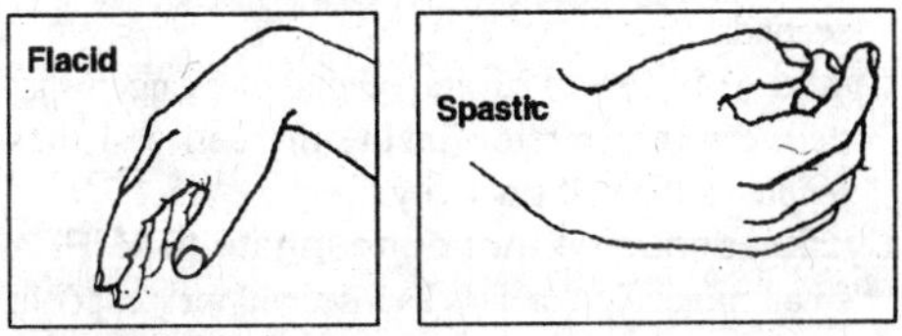

warning signal. A person may loose consciousness. The most common effects are hemiplogia and aphasia. The type of paralysis affecting the extremities especially the hand and foot may be spastic or flaccid.

Cyanide It is a non-drug chemical causing tissue anoxia by chelating the ferric part of intracellular respiratory enzyme. Poisoning may result as an accidental exposure through inhaling smoke or by self-administration. The symptoms of acute poisoning are due to tissue anoxia with dizziness, palpitation and feeling of chest constriction. Breath smells of bitter almonds. In severe cases there is acidosis and coma. Inhaled hydrogen cyanide may cause death within minutes. Kelocyanor in doses of 300 to 600 mg IV given over one minute is the drug of choice if diagnosis is confirmed.

Cyanide poisoning The commonly accepted lethal dose for postassium and sodium cyanide is 50 to 200 mg. Cyanide poisoning can occur via inhalation. Death can occur within minutes. When inhaled symptoms develop within seconds.

Involvement of CNS leads to vertigo, sweating, confusion, syncope, hyperthermia, seizures, paralysis, coma and death reults consequently. There will be acidic and burning taste and froathing at mouth. Dyspnoea develops hypotension and tachycardia. Patient develops severe lactic acidosis.

Cyanosis Bluish discoloration or skin color changes, particularly around the mouth and in the nail beds due to lack of oxygen.

Cyanotic Pertaining to cyanosis.

Cyclamates The sodium or calcium salts of cyclohexylsulfumic acid. It is water-soluble with sweet taste 30 times that of sucrose.

Cycle succession of events.

Cycle ergometer testing An exercise performed on a stationary bicycle.

Cycle time (stride time) The amount of time required to complete a gait cycle; measured in seconds.

Cyclic AMP One of several second messengers that delivers information inside the cell and thus regulates the cell's activity.

Cyclic adenosine monophosphate (CAMP) A small molecule that acts as a second messenger in nuerons.

Cyclic AMP One of several second messengers that delivers information inside the cell and thus regulates the cells activity.

Cyclic feeding Continuous instillation of liquid nourishment for 8 to 12 hours.

Cyclic guanosine monophosphate A nucleotide that facilitates smooth muscle contraction and may enhance mast cell release of histamine and other mediators to cause bronchoconstriction.

Cyclic nucleotide phosphodiesterase An enzyme that breaks the bonds between the diesterified orthophosphoric acids that constitute the components of nucleic acids.

Cyclical parthenogenesis An alternation between parthenogenesis and sexual reproduction.

Cyclical vomiting It is due to acidosis in children. Constipation, over eating of fatty foods, eggs and chocolates may precipitate it. Throat infection, over strain in school, journey on hills may precipitate it. Attack comes on suddenly with headache, vomiting, drowsiness, dehydration and rapid thready pulse.

Cyclophosphamide Cytotoxic drug used as an immunosuppressive.

Cycloplegia Paralysis of accommodation is usually seen following use of cycloplegic drugs, contusion injury or due to paralysis of third nerve. It is often unilateral. Bilateral paralysis of accommodation follows after diabetes, alcoholism and meningeal disease. In a case of complete paralysis there is widly dilated pupil.

Cyclopropane BP It is a colourless gas with sweat smell. Molecular weight is 42. Boiling point is 34°C. It is one and half times heavier than air. Critical temperature is 175°C. Critical pressure is 54 atmospheres. It liquefies at ordinary temperature. It is taken up and excreted via the lungs with little metabolism. It is a powerful respiratory depressant, Cardiac output is increased with arterial pressure well maintained. As an anaesthetic it is always used in a closed system. Its action is rapid. It is comparatively safe and can be used for a wide range of operations. Drug is excreted largely unchanged and recovery is rapid so is useful in old patients.

Cyclosporin It is a polypeptide obtained from a soil fungus. It does not depress haemopoiesis. 40 per cent of it is absorbed in GIT and is metabolised in liver. Half-life is 27 hours. It is used to prevent and treat rejection of organ transplants. It may be given orally. It can be given to psoriasis patients also. It is nephrotoxic. Hypertension develops in about 50 per cent cases.

Cyclosporine A-T cell specific immunosuppressive drug used to prevent graft rejection.

Cyclothyrnia A milder version of a cyclical mood disorder in which mood swings can occur but are not as intense as in bipolar disorder.

Cyesis Pregnancy

Cylinder cast Rigid mold that encircles an arm or leg.

Cylindric bronchiectasis A dilatation, of uniform caliber, of the bronchi and brochioles that results from chronic inflammation or obstruction.

Cylindrical grip It has all the fingers flexed around the object.

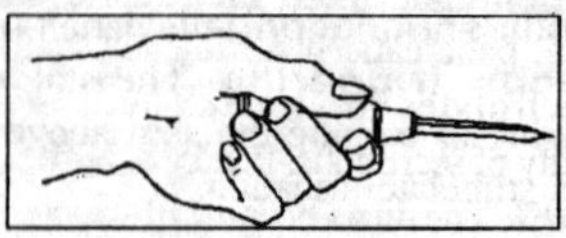

Cynical beliefs Beliefs that others are motivated by selfish concerns.

Cynodont Canine tooth.

Cyst Pathologic space in bone or soft tissue containing fluid or semifluid material, generally lined by epithelium.

Cyst branchial It is a cystic swelling arising in connection with the persistent cervical sinus which is formed due to the fusion of overgrowing second brachial arch with the 6th brachial arch. The lump lies below the angle of the jaw beneath the middle of sternomastoid muscle and bulges into the carotid angle. Size is ovoid and varies from 5 to 10 cm in width. The fluctuation is not always easy to elicit. It is not tender. Lump is not very mobile as it is closely tethered to the surrounding structures. Due to thick content transillumination test is negative. The local deep cervical lymph nodes should not be enlarged. Aspirated material may show fat globules and cholesterol crystals secreted by sebaceous glands.

Cyst ovarian It is centrally situated and grows from below upwards. It can be moved laterally not upwards. Enlargement is fairly uniform and gives all signs of fluid. Level does not alter with the position of patient. There will be menstrual irregularities. Cyst may be clearly felt by bimanual examination. When cyst contains pus there may be fever. Attack of pain indicates adhesions. Malignant papilliferous cyst is indicated by presence of nodules on wall, emaciation, ascites and oedema of legs.

Cystadenolymphoma Main symptoms are soft, mobile, painless, slow growing, frequently bilateral mass most commonly occurring in the parotid gland.

Cystadenoma of prostate These are multicystic septated lesions originating from the prostate gland and displacing the seminal vessels.

Cystectomy The surgical removal of the bladder.

Cystic duct Duct from the gall bladder; it joins the common hepatic duct to form the CBD.

Cystic fibrosis It is an autosomal recessive condition. The main manifestations are lung disease, pancreatic insufficiency and an increase in electrolytes in sweat. There is increase in viscosity of secretions. Pancreas is affected in more than 90%. The ducts become obstructed and dilated and acini disappear. Similarly obstruction of small bronchioles leads to obstructed bronchi ending with chronic bronchitis, atelectasis and bronchiectasis. In liver small bile duct becomes blocked. Patchy pericholangitis may develop.

Cystic hygroma It is congenital multiloculated cystic mass arising from Jugular lymph sac. It illuminates well usually present soon after birth. Tongue and pharynx may be involved so surgery is difficult.

Cystic lesion An injury or wound caused by the formation of cysts.

Cystic renal dysplasia It is sporadic, non-familial disease resulting from abnormal metanephrotic differentiation. It is associated frequently with abnormalities of ureter and lower urinary tract. Affected kidneys are enlarged and multicystic. There may be focal cartilage formation.

Cysticercosis Causative factor is *Taenia solium.* Dead larvae may cause muscle pain, weakness, and fits. Ocular features include endophthalmitis, optic atrophy, papilloedema and retinal haemorrhage.

Cysticercus A tapeworm larva, developing from the oncosphere of some cyclophyllideans, that is characterized by a fully developed scolex invaginated into a fluid-filled vesicle, or bladder; also called bladderworm.

Cystid In colonial animals, living and nonliving parts of the body wall of an individual colony member.

Cystinosis It is a rare disorder. It is characterised by intralysomal accumulation of free cystine in tissues like cornea, conjunctiva and bone marrow. It has 3 forms : *infantile form* leading to *Fanconi syndrome* and renal insufficiency in first decade, *juvenile* form with renal disease, and in *adult form* in which cystine is deposited in cornea and not in kidneys. Hexagonal or rectangular cystine crystals can be detected in cornea. Adult form does not require any treatment while in infantile and juvenile form adequate fluid intake and vitamin D helps. Glomerular damage is progressive. Death occurs due to renal failure. Children show blonde hair. Depigmented patches over the temporal fields of retina permit an early diagnosis of cystinosis.

Cystitis The catheter is the most common cause of lower urinary tract infection. There may be descending infection from kidney or adjacent structures. The symptoms are painful and frequent micturition, pain over bladder, and passage of pus in urine. Pain may be felt at the end of micturition. In urethritis, also pain is felt once urine has been voided. Frequency of micturition may be extreme. Patient may develop fever. In chronic cystitis, pain and strangury are less prominent, but frequency of micturition and pyuria are always present. Chronic cystitis may persist for months without symptoms.

Cystocele The pouching down-ward of the bladder through the vaginal wall.

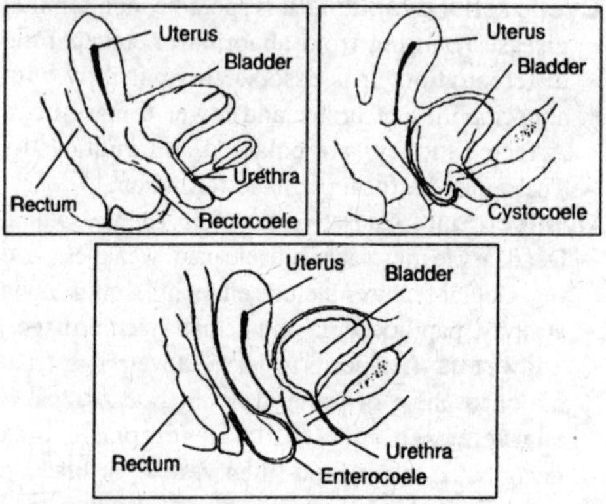

a. Rectocele b. Cystocelec Enterocele

Cystochrome oxidase system Series of iron containing enzymes within mitrochondrial inner membrane.

Cystogenous glands In some cercariae of digenetic trematodes, secretory cells that give rise to metacercarial cysts.

Cystoid macular oedema Cystoidmacular oedema is a condition in which there is accumulation of fluid at the macula. It is a common disorder of macula seen in uveitis, retinitis pigmentosa and retinal vein occlusion. There develops cystoid areas at the posterior pole. These multiple microcysts may coalesce to form a larger cyst filled with fluid. It leads to formation of lamellar hole at macula. Fluorescein angiography shows a flower petal pattern and hyper-fluorescence.

Cystokines Signal molecules released from immunocytes, supporting cells or other cell type that can interact with other cells of immune system.

Cystosolic Pertaining to cytosol.

Cytoarchitectonic map Map of the neocortex based on the organisation, structure, and distribution of the cells.

Cytochrome A hemoprotein in which one or more heme is alternately oxidized and reduced in electron transfer process. Heme proteins serve as electron carriers in respiration, photosynthesis, and other oxidation-reduction reactions.

Cytocidal Causing or capable of causing death to cells.

Cytodifferentiation The process through which a cell or tissue acquires its characteristic biochemical phenotype.

Cytogamy A self-mating process in paired cells that yields whole genome homozygotes.

Cytogenetics The study of chromosomal structure.

Cytoid bodies Cytoid bodies are cotton-wool spots on retina resulting from degeneration of nerve fibres due to occlusion of retinal vessels. These are found in cases of systemic lupus erythematosus (SLE) and polyarteritis.

Cytokine receptor A membrane-bound protein or glycoprotein that binds a specific cytokine and triggers intracellular signal transduction.

Cytokines Protein mediators released by many cells including monocytes. lymphocytes, macrophages and endothelial cells.

Cytokinesis Distribution of the cytoplasm into two separate cells during cell division; coordinated with nuclear division (mitosis)

Cytoking Any of several soluble chemical mediators that are secreted by cells and react with other cells.

Cytology It is done to detect abnormal cells specially cancer. Best known cytology is for screening cancer cervix. Cytology is valuable in detecting recurrent tumours in people who have already been treated for cancer. Cytology can be helpful in determining the cause of pleural effusion and ascites.

Cytology exfoliative Science of examining cells obtained by wiping or scrapping surface of lesion.

Cytolysis The rupture of living cells in which the contents leak out.

Cytolytic lymphocyte WBCs which have capacity by means of direct cell to cell contact to cause lysis and subsequent death of target cells.

Cytometer A device for counting and measuring cells.

Cytopathic Causing or capable of causing disease in cells.

Cytophilic Binds to cells.

Cytoplasm In a cell, the protoplasm located outside of the nucleus.

Cytoplasmic maturation The process that accompanies oocyte nuclear maturation to prepare the cytoplasm for fertilization and embryo development.

Cytoplasmic stress Conditions associated with accumulation of misfolded or damaged proteins in the cytoplasm.

Cytoskeleton The collection of microtubules, microfilaments, and intermediate filaments that support the cytoplasm and organelles; also involved with cell movements. The filamentous network providing structure and organization to the cytoplasm.

Cytosol Cytoplasm, with the exception of the mithochondria and endoplasmic reticular components.

Cytostome In dinoflagellates, the buccal aperture, permanently opens but able to dilate. It allows the prey to be transported into the cell.

Cytotoxic antibiotics These antibiotics interfere with DNA/RNA synthesis. These include bleomycin, dactinomycin, plicamycin, mitomycin and streptozotocin. Antibiotics depress the bone marrow.•These cause alopecia, cardiomyopathy and pulmonary fibrosis.

Cytotoxic drugs It is a group of drugs that kills or damages cells, i.e. anticancer drugs. These can kill healthy cells too which are multiplying fast as hair, nails and noncancerous cells in bone marrow causing anaemia.

Cytotoxicity The capacity for an agent or metabolic product to exert a specific destructive action on certain cells, or the degree of such action.

Cytotoxin A substance or agent that damages cells.

D

D & E Abbreviation for dilatation and evacuation.

D and C It is a short form for dilatation and curettage. It is mostly done in case of irregular bleeding or to terminate early pregnancy. Under anaesthesia cervix is dilated and with the help of curettage, endometrium is being scraped out.

D.O.M.S. Delayed onset of muscle soreness is essentially limited to uncoditioned individuals undertaking unaccustomed exercise having more of eccentric component in it. It is mildly disabling and transient and resolves within 3-5 days.

D2 receptor A receptor for the neurotransmitter dopamine; target for major tranquilizers.

Dacroadenitis It occurs occasionally in general infections like mumps, influenza and infectious mononucleosis. It may suppurate also. There is painful swelling at the outer third lid. It will be associated with follicular conjunctivitis, periorbital oedema and optic neuritis. Antibiotics help.

Dacrocystitis It is the inflammation of tear sac. It lies between the inside corner of eyelid and nose. It develops due to blockage of the duct. Duct carries tears from the tear sac to the nose. There may be pain, redness and swelling of the inner corner of eyelid. There may be watery eye.

Dacrocystography It is a radiographic examination of lacrimal sac and duct with injection of contrast medium.

Dactyl A digit or hand or foot.

Dactylitis An inflammatory condition of digits.

Dactylography Impression of thumb and fingers is used as a scientific method to identify a person. This is usually recorded in case of a criminal and in society who are uneducated put their thumb impression in lieu of signature. It is based on the principle that individual peculiarities or patterns of arrangement and distribution of papillary ridges and pores of sweat glands on fingertips are absolutely constant and persist throughout one's life from birth to death. The chance of finger prints of two different individuals being same are 1 in 64,000 millions.

Dactyloscopy The study of fingerprints and fingermarks.

Daily journal sheet Financial record used as a legal document to indicate the listing of activities for each patient seen in the office during the day.

Dakin's solution A solution for cleansing wounds composed of sodium hypochlorite and sodium bicarbonate.

Dalrymple's sign The sign is marked by staring appearance with markedly widened palpebral fissure and retraction of upper eyelid, and is seen in hyperthyroidism.

Dalton The weight of a single hydrogen atom (1.66 x 10^{-24} g).

Dalton's law The pressure exerted by fixed amount of gas in a mixture equals the pressure it would exert if alone.

Damages The amount of money necessary to compensate a plaintiff for injuries caused by the defendant's conduct.

Dance therapy The goals of dance therapy include decreasing physical and psychological tension through expressive movemnet. Result involves stress relief, pain reduction and increased circulation.

Dandruff It has two forms of presentation, dry and oily. The dry form presents with fine, thin powdery, whitish or greyish, dry or slightly greyish scales which becomes loose and fall on shoulders. Lesions do not cause erythema. Hair appear dry and lustreless but they do not fall. There may be itching. Oily form of dandruff may accompany erythema and produce well-defined circumscribed patches or diffuse distribution of greasy, yellowish thick scales and crusts. There is slight itching. Hair may be matted and start falling and may lead to premature baldness. Suitable shampoo should be used.

Dandy-Walker cyst There is cystic dilation of fourth ventricle with hypoplasia of cerebellar hemisphere and vermis. There may be agenesis of corpus callosum, aqueduct stenosis or leptomeningeal cyst. Occiput of head is prominent. Fourth ventricle never appears normal in size or location.

Dangling To sit on the side of a bed with legs dependent or feet on the floor.

Dantrolene sodium Skeletal muscle relaxant which acts by interfering with calcium ion release from sarcoplasmic retinculum. It is useful in muscle spasm.

Dapre The daily adjustable progressive resistive exercise technique may be more effective as progression is made daily. A weight of 6 RM is the starting load and daily progression is made based on the previous session.

Dark adaptation Increasing visual sensitivity as one remains in darkness or low illumination.

Darkfield A type of microscopy wherein the magnified image brightly colored features on a dark background.

Dartos fascia The fascial support structure of the penis, intimately associated with the skin and vascularity to the skin.

Dartos muscle The layer of smooth muscle beneath the skin of the scrotum.

Data Pieces of information collected in a study to answer research questions.

Data base assessment Initial information about the the patient's physical, emotional, social, and spiritual health.

Data compression The compression of data to alleviate the problem particularly prevalent in imagery of the quantity and intensity of the data that are required to be processed and communicated.

Database All the information available that contributes to therapeutic interaction.

Databasing Collection of DNA types from a large, diverse population for the purpose of determining the frequency of occurrence of a particular DNA type.

Date dredging The alalysis of large data sets with modern computer techniques, permitting the assessment of hundreds of possible associations among the study variables. Unless alpha is adjusted, the testing of multiple hypotheses raises the risk of false-positive error.

Date rape Rape involving a perperator who has some level of romantic relationship with the victim ranging from having just met to being established partner.

Davenport diagram It is a graph of plasma bicarbonate concentration against pH useful in interpreting and explaining acid-base disturbance.

Davis Law It states that ligaments or any soft tissue when put under a moderate degree of unremitting tension will elongate.

Day blindness It may occur in central opacities of cornea or of the lens associated with glare and photophobia. Pupil does not constrict to light. Total colour-blindness and degenerative retinal diseases may result it.

Day residue Any element of a dream that is clearly derived from some event of the previous day. The day residue is often useful in deciphering meaning from the dream.

Day-case surgery Surgery in which patient comes to hospital and returns on the same day after surgery.

DCA Diffuse axonal injury.

DDS Doctor of Dental Science; Doctor of Dental Surgery.

DE Double-ended, as in a double-ended hand-cutting instrument.

De Facto A right or obligation that is recognized because of existing custom, rather than a statute or court decision.

De Quervain's disease It is tensosynovitis of first dorsal compartment. The tendons of extensor pollicis brevis and longus are housed within the compartment. The condition is related to excessive mechanical stresses. Pain, swelling and decreased range of motion of thumb are characteristic of the disease. It may be radiating to arm, clinical signs include swelling localised in the area of radial styloid, decreased grip and pinch strength and local tenderness

De Quervainis Syndrome This is the most common tendinopathy arising at wrist. It is seen

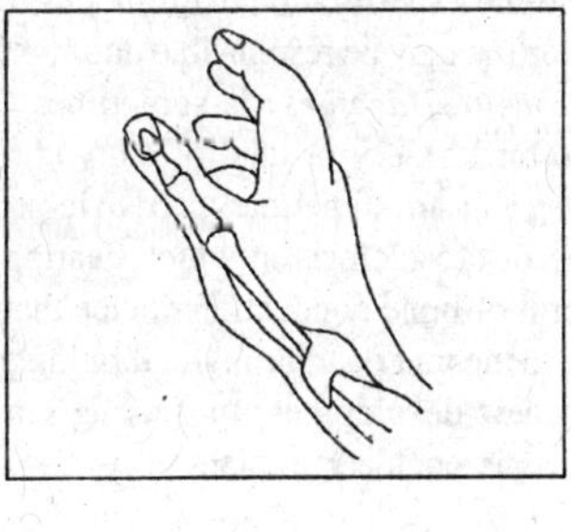

in players of golf and baseball player. There is inflammation of first dorsal extensor compartment. There develops pain along dorsoradial side of wrist. With motion of thumb crepitus may be felt.

Dead Without life.

Dead space Volume of inspired air that takes no part in gas exchange.

Dead-end host A term for a host that can be infected by a pathogenic agent—but that is not part of the cycle of transmission of agent to other organisms.

Deaf language British scientist developed language for the deaf people with the help of two fingers.

Deamination A process through which an amino acid group breaks off from an amino acid molecule, resulting in molecules of ammonia and keto acid.

Diaphragm A sheetlike dome of muscle and connective tissue that separates the thoracic and abdominal cavities.

Death It is the permanent cessation of vital function. Heart, lung and brain stop working. If person is not on ventilator, the diagnosis of death is based on absence of spontaneous breathing, absence of heart beat and fixed pupils unresponsive to light. An EEG showing absence of electrical activity in the brain cerebrum is not required.

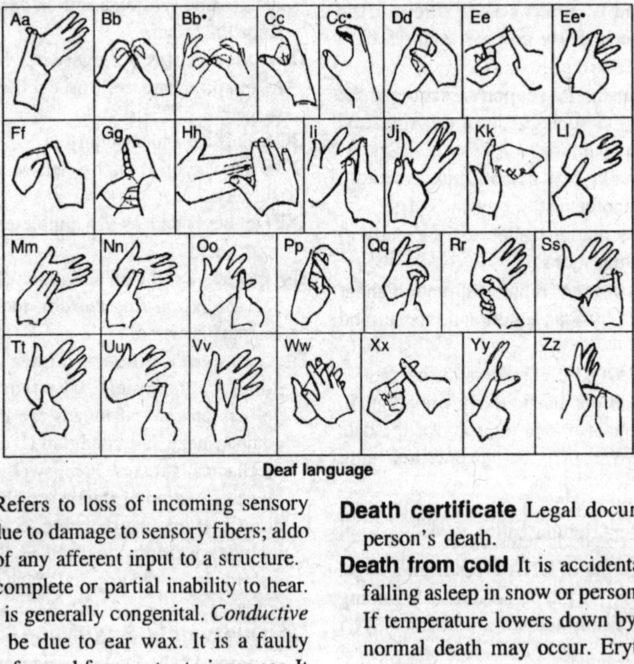

Deaf language

Deafferented Refers to loss of incoming sensory input usually due to damage to sensory fibers; aldo refers to loss of any afferent input to a structure.

Deafness It is complete or partial inability to hear. Total deafness is generally congenital. *Conductive deafness* may be due to ear wax. It is a faulty transportation of sound from outer to inner ear. It may be due to perforation of drum. Less commonly otosclerosis may be responsible due to otitis media. *Sensorineural deafness* is sometimes congenital due to birth injury or due to faulty chromosome. Hearing aids are sometimes used to lessen deafness caused of otosclerosis in which hearing aid takes the form of bone conducting device that transmits sound to the inner ear through vibrating pad behind ear. A new development in treating sensorineural deafness is cochlear implant.

Death certificate Legal document confirming a person's death.

Death from cold It is accidental such as drunken falling asleep in snow or person lost in snow drips. If temperature lowers down by 15 to 20°F below normal death may occur. Erythematous patches will develop on skin, heart's action will become feeble and pulse weak. Gradually stupor and coma may develop.

Death instinct In psychoanalysis, one of the basic forces of the id and therefore assumed to be inborn. An impulse or motivation towards destructive behaviour, manifest in various aggressive reactions towards others and towards oneself.

Death, dying The cessation of all physical and chemical processes that invariably occurs in all living organisms; a stage of life.

Debride To remove mechanically.

Debridement Removal of foreign material and devitalized tissue from a vicinity of a wound.

Debriefing Discussing an experiment and its purpose with subjects after its completion; required if the experiment involved deception.

Debris Foreign material or particles loosely attached to surface.

DEC Program Drug Evaluation and Classification Program.

Decadactylar Made from ten fingers, as in 'ten prints cards' used to register known offenders.

Decalcification The withdrawl of calcium from the bones where it has been deposited. It may be due to inadequate supply of calcium in diet so that calcium has to be taken out from bones.

Decalcification dental It is a dissolving of minerals in a tooth. After prolonged exposure of bacteria, acid causes changes on the surface of tooth. When plaque is brushed away decalcified area is seen as chalky white area. Decalcification penetrates the enamel to the dentin. Pulp once infected tooth may die.

Decay theory A theory of forgetting based on the premise that the engram deteriorates during an interval when it is not activated.

Deception A communicative activity of the person who deliberately tries to create in others a belief or understanding which he or she considers to be false.

Decerebrate posture It is composed of internal rotation and hyperextension of all limbs with hyper extension of all limbs with hyper extension of neck and spine and absent righting reflex. It results from transection of upper brainstem.

Decibel A unit for expressing the relative intensity (loudness) of sound

Decidua The structure of thickened endometrium that develops after conception and, except for the deepest layer, sheds during childbirth.

Decidua basalis The part lying directly under the embedded ovum that forms the maternal component of the placenta.

Decidua capsularis The portion that overlies the ovum, separating it from the rest of the uterine cavity.

Decidua vera The remaining portion that is not in immediate contact with the ovum. Sometimes called the *d. parietalis*.

Decidual Relating to the decidua or decidualization.

Deciduous Falling off or being shed seasonally or at a particular stage of development. In the body, referring to the first set of teeth.

Deciduous dentition That which will be shed. Term pertains specifically to the first dentition of humans or animals. The teeth constituting the first dentition.

Deciduous teeth The primary teeth that fall out to be replaced by the permanent teeth.

Decision analysis A systematic approach to decision making under conditions of uncertainty. Decision analysis focuses on structuring the management alternatives and consequences, the uncertainties, and the preferences of the decision makers.

Declaration of Geneva A medical person is supposed to take an oath

- I solemnly pledge myself to consecrate my life to the service of humanity.
- I will practise my profession with conscience and dignity.
- I will respect the secrets which are confined in me.
- I will maintain by all means in my power the honour and noble tradition of medical profession.
- My collegues will be my brothers and I will pay respect to my teacher.
- I will not permit consideration of religion, nationality or race, party politics or social standing to intervene my duty and my patient.
- I will not use any of my medical knowledge contrary to the laws of humanity.

Declarative memory A type of memory illustrated by the ability to recount the details of events, including time, place, and circumstances, in contrast with the ability to perform some act or behavior. Literally, declarative memory refers to the ability to recount what one knows, which is lost in many types of amnesia.

Decomposition It begins when rigor mortis ceases and is most sure sign of death. It develops due to mainly *Clostridium welchii*. Shortly after death these pass into bloodstream from bowel. Richly vascular organs putrefy first. These bacteria liberate various proteolytic, saccharolytic and lipolytic enzymes and destroy various tissues. Lecithin are from *Cl. welchii* dissolves the lecithin of cell membrane including those of RBCs and causes postmortem haemolysis.

Decomposition reaction The break-down of a larger molecule into smaller molecules, ions, or atoms.

Decompression Removal of gas and secretions from the stomach or bowel.

Decompression sickness Decompression sickness results from the formation of gas bubbles in the diver's tissues during ascent from depth. At depth divers accumulate large quantities of nitrogen due to high pressure gas mixture they breathe. When divers ascend pressure falls and gas can no longer be hold within the tissues and bubbles may block blood vessels. Common symptoms include skin itching and mottling and severe pain in and around joints. There may be weakness, visual disturbance and loss of balance. Decompression chamber helps the patient. Repeated episodes lead to degenerative disorders of bone and joints.

Decongestant An agent that possesses the property of reducing congestion.

Decongestant drugs These are the drugs used to relieve nasal congestion. These are used in upper respiratory infection. If decongestant nasal drops are continued and then stopped, there may be withdrawal symptoms worse than before. Hence these drops should not be continued for long.

Decorticate posture It is caused from lesions of carebral cortex with preservation of basal ganglion and brainstem function. Abnormal flexion of upper extremities and extension of lower extremities.

Decorticate rigidity Sustained contraction of extensor muscles in the lower limbs and flexor muscles in the upper limbs as a result of a brainstem lesion.

Decreased breath sounds Difficult to hear; caused by reduced inspiration or hyperinflation.

Decubitus An act of lying down;

Decubitus ulcer It is a condition of ischaemic necrosis and ulceration of skin resulting from prolonged pressure from bed, wheelchair, etc. or in case of paralysis. It usually involves area of bony or cartilaginous prominence. Condition usually presents with erythema over the pressure points of body. The erythema blanches or disappears on pressure. Later, erythematous area shows oedema and induration. There may be evidence or epidural blistering or desquamation. Progression of condition leads to superficial necrosis and ulceration of the area which may become deeper involving whole extent of skin, fat and muscle.

Decubitus views Refers to radiographic images obtained while the patient is lying down.

Decuspation Removal or complete reduction of the cusp of a tooth.

Decussation A crossing of nerve fibers from on side of the CNS to the other.

Dedicated pathway A term for the entire series of biosynthetic steps, beginning with the first committed step, that converts a common metaboilite to a specific metabolite.

Deduction A type of logic by which one draws a specific conclusion from one or more known truths or premises; often formed as an "if/then" statement.

Deductive reasoning Thought processes aimed at deriving a specific conclusion from certain premises; reasoning from the general to specifics. One form of deductive reasoning is based on the syllogism, a three-part statement consisting of two premises and conclusion.

Deep Farther away from the body's surface.

Deep bronchial veins An intrapulmonary bronchiolar plexus of veins that communicates freely with the pulmonary vein and eventually coalesces into a single trunk that ends in a main pulmonary veins or in the left atrium.

Deep cardiac plexus The dorsal part of the network of nerves that constitutes the cardiac plexus; formed by branches from the cervical and upper thoracic sympathetic ganglia and from the vagus and recurrent laryngeal nerves; located anterior to the tracheal bifurcation, superior to the division of the pulmonary trunk, and posterior to the arch of the aorta.

Deep chordae Chordae tendineae that attach to the more peripheral aspects of the rough region of a valve leaflet.

Deep dorsal vein The major component of the intermediate venous drainage of the penis, beginning subcoronally as the retrocoronal plexus extending proximally to join the preprostatic plexus.

Deep fascia A sheet of connective tissue wrapped around a muscle to hold it in place.

Deep muscle relaxation A procedure in behaviour therapy. The patient learns to control various muscle groups in the body and therefore to gain a state of relaxation, which is incompatible with anxiety; usually employed to relieve anxiety and various phobic reactions.

Deep peroneal nerve Anterior tibial is one of the two terminal branches of common peroneal nerve

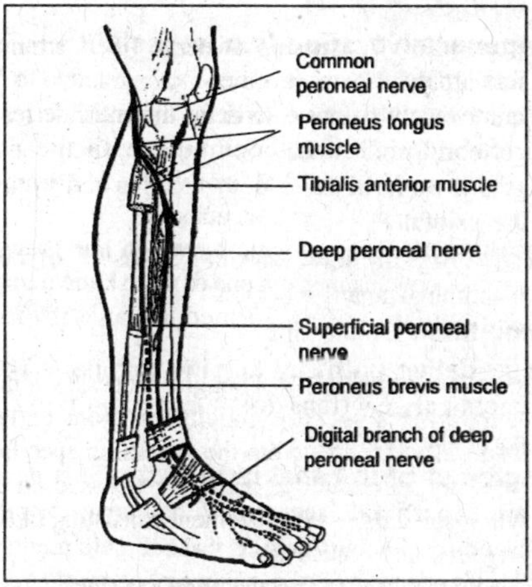

which divides in peroneus longus muscle. It supplies extensor digitorum longus, peroneus tertius, extensor hallucis longus and tibialis anterior.

Deep stroking Deep stroking is given with much greater pressure and is usually perfomed rather slowly. Given in this manner, it tends to stimulate the circulation to the deeper muscle tissue.

Deep vein thrombosis A thrombosis, most often in the legs or pelvis, that results from phlebitis, vein injury, or prolonged bed rest.

Defaecation It is the process and action of evacuating faeces from rectum. Normal process relies on peristalsis within colon and relaxation of sphincter of anus. Impaction of faecation of 48 hours is known as constipation while frequent liquid defaecation is called diarrhoea. Discharge of faeces from the rectum.

Defalcation Root canal, C-shaped.

Defamation An act in which untrue information harms a person's reputation.

Defamation of character False communication of information about a person that results in injury to a person's reputation by verbal (slander) or written (libel) word.

Defecation The elimination of feces from the rectum through the anal canal and out of the anus.

Defect, osteoporotic In some patients foci of red bone marrow large enough to present as radiolucencies develop in certain areas of jaws. Because these are asymptomatic, are found only on routine examination. Mandible is more involved than maxilla. Microscopically specimen reveals haemopoietic marrow including fat and immature cells of polymorphonuclear and erythrocytic series.

Defenant The person accused of committing a crime in a criminal case; or the party against whom suit is brought seeking either damages or relief in a civil case.

Defence mechanisms Behaviour patterns primarily concerned with protecting the ego. Presumably the process is unconscious and the aim is to fool oneself. It is intrapsychic processes serving to provide relief from emotional conflict and anxiety. Conscious efforts are frequently made for the same reasons, but true defence mechanisms are unconscious. Some of the common defence mechanisms defined in this glossary are : compensation, conversion, denial, displacement, dissociation, idealisation, identification, incorporation, introjection, projection, rationalisation, reaction formation, regression, sublimation, substitution, symbolisation, and undoing.

Defendant Party against whom relief or recovery is sought in a lawsuit.

Defense The defendant's answer to the plaintiff's complaint. A defense may contest the truth of the plaintiff's allegations, or claim a legal privilege to commit the act complained of.

Deferred sexual maturation In birds, the delaying of the first breeding attempt for one or more years, and up to 12 years after hatching.

Defibrillation It is an application of an electric current across the heart to convert ventricular fibrillation to sinus rhythm.

Defibrillator An agent or measure, for example an electric shook, that arrests fibrillation of the ventricular muscle and restores the normal beat.

Definitive host The host in which a parasite having an indirect life-history pattern attains maturity and participates in sexual reproduction.

Definitive zone A term for the narrow cortical zone that surrounds the fetal zone of the fetal adrenal gland.

Deflation reflex Stimulation of inspiration by lung deflation It is initiated by pulmonary stretch receptors.

Deflection attitudes The normal attitude of fetal vertex during labour is one of full flexion on the

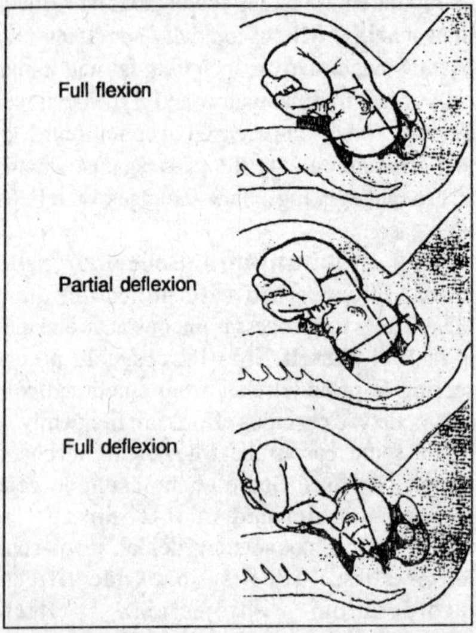

neck. Fetal chin is against the upper chest. Deflection attitudes include various degrees of deflection or even extension of fetal head on the neck.

Deformation Distortion; disfigurement.

Deformity A permanent change in the shape of a bone, usually at or near a joint, that limits movements and function.

Degeneration of placenta Fatty, calcareous or cystic change is seen within placenta. Fatty and calcareous degenerations are usually combined and are constantly found in long-standing infarcted areas. Calcification in placenta may be seen in good X-ray. Cystic degeneration results in formation of small, amniotic cysts upon the fetal surface of placenta. They are frequently multiple but never large. They do not affect the functional capability of organ.

Degenerative Deterioration or breaking down of a part or parts of the body.

Degenerative disorders Many of features of aging, i.e. wrinkles of skin, joints pain are due to degenerative changes. Amongst CNS disorders, the most common is Alzheimer's disease. Retinitis pigmentosa is another degenerative disease and may cause blindness. In blood vessels degenerative changes in muscle coat of these blood vessels are unusually severe and calcium deposits may be seen on X-ray.

Degenerative spondylolisthesis There is a forward displacement of vertebra in relation to one immediately below with degenerative changes in certebral bodies. Discomfort is brought on by getting up from chair. Both standing and walking are painful.

Degloving Intraoral surgical exposure of bony mandibular anterior region.

Deglutition Swallowing.

Degradative pathway Specific enzymecatalyzed chemical reactions for the metabolism of a particular substrate.

Degree of birth canal lacerations First degree are superficial lacerations that have minimal bleeding. Second degree include subcutaneous tissues or fascia of perineal body but not the rectal sphincter.

Third degree lacerations extend through skin, mucous membranes including rectal sphincter. Fourth degree lacerations extend through rectal sphincter and expose the lumen of rectum. This has to be repaired in layers using interrupted sutures.

Degree of conversion The percentage of carbon -carbon double bonds reacted or converted to single bonds during a polymerization reaction; abbreviated as DC; appropriate for describing the degree of polymerization of a cross-linked polymer.

Degree of cure The extent to which a polymer, such as a dental composite, has reacted; essentially the same as degree of conversion.

Degree of polymerization The average number of monomers that reacted to form each polymer chain in a linear polymer system.

Degrees of freedom The number of ovservations in a data set that are free to vary once the parameners of the data set (e.g., the mean) have been established.

Degrowth In some invertebrates, the ability to shrink or reduce in size when nutrients are scarce.

Dehiscence A splitting or peeling down along a natural line. Separation of the layers of a surgical wound. Isolated area in which a root is denuded of bone when the denuded area extends to the margin of the bone.

Dehydration Removal of water, the condition that results from undue loss of water. Total human male body contains 60 per cent water and 50 per cent in case of female. Normally dehydration is prevented by sensation of thirst. This mechanism may fail when sufficient water is not available and there is high loss of fluid in body due to vomiting and diarrhoea. In temperate climate, about 1500 ml of water is lost due to sweating and from lungs. Symptoms of dehydration includes severe thirst, dry lips and tongue, increase in heart rate, dizziness and confusion. There will be scanty urine, and person may develop cramps and pallor. One should consume as much fluid as possible. Salt losses from heavy sweating need to be replaced either in diet or to be mixed in fast drip of glucose saline will help.

Dehydroascorbic acid A toxic, oxidized form of ascorbic acid or vitamin C.

Dehydrogenases Enzymes catalyzing the removal of pairs of hydrogen atoms from their substrates.

Delamination In implant dentistry, the separation of a coating from its substrate.

Delayed Hypersensitivity An allergic response in which the onset of symptoms may not occure until 2 or 3 days after exposure to an antigen. Produced by T cells, it is a type of cell-mediated immunity.

Delayed conditioning A method of classical conditioning in which the conditioned stimulus remains present until the appearance of the unconditioned stimulus.

Delayed hypersensitivity Allergic reactions have been divided into two types. *Immediate hypersensitivity* which develops rapidly after administration of antigen, delayed hypersensitivity in which the response occurs 24 to 48 hours later. Immediate reactions are mediated by specific circulating antibodies while *delayed hypersensitivity* reactions are mediated by sensitised lymphocytes and are dependent on serum antibodies.

Delayed involution of uterus Immediately after parturition, uterus measures 15cm long, 12cm broad and 7.5cm thick and weights about 1000gm.

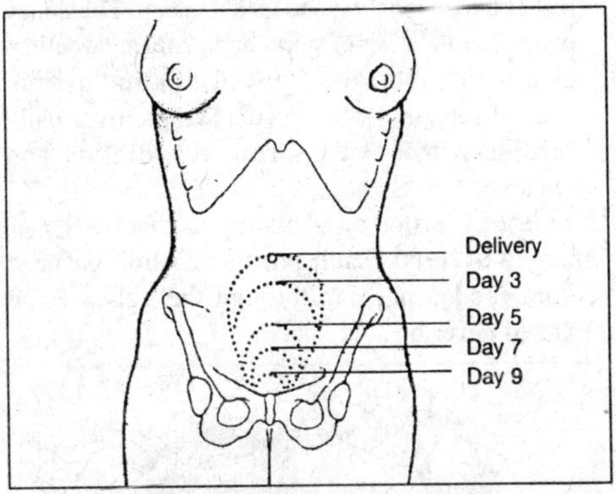

It gains its non pregnant (7.5 x 5 x 2.5 cm) size after five or six weeks. Delayed involution results in chronic stage of enlargement of uterus. Lochia discharge is prolonged and there may be prolonged vaginal bleeding.

Delayed union, fracture Compound fractures are most likely to develop delayed union. Extensive soft tissue damage also produces further impairment of blood supply of bone fragments. Infection of fracture haematoma usually leads to nonunion. Interposition of soft tissues between fracture fragments makes difficult them to unite. Poor blood supply at fracture site interferes with healing since the invasion of the haematoma by blood vessels is slow or absent. Low oxygen tension produced by a poor blood supply interferes with production of bone by undifferentiated mesenchymal cells. Inadequate immobilisation leading to excessive movement not allowing callus to form a bridge may delay union. Diabetes interferes in healing.

Deleterious Injurious : hurtful.

Delinquency Antisocial, illegal, or criminal conduct.

Delirium It is a state of mental confusion. Symptoms are those of disordered brain function. Failure to understand events or remember what is happening, increased anxiety, physical restlessness and sudden swings of mood occur. Even high fever may result it. Children and old people are most liable to develop it.

Delirium tremens It is a state of hallucination and trembling along with confusion. It generally develops in alcoholics. The symptoms include restlessness, agitation and lack of sleep. There may be fever, dilatation of pupil and profuse sweating. Confusion follows visual hallucination. Convulsions may also occur. Symptoms usually subside within 3 days rest, rehydration and sedation.

Delivery Expulsion of a child by mother.

Delivery of head Gentle pressure controls the head from sudden pushing through the vulva. Head should never be held back.

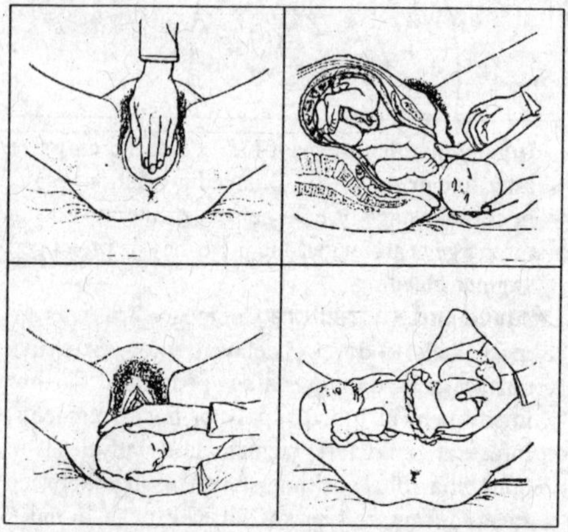

Delivery of placenta It will be wrong to interfere by rubbing the uterus roughly because it may set up irregular contraction. Controlled cord traction will reduce blood loss and to shorten the third stage.

Delivery position Comfortable positions are lithotomy and knee chest positions.

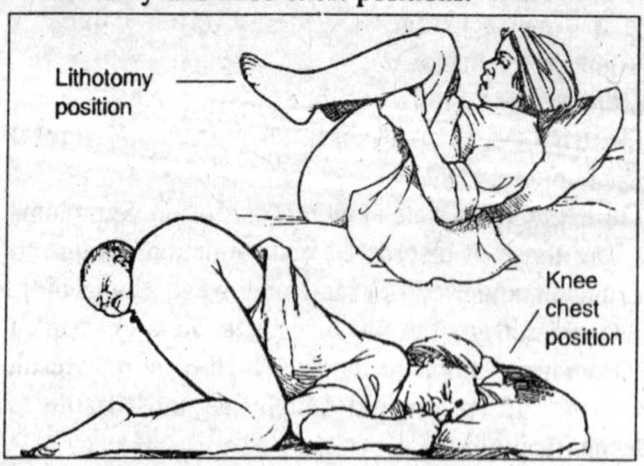

Delta endotoxin A protein toxin produced by the bacterium I that is lethal whan ingested by insects of a specific order.

Delta rhythm A rhythmic electroencephalographic waveform with a frequency ranging from 0 to 3 hertz that can be recorded from the scalp of a subject who is sleeping.

Deltoid Triangular muscle over the shoulder; inserts onto the humerus; abducts the arm.

Deltoid site Injection area in the lateral upper arm.

Delusion It is the belief and insistence that something exists when it does not exist. It differs from illusion which is an impression that something exist but is quickly corrected. It differs from hallucination which is an impression that something exists because there is sensory evidence of it.

Dementia It is due to brain disease and there is decline in all areas of mental ability. Person with dementia may not remember recent events. He becomes confused over days and dates. Sudden emotional outbursts or embarssing behaviour may be the first signs of illness. In severe case psychotic delusion may develop. Person becomes like a child and he is to be looked after like a child only. Not very effective treatment is available so far.

Dementia precox (schizophrenia) There is an abnormal emotional reaction accompanied by apparent deterioration in the personality. There is family history of nervous illness. Onset is insidious and no proper cause can be demonstrated. There is gradual loss of interest in environment. Delusions and hallucination may be prominent. Hallucinations are both auditory and visual. Attacks of depression alternating with outbursts are common.

Demethylation A microbial process which removes the methyl groups from volatile forms of selenium, such as dimethylselenide or methane selenol.

Demineralization Loss of calcium and phosphorus from bones.

Demographic Characteristic such as age, income, education, race, sex and so on which can be used to describe individual or a group.

Demyelination Every nerve is having a covering of fatty sheath. The sheath provides nutrition to nerves. Demyelination results in loss of functioning of nerve, causing loss of sensation, coordination and power in specific areas. In multiple sclerosis patches of demyelination are seen. Symptoms include blurred vision, muscle weakness and loss of coordination.

Denaturation The change in shape of a protein caused by breaking hydrogen bonds; agents that cause denaturation include heat and changes in pH. Partial or complete unfolding of the specific native conformation of a polypeptide chain, protein, or nucleic acid.

Denatured A change in the shape of protein structures caused by heat, light, acids, or alcohol.

Dendrite A branch of a neuron that consists of an extension of the cell body, thus greatly increasing the area of the cell.

Dendrodendritic synapse A synapse between two dendrites.

Denervation hypersensitivity Increased sensitivity of denervated skeletal muscle to acetyl choline. It develops after 4-5 days of denervation.

Dengue A disease caused by a mosquito-transmitted virus; also known as blackwater fever.

Denial A defence mechanism, operating unconsciously, used to resolve emotional conflict and allay anxiety by disavowing thoughts, feelings, wishes, needs, or external reality factors that are consciously intolerable.

Denitrification The biochemical reduction of nitrate or nitrite to nitrogen gas and nitrous oxide during microbial respiration without oxygen present.

Denominator data Data that define the population at risk.

Denonvillier's fascia Rectovesical septum.

Dens in dente There is tooth within a tooth. There are 2 types of it. *Coronal type* is caused by invagination of all layers of enamel organ into the dental papilla. When hard tissues are formed the invaginated enamel organ produces a small tooth within the future pulp chamber.

The maxillary lateral incisor is most frequently involved. Pulp is usually exposed and becomes inflamed or necrosed. Periapical lesion may be associated. In *radicular type* dens invaginatus is a folding of Hertwig's sheath into the developing root. These tooth often contains pulp necrosis and apical lesions.

Dense bone Bone Where the outer layer is hard and dense.

Densitometry Determination of variations in density by comparison with that of another material, or with a certain standard.

Density The overall darkness or blackness of a dental radiograph. With respect to population, a measure of the number of people in relation to a certain space.

Dental amalgam Alloy, one of the constituents of which is mercury, used for dental restorations and dies.

Dental anomally An aberration or deviation from normal anatomic growth, development or function.

Dental assistant Auxiliary to the dentist.

Dental biophysics The branch of biophysics that deals with biologic behavior of oral structures as influenced by dental restorations.

Dental caries It is a decalcification and disintegration of hard dental tissues. Certain species are more susceptible to caries than others. Sticky, sugary diet causes more of it. Caries is initiated by demineralisation of enamel by organic acids produced locally by bacteria. In addition to mineralisation bacteria destroy the dentin. In the development of caries certain oral bacteria colonise the surface of teeth in the form of sticky gelatinous film that besides the bacteria contain mucus, desquamated cells and food debris known as dental plaque. *Streptococcus mutans* is the common causative factor. The stickiness of the plaque is caused by dextran which is produced by fermenting of dietary sucrose. Finally, the rate of caries initiation and extension depends on the susceptibility of enamel. In acid to acid production, some of the bacteria produce proteolytic enzymes which break the organic portions of enamel and dentin. The clinical appearance of caries varies from a chalky white area on enamel to a deep lesion. Acute caries grows faster while in chronic caries the pulp responds by forming secondary dentin and is exposed only in the late stage of disease

- In arrested caries it cease to progress.
- The term recurrent caries is used for carious lesions that begin around the margins of defective restorations.
- Radiation caries begins a few weeks to few months after radiation and looks like a decalcification process around the cervical area of

teeth. This caries can surround the entire crown and result in its amputation.

Dental cast A positive likeness of a part of parts of oral cavity produced into durable hard material.

Dental casting It refers to the process of pouring a liquid material into a cavity in a mold to produce a restoration or appliance.

Dental chair Great revolution has come in dentistry in last 2 decades as regards equipment and scientific development is concerned. Now very sophisticated, hydrolic dental chairs are available

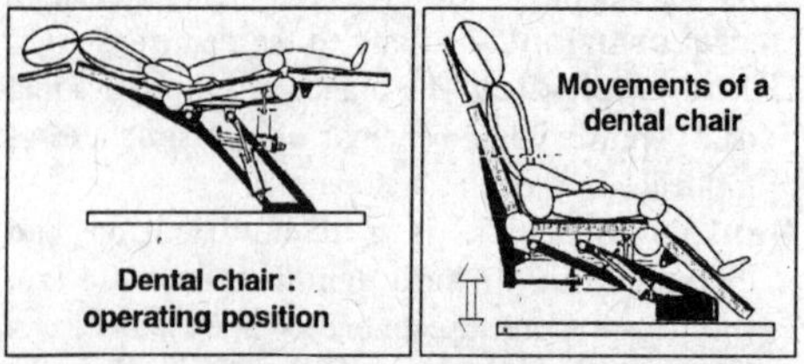

Dental chair : operating position

Movements of a dental chair

with multiple movements and tilts. Now it can be used for minor surgical operations also.

Dental chart A diagrammatic chart of the tooth on which the findings of X-Ray and clincial examination are recorded.

Dental elevator One of the blades used for engaging teeth and or roots to remove them from alveoli.

Dental engine Electric motor that by means of a continuous cord drive over pulleys, or other styles, actuates a handpiece that holds a rotary instrument.

Dental hygiene armamentarium All the instruments and equipment used during a dental hygiene procedure.

Dental hygienist Person educated in an accredited school and licensed by the state where residing to provide health services, such as scaling and polishing teeth, health education and training, and radiography, under the direction of a licensed dentist.

Dental laboratory technician One skilled in the art of executing the dentist's prescriptin for the mechanical fabrication of dental appliances.

Dental lathe Machine for producing rotary motion that uses a grinding or polishing wheel. The object that is revolved by it may be fashioned to a circular pattern with the instrument, which is stationary.

Dental materials The science surrounding the study and development of the materials used to restore and replace oral tissues.

Dental napkin Disposable bid placed on patient during dental operation.

Dental practice act Legal standards for the practice of dentistry developed through legislative action within the state. Defines minimum education standards, requirements for licensure/registration and the criteria for license revocation or suspension for a dentist, hygienist, and in several states the dental assistant.

Dental prosthetic laboratory procedures The steps in the fabrication of a dental prosthesis that do not require the presence of a patient for their accomplishment.

Dental public health Speciality of dentistry concerned with preventing the controlling dental diseases and promoting dental health on a comunitywide basis.

Dental stools Seat with four or five casters and some from of back or abdominal support used by dental health care workers at chairside.

Dental surgeon Doctor who treats diseases of teeth and oral cavity and repairs, fills and replaces teeth.

Dental unit Piece of equipment in which are assembled various dynamic instruments used in dental treatment, such as dental handpieces, operatory light, bracket table, saliva ejector, water supply, electric outlets, compressed air, and miscellaneous instruments.

Dentate Dentate nucleus of cerebellum denate gyrus in the temporal lobe.

Denticle A pulp stone; relatively large body of calcified substance in the pulp chamber of a tooth.

Denticulate Denticulate ligament of pia mater anchoring the spinal cord.

Dentifrice A paste used to clean the teeth; toothpaste.

Dentin Portion of the tooth that lies subjacent to the enamel and cementum. Consists of an organic matrix on which mineral (calcific) salts are deposited; pierced by tubules containng filamentous protoplasmic processes of the odontoblasts that line the pulpal chamber and canal. It is of mesodermal origin.

Dentinal Pertaining to dentin.

Dentinal dysplasia It is related to dentinogenesis imperfecta. It is a hereditary disease transmitted as an autosomal dominant characteristic. Both the deciduous and the permanent dentitions are affected. The teeth appear clinically normal but are lost prematurely. X-ray shows short pointed roots, periapical lucencies and obliteration of pulp chambers and root canals. There is no treatment.

Dentinal tubules Space in the dentin in which odontoblasts are found and are active.

Dentinocemental junction Line of union of the cementum and dentin of the tooth.

Dentinoenamel junction (DEJ) The junction between the dentin and enamel of a tooth.

Dentinum Dentin.

Dentist One whose profession is to treat disease and injuries of the teeth and oral cavity and to construct and insert restorations of and for the teeth, jaws, and mouth.

Dentistry It is the scientific branch dealing with teeth and associated structures of mouth. It deals with prevention, diagnosis, and treatment of diseases, fitting crowns and making bridges *Orthodontics* concerns with the moving of improperly aligned teeth to improve function. *Prosthodontcst* makes bridges and dentures. *Endodontics* involves the treatment of diseases of pulp. *Periodontics* treats disorders of gums and supporting structures of teeth.

Dentition Natural teeth in position in the dental arches.

Dentition primary Twenty teeth that compose normal childs's set of teeth.

Dentode An exact reproduction of a tooth on a gnathographically mounted cast.

Dentofacial Pertaining to both the teeth and the face.

Dentolegal Pertaining to dental jurisprudence.

Dentrifrice A pharmaceutical compound used in conjunction with tooth brush to clean and polish the teeth. In contains mild abrasive, a detergent, flavouring agent, binder and a deodorant.

Dentulous Having the natural teeth.

Denture It is an appliance to replace missing natural teeth. These dentures are made of acrylic on metal base. Nowadays porcelain teeth matching with original colour of teeth are available. These closely resemble original teeth. These blend well with the contour of the face.

Denture induced stomatitis A well fitting upper denture cuts off the underlying mucosa from the protective action of saliva. It can promote candidosis.

Dentures Artificial teeth.

Denudation Laying bare; surgical or pathologic removal of epithelial covering.

Deontologic theory Ethical theory holding that the right course of action is one dictated by ethical principles and moral rules.

Deontology Ethical study based on duty or moral obligations.

Deoxyribonucleic acid Type of nucleic acid containing the sugar deoxyribose; the genetic material of cells; DNA.

Dependency hypothesis A hypothesis of drug addiction that postulates that drug use is maintained to prevent withdrawal symptoms.

Dependency needs Vital needs for mothering, love, affection, shelter, protection, security, food, and warmth. May be a manifestation of regression when they reappear openly in adults.

Dependent edema Edema of the lower body parts.

Dependent position The lowest position of an extremity or body.

Dependent variable An aspect of behaviour or experience which depends upon changes in or changes with the independent variable, e.g. speed of reaction is partly dependent upon the intensity of the stimulus to which the response is made.

Depersonalisation It is a state of anxiety in which an individual feels as if the mind is separating from body. It indicates anxiety and psychological disorder.

Depoarize Make the membrane potential of the neuron less negative.

Depolarisation A decrease in the magnitude of the electric potential across a cell membrane; the neutralisation of polarity.

Depolarization A decrease in the electrical charge across a membrane, usually due to the inward flow of sodium ions.

Depolarization block Conduction block produced by high frequency stimulation.

Depolarize Make the membrane potential of the neuron less negative.

Depositions Oral or written testimony taken under oath but outside of a courtroom. A verbatim transcript is made and can be used as evidence in a trial.

Depot injections This is given intramuscular. It provides slow, steady absorption into the bloodstream. These injections are of very high dose than normally given dose. Inclusion of oil or wax makes its absorption slow. The release of drug may be made for days and months. Disadvantage of such injection is that uneven release of drugs prolongs side effect.

Depression There develops a feeling of hopelessness. Everyone atleast once in life develop such feelings in specific circumstance when near and dear one dies. But certain people without sufficient stimuli develop such sadness. Symptoms vary with severity of disease. In mild form anxiety and variable moods are presenting features. Person may laugh or have fits of crying off and on without any cause. Person becomes withdrawn and unable to sleep. Movements and thinking process become slower. Early morning they are more depressed and as sun arises, feels better. Causative factors may not be obvious, women suffer more than men. Psychotherapy, antidepressant type of drugs are effective in over two-third of patients. If they are suffering from delusions ECT is effective and safe.

Depressive state A melancholic mood, a feeling of hopelessness, an attitude of dejection. In serious cases, a symptom of mental illness.

Deprivation dwarfism Physical under-development found in children reared in isolation or in institutions. Thoughts to be an effect of the stress associated with emotional deprivation.

Deprivation, emotional Lack of adequate and appropriate interpersonal and/or environmental experience, usually in the early developmental years.

Depth In implant dentistry, the dimension of an implant measured coronoapically, or of available bone measured apically from the ridge crest to the nearest limiting anatomic landmark.

Depth Drill In implant dentistry, a bone drill designed to establish the angle and depth of an osteotomy.

Depth of charring A measurement of the depth to which an object, often wood, has been burned or charred by a fire.

Depth of field In microscopy, the slice of the specimen that contributes to the infocus image at a particular focus level.

Depth of pressure Compressive stress that can be light, moderate, deep, or varied.

Depth perception The ability to see three-dimensional features, such as the distance of an object from oneself and the shape of an object.

Depth psychology The psychology of unconscious mental processes. Also a system of psychology in which the study of such processes plays a major role, as in psychoanalysis.

Depth, psychological Related to unconcious psychological process.

Derealization An alteration in the perception of ones surroundings so that a sense of reality of the external world is lost.

Derived sugars Sugars in which the aldehyde group is oxidized or reduced, or a hydroxyl group is substituted or derivatized.

Derivitization The process of chemically modifying a substance to render more amenable to chromatography and/or detection.

Derma Skin.

Dermal papilla Fingerlike projection of a papillary region of the dermis that may contain blood capillaries or corpuscles of touch (Meissner corpuscles).

Dermal papillae Upper region of the dermis that forms part of the dermalepidermal junction and forms the ridges and grooves of fingerprints.

Dermal-epidermal junction Junction between the thin epidermal layer of the skin and the dermal layer providing support for the epidermis.

Dermatitis It is an inflammation of skin, may be due to allergy. In addition of eczema three forms of skin dermatitis are seborrhoeic dermatitis, contact dermatitis and photodermatitis. *Seborrhoic dermatitis* is red, scaly, itchy rash that develops on the face, scalp and chest. It may cause dandruff. *Contact dermatitis* is a reaction to some allergens that comes in contact with skin. Detergents, rubber, metals are the common cause. There may be itching blister. Avoiding of irritant and corticosteroids are useful remedy.

Dermatitis herpetiformis It is a rare, chronic, relapsing inflammatory eruptions of skin occurring due to several immunological abnormalities. Condition shows a positive association with glutensensitive enteropathy. There is an increased incidence of thyroid disease. It gives rise to vesicular, bullous and pustular lesions on an erythematous base. Lesions tend to form clusters and distributed symmetrically. Mucous membrane is generally not involved. Lesions are heavily excoriated and condition may be associated with coeliac disease. Skin biopsy helps in diagnosis. It is treated with dapsone 50 to 200 mg daily orally.

Dermatoglyphics Pictures made from arrangements of ridges on the skin surface.

Dermatology The medical specialty dealing with diseases of the skin.

Dermatomyositis It is an inflammatory degenerative disease leading to muscle atrophy. There develops weakness of pharyngeal and palatal muscle which causes dysphagia and nasal speech. There will be difficulty in chewing. Involvement of oral mucosa is not diagnostic. On face butterfly lesions may develop. Swelling of eyelids, face and lips are noted. Calcinosis of soft tissue is seen. Calcified nodules may appear on face. Tongue may also become rigid owing to severe calcinosis.

Dermis Dense connective tissue that forms the deep layer of the skin; responsible for the structural strength of the skin. The deeper of the two major layers of the skin, composed of dense fibrous connective tissue interspersed with glands, nerve endings, and blood vessels; sometimes called the true skin.

Desaturate The act of desaturating; an increase in the percentage of total oxygen-binding sites on the hemoglobin molecule that is unfilled.

Descemetocele It is the herniation of Descemet's membrane through the base of corneal ulcer. It is seen in cases wherein whole thickness of substantia propria has been destroyed and cast off. Descemet's membrane forms the base of ulcer. It becomes unable to withstand the normal intraocular pressure and therefore bulges through the base of ulcer, herniating and appearing as transparent vesicle.

Descending aorta The part of the aorta between the arch and the bifurcation into the iliac arteries; it includes the thoracic and abdominal aortae.

Descent Passage of the presenting part of the fetus into the birth canal; it begins at the onset of labour and proceeds during effacement and dilatation of the cervix.

Descogenic Pain originating form a disc.

Descriptive epidemiology Activities releated to characterizing patterns of disease occurence.

Descriptive theory The least restrictive form of theory, simply describing the phenomenon of interest.

Desensitisation It is a method in which patient is exposed repeatedly to which he or she is sensitive until a degree of tolerance is established. It is most useful in case of allergies.

Desflurance It is a colourless liquid with pungent vapour whose boiling point is 23°C and is used as inhalational anesthetic agent.

Desiccation The act or process of drying up.

Designer drugs Addictive drugs that are synthesised or manufactured to give the same subjective effects as well-known illict drugs. Since the process is a covert operation there is great difficulty in tracing the manufacturer to check the drugs for adverse effects.

Desistence Cessation of criminal activity in a person who has previously committed illegal acts.

Desmoid tumour It looks like a tendon in its appearance and texture. It is a benign fibrous tumour arising in the musculoaponeurotic structures below the level of umbilicus. It is notorius for recurrence so it is also known as recurrent fibroid of Paget. It is common is multiparous women and may occur in scars of old hernia or other abdominal operation wound. A small haematoma of the abdominal wall due to trauma may be a precipitating factor. It is essentially a benign, hard fibroma. It is completely uncapsulated fibroma and is so hard that it cracks when it is cut. There may be myxomatous change. Recurrence is very common. There is no tendency to metastasise. Very rarely it may undergo low-grade sarcomatous change. Diagnosis is confirmed by excision biopsy. Excision includes wide margin of surrounding healthy tissue of at least 2.5 cm.

Desmolysis Destruction and disintegration of connective tissue.

Desmosome A point of adhesion between two cells.

Desmosome-gap junctions Site of adhesion and likely intercellular communication between sertoli cells and germ cells.

Desone Trademark for a soft dental casting gold alloy.

Desorption The non-destructive elution and recovery of, for example, metal of metalloid species, radionuclides, and organometal compounds from loaded biological material by physicochemical treatment.

Desquamatic gingivitis It is a rare condition. Irregular areas on the entire gingiva are fiery red, smooth and shiny. Stroking the gingiva with finger, cotton or blast of air may peel away the surface epithelium exposing the painful bleeding. In severe cases gingiva is covered by multiple raw bleeding areas. These lesions may begin as blister like eruption that break.

Desquamation Shedding or casting off, as of the superficial epithelium of mucous membrane or skin; a normal physiologic process.

Dessicated liver It is a dehydrated liver.

Dessigation The act of drying.

Desurgency Those scoring high on cattell's sixteen personality factor questionnaire are interospective, restrained and solemn.

Detergent A molecule with polar and nonpolar portions that can disrupt membranes by stabilizing the dispersion of hydrophobic lipids and proteins in water.

Deteriogenic Describing organisms causing or capable of causing biodeterioration.

Determinism The doctrine that for every effect there is a cause, in psychology, the view that every aspect of behaviour or experience is related to an antecedent event, external or internal to the individual.

Detoxification Treatment by the use of medication, diet, rest, fluids, and nursing care to restore physiologic functioning after it has been seriously disturbed by the overuse of alcohol, barbiturates, or other addictive drugs.

Detritus Debris that adheres to tooth, gingival, and mucosal surfaces.

Detrusor instability 'Unstable ladder' characterized by spontaneous expulsion of urine despite conscious attempts at restraint.

Detrusor muscle Muscle in the wall of the urinary bladder.

Detumescence The subsidence of swelling, congestion, or turgor; the period in which the brgan or passage decreases in size and returns to its original state.

Developer cut-off An artefact seen on dental radiographs that results from a low level of developer solution and represents an undeveloped portion of a film; a straight, white border appears on the processed radiograph.

Developer spots An artefact seen on dental radiograph caused by developer solution coming in contact with the film before processing; dark spots appear on the processed radiograph.

Development All of the processes involved in the differentiation of specific tissues plus growth in body mass.

Development age Age based on functional behavior and ability to adopt the environment.

Development anatomy The study of development from the fertilized egg to the adult form. The branch of anatomy called embryology is generally restricted to the study of development from the fertilized egg through the eighth week in utero.

Development of local anesthetics Cocaine was introduced in 1884, stovaine in 1904, cinchocaine in 1925, amethocaine in 1931, lingocaine in 1947, Chloroprocaine in 1952, prilocaine in bupi vacine in 1963, etidocaine in 1972 and ropivacaine in 1977.

Developmental Pertaining to the process of human growth and development.

Developmental cataract It is commonly seen in its minor form. Most people show some kind of minute opacity of lens. It is seen in many forms, shapes and sizes at varied locations. Developmental cataract has a tendency to affect a particular zone which got disturbed during its formation.

Developmental disorder A handicap or impairment originating before the age of 18 years which may be expected to continue indefinitely and which constitutes a substantial impairment. The disability may be attributable to mental retardation, cerebral palsy, epilepsy, or other neurologic conditions and may include autism.

Developmental dyslexia Pronounced reading difficulty in children who are the match of their peers in other respects.

Developmental groove Fine depressed line in the enamel of a tooth that marks the union of the lobes of the crown in its development.

Developmental migration The movement of animals from one area to another as animal size and feeding preferences change. This is often a one-way migration.

Developmental or normative transitions Predictable family changes related to the oldest child's development that occur in an expected time line congruent with movement through the eight family stages. Even though families have children in more than one developmental stage, it is assumed that parents have some experience with the earlier stages of family development because of the parenting of the first child.

Developmental process Changes and functions occurring during a human's early years as the body becomes more efficient and more effective.

Developmental psychopathology A field of study that focuses on the developmental and longitudinal course of psychiatric disorders across the life cycle.

Developmental task Psychological and social tasks associated with growth and change or transition. Specifically, the developmental tasks of pregnancy are those associated with transition to parenthood and the psychosocial assimilation of the expected baby into the life of the mother and father.

Developmental toxicity A general term for adverse effects on development, manifested as death, malformation, growth retardation and functional deficit.

Deviancy The quality of having a condition or engaging in behavior that is atypical in a social group and is considered undesirable.

Deviant Those people or things that do not fit in social norms are "deviant". The term "deviation" was originally from the field of statistics, describing the data that lay outside of the bell curve.

Deviation IQ A statistically derived IQ, not determined by the traditional MA/CA method. It is determined instead by the standard deviation of MA scores at a given CA and the deviation of the individual's score from the mean of this distribution.

Deviation score Calculated by subtracting the mean of a data set from each raw score.

Devil model An earlier view of the origin of mental disorders, suggesting that the cause was the devil, inhabiting the individual's body. The proposed treatment ranged from dunking to starvation to other forms of torture, all with the purpose of driving out the devil.

Devital Deprived of life.

Devital tooth Pulpless tooth.

Devitalise To deprive of vitality or of life; in dentistry, to destroy the vitality of the dental pulp.

Dexamethasone In tablet form it is useful in asthma, stroke or brain tumour, multiple sclerosis, etc. As nasal spray it is useful in allergic rhinitis and as eyedrop in iritis. A potent synthetic glucocorticoid that does not bind to transcortin.

Dextran Water soluble polymer of glucose of high molecular weight.

Dextran 40 Average molecular weight is 40,000. Half-life *in vivo* is only 3 hours. Duration of useful plasma expansion is about 1 hour. It is used to increase intravascular volume and to reduce blood viscosity. It prevents intravascular aggregation of red cells, and to reverse peripheral ischaemia. It does not interfere with cross-matching. It should not be given in dehydrated patients.

Dextran 70 Its molecular weight is 70,000. It is used to reduce thrombosis. It is nontoxic, electrically neutral and chemically inert. It has acidic pH. 25 % is excreted within 3 hours. Only 50% can be recovered from urine. It is useful as plasma substitute in case of burns and surgical shock. It increases venous return to heart. These should not be used in asthmatic and allergic patients. Platelet stickiness is increased. Large volume can cause bleeding. 500 ml of it increases the circulatory plasma volume by 750 ml.

Dextrins Starch is quickly hydrolysed to glucose by boiling with dilute acids.

When hydrolysed by ptylin ill-defined substances dextrins are formed. They have a faint sweet taste. They form sticky solutions in water and are used as adhesives.

Dextro Prefix designating an aqueous solution.

Dextrose drip Five per cent of solution is isotonic and may be used from drip to replace and to keep open an intravenons route for medication. It has an acid pH. If a combination of saline and glucose is to be employed the proportion should be 1/5 normal saline and 4.3 % glucose. This mixture is isotonic. Thrombophlebitis can be minimised by neutralisation of pH of 6.8. Glucose of 10 % or more may produce thrombophlebitis. Levulose is better. Dextrose 5 % is ineffective replacement in case of trauma.

Dextrose equivalent (DE) An indication of total reducing sugars as glucose percentage. Unhydrolyzed starch has a DE of zero and glucose has a DE of 100.

Dhatura There are two varieties one with white flowers and another with black ones. Flower is bell-shaped and bulb is spherical. Each fruit has 400-500 seeds. Ingestion of 4 to 6 seeds may be fatal. Symptoms of toxicity develops within 30 minutes of ingestion. Vomiting immediately develops due to gastric irritation. It is bitter in taste. Patient develops dryness of mouth, burning pain in mouth and dysphagia. Pupils will be dilated. There will be hyperthermia, urinary retention and decreased bowel sounds. Delirium is quiet frequent. Patient tries to pull imaginary threads from tips of his or her fingers. Ataxia, disorientation, frank psychosis develop. In fatal cases, stupor, coma and convulsions develop.

Diabetes in pregnancy During first half of pregnancy, maternal hypoglycemia occurs due to rapid transfer of maternal glucose to fetus. Nausea and vomiting in early pregnancy may produce a decreased demand in insulin requirement. Maternal hypoglycemia in early pregnancy may pose a problem in differentiating a starvation ketosis from diabetic ketosis. In second half of pregnancy insulin requirement is increased by 70%.

Diabetes insipidus There is an excessive thirst and passing of enormous quantity of urine. Diabetes insipidus results from a failure of pituitary gland to secrete antidiuretic hormone (ADH). A person may pass 10 to 30 pints of urine within 24 hours provided sufficient water is consumed. If sufficient water is not taken dehydration may take place. Treatment includes administration of ADH. Low sodium diet should be consumed.

Diabetes mellitus In this condition pancreas is not able to produce sufficient insulin to neutralise sugar. As a result the level of glucose in blood becomes higher. It results in fatigue due to excessive urination, thirst and hunger. Insulin-dependent diabetes is more severe appearing before the age of 35. It develops very rapidly. Insulin secreting cells known as beta cells are being destroyed without regular insulin injection person may go under coma and dies. The other which is common develops after the age of 40 and is known as non-insulin dependent type II. It develops slowly and is generally discovered during routine medical examination. In such cases insulin is not required and mostly dietary measures, weight reduction and oral tablets keep the person fit. It runs in families. Obesity is the predisposing factor, certain illness, i.e. pancreatitis, corticosteroids and some diuretics, infections, pregnancy may also precipitate it. The aim of treatment is to prolong life, relieve symptoms and prevent long-term complications. Regular physical activity will help. Commonest complications are retinopathy, neuropathy and nephropathy.

Diabetic amyotrophy During poor control of diabetes person may complain of it. The clinical symptoms are of severe constant pain in one thigh accompanied by wasting and weakness of quadriceps muscles. There are no sensory findings. Many patients recover when control of diabetes improves. Electromyography shows that more muscles than are denervated. Paraspinal muscles have potential of fibrillation and fasciculations.

Diabetic cardiomyopathy Myocardial dysfunction attributable to the effects of diabetes.

Diabetic gangrene It may develop due to trophic changes resulting from peripheral neuritis and atheroma of arteries. It may result in ischaemia and excess of sugar lowers resistance to infection. Neuropathic factors impair sensation and thus favours minor injuries. Muscular involvement is frequently involved by loss of reflexes and deformities. Thick callosities develop of soles.

Diabetic neuropathy Males are more affected. There is close relation between degree of hyperglycaemic control and duration of diabetes. Most common is sensory distal neuropathy with painful burning sensation in feet and toes. Motor features are slight or absent. Ankle jerks may be absent. Loss of skin sensations may result in deep indolent ulcers. Repeated minor injuries may result in gross hypertrophic osteoarthropathy.

Diabetic retinopathy It occurs due to lack of insulin which causes increase in blood glucose concentration. The diabetic retinopathy is a microangiopathy in which retinal blood vessels affected are precapillary arterioles. Microaneurysm appears as small round dot usually situated on

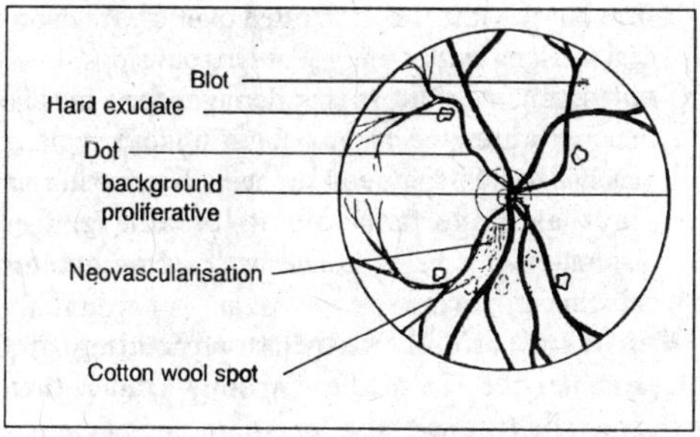

temporal side of macula. Haemorrhage may be of flame shaped or round dot haemorrhages. Round dot haemorrhages are deeper in middle layers of retina. Retinal vessels appear dilated, full and tortuous. There may be looping. There will be visual loss. The macular oedema can be diagnosed by slit-lamp examination. The macula assumes a cystoid appearance.

Diabetogenic Condition such as pregnancy which produces the effects of diabetes.

Diabetogenic hormones Chemical messengers that antagonize the actions of insulin on peripheral tissues and indirectly promote an increase in pancreatic insulin secretion.

Diabetogenic tending To cause diabetes mellitus, including insulin resistance and glucose intolerance.

Diagnosis Distinguishing one disease from another or determining the nature of a disease from signs and symptoms by inspection, palpation, laboratory tests, and other means.

Diagnosis, definitive A final diagnosis.

Diagnosis, differential The recognition of a specific disease, syndrome, injury, or condition based on the scrutiny of clinical information, including data from a patient's history, physical examination, laboratory testing, and response to treatment.

Diagnostic Useful in determining a diagnosis; pertaining to the art and science of distinguishing one injury, disease, or dysfunction from another.

Diagnostic examination Procedure that involves physical inspection of body structures and evidence of their function.

Diagnostic interview schedule A standard mental health diagnostic interview based on DSM that is used in population survey.

Diagnostic model Reproduction of the dental arches and surrounding tissues; produced from impressions.

Diagonal artery The first, and generally largest, of the left anterior ventricular branches of the anterior interventricular coronary artery; it sometimes arises directly from the trunk of the left coronary artery.

Diagonal conjugate The distance between the promontory of the sacrum and the lower margin of the pubic symphysis, which can be measured clinically.

Diagonal conjugate measurement The chief internal pelvic measurement made to determine the actual diameter of the pelvic passage. It is the distance between the sacral promontory and the lower margin of the symphysis pubis.

Dialysate The portion of a solution that can pass through a dialyzing membrane; diffusate.

Dialysis Diffusion through a membrane.

Dialysis encephalopathy It is also known as dialysis dementia and is a complication of haemodialysis. Clinical features include progressive aphasia, personality changes, myoclonus, convulsions and intellectual deterioration. EEG shows frontal slow wave discharge with spikes and sharp waves. After some time these features become permanent.

Diameters of fetal skull :

Suboccipitobregmatic	9.9cm
Suboccipitofrontal	10.5cm
Occipitofrontal	12cm
Mentovertical	13.8cm
Submentobregmatic	9.9cm

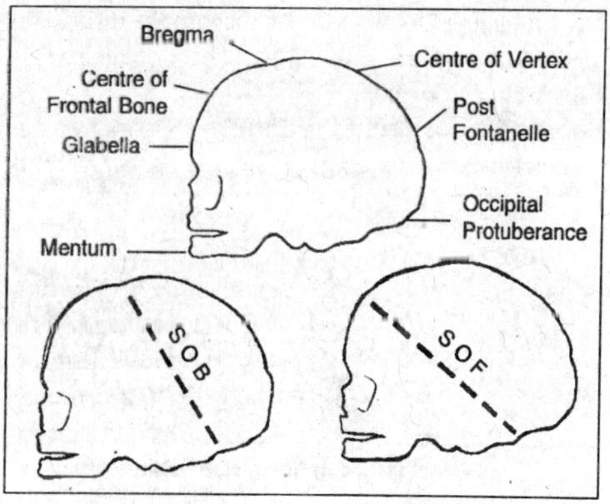

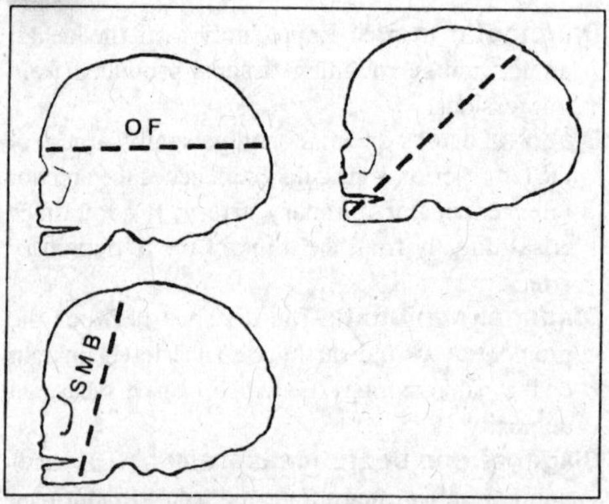

Diamorphine hydrochloride (Heroin) This is a diacetyl ester of morphine and is most likely drug to cause addiction because of euphoria it produces. It depresses the respiratory centre and cough reflex more than morphine and is twice potent as pain reliever. Diamorphine 5 mg has a quicker onset of activity, more marked sedation, fever and emetic sequelae than 10 mg morphine. It is an excellent post-operative analgesic although its effect does not last long. Usual dose is 2.5 to 5 mg of hydrochloride.

Diapedesis The migration of white blood cells through the endothelial walls of blood capillaries into the surrounding connective tissues.

Diaphoresis Profuse sweating. In obstetrics, it is part of the reversal of water metabolism, in which excess fluid accumulated during pregnancy is eliminated.

Diaphragm It is a strong, thin, domed sheet of muscle that separates chest from abdomen. Through it passes several blood vessels and oesophagus. Contraction of diaphragm results in inhalation of air into lungs. Through it hiatus hernia may develop.

Diaphragm for family planning Diaphragm is a saucer-like appliance made of thin rubber with a firm but flexible rim. It is fitted over the mouth of cervix along with family planning jelly.

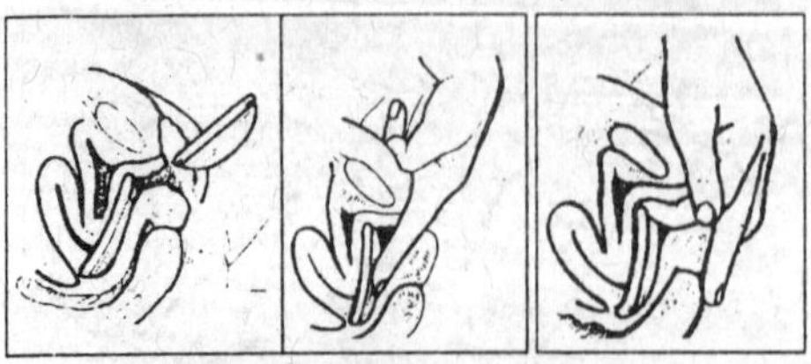

Different stages of fitting diaphragm

Diaphragm muscle It is a dome-shaped muscle that separates the thorax from abdomen. It is attached to ribs, spine and sternum. The diaphragm plays an important role in breathing. For inspiration it is being drawn in the lungs and for exhaling it relaxes.

Diaphragmatic breathing Breathing that promotes the use of the diaphragm rather than upper chest muscles.

Diaphragmatic hernia Hiatus hernia occurs at the the point where the oesophagus passes through diaphragm. Hernia may be sliding or non-sliding. There may not be any symptoms. Due to regurgitation of acid, heart burn or acid eructation may be complained of. This is felt after a heavy meal or after stooping forward or lying down. After hot drinks it may be aggravated. Due to pressure of gastric pouch there may be cough, precordial distress, anginal pain, hiccough, etc. In strangulated condition there will be severe retrosternal pain.

Diaphragmatic paralysis Loss of function of the diaphragm or hemidiaphragm as the result of a disease or injury to the nerve supply.

Diaphragmatic pleura The serous membrane lining the diaphragm.

Diaphysis Shaft of a long bone.

Diarrhoea It is an increased liquidity, frequency or volume of movements as compared to normal for that person. Acute diarrhoea develops time to time due to contaminated food or water. Such episode clears within 2 to 3 days even without treatment, only from fluid balance. While chronic diarrhoea is due to some diseases and requires treatment and investigations. In normal person it is colon which absorbs water from food residues and making contents semisolid. But if intestinal contents anyhow pass too quickly from it may result in diarrhoea. It may take the form of repeated attacks of acute diarrhoea such as Crohn's disease and ulcerative colitis. It does not require drug treatment, fluid balance is to be maintained.

Diarthroses Freely movable joint.

Diastasis The late portion of diastole when blood is entering the ventricles slowly and the venous pressure tends to rise.

Diastasis recti Separation of longitudinal muscles of abdomen during pregnancy.

Diastasis Rectus The bellies of rectus abdominis muscles held together by the linea alba are separated in this condition. The lines alba my have thinned, separated or severed completely. The muscle is also stretched.

Diastema A space or separation between two teeth, most noticeably between the upper central incisors.

Diastereoselectivity The ability of a catalyst of reagent to distinguish between stereoisomers other than enantiomers.

Diastole Relaxation of the heart, interposed between its contractions; opposite of systole. The sequence of the cardiac cycle during which a heart chamber wall is relaxed. The period of the cardiac cycle when the ventricles of the heart are not contracting. Relaxation of the heart chambers during which they fill with blood; usually refers to ventricular relaxation.

Diastolic blood pressure The lowest arterial blood pressure reached during a given ventricular cycle.

Diastolic dysfunction An inability of the ventricles to accept the blood ejected from the atria.

Diastolic hypertension It results due to an excessive constriction or narrowing of arterioles throughout the body. Greater is the narrowing, greater will be the diastolic blood pressure.

Diastolic interval Duration of diastole. It is shortened when heart rate is increased and normally is 0.62 seconds at 65 beats/minute.

Diastolic pressure Pressure in the arterial system when the heart relaxes and fills with blood.

Diathermy The therapeutic use of high frequency electric current to generate heat within some part of body. The frequency is greater than the maximum frequency for neuromuscular response and ranges from several hundred thousand to millions of cycles per second. It is used to increase blood flow in certain areas.

Diathesis An inherited susceptibility or predisposition to a particular disease.

Diathrosis A type of functionally classified joint in which the articulating bones are freely movable; also called a synovial joint.

Diatoric A metal retention pin used in anterior porcelain denture teeth; appears radiopaque.

Diazepam It is used to treat anxiety and loss of sleep. It has also role as muscle relaxant to treat back pain. It is used in alcohol withdrawal also.

Diazotroph An organism capable of biological nitrogen fixation. Thus, diazotrophic.

DIC Disseminated Intravascular Coagulation.

Dichotic listening A procedure whereby two different auditory stimuli are played simultaneously to each ear.

Dichotomous variable A variable that can take only two values, such as male/female or present/absent.

Dick test The test consists of an intradermal injection of 0.1 ml of standardised diluted erythrogenic toxin and a control, and the test is considered to be positive, when it produces erythema and oedema measuring more than 10 mm in diameter after 8 to 24 hours, and no reaction on the control site. The test becomes positive in scarlet fever but has now largely been abandoned.

Dick-Read approach to childbirth The approach that is based on the understanding that fear of pain produces muscular tension, which produces pain and greater fear. This approach includes an educational programme to teach physiological processes of labour, exercise to improve muscle tone, and techniques to assist in relaxation and prevent the fear-tension-pain mechanism. Also called Read method of childbirth preparation.

Dicrotic pulse A pulse that feels double on palpation; caused by prolonged ending of the pulse wave; also may be perceived as a weak wave between two beats.

Dicta The writings of a judge in an opinion that do not specifically affect the resolution or determination of the case and are not part of the common law resulting from the decision. Dicta are important when used to indicate how the court might rule in future cases with related facts.

Diencephalic amnesia Amnesia associated with shrinkage of the mammillary bodies.

Diencephalic syndrome It is a cause of short stature. The cause is usually a tumour at the optic chiasm, in the third or fourth ventricle. The symptoms start before the age of 6 months or upto 3 or 4 years. Signs of increased intracranial pressure are there.

Diencephalon It is developed from forebrain. It is made up of the thalamus, hypothalamus, epithalamus and subthalamus. In the intact adult brain only ventral surface of diencephalon is visible. This is the area which lies behind the optic chiasma and shows pituitary stalk and mamillary bodies.

Diestrus In veterinary species, the period of ovarian cycles dominated by corpus luteum secretion of progesterone.

Diet The customary allowance of food and drink taken by a person from day to day.

Diet analysis Documentation of food intake that is analyzed for quality and content to ensure a balanced diet and controlled oral health.

Diet history Assessment technique used to obtain facts about a person's eating habits and factors that affect nutrition.

Dietary standards A guide to adequate nutrient intake levels against which the nutrient values of foods consumed are compared.

Diethylstilbesterol It is similar to natural oestradiol. It is used to supplement or replace oestrogen. It is used to treat hypogonadism and symptoms of menopause. In high doses it can be used as postcoital contraceptives. In males it treats prostate cancer. It should not be taken during pregnancy.

Dieting Deliberate modification of food intake in order to lose weight.

Differential amplifier An amplifier that processes the voltage difference between two input terminals, effectively rejecting common mode voltage that appear between each input terminal and the common ground.

Differential conditioning Conditioning in which the organism discriminates between stimuli, giving a conditioned response to one stimulus and not to a similar but different one.

Differential diagnosis The determination of which one of two or more diseases or conditions a patient has, by systematically comparing and contrasting their clinical findings.

Differential error Nonrandom, systematic, or consistent error in which the values tend to be inaccurate in a particular direction. Same as Bias.

Differential loss In the context of trace evidence, differential loss may occur following transfer from a donor or more than one trace component or material. Differential loss occurs when the persistence properties of the two or more trace components differ.

Differential validity When the coefficients for different samples of person, such as majority and minority groups, are unequal. The test is therefore viewed to be less appropriate for some groups than for others.

Differentiate A process by which daughter cells become different in structure and function (by using different genes from the genome-all cells of the body share), as when some of the original cells of early developmental stages differentiate to become muscle cells and other cells become nerve cells, and so on. (Differentiation is another form of this term).

Differentiation Specialization of cell structure and function during embryonic growth and development.

Differentiation antigen A cell surface molecule expressed at a particular stage of development or on cells of a given lineage.

Difficult coitus Causes include of painful coitus. Other causes may be bony ankylosis of hip in extreme adduction making sex play impossible. There may be developmental defects of vagina and failure of canalisation.

Diffraction The spatial distribution of waves that are scattered from an object and recombine interfering with one another.

Diffuse Not definitely limited or localized; usually involving several areas of the brain.

Diffuse active otosclerosis There is abnormal vascularity with a great increase in size and number of marrow spaces.

Most of these spaces are lined by osteoblasts. Between the marrow spaces the ground substance stains blue or dark bluish red and cement lines between plates of bone are irregular. Number of osteocytes is greatly increased.

Diffuse brain damage Widespread, generalized deficits in the brain.

Diffuse noxious inhibitory controls Appropriate neural connections whereby painful stimulations of one part of the body may produce pain relief in all other parts.

Diffuse otitis externa Main symptoms include tragal tenderness, diffuse swelling of skin of external auditory canal.

There may be complete luminal obstruction resulting in hearing loss.

Diffusion The movement of molecules from an area of high concentration to an area of low concentration due to random thermal motion. Tendency for solute molecules to move from an area of higher concentration to an area of lower concentration in solution; the product of the constant random motion of all atoms, molecules, or ions in a solution.

Diffusion bonding Relative movement of atoms across an interface, leading to unification of one part with another. In some situations, may be used to enhance the strength of porous surface layers intended for biological ingrowth.

Digeorge syndrome Immuno-deficiency caused by a congenital failure in thymic development resulting in a lack of mature functional T cells.

Digestion The process whereby ingested food is broken down to form that can be absorbed across the intestinal wall. The breakdown of carbohydrates, lipids, proteins, and other large molecules to their component parts.

Digestive system Organs that work together to ensure proper digestion and absorption of nutrients.

Digestive tract The tract from the mouth to the anus, including the stomach and intestines, where food is taken in, broken down, and absorbed.

Digit A single symbol or character to represent a quantity.

Digital Of pertaining to, or performed with a finger.

Digital clubbing A proliferative change in the soft tissues of nail beds resulting in a broadening of their ends; the nails are abnormally curved.

Digital image Discrete representation of information on a regular grid. Each point on the grid is called a pixel and the value of the pixel often represents a color.

Digital nerve block Each digit is supplied by two palmar and 2 dorsal nerves. Two-three ml local anaesthetic agent is given with the help of fine needle.

Digital number It is the value of a number stored in digital form for example in a computer. Digital numbers are stored by a number of bites and can assume finite set of values over a finite dose.

Digital radiography It is a system that generate digital images which can be displayed using computers and high-resolution cathode ray monitors. There is important difference between conventional analogue film image and a digital image. In conventional image, grey scale is made up of number of black silver grains per unit area and grains are not visible to eyes. While digital image consists of square (pixels) with eyen density within each square. Hence viewing a digital image the viewing distance should be long enough.

Digital subtraction angiography (DSA) It is a relatively non-invasive computer-assisted imaging modality, principally used for assessment of extracranial carotid and vertebral artery disease, peripheral vascular disease and pulmonary angiography. It can also evaluate intracranial aneurysm and vascular tumour with a prominent venous component.

Digitilized radiography Use of a small camera and computer to record an image electronically.

Dilatation The condition of being dilated or stretched.

Dilatation of cervix and curettage It is the conventional operation for terminating early

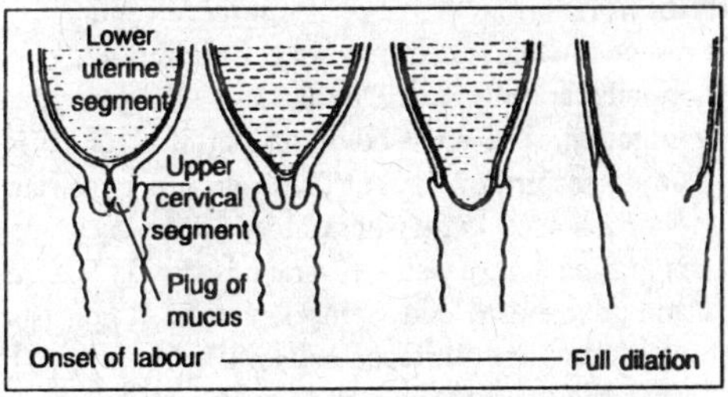

pregnancy. Operation should preferably be performed under general anaesthesia.

Dilated cardiomyopathy A disease of the myocardium characterized by ventricular dilatation and cardiac muscle contractile dysfunction.

Diltiazem It is a calcium channel blocker used in the treatment of hypertension and angina. It reduces the frequency of angina. As side effects, it may cause headache loss of appetite, nausea, and swelling of ankles.

Diluent Specified fluid to dissolve the solute.

Dimaxillary Pertaining to right and left maxillae.

Dimensional change Percentage of shrinkage or expansion of a dental material or other substance.

Dimensional variables Same as continuous variables.

Dimorphism The manifestation in the same species of two forms, such as male and female; refers to both bodily form and appearance and to sex differences in behaviour and language.

Din genes Genes regulated as part of the DNA inducible network of gene regulation; a term usually only applied to genes of unknown function; when function is identified, the "din" designation is then replaced by a more appropriate function-related name.

Dinomitosis Mitosis of the dinokaryon, characterized by the presence of an extranuclear mitotic spindle crossing the nucleus via cytoplasmic channels.

Diochroic As in pleochroic, but commonly used to denote a color change between only two viewing axes.

Dioecious Describing species in which there are individuals of two separate sexes, male and female.

Dipeptidase An intestinal peptidase that completes the hydrolysis of proteins to amino acids.

Diphtheria It is an acute infection caused by *C. diphtheriae*. It is characterised by pseudomembrane in pharynx. Children above 6 months are affected. Disease spreads by droplet infection. The most common portal of entry is upper respiratory tract. These do not penetrate deeper tissues, lymphatics or blood. Primary lesion is glistening. Greyish membrane is firm in texture and adherent to underlying structure. It consists of exudate and fibrinous network.

Tonsils, pillar of fauces and larynx are commonly affected. Incubation period is 2 to 7 days. Onset is sudden, fever is moderate, general weakness is present. Swallowing becomes painful. Pharynx becomes dull and red. Tonsils are enlarged and glands become prominent. There may be palatal palsy with nasal voice and nasal regurgitation of food.

Diphtheria carriers When diphtheria bacilli are present in the nose and throat without any manifestation of infection the condition is called carrier stage. In convalescent carriers, the organisms are present for 6 to 8 weeks. During outbreaks of disease contact carriers are seen. In swab-positive cases antitoxins are given.

Diphyllobothrium latum It is a broad fish tape worm of 10 meters and 1020 m.m. wide. It consists more than 3000 proglottids. It attaches to mucosal lining of ileum.

Diplegia Paralysis of like parts on either side of the body. In cerebral palsy, diplegia describes involvement of the lower extremities predominantly, with only mildly affected upper extremities.

Diploe The spongy layer of bone positioned between the inner and outer layers of compact bone.

Diploid Having two sets of genetic information; describing a cell with two chromosomes of each type. Having a pair of chromosome 46 or 23 pairs that represents one copy of every chromosome from each parent.

Diplopia The perception of two images of a single object.

Diplotene A stage in the first meiotic prophase in which DNA is duplicated, after which the oocyte enters a resting phase,

Dipole A molecule having both positive and negative charges.

Dipyridamol testing It is an alternative to exercise testing. In it, coronary dilator dipyridamole is used. This drug uses myocardial blood flow in normal coronary artery but not in arteries distal to stenosis. $^{201}T_1$ uptake in the normal distribution or decreased activity in stenotic area is increased. The resulting image will appear similar to one following exercise. Imaging of $^{201}T_1$ injected 3 to 5 minutes after IV dipyridamole 0.56 mg/kg has a sensitivity for CAD similar to that of exercise testing.

Dipyridamole An agent that reduces platelet aggregation and causes coronary vasodilation.

Direct ophthalmoscopy Make the patient sit comfortably and ask him to look at a distance spot light. A dilated pupil allows better view of the fundus. For examination of the right eye fundus, stand on the right side of the patient with ophthalmoscope in the right hand and view through the right eye. For examination of the left eye fundus, stand on the left side of the patient with ophthalmoscope in left hand and view through the left eye. Viewing through the sight hole of the ophthalmoscope, approach the patient, focusing the light on the pupil until you see a red glow and thereafter the fundus. Interpose the lens in the ophthalmoscope if the retina is not visible clearly. It is handy, portable and self-luminous. Image is erect, and magnified to 15 times. Opacities in vitreous and lens can be examined. Refractive error can be assessed.

Direct calorimetery The direct measurement of actual energy expanded by the body throughout a given period. It is measured by placing a human subject in a special calorimeter. The heat given off by the subject is absorbed by the water in the coils surrounding the well insulated chamber where by, the total heat can be measured directly.

Direct causality The factor under consideration exerts its effect without intermediary factors.

Direct Comb's Test RH positive fetal cord red blood cells become coated with RH antibody from the rhesus negative mother. With the addition of coomb's reagent these red cells from the fetal cord blood become agglutinated.

Direct contact Method of disease tranmission caused by coming into contact with the infected person.

Direct contact victims Emergency and rescue workers who search the rubbles for survivors and dead bodies.

Direct development A type of life cycle that includes neither a distinct larval form nor a dramatic metamorphosis. In direct development, the embryo develops directly into a juvenile by a series of gradual changes.

Direct diagonals When muscles contract in proper sequence, the stressed muscle group overcomes the demand made on it. The correct timing plays an important role both in complex motion and in sports. In direct resistance, maximal resistance occurs over the entire cause of motion.

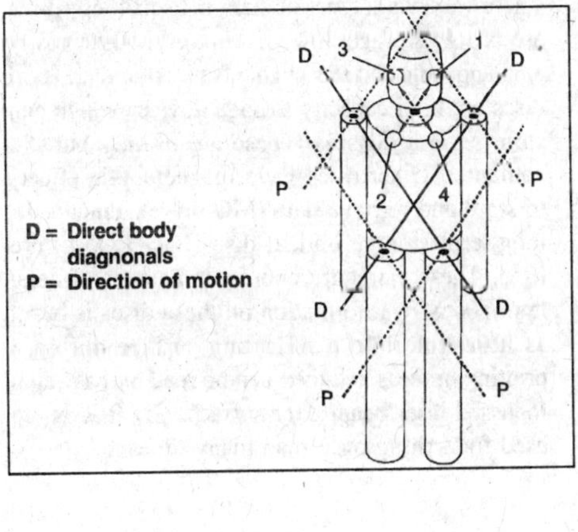

Direct gold A restoration made from essentially pure gold in the form of sheets or pellets; it is condensed directly into a cavity preparation.

Direct inguinal hernia The hernia protrudes directly through the posterior wall of inguinal canal in the Hesselbach's triangle. The direct hernial sac lies outside the cord. Direct hernias are mostly acquired in nature. It seldom comes out through the superficial inguinal ring. The neck of direct harnial sac is wide and therefore hernia appears immediately on standing and disappears again immediately when patient lies down.

Direct laryngoscope It is a U-shaped instrument consisting of laryngoscopic tube. There is a strong horizontal handle to control the tongue and a vertical handle to manipulate. These are of two types : distal illuminating laryngoscope or proximal illuminating or Negus type.

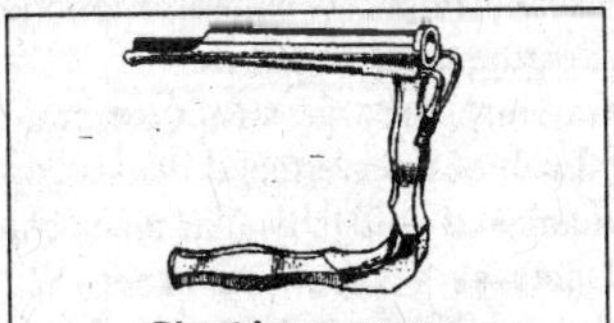

Direct laryngoscope

Direct motor pathways Collections of upper motor neurons with cell bodies in the motor cortex that project axons into the spinal cord, where they synapse with lower motor neurons or association neurons in the anterior horns.

Direct supervision Dentist has designated a patient of record upon whom services are to be performed and has described the procedure to be performed.

Direct vision Ability to see an object with the naked eye without the use of a mirror to reflect the image.

Directed donors Relatives and friends who donate blood for a patient.

Directed verdict When a trial judge decides that the evidence of law is so clearly in favor of one party that it is pointless for the trial to proceed, the judge may direct the jury to return a verdict for that party.

Direction of flight The trajectory of a blood drop which can be established by its angle of impact and directionality angle.

Directional coronary atherectomy A procedure in which atherosclerotic plaque is removed from the lumen of a coronary artery.

Disability An inability to perform an activity in the manner or range considered normal for that individual; the result of an impairment.

Disability limitation Medical and surgical measures aimed at controlling or correcting the anatomic and physiologic components of disease in symptomatic patients and precenting resultant limitations in functional ability.

Disablement Within this text the term is used to describe the actual, objective loss of function as a result of illness or accident.

Disaccharide Any of a class of carbohydrates, including lactose and sucrose, that yields two monosaccharides on hydrolysis.

Disaster Usually refers to natural calamities such as floods, earthquakes and fires.

Disc It is a flat, circular structure containing cartilage. Each of intervertebral disc is composed of outer hard and soft jelly like inner core. The material acts as a shock absorber. With age intervertebral disc is wore out and becoming susceptibe to more damage due to injury. In old age disc may prolapse and put pressure on nerve and result in pain along the distribution of nerve. Disc prolapse generally develop in lower spine.

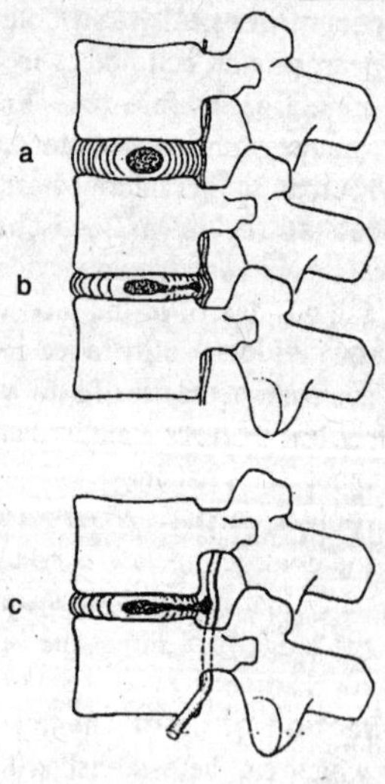

a. Normal disc
b. Bulging disc
c. Herniated disc

Disc calcification Calcification of intervertebral disc is not uncommon specially in dorsal spine of adults in annulus fibrosus and secondary to degenerative process. Multiple disc calcifications also occur with ochronosis. It is an incidental finding. It may cause stiffness of vertebral and localised tenderness. A mild torticollis may be noted.

Disc herniation pain Back pain disappears with onset of leg pain. Pain becomes worst on forward bending, coughing or sneezing and is relieved by lying with knees flexed. Numbness can be detected over one dermatome. Muscle weakness may be noted on heel walking.

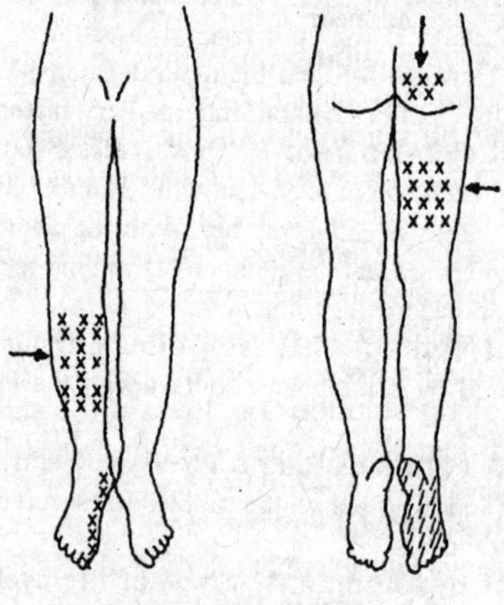

L4 disc prolapse pain
xx - aching pain /// - stabbing pain

Disc, computer It is a storage device for computer. There are several types of disks in use. Floppy discs are of low storage, low cost upto 2 MByte easily exchangeable and removable from computer. Hard discs are high capacity storage devices which can store several GBytes. These are usually built in computer. Other discs have magnetooptic effects to store and retrieve data (MO drive). Finally for long-term storage optical discs (CD ROMs) are used. These can store enormous amount of data, upto 700 MB. Information on these discs is burnt as little hole into a reflecting surface during a printing process and then can be read by passing a focussed laser beam over surface. CD ROMs are used for writing once read many times.

Discchari.de A sugar formed by two single carbohydrate units bound together; sucrose, maltose, and galactose are disaccharides.

Discectomy Partial or complete removal of an intervertabral disc.

Discent Passage of the presenting part of the fetus into and through the birth canal; it begins at the onset of labour and proceeds during effacement and dilatation of the cervix.

Discharge Termination of care from a healthy care agency.

Discharge instructions Directions for managing self-care and medical follow-up.

Discharge planning Managing transitional needs and ensuring continuity.

Discharge summary A written summary of the client's treatment and the results obtained prior to discharge from a service program.

Discharging chambers The two lower chambers of the heart called ventricles.

Discitis Infection or inflammation an intervertebral disc or disc space.

Disclosing solution Some form of dye applied to teeth stain bacterial and mucinous plaque on the tooth surface.

Disclosure Making known that which is not apparent. Often used in respect of the first making known of a sexual violation by a victim.

Discography It is the examination of intervertebral disc involving injection of contrast medium directly into disc space. It is performed to disclose rupture of annulus fibrosus specially in lumbar region. About 1 to 2 ml water soluble contrast is injected into nucleus pulposus.

Discoid lupus erythematosus It is a chronic recurrent disorder of collagen of unknown origin. It presents with single but may be multiple and asymptomatic, sharply marginated, localised erythematous papule with smooth surfaces but later covered with grey scales. Margins of lesions usually show hyperpigmentation. On the face lesions may produce butterfly appearance due to coalescence of lesions. Involvement of scalp may cause irreversible scarring alopecia, condition is usually asymptomatic. Lesions are treated with Calamine lotions with 3% ichthammol applied locally but tropical corticosteroids are more effective.

Discopathy Any pathological changes in a disc of a joint or of any organ from the original position.

Discount rate of pain A measurement of the difference between fear of pain experienced now and of that experienced in furture.

Discounting A reduction in the present value of delayed benefits.

Discovery The pretrial investigation by an attorney to determine the relevant facts of a case.

Discovery approach Learning situations in which the subject must discover the chief contents or principles and then incorporate them into his or her behaviour and thinking.

Discovery of inhaling anesthetic agent Various agents were discovered as diethyl ether (1842) N2O (1844) chloroform (1847) ethyle choloride (1848) ethylene (1923) cyclopropane (1930) trichloroethylene (1935) halothene (1956) Methoxyflurance (1960) enflurane (1966) isoflurance (1971) desflurane (1994) and sevoflurane (1996).

Discovery rule A rule tolling the statute of limitations unit the plaintiff knew or should have known of the injury. This is important for conditions such as cancer due to a toxic exposure that take years to become manifest.

Discrete variables Dichotomous variables and nominal variables are sometimes called discrete variables because the different categories are completely separate form each other.

Discrimination Showing of partiality or prejudice in treatment; specific action or policy directed against the welfare of a certain person or group of persons.

Discrimination question In sensory psychology, a condition which concerns the difference threshold. The focus is upon an organism's ability to notice a change in stimulation. For example, a light appears in a dark room and then it is presented again. The individual may ask whether the second light is brighter, dimmer, or the same as the first one. In general terms, the problem is to notice a change in stimulus intensity.

Discriminative stimulus A stimulus that signals the availability of a consequence, given that a response occurs.

Discriminative touch It is the ability of the body to differentiate between two stimuli, presented simultaneausly. Tip of fingers have the highest power of discrimination, while the pack has lowest.

Disease Any departure from health of a structure, organ, or system. A clinical syndrome with characteristic signs and symptoms related to dysfunction in a bodily organ caused at least in part by biological forces.

Disease cycle The chain of events involved in disease development, including the stages of development of the pathogen and the effects of the disease on the host.

Disease outbreak A sudden, unexpected increase in the occurence of a disease within a relatively limited geographical area.

Disease perevention The recognition of a danger to health that could be reduced or alleviated through specific actions or through changes in lifestyle behaviors.

Disease vector A carrier such as the mosquito that transmits disease to humans.

Disequilibrium syndrome In intracranial pathology or severe acidosis after dialysis patient develops tremors, convulsions and coma.

Dishabituation Facilitation of habituated stress response following exposure to an intense or a novel stressor.

Disinfect To carry out a process of disinfection; destroy or otherwise inactivate pathogenic microorganisms.

Disinfectants Chemicals that destroy active microorganisms but not spores.

Disinfection Act of destroying some pathogenic microorganisms.

Disinhibition Freedom to act according to one's inner drives or feelings, with less regard for restraints imposed by cultural norms or one's superego; removal of an inhibitory constraining, or limiting influence, as in the escape from higher cortical control in neurologic injury, or in uncontrolled firing of impulses when a drug interferes with the usual limiting or inhibiting action of GABA within the central nervous system.

Disinhibition theory A theory to explain the effects of alcohol in which intoxication is associated with the loss of moral and social values in favor of instinctual behaviors.

Dislocated jaw Mouth is open but patient is unable to close. Procedure to help patient, thumbs wrapped in guaze piece are placed on the occlusal surface of mandibular teeth. Fingers are curved under the body of mandible. Jaw is pressed down and back with thumb while pulling up and forward with the fingers. It permits condyle to pass over the articular eminence in normal position.

Dislocation acromioclavicular joint It becomes hypermobile and dislocates due to fall. The lateral end of clavicle is displaced superiorly and shows a lump over the joint. There will be pain initially but on repair, instability does not restrict movements.

Dislocation Hip In can be anterior and posterior causing pain. Anterior dislocation can take place

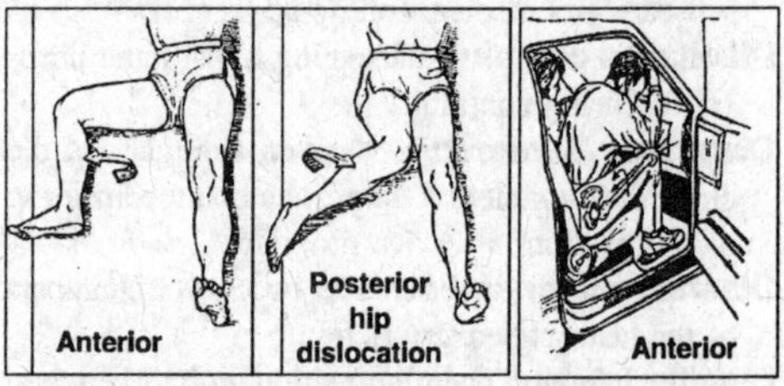

while driving car and leg is held in flexed, abducted and externally rotated position. With posterior dislocation, the leg is shortened, adducted and internally rotated.

Dislocation joint Two bones of joint do not remain in contact may be due to injury. When bones remain in partial contact, it is known as subluxation.

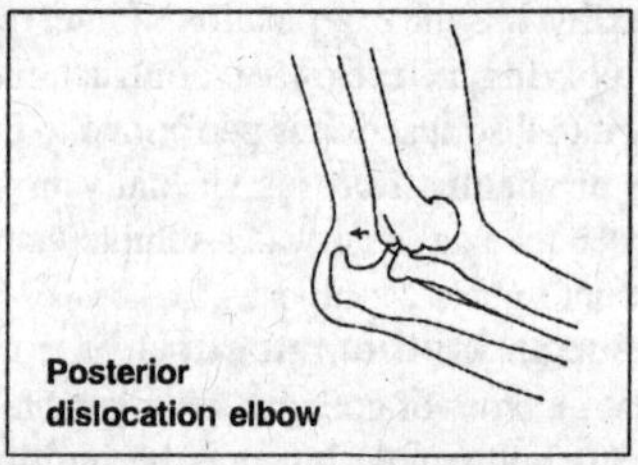

Dislocation takes place when joint ligaments or capsule gives way. It results in restriction of movements. After getting X-ray done bones are manipulated back into their proper position. If not possible operation may be required.

Disorder A derangement or abnormality of function; a morbid condition.

Disorder of behaviour Over-activity is characteristic of all forms of excitement, mania, schizophrenia and general paralysis. Activity is purposeful but not productive. In state of mania person becomes talkative, exaggerated in form of flight of ideas. In schizophrenic behaviour repetition of movement or speech may occur over a prolonged period. Retardation of psychomotor activity is seen typically in melancholic depression. It may be accompanied with negative thoughts. Morbid impulses are the result of urge to carry out some action. Kleptomania is impulse to steal.

Disorder of perception Hallucinations are sensory perceptions without any external cause. In illusion, real perceptions are misinterpreted. Clouding of consciousness may be produced. Hallucinations are present in early stage of mental illness. Hallucination affects all senses, hearing the most. Therefore, avditary hellucinations are most common. These include indeterminate noises but more often consist of words spoken. In schizophrenia voices may be said to arise from within and may be attributed to one of internal organs. Hallucinations of night are less frequent. Hallucination of smell is found in more chronic type of illness. Hallucination of touch occurs specially delirium tremens and cocaine addiction.

Disorder of personality In deper-sonalisation the patient ceases to believe in his own existence. Person feels that he has lost his own reality. Splitting of personality is seen in schizophrenia. Dissociation is a mental mechanism to avoid conflict seen in somnambulism. More complete degree of dissociation gives rise to double or multiple personality.

Disorder of thought It is a false belief, quiet impervious to argument or reason. In certain cases significance of delusional idea and its method of elaboration are obvious, in many they remian a method of speculation. Hallucinations may form the basis of subsequent delusional idea. Insight is degree of conscious appreciation. An obsession is an idea that obtrudes into the mind, the individual being perfectly aware of its absurdity and control over his will. Passivity feelings are found in schizophrenia.

Disorders of consciousness Consciousness implies ability to be aware of ourselves and our environment involving the ability to synthesise and evaluate new experience. It is dependent on attention. If power of attention is impaired there develops confusion, perplexity and bewilderment. It is found in acute stages of mental illness and in toxic infective group of psychosis. Dream state is of psychogenic origin. Delirium is psychogenic but may be of toxic in origin. Proufound degree of delirium is followed by complete amnesia.

Disorders of emotions Emotional disturbances are assessed by the intensity, duration and degree of harmony between mood and content of thought. Exhalation is an exaggerated degree of elation, typical of mania. Euphoria is abnormal feeling of wellbeing. Feeling of depression, i.e. hopelessness is severe in melancholia and mild in neurosis. Anxiety implies more than fear. Apathy indicates no pleasure, no sorrow. Emotional instability is seen as rapid variation in the effective state without any apparent cause. It occurs in organic condition.

Disorders of memory Loss of memory is known as amnesia. It is a common sequelae of head injury, a seizure or a hysterical attack. Anterograde amnesia denotes a loss of memory for recent events— retrograde is for remote events. An antegrade amnesia not accompanied by any disorder of consciousness, and is usually indicative of an organic syndrome. In secondary dementia, generalised loss of memory is found. Paramnesia indicates a falsification of memory. Hyperamnesia denotes an abnormally acute memory.

Disorganization The process of destruction of any organic tissue; any profound change in the tissues of an organ or structure which causes the loss of most or all of its proper character.

Dispar Unequal.

Dispersoid A colloid in which the dispersity is relatively greater.

Displacement A defence mechanism, operating unconsciously, in which emotions, ideas, or wishes are transferred from their original object to a more acceptable substitute; often used to allay anxiety.

Display matrix It denotes the number of addressable pixels on computer monitor. It ranges from 640 to 480 to 1280 to 1600 and even more.

Disposable endorectal coils Such coils are recommended for high resolution magnetic resonance imaging for the human colon, cervix and surrounding prostatic pelvic tissue. One time use, disposable endorectal coil has been designed to be inserted into the human rectum. It should not be used in case of recent major surgery, inflammatory bowel disease and severe hemorrhoids.

Disposition A term describing the orientation of the fetal axis and extremities, in addition to presentation and position.

Dispositional Relating to disposition or personality rather than to situation.

Disputed utterance Audio recording of an anonymous call or of a wiretapping procedure, generally collected through the telephone.

Dissect To separate tissues and parts of a cadaver (corpse) or an organ for anatomical study.

Dissecting aneurysm A dissecting aneurysm is one in which the blood dissects its way along a tunnel between the medial coat and the adventitia. It is not a true aneurysm because the vessel is not dilated, but rather a haematoma of arterial wall. Leakage of blood may occur at the site of an atheromatous ulcer of the intima or at the site where intima has weakened. It usually occurs in elderly hypertensive patients and affects commonly the ascending aorta or near the origin of subclavian artery.

Dissecting aneurysm of aorta Cystic medial necrosis of aorta is the most common cause of dissection. Onset is sudden. There is severe precordial pain which may extend backwards in paravertebral region or downwards in abdomen. It is accompanied by severe shock and collapse. Pulse is weak, quick or may be unequal. BP is low. If iliac arteries are involved lower limb becomes pulseless and cold. If dissection extends upwards there may be pain in neck, hemiparesis and appearance of systolic or diastolic murmur.

Dissection Cutting technique used to separate body parts for study.

Disseminated intravascular coagulation An acquired disorder in which there is acceleration of thrombi formation and also increasing fibrinolytic activity resulting in haemorrhage. The disorder can be either chronic or acute. In obstetrics, it is usually acute and considered a medical emergency.

Disseminated lupus erythematosus It is an inflammatory, multisystem connective tissue disorder of unknown aetiology. Condition causes acute necrotising vasculitis of small vessels of skin. It may begin insidiously with symptoms of rheumatic pain. When it involves skin, it produces bright red coloured and less demarcated macules which are often precipitated by exposure to sunlight or UV rays. Atrophy, scarring and pigmentary changes may occur. It presents with butterfly rash or dusky red discolouration of skin of nose and cheeks. There may be ulcers on legs and dilatation of nail bed capillaries condition can also involve mucous membrane erosions. Patients are treated with corticosteroids.

Dissimilatory reduction The reduction of a compound in an energy-yielding reaction. The reduced product does not become incorporated into cellular material.

Dissociate The separation of positive and negative ions when they dissolve in water and are surrounded by water molecules.

Dissociated sensory loss Loss of one sensory modality with preservation of others.

Dissociation The splitting off of clusters of mental contents from conscious awareness, a mechanism central to hysterical conversion and dissociative disorders; the separation of an idea from its emotional significance and effect as seen in the inappropriate effect of schizophrenic patients.

Dissociation viewpoint The viewpoint that the hypnotic condition is brought about through a shift from the higher to lower brain centres. Certain voluntary activities, it is hypothesised, become involuntary. The normal brain controls are reduced or split off from consciousness—hence the term "dissociation".

Dissogony The ability to exhibit two periods of reproductive, larval and adult separated by a period of gonadal regression.

Distal Away from the median sagittal plane of the face and following the curvature of the dental arch.

Distal convoluted tubule Convoluted tubule of the nephron that extends from the ascending limb of the loop of Henle and ends in a collecting duct.

Distal end Most posterior part of a removable dental restoration or denture flange.

Distal stimulus An object or other sensory element in the environment.

Distal tibiofibular syndesmosis The interosseus membrane and four other ligaments combine to form the distal tibiofibular syndesmosis. This include anterior tibiofibular, posterior tibiofibular, transverse tibiofibular and thickest, strongest part of interosseus membrane.

Distichiasis In this condition there is an extra row of eyelashes. These may be misdirected and rub against the cornea. These may be removed by electrolysis.

Distal Farther from the point of attachment to the body than another structure.

Distilled water Water that has been subjected to a process of vapourisation and subsequent condensation for purification.

Distocclusion In which the mandibular first molar is in a position distal to that of class I occlusion. The mesical buccal cusp of the maxillary first molaris anterior or mesical to the buccal groove of the mandubular first molar.

Distortion Any mechanical departure from ideal or normal symmetry in the body framework.

Distortion (radiographic) Deviation of a radiographic image from the true outline or shape of an object or structure.

Distractibility Inability to maintain attention; shifting from one area or topic to another with minimal provocation. Distractibility may be a manifestation of organic impairment or it may be a part of a functional disorder such as anxiety states, mania, or schizophrenia.

Distraction A painreduction technique that diverts an individual's attention away from the pain sensation.

Distraction osteogenesis In vivo surgical sectioning of a selected area of bone, which through slow and controlled separation allows for incremental bone formation to increase volume and/or changed configuration.

Distress fetal The signs imply metabolic abnormalities and may reflect fetal hypoxia and acidosis Fetal distress is a term applied to a set of signs indicating that if fetus is not born may die. There may be meconium staining of amniotic fluid and intrauterine growth retrardation.

Distribution of blood Total blood is 70 ml/kg in adults and 80 mL/kg in children and 90 mL/kg in neonates.

Disulfiram In alcoholism it inhibits the metabolism of alcohol with production of acetaldehyde causing unpleasant sensations.

Disuse atrophy When prolonged inactivity results in the muscles getting smaller in size.

Disuse syndrome Signs and symptoms that result from inactivity.

Diuresis renography It is carried out to distinguish true from false obstruction of pelviureteric junction. It is conveniently performed at the end of standard 16 minute renogram by injection of frusemide 0.5 mg/kg. Rising renogram curve at this stage is due to relatively slow flow through a dilated but not obstructed renal pelvis, a prompt fall in curve will be shown in response to diuretics.

Diurnal Occurring in a 24-hour cycle.

Diurnal rhythm A biological rhythm based on 24 hours a day.

Divergent thinking Thought which is directed toward finding many different answers or novel answers to a problem, the goal is to seek numerous possible solutions rather than the single answer.

Divergent outlet forcep These were introduced in 1968. Now a days it is very popular to be used.

Divergent thinking A form of thinking in which there is a search for multiple solutions to a problem (such as, How many different ways can a pen be used?); contrasts with convergent thinking.

Diversified technique Adjustive technique designed to correct vertebral and extravertebral subluxations. In general, each college teaches its own version of diversified technique.

Diverticulitis Inflammation and perforation of diverticula cause fever, pain, tenderness. Abdomen becomes rigid. Perforation may lead to peritonitis. In some cases, it may result in narrowing. Bed rest and antibiotics may help. In case of perforation surgery may be needed.

Diverticulosis The presence of diverticula

Diving bradycardia The slowing or stopping of the heart displayed by most diving animals during immersion in water.

Diving reflex There develops decreased respiration, vagal bradycardia and muscle bed constriction following immersion of face in water. Cerebral and cardiac circulations are preserved.

Division The largest phylogenic grouping within a domain. This grouping can be considered analogous to the kingdom and includes one or more phyla.

Divisome In prokaryote cell division, the macromolecular complex that carries out division at the cell center.

Dizygotic twin There is fertilization of two ova, two implantation, two placenta, two chorions and two amnions.

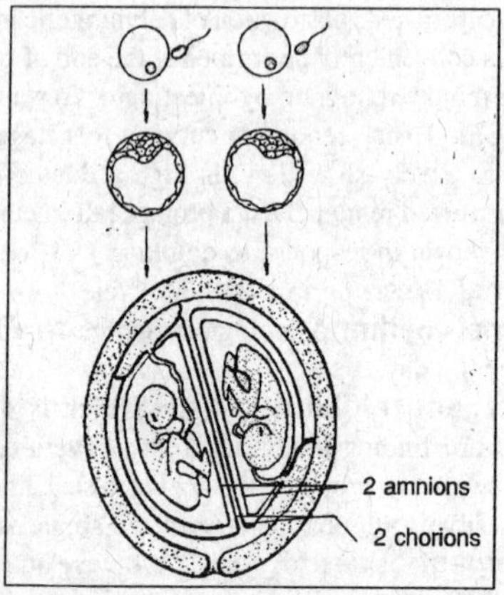

Dizziness It is a sensation of spining either of oneself or of surrounding. There may be nausea, vomiting, sweating or fainting. Lowering of BP is more common. Tiredness, stress, fever, anaemia may cause it. Dizziness as part of vertigo is usually due to a disorder of the inner ear, acoustic nerve or brainstem. Antiemetic or antihistamine drugs may be helpful.

DJP Degenerative joint disease.

DMD Doctor of Dental Medicine.

DNA It is deoxyribonucleic acid. The bases in DNA are the same as RNA except that thymine occurs in place of uracil. DNA is a substance of genes, chromosome and inheritance. In all higher cells DNA is confined to the chromosomal structures inside the nuclear membrane. DNA undergoes mutation. The most important features of DNA is the pairing of purine and pyrimidine bases to each other. A given individual of species may have a different set of genes from another individual of same species and may have different eye and hair colours.

DNA chimera A DNA containing genetic information derived from two different species.

DNA hybridization The process by which two complimentary strands of DNA bind to each other in a mixture of DNA strands.

DNA library A random collection of cloned DNA fragments that includes all or most of the genome of a given organism; also called a genomic library.

DNA looping The interaction of proteins bound at distant sites on a DNA molecule so that the intervening DNA forms a loop.

DNA microarray A miniaturized array containing thousands of DNA fragments representing genes in an area of a few square centimeters. These "chips" are used mostly to monitor the expresson of genomes at the level of messenger RNA.

DNA microinjection A technique for introducing nucleic acids into cells such as the oocytes of *Xenopus*, mamalian cells in culture of fertilized mammalian eggs via a small bore glass needle using a micromanipulator.

DNA polymerase An enzyme that catalyzes the synthesis of DNA from a DNA template.

DNA replication The unique ability of DNA molecules to make copies of themselves.

DNA-directed RNA polymerase An enzyme that synthesizes RNA using a DNA template.

DNR orders Do not resuscitate orders are explicit instructions that are written by a physician directing care providers not to revive or sustain the vital functions of persons in respiratory or cardiac arrest.

Doctor's consultation charges Medical profession is a service to the society but in return he or she is authorised to have reasonable fee which patient is obliged to pay.

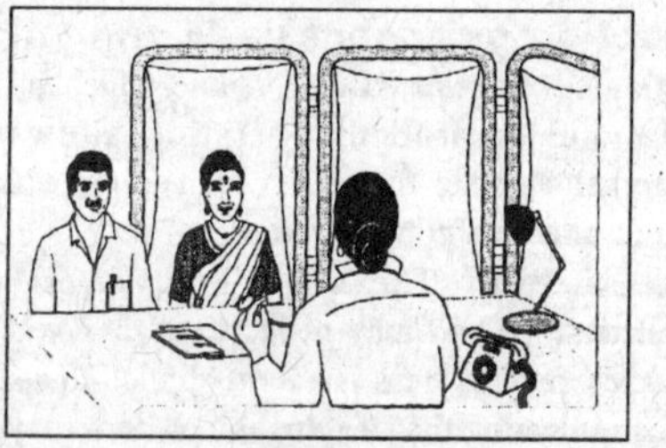

Doctrine A theory supported by authorities and having general acceptance.

Documenting Process of writing information.

Doll's eye movements Reflex elicited in unconscious patients by quickly turning the patients head to one side and hold it.

Dolobid It is a fluorophenyl derivative of salicylic acid. Its half-life increases from seven hours when dose is 250 mg/d to 15 hours when it is 500 mg/d. It is useful in osteoarthritis and results in a fewer gastric adverse effects. Diarrhoea is more common. It is also uricosuric. There may be cross allergy with aspirin.

Dolorific Producing of causing pain.

Domain A region of a protein with a defined function.

Doman-Delacato System It recommends periods of inhalation of CO_2 from a breathing sack, restriction of fluid intake and development of cereral hemispheric dominance. Cerebral dominance is attempted by principal use of dominant eye, hand, foot and arm and other methods. Children are also turned upside down and whirled around to stimulate vestibular apparatus.

Dominance A predisposition to play a prominent or controlling role when interacting with others. In *neurology*, the (normal) tendency of one-half of the brain to be more important than the other in mediating various functions (cerebral dominance). In *genetics*, the ability of one gene (dominant gene) to express itself in the phenotype of an individual, even though that gene is paired with another (recessive gene) that would have expressed itself in a different way. Two recessive genes must be present to express the recessive trait. Cortical dominance refers to the dominance of one side or hemisphere of the brain in control of handedness and speech.

Dominant allele An allele that overrides the influence of alternate alleles on the homologous chromose; the allele that is expressed.

Dominant follicle Of the cohort of follicles that begins final maturation, a follicle that is destined to ovulate.

Dominant inheritance The acquiring of a characteristic by transmission in a gene from parents to their offspring regardless of the state of the corresponding allele.

Domoic acid A glutamate analogue that, in small amounts, stimulates glutamate receptors and in higher amounts induces death of the neuron.

Domperidone Half-life is 7 hours. It enhances contractions of the gastric antrum and relaxes pyloric sphincter. It crosses the blood-brain barrier poorly. It is used for nausea or vomiting associated with GIT disorders. Dystonic reactions with domperidone are much fewer than metachlorpramide.

Don To put on.

Donath-Landsteiner syndrome When blood of the patients of paroxysmal haemoglobinuria is cooled to 5°C and then warmed, haemolysis occurs due to the presence of circulating haemolysin, and this reaction constitutes Donath-Landsteiner phenomenon.

Donee One who receives a gift.

Donor A female from whom embryos are recovered, or a male provider of spermatozoa used for insemination.

Donor site The area from which skin has been harvested to use an autograft to cover an open wound.

Donor tissue Tissue gingiva, mucosa, or bone moved to a new location in a grafting procedure.

Dopa Dihydroxyphenylalannine, a precursor of dopamine, notepinephrine, and epinephrine.

Dopamine It is a naturally occurring precurssor of norephinephrine. It has potent inotropic effect and vasoconstrictive effect. It constricts cutaneous and muscular vessels but dilates renal and splanchnic vessels. At a dose of 2-5 mg/kg/minute, the vasodilatation is maximum but in dose exceeding 20 mg/kg/minute it raises systemic vascular resistance due to intense vaso-constriction. It is a physiological derivative of noradrenaline. It improves cardiac contractility without increasing its rate. Improvement in renal blood flow is seen. Diuresis takes place. It raises blood pressure. Side effects include dyspnoea, headache, angina, hypertension and dysrrhythmia.

Dopamine hypothesis A theory that attempts to explain the pathogenesis of schizophrenia and other psychotic states as due to excesses in dopamine activity in various areas of the brain. This theory is, in part, based on biologic observations that the antipsychotic properties of specific drugs may be related to their ability to block the action of dopamine.

Dopamine hypothesis of schizophrenia A hypothesis proposing that schizophrenic symptoms are due to excess activity of the neurotransmitter dopamine.

Dopaminergic Relating to those nerves or receptor sites that employ dopamine as their neurotransmitter.

Doppler angle It is the Doppler ultrasound blood flow velocity measurement, the angle between the

Doppler ultrasound beam and direction of blood flow in the vessels being examined. Doppler instrument 'sees' only the blood flow velocity component being directed straight towards the transducer.

Doppler effect Increase in observed frequency of a signal when the signal source approaches the observer and decrease when the source moves away.

Doppler stethoscope Device that helps detect sounds created by the velocity of blood moving through a blood vessel.

Doppler ultrasound Measurement of blood flow is a sharper hemodynamic assessment of fetal condition. Doppler imaging helps in knowing index of A=peak systolic, B=diastolic and ratio of umbilical artery. Greater the diastolic flow lower the A/B ratio.

Doppler velocimetry The use of Doppler ultrasonography techniques to determine both direction and velocity of blood flow.

Dorendorf's sign The sign identifies fullness of one supraclavicular fossa, and occurs in aortic arch aneurysm.

Dorsal Pertaining to the back or to the posterior part of an organ.

Dorsal body cavity includes the cranial and spinal cavities.

Dorsal body cavity Cavity near the dorsal (posterior) surface of the body that consists of a cranial cavity and vertebral canal.

Dorsal column stimulation It is a technique used in intractable pain management.

Dorsal position This position is used for examination of chest and abdomen. Patient lies on back with one pillow under the head. Arms lie on side. Knees are slightly flexed. Head may be turned to one side.

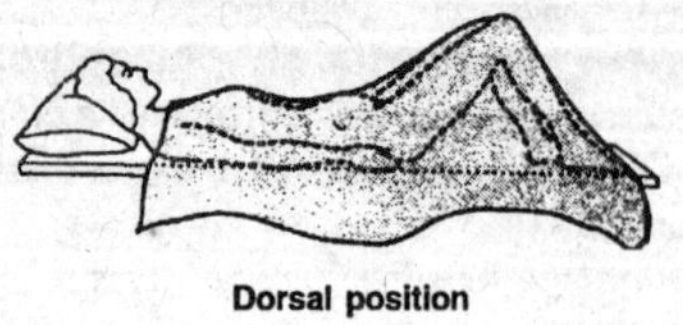

Dorsal position

Dorsal recumbent position Reclining posture with the knees bent, hips rotated outward, and feet flat.

Dorsal root ganglion Area where posterior and anterior branches marge to form pleripheral nerve.

Dorsal spinothalamic tract In the dorsal part of the spinal cord, a pathway that carries fine touch and pressure fibers.

Dorsal surface The posterior surface of the body, except that the front or top of the foot is the dorsal surface.

Dorsal-column nuclei Nuclei in the brainstem that receive fine touch and pressure fibers from the dorsal spinothalamic tract of the spinal cord.

Dorsalis An anatomical term denoting a position closer to the back surface.

Dorsiflexion Movement at the ankle or wrist as the dorsum of the foot or hand is elevated.

Dorsogluteal site Injection area in the upper outer quadrant of the buttocks.

Dorsomesial Pertaining to the mesial or median aspect of the back.

Dorsonasal Pertaining to the bridge of the nose.

Dose Amount of drug.

Dose limit It is the limit of irradiation dose from ionising radiation to which public can be exposed. The dose limits for public at large are lower than those for people working in an environment where radioactivity is present.

Dose-effect curve A curve related to dose of radiation and its effect.

Dose-response relationship Exists when an increase in the intensity or duration of exposure increases the risk of an adverse outcome.

Dosia Dose.

Dosimeter It is the device used to measure the radiation dose to which an individual has been exposed. There are two types : dosimeter badges which are worn to measure cumulative doses over periods of weeks, and pocket dosimeter which are generally used for monitoring shorter term exposure.

Dossier A collection of documents concerning the same subject or individual such as the accumulated records of patient's case history.

Double-blind In psychological experiment, any method which prevents both the experimenter and the subject from knowing which treatment the subject receives. Often used in drug experiments.

Double blind study A research study in which both the research patient and the research clinician are 'blind' to the type of medication or other manuever being used to treat the patient. This prevents the expectations of the patient and researcher from biasing the research result.

Double contrast barium enema The barium enema is combined with insufflation of air for a much better see through effect, than single contrast method. The barium suspension should only coat the mucosa in a thin layer.

Double helix The natural coiled conformation of two complementary, antiparallel DNA chains.

Double loops Fingerprints with two loop formations each consisting of at least one free recurving ridge and two deltas.

Double lung tranplantation Early technique for lung tranplanation using a tracheal anastomosis and a double lung en bloc.

Double support time The period of the gait cycle when both lower extremities are in contact with the supporting surface double support; measured in seconds.

Double vision It is diplopia. It may be a result of deviation or malalignment of two eyes. In strabismus movement of eye in a particular direction due to paralysis of one or more of muscles. Double vision may be caused by a tumour or blood clot behind the eye. The onset of double vision in adult life requires immediate attention to rule out tumour, aneurysm or neurological disorder.

Double-bagging Infection control measure in which one bag of contaminated items, such as trash or laundry, is placed within another.

Double-bind situation A situation in which contradictory demands or meanings are communicated in the same message or environment. The father, for example, may encourage his sons to be competitive and follow the "law of the jungle" while the mother urges him to cooperate with other people and "turn the other cheek." On this basis, the sone is in a double bind.

Double-blind study A study in which neither the subjects nor the investigators are anware of the treatment assignment until the trial is terminated.

Doublevold A procedure of discarding the first urine specimen and testing the second urine specimen that was obtained 30 to 45 minutes later; this procedure gives a more accurate amount of glucose being spilled into the urine at that particular time.

Douche Previously douche was used as a means of contraception after intercourse and it was used in cases of vaginal infection also but now it has been proved that douche may introduce infection.

Douglas, cavity or pouch Rectouterine excavation or pouch.

Doula An experienced woman in childcare who provides continuous physical, emotional, and information support to the woman in labour.

Down's syndrome It happens due to chromosomal abnormality resulting in mental handicap; child has 47 chromosomes instead of 46. In most cases extra chromosome is 21. The face and features are small, the tongue is large and tends to protrude. Hands are short and broad. IQ of child may be between 30 to 70. But these children are affectionate, friendly and cheerful. They fit well in family. There is no cure of mental handicap.

Doxapram An analeptic that stimulates respiration more than it activates the cortical or spinal neurons.

Doyen's mouth gag It is a self-retaining tube retractor with locking system. It is used to keep mouth open during surgery. It is useful during stomach wash.

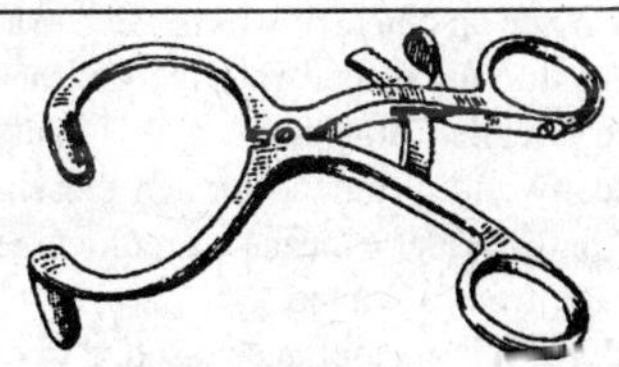

Doyen's mouth gag

Dr. Black J.V. classification of cavities It is used to prepare and for dental cavity restoration as well :

Class I—Pit and fissure cavities on occlusal surfaces of premolars and molars and lingual surfaces of maxillary incisors.

Class II—Cavities on proximal surfaces of premolars and molars.

Class III—Cavities on proximal surfaces of incisors and canines. It does not involve incisal angle.

Class IV—Cavities on proximal surfaces of incisors and canines. Incisal angle is involved.

Class V—Cavities on gingival third of facial or lingual surfaces of all teeth.

Class VI—Cavities on incisal edge of anterior teeth or on occlusal cusp height of posterior teeth.

Dr. Maignes examination table This table is useful for lumbar traction in which thorax and pelvis have to be fastened.

Dracunculiasis It develops due to worm, *Dracunculus mendinesis* worm inhabits in the subcutaneous tissue and body cavities. It measures about 40-80 cm in length. It has cylindrical, smooth, white body with pointing tail. In human beings, gravid female worm migrates to the skin surface especially of legs and feet. When come in contact with water the worm penetrates through the subcutaneous tissue and produces a cutaneous blister that ulcerates later. Worm then discharges large number of larvae which are ingested by cyclops. Penetration by female gravid worm causes formation of cutaneous blister that ulcerates in absence of secondary infection which heals in 4 to 6 weeks. Formation of blister gives rise to urticaria, nausea, dyspnoea. As blister ulcerates the symptoms subside.

Drag The amount of pull on the tissue.

Drag force When an object moves relative to a fluid, it is subjected to the resistitive effects of the fluid. This force is called drag force and is caused by fluid viscosity and turbulence, when present.

Drain Tube that provides a means for removing blood and drainage from a wound.

Drain, surgical It is an appliance inserted into body cavity to permit drainage of fluid. The most common drains are soft rubber tubes whose other end is connected to a collection of bag or bottle. A valve prevents fluid from refluxing back. There are also corrugated drains available. Suction drains consist of thin tubes with many small holes to collect fluid.

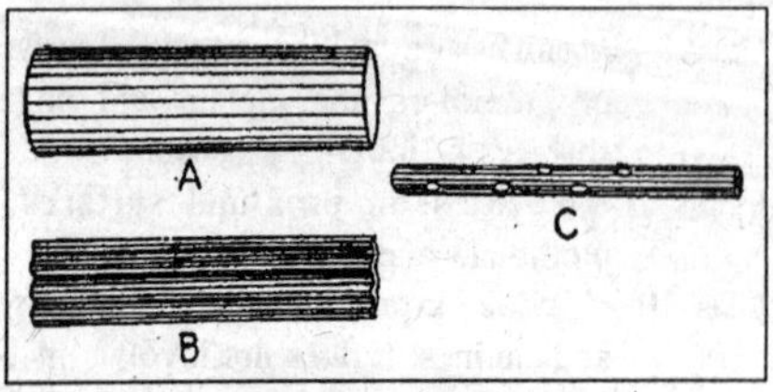

Surgical drains

Drainages There are two types of drainages : corrugated drainage and closed tube type drainage. Closed tubes may be of perforated type. Drainages are used during surgery to encourage removal of pus. These are properly sterilised before putting in.

Drape Tube that provides a means for removing blood and drainage from a wound.

Draping The procedures of covering and uncovering areas of the body and turning the client during the massage.

Draw-back effect Blood in the barrel of a firearm that has been drawn backward into the muzzle.

Drawdown effect Cooling of the ear when it comes in contact with a thermometer probe.

Drawer sign The patient sits hanging his legs. The examiner holds the upper end of the leg with one hand and grasps the heel with the other, and apply forces to move the talus anteriorly and posteriorly. In this sign if there is distal displacement of the talus it indicates rupture of anterior ligaments of the ankle but of posterior ligament if the movement is proximal. It is seen in the cases of ankle sprain.

Drawsheet A special sheed placed over the regular sheed on a bed and used to move a person in bed.

DRE Drug recognition examiner.

Dream interpretation A fundamental technique in psychoanalysis in which dreams are studied in terms of underlying meaning.

Dreaming An imagined, visual, hallucinated event that occurs during sleep.

Dressing Cover over a wound.

Dressing apraxia An inability to dress oneself properly owing to a disorder in body scheme or spatial relations, rather than difficulty in motor performance or incoordination.

Dressing material cabinet Dressing room should be neat, clean and flies proof. Certain dressing material may be kept in open and certain in closed cabinet only.

Dressings These are cotton rolls used to control bleeding, absorb secretions or prevent contamination. These should be sterile to avoid introduction of bacteria from outside. It should have the property to absorb, otherwise bacteria will get an opportunity to multiply. Nowadays adhesive

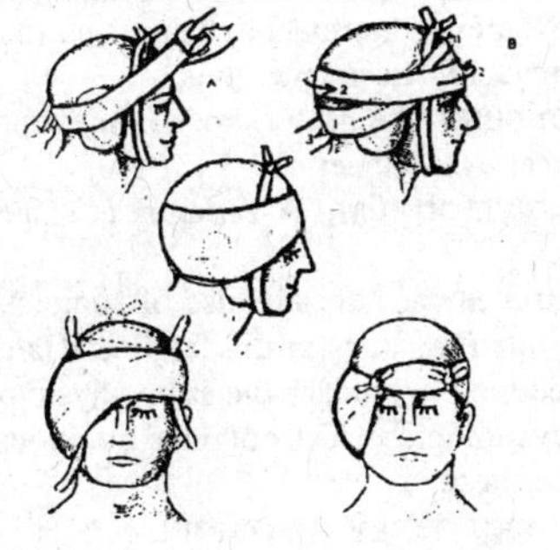

Dressings

bandages are available in different sizes, ready to use; and to protect small wounds such as cuts and abrasions. Gauze is applied in layers and for packing wound.

Nowadays, non-sticking dressings are also available. Such dressings can be removed without disturbing granulation tissues.

Dressler's syndrome The syndrome includes fever, pericarditis with frictional rub, pericardial effusion, pleurisy with effusion, pneumonitis, and joint pains following myocardial infarction.

Dried fruits In drying over 50% water is removed but all nutrients remain. Calorie value increases by 4-5 times.

Drip pattern A bloodstain pattern which results from blood dripping into blood.

Drive Basic urge, instinct, motivation; a term used to avoid confusion with the more purely biologic concept of instinct. A physiological condition involving sensitivity to certain types of stimulation. Usually it impels the organism to become active. Distinguished from a motive in being initially indiscriminate, without an appropriate direction.

Drive-reduction theory A motivational concept emphasising that the behaviour of organisms is concerned primarily with reducing bodily or physiological tension. For example, an organism is motivated to reduce tension by turning towards the sunlight, obtaining water, or seeking rest.

Dromotropic Possessing the ability to influence the conduction velocity of a nerve or muscle fiber.

Drop arm test A test used to assess the integrity of automatic proprioceptive reactions; the limb is raised to a new position and suddenly dropped.

Drop attack Sudden loss of tone in the lower limbs; associated with ischemia of the medullary pyramids. Subject is usually a middle-aged woman who complains of repeated falls on her knees without warning. Such patients have not tripped and there is no loss of consciousness. Drop attacks usually occur while walking. Such patients have no symptoms of brainstem involvement such as double vision or dysarthria in relation to drop attacks.

Drop factor Number of drops per milliliter in intravenous tubing.

Drop method Examination of blood by a single drop of blood.

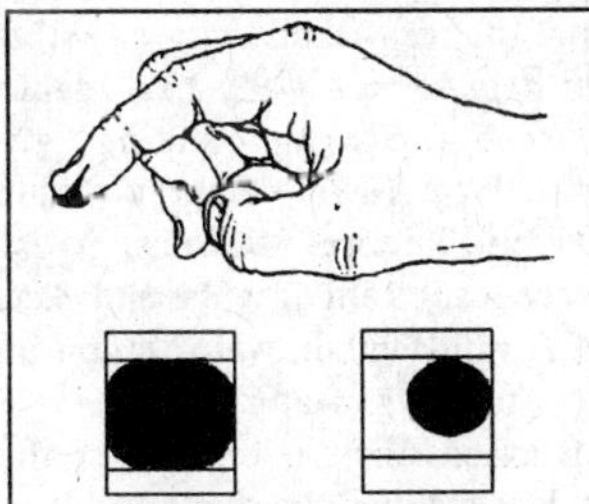

Drop shot Lead shot containing less than 0.5% alloying metal also called soft shot.

Droplet nuclei Dried residual of largest respiratory droplets which may carry infectious microorganisms. Droplet nuclei of clinical importance are in the 1 to 5 micro millimeter diameter range.

Droplet precautions Measures that block pathogens in moist droplets larger than 5 microns.

Drowning It may result in death due to suffocation as a result of hypoxia being immersed in fluid media. To start water gets entrance into oesophagus. Laryngeal reflex prevents water entering to lungs but this process impairs breathing leading to hypoxia and death. If person floats face up may survive but if he floats face down will sink. 75 per cent persons die due to fluid in lungs while 25 per cent die due to pure suffocation.

Drug It is chemical substance which can alter the function of some organs. These include prescribed as well as over the counter remedies. These are naturally occurring substances extracted from plants and minerals. Insulin and growth hormone are synthesised using engineering procedure. All new drugs are tested for their efficiency and safety. First laboratory experiments are done, then human volunteers are tested, and finally clinical trials on patients are done. It has four distinct phases. Phases-1, 20-25 patients are taken to study pharmacokinetic data. In phase-2, 50-200 patients are studied for safety, efficacy and pharmacokinetic study. In phase-3, 200-500 patients are studied for tarther evaluation of safety & effiacy. In phase-4, more than 1000 patients are needed to show the 'real life' effiacy of the drug.

Drug dependence It is the compulsion of taking drug. Drug dependence is of two types. In *psychological dependence* person feels craving or emotional distress when drug is withdrawn. In *physical dependence* body has adapted to the presence of the drug causing withdrawal symptoms. Withdrawal symptoms cause severe physical and mental distress. Mostly drug dependence results after regular and excessive use of drug. A mild withdrawal reaction may cause yawning, sneezing, watery eyes and sweating. Severe reactions include cramps, confusion and seizures. It is note worthy that all CNS stimulants cause psyenogenic dependence while all depressant cause physical dependence.

Drug eruptions These are of sudden onset, wide and symmetric dissemination with pruritus. These may be papular, vesicobullous or pustular. Fixed drug eruptions occur persistently at the same site the drug is given. These are often bullous and eczematous initially and later on hyperpigmented in colour.

Drug Fast Drug-resistant.

Drug holiday Discontinuance of a therapeutic drug for a limited period of time. Sometimes used as a way of evaluating baseline behaviour or as a means of controlling or reducing the dosage of psychoactive drugs and side effects. It is not popular now. Earlier, it was used in the treatment of Parkinson's disease.

Drug interaction The effects of two or more drugs taken simulataneously; producing an alteration in the usual effects of either drug taken alone. The interacting drugs may have a potentiating or additive effect and serious side effects may result. An example of drug interaction is alcohol and sedative drugs taken together, which may cause central nervous system depression. They are of two main types : pharmaeodynamic interactions or pharmacokinetic interactions.

Drug misuse The use of drugs in an unprescribed or excessive manner.

Drug polymorphism A variation in response to a drug.

Drug tolerance Repeated use of some substance, drug, often narcotics, so that larger and larger doses are required to produce the same physiologic and/or psychologic effect obtained previously by a smaller dose.

Drug-dependency insomnia A condition that results from continuous use of "sleeping pills" in which a person becomes tolerant of the drug while the drug also results in deprivation of either REM (rapid eye movement) or NREM (nonrapid eye movement) sleep, leading the person to increase the drug dosage.

Drug-induced myopathies Number of drugs cause diffuse muscle aching and mild weakness without progression to a severe myopathy with salbutamol, cytotoxic agents, cimetidine and lithium more severe necrotising myopathy has been reported. Abuse of heroin and alcohol may also result it.

Drug-induced parkinsonism (pseudoparkinsonism) A reversible syndrome resembling the disease parkinsonism, resulting from the dopamine-blocking action of antipsychotic drugs. Pill-rolling movements are less common than in the naturally occurring disorder. Anti-cholinergic drugs are used as first time treatment.

Drug-resistant Resistant to the action of drugs.

Drusen Drusen are deopsits of a hyline-like calcific material within optic disc. Presence of drusen may give a false appearance of papilloedema. Except the full physiological cup, all the fundus findings are against papilloedema. Presence of venous pulsation further helps to diagnose a drusen. On ophthalmoscopy there may appear waxy pearl-like irregular bodies on the surface of optic disc. Fluorescein angiography shall be helpful in differentiating it from papilloedema. In papilloedema there is an early leakage of dye.

Dry beriberi Thiamin deficiency affecting the nervous system producing paralysis and extreme muscle wasting.

Dry body weight An estimate of actual weight without the weight of ascites fluid.

Dry heat It is believed to kill the microorganism by promoting a destructive oxidation of essential cells required a temperature of 160°C for 60 minutes. It is used to sterilise glass syringes. The lethal effect of dry heat is attributed to denaturation and coagulation of protein. One of primary site of thermal injury in the cell is cytoplasmic membrane. Cell membrane is site of respiration and protein synthesis. It is employed mainly for sterilisation of glassware, all glass syringes and other goods which are not spoiled by high temperature. It is the application of heat to the body or part of body without any contact by moisture of water vapours to the body. Infrared lamp, short-wave diathermy, hot compress, hot water bottle, electric pad and electric light are the sources of dry heat.

Dry heat sterilisation It is believed to kill the microorganism by promoting a destructive oxidation of essential cell requiring a temperature of 160°C for 60 minutes. It is used to sterilise glass syringes.

DSM-IV Official classification system of mental disorders published by American Psychiatric Association.

Dual role Overlap in the scope of practice, with one professional providing support in more than one area of expertise.

Dualism A philosophical position that holds that both a nonmaterial mind and the material body contribute to behavior.

Dualistic thinking A type of thinking which assumes that something is either right or wrong; the truth or falsity of something can always be determined. This type of thinking, common in some students, may be followed by two later stages.

Duchenne muscular dystrophy It is an allelic X-linked disorder. The location of the gene on X-chromosome and gene product are known. Development of affected child is very slow. Milestones are delayed of 6 months. There is an associated mild intellectual retardation. Even at the age of 4 child cannot get up after falling on floor. There is some hypotonia of muscles and shoulders. There is pseudohypertrophy of calf muscles. Level of phosphate kinase is raised. Death usually occurs by the age of 18.

Ducrey's skin test It consists of an intradermal injection of suspensions of killed *Haemophilus ducreyi* which when positive produces an indurated area of more than 5 mm in diameter after 48 hours. The test is used for the diagnosis of chancroid, but a positive result may also indicate a past infection.

Duct A passge with well-defined walls; especially a tube for the passage of excretions or secretions.

Ductal Pertaining to a duct.

Ductal carcinomal in situ Cancer cells that develop from the lining of the milk duct but are confined to the ducts of the breast. DCIS is considered to be a prescursor to invasive cancer.

Ductile Ability of a material to be stretched or elongated without fracture.

Ductility The characteristic of a material, allowing it to undergo significant plastic or permanent deformation under stress before fracturing; the opposite of brittleness.

Ductless Having no exretory duct.

Ductless gland Specialized gland that secretes hormones directly into the blood.

Ducture A minute duct. Called also ductulus.

Ductus The duct that carries sperm from the epididymis to the ejaculatory duct. Also called the seminal duct.

Ductus arteriosus In fetal state with constricted pulmonary arterioles, the pulmonary blood pressure exceeds the aortic blood pressure and there is right to left shunting. When ventilation is established the pulmonary BP will fall, so the direction of flow through ductus reverses. Closure of ductus is mainly dependent on the oxygenation of blood perfusing it. Oxygen appears the main stimulus of closure of ductus.

Ductus deferens A thick, smooth, muscular tube that allowed sperm to exit from the epididymis and pass from the scrotal sac into the abdominal cavity; also known as the vas deferens.

Ductus venosus A continuation of the umbilical vein that shunts blood returning from the placenta past the fetus's developing liver directly into the inferior vena cava.

Due care The degree of care that would or should be exercised by an ordinary person in the same position.

Dumb rabies Animal looks profoundly depressed and unaware of its surroundings. Paralysis of muscles of head and neck occurs and dog becomes unable to chew food. Disease is fatal within 10 days. Virus is present in brain, spinal cord and salivary and lacrimal glands. Infection is diagnosed by the presence of Negri bodies. There is shorter incubation period in persons bitten on face and head due to vascularity and proximity to brain.

Dumping syndrome It is characterised by epigastric fullness, abdominal cramps, nausea, vomiting, tachycardia, sweating, pallor, flushing, giddiness, or even syncope, all after meals occurring generally in persons who had gastrectomy or similar other operations.

Duodenal atresia There is a strong association with Down's syndrome. Chromosomal analysis for trisomy 21 is desirable.

Duodenal drainage test A test in which an inestinal specimen is obtained via a swallowed tube and examined for diagnosis of gallbladder and pancreatic diseses.

Duodenal papillae Ducts located in the middle third of the duodenum that empty pancreatic digestive juices and bile from the liver into the small intestine; there are two ducts, the major duodenal papillae and the minor papillae.

Duodenal ulcer It is an ulcer in the area of duodenum. Person feels pain when stomach is empty, specially at night. This is due to acidity. At that time even if you take two biscuits pain will subside. While in gastric ulcer pain is increased on consuming food.

Duodenitis It is an inflammation of the duodenum resulting in vague symptoms. There is no ulcer but diffuse area of inflammation is seen. There is redness and swelling of cells in the duodenal lining.

Duodenum The first subdivision of the small intestine where most chemical digestion occurs.

Dupuytren's contracture In this palmar aponeurosis is thickened and contracted. It affects generally the ring finger. First the proximal phalanx remains unaffected since the palmar aponeurosis does not extend to that phalanx. The finger can neither be straightened actively nor passively even of flexing the wrist.

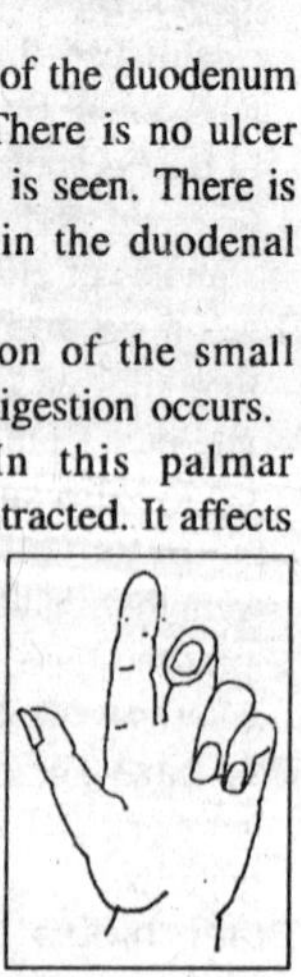

Dura mater The spinal dura mater represents only the inner or meningeal layer of the cerebral dura mater. It is connected by fibrous slips to the posterior ligament, especially near the lower end of vertebral canal. The dural sheaths of spinal nerves fuse with connective tissue. A strong fibrous layer forms tubular sheath attached above the margin of foramen magnum and ending below at lower border of second sacral vertebrae. Tough, fibrous membrane forming the outermost meningeal covering of the brain and spinal cord.

Durable power of attorney A document that names a person who would make treatment decisions for a patient if they were not able to make them for themselves. Generally it is a person who knows the patient and his or her values well and is in a good position to represent their wishes to the patient's physician.

Dural tap Accidental puncture of dura while performing extradural anesthesia.

Duration The length of time a method lasts or stays in the same location.

Duration of 3rd stage labour Duration is five to 10 minutes and consist in 2 phases, the phase of placental separation and phase of placental expulsion.

Duration of action Length of time during which a drug is present in a concentration great enough to produce a therapeutic effect.

Duration of drowning Body heat is lost about twice as rapidly in water than in air. Wrinkling of skin begins shortly after immersion. Bleaching of cuticle begins after 12 hours. Sodden appearance of epidermis is seen in 24 hours. Epidermis and nails are loosened and skin of hand and feet are peeled off within a week.

Durran's sign Increased rate and depth of breathing following rapid injection of solution into extradural space.

Dust cells Macrophages the at ingest particulate matter in the small air sacs of the lungs.

Duty cycle The relationship between magnitude of force absorption by alveolar bone and time, within or without an interposing, shock-absorbing ligament.

Duty of patient Patient should furnish the doctor with complete information about facts desired by doctor regarding disease and causative factors. Patient should have faith in doctor and obey his or her direction and pay a reasonable fee for doctor's service. He or she should not exploit the doctor in any way.

Dwarfism It is an abnormally restricted growth of body such as seen in achondroplasia, It may occur due to deficiency of growth hormone produced by pituitary gland. Mental development is usually normal.

Dying declaration Dying declaration is a statement verbal or written made by a person related to cause his or her death or any of circumstances of the transactions related to death. Dying declaration is accepted in court of law in case of death of a person but if he or she survives it has no legal value. Should the person be alive, an accused gets a chance of cross-examination of a person.

Dying with dignity Treating a terminally ill person with respect regardless of his or her emotional, physical, or cognitive state.

Dynamic equilibrium The maintenance of body position, mainly the head, in response to sudden movements such as rotation.

Dynamic labyrinth The semicircular canals.

Dynamic posturography A computerized test of sensory organization and movement coordination during standing balance.

Dynamic splint A splint that allows for and enables movement.

Dynamic weight transfer rate The speed at which an individual standing in the parallel bars can transfer weight from one extremity to another; measured in seconds from the first lift off to the eighth lift off.

Dynamics Study of motions of bodies and forces acting to produce the motions.

Dynamometer A device that quantitatively measures muscle strength.

Dysaesthesia A feeling of fullness, pressure or itching about the ear are with pathologic sensations develop. Compared with otalgia, patients tend to be less precise in describing the character and location of dysaesthesia.

Dysafferentation Abnormal afferent input as a result of joint restriction, involving a functional decrease in the activity of large-diameter mechanoreceptor afferent fibers and a simultaneous functional increase in activity of nociceptive afferent nerve fibers.

Dysarthria Lesion in or adjacent to Broca's area may disturb cortical pattern of lip and tongue movements to make speech dysarthric. A lesion of one internal capsule produces little dysarthric. Lesions in both internal capsule result in severe loss of control of speech which becomes slow, strained known as spastic dysarthria. It is accompanied by a brisk jaw jerk and pout reflex. Lesion in brainstem may result in palatal palsy and nasal voice. Acute intoxication with alcohol or barbiturates produce a slurring and slowing of speech.

Dysarthriaclumsy hand syndrome Syndrome associated with a vascular lesion of the genu of teh internal capsule.

Dyscontrol syndrome Causes include tumours of limbic system and/or localised atrophy of brain. Person will have manic behaviour, physical bruitality without motive, sexual assaults, seizures, lack of memory, hallucinations, depression and speech difficulties. There will be visual field defects.

Dysentery It is a severe infection of intestine causing diarrhoea mixed with blood, pus and mucus. There is an abdominal pain too. Faecal matter is little but blood-stained and watery mucus is there. *Bacillary dysentery* is caused by *Shigella*. Diarrhoea is watery. *Amoebic dysentery* is caused by parasite *Entamoeba histolytica*. It starts more gradually and often has a chronic course.

Dysfunction An in-between state of which one is "not healthy" but also "not sick".

Dysfunctional labour Abnormal uterine contractions that interfere with the normal progress of labour.

Dysgenesis The abnormal formation of an organ.

Dyskinesia Movements that are abnormal or involuntary or both.

Dyskinetic cerebral palsy Movement problems associated with damage to the basal ganglia associated with cerebral palsy.

Dyslexia It is a disorder manifested by difficulty in learning to read in spite of conventional instruction, adequate intelligence and adequate opportunity. Children may have been late in starting to talk and may show deficits in spoken as well as written language. There is some evidence of a neurobiological disturbance in dyslexia.

Dysmaturity Low birth weight is used for a baby whose birth weight is low in relation to its gestation age. This is expressed as birth weight below the tenthcentile for their gestational age as per graph. There is loss of subcutaneous fat and such babies have thin bodies and large heads. Skin is dry and wrinkled.

Dysmenorrhoea It is a pain or discomfort during or just before a menstrual period. It usually starts two or three years after the first period and generally diminishes after the child birth at about the age of 25. Dysmenorrhoea may be due to excessive production of or undue sensitivity to prostaglandin which stimulates muscular spasm. Girls develop cramp-like pain in lower abdomen in waves. It starts 12 hours before menses and lasts for half a day. It is relieved by analgesics.

Dysmeteria Refers to reduced motor control in cerebellar disease.

Dysmetria Loss of ability to guage distance, speed or power of movement.

Dysostosis Defective ossification.

Dysphasia Mild/moderate expressive aphasisa.

Dysphonea Hoarseness of speech.

Dysphonia It is a disorder of vibrating vocal cords. Vibrating cord may be paralysed by a recurrent laryngeal palsy so that voice becomes hoarse. There may be simple mechanical cause for dysphonia such as vocal cord polyp distorting the flow of expired air. Patients of parkinsonism often shift their expired gases very slowly so their voice is quiet or soft. Speech becomes monotonus.

Dysphoria Exaggerated feeling of depression of anxiety.

Dysphoric mood One symptom of depression in which patient feels sad, despondent, discouraged or unhappy. Significant anxiety and irritability is also indicative of dysphoria.

Dysplasia Change in the size, shape, and organization of cells due to chronic irritation or inflammation; may either revert to normal if stress is removed or progress to neoplasia.

Dysplasia, ectodermal It is a hereditary disease that involves all structures derived from ectoderm. It is a recessive mutation and males are mostly affected. General and oral manifestations include absence of sweat glands and sebaceous glands, depressed bridge of nose, protrusion of lips, defective mental development. There is complete or partial anodontia of both the deciduous and permanent dentitions with malformation of any teeth.

Dyspnea Difficult or laboured breathing.

Dyspnoeic index Difference between maximal voluntary ventilation and maximum minute ventilation reached during exercise.

Dyspraxia A partial loss of ability to perform coordinated movements.

Dysrhythmia Irregular pattern of heart beats.

Dyssocial behaviour The behaviour of persons who are not classifiable as antisocial personalitic, but who are predatory and follow criminal pursuits. Formerly called sociopathic personalities.

Dystocia Difficult, slow, or painful birth or delivery. It is distinguished as maternal or painful birth or delivery. It is distinguished as maternal or fetal ie, the difficulty may be due to some deformity on the part of the mother or on the part of the child.

Dystonia Acute tonic muscular spasms, often of the tongue, jaw, eyes, and neck, but sometimes of the whole body. Sometimes occurs during the first few days of antipsychotic drug administration. These are sustained muscle contractions causing twisting and repetitive movements or abnormal postures. Dystonia movements may be rapid or so slow that one abnormal posture slowly changes to another. These can be modified by putting sensory input. Muscles going into dystonic spasm during some movements may function entirely normal in others.

Dystonic gait Dystonic gait is commonly found in chorea, athetosis, ballismus and torsion dystonia. In Parkinsonian patients successfully treated with high doses of levodopa, definite dystonia can found.

Dystonic posturing Sustained twisting deformity that may last for several minutes or permanently.

Dystonic reaction Consist of involuntary muscle contraction involving face, side effect of many antiemetic drugs.

Dystress A harmful form of stress, the level of which must be low in order for an individual to have good health.

Dystrophia myotonia There develops increase in muscle tone following contraction and is exacerbated by cold. There maybe cardiomyopathy with conduction defect. Mental retardation may be there with sleep apnoea.

Dystrophia myotonica The features of this autosomal dominant inherited condition include distal myopathy, myotonia, cataracts, frontal boldness and hypogonadism. Vault may be thickened and myocardium may be involved. There will be progressive intellectual impairment. Pharyngeal dyscordination produces dysphagia and oesophageal dysmotility and dilation may occur. Unexplained diarrhoea and malabsorption have been described. Gall stones are formed.

Dysuria Difficult or uncomfortable voiding.

E

Ear It is an organ of hearing and balance. It consists of three parts. *Outer ear* consists of pinna made of muscle and cartilage. The eardrums separate the outer ear from middle ear. Ear drum is a thin, fibrous, circular membrane covered with a thin layer of skin when air pressure changes drum vibrates. *Middle ear* is a small cavity between the eardrum and inner ear.

It conducts sound to inner ear by means of tiny three linked movable bones called ossicles. The malleus is joined to the inside of ear drum. Eustachian tube runs forward and down into the back of nose. Generally it remains closed but it opens by muscular contraction. The *inner ear* is an extremely intricate series of structures. The front part is cochlea concerned with hearing. Rear part is of three semicircular canals concerned with balance.

Ear wax It is a deep yellow secretion known as cerumen, produced by glands in outer ear canal. In some cases it forms in excess and may even cause temporary loss of hearing. Excess of wax gives feeling of fullness in ear. Wax can either be removed with ring probe. If wax is hard, it can be softened with oil or mild hydrogen peroxide and then can be flushed with ear syringe with lukewarm water.

Earache Pain in otitis media is likely to be severe and stabbing. There may be loss of hearing. Otitis externa may also cause earache. Infection may be localised or may affect whole of canal. Intermittent earache may develop due to dental problem. Antibiotics and pain killer may be useful.

Eardrum It is a delicate septum of skin and membrane that separates outer ear to the middle ear. Sound vibrations are transferred from the eardrum to the malleus. Perforation of it may result in otitis media and result deafness.

Eardrum, perforation Rupture of eardrum in children takes place due to otitis media. Then inserting a sharp pin, pencil to clean ear may rupture the diaphragm. Those are inserted to relieve irritation. Antibiotics are better to treat perforation along with anti- inflammatory drugs. Do not put eardrops.

Early deceleration Transient slowing of the fetal heart rate in a pattern that is almost a mirror image of the contraction.

Early fetal death Delivery of a dead fetus during the first 20 weeks of gestation.

Eating disorders A group of behaviors fueled by unresolved emotional conflicts symptomized by altered food consumption.

Ebola virus infection A virulent hemorrhagic disease with a high case fatality ratio.

Eburnation Increase in bone density.

EBV Epstein-Barr virus.

Eccentric A lengthening contraction.

Ecchymosis Black and blue discoloration of the skin caused by the escape of blood from the vessels into the tissues; bleeding into the subcutaneous tissues.

Eccrine Small sweat glands distributed over the total body surface.

Eccrine gland Gland that secretes directly on the outside skin while apocrine glands secrete to the surface through short ducts. All the sweat glands of palm, soles and hands are like that.

Eccrine sweat glands Secretory glands distributed over the body that secret sweat.

Eccrinic Concerning the eccrine gland; a small sweat gland which occurs all over the human body; they secrete clear water-soluble sweat.

Ecdysiostatin A hormone that inhibits the production of ecdysteroids by endocrine glands.

Ecdysone A steroid hormone produced by an endocrine gland in insects and other arthropods such as crustacea as a precursor to the active form, 20-hydroxyecdysone, which controls molting.

ECG (Electrocardiogram) It is a linear graph of voltage fluctuations produced by the myocardium.

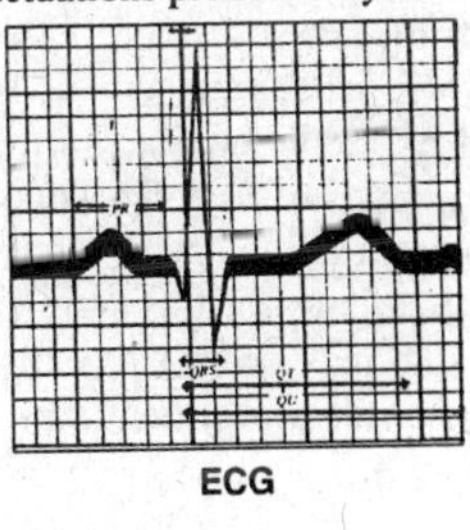

ECG

The heart muscle possesses the property of automatic rhythmic contraction. The impulses that arise in the conducting system spread through out the myocardium resulting in excitation of muscle fibres. Result is weak electric currents, which spread throughout the entire body. These can be recorded by placing electrodes at various positions on the body and connecting them to an electrocardiographic apparatus.

ECG/EKG Electrocardiogram; electrocardiograph.

Echinococcus granulosus These are smallest amongst tapeworms measuring 2-8 m.m. long containing 3 proglottids. Scolex bears 28-50 hooks, four prominent suckers and a short neck. Once swallowed, eggs pass through the stomach and hatch in small intestine. Hydatid cyst grows slowly reaching a diameter of 10 m.m. in 5 months.

Echinocytes Contracted red blood cells with spiny projections.

Echo In the study of memory processes, a fleeting sensory image of an auditory stimulus. The stimulation, after a sound has occurred, is still in the sensory register, which is part of the peripheral nervous system.

Echocardiography It is the ultrasound examination of heart and great vessels. It provides a variety of techniques including M-mode, two-dimensional B mode real-time scanning. Even 3D images are possible.

Echography Soft tissue examination that uses sound waves in ranges beyond human hearing.

Echolalia Automatic repetition by an individual of what is said to him/her.

Echolocation The ability to identify and locate an object by sound that bounces off the object.

Echopraxia The spasmodic and involuntary imitation of the movements of others.

Eclampsia Symptoms of preeclampsia are severe headache, dimness of vision or temporary blindness, severe epigastric pain and vomiting. Urine contains albumin. Convulsions are epileptiform in character and consist of tonic followed by clonic contractions. There may be marked cyanosis of face, lips are drawn back and tongue protruded. Varying amount of mental disturbance follows the fit. Convulsions are always multiple and may occur every hour. High blood presure is a rule and patient may develop fever. Anuria is of grave significance. Jaundice is rare. Puerperal sepsis may prove to be a cause of death.

Eclectic Literally, "choosing" Eclecticism in therapy, for example, occurs when the therapist espouses no single approach but chooses among the viewpoints available.

Eclipse In virology, a term for the period between the entry of a virus into a cell when it loses its infectivity as an independnet particle to the appearance inside the cell of fully infectious progeny virus particles.

Eclipse blindness It occurs due to looking solar eclipse. There develops damage to macula due to concentration of infra red rays at macula. It is usually bilateral but may be unilateral too. Patient complains of photophobia, chromatopsia and positive scotoma. On ophthalmoscopy there are changes at the macula in the form of oedema, fine haemorrhages, degenerative changes as yellow spots.

Ecology The science that deals with the study of the environment and the life history of organisms. The study of relationship between human organisms and their physical habitats including their biological, cultural and psychological adjustments.

Ecotone An ecological interface; a zone of transition between two habitats.

ECT (Electroconvulsive therapy) It is an anticonvulsive therapy using electric shock. Muscle relaxants are given. The patient is given anaesthesia before, and two electrodes are applied on temples and controlled electric pulse is passed to cause seizure. Seizure is indicated by brief muscular rigidity, followed by twitching of eyelids and limbs. Course of ECT consists of 6 to 12 seizures and patient starts improving after third session.

Ectadenia Accessory glands of male insects derived from ectoderm.

Ecto Prefix denoting outer or outside.

Ectoderm The primary germ layer that gives rise to the nervous system and the epidermis of skin and its derivatives.

Ectoderm stage Layer of cells that develops into the nervous system, speciality organs, epidermal tissue, and mucous membranes.

Ectomy Suffix used to denote the removal of/or excision of an anatomic structure.

Ectoparasite A parasite that lives on the exterior surface of the host.

Ectopia vesicae It is more common in females. There is an absence of anterior wall of bladder and of lower part of abdominal wall. Symphysis pubis also fails to develop as does the anferior wall of urethra. The red mucous membrane of bladder projects forwards in from anterior abdominal wall and two ureteric orifices. Treatment is closing the bladder and repairing abdominal wall.

Ectopia lentis It is a condition where lens is displaced in the direction away from poorly developed segment of zonule. There is strong hereditary tendency. Edge of lens may be seen in pupillary area. The edge appears as a dark cresent on ophthalmoscopy due to prismatic reflections. Iridodonesis is there. Anterior chamber becomes irregular. Slit lamp may show zonular fibres. Lens becomes smaller than normal and more spherical. Lens may dislocate and secondary glaucoma may occur. There may be unilocular diplopia. Removal of lens is suggested if there is diplopia and dim vision.

Ectopic Arising or produced at an abnormal site or in a tissue where it is not normally found.

Ectopic ACTH syndrome Syndrome occurs from excessive production of glucocorticoids from non-endocrine tissues at ectopic sites other than adrenals, like carcinoma of lung, thymoma and medullary carcinoma of thyroid. Clinical features resemble to that of Cushing's syndrome. There will be moon face, buffalo hump and protruded abdomen. There will be hirsutism, amenorrhoea, glycosuria, acne and cubitus valgus. Osteoporosis of vertebral body will be seen along with collapse and rib fracture.

Ectopic bone Bone that is situated elsewhere than in the normal place.

Ectopic expression The aritifcial expression of a gene under conditions where it would not normally be expressed.

Ectopic foci Multiple aberrant points of origin; the locations from which abnormal myocardial depolarizations originate.

Ectopic ossification The formation of bone outside its usual location.

Ectopic pregnancy It is the pregnancy which develops outside the uterus. It develops commonly in fallopian tube. The fertilised ovum stuck up in fallopian tube. It is more common in previously infected or operated tubes or if woman has an IUD. There will be a severe pain in abdomen and vaginal bleeding. After rupture female may develop pallor, sweating and faintness. Female may undergo shock and life becomes threatening. Operation is the remedy.

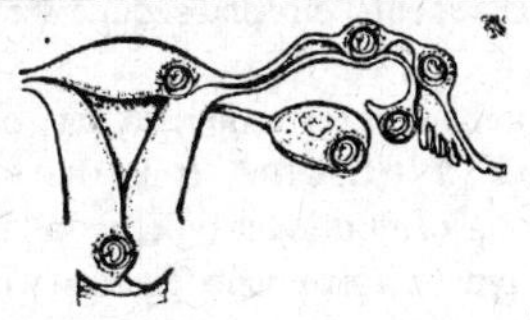

Sites of ectopic pregnancies

Ectopic site Abnormal or unexpected site of infection.

Ectopic testis Testis that has exited the inguinal canal but is not in the scrotum.

Ectothermic Having body temperature that varies according to the surrounding environmental temperature.

Ectotrophic Obtaining nutrients from an external or surface source; e.g., certain parasitic plant fungi located on the surface of a root.

Ectropion Eversion of an edge or margin, as of the columnar epithelium of the endocervical canal onto the ectocervix. The tissue appears darker pink-red and bumpy compared with the smooth pink squamous epithelium of the ectocervix. It is a condition of rolling outward of lid margin. In old age there is sagging of lid in the inner aspect causing eversion of lower punctum. Paralytic ectropion is seen in cases of facial nerve paralysis. In it mostly lower lid is involved. Cicatricial ectropion is seen in case of injury, burns and scarring of lids. Due to sagging lower conjunctiva, lower fornix and lower bulbar conjunctiva are exposed. There can be keratinisation and xerosis of exposed conjunctiva.

Eczema It causes thickening of skin, itching with scaling or blisters. Allergy and contact dermatitis may be the predisposing factors. *Atopic eczema* is common in babies appearing between the ages of 2 to 18 months. Skin scales up with mild blisters.

In severe cases cortisone ointments and antihistaminic drugs may be helpful. In adults hands and legs are commonly involved, may be due to detergents, etc. and require the same line of treatment.

EDD Abbrebiation for estimated date of delivery.

Eddowes' syndrome It is the osteogenesis imperfecta of dominant type, a collagen disorder of autosomal involvement. It is seen with blue sclera and skeletal anomalies of variable types with increased fragility of bones. Osteoporosis and dental deformity is noted. Bones are deformed due to multiple fractures. Multiple soft tissue swelling over extremity and deafness is noted.

Edema Abnormal swelling due to large amounts of fluid in the tissues.

Edentulous Without any natural teeth. The state of the oral cavity afterall teeth have been lost.

Edentulous zone An area without teeth.

Edge angle The angle formed between the clearance face and the rake face of a bur.

Edible portion The term refers to that part of food which is eaten.

Edrophonium test Following a test dose of 2 mg, 8 mg of edrophonium chloride, an antagonist of skeletal muscle relaxant, is administered intravenously, which produces a short but immediate muscle function improvement in cases of myasthenia gravis.

The test is used for diagnosis of myasthenia gravis, and also for the differentiation between myasthenic and cholinergic crises in which case the agent worsens cholinergic crisis but improves myasthenic.

Edwards' syndrome It is a chromosomal disorder. An extra chromosome is found in 17-18 (E) group. An autosomal disorder characterised by abnormal skull, small mandible, malformed ears, short sternum, congenital heart diseases, diaphragmatic or inguinal hernia, and mental retardation. Average life span is 90 days.

EEG Electroencephalogram.

Efector cell Cells that have differentiated to a mature form and become activated following exposure of its precursor to an antigen.

Effect modification Occurs when the strength of the influence of a causal factor on outcome is altered bya third variable, the effect modifier.

Effective cough Four-stage cough consisting of a deep inspiration, glottis closure, abdominal muscle contraction, and forceful exhalation.

Effectiveness Usefulness of a particular treatment to the individuals receiving it under typical clinical conditions, usually determined by nonexperimental methods in outcomes research; contrast with efficacy.

Effector An organ of the body, either a muscle or a gland, that responds to a motor neuron impulse.

Effector cells Cells which carry out an immune function, e.g. cytokine release, cytotoxicity.

Efferent arteriole A vessel of a renal vascular system that transports blood from a glomerulus to a peritubular capillary.

Efferent ductule Small duct that leads from the testis to the epididymis.

Efferent fibre Nerve fibre going from the central nervous system toward the peripheral nervous system; motor fibre.

Efficacy In pathology, the maximum possible reduction in incidence of a disease attributable to an intervention designed to prevent and control the disease.

Effleurage It is a movement which is done with the flat of a hand with the fingers close together. Tip of the fingers turn inside. Effleurage precedes all other

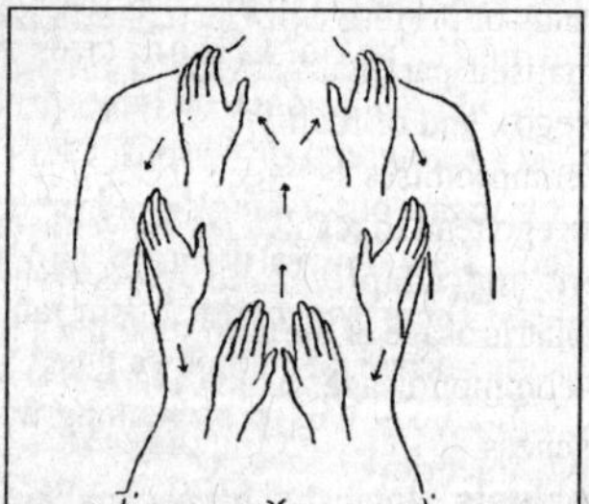

movements because of its relaxing effect. These movements are generally towards the heart. Movement should be slow and rhythmic. Patient should feel one continuous movement of different pressures. Massage of abdomen or other parts performed during labour.

Effluent 1. Flowing out or away. 2. liquid waster resulting from sweage treatment or industrial process, especially such matter released into waterways.

Effort syndrome It is the name given to a clinical picture developing in variety of nervous conditions. The symptoms comprise breathlessness, giddiness, palpitation, tachycardia and exhaustion. All these symptoms are exaggerated by exercise. They may be superadded to a hysterical or a psychopathic personality. Prognosis is better.

Effusion Excess fluid in the joint indicating irritation or inflammation of the synovium; excess of fluid in a body cavity.

Egg A female gamete involved in sexual reproduction; ovum. In certain animals, e.g., birds, an external shelled body expelled from the female's body, consisting of this reproductivie element and protective and nutritive materials.

Egg cell The female germ cell arrested in metaphase of the second meiotic division.

Egg-laying hormone (ELH) In certain animals, e.g., gastropods, peptides of approximately 4,500 daltons in size, found in clusters of neurons in the nervous system. Upon secretion into the circulation, these peptides activate egg laying and related egg-release behavior.

Ego In psychoanalytic theory, one of the three major divisions in the model of the psychic apparatus, the others being the id and superego. The ego represents the sum of certain mental mechanisms, such as perception and memory, and spoecific defence mechanisms. It serves to mediate between the demands of primitive instinctual drives (the id), of internalised parental and social prohibitions (the superego), and of reality.

The compromises between these forces achieved by the ego tend to resolve intrapsychic conflict and severe and adaptive and executive function. Psychiatric usage of the term should not be confused with common usage, which connotes self love or selfishness.

Ego analysis Intensive psychoanalytic study and analysis of the ways in which the ego resolves or attempts to deal with intrapsychic conflicts, especially in relation to the development of mental mechanisms and the maturation of capacity for rational thought and action. Modern psychoanalysis gives more emphasis to considerations of the defensive operations of the ego than did earlier techniques, which emphasised instinctual forces to a greater degree.

Ego ideal The part of the personality that comprises the aims and goals for the self; usually refers to the conscious or unconscious emulation of significant figures with whom one has identified. The ego deal emphasises what one should be or do in contrast to what one should not be or not do.

Ego psychology The study and elucidation of those slowly changing functions known as psychic structures which usually shape, channel, and organise mental activity into meaningful and tolerable patterns of experience. The usual structures referred to in his or her sense are memory, speech, locomotion, cognition, drive, restraint, discharge, and the capacity to make judgements and decisions.

Egocentrism Complete absorption with self, an inability to understand that others have a different point of view.

Interest centered on self rather than needs of others.

Egophony An auscultatory finding denoting an increased density of the underlying lung tissue; demonstrated when the vowel sound "e" is spoken but is heart through the stethoscope as "a".

Egyptian foot Big toe is longer than second toe.

Ehlers-Danlos syndrome It is an autosomal dominant disorder. There is absence of elastic and collagen fibres in the skin. Skin becomes thin and atrophic. There will be delayed healing of wound and hypermobility of joints and subluxation. Patient will develop ptosis, epicanthus and subluxation of lens.

EIA Enzyme immunoassay.

Eicosanoids Local hormones derived from a 20-carbon fatty acid (arachidonic acid); two important types are prostaglandins and leukotrienes.

Eicosapentaenoic acid (EPA) The main omega-3 fatty acid in fish.

Eisenmenger's syndrome Pulmonary hypertension with reversal at arteriovenous shunt is called Eisenmenger's syndrome.

It is seen in cases of VSD and PDA. Clinical features include tiredness, central cyanosis, polycythemia, clubbing, prominent 'a' wave in neck, right ventricular hypertrophy and very loud second heart sound. X-ray shows dilated pulmonary artery, right ventricular enlargement and increased vascularity of lung fields.

Ejaculation Ejaculation is experienced by males after puberty when the prostate and accessory glands become functional. Females have nothing to ejaculate. The fluid that lubricates the vagina is produced during arousal and does not correspond to seminal fluid which is thick and has glue-like consistency. In males, first there is strong sense that ejaculation is imminent and person cannot stop it. Secondly, person feels contracting urethra followed by fluid moving out under pressure.

Ejaculation stage Prostate, seminal vesicle, vasdeferens and penis contacts. Seminal fluid comes out as jerks.

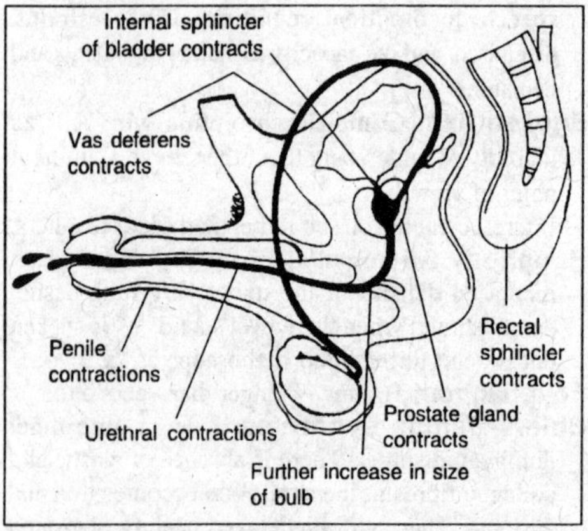

Ejaculatory duct Duct formed by the joining of the ductus deferens and the duct from the seminal vesicle that allows sperm to enter the urethra.

Ejaculatory incompetence The term is used for ejaculation deficiency. Conditions resulting it include fear of impregnating the partner, traumatic experience and unconscious feelings as being rejected.

Ejaculatory urge It is the impulse of male to expel semen through urethra during orgasm. In the sexual response cycle man arrives at a point of ejaculatory inevitability when the ejaculation reflex is abruptly triggered.

Ejection fraction The portion of the stroke volume pumped from the left ventricle.

Ejection sound It is a sharp, high pitched sound heard in early systole at the time of ejection of blood from left ventricle into aorta or from right ventricle into pulmonany artery. Pulmonary ejection sound is best heard in pulmonary area over left third intercostal space close to sternum. It is best heard during expiration and diminishes during inspiration. It is poorly heard at apex. Aortic ejection sounds are common in patients of bicuspid aortic valve and in aortic stenosis. It disappears when valve is calcified. Aortic ejection sound can also be heard with aortic regurgitation, coarctation of aorta, aneurysm of ascending aorta and in Fallot's tetralogy.

Elastase A serum proteinase that hydrolyzes elastin.

Elastic deformation Any recoverable deformation.

Elastic bandage Bandage of elasticized fabric that provides srpport and allows movement.

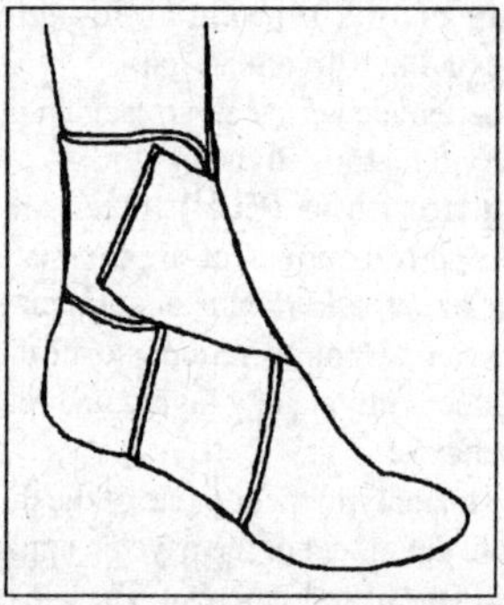

Elastic cartilage A type of nonhyaline cartilage in which matrix contain a high proportion of elastic tissue as seen in epiglottis, external ear and ligamentum flavum.

Elastic deformation Deformation of a material or tissue such that it recovers to its original form from stretching, compression, or shear distortions.

Elastic fibers Prodein strands that are found in certain connective tissue that have contractile properties.

Elastic limit The maximum amount of stress that a particular material can withstand before undergoing a permanent change in shape.

Elastic modulus The stress divided by the strain in the linear portion of a stress- strain diagram; a measure of a material's stiffness of flexibility.

Elastic tissue These contain large number of elastic fibres. Elastic fibres outnumber collagen fibres. Tissue has a springly, resilient nature. The ability to stretch and rebound allows it to tolerate cycles of expansion and contraction. It is found in the walls of blood vessels, and it surrounds the respiratory passage.

Elasticity The ability of tissue to return to its original shape after contraction of extension.

Elastics Rubber bands used to apply force to the tooth during orthodontic treatment.

Elastin A fibrous and stretchy protein found in tissue. It gives skin its elasticity.
Insoluble protein uniting muscle fibres in meat. It is not changed on heating and is a cause of tough meat.

Elastosis Degeneration of elastic tissue.

Elbow The synovial joint between the brachium and the antebrachium.

Elbow dislocation Elbow dislocations in children are more often posterior but may be anterior, medial or lateral. Reduction under general anaesthesia is recommended within 6 hours. Then elbow is immobilised in 90 degrees or more of flexion.

Elbow restraints Elbow restraints are used to prevent flexion of the arm when a child receiving IV therapy or has dressings which are not to be disturbed. Both elbows are usually restrained.

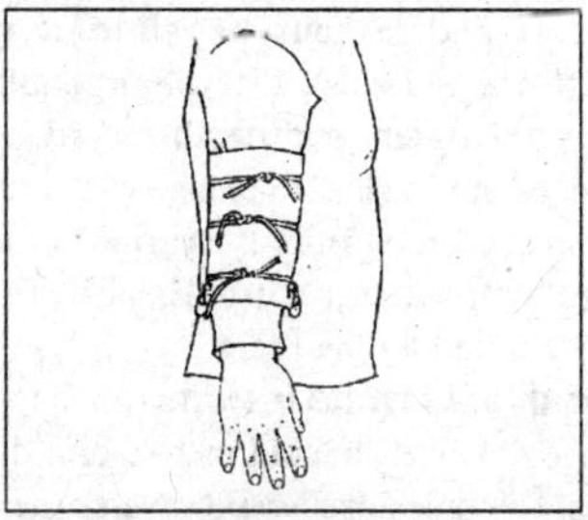

Elbow-Carrying Angle This angle is the lateral deviation of the radius and ulna from the humerus at the elbow joint; 10 to 20 degrees is its normal measurement, especially in women.

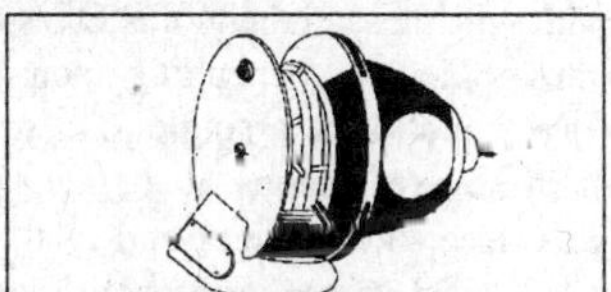

Eldridge-Green lamp

Eldridge-Green lamp In this lamp, various colours are shown to the patient through an observation hole. His or her answers shall label him or her either normal or colour deficient or colour blind. He or she can be labelled either colour deficient or colour blind based upon the answers.

Elective abortion Deliberate termination of a pregnancy.

Elective amputation Elective amputation may be performed when the hand or the entire limb is sensationless and functionless. The hand may be swollen, painful and limited in range of motion. The most frequent cause is brachial plexus injury or multiple cervical root avulsions.

Electra complex An infrequently used term describing the pathologic relationship between a woman and a man based on unresolved developmental conflicts partially analogous to the oedipus complex in a man.

Electric injury It is the damage caused by the passage of an electric current. The tissues of body being moist and salty are good conductor of electricity. Dry skin provides a high resistence. Person in bathroom or standing on a good conductor of electricity may prove fatal. AC is more dangerous than DC.

Electric light Electric light as a source of heat is used for application of heat on body specially for an extensive area of body. So it is used for an extensive burn or for drying casts or extensive wounds. For generalised heat application to the body, 200 watt bulb is used.

Electric pad Electric pads may be used in place of hot water bottle. With the help of it one can apply evenly released heat to a part of body. Electric pad should not be used for commatose patient or a patient while he or she is asleep. It should never be used over moist area to avoid short circuit.

Electric shock-treatment Do not touch the patient directly. If his body is touching water, body salt will make the water conduct the electricity causing you to be shocked. Turn off electricity. Break the person's contact with electric source without directly touching him. Use an object that will not

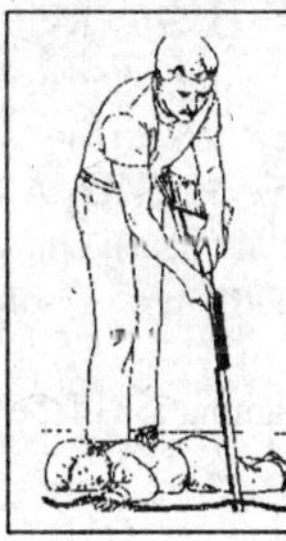

Electric shock-treatment

conduct electric charge, i.e. rubber, dry wood, paper, broom handle. Monitor CPR.

Electric stimulation of bone The applicaton of an electric current to stimulate osteogenesis.

Electrical otoscope It is an aural speculum with a self-illuminating electrical device. It is commonly used to examine minute perforation in tympanic

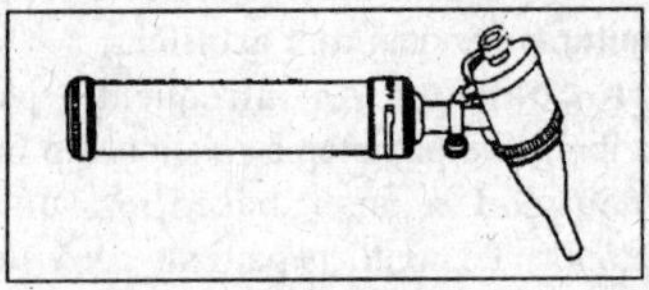

membrane. It helps in otosclerosis to see honey-combing of tympanic membrane. This has fixed focus.

Electrical potential An electrical charge; the ability to do work through the use of stored potential electrical energy.

Electrical properties Two properties, corrosion and galvanism, are found in dental materials. When two metals come in contact with each other in the oral cavity an electrical reaction occurs.

Electrical shock Discharge of electricity through the body.

Electrical silence The absence of measurable electromyographic activity, typically recorded at rest in normal muscles.

Electrical stimulation The flow of electrical current from the tip of an electrode through brain tissue, resulting in changes in the electrical activity of the tissue.

Electrical symbols These are used to denote components of electrical circuit. Specific symbols are used to indicate safety features.

Electrical synapse Synapse consisting of gap junctions.

Electricity The flow of electrons from a body that contains a higher charge to a body that contains a lower charge.

Electro surgery A technique that uses a high frequency alternating electric current.

Electrocardiogram (ECG or EKG) A record of the electrical activity of the heart; shows certain waves called P, Q, R, S, and T waves; sometimes a U wave.

Electrocardiography Examination of the electrical activity in the heart.

Electrochemical neutrality Balance of cations with anions.

Electrochemical potential The energy required to maintain a separation of charge and of concentration across a membrane.

Electrocoagulation It is used to stop bleeding. It can be used during operation to close freshly cut blood vessels. The current is applied through a fine needle or through a knife.

Electrocyte One of the cells of the electric organ of electric fist that generate the electric organ discharge.

Electrode An insulated wire or a salt-filled glass tube that is used to stimulate or record from neurons.

Electroencephalogram (EEG) A graphic (voltage vs. time) depiction of the brain's electrical potentials recorded by scalp electrodes. It is used for diagnosis in neurologic and neuropsychiatric disorders and in neurophysiologic research. Sometimes used interchangeably with electrocorticogram and depth record, where the electrodes are in direct contact with brain tissue, the brain, recorded from the surface of the scalp.

Electroencephalography Examination of the energy emitted by the brain.

Electrogalvanic white lesions Such lesions may be leucoplakial, lichenoid or like oral discoid LE lesions. White lesions would reverse the causative metal restoration were replaced.

Electrogenic Contribution to an electrical potential across a membrane.

Electro-Goniometer It is a deviece which converts angular motion of the joint into an electric signal and enables the measurement of R.O.M. of a joint. An electro goniometer depending upon the design can measure motion at a single joint or measure motion in several planes at a time. The skill required to use such devices and relatively high cost have limited its use in research field.

Electrokinetic separation Separation mode in which the electric field is the driving force, but where the selectivity is not based onto electro phoretic mechanisms.

Electrolysis It is the process of permanent removal of unwanted hair by means of a short wave electric current destroying the root of hair. Unwanted hair over face and legs, etc. may be removed temporarily by shaving or plucking and wax preparations. To remove each hair a fine needle is inserted into follicle and a small electric current is passed through root to destroy it.

Electrolyte Any substance that, when placed in solution, conducts and is decomposed by electricity.

Electrolyte balance Homeostasis of electrolytes.

Electrolyte sialadenitis There becomes transient swelling of the submandibular gland during and after eating usually with tension pain. Glandular discharge is milky or purulent with increased viscosity. Electrolyte sialadenitis is on a continuum with sialolithiasis. Changes in the composition of salivary electrolyte with ductal inflammation may cause it.

Electrolytes Chemical compounds, such as sodium and chloride, that are dissolved, absorbed, and distributed in body fluid and possess an electrical charge.

Electromyogram Electrical activity of whole muscles recorded by surface electrodes, or that of single motor units recorded by intramuscular needle electrodes.

Electromyograph The instrument used to record and study the intrinsic activity of skeletal muscle.

Electromyography (EMG) It is the study of voluntary and spontaneous electrical activity of muscles. The single motor neuron along with the muscle fibres it supplies constitutes a motor unit. If the motor unit loses muscle fibres some fibres cannot be activated as in myaesthenia gravis. In neuropathy axons are lost resulting in longer EMG record. Resting muscles are usually silent in EMG.

Electromyogrpahic Pertaining to the graphic record of the electrical activity of active muscle or the apparatus used to obtain it.

Electron One of three parts of an atom, an electron is a negatively charged particle that moves about the nucleus of an atom.

Electron acceptor A low molecular weight inorganic or organic species, compound or ion that is oxidized in the first step of an electron transfer process.

Electron microscope A microscope that uses an electron beam, instead of light beam to produce an image.

Electron multiplier The electron multiplier is a device that transforms the ion beam of charged fragments into an electrical signal to be sent in a wire and monitored by a recorder or data system.

Electron transfer Movement of electrons from substrates to oxygen via the carriers of the respiratory chain.

Electron transport chain A sequence of electron carrier molecules on the inner mitochondrial membrane that undergo oxidation and reduction as they synthesize ATP.

Electron transport system Cellular process within mitochondria that transfers energy from high-energy electrons from glycolysis and the citric acid cycle to ATP molecules so that the energy is available to do work in the cell.

Electronic fetal monitor A system for monitoring fetal heart rate and uterine activity by electrically operated instruments.

Electron-transport chain Series of energy transfer molecules in the inner mitochondrial membrane; they receive energy and use it in the formation of ATP and water.

Electroosmotic flow Flow of liquid generated in an electrophoretic system under the driving force of the electric field, by the migration of buffer ions dragging water osmotically.

Electrophoresis A biochemical technique in which different molecules can be separated and identified by their rate of movement in an electric field.

Electroplating An electrical process by which a metallic surface is "plated" or coated on to a substrate by applying electric current through a solution containing metallic ions.

Electropure process Method of pasteurising milk by passing a low frequency alternating current.

Electrosurgery unit High-frequency electrical source used to cut or alter tissues in the oral cavity.

Electrotonus A decremental voltage change passing over the neuronal soma following receptor activation.

Element Any of more than 100 substances that consist of only one kind of atom and cannot be decompsed into simpler substances.

Elemental formula A dietary solution that provides ready-to-absorb basic nutrients, requiring minimal digestion.

Elements of a fingerprint Two separate groups of ridges appear in all patterns except arches and tented arches, the recurving or core elements, and the nonrecurving or delta elements. Delta and core elements are critical reference points in pattern determination.

Elephantiasis neurofibromatosa It is a rare and congenital condition. It is a severe form of plexiform neurofibromatosis. Limbs are common sites, specially lower limb. Clincally, skin becomes coarse, dry and thickened and looks like an elephant's hide.

Subcutaneous tissues become greatly thickened and fat is replaced by fibrous tissue usually it may be confused with the filarial elephantiasis but the lymphatics remain normal.

Elephantitis gingivae It may occur after use of dilantin in hereditary fibromatosis gingivae or in association with mouth breathing problems. In all patients gingiva is firm and fibrous and covers crowns of teeth. Since the gingiva is enlarged it leads to the formation of deep sulcus or a pseudopocket.

Elevator Hand instrument used for lifting teeth during extraction.

ELISA Enzyme-linked immunosorbent assay, a highly sensitive serological technique that is widely used to detect and measure the levels of various specific antibodies and antigens.

Ellipsoid joint In it convex ellipsoid surface is recieved into a concave ellipsoid surface. Wrist joint is ellipsoid type.

Ellis-van Creveld syndrome It is characterised by ectodermal dysplasia affecting the nails, hair and teeth, polydactyly, shortened distal limbs, and congenital cardiac defect.

Ellsworth-Howard test It is a test for the diagnosis of pseudohypoparathyroidism but can also be used to differentiate it from true hypoparathyroidism. It is done by intravenous administration of parathyroid extract and then by measuring the serum and urinary phosphorus.

Elongation A radiographic error resulting from insufficient vertical angulation; the teeth on the film appear longer than their actual length.

ELPS Abbreviation for excessive lateral pressure syndrome.

Eluate The effluent from a chromatographic column.

Elute To wash off or to remove.

Emaciation There is wasting of body's muscles after using up all its store of energy in form of fat. Condition is caused primarily by malnutrition. Condition of excessive leanness or wasted body tissues.

Emancipated minor A minor who can be considered to have the rights of an adult when it can be shown that he is, in fact, exercising general control over his life.

Embolectomy Surgical removal of a lodged arterial embolus.

Emboli The plural of embolus; multiple plugs that occlude a vessel; composed of detached thrombus, bacterial mass, vegetation, of other foreign bodies.

Emboliform Emboliform nucleus of cerebellum.

Embolisation Occlusion of vascular structures by transcatheter approach or percutaneous puncture using liquid or particulate embolisation material. Main indications include treatment of haemorrhage, AVM and tumour ablation.

Embolism The sudden blocking of an artery or vein by a blood clot or other obstruction that was brought there by the blood current.

Embolus A clot or other obstruction brought to a vein or artery by the blood from a larger vessel. A detached clot or other foreign body that occludes a blood vessel.

Embossing Embossing is the process of putting raised letters and numbers on plastic cards.

Embrasure Opening, as in a wall. The space between the curve proximal surfaces of the teeth.

Embryo The fetus in its earlier stages of development, especially before the end of the second month.

The product of conception *in utero* from the third through the fifth week of gestation; after that length of time it is called the fetus. In prenatal development, the developing human between 14 and 56 days of development.

Embryology Study of the development of an individual from conception to birth.

Embryonic Relating to, describing, or involving the embryo.

Embryonic disc The flattish portion of a fertilised ovum in which the first traces of an embryo are seen.

Embryotoxins Substances that kill or alter the embryo.

Embryotropic Relating to or describing conditions supportive of or stimulatory to growth and development of the embryo.

Emergenesis The inheritence of characteristics that require the cooccurence of multiple genetic traits.

Emesis Substance that is vomited.

Emesis basin A basin, usually kidney-shaped, used for receiving material expectorated or vomited.

EMG Abbreviation for electromyelogram.

Emigration Process whereby white blood cells (WBCs) leave the bloodstream by slowing down, rolling along the endothelium, and squeezing between the endothelial cells. Adhesion molecules help WBCs stick to the endothelium.

Eminence, iliopectineal Iliopubic eminence.

Emission Deposition of seminal fluid into posterior urethra.

Emmetropia It is a condition in which incipient parallel rays of light coming from infinity come to focus on the light sensitive layer of retina when the eye is at rest. In it axial length and curvature of the cornea may vary a little. A minor degree of low ametropia should be considered a biological variant and not pathological.

Emolients These are fatty or oily substances which soften the skin. These are bland oily substances which when applied to the skin protect it from irritation and render it softer and more elastic. These induce vasodilation by the heat of the material. Linseed poultices are well known. It is used to relieve itching and irritation over skin and to soften and remove crusts and scabs.

Emotion A complex condition underlying such feelings, actions, and physiological changes as occur in fear, rage, excitement, and so on. In its most obvious manifestations, it is an acute condition characterised by disruption of routine experiences and activities. It is temporary and subjective mental disposition that is different from normal and is the focus of mood. Emotion may be pleasant or unpleasant and may result in stress. Lack of emotional development also indicates mental disorder.

Emotion focussed coping Attempts to manage one's emotions during stressful periods.

Emotional deprivational dwarfism Child who lacks security and emotional warmth of home. These are brought up in orphanages and broken homes and remain small in size. Child may be neglected physically. Facies are immature. Bone age may be delayed. Levels of human growth hormone and somatomedin may also return normal.

Emotional anesthesia Feelings of being detached or estranged from others, a loss of ability to enjoy or feel interest in previously enjoyable activities, or the lack of any emotions or feelings.

Emotional circumflex A circular arrangement of facial expressions defined by two dimensions. Pleasant-love, happy to unpleasant anger.

Emotional control Ability to regulate or control emotional communication.

Emotional dysregulation syndrome Pathologic laughing and weeping.

Emotional eating Eating in response to emotional cues.

Emotional exhaustion Feelings of being emotionally overextended and drained by others.

Emotional expressivity The ability to convey emotions and feelings, the most visible component of charisma.

Emotional focussed coping Coping responses that are geared toward managing one's emotions during stressful episodes.

Emotional health The capacity to easily express or suppress emotions appropriately.

Emotional Intelligence The ability of an individual to adoptability and effectively regulate his or her emotional behaviour in a social context.

Emotional lability Changeable moods, with rapid mood swings. Unstable or changeable emotional state.

Emotional load Psychosocial causes of unpleasant and during emotions induced by percieved or extrinsic nature of work load inducing psychobiological changes

Emotional maltreatment Verbal or nonverbal parent to child communications that may be psychologically injurious to child given the child's age and developmental status.

Emotional memory Memory for the affective properties of stimuli or events.

Emotional rehearsal The tendency to persist in thinking about emotionally upsetting events which have happened in the past or might occur in future.

Emotional sensitivity Skill in receiving and interpreting the emotional messages of others.

Emotions in labour Woman in love is very sensitive, childbirth is considered a personal achievement. She readily over reacts to any critical remarks. Many woman have exhilarating experience of childbirth.

Empathy Insightful awareness, including the meaning and significance of the feelings, emotions, and behaviour of another person. The projection of one's own consciousness into that of another. Empathy may be distinguished from sympathy in that the former state includes relative freedom from emotional involvement.

Emphysema In this the alveoli in the lungs become damaged. It is more exaggerated by smoking. Through this walls of alveoli inhaled oxygen is passed into the blood stream. Pollutants release chemicals which damage the alveolar walls. Emphysema is accompanied with chronic bronchitis. To start with there may not be any symptoms, but later on it results in shortness of breath. Chest becomes barrel shaped.

Emphysematous pyelonephritis It is a rare form of acute necrotising pyelonephritis, characterised by gas formation either within renal parenchyma or perirenally. Symptoms include fever, shaking chill and flank pain. Predisposing factor is diabetes mellitus in over 80 % cases. Sonography reveals dirty shadows caused by air-tissue interface.

Empirical Based on experience and observation.

Empiricism Seeking evidence through direct experience rather than through reasoning or intuition.

Employee A person who works for another for a wage.

Empowerment The process of providing information and resources to help others to reach a goal.

Empty sella syndrome It is a condition in which a subarachnoid recess extends into the sella causing compression to the pituitary gland. It may be primary or secondary. Primary sella syndrome is associated with hypertension and obesity. Usually there is a defect in diaphragm sella which transmits CSF flow. Secondary type is due to surgery, radiotherapy or infarction of pituitary. Optic disc becomes pale with reduced visual acquity. Cortex of sella remains intact.

Emptying reflex The reflex that causes the contraction of the bladder wall and relaxation of the internal sphincter to allow urine to enter the urethra, which is followed by urination if the external sphincter is voluntarily relaxed.

Empyema It is accumulation of pus in pleural cavity. It may be secondary to pneumonia, or by rupture of lung abscess or subphrenic abscess in the pleural space. Common organisms responsible for empyema are *Staphylococcus aureus*, coliform organisms and *Pseudomonas*. Clinical findings are similar to pleural effusion. There may be bulging of intercostal spaces and burrowing of subcutaneous tissue.

EMS Emergency Medical Service.

EMT Abbreviation for emergency medical technician.

Emulsification The dispersion of large lipid globules to smaller, uniformly distributed particles in the presence of bile.

Emulsifier A substance that works by being soluble in water and fat at the same time.

Emulsify To form an emulsion, which is one liquid dispersed in another liquid.

Emulsifying agents Substances such as gums, egg yolk, albumin, casein, soaps, lecithin and glycerol monosterate.

Emulsion Mixture of two liquids, one of which is insoluble in the other.

Enalapril An antihypertensive agent.; an angiotensin-converting enzyme inhibitor.

Enamel Glistening tissue covering the anatomic crown of the tooth composed primarily of hexagonal rods of hydroxyapatite, sheathed in an organic matrix and oriented with the long axis approximately at a right angle to the surface.

Enamel adhesives These materials are essentially unfilled composites are pit and fissure sealants applied to enamel surface with a brush. They have excellent flow properties which coat and fill in the small irregularities of acid-etched enamel surface. These are also used for intra oral repair of fractured composite restorations.

Enamel wares cleaning These should not be scraped by any sharp or rough object as the enamel coating is easily chipped off leaving an ugly surface. It can be cleaned with detergent and washed with soap water and dried. If aseptic enamel items like kidney trays or small bowls are required for any surgical or sterile use, these can be boiled in big bowls for 20 to 30 minutes. Phenol or lysol treatment by dipping it for 4 hours also make these sterilised.

Enamlum Dental ENAMEL.

Enantiomer A molecule whose spatial orientation is such that its mirror image is nonsuperimposable, as in a person's left and right hands. There must be at least one chiral center in the molecule for this to occur.

Encephalitis It is an inflammation of brain specially by viral infection. Meninges may also be infected. Herpes simplex virus type I is generally responsible. It often starts as a headache, fever and prostration. Later on hallucinations, confusion and paralysis of one side may take place. There is gradual loss of consciousness. Neck may become rigid. CT imaging will be useful. Acyclovir IV will prove effective for treatment.

Encephalization quotient (EQ) A measure of brain size obtained from the ratio of actual brain size to the expected brain size for an animal of a particular body size.

Encephalopathic syndrome A syndrome characterised by congenital rigidity of the extremities, uncontrollable sucking and grasping reflexes, and clouding of consciousness.

Encephalopathy Any of the metabolic toxic, neoplastic, or degenerative diseases of the brain.

Enchondroma Single tumors are common and are found mostly in hand within the medullary cavity

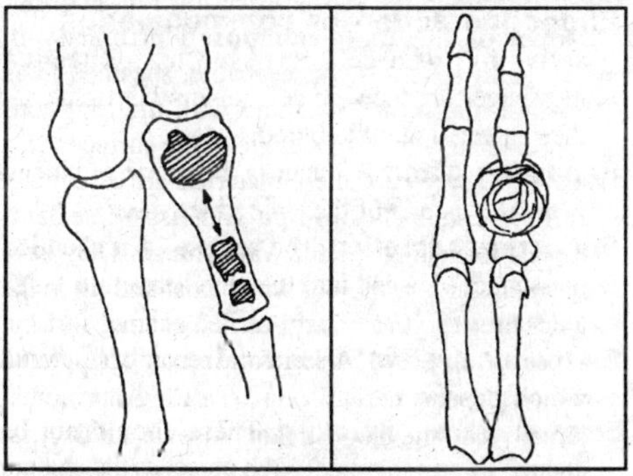

of phalanges. these are slow growing and there is no destruciton of cortex and no periosteal reaction is seen. Flecks of amorphous calcification may be seen in neoplastic tissue.

Encoding The process of preparing information in such a way that it can be readily stored and retrieved. An individual hearing the telephone number 235-1010 might encode it as 5,5, 10,10, remembering that the first of the two fives, a combination of two fives is a combination of two smaller numbers.

Encopresis Soiling in ones pant due to faulty toilet training.

Encounter group Meeting of individuals with trained leaders for the purpose of relating to one another in an affective manner, thereby achieving greater understanding of oneself and interpersonal relationships. Sometimes called T-groups.

End artery The terminal branch of an artery.

End bulbs hese are encapsulated, peripheral sensory receptors. Each one is about 50 mm in diameter and contains an axon which is branched and coiled. The bulbs of Krause are found in skin of the forearm.

Ruffini endings are found in deeper part of corium and joint capsule. Golgi-Mazzoni endings are found in corium. Genital corpuscles are found in glans penis and clitoris. Articular corpuscles are found in joint capsules.

End corn A hyperkeratotic area seen on tip of toe just plantar to the end of nail.

End foot The terminal part of an axon that conveys information to other neurons; also called terminal button.

End plate On a muscle, the receptorion complex that is activated by the release of the neurotransmitter acetylcholine from the terminal of a motor neuron.

End to end anastomosis Direct anastomosis of the two remaining segments of artery is used.

Endemic Describing a disease or condition that occurs constantly over an extended period of time in a given population or geographic area describing a pathogen that is native to the environment in which its host occurs.

Endemic disease Disease that is occurring regularly in a defined population.

Endemiology The field of study dealing with the occurrence of endemic diseases.

Enderine It is a polychlorinated hydrocarbon used as an insecticide.

It has bitter taste and is insoluble in water. In acts against most insect pests used for cotton and sugar cane. Symptoms of poisoning include tremor, ataxia, convulsion and death occurs due to respiratory failure. Gastric lavage, purgatives and sedation are useful.

Endocardial biopsy A sample of the endomyocardium taken to determine myocardial rejection in cardiac transplant patients.

Endocardial cushions The epithelial outgrowths of the dorsal and ventral walls of the atrioventricular division of the heart tube.

Endocardial leads Electrical connection, usually of a pacemaker, attached to a innermost epithelial lining of the heart.

Endocardial viability ratio Ratio of diastolic pressure time index to tension time index.

Endocarditis It is the inflammation of endocardium chiefly involving the valve structure. It may be infective or non-infective. Infective may be due to bacteria and fungi. Non-infective may be systemic lupus erythematosus (SLE), rheumatic fever and postmyocardial. Left side of heart is affected in 80% cases. Clinical features include malaise, fatigue, arthralgia, anorexia, pain in loin, coma and convulsions. Petechial haemorrhages and Osler's nodes are present.

Endocardium The layer of the heart wall, composed of endothelium and smooth muscle, that lines the inside of the heart and covers the valves and tendons that hold the valves open.

Endocervical polyp Under the influence of oestrogen, the endometrial or endocervical glands hypertrophy until the tissue is thick and polypoidal.

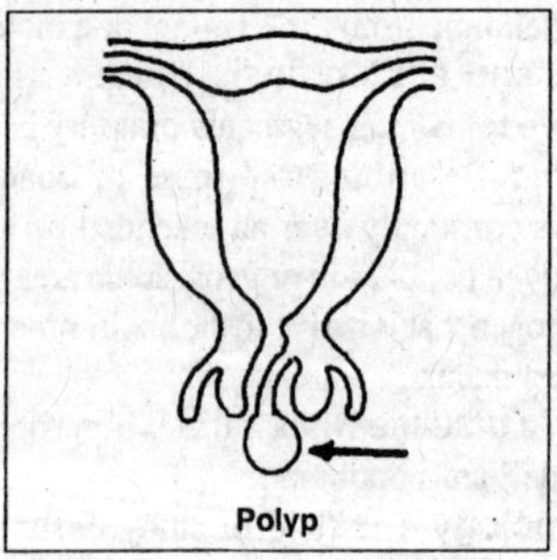

Polyp

These polyps usually develop stalks and protrude out through the cervical os. Majority are less than 0.5 cm in size. These cause abnormal bleeding, menorrhagia or postcoital bleeding. Treatment includes twist and cauterisation.

Endocervical smear Mostly it is taken for a Pap smear by inserting an endocervical brush, the longer serrated edge of a spatula or a cotton swab

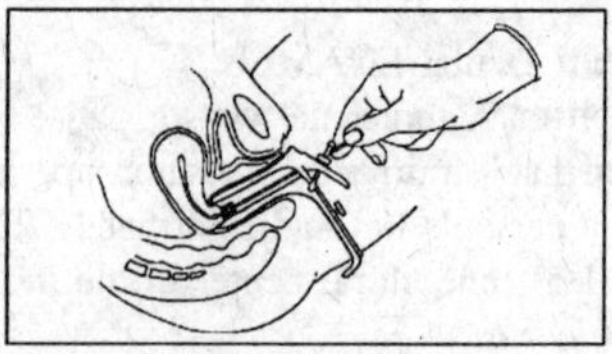

or a cotton swab about 1/8 inch into the cervical os and rotating the instrument 360 degrees clockwise. Then smear the specimen onto a glass tube. Spray the slide with cytological fixative agent immediately.

Endocervix The membrane lining the canal of the cervix; the region of the opening of the cervix into the uterine cavity.

Endochondral bone Bones that develop as hyaline cartilage models first and are then ossified.

Endochondral growth Growth of cartilage, which is then replaced by bone.

Endochondral ossification The process in which most bones are formed from cartilage models.

Endocrine Ductless gland that secretes internally, usually into the circulatory system.

These emit their hormone secretions directly into blood stream while exocrine glands use ducts to convey their secretions to particular site. Endocrine glands include pituitary, adrenal, thyroid and parathyroid glands and gonads.

Endocrine action or communication The activation of a cell or tissue by a chemical messenger produced in cells of another tissue and then secreted into the blood.

Endocrine gland A ductless, hormone-producing gland that is part of the endocrine system.

Endocrine secretion The release of a chemical messenger by a cell into the bloodstream to act on a distant site.

Endocrine system A series of interlocking glands which deposit their products, called hormones, directly into the bloodstream. Also called ductless glands.

Endocrinology The discipline in which hormones are studied.

Endocytosis The uptake into a cell of large molecules and particles in which a segment of plasma membrane surrounds the substance encloses it, and brings it in; includes phagocytosis, pinocytosis, and receptormediated endocytosis.

Endoderm The inner of three layers of cells during early embryonic development; the embryonic tissue type from which digestive and respiratory epithelial tissues differentiate.

Endodontia The division of dental science that deals with etiology, diagnosis, and treatment of diseases of dental pulp and their sequelae.

Endodontic file Small metal hand instrument with tightly spiraled blades used to clean and shape a root canal.

Endodontic instrument When an instrument is used with a complete rotating action in a canal with apical curvature instead of round shape a gouged cavity will be created.

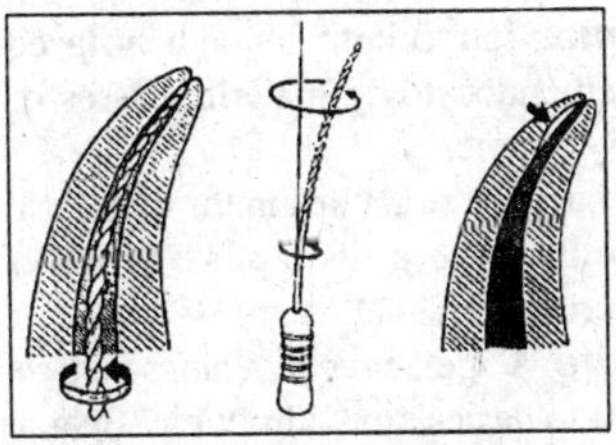

Endodontics The branch of dentistry concerned with the prevention, diagnosis, and treatment of diseases that affect the pulp. root, periodontal ligament, and alveolar bone.

Endodontist A dentist who specializes in or limits his practice to endodontics.

Endodontoma Tooth resorption, internal;

Endodyogeny A process by which tachyzoites and bradyzoites divide involving creation of two daughter cells wholly within a mother cell.

Endoflifecare Care given to a terminally ill client.

Endogenous Denoting a product or process arising from within the body as opposed to exogenous products or influences from external sources.

Endogenous infection An infection caused by microbes from the hosts own flora.

Endogenous ochronosis The condition is associated with alkaptonuria. Greyish-brownish discolourations can be seen in sclera and symmetrically oil droplets brownish superficial corneal dots lie closely to limbus.

Endogenous opioid peptides Peptides released both with the brain and from pituitary cells that inhibit binding of morphine like compounds to receptors.

Endogenous opioids Naturally produced morphine-like chemicals.

Endogenous rhythms Biological processes ulitmately controlled from within the organism by some kind of physiological time keeping mechanism i.e. biological clock.

Endogenous selection Natural selection that acts against genotypes regardless of the environment.

Endognathion The inner segment of the incisive bone.

Endolithotrophic Describing organisms living inside rocks, as some fungi.

Endolymph A fluid within the membranous labyrinth and cochlear duct of the inner ear that aids in the conduction of vibrations involved in hearing and the maintenance of equilibrium.

Endomastoiditis Inflammation within the mastoid cavity and cells.

Endometrial biopsy It is done in later half of menstrual cycle, at about 21st or 22nd day. It helps to evaluate corpus luteum and to determine

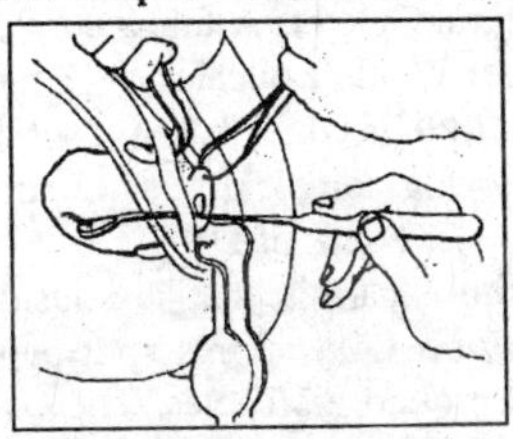

whether or not patient is ovulating by the presence or absence of secretory endometrium. It may also know about malignancy.

Endometrial biopsy curette This is a blunt hollow instrument. It has got a notch with cutting edge near the blunt tip, 5 cm earlier to end there is a slight angulation. This has a stylet for removing the biopsied tissue. Endometrial biopsy is done after giving cervical block. A specimen of cervical canal or the endometrium is then obtained using the curette.

Endometrioma of umbilicus It is a pathological condition, where there is presence of ectopic endometrial glands in the umbilicus It occurs in women between 20 and 45 years of age. Umbilicus becomes painful and bleeds at each menstruation. There is a small fleshy mass at the umbilicus. There may be an associated endometrioma in uterus or ovary. When single umbilectomy will cure the condition.

Endometriosis It is most common between the age of 25 and 40 and may result in infertility. The exact cause is unknown. But during menses, all of the endometrium is not shed out and may adhere and grow on any of the pelvic organ.There may be heavy menstrual bleeding. There will be pain in abdomen and lower back during menses and pain during intercourse. As a treatment contraceptive pills may be useful.

Endometrium Mucous membrane comprising the inner layer of the uterine wall; consists of a simple columnar epithelium and a lamina propria that contains simple tubular uterine glands.

Endomysium The connective tissue sheath that surrounds each skeletal muscle fiber, separating the muscle cells from one another.

Endoneurine The thin wrapping of fibrous connective tissue that surrounds each axon in a nerve.

Endoneurium The connective tissue sheath that surrounds each nerve fiber, separating the nerve fibers one from another within a nerve.

Endonuclear Within a nucleus.

Endonucleases Enzymes that have specific binding sites of varying complexity at which they break phosphodiester bonds of DNA.

Endoparasite A parasite that lives inside the host.

Endopeptidase Enzyme that split peptide bonds inside the protein molecules. These are pepsin, trypsin and chymotrypsin.

Endophlebitis Inflammation of the intima of a vein.

Endoplasmic reticulum A cytoplasmic organelle composed of a network of canals running through the cytoplasm of a cell.

Endoplasmic reticulum Membranous network inside the cytoplasm; rough endoplasmic reticulum has ribosomes attached to the surface; smooth endoplasmic reticulum does not have ribosomes attached.

Endoprosthesis An artificial internal body part that is surgically implanted.

End-organ One of the larger, encapsulated endings of the sensory nerves.

Endorphin A naturally produced chemical with morphine-like action; usually found in the brain and associated with the relief of pain. May be the body's own protection against pain. Chemical in central nervous system that influences pain perception; a natural painkiller.

Endoscope It is an instrument for looking inside the body. Mostly used nowadays is fibreoptics and consists of a long tube which when inserted through a body orifice or small surgical incision connected to a binocular eyepiece or camera. Some may have attachment for biopsy and diathermy.

Endoscopic ultrasonography It is performed via an ultrasound probe mounted at the tip of an endoscope.

Newer versions have high frequency (7.5-12 MHz) linear array transducer incorporated into tip of fibreoptic endoscope.

Endoscopy An operative procedure in which a fiberoptic camera is used to visualize any potential body cavity.

Endosomes Intracellular smooth surfaced vesicles in which endocytosed material passes on its way to the lysosome.

Small, bag-like structures in the cytoplasm of cells that are involved in the uptake of material from the exterior of the cell.

Endospore A metabolically quiescent cell that is resistant to desiccation, ultraviolet light, and other environmental insults; formed by certain genera of bacteria including bacillus and clostridium.

Endosseous implant An implant placed directly within the maxilla or mandible.

Endosteum The membrane that lines the medullary (marrow) cavity of bones, consisting of osteoprogenitor cells and scattered osteoclasts.

Endosymbiosis The condition of an organism living inside a member of a different species.

Endosteum The membranous layer of connective tissue that lines the medullary cavity.

Endothelial cell A cell that forms blood vessels.

Endothelin Vasoconstrictor peptide derived from vascular endothelium regulating the vascular tone and B.P.

Endothelium It covers surfaces not communicating with the atmosphere. The cells are connected with one another by intercellular protoplasmic bridges. It is distributed as lining of interior of heart, blood vessels and lymphatics.

It lines the cavities of serous membranes as pleura, pericardium, peritoneum and dura. It lines the cavities which surrounds the joints and bursae. As regards its functions, it provides smooth and moist surface. In kidneys, it allows blood plasma to be filtered. In capillaries it allow passage of gas and nourishment and waste materials in and out of vessels.

Endotherm Animal e.g., mammals, birds that has a high and relatively constant body temperature produced by internal heat production and relatively unaffected by changes in the ambient temperature.

Endothermic Having body temperature determined by heat energy generated internally.

Endotonic implant It is a metallic implant extending through root canal into periapical bone to increase support and retention of teeth.

Endotoxins These are derived from structural component of microorganism. Typical endotoxins are associated with gram- negative bacteria. Endotoxins are antigenic but poor antigens as compared to exotoxins. They are toxic but much less potent and less specific in their cytotoxic effect than exotoxins. Lipid fraction is mainly responsible for their toxicity. Endotoxin shock also occurs as a fatal, terminal condition in gram-negative infection in man.

Endotracheal Within the trachea.

Endotracheal goitre This is not a true neoplasm but a dystopic lesion that is associated with thyroid gland and is involved by changes in the gland. Usual site involved is posterior wall of upper trachea.

Endotracheal intubation The insertion of a tube into the trachea to be used to administer

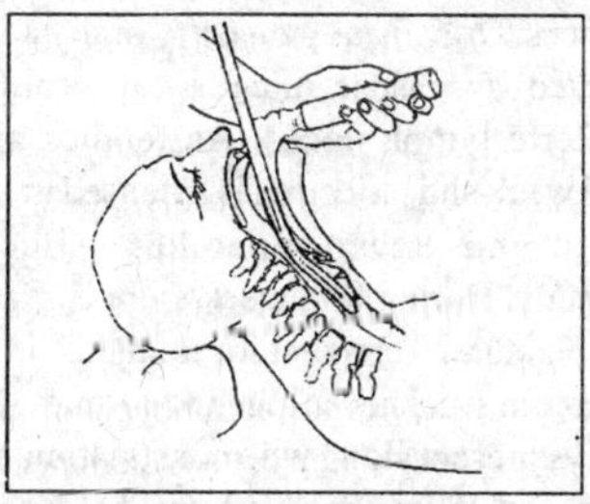

anaesthesia, maintain an airway, or ventilate the lungs.

Endotracheal tube A flexible, hollow cylinder inserted nasally or orally into the trachea to provide an airway.

These maintain an airway in those who are unconscious or unable to ventilate at their own. Tube is inserted by a physician. It is generally

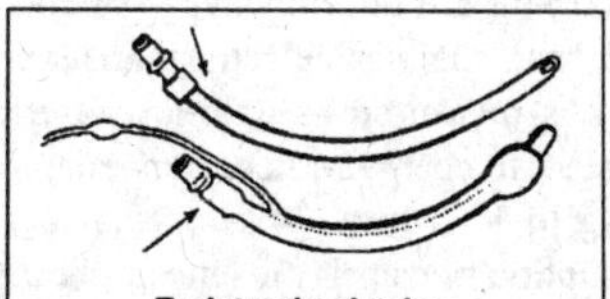

Endotracheal tubes

removed after 48 to 72 hours. If required for longer time then tracheostomy should be done.

Endotrophic Obtaining nutrients from an internal source; e.g., certain parasitic plant fungi living inside the plant root.

End-stage renal disease Any condition that impairs the function of the kidneys to such an extent that the patient exhibits kidney failure, hypertension, excessive glomerular permeability to proteins, and others specific tubular abnormalities.

Endurance training Continuous vigorous exercise requiring the body to increase its consumption of oxygen and developing the muscles; ability to sustain activity over a prolonged period of time.

Enema It is the introduction of fluid into rectum either to empty lower bowel or to introduce a

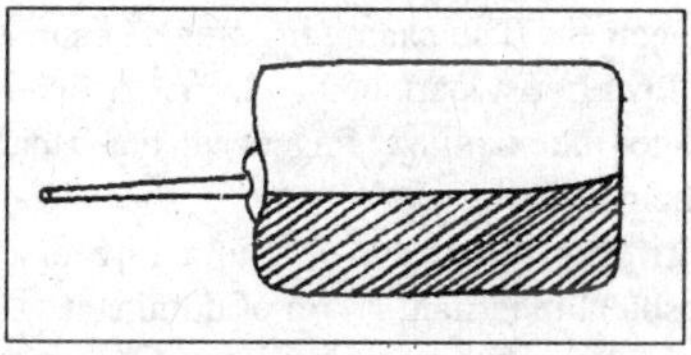

medicinal substance for its general or local effect or for diagnostic purpose. For emptying purpose, soap solution enema is given. For diagnostic enema barium is used. Cold enema is given to reduce temperature. Sedative enema is given to quieten patient while starch or opium enema is for soothing of irritated mucosa of colon. Carminative enema is used to relieve gaseous distension, starch to check diarrhoea, hypertonic enema to destroy parasites and oxytocic enema to stimulate uterine contraction and labour.

Energized family A family unit that responds to the needs and interests of all members, while coping effectively with life transitions and problems. An energized family is flexible, has an equal distribution of power, and has a health-promoting lifestyle.

Energy There are different types of energy, light, sound, heat, chemical, electrical and kinetic. Food energy is measured as calories. One calorie is equivalent to energy to raise temperature of water of 1 kg to 1°C, from 14.5 to 15.5°C. Excessive consumption of calories results in obesity. Energy is needed to keep the heart beating and lungs functioning and to keep body temperature maintained. This minimum requirement of calories without body activity is known as basic metabolic rate (BMR). It is about 1700 calories in young adult depending on body surface.

Energy coupling The transfer of energy from one process to another.

Energy spilling A term for the process microorganisms used to dissipate excess energy.

En-face Position that allows eye to eye contact.

Engagement 1. In clinical obstetrics, applies to the entrance of the presenting part into the superior pelvic strait and the beginning of the descent through the pelvic canal. 2. Also relating to parent-infant interaction: behaviours designed to induce and sustain social changes.

Engagement of head When the biparietal plane of the fetus has passed through the pelvic inlet as in engagement. The examining fingers cannot get to the lowermost part of head. When head is not engaged the examining fingers will reach the bottom of the presenting part.

Engelmann syndrome It is a rare disease of autosomal inheritant group of dominant variety. It is known as diphyseal dysplasia. Clinically, there will be diminished muscle mass, leg pain and muscle weakness. There will be delayed walking and delayed dentition. Deafness and hypogonadism may be noted with exophthalmos.

Engineering In implant dentistry, the planning or function of abutment support in terms of strength, number, and positioning, influencing long-term function of a prosthesis within physiological limits of health.

Engorgement Hyperemia; local congestion; excessive fullness of any organ or passage. In obstetrics, refers to an exaggeration of normal venous and lymph stasis of the breasts, which is caused by increased amounts of milk in the lobules and ducts and circulating blood and lymph in the mammary glands.

Engorgement of breast This commonly occurs between third and fifth day after childbirth. Venous and lymphatic oedema are common. Milk ejection is inhibited. Cold compression helps the patient.

Engram A memory trace; a neurophysiologic process that accounts for persistence of memory

Enhancer A region of genomic DNA, more distant upstream or downstream than the promoter sequence, that up-regulate expression of a gene

Enkephalin Peptide chemical in the central nervous system that acts as a natural painkiller.

Enmeshment The close emotional involvement of two or more people.

Enostosis A dense bony focus inside a bone composed of lamellar bone.

Enriched A food may be labelled enriched if it contains added nutrients in kinds and amounts meeting standards.

Enrichment Returning nutrients that were lost because of processing to their original levels

Enteral feeding Nutrients supplied to the gastro intestinal tract orally or by feeding tube.

Enteral nutrition Administration of nurishment via the gastrointestinal tract.

Enteric The term referring to the small intestine.

Enteric coated Tablets coated with a substance that does not dissolve until reachhing the intestime. Used when drug constituents are irritating to oral and gastric mucosa.

Enteric fever It is caused by *Salmonella typhi* and *paratyphi*. Infection spreads by food, flies, fingers and faeces. Organisms gain entry orally and are not destroyed by gastric juice. They proliferate in mesenteric lymph nodes. Antibodies appear in second week and, infection is localised in liver, gall bladder and Peyer's patches. Ulcers heal completely. During first week there is gradual rise of temperature. Temperature is higher in evening than morning and never touches normal. Headache is always present along with constipation, lassitude and malaise. Pulse shows relative bradycardia and dicortism. Tongue is always coated with red margins and clean tip. Abdomen is tumid, caecal gurgling is present due to fluid, faeces and gas. Spleen is soft and palpable. Rashes may develop at the end of first week. During second week continuous fever is there. Headache disappears and patient becomes mentally dull, weak and stuprose. Constipation is replaced by looseness of bowel. Cough may persist. Pulse shows tachycardia. Tongue is dry and coated. Spleen is 4 to 5 cm enlarged while liver may be just palpable. There may be muttering delirium. In third week temperature comes down and become delirious. Patient becomes dull.

Enteric microorganism A microorganism that replicates in the intestinal tract of humans and other warmblooded animals and is shed in fecal material.

Enteric-coated tablet Tablet covered with a substance that does not dissolve until it has passed the stomach.

Enteritis Any disease of intestine.

Enterobacteriaceae a family of the Gamma-Proteobacteria that includes Escherichia coli and related gram negative bacteria.

Enteroception Refers to stimuli transduced within the alimentary tract.

Enterocytoma It is a pathological condition arising from the patent central portion of the vitello-intestinal duct. It gives rise to intra-abdominal cyst. Through a band it is fixed to the umbilicus and to small intestine. Patient presents with a small, spherical, mobile swelling deep to the umbilicus. Treatment includes excision of cyst along with band.

Enterogastric reflex A reflex that inhibits gastric secretion; initiated by food in the small intestine.

Enterohemorrhagic Acting as an intestinal pathogen.

Enterokinase An ingredient of intestinal juice which activates the trypsinogen and chymotrypsinogen of pancreatic juice to form trypsin and chymotrypsin, the active enzyme.

Enteropathy Any disease of intestine.

Enterotoxin An organism or substance able to induce damage to the intesitine, generally leading to fluid accumulation.

Enterovirus One of a group of viruses infecting the intestinal tract.

Enthesis The site of attachment of a tendon or ligament into the periosteum of bone.

Enthesitis Inflammation resulting from stress on muscle or tendon attached to bone.

Entoleter Machine used to disinfest cereals and other foods.

Entorhinal Refers to entorhinal cortex of the temporal lobe.

Entorhinal cortex Located on the medial surface of the temporal lobe, the entorhinal cortex provides a major route for neocortical input to the hippocampal formation; often degenerates in Alzheimer's disease.

Entrain The make one even take place within the same period as another event takes place. Literally, to get on a train.

Entrainment The coordination of movements or their synchronization to a rhythm.

Entrapment Pathologic pressure placed on a nerve or vessel by soft tissue.

Entrapment neuropathy (carpal tunnel syndrome) Classical symptoms include nocturnal awakening by painful paraesthesia in affected hand. Tingling will be in lateral three and half digits. Patients try to get relief by shaking his or her hand or by hanging it down out of bed. Affected woman has carpal tunnels of smaller cross-section. Some thickening of synovial sheath of tendon is seen in rheumatiod tenosynovitis.

Entropion clamp This clamp also has a plate on one side and a rim on the other side. There is a separate clamp for each eye. Different sizes are available to fit properly in the lid as the size of the lids varies with each person. In this the plate is towards the conjunctival side and the rim on the skin side. It also acts as a haemostat. The plate protects the underlying eye.

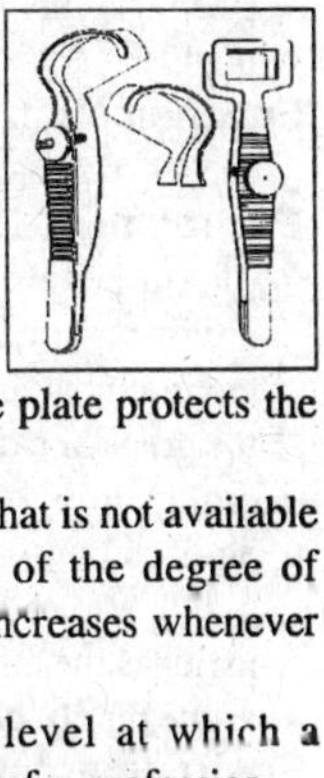

Entropy The energy of a system that is not available to perform work. A measure of the degree of disorder in a system, entropy increases whenever energy is transformed.

Entry level The educational level at which a practitioner enters the practice of a profession.

Enucleate To remove a lesion in its entirety.

Enucleation Removal of the eyeball, performed in cases of malignancy,server infection, extensive trauma, or to control pain in glaucoma.

Enucleation scissors It is used to cut the optic nerve in the surgery of enucleation. Along with the optic nerve other structures cut are central retinal artery and vein, short and long posterior ciliary arteries and nerves. In cases of retinoblastoma, the nerve should be cut at least

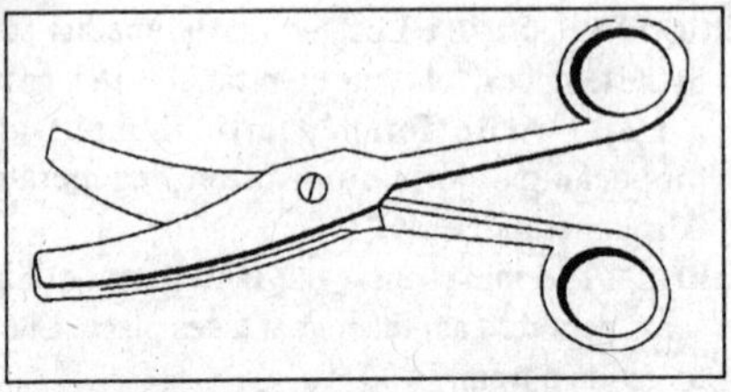

1.5 cm behind the sclera so that later histopathology performed on the nerve may indicate any extraocular extension if any.

Enuresis Some children lose control and empty the bladder and wet the bed. When bed wetting occurs frequently it is known as enuresis. In primary enuresis there is delay in maturation of neurological control of sphincter and children are never dry at night. There is mental subnormality. In secondary enuresis causative factor is emotional disturbance and child-parent maladjustment. Patient may apprehend parents. These children sleep very soundly and may be difficult to arouse them. The signals of distended bladder to empty the bladder do not reach to conscious level of their mind during sleep and this may cause involuntary emptying of bladder.

Envenomation Injection of venom by an animal snakes, scorpions into human body.

Environment Everything which surrounds the units of inheritance. There is the intracellular environment, within the cell, the intercellular environment, involving the effect of cell upon cell, the prenatal external environment, surrounding the embryonic or fetal organism: the internal environment, within the organism, such as the blood, and the external environment, and which includes the social or cultural environment as well as the purely physical environment.

Environmental hazards Potentially dangerous conditions in the physical surroundings.

Environmental psychologists Specialists who study how the environment affects behavior.

Environmental psychology The area psychology dealing with the relationships between the physical environment and psychological processes. These psychologists attempt to design environments most appropriate to human activities.

Enzootic disease Disease that is occurring regularly in animal populaitons.

Enzyme An organic compound, frequently protein in nature, that can accelerate or produce by catalytic action some change in a specific substance. It is a protein that regulates the rate of a chemical reaction in the body. Every cell in the body produces some or other enzyme reflecting their specific activity. Pancreas produces digestive enzyme lipase, protease and anylase. Many inherited metabolic disorders, G6PD deficiency are caused by defects of specific enzymes. Lack of streptokinase may lead to coronary thrombosis. Many drugs inhibit or block enzyme and some antibiotics destroy bacteria by blocking bacterial enzymes. Some anticancer drugs act by blocking some of enzyme.

Enzyme induction Synthesis of new enzyme protein in response to some stimulus such as hormone or substrate.

Enzyme repression Reduction in synthesis of enzyme protein in response to some stimulus such as hormone.

Eosimophilia-myalgia sysdrome A syndrome of muscle pain and hypereosinophilia caused by a contaminant in one commercially prepared brand of the amino acid L-tryptophan.

Eosin An acidic dye used a counterstain in histology.

Eosinophil A type of white blood cell characterized by the presence of cytoplasmic granules that become stained by acidic eosin dye. Eosinophils normally constiture about 2% to 4% of the white blood cells.

Eosinophilia granuloma Headache is generally diffuse and unilateral. There develops flat or crater-like retracted tumour with a tense consistency. Tender cerebral deficiency also occurs. Multifocal lesions are common affecting numerous bones.

Eosinophilic gastritis Thickening is mainly in antrum. There is mucosal oedema and eosinophilic infiltration and this extends to the small bowel. The presentation with nausea, vomiting and pain together with antral thickening is seen on X-ray.

Eosinophilic gastroenteropathy There are large numbers of eosinophils infiltrating part or all of gastrointestinal tract. Known causes are parasites, eosinophilic leukaemia and lymphomas. Clinical features are diarrhoea and abdominal pain. There is usually blood eosinophilia. Extensive mucosal infiltration with eosinophils is associated with malabsorption syndrome. GIT bleeding is rare and wall of intestine is severely thickened. Intestinal obstruction may be there. If serosa is infiltrated ascites can occur.

EPA Environmental protection Agency.

Ependymal The neuroglial cell layer lining the ventricles of the brain.

Ependymal cell A glial cell, found on the walls of the ventricles of the brain, that makes and secretes cerebral spinal fluid.

Neuroglial cells that cover choroid plexuses and produce cerebrospinal fluid they also line the ventricles of the brain and probably assist in the circulation of CSF.

Ephebodontics Dentistry for the individual undergoing the transition from childhood to adulthood; that is, the period of life known as adolescence.

Ephedrine It delays the destruction of adrenaline to maintain a high blood catecholamine level. It releases stored noradrenaline from nerve endings in the vessel walls. It is a potent sympathetic stimulant. The rate and force of cardiac contraction are increased and blood pressure raised. Arterioles are constricted. Duration of effect is 30 to 40 minutes. It dilates pupil. It can be used in state of hypotension, bronchospasm, heart block, carotid sinus syndrome, urticaria, enuresis and myasthenia.

Ephelis It is circumscribed macular collection of pigment in epidermis or oral mucosa. Increased amount of melanin pigment in the region of basal layer of cell.

Epiblast The outer layer of the blastoderm, which will later segregate into ectoderm and mesoderm.

Epicanthus Epicanthus appears as a semilunar fold of skin extending from the foot of nose to the inner end of lower eyelid. The concavity of fold is toward the eye and it tends to conceal the inner canthus and carbuncle. It is characteristic of Mongolian race. Fold may exist in fetal life and it may disappear with the development of bridge.

Epicardial lead Electrical connection, usually of a pacemaker, attached to the innermost epithelial lining of the heart.

Epicardium The outermost layer of the heart ; the visceral layer of the pericardium; formed from the outer layer of the myoepicardial mantle.

Epicondyle Projection on (usually to the side of) a condyle.

Epidemic The occurrence in a community or region of a group of illnesses of similar nature, clearly in excess of normal expectancy and derived from a common source.

Epidemic threshold The necessary degree of variation from usual patterns required for a disease to qualify as an outbreak.

Epidemiological transition The changing pattern of most prevalent diseases from infections to chronic degenerative disease.

Epidemiology The science that is concerned with health events in human populations.

Epidermal growth factor (EGF) A neurotrophic factor that acts to stimulate mitosis in stem cells.

Epidermal naevus It is also known as hard naevus. There is hyperplasia of epidermis specially in stratum corneum. Lesions do not show any presence of naevus cells. These are elevated, sharply demarcated, hard, rough surfaced papules or nodules. Lesions are localised and generally distributed unilaterally. These are hairless and are symptomless. These may resemble like acne known as acneform naevus. Application of electrocoagulation or cryosurgery helps.

Epidermis Outer portion of the skin formed of epithelial tissue that rests on the dermis; resists abrasion and forms a permeability barrier.

Epidermoid carcinoma It is a malignant tumour arising from squamous cells. In the case of skin, it is the prickle cell layer from where squamous cell carcinoma arises. Occasionally it may arise from the columnar cells undergoing metaplasia, e.g. gall bladder, bronchus, and cardiac end of stomach. Any part of skin and its appendages in face, dorsum of hands, palms and soles may be affected. These are of two types, ulcerative and proliferative.

Epidermolysis bullosa It is a rare, inherited, mechanobullous disorder occurring at birth. Epidermolysis bullous simplex is the benign and simple type presenting with vesicle, bullae and epidermal cysts involving skin surface only. Lesions are sparce while epidermolysis bullosa junctional is an uncommon but lethal conditon. It presents with severe blistering all over body without scarring, while epidermolysis bullosa dystrophica is the severe form which is characterised by blister formation which may be haemorrhagic followed by scarring. No effective therapy is available.

Epididymal Relating to or involving the epididymis.

Epididymal sperm Mature or immature sperm contained within the epididymal canal.

Epididymoorchitis Inflammation of the testis and epididymis, representing usually a complication of a sexually transmitted disease, such as gonorrhea or syphilis.

Epidural anaesthesia Anaesthesia produced by injecting between the vertebral spines and beneath the ligamentum flavum into the extradural space. It is used in obstetric anaesthesia to alleviate maternal pain with minimal danger to the infant. It requires the expertise that is afforded to a surgical patient.

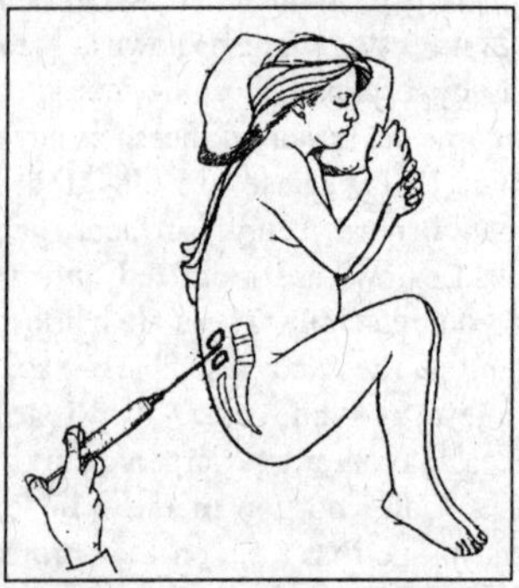

Epidural block It provides the most effective relief in labour but it requires professional skill.

Epidural haematoma Thick bone covering of skull is the first line of defence against injuries but on occasions skull fracture tears the middle meningeal artery which lies between skull and dural sac. The ruptured artery pours blood, which collects in a large pool. Pooling of blood is called haematoma. Epidural haematoma is a serious condition. Vomiting, pulse slowing make person unconscious. Even during lucid interval person will be confused. CT scan helps in diagnosis.

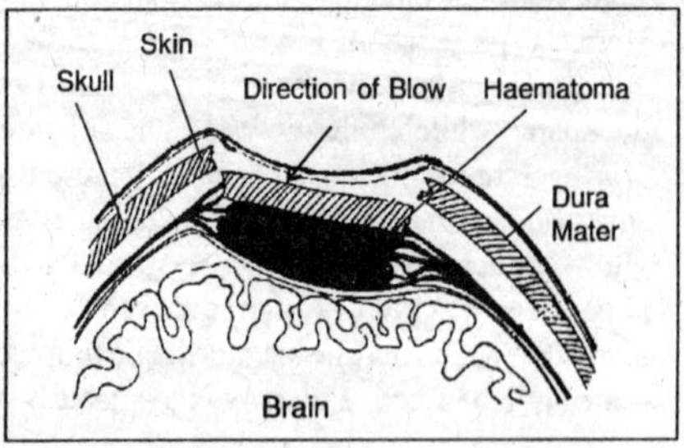

Epidural space A space between the spinal dura mater and the bone of the vertebral canal.

Epigastric pain in toxemia It occurs due to stretching of capsule of liver by hemorrhage and acute liver pathology. Increasing SGOT provides a poor diagnosis.

Epigenetic Describing gene activity that produces phenotypic but not genotypic change.

Epiglottis Cartilage in the throat which guards the enterance to the trachea. It prevents food and fluid from entering it and lungs when a person swallows. A leaflike structure positioned on top of the larynx. It covers the glottis during swallowing. Plate of elastic cartilage, covered with mucous membrane, that serves as a valve over the opening of the larynx during swallowing to prevent materials from entering the larynx.

Epilepsy It is a seizure caused by abnormal electrical activity in brain. It is a symptom of brain dysfunction. Seizure may occur due to head injury, birth trauma, brain infection, tumour and stroke. It is classified into two generalised and partial seizures. *Generalised seizures* cause loss of consciousness, affect the whole body while temporal lobe epilepsy is a type of partial seizure. It is caused by damage to a limited area of brain. Generalised epilepsy has been classifed into two types : *Grand mal* seizure results into unconsciousness, entire body stiffens and jerks uncontrollably. There may be cry, breathing becomes irregular. Muscles relax and control over bowel and bladder is lost. Prolonged seizures may be proved fatal. *Petit mal* seizures cause momentary loss of consciousness without abnormal movements. These generally develop in children. There is blank period from seconds to minutes. It is like a day dreaming. *Partial* seizures are divided into simple seizures in which consciousness is maintained and complex seizures where consciousness is lost. In simple seizure there will be tingling sensations or hallucination of smell and vision.

During complex partial seizures person becomes dazed and may not respond if addressed. EEG and CT scan or MRI may be helpful. Anticonvulsant drugs are the main line of treatment. Such drugs have side effects of drowsiness and impaired concentration.

Epileptic insanity It is characterised by transitory fits of mania followed by recovery. The attacks recur more and more frequently. There is laxity of morals, hallucinations, loss of memory and sexual excesses. True epileptic fits are always accompanied by fits.

Epimastigote In this kinetoplast, basal body complex is situated more posteriorly but anterior to nucleus.

Epimerases Enzymes that catalyze the reversible interconversion of two epimers.

Epimural Describing bacteria attached to the epithelial cells lining the gut.

Epimysium The fibrous connective tissue layer surrounding a skeletal muscle.

Epinephrine Hormone secreted by the adrenal medulla that stimulates hepatic glycogenolysis, causing an elevation in the blood sugar, vasodilation of blood vessels of the skeletal muscles, vasoconstriction of the arterioles of the skin and muscles, and stimulation of heart action. Used as local anesthetics for its vasoconstrictive action.

Epineruium The outer layer of a sheath which surrounds and holds together nerve trunks, composed of connective tissue and collagenous fibers.

Epiphora It is a passive process in which though the secretion of tear fluid is normal, yet the lacrimal drainage system is not able to drain the tear fluid resulting in overflow of tear fluid. It can occur in dacrocystitis—acute and chronic, eversion of lower punctum and occlusion of canaliculi.

Epiphyseal fracture When the epiphyseal plate is separated from the epiphysis or diaphysis; this type of fracture can disrupt the normal growth of the bone.

Epiphyseal line Dense place of bone in a bone that is no longer growing, indicating the former site of the epiphyseal plate.

Epiphyseal plate A hyaline cartilaginous layer located between the epiphysis and diaphysis of a long bone. It functions as a longitudinal growing region.

Epiphyseal scar A radiodense line present at the ends of mature long bone.

Epiphyseal stapling A surgical technique for the correction of a limb length discrepency.

Epiphysis The end segment of a long bone, separated from the diaphysis early in life by an epiphyseal plate but later becoming part of the larger bone.

Epiploic appendage One of a number of little, fat-filled processes of peritoneum projecting from the serous coat of the large intestine.

Episcleritis It is an inflammation of superficial scleral lamellae and deep subconjunctival tissue. It is more common in elderly females. It is an allergic reaction to an endogenous toxin from any septic focus of body. Most of the cases suffer rheumatoid arthritis. It is a collagenous disease. There is localised redness of sclera with little or no pain. Localised swelling is tender to touch. There will be localised congestion around the nodule. Localised congestion results due to involvement of deeper scleral vessels. Congestion appears purple. Similarly one or more small nodules of dense leucocyte infiltration are seen near limbus. Conjunctiva moves freely over nodules. If not treated well may result in scleritis.

Episiotomy It consists of an incision in the perineum in order to enlarge the vaginal introitus to provide enough room for the head or breech to escape more safely. It is done when there is delay in delivery and when head is distending the perineum. It may be done as part of forceps delivery and when there is a threat of perineal tear in normal delivery. Operation is done under usual aseptic and antiseptic condition. Anaesthesia is given by local infiltration.

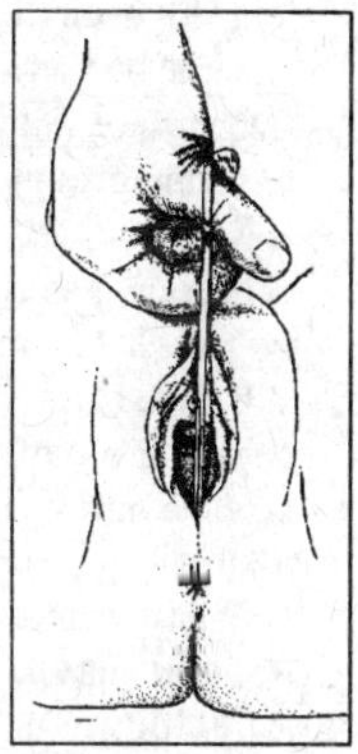

Episode A noteworthy happening occurring in the course of a continuous series of events.

Episodic memory A memory which occurs in the context of a particular episode, event, or experience. It pertains to a specific situation in one's life.

Episome An extrachromo-somal element in cells which can sometimes become associated with the chromosome.

Epispadias A congenital anomaly in which the urethra opens on the dorsal surface of the penis. In severe cases, the upper wall of the urethra may be absent.

Epistatic Describing differential genetic effect on phenotype in which an antibody can bind.

Epistaxis Nasal bleeding following trauma, excessive heat or hypertension. It is usually managed by packing.

Epithalamus It is made up of pineal body, habenular nuclei, stria medullaris thalami and epithelial roof of third ventricle.

Epithelia membrane Membrane composed of epithelial tissue with an underlying layer of specialized connective tissue.

Epithelial tissue Covers the body and its parts; lines various parts of the body; forms continuous sheets that contain no blood vessels; classified according to shape and arrangement.

Epithelialization The healing of a wound by growth from the epithelium.

Epithelise To cover or become covered with epithelium.

Epithelium It is a tissue composed entirely of cells joined together by minimal amount of cementing material and arranged as an expansion covering a free surface lining the interior of a hollow organ or forming solid masses.

It is not supplied with any blood vessels, except in endocrine glands. It is nourished by imbibition of lymph. It has minimal amount of intercellular substance. Its cell substance often undergoes chemical modifications and the whole cell may become horny or keratinised.

Epitope That part of an antigen recognized by antigen receptor.

Epizootic disease Disease outbreak in animals.

Eponychium The thin layer of stratum corneum of the epidermis of the skin that covers or lines all exposed body surfaces.

Epsoin salt Magnesium sulphate acting as purgative.

Epstein's pearls Small white cysts on the hard palate or gums of the newborn. They are not abnormal.

Epstein-Bar virus (EBV) infection Variety of neurological syndromes have been associated with (EBV) including aseptic meningitis, transverse myelitis, acute psychosis and an acute cerebellar ataxia.

Epuloid Resembling an epulis.

Epulosis Cicatrization.

Epulotic Pertaining to, characterized by, or promoting cicatrization.

Equianalgesic dose Oral dose that provides the same level of pain relief as a parenteral dose.

Equidae An animal family of the order perissodactyla. Members include horses, zebras, and mules.

Equilibrium State in which a body is at rest with neither translatory nor rotatory motion (static equilibrium), or in which a body is in constant motion with no acceleration or deceleration (dynamic equilibrium).

Equilibrium reactions Total body automatic responses that serve to maintain or regain balance during posture and movement.

Equity A historic term for courts dealing with situations where there was no specific legal remedy. Tending to disprove or excuse a charge of fault of guilt.

Equity theory In interpersonal relationships, the view that people develop and maintain a relationship when the gain is at least equal to what they feel they deserve.

For example, an extremely wealthy person and an extremely popular person may maintain a relationship because each is receiving from the other what he or she feels is deserved.

Equivalence The ratio of antibody to antigen at which immunoprecipitation of the reactants is virtually complete.

Erb phenomenon The finding of increased electric irritability of motor nerve in tetany.

Erb's paralysis Partial paralysis of the brachial plexus, affecting various muscles of the arm and the chest wall.

ERCP Endoscopic retrograde cholangiopancreatography is the method to evaluate biliary tree and pancreatic ducts.

ERCP is done with papillotomy as therapeutic intervention for biliary calculi. Diagnostic ERCP is indicated in jaundice.

Erectile Tumescence or engorgement of corporal bodies leading to elongation, widening and rigidity of penis.

Erectile dysfunction Failure to maintain an erection long enough for sexual intercourse. Also known as impotence.

Erection Engorgement of erectile tissue with blood such as in the erectile tissues of the penis causing the penis to enlarge and become firm.

Erector spinae Common name of the muscle group of the back; holds the back erect.

Erepsin Name given to mixture of enzymes contained in the intestinal juice.

Erg A unit of energy equal to a force of one dyne acting through a distane of 1 cm. It is equal to 2.4 X 10^{-8}.

Ergogenic aids Drugs and dietary regimens believed by some, but not proven, to increase strength, power, and endurance.

Ergometer A calibrated instrument used to accurately determine work load during an exercise challenge; commonly a treadmill or stationary bicycle.

Ergonomic load Physical causes of biomechanical strain induced by frequent or postural work demands.

Ergonomics Field of engineering science devoted to promoting comfort, performance, and health in the workplace.

Ergonovine stimulation A test of cardiac performance in which a pharmacologic stimulant is administered to the patient; ergonovine is an alkaloid of ergot used as a stimulant of smooth muscle.

Ergotamine Half-life is 2 hours. It constricts all peripheral arteries and not just those affected. Due to tissue binding it affects on arteries. Patients with vascular disease, coronary and peripheral are particularly at risk. It is extensively metabolised by liver. It may be given orally, sublingually or by inhalations. Total dose in acute attack should not increase 6 mg. Mild overdose causes nausea and vomiting. It is powerful oxytocic and is dangerous in pregnancy.

Erogenous zones These are different external areas of the body which are exceptionally sensitive to sexual stimulation, including breasts, buttock, thighs, ear lobules, area adjacent to sex organs, etc.

Erosion It is a loss of hard dental tissues along the gingival margins of teeth. The lesions are shaped like a dish, wedge or crescent. These generally develop on buccal surface and have sharp margins. These present hard, polished, shiny base. The cause of erosion is not known. Method of daily brushing may play a main role.

Hyperthyroidism, abnormal secretion from mucosal glands and discharge from gingival pockets may cause it. There is no known treatment for erosion.

Erotic Consciously or unconsciously invested with sexual feeling; sensually related. It is particular literature, plays, films, illustrations, painting and acts dealing with erotic themes which are capable of strongly stimulating sexual responses.

Eructation The process by which ruminants let fermentation gases escape from the rumen.

Eruption The act of breaking out, appearing or becoming visible; a visible pathologic lesion of the skin, marked by redness, swelling, or both.

Erysipelas It is an acute inflammatory condition of skin and of subcutaneous tissue. Group A Beta haemolytic *Streptococcus*, *Staphylococcus* and pneumococcus are causative factors. It produces acute inflammation with swelling of lymphatics of skin and presents with intense oedema, vascular dilatation and enlargement of lymphatics. In severe cases deeper tissues are involved with thrombosis, cellulitis and suppuration.

There may be itching or discomfort at the site of inoculation followed by formation of small area of erythema.

It spreads to form tense, sharply demarcated, glistening, tender, hot oedematous area with elevated margins, often on cheeks. The affected skin appears hot and firm. Local lymph glands are enlarged and painful. The condition however seldom causes any complication except lymphoedema. Antibiotics and analgesics become helpful.

Erysipeloid It is caused by gram-positive microaerophilic bacteria.

It is very common in fishermen, butcher and meat handlers.

It presents with erythema and less marginated swelling on fingers and back of hands. It slowly progresses to form sharply demarcated, purplish red coloured, indurated maculopapules which are raised but not vesiculated.

The affected area appears swollen and tender. Patient also complains of pain and itching and burning sensation. Burning condition is self-limiting but may lead to bacteraemia. Antibiotics are useful.

Erythema Patchy, circumscribed, or marginated macular redness of the skin or mucous membranes due to hyperemia or inflammation.

Erythema induratum It is a chronic, benign tuberculous vasculitis. It gives rise to indolent recurrent, bluish red, soft nodules distributed symmetrically.

The nodules usually persist for a few months, then tend to dry up and heal, and then recur. Later on skin becomes dusky or bluish in colour and nodule softens at the centre.

Ulcer has deep or undermined edges. Antituberculous treatment is to be given.

Erythema nodosum Erythema nodosum is an inflammatory reaction of dermis and subcutaneous tissue. Prior to development person may develop fever, malaise and bone pain.

This is followed by hot, red, painful tender, multiple nodule. The lesions tend to be distributed symmetrically and appear in crops.

The nodules vary in size from 1 to 10 cm in diameter. Nodules do not suppurate nor cause any ulceration. Lesion lasts about 6 weeks and resolve without scarring.

Erythema toxicum A blotchy rash that may appear in the first few days of life. It develops more frequently on the back, shoulders, and buttocks. No treatment is necessary and it will disappear in a day or so. It is also called "newborn rash."

Erythematous Of the nature of erythema.

Erythematous candidosis It is patchy red mucosal macules due to C albicans infection in HIV positive cases. Hard palate, dorsum of tongue and soft palate are favoured sites.

Erythralgia Redness and pain of the skin.

Erythrasma It is caused by gram-positive rods, *Corynebacterium minitissimum.*

It presents with well-demarcated dry, brown or reddish, slightly scaly patches. Lesions generally develop on moist areas of body such as toe webs. In groin it develops irregular and pink patches which later become brown with thin scales.

The lesions tend to show fissuring and slight maceration. Diagnosis is made from identification of causative organism from smear culture. Exposure to light causes coral red fluorescence of lesions.

Erythromycin is effective against lesion.

Erythremia Presence in the blood of excessive numbers of erythrocytes;

Erythroblastosis fetalis Hemolytic anemia in an Rh positive newborn caused by maternal antibodie against the Rh factor that have crossed the placenta.

Erythroblastosis fetalis A haemolytic anaemia of the fetus caused by the transplacental transfer of maternally formed Rh antibodies against an Rh-positive fetus.

Erythrocytes Red blood cells.

Erythromycin It binds to bacterial ribosomes and interferes with protein synthesis. It is bacteriostatic. It is effective against gram-positive organisms. It is useful against infection of upper respiratory tract specially in pertussis. Erythromycin is destroyed by the acid in stomach. Excretion is in bile and faeces. It is useful in patients who are allergic to penicillin. Effective dose is 250 mg 6 hourly. It may cause cholestatic jaundice with abdominal pain and fever. GIT disturbances are rare. Long use may affect liver.

Erythroplakia These are bright red velvety plaques on the oral mucosa. These are irregular in outline but well defined. There may be nodule formation and may have white or yellow spots on a red background. Microscopically, these show epithelial atrophy and varying degrees of epithelial dyskeratosis condition and is similar to leucoplakia.

Erythroplasia of Querat It appears as dark red, velvity and well marginated. It is flat or slightly raised indurated patch on glans penis or inner side of prepuce. If it develops ulcer and discharge is there, may become painful. It is similar to carcinoma *in situ*. Local excision of lesion is adequate.

Erythropoiesis Formation of red blood cells.

Erythropoietin Protein hormone that stimulates erythrocyte formation in red bone marrow.

The growth factor required for the generation of erythrocytes from the pleuripotential stem cell.

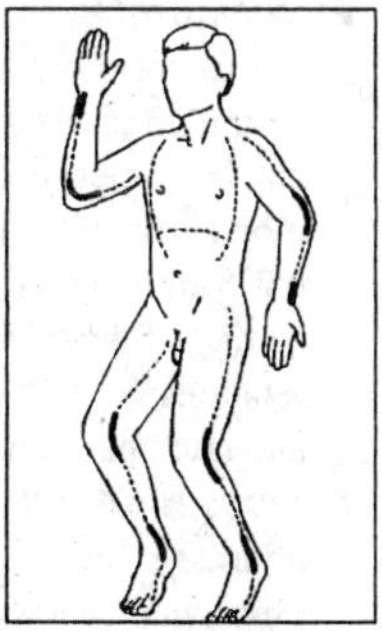

Eschar The thick, coagulated crust that forms after a chemical or thermal burn.

Escharotic Corrosive; capable of producing sloughing.

Escharotomy An incision made through the eschar.

Esherich's sign In tetany a muscular contraction of the lips that resembles a goat's snout.

ESO Abbreviation for electrospinal orthosis.

Esophageal stricture It may cause difficulty in swallowing. Most common cause is cancer. Reflux oesophagitis may also cause it. There will be pain while eating food, weight loss and regurgitation. Barium swallow examination and endoscopy will help in diagnosis.

Esophagogastroduodenescopy It is done in upper gastrointestinal bleeding, evaluation of healing of gastric ulcer, evaluation of stomach and duodenum after gastric surgery. It helps in finding out the cause of dysphagia, dyspepsia, gastric outlet obstruction or epigastric pain.

Esophagus A tubular portion of the GI tract that leads from the pharyns to the stomach as it passes through the thoracic cavity.

Espundia A disease caused by *Leishmania braziliensis,* also known as mucocutaneous leishmaniasis.

ESR It is the abbreviation for erythrocyte sedimentation rate. It is the rate at which red blood cells sink toward the bottom of a test tube. Whole blood from the patient is mixed with anticoagulant in a test tube and left undisturbed for one hour. The RBCs which can be seen as a dark red clump settle down leaving a clear fluid above. ESR is raised in pulmonary tuberculosis, gout, acute infections, acute myocardial infarction, anaemia and pregnancy.

ESR increases very rapidly in kala-azar, multiple myeloma, rheumatoid arthritis and haemolytic anemia. It decreases in polycythemia vera, CCF and dehydration.

Essential amino acids Protein components that must be obtained from food beacuse they cannot be synthesized by the body.

Essential fat Certain components of body fat that are essential for life.

Essential fatty acids The group of polyunsaturated fatty acids produced by plants; but not by humans; required in the human diet.

Essential nutrients Nutrients that cannot be made by the human body and must be provided by foods.

Essential organs Reproductive organs that must be present for reproduction to occur and are known as gonads.

Essential touch Vital, fundamental, and primary touch that is crucial to well-being.

Essentialism Reducing the cause of a characteristic or behavior to one cause. Biologic essentialism explains everything as a product of genes or blood.

Established uraemia There develops considerable biochemical changes along with toxaemia. There is retention of nitrogenous bodies causing respiratory symptoms; rising of blood phosphate and lowering of calcium product neuromuscular irritability. Excessive loss of potassium takes place. Even may cause weakness and paralysis. Cerebral oedema, vascular spasm or occlusion produce convulsions, headache and drowsiness. The term uraemia therefore is used to indicate a symptom complex, which show different features depending on chemical state of blood and cerebral abscess. Persistent headache, restlessness, twitching, muscular cramps and tremors are frequent.

Esthetic Pertaining to beauty, or the improvement of appearance.

Esthetics In dentistry, a philosophy concerned with the appearance of a dental restoration, as achieved through its color and/or form.

Estimated average requirement The amount of a nutrient needed to meet the basic requirements of half the individuals in a specific group, the basic for setting the RDAs.

Estriol The most abundant estrogen in pregnancy; its measurement can be used as an index of fetal/placental functions.

Estrogen replacement therapy (ERT) A technique for relieving various symptoms associated with estrogen deficiency; e.g., as experienced followed menopause.

Estrogen response element A palindromic nucleotide sequence that is specifically recognized and bound by the DNA binding domain of estrogen receptors.

Estrus The period of sexual receptivity in the female; the portion of the estrous cycle characterized by high levels of follicular estrogen production, during which time the female will accept the male for mating.

Etching 1. The act or process of selective dissolution 2. In dentistry, the selective dissolution of the surface of tooth enamel, dentin, porcelain, or a dental implant through the use of acids or other agents to create a retentive surface.

Ethambutol Half-life is 4 hours. It is bacteriostatic. It is used with other drugs to delay or prevent the emergence of resistant bacilli.

It is well absorbed from GIT. It reaches CSF to inhibit mycobacterial growth. In recommended doses of 15 mg/kg/day it is nontoxic. Main problem is optic neuritis. Excretion is through kidneys. It may cause loss of visual acuity and peripheral vision loss. Red and green colour blindness may also result.

Ethambutol amblyopia It has been noted that ethambutol affects the optic nerve if the daily dose exeeds more than 15 mg per kg body weight per day. Drug may affect the nerve directly or by interfering zinc metabolism. There is bitemporal hemianopia indicating that the site of lesion is chiasma. There is impaired colour vision for red and green ophthalmoscopy shows a swollen disc with hyperaemia and splinter haemorrhages.

Ethclass The intersection of social class and ethnicity. This intersection produces identifiable dispositions and behavioral patterns in families.

Ether It is a safe inhalation agent in untrained hands and a reliable and potential anaesthetic agent. It is inflammable and explosive also. Ether is now rarely used.

Ether intoxication The fatal doses of ether by ingestion and inhalation are 30 ml and 400 ppm respectively. The patient may develop varying degress of CNS depression producing delirium, confusion, agitation and cardiac arrest.

Ethical Rules or principles that govern right conduct and distinctions between right and wrong.

Ethical behavior Right and good conduct that is based on moral and cultural standards as defined by the society in which we live.

Ethical dilemma A situation in which no solution seems completely satisfactory.

Ethical principles General action guides specifying moral actions that are prohibited, required, or permitted in certain circumstances.

Ethics 1. Science of moral obligation; a system of moral principles, quality, plus practice. 2. The moral obligation to render to the patient the best possible quality of dental service and to maintain an honest relationship with other members of the profession and humankind in general.

Ethics, medical It is a code of behaviour that addresses the relationship between patient and physician. Medical ethics covers a wide range of behaviour including physicians involvement with patient, public image and commercial behaviour. Physician should not exploit the relationship they develop with patients and their families. Physicians are expected to keep up their knowledge and standard of procedures.

Ethmoid bone Spongy bone that forms the roof of the nasal fossae and a portion of anterior fossa of the skull that opens into the nasal cavity.

Ethnic group A group that is socially distinguished by it self or by others on the bases of nationality, culture or language.

Ethnicity Different from racial groups, ethnic groups are those people who share cultural practices and characteristics, such as a food, clothing, religion, music, and the like, in any combination. A group's sense of "peoplehood" based on a combination of race, religion, ancestral history, and nationality.

Ethnocentrism Opinion that the beliefs and customs of one's own ethnic group are superior.

Ethnography Descriptive anthropology.

Ethnology A science that concerns itself with the division of mankind into races and their origin, distribution, relations, and characteristics.

Ethnorgraphy A qualitative research methodology primarily used to study cultures.

Ethology The study of the whole animal, focusing on observable patterns of behaviour and their functions. It is a biological approach which, unlike psychology, does not deal with emotions or mental process- which makes it particularly suitable for studying infants and animals who can't tell you what they feel.

Ethyl alcohol poisoning Ethamol is used as solvent, antiseptic, chemical intermediate and beverages. The alcoholic content in various types of drinks are : beer 4 to 8 %; wines and champagne 10 to 20 %; whisky, rum, gin and brandy 40 to 55 %. The fatal dose is 300 to 400 ml of absolute alcohol. Serious toxicity occurs in children if more than 1 to 2 ml/kg is ingested.

Mild intoxication produces disinhibition, slight visual impairment, incoordination and a slowing of reaction time. In severe cases, depression of CNS takes place. It may be followed by hypothermia, hypotension, respiratory failure and death. Breath has characteristic odour.

Mild metabolic acidosis is common. Blood level of 50 to 100 mg/dl are associated with mild features while levels above 300 mg/dl lead to serious features.

Ethyl chloride It is a colourless liquid which is flammable and is used as a local anaesthetic. It is applied as a spray to skin. It evaparates easily and quickly. It is useful to spray before a minor surgery of boil, etc.

Ethylation The act or process of introducing an ethyl group.

Ethylene It is a colourless gas of slightly sweet odor and taste used in inhalation anaesthesia.

Etiology 1. Causative factors. 2. The factors implicated in the causation of disease. 3. The study of the factors causing disease.

Etorphine hydrochloride It is an analogue a naturally occurring opioid, 400 times as potent as morphine and is used to immobilise large animals.

Eubacteria Another name for the domain 'bacteria, which is now the preferred term.

Eucestode Body of adult eucestode consist of three distinct regions, scolex, neck and strobila. The lifecycle usually requires one or two intermediate hosts in each of which it undergoes a specific development phase.

Eudiamonistic family health model Professionals who use this model as their philosophy of practice focus on efforts to maximize the family's well-being and to support the entire family and individual members in reaching their highest potential

Euganthia The normal or proper relationship of jaws to each other.

Eukaryote A cell containing a membrane bound nucleus with DNA and RNA chromosomes.

Eukaryotic Generally, describing a cell in which DNA is housed within a nuclear envelope, or an organism having this cellular feature.

Eukinesia Good movement.

Euphoria An exaggerated feeling of physical and emotional well-being, usually of psychologic origin. Also seen in organic mental disorders and in toxic and drug-induced states.

Eupnea Easy or normal respiration.

Euprolactinemic Having a serum or plasma prolactin concentration within the normal range.

Euspermatozoa Sperm that fertilizes the egg and therefore contribute to the zygote genome.

Eustachian Canal Auditory tube.

Eustachian tube It is a passage which connects the middle ear and back of nose. Tube is 36 mm long. Smooth, wet mucous membrane lines the tube. Lower end of eustachian tube opens during swallowing and yawning. Suddén change of pressure outside or inside it may result in ear pain as in aeroplane taking off.

Eustress A helpful form of stress that must have been present in order for an individual to have good health.

Euthanasia This is the procedure of killing a human being whose suffering is very painful and incurable. It is against all the laws.

Euthyroid sick syndrome (ESS) It is a complex of abnormalities in serum thyroid hormone level, which occur in patients with non-thyroidal illness. TSH level is normal. T_3 is low because of impaired conversion of T_4 to T_3 in peripheral tissue. In ESS, free T_4 is normal and reverse. T_3 is increased; in hypothyroidism, both free T_4 and T_3 are decreased.

Eutroph An organism that grows well when the presence of nutrients is ample or high.

Evaluation Interpretation of objective and subjective data for the purpose of determining a musculoskeletal diagnosis and the appropriate course of treatment.

Evaporation Heat being lost from the skin by sweat being vaporized.

Evaporite A residue of salts left behind after brines evaporate to dryness.

Event-related potential (ERP) A change in the slow-wave activity of the brain in response to a sensory stimulus.

Eversion Truning outward or inside out, such as truning the food outward at the ankle.

Eves tonsillar snare It is the most common and powerful snare used in ENT surgery. It crushes the tissue before cutting it.

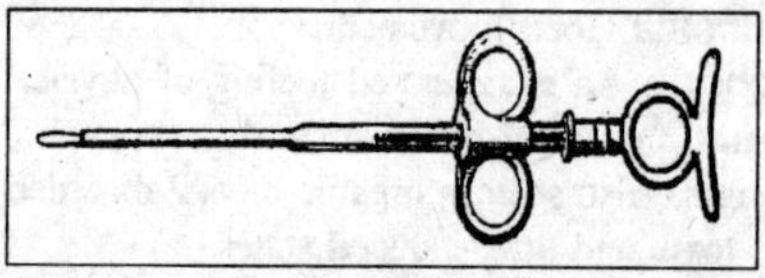

Evisceration The separation of wound layers with the protrusion of abdominal organs through the wound layers.

Evisceration scoop It is used to scoop out the contents of the eyeball during evisceration. After cutting the corneas, the scoop is introduced

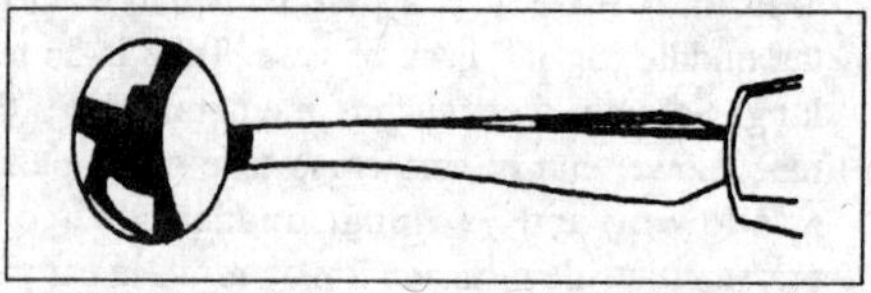

between the sclera and uvea and moved around to separate the structure from the sclera and then scoop out the contents.

Evoked potential Waveform elicited by a stimulus.

Evoked potential Electrical activity produced by the brain in response to any sensory stimulus; a more specific term than event-related potential.

Evolutionary psychology The study of behavior that uses principles of natural selection to account for human behaviors.

Evoporative heat transfer The loss of heat energy from the body to the ambient by evaporation of water from the skin to the surfaces to the respiratory tract.

Ewing's tumour, jaw It is rarer tumour of jaw and involves mandible more than maxilla. Patients are generally below the age of 20. Tumour grows rapidly with pain, fever and swelling. Teeth become loose and migrate, cortical bone is destroyed. Tumour is radiosensitive and surgical excision is also possible followed by chemotherapy.

Exacerbation An increase in severity of a disease or any of its symptoms.

Examination A procedure that includes more than one type of test; e.g., a postural examination that includes a variety of tests.

Examination, cervix Insert your fingers deeper until the cervix is located with the palmar surface of fingers. Feel its surface and run fingers around its circumference. Gently move the cervix from side to side. Assess the shape, position and consistency of cervix. It should feel smooth, mobile and nontender. Cervix of pregnant woman is usually softened and enlarged by third trimester.

Examination, uterus Insert the index and middle finger in vagina and position the second hand for examination of uterus on abdomen. Bring the external hand down toward the symphysis pubis and

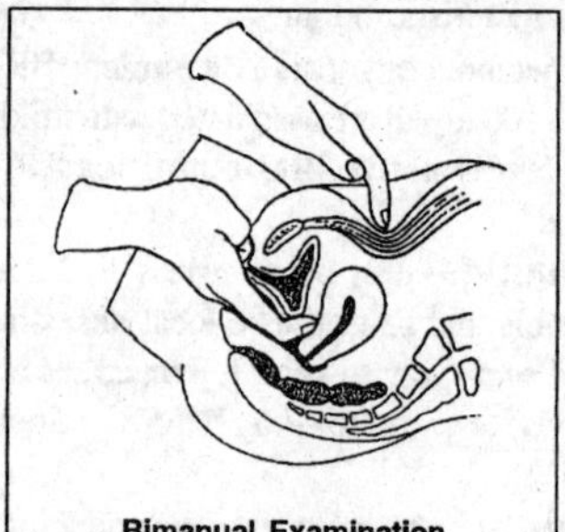

Bimanual Examination

inward toward the external hand to trap the uterus for examination.

Examine the uterus for position, shape, consistency, tendernes, mobility and surface regularity. Flexion indicates that the uterus is bent upon itself. Also note whether uterus midline or deviates to the left or right of pelvis. Non-pregnant uterus is small fitting comfortably under symphysis pubis in pelvis.

Exanthem An eruption or rash on skin.

Excavation Removal of carious material from a tooth in preparation for restoration.

Excavator Hand instrument with a small spoon on both side-ends for a variety of manipulative task.

Excementosis Hyperplasia of the cementum of the root of a tooth.

Exceptional intelligence A person with an IQ above 130, called gifted, or below 70, known as retarded. Exceptional individuals comprise the upper and lower 2 per cent of the population with respect to general intellectual ability.

Excessive overjet The anterior teeth are observed for overjet overbite relationship. In normal overjet relationship the mandibular teeth lie just lingual to the maxillary teeth. In class II malocclusion the overjet is excessive.

Exchange reaction A combination of a decomposition reaction, in which molecules are broken down, and a synthesis reaction, in which the products of the decomposition reaction are combined to form new molecules.

Exchange theory The viewpoint that interpersonal relationships are maintained whenever the individuals perceive the gain to be greater than the overall expense.

In short, the relationship is regarded in terms of profit and loss. A woman enjoys a man's cooking, but she dislikes his incessant talking. In deciding whether to continue the relationship, she compares her satisfaction with his cooking and her dissatisfaction with his verbal style.

Exchange transfusion It becomes imperative if jaundice appears early and rapidly progresses. If the coomb's test is positive, the cord hemoglobin is less than 14 gm% and if unconjugated bilirubin is 7 mg per 100 ml exchange transfusion is needed. A rising unconjugated serum bilirubin approaching 20 mg per 100 ml is a further indication of exchange transfusion.

Exchange vessels The capillaries, sinusoids, and postcapillary venues where the exchange of gases, nutrients, and metabolic products occurs.

Excimer laser A gas laser which emits pulses of light in the ultraviolet region at 193 n.m.

Excise Cut away entirely.

Excision Process of taking out.

Excision The removal of damaged nucleotides from incised nucleic acids.

Excisional biopsy It is accomplished by removing the entire lesion for microscopic examination. This is a preferable approach in most cases and treatment can be started at earliest.

Excitability The ability of muscle tissue to receive and respond to stimuli; the ability of nerve cells to respond to stimuli and convert them into nerve impulses.

Excitant An agent that produces excitation of the vital functions, or of those of the brain.

Excitation A process that increases the likelihood that neurons will be activated.

Excited state An energy-rich state of an atom or molecule; produced by the absorption of light energy.

Excitement sexual stage In males, the smaller flaccid penis tends to enlarge proportionately. There

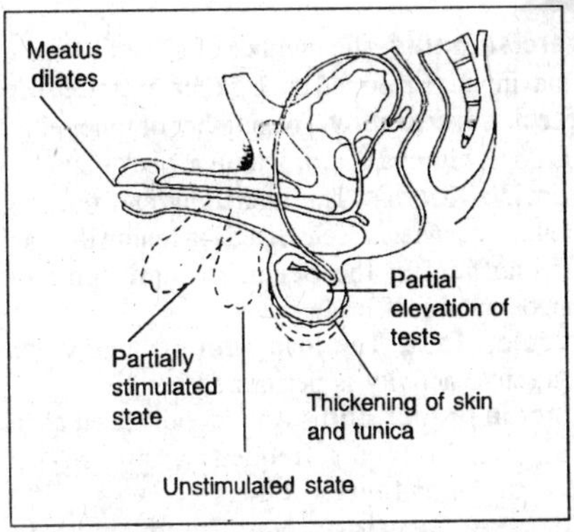

is partial elevation of testes and thickening of scrotal skin.

Excitotocicity Toxic effects on target neurons, of excessive glutanmatergic activity.

Excoriation Chemical skin injury.

Excrement Material eliminated from the body as waste, especially fecal matter.

Excrescence The abnormal outgrowth of structure.

Excretory system cestode It consist of two components collecting canals and flame cells. Four laterally aligned collecting canals two dorsal and two ventral extending the entire length. Ventral canal carries fluid away from scolex.

Execute To sign, and deliver a written legal instrument.

Exemption A situation in which a professional is not required to comply with an existing law because of educational or professional standing.

Exercise The performance of physical activity for the purpose of training or developing the body or mind.

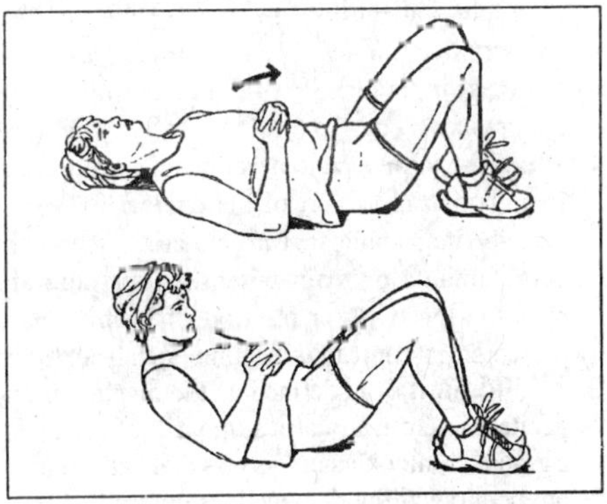

Exercise bouts The number of sets of a repetition maximum performed during each exercise session.

Exercise frequency The number of times exercise is done within a day or within a week.

Exercise Kegel's The tightening and relaxing of pubococcygeal muscle. It aids in toning the vagina, strengthening the perineum and controlling incontinence of urine.

Exercise load The load with or against which muscular activity is performed.

Exercise prescription An individualized exercise program involving frequency, intensity, time (duration), and type.

Exercise testing Monitored, multilevel cardiovascular or pulmonary evaluation of the patient's responses to controlled stress.

Exercise tolerance The capacity of both aerobic and anaerobic combined to perform exercise; also, the components of the oxygen transport system and their capacity to provide oxygen.

Exergonic Denoting chemical reactions that liberate energy.

Exfoliate To fall off in scales or layers; in dentistry, to shed primary teeth.

Exfoliation Shedding of primary teeth.

Exhalation Moving air out of the lungs; also known as expiration.

Exhaustion Great lassitude accompanied by muscle pain and vertigo, nausea, headache, faintness, dilated pupils, weak pulse, shallow respiration. The collapse supervenes and death ensues from heart failure.

Exhaustion psychosis This results from exhaustion of nervous system usually in old age. Onset is insidious. Insomnia is always the first symptom. Patient loses his or her self-control and memory deteriorates. Later, mental confusion and depression occur. Visual hallucinations are common.

Exhibit The term used to describe an item presented in a court trial as part of the evidence. The term describe items collected from a crime scene, from complainants or from witensses for laboratory examination. Only a fraction of such items are presented in court thus become actual 'exhibits'.

Exhibitionism It is defined as the display of one's genitals or erotically arousing parts of the body to a group of onlookers or viewers that had not invited or encouraged the display. It is committed for the purpose of getting gratification through the exhibition itself. Normal exposure of body is commonly used in advertisement while exhibitionism is pathological.

Exhumation Body is taken out when a suspicion of foul play arises in connection with a death under obscare circumstances. Sometime done after the burial of body to establish the identity of the diseased, when dead body is taken out it is done under the supervision of police. There is practically no limit of time in English law to the utility of an exhumation. As long as bones remain intact, these may afford valuable evidence by which murder by arsenic or other minerals may be recognised.

Existential neurosis A condition in which an individual is disturbed chiefly because he or she can find little or no meaning in life. It is the chief difficulty of most individuals who seek some sort of psychotherapeutic treatment.

Existential psychiatry (exis-tentialism) A school of psychiatry evolved from orthodox psychoanalytic thought; stresses the way in which a person experiences the phenomenologic world and takes responsibility for existence. Philosophically, it is holistic and self-deterministic in contrast to biologic or culturally deterministic points of view.

Existential therapy An approach to psychotherapy which emphasises that human existence is a process of emerging, developing, or becoming, not a static condition. Many of the techniques in existential therapy are not clearly differentiated from those in other forms of psychotherapy.

Existentialism A philosophically oriented approach to personality and therapy which stresses subjectivity, the individually of experience, and consequently, a spontaneous approach to life.

Exit route Means by which microorganisms escape from their original reservoir.

Exit site Point at which a catheter leaves a body site.

Exocervix The portion of the cervix lined with squamous epithelial cells.

Exocrine Secreting into a duct; opposite of endocrine.

Exocrine gland These are glands that use a duct to convey its secretion to the desired site. Exocrine glands include sweat glands.

Exocytosis The process of cellular secretion in which the secretory products are contained within a membrane enclosed vesicle. The vesicle fuses with the cell membrane so that the lumen of the vesicle is open to the extracellular environment.

Exodontia Practice of removing teeth from oral cavity.

Exodontics The science and practice of removing teeth from the oral cavity.

Exogenous Originating outside the body or produced from external sources.

Exogenous DNA "foreign" DNA sequence that are not homologous to the host genome..

Exogenous rhythms Biological processes that arise solely, or mainly, as a direct response to transient environmental signals or conditions.

Exolever The instrument which uses principal of leverage for extracting and removing teeth.

Exons Sequences that flank introns in precursor RNA molecules prior to splicing, and that are joined together in the mature RNA.

Exonuclease An enzyme that degrades DNA from a terminus.

Exophoria It is a condition of an outward duration of eyes when fusion is disturbed. In exophoria due to convergence weakness defect is greater for near vision than for distance vision. While in exophoria due to divergence excess the defect is greater for distance vision than for near vision.

Exophthalmia Bulging of the eyes that frequently accompanies Graves' disease, due to accumulation of a type of connective tissue behind the eye.

Exophthalmic goitre Thyroid gland is greatly enlarged and basal metabolic rate is grossly increased. The rate and output of heart increases and even auricular fibrillation may supervene. A fine tremor of skeletal muscles may present, eyeball is protruded. Skin becomes moist and flushed. There may be hyperglycaemia and appetite may increase with acute nervousness and irritability.

Exostosis These are most common oral exophytic lesions. These are readily recognisable, peripheral, benign, slow growing bony protuberances of jaws. These have smooth contours and covered with normal mucosa. These are bony hard on palpation and are attached by broad bony base to mandible. Removal is not very necessary unless it is causing physical or psychological problem.

Exothermic reaction Chemical reaction that gives off heat as the chemicals react.

Exotoxins These are proteins in nature and are sensitive to temperature above 70°C, 50% alcohol, formaldehyde and dilute acids. They can be easily denatured after which they lose their toxicity irreveribly but retain their antigenic character and become toxoids. Some exotoxins such as those of *Cl. botulinum* and enterotoxins of *Staphylococcus* are harmful only when ingested. Whereas diphtheria toxins if taken orally has no effect unless it is injected.

Expectancy value theories Models of motivation in which expectancies and values interact to determine behaviour.

Expected date of confinement Most infants will deliver 280 ±14 days after the first day of last normal period. Easy reckoner is achieved by adding 9 months and 7 days to the date of last menstral period to determine EDC.

Expected value of pain The product of multiplying the likelihood of experiencing a painful event by amount of pain it would inflict.

Expectorant An agent that facilitates removal of bronchopulmonary secretions.

Expectorate The act of coughing and spitting out musous from the respiratory tract.

Expectoration Expulsion of mucus or sputum from the mouth or lungs.

Experiential group A group whose main purpose is concerned with sharing whatever happens in a spontaneous fashion.

Experiment A method of testing a hypothesis.

Experiment, classical The control or manipulation of stimulus and/or organism condition in order to determine their causal influence on aspects of experience and behaviour of the organism. In the classical experiment variable, is manipulated at any given time in order to determine its influence on the dependent variable, which is usually some reaction of the organism. Thus, the classical experiment is sometimes called the single-factor experimental design. Compare with multifactor studies.

Experimental condition The portion of an experiment in which the subjects are exposed only to the factor under study, usually called the independent variable. The subjects in this condition are usually given some special treatment, as opposed to the subjects in the control condition, who generally are not exposed to the independent variable.

Experimental design The logical framework of an experiment which maximises the probability of obtaining or detecting real effects and minimises the likelihood to ambiguities regarding the significance of the experimentally observed differences.

Experimental psychology Experimental investigation of psychological problems. Not limited of physiological processes.

Expert witness A status conferred on a witness based on appropriate qualifications, training, and experience which acknowledges that competence and authority of the witness in a particular area of expertise. Expert witnesses are permitted to offer opinions in court related to their area of expertise which would not be permitted to a witness without such status.

Expirated blood Blood that is blown out of the nose, mouth, or wound as a result of air pressure and/or air flow which is the propelling force.

Expiration The process of expelling air from the lungs through breathing out; also called exhalation.

Expiratory center One of the two most important respiratory control centers, located in the medulla.

Expiratory muscles Muscles that allow more forceful expiration to increase the rate and depth of ventilation; the intercrease the rate and depth of ventilation; the internal intercostals and the abdominal muscles.

Expiratory reserve volume (ERV) The amount of air that can be forcibly exhaled after expiring the tidal volume.

Expiratory retard An orificial resistance applied during exhalation that permits the ventilatory circuit pressure to drop slowly to atmospheric pressure as the flow of expiratory gas ceases.

Explicit memory Memory in which subjects can retrieve an item and indicate that they know that the item they have retrieved is the correct item (that is, conscious memory).

Exploration Examination by touch with or without instruments.

Exploratory laparotomy The surgical exploration or examinatino of an abdominal organ or part.

Explorer Instrument with fine, sharp tip used to feel the surface characteristics of a tooth.

Explosive A substance that reacts with oxygen essentially instantaneously to produce a violent, exothermic reaction that produces rapidly escaping gases.

Explosive limits These are the upper and lower concentrations of a flammable vapor in air at which the mixture can explode. These limits can be relatively wide, as in the case of hydrogen (4.1 % vapor to 74.2% vapor in air), or more restricted, as in the case of petrol i.e. 1.3% vapor to 6% vapor in air.

Exposure keratitis It occurs due to improper wetting or polishing of corneal surface even though there is normal secretion of tear fluid. This is due to inability of the lids to polish the cornea with each blink. It may be caused by exophthalmos, proptosis, Parkinson's disease and seventh cranial nerve palsy. The exposed corneal epithelium becomes desiccated and substantia propria becomes hazy. There may be superficial erosions on the exposed cornea or an ulcer.

Express Manifestation using direct, clear language, either spoken or written.

Express contract A contract that is an actual agreement between the parties. Terms are beng declared at the time of making.

Expressed emotion Attitudes and feelings expressed by relative during family interaction to an individual with a psychotic disorder that will be described as critical comment, overt or subtle hostility or emotional over involvement in the individual affair.

Expression The appearance of the face as determined by the physical or emotional state.

Expressive aphasia Loss of motor speech.

Expressive aphasia Loss of motor speech.

Expressive behaviors Actions designed to provide affective support.

Expressive touch Touch applied to support and convey awareness and empathy for the client as a whole.

Exsanguination Extensive loss of blood.

Exsufflation Forced discharge of breath.

Extended care Services that meet the health needs of patients who no longer require acute hospital care.

Extended care facility Health care agency that provides longterm care.

Extended family All members of a kin network as defined by either biological or legal connections.

Extensibility The property of muscle that permits it to lengthen or be elongated.

Extension A movement that increases the angle between parts of a joint.

Extension for prevention To prevent the recurrence of decay, extension of the preparation subgingivally and axially and occlusally into an area that is readily polished and cleaned.

Extension of hip It is only tested when patient is lying prone. The examiner uses one hand to fix the pelvis and the other to extend the leg.

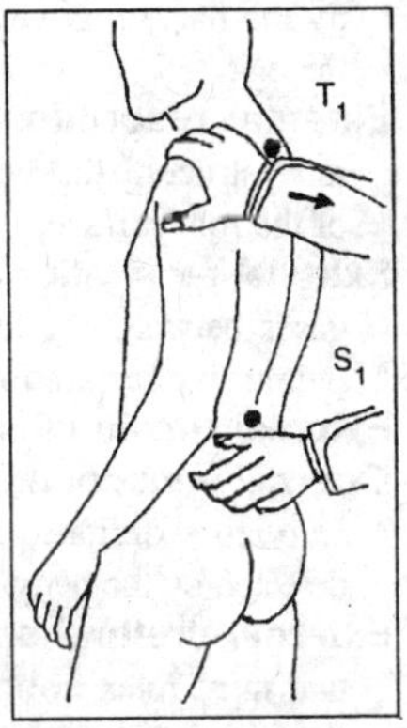

Extension of spine It can also be done in standing position. It is best to anchor the spine by placing the palm of the hand over the posterior iliac spines. Extension of spine is decreased in polymyositis myopathy and myasthenia gravis. It should be tested actively and passively.

Extensor reticulum It is a fibrous band which extends across the back of wrist under this reticulum. There are six tunnels for the passage of extensor tendons. Each passage has a synovial sheath.

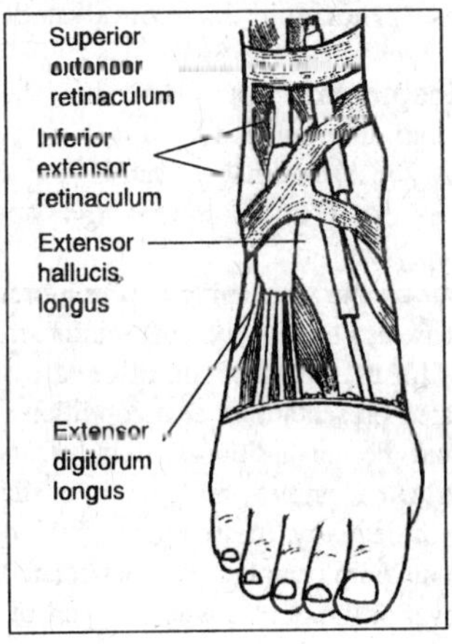

External Located on or toward the surface.

External auditory meatus A hole or opening in the temporal bone located superior and anterior to the mastoid process; appears radiolucent.

External acoustic meatus An opening through the temporal bone that connects with the tympanum and the middle era chamber and through which sound vibrations pass; also called the external auditory meatus.

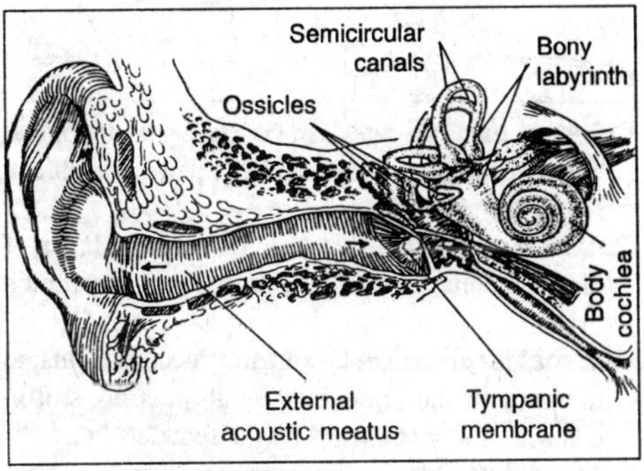

External air leak The presence of air originating from outside of the closed chest drainage system.

External ballotment One hand placed on the abdomen taps the abdomen and displaces the fetus to the other side across the uterine cavity, the other hand placed on the opposite side of abdomen feels the impact of the displaced fetus. It is positive at 24th to 26th week of pregnancy.

External carotid steal syndrome It is due to vertebrobasilar artery insufficiency resulting from siphoning of blood from vertebral artery to external carotid artery.

There may be blockage of external carotid at its origin. Clinically, there will be brief ischaemic attacks causing dizziness, diplopia, blurred vision, dysphagia and ptosis.

External catheter Urine collecting device applied to the skin.

External cephalic version Version is turning the fetus either by an external manipulation on the abdomen or an internal manipulation in uterine cavity.

By external version breech is converted to a favourable cephalic presentation. Transverse lie if left alone, may lead to obstructed labour. It is contraindicated in twins.

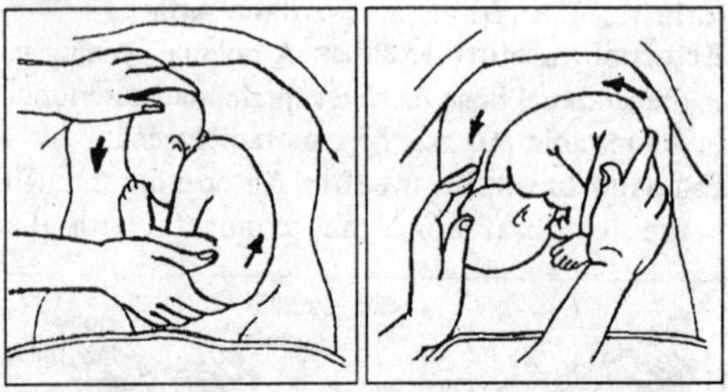

External ear The outer ear, consisting of the pinna, external auditory canal, and tympanic membrane (eardrum).

External elastic lamina A fenestrated layer of elastic connective tissue that covers the tunica media.

External fertilization Fertilization occuring outside the body of the female, although possibly still in contact with or sheltered by the female's body.

External fixation It is a means of fracture treatment that utilises multiple pins usually placed above and below the fracture site. The fracture is reduced and the pins are incorporated into an out rigger or plaster

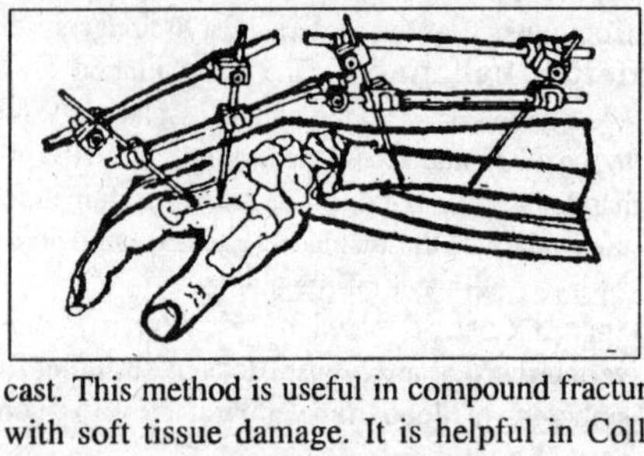

cast. This method is useful in compound fractures with soft tissue damage. It is helpful in Colles fractures that are loosing positions.

External fixator Metal device inserted into through one or more bones.

External genitalia External reproductive organs.

External intercostal muscles Eleven pair of muscles; each attaching from the inferior border of a rib to the superior border of the rib below; acts to pull the ribs together.

External intercostals Inspiratory muscles that enlarge the thorax, causing the lungs to expand and air to rush in.

External jugular vein One of a pair of lare vessels in the neck that receive most of the blood from the exterior of the cranium and the deep tissues of the face.

External nares The external nostrils, or the openings into the nasal cavity on the exterior of the body.

External oblique The Outer most layer of the anterolateral abdominal wall.

External oblique ridge A linear prominence of bone located on the external surface of the body of the mandible; appears radiopaque.

External os The vaginal opening of the cervix.

External otitits A common infection of the external ear; also known as swimmer's ear.

External pipping The first break of the eggshell by the hatchling when it begins to emerge from the egg.

External resorption A regressive alteration of tooth structure that takes place along the periphery of the root surface.

External respiration The exchange of respiratory gases between the lungs and blood. Also called pulmonary respiration.

External rotation Rotation of a joint outward.

External sensory information Stimulation from an origin exterior to the surface of the skin that is detected by the body.

External urethral sphincter Voluntary muscle that must relax in order for the client to void or completely empty the bladder

External validity Is presint when the results of study are true and meaningful for a larger populatin ant not just for the study participants.

Exteroception Refers to stimuli transduced at the body surface, rather than within the body wall/ limbs (proprioception) or alimentary tract (enteroception).

Exteroceptor A receptor adapted for the reception of stimuli from outside the body.

Sensory receptors that are sensitive to changes in the external environment (as opposed to interoceptors).

Extinction The weakening of a reinforced operant response as a result of ceasing reinforcement. Also, the elimination of a conditioned response by repeated presentations of a conditioned stimulus without the unconditioned stimulus.

Extirpation Complete removal or eradication of a part; in dentistry, the removal of the dental pulp from the pulp chamber and root canal. In surgery, removal of tumor as a whole or part of it.

Extra oral Outside of mouth.

Extracellular Refers to the outside of the cell.

Extracellular fluid (ECF) The water found outside of cells located in two compartments between cells (interstitial fluid) and in the blood (plasma).

Extracellular matrix Nonliving chemical substances located between cells; often consisting of protein fibres, ground substance, and fluid.

Extracellular parasite An organism that lives in derives nourishment from another organism without invading the host's cells.

Extracoronal dressing Temporary restoration that encircles all or part of the remaining tooth.

Extracorporeal shock-wave lithotripsy (ESWL) This technique was first developed in Germany in 1982. It was devised to avoid use of any sort of operative intervention. It involves shockwaves from a spark generator piezoelectric dish or electromagnetic plate directly onto the stone under X-ray/ultrasound control. The shockwaves generated in water cushion pass through the skin into the kidney and disintegrate the stone *in situ.* Twenty per cent develop sepsis and ureteric colic due to passage of fragments.

Extracorporeal ultrafiltration A process by which large molecules are separated from small molecules in a solution outside the body.

Extraction Removal of a tooth from the oral cavity by means of elevators and/or forceps.

Extraction vacuum In assisted childbirth, the use of a metal cup applied to the fetal head by creating a vacuum between it and the head to assist in the delivery of a fetus. Traction is exerted by means of a short chain attached to the cup, with a handle at its far end.

Extradural abscess It is usually caused by extension of infection from frontal sinuses, or from mastoid cavity. There is intense local pain and oedema of scalp. Extradural abscess can also occur in spinal column secondary to infection in vertebra.

Extradural haematoma It is the collection of blood located between the inner table of skull and dura. It may result from middle and posterior meningeal artery. Clinical pattern includes initial period of unconsciousness, hemiparesis, pupillary dilatation followed by a lucid interval of unconsciousness followed by lucid interval after which rapid neurological symptoms of hemiparesis

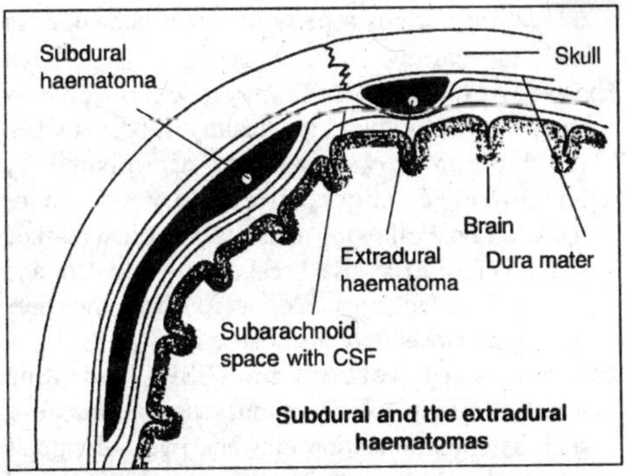

Subdural and the extradural haematomas

and pupillary dilatation develops. However lucid interval is seen only in 20% cases.

Extradural haemorrhage It is the bleeding between the inner surface of skull and the external surface of the dura mater. It generally results from a blow. The person may lose consciousness. Headache may gradually increase in severity with drowsiness, vomiting and paralysis of one side. CT or MRI is very helpful.

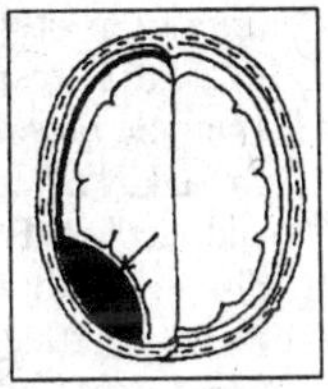

Extragonadal reserve The sperm stored in the epididymis, amounting to several days' worth of testicular production, available for ejaculation.

Extramedullary Outside the bone marrow.

Extraocular movements Eye movements controlled by several pairs of eye muscles.

Extraoral Outside the mouth; outside the oral cavity.

Extraoral radiography Examination of oral and paraoral structures by exposing films placed extraorally.

Extrapyramidal Outside or other than the pyramidal tract.

Extrapyramidal syndrome A variety of signs and symptoms, including muscular rigidity, tremors, drooling, shuffling gait (parkinsonism); restlessness (akathisia); peculiar involuntary postures (dystonia); motor inertia (akinesia) and many other neurologic disturbances. Results from dysfunction of the extrapyramidal system. May occur as a reversible side effect of certain psychotropic drugs, particularly phenothiazines.

Extrapyramidal system The portion of the central nervous system responsible for coordinating and integrating various aspects of motor behaviour or body movements.

Extrarenal uraemia It may occur in elderly subjects when kidneys are healthy. It occurs when renal blood flow is greatly diminished by haemorrhage, shock, circulatory failure or dehydration. Following maelena, it is often marked as a result of excessive breakdown of protein and absorption of nitrogenous material from intestine. Severe alkalosis may also cause it.

Extrasensory perception (ESP) Perception which allegedly occurs without sensory awareness, such as communication between two individuals when there appears to be no channels of information exchange.

Extrastriate cortex Visual cortical areas outside the striate cortex; also called secondary cortex.

Extrasystoles These are ectopic impulses which arise from sites other than SA node and give rise to ventral response, whenever they reach the ventricle outside its refractory period. It may be caused by excessive intake of tea, coffee, cigarette and alcohol. Pregnancy, anxiety, coronary artery disease and thyrotoxic heart disease may also result it. Extrasystoles may cause palpitation, irregular heart beat, vertigo and syncope. Small beat following a short pause and big beat following a long pause may be felt at wrist.

Extravaginal intercourse It is an intercourse in which erect penis is inserted in a body area other than vagina. Anus is the most common dite of extravaginal sex. It is known as anal sex. Other extravaginal intercourses includes coitus interfemora, coitus intramammas and coitus in umbilicus or axilla.

Extravasation The inadvertent infiltration of intravenous fluids or medications into the subcutaneous tissues surrounding the infusion site.

Extravascular lung water Volume of water contained within pulmonary interstitium and alveolar space. It is usually 4-5 mL/kg.

Extreme acidophile An organism with a pH optimum for growth at, or below, pH 3.

Extremity restraints Restraints used to immobilize one or all extremities.

Extremophilic Requiring, or growing optimally in, extreme environmental conditions; e.g., extremes of temperature or pressure.

Extrinsic Pertaining to an outside or external origin.

Extrinsic regulation Regulation of the heart that does not require ATP and moves substances into or out of cells from a higher to a lower concentration.

Extrinsic asthma A narrowing of the bronchial airways as the result of an allergic reaction to foreign substances.

Extrinsic muscle Muscles attached to the trunk and a limb.

Extrovert Person who does not like to remain alone and is talkative. He or she enjoys company. These are qualities to become leaders. Extroverts do not enjoy routine activity.

Extrus cycle Cyclic changes in the structure and functions of the ovaries and female reproductive tract of mammals other than humans, accompanied by periods of "heat"(estrus) or sexual receptivity. Estrus is the equivalent of the human menstrual cycle but differs from the human menstrual cycle in that the endometrium is not shed with accompanying bleeding.

Extrusion Abnormal displacement of teeth out of bone.

Extrusion reflex The response that causes an infant to push anything solid out of mouth.

Exudate The material composed of serum, fibrin, and white blood cells in variable amounts, formed as a reaction to injury of tissue and blood vessels.

Exudate ascites It is often deeper yellow, sometimes obviously blood stained with a high protein content of more than 25 gm/L, the fluid may clot spontaneously and often contains inflammatory or neoplastic cells. It is characteristic of inflammatory or neoplastic disease of the peritoneum. Such type of ascites is seen in primary hepatoma of liver, chronic right sided heart failure, pancreatitis and peritoneal tuberculosis.

Exudative infiltrate Fluid that has permeated or penetrated into the tissues.

Exudative retinal detachment There is damage to retinal pigment epithelium. It allows fluid from choroid to gain entry and causes detachment. It is common in posterior scleritis and choroidal tumours. There is no photopsia. There are symptoms of floaters mainly due to associated uveitis. There is loss of peripheral visual fields which is fast progressive.

Exuviation The shedding of any epithelial structure, as of the deciduous teeth.

Eye It is an orgen of sight and focuses an image onto the retina. Two eyes work in coordination under control of brain. Each eyeball moves by six delicate muscles. Eyeball has a tough outer coat the sclera. Sclera is a white portion of an eye. The circular part of cornea is transparent and protrudes slightly. Cornea is main lens of eye and performs most of focussing. Behind cornea is shallow chamber full of aqueous humour at the back of

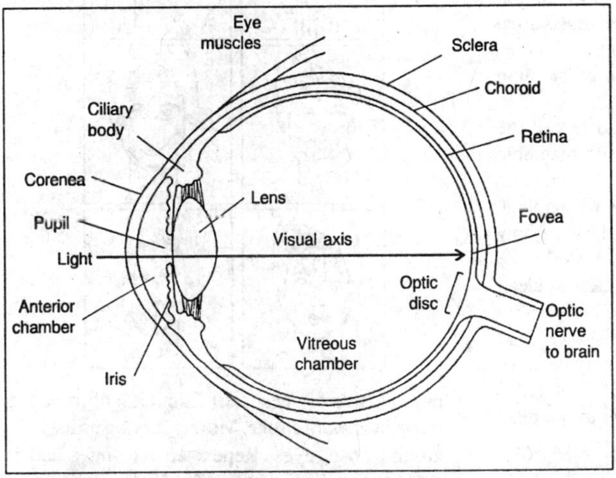

which is iris with its central hole, pupil. Pupil looks black and its size is altered with changes in light intensity. On the inside of the back of eye is retina, a complex structure of nerve tissue on which image is formed by the cornea. The eyeball is sealed off from the outside by a flexible membrane called conjunctiva. The conjunctiva contains many tiny tear secreting and mucus producing glands. Each eyelid contains about 30 Meibomian glands opening along the lid margin behind the roots of lashes.

Eye changes in pregnancy There is increased thickness of cornea and decreased intraocular pressure. Edema causes a 3% increase in corneal thickness. It may create problem with contact lenses. Intraocular pressure falls by 10%.

Eye injury during birth Subconjunctival hemorrhage presents as a red ring around the cornea. It disappears in a week or two without causing any trouble. In some cases forceps injury may cause hemorrhage in anterior chamber of eye with traumatic glaucoma.

Eye speculum It is used to keep the eye open during surgery on the eye. Various types are available. The best and most commonly used speculum is the universal eye speculum. The lid sutures have replaced the use of the speculum, in intraocular surgery. It is useful for minor surgical procedures requiring separation of lids.

Eyebrown The hairy ridge superior to the eye.

Eyelet A hole in metal ring or shoes that is used for lashing.

Eyelid These are membrane lined covering of skin, muscle and connective tissue over the front of eye. Protective eyelashes are attached to it. Lacrimal glands keep the mucous membrane neat and clean. Diseases of eyelids include blepharitis, chalazion, conjunctivitis and stye.

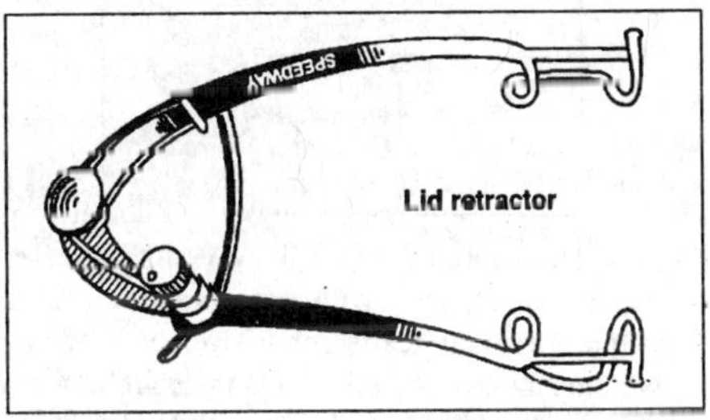

F

Fabere sign The patient lies supine on the table with thigh and knees flexed. The heel of one leg to be tested is then placed above the patella of the opposite leg and the knee is pressed downward and laterally. There will be limitation of motion due to resistance in cases of lumbagosciatica syndrome but pain in cases of the hip.

Fabrication in dentistry, construction or building up, as of dental restoration.

Face bow Caliper-like device used to record the relationship of the maxillae and/or the mandible to the temporomandibular joints.

Face bow fork Part of the face bow assemblage used to attach the occlusion rim to the face bow proper.

Face mask These should be simple, easy to clean and sterilise. They should provide good fit with a patient's face and add, minimal dead space. Dead space may be 78 to 198 ml and this may equal or exceed the anatomical dead space of an average adult. Face mask connectors also add to the dead

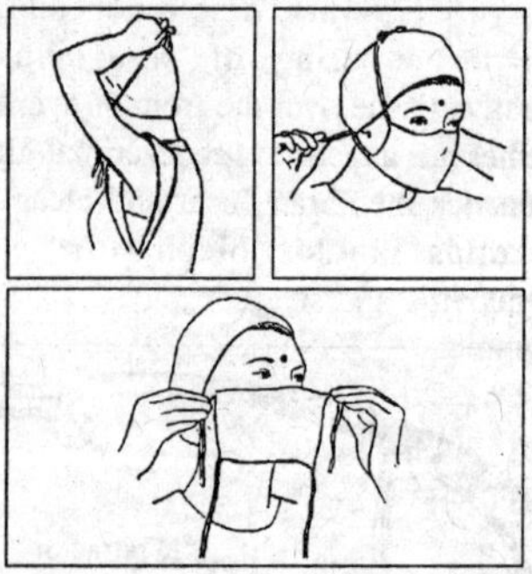

space. Disposable face masks are suitable. Face mask is put on by all theatre personnel before beginning the surgical scrub. Cover both of your nose and mouth. Avoid sneezing, coughing and excessive conversation, all of which load the mask with bacteria or other micro-organism. Change the mask with each patient.

Face massage It is very essential to do face massage to improve the blood circulation. Take a bit of cream and spread it gently all over the face and do not forget the neck. Both hands cupped and crossed

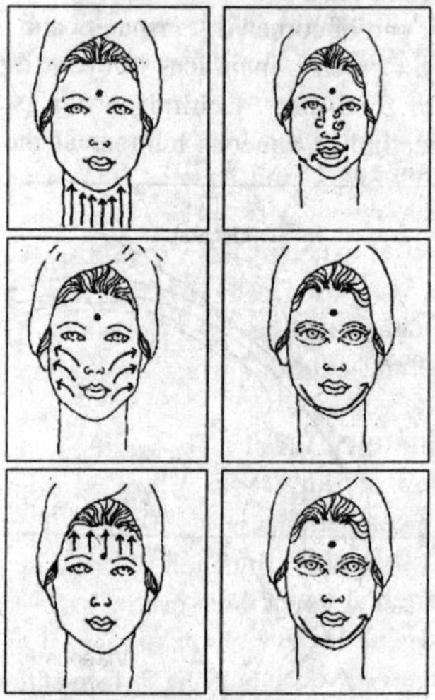

on each side of neck, start from base of neck and move in upward stroke. Move your fingers in circle around nose, eyes. Repeat all ten times and it should not take more than 5 minutes.

Face presentation It is characterised by a longitudinal lie and full extension of fetal head on

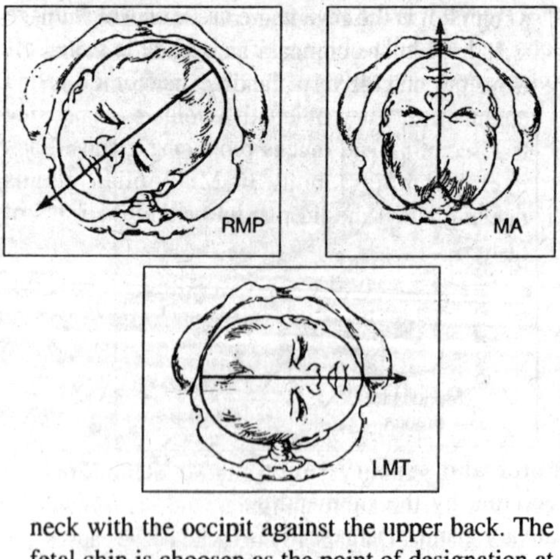

neck with the occipit against the upper back. The fetal chin is choosen as the point of designation at vaginal examination.

Face tent Device that provides oxygen in an area around the nose and mouth.

Face-lift It is a cosmetic operation. In it, wrinkles of face are smoothened out and sagging skin is lifted. Most of cases scars fade within a year and are hidden in natural crease line.

Face-nerve supply The trigeminal nerve supplies the skin of the front and side of scalp, forehead, eyelids, external nose, cheeks, lips and chin. It has three branches : ophthalmic, maxillary and mandibular.

Faces Material expelled from the GI tract during defection, composed of undigested food residue, bacteria, and secrections; also called stool.

Facet A small, smooth surface of a bone where articulation occurs.

Facet asymmetry Vertebral structure in which the orientation of the facets is not anatomically bilaterally comparable.

Facet joint injection Injection of posterior facets of intervertebral joints done in low back pain not associated with leg symptoms or signs.

Facial Term used to designate the surface of the tooth toward the face.

Facial clefts Fissures along the embryonal lines of the junction of maxillary and lateral nasal process.

Facial myokymia Symptoms include involuntary periorbital muscle contractions of varying location and intensity. It may affect entire half of face. These are not limited to muscles supplied by facial nerve.

Facial nerve It is the seventh nerve and arises from pons and medulla oblongata and sends branches to face, neck and salivary glands. It performs both

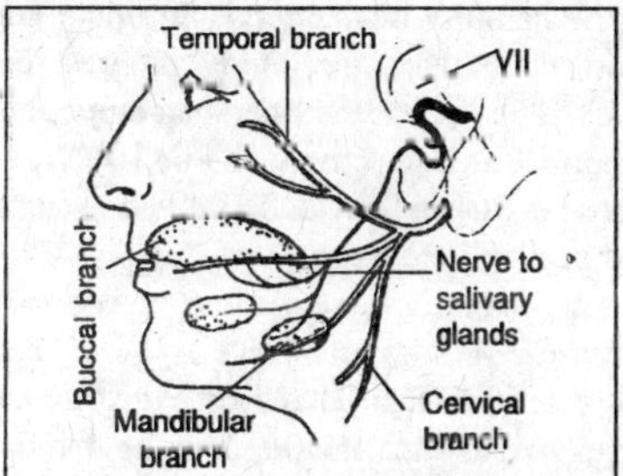

motor and sensory functions. It stimulates secretion by the submandibular and sublingual salivary glands. Damage to the facial nerve causes weakness of facial muscles.

Facial nerve block It is performed to prevent blephrospasm during eye surgery with retrobulbar block.

Facial pain Pain may be localised or may be referred from elsewhere or may occur for unknown reason. Amongst infection sinusitis can cause pain around eyes and cheek bones. Mumps cause cheek pain before any swelling appears. Trigeminal pain is unilateral and is severe. Knife like pain may be due to herpes. Referred pain may be felt in jaw due to angina pectoris.

Facial palsy during birth Condition is caused by blade of forceps pressing on the facial nerve. Such injury may also develop in spontaneous delivery. Facial nerve may also be injured during skull fracture. Very rarely, facial nerve palsy may be bilateral which is manifested by lack of expression during crying.

Facial paralysis Bell's palsy is the paralysis of muscles supplied by the seventh cranial nerve. Causes include from exposure to cold to malignant tumour of parotid gland. Some cases are believed to be caused by herpes simplex type I virus. Paralysis is unilateral.

On the affected side, eye cannot be closed. The mouth droops and saliva escapes from corner of mouth. Patient becomes expressionless due to paralysis of muscles. There develops difficulty in speech and mastication.

Facial spasm Paroxysmal, spasmodic tonic clonic muscle twitches limited to mimetic muscles supplied by facial nerve. Bilateral occurrence is not uncommon. Symptoms tend to increase over time. There may be long remissions. Cause is not definitely known.

Facies The features, general appearance and expression of face.

Facilitaton Increasing the likelihood of depolarization.

Facilitated diffusion Movement of molecules through a membrane in combination with a carrier molecule; not linked to metabolic use of energy. Net movement always occurs down a concentration gradient from high to low concentration.

Facilitation Lowered threshold for firing in a spinal cord segment, resulting from afferent bombardment associated with spinal dysfunction.

Facioplasty Plastic surgery of the face.

Fact witness Witness who must provide only firsthand knowledge, not hearsay.

Factor analysis A statistical technique that examines population clusters to extract patterns of commonality.

Facultative Able to grow in the presence of a given environmental factor, but not restricted only to the presence of that factor; e.g., bacteria that can grow in the presence or absence of oxygen.

Facultative anerobe Microorganisms that can exist under either aerobic or anaerobic conditions.

Facultative cells Cells that can live in the presence or absence of oxygen.

Facultative parasite An organism that lives in and derives nourishment from another organism under more than one specific set of environmental factors.

FAD Flavin adenine dinucleotide; a coenzyme derived from riboflavin that participates in electron transport within mitochondria.

Fad batch processing In bioreactor technology, a process in which liquid media is fed to the reactor continuously.

Faecal fat This is an overall indicator of digestive and absorptive function. It is a measure of faecal fat output and comparison of this with the dietary fat intake, the fat balance.

Absorption of about 93% or more of fat is regarded normal. Thus a test requires a measured and constant dietary fat intake with complete collection of stool. At least 5 days collection and study is necessary. This test gives a good overall assessment of adequacy of bile salts level in upper small intestine and of the function of the pancreas and small intestine.

Faeces It is a waste material from digestive tract that is expelled through anus. Faeces contain dead bacteria, deadells from intestinal lining, secretions from intestine and bile from liver. Liquid or very loose, frequent motions are called diarrhoea. It may be due to malabsorption. Pale faeces may be due to lack of bile in intestine due to bile duct obstruction. Dark faeces may be due to large amount of iron. Black faeces may be due to bleeding in stomach, duodenum and small intestine. Slimy faeces may be due to excessive mucus. Blood in stool may be due to dysentery.

Faget's sign According to this sign though the pulse remains rapid initially, but soon becomes increasingly slow for the degree of body temperature as it is seen in yellow fever.

Fahenheit scale Scale that uses 32°F as the temperature at which water freezes and 212°F as the point at which it boils.

Fahrenheit It was first made by German scientist Gabriel Fahrenheit (1686-1736). In Fahrenheit freezing point is 32°F, the boiling point is 212°F and normal body temperature is 98.4°F.

Fahrenheit/centigrade temperature These are two different scales of measuring temperature. Nowadays, centigrade scale is more commonly used. For changing Fahrenheit to centigrade temperature and *vice versa* the formula is as F–32–5/9=C or Cx9/5+32°=F.

Failed forceps An unsuccessful attempt to deliver by injudicious and faulty employment of forceps in an unsuitable environment.

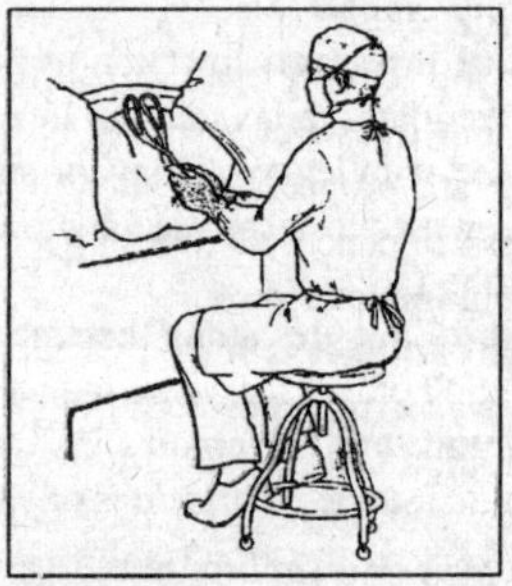

Failure of descent Absence of descent during the first stage, deceleration phase, or second stage of labour.

Failure to progress The cessation of labour due to the inability of the cervix to dilate normally. This occurs when the rate of progress in active labour falls below the Friedman curve, but there is normal uterine activity and no CPD.

Failure to thrive Growth delay with postural signs and poor muscle tones.

Fainting It is a temporary loss of consciousness because brain does not receive oxygen. Commonest cause is vasovagal attack or overstimulation of vagus nerve. Such fainting may be due to severe pain, stress or fear. Standing still for long may cause fainting, which is due to blood pooling in veins of legs. It is more common in old diabetics. Vertebrovestibular insufficiency may be associated with temporary difficulty in speaking or weakness in limbs. Fainting may be due to lack of blood flow in arrhythmia resulting from heart attack/ block.

Faith healing The healer usually transmits this healing force to the sufferer by placing hands over head. Often both healer and sufferer have a deep religious faith. Allopathy believes that such cures are not due to divine power but to the fact that the disorders were hysterical in origin.

Falciform ligament An extension of parietal peritoneum that separates the right and left lobes of the liver .

Fallen arch When the tendons the ligaments of the foot weaken, allowing the normally curved arch to flatten out.

Falling foot arch Weakness of muscles causes a condition calling falling arches and suggests that the ligaments alone cannot support the arches over a long period of time. The usual treatment is exercising the muscles and treatment is not always successful. Putting metal support in shoes relieves pain, but does not restore the muscle. Falling arches are progressive and fully developed are painless. Foot does not function well when walking or running along distance.

Fallopian tube It is a tube extending from uterus to ovary. It transports eggs and sperms where fertilisation takes place. It is about 3 inches long. Narrow end opens in uterus while expanded end is divided into fimbria near ovary. It sweeps up egg once it is expelled from ovary. Ectopic pregnancy usually occurs in fallopian tube.

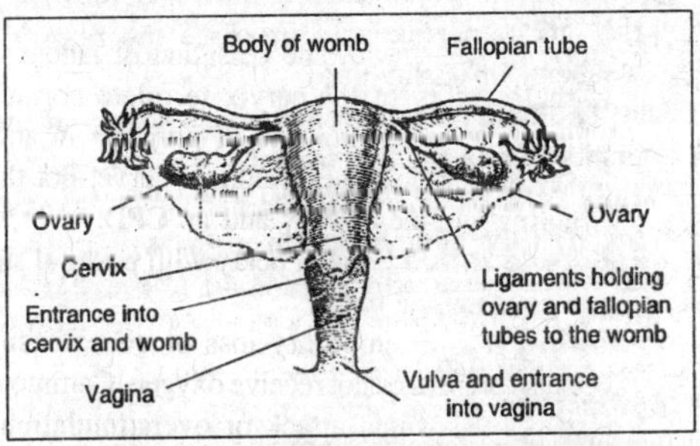

Salpingitis is inflammation of the fallopian tube by bacterial infection It lies in the upper borders of broad ligament enclosed in peritoneum. Each tube is of 10 cms. It has four parts, interstitial, the isthmus, the ampulla and fimbrial portion. The blood supply is derived from the uterine and ovarian arteries. Nerves are branches of pelvic plexus. T_{11}, T_{12} and L_1.

Fallot's tetralogy This is the most common congenital cyanotic disease. The defects consist of pulmonary stenosis, hyperventricular septal defect, right ventricular hypertrophy and dextroposition of aorta overriding the ventricular septum. Clinical features include dyspnoea and fatigue, severe cyanotic spells, central cyanosis, loud systolic murmur on left second space and single and loud sound at A1. ECG shows moderate right ventricular hypertrophy.

False negative In a diagnostic test, a negative reaction in the presence of disease.

False aneurysm It is a sac formed by condensed periarterial fibrous tissue and it communicates with the lumen of artery through an opening in its wall. It may develop commonly due to penetration or rupture of the arterial wall.

False chordae A fibrous collagenous cord passing from the papillary muscles to one another or the ventricular walls.

False cyst It is walled off collection of fluid. These are usually exudation or degeneration cyst Pseudocyst of pancreas is an encysted collection of fluid in lesser sac. Fluid may collect in centre of a tumour due to haemorrhage or colliquative necrosis.

False imprisonment Interference with a person's freedom to move about at will without legal authority to do so.

False labour A condition in the latter weeks of some pregnancies in which, irregular uterine contractions are felt but the cervix is not affected.

False negative In a diagnostic test, a negative reaction in the presence of disease.

False pelvis The part of the pelvis superior to a plane passing through the linea terminalis, which supports the uterus during late pregnancy and directs the fetus into the true pelvis at the proper time.

False pocket Excessively deep sulcus caused by gingival swelling without apical migration of the epithelial attachment.

False positive An incorrect result of a test or procedure that falsely indicates the presence of finding, condition or disease.

False ribs The eighth, ninth, and tenth pairs of ribs that are attached to the cartilage of the seventh ribs rather than the sternum.

False vocal cords The supporting folds of tissue for the true vocal cords within the larynx.

Falx carebri A fold of dura mater anchored to the crista galli of the ethmoid bone. It extends between the right and left cerebral hemispheres.

Falx cerebelli A fold or the dura mater anchored to the occipital bone. It projects inwards between the right and left cerebral hemispheres.

Familial Presence of a trait or condition in a family often than would be expected by chance alone.

Familial tremor Benign essential tremor.

Family Collection of individuals usually of at least two generations, sometimes connected by marriage or biology sharing the functions of providing food, shelter and raising children.

Family appraisal of the illness The way the family sees the illness.

Family as a component of society Focus of assessment and intervention is on the family as an institution in society. The family as a whole interacts with other institutions educational, religious, economic, health to receive, exchange, or give communication and services.

Family as a system Focus of assessment and intervention is on the interactions between family members. The family is viewed as an interactional system, in which the whole is more than the sum of its parts. The focus is on the individual and family simultaneously.

Family as the client Focus of assessment and intervention is on all individual family members. The family is in the foreground and the individuals are in the background. The family is the sum of individual family members.

Family as the context Focus of assessment and an intervention is on the individual person. The individual is in the foreground and the family is in the background. The family is the context for the individuals as either a resource or a stressor to their health and illness.

Family career The dynamic process of change that occurs during the life span of the unique group called the family. American families are diverse and are created through marriage, remarriage, adoption, and partnerships. Family careers include family stages and transitions that can occur in a nonlinear fashion.

Family child care The care provided for a small number of children in care giver's home.

Family child health nursing Focuses on the relationships, family tasks, and nursing care related to children's health.

Family coping Family strategies, patterns, and behaviors designed to maintain or strengthen the family as a whole, maintain the emotional stability and well-being of its members, and initiate efforts to resolve family hardships created by a stressor, maintain the well-being of its members, and use family and community resources to manage stress and hardship.

Family function The purpose that the family serves for: (1) its members and (2) for the society in which it exists.

Family health A dynamic, changing relative state of well-being that includes theological, psychological, spiritual, sociological, and cultural factors of the family system. A holistic term referring to functional and dysfunctional families. The term further encompasses the biological and spiritual aspects of family life.

Family health care nursing The process of providing for the health care needs of families that are within the scope of nursing practice. Family health care nursing can be aimed at the family as context, the family as a whole, the family as a system, or the family as a component of society.

Family health promotion Behaviors of the family that are undertaken to increase the family's wellbeing or quality of life.

Family life cycle Developmental phases of the family from beginning to end.

Family process The ongoing interaction between the family members through which they accomplish their instrumental and affective tasks.

Family Quantitative data Derived from family assessment and measures, counts, or compares properties or aspects of the family. This information is usually derived from closed-ended questions that assign a value to the answers that are then submitted for analysis through descriptive or inferential statistics.

Family resources The physical, social, or financial support available to a family.

Family rules The spoken or unspoken patterns that define order in the family.

Family stages Refers To Duvall's eight stages of family development, These are marriage without children, childbearing, preschool children, school children, adolescents, launching of young adults, middle age of parents and ageing of family members.

Family structure The ordered set of relationships among the parts of family and between the family and other social systems.

Family therapy A therapeutic technique which assumes that the basis of an individual's disorder lies within the family of which that individual is a member. The family is treated as a group of related individuals, all of whom have a problem, embodied in the identified patient and other conditions. Therefore, the treatment should involve the entire family.

Family transitions Family developmental and situational events that signal a reorganization of family roles and tasks during family careers.

Family types Predictable and discernible patterns of family functioning.

Family values A family's system of ideas, attitudes and beliefs about the worth or priority of entities, or ideas that bind together the members of a family in a common culture.

Family-centred care Maternity care that takes into account other members of the family, particularly fathers and children, in prenatal, intrapartum, and postpartum care of pregnant women.

Fanconi syndrome There is generalised aminoaciduria, glycosuria, mild proteinuria, hyperphosphaturia and reduction of urinary concentrating capacity. Systemic metabolic acidosis, hyperchloraemia, hypokalaemia and hyperphosphataemia are the results. In children, one may develop failure to thrive, fever and dehydration. Child may be stunted and rickets will be prominent.

Fantasy An imagined sequence of events or mental images, e.g daydreams, that serves to express unconscious conflicts, to gratify unconscious wishes, or to prepare for anticipated future events. It is a mental image that may take the form of imagined events, day dreams or night dreams based on imagination, wishes and unfulfilled impulses. Sex is composed of fiction and fantasy. Actually physcial and mental stimulation is necessary for adequate arousal and functioning in sex. Required physical stimulation is well known but mental component is more important. Fantasy serves as substitute for action and provides temporary satisfaction till physical satisfaction. Fantasy allows partial expression of forbidden wishes. Male fantasies have a strong visual emphasis, while females emphasise the emotional and romantic aspects of sex in their fantasies.

Far response Sympathetic activity causing flattening of the lens for far vision.

Faradism It is used as a muscle exerciser because of readiness of muscle fibres to accept this form of stimulation. It is most efficient when pads are kept at point of origin and point of insertion of muscle.

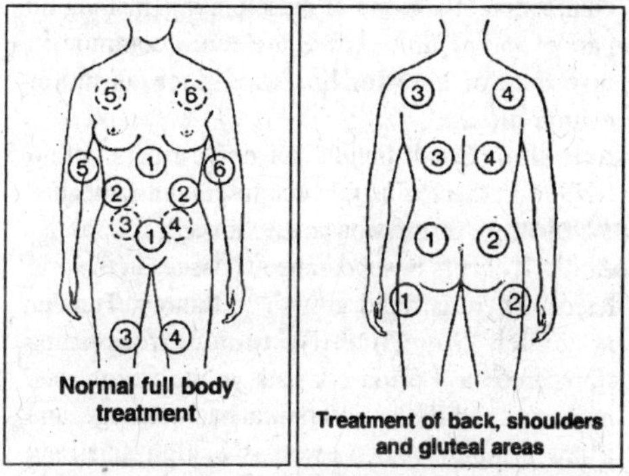

Normal full body treatment

Treatment of back, shoulders and gluteal areas

In general two pads or pair of pads which complete the circuit should be placed at either end of muscle or group of muscles which are to be activated. A healthy person could have 15 minutes for first treatment, 20 minutes second time, and 25 minutes third time.

Farina A cereal made from hard wheat, from which the bran and most of germ have been removed. It is creamy coloured rich in protein and easily digestible.

Farrowing The birth process in swine.

Fas A member of the TNF receptor gene family. Engagement of Fas (CD95) on the surface of the cell by the Fas ligand present on cytotoxic cells can trigger apoptosis in the Fas-bearing target cell.

Fascia A tough sheet of fibrous tissue binding the skin to underlying muscles or supporting and separating muscles.

Fascia bulbi Vagina bulbi.

Fascia lata The external investing fascia of the thigh.

Fascial sheath A flat sheet of connective tissues used for separation, stability, and muscular attachment points.

Fascicle A small bundle or cluster, especially of nerve or muscle fibers (cells). Also called a fasciculus.

Fasciculation Abnormal, spontaneous twitch of all skeletal muscle fibers in one motor unit that is visible at the skin surface; not associated with movement of the affected muscle; present in progressive diseases of motor neurons, for example, poliomyelitis and amyotrophic lateral sclerosis.

Fasciculations It is an involuntary, spontaneous contraction of a group of muscle fibres making up part of motor unit. These are more common in disorders of anterior horn cell such as motor neuron disease.

Fasciculus 'Small bundle' of nerve fibers within CNS, e.g., fasciculus gracilis, fasciculus cuneatus.

Fasciotomy An incision made through the fascia.

Fascitis It occurs in subcutaneous tissues in the oral lesion. There is rapid growth of tumour. Tumour is tender. Superficially, tumour resembles fibrosarcoma. Lesion consists young fibroblasts, numerous capillaries, interstitial haemorrhage, and a few lymphocytes. Lesion is benign and may regress spontaneously.

Fastigial Fastigial nucleus in roof of fourth ventricle.

Fasting Abstaining from food and drinking only liquid. Fast metabolism is maintained by energy supplied from substances stored in the body. About 6 hours after the last meal, body starts using glycogen stored in liver for 24 hours. After it body gets energy from stored fat in body, protein from the breakdown of muscles is also used as an energy source. If fasting continues body's metabolism is also slowed down, the fat and protein from muscles are consumed more slowly. To start weight loss is rapid, later it is slowed down. Water that would normally have been excreted is absorbed by tissues. Thus accumulated fluid causes oedema of legs and abdomen. In prolonged fast digestive power is impaired because stomach gradually stops secreting digestive juices. Prolonged fasting also halts the production of sex hormones causing amenorrhoea. Body's immunity is also lowered down. To reduce weight long fasting is not necessary and reduction of quantity and quality of food will help.

Fasting blood glucose Level of glucose circulating in blood serum agter an 8-hour fast; also called fasting blood sugar (FBS).

Fasting blood sugar No food is given 12 hours of taking the blood. During evening meal and prior day of that patient should take 300 gm of carbohydrate. In the morning 3 ml blood is taken in oxalate tube. Tube with blood is labelled as fasting blood sugar.

Fat Adipose tissue of the body; fatty acids, or lipids, are the most concentrated form of the energy-releasing nutrients, providing 9 kcalories per gram.

Fat embolism It is often associated with fractures of lower limb bones. Onset of symptoms may rapidly follow the injury or may be delayed for 2 to 3 days. Pulmonary signs and symptoms include dyspnoea, pallor, cyanosis, pyrexia and frothy sputum. Fat globules may be seen in sputum and urine. Cerebral changes develop within 24 hours with pyrexia and restlessness leading to coma, convulsions and paralysis. Skin changes includes purpuric eruptions. There may develop hypoxaemia, acidosis, hypocalcaemia, anaemia and thrombocytopenia.

Fat pad sign Joint effusion due to hemorrhage or fluid displaces the extracapsular fat pads away from the bone creating fat pad sign. It is useful in assessing trauma involving wrist and elbow.

Fat soluble Soluble in fats or solvents for fats; in nutrition a group of vitamins classified according to their method of metabolism.

Fat tissue Adipose tissue; specialized to store lipids.

Fatal Causing death; deadly; mortal.

Fatal period of drowning This varies with mode of death and it could be almost instantaneous in vagal inhibition. Asphyxia supervenes in 2 minutes and will take another 2 to 5 minutes before the heart stops. Death is sure if body remains submerged more than 5 minutes.

Fatal suicide A suicide act that results in death of an individual.

Fatigue The state of increased discomfort and decreased efficiency resulting from prolonged or

discomfort and decreased efficiency resulting from prolonged or excessive exertion; loss of power or capacity to respond to stimulation.

Fatigue fracture A fracture of bone or implant caused by cyclic loading that may or may not result in permanent deformation.

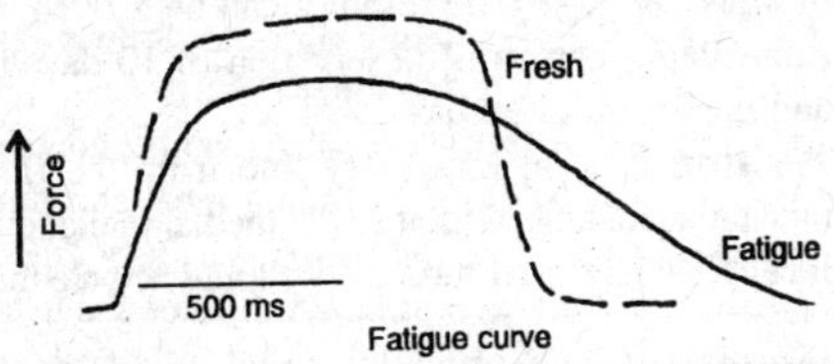

Fatigue curve

Fatigue limit The load a material can endure indefinitely on subjection to cyclic loading.

Fatigue strength The point at which a material will fracture in response to cyclical loads at magnitudes below the yield strength.

Fats These are rich source of energy and each 1 gm gives 9.1 calories. These are compounds containing carbon, hydrogen and a small amount of oxygen. These are mostly composed of fatty acids and glycerol. These are of two types : saturated and unsaturated.

If hydrogen content is maximum it is known as saturated. If there are some sites of carbon atom unoccupied by hydrogen then it is known as polyunsaturated. Saturated fats are solid and oils are liquid at room temperature.

Fat-soluble vitamins Those carried and stored in fat; vitamins A,D, E, and K.

Fatty Pertaining to fat.

Fatty acid Straight chain of carbon atoms with a learboxyl group (–COOH) attached at one end; a building block of fats.

Fatty infiltration There is a unilateral or bilateral enlargement of major salivary gland specially parotid gland due to fatty infiltration. Although specific cause is not known but condition is seen in protein deficiency, alcoholism, cirrhosis of liver, tuberculosis and diabetes mellitus. There is infiltration of lobules with normal fat cells. No treatment is indicated.

Fatty liver It results from excessive entry of free fatty acids into liver or enhanced fatty acid synthesis. Causes of fatty liver include alcohol abuse, protein malnutrition, diabetes mellitus and obesity.

Fauces The passageway between the mouth and the pharynx.

FDI system It is a more recent and it combines the palmer system with numbers used to designate the various quadrant. This result in two digit representing quadrant and second representing tooth.

F-distribution A distribution of squared t statistic that is sometimes used if the dependent variable consists of only two categories.

Fe receptors Cell surface receptors which bind the Fe portion of particular immunoglobulin classes.

Fear conditioning The learning of an association between a neutral stimulus and a noxious event such as a shock.

Feature extraction Separate simultaneous analysis of individual features of the scence by the visual associaltion cortex.

Febella A small sesamoid bone often found in the tendon of lateral head of the gastronemius muscle.

Febrile Pertaining to fever; feverish.

Fecal impaction Condition in which it is impossible to pass feces voluntarily.

Fecal implication A collection of compressed or hardened feces in the colon or rectum that cannot be moved voluntarily.

Fecal incontinence Inability to control the elimination of stool.

Feces Material expelled from the GI tract during defecation, composed of food residue, bacteria, and secretions; also called stool.

Fecundability The fact or probability of achieving a live birth within one menstrual cycle. More generally, the production of sperm or eggs and of viable embryos.

Fecundation The act of impregnating or the state of being impregnated; the fertilisation of the ovum by means of the male seminal element.

Fecundity The fact or probability of achieving a live birth within one menstrual cycle. More generally, the production of sperm or eggs and of viable embryos.

Federal Dentaire International International organization that produced a tooth identification system (FDI Tooth Numbering System) based on a two-digit system; the first digit indicates the arch, dentition, and location and the second digit refers to the specific tooth.

Feedback A reciprocal process in which a chemical agent produces a change or activity, which in turn regulates the further action of that agent.

Feed back inhibition A process whereby the end product of the system is able to inhibit the activity of higher order stimulating events.

Feedback control A control mechanism in which the product of a transcription unit can negatively control its own expression.

Feedback inhibition The inhibition of enzyme activity by a product of a reaction or a pathway. The first enzyme of a pathway is usually the only target of such control.

Feedback loop Mechanism by which hormone production is turned off an on.

Feedback system A sequence of events in which information about the status of a situation is continually reported (fed back) to a control center.

Feeding Supplying nourishment; giving food to.

Feeding artificial A process of feeding those who can not take food by oral route. Generally Ryles tube is used. In some cases intravenous infusion is done. Premature babies often require tube feeding if their sucking reflexes are underdeveloped.

Intravenous feeding done if small intestine is damaged. There are two methods of feeding, bolus feeding and continuous feeding. In bolus feeding rapid administration of set amount of nutrients at fixed intervals are done. Continuous drip feeding is tolerated better. Intravenous drip is given when orally it is not feasible and tube feeding is impracticable.

Feeding relationship The interactions or patterns of behaviors surrounding food preparation and consumption within a family.

Feeding through gastrostomy tube Sometimes surgeon performs gastrostomy operation for feeding a patient in case of operation over oesophagus or soft palate or tumours/strictures of oesophagus.

Nurse has to feed the patient carefully through the gastrostomy tube. The tube is inserted through an abdominal wall going into the stomach by piercing stomach wall. Catheter of tube is of self-retaining type. Tube is taken out periodically and is replaced by new one.

Fee-splitting The division of money received by a specialist between himself and the practitioner who referred the patient to him.

Feigned insanity There is always a motive for feigned insanity. People become insane to escape punishment. A definite diagnosis between a true insanity and a feigned insanity can be arrived by subjecting a person of observation of 10 days to and maximum of 30 days.

Feiss line It is an imaginary line from the first metatarsophalangeal joint to the medial malleolus. Ideally the navicular tuberosity should be palpable

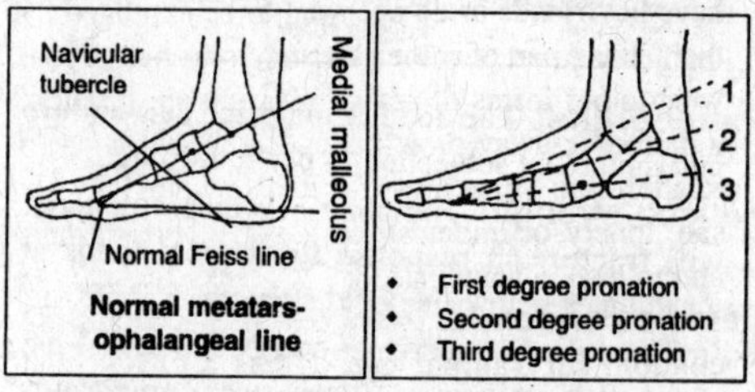

along this line, both while a person is bearing weight or not. Dropping of this bony landmark with weight bearing below the line leads to suspicion of flexible pes planus.

Felcon's infection It is the pulp space infection. The index finger and thumb are affected. Origin of infection may be a prick. It will have dull pain becoming worse when hand is depdendent. There develops swelling and 40 hours after it, there develops a throbbing pain interfering with sleep. Light pressure may increase the pain. Corresponding regional lymph nodes are enlarged and tender. If untreated, abscess tends to point towards the centre of the pulp. Then collar stud abscess may develop.

Felon It is an infection of closed space of the pulp of the distal phalanx. It is secondary to a local

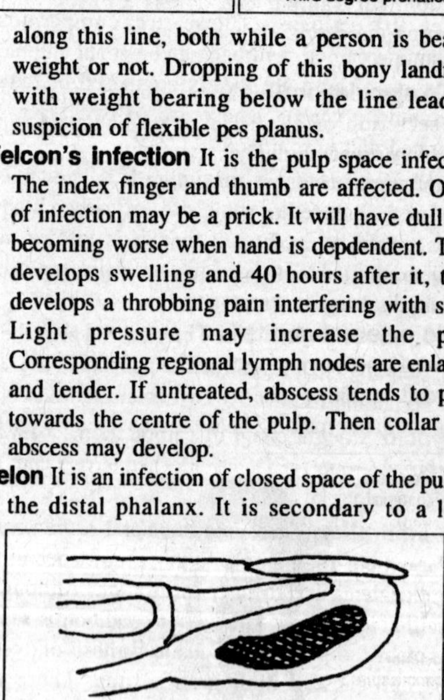

Felon—pus accumulation in pulp

puncture wound and is characterised by rapidly increasing pressure and pain. Osteomyelitis of distal phalanx and extension of infection into flexor sheath or adjacent joint may result. Early incision and drainage are indicated.

Felony Serious criminal offense.

Felty's syndrome It is characterised by rheumatoid arthritis, wasting of muscles, easy fatiguability, low-grade fever, splenomegaly, lymphadenopathy, leucopenia, sometimes ulcertation in the legs, and increased susceptibility to infections.

Felxion A movement that decreases the angle between parts of a joint.

Female masturbation Some young girls masturbate before marriage because they do not have boyfriends or do not want to be exploited by them. It is a part of autoeroticism. Some masturbate when other forms of sexual pleasure are missing, a partner is away or something going wrong in a relationship. Some may masturbate when they are sad, lonely or under stress using it a last resort and to have a sound sleep.

Female condom A prelubricated polyurath are condom for vaginal use. It has a closed end covering the cervix and an open end fitting into introitus.

Female ejaculation This is not a correct term used for secretion of a lubricating fluid by glands adjacent to vagina during sexual stimulation. As sexual stimulation and excitement build up, the flow of the lubricating fluid increases. In certain cases sudden contraction of vaginal wall causes fluid to spurt which is commonly mistaken as female discharge.

Female external genitalia The external genitalia of female is known as vulva. The pudendal cleft is guarded on either side by two rounded folds of skin, the labia majora. These are covered by hair

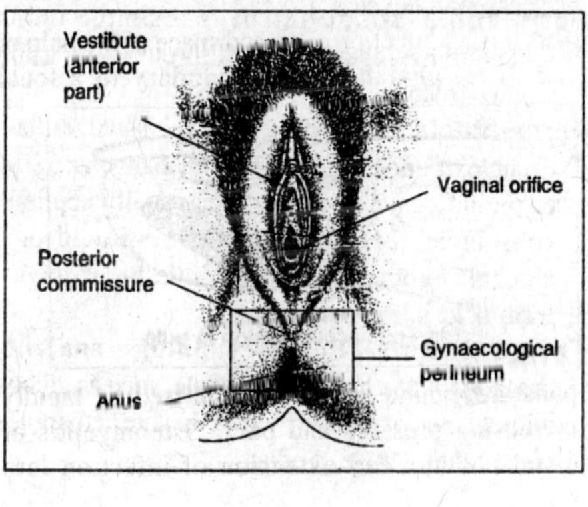

on their lateral aspect. Between the labia majora are two smaller folds, the labia minora. Between the labia minora and the clitoris in front is the area known as the vestibule of the vagina. The two labia minora unites behind to form a prominent fold known as the fourchette.

Female genital flora The fallopian tubes, the cavity of uterus and upper one-third of cervical canal are free of microorganisms. Lower one-third of cervical canal always contains microorganisms as does vagina. In healthy woman Doderlein's bacillus is the only organism which is found in upper two-third of vagina. During puerperium acidity of vagina is reduced and colliform bacilli may develop. After menopause Doderlein's bacillus are reduced, otherwise these produce lactic acid which does not allow other organisms to grow.

Female reproductive cycle (FRC) The combination of the menstrual and ovarian cycles

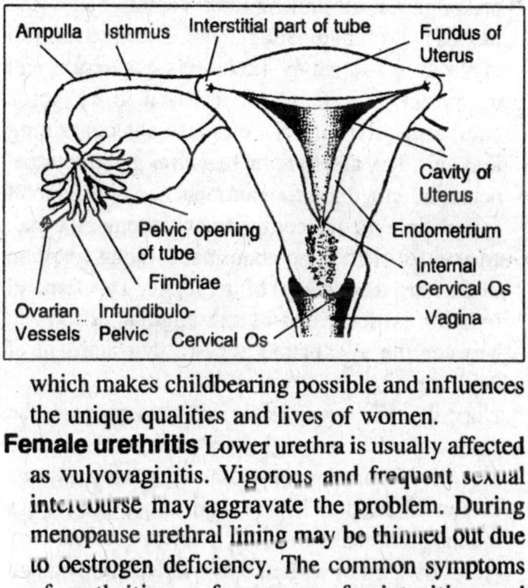

which makes childbearing possible and influences the unique qualities and lives of women.

Female urethritis Lower urethra is usually affected as vulvovaginitis. Vigorous and frequent sexual intercourse may aggravate the problem. During menopause urethral lining may be thinned out due to oestrogen deficiency. The common symptoms of urethritis are frequency of micturition and dysuria. Patient complains of pain during micturition and not at the end. Examination may reveal red urethral orifice.

Female urethral stenosis Common sites of narrowing are bladder neck and meatus. It may be congenital or as a result of infection, injury and neoplasm. Patient complains of poor stream, and repeated urinary infections. Treatment includes control of infection and removal of cause surgically.

Femoral Pertaining to femur.

Femoral anteversion Internal rotatory angulation of the femur due to anterior angulation of the femoral neck causes femoral anteversion.

Femoral canal It is the inner most, medial compartment of femoral sheath. Canal is about 2 cm, long end is conical in shape with the base directed upwards. At the base lies the femoral ring above up to saphenous ring below. All the boundaries are rigid except the fibrous septum laterally. The ring is closed above by the septum cruale. Contents of femoral canal are fibrofatty tissue, lymph nodes and lymphatics.

Femoral retroversion External rotatory angulation of the femur due to posterior angulation of the femoral retroversion.

Femoral shaft line The line seen on X-Ray running parallel to the long axis of femur.

Femoral sheath This is a funnel-shaped fascial prolongation around femoral vessels below the medial half of inguinal ligament. The anterior wall of sheath is formed by the fascia transversalis and the posterior wall by fascia iliaca. It has three compartments: lateral compartment containing femoral artery and femoral branch of genitofemoral nerve; Intermediate compartment contains femoral vein ; while medial compartment is femoral canal.

Femoral torsion Is an abnormal twisting (rotation in the transverse plane) of the femur. This femoral twisting is described as the angular difference between the axis of the upper femur and that of the knee.

Normally, the upper femur is anterverted i.e. the head and neck are angled forward relative to the rest of femur. Increased anterversion allows increased medial hip rotation equivalent to a medial rotational deformity. The upper femur may be retroverted or angled posteriorly. Retroversion is uncommon and results in increased lateral rotation of the hip. An abnormal increase in anterversion or retroversion is sometimes called antetorsion and retrotorsion. The terms medial femoral torsion and lateral femoral torsion are used more common.

Femoral-popliteal bypass A surgical procedure in which a vascular prosthesis is placed to bypass an occlusion of the distal femoral artery or proximal popliteal artery, or both

Femur It is the longest bone in the body. Lower end forms a knee joint. Upper end is a ball shaped fitting in acetabulum of hip bone forming a hip

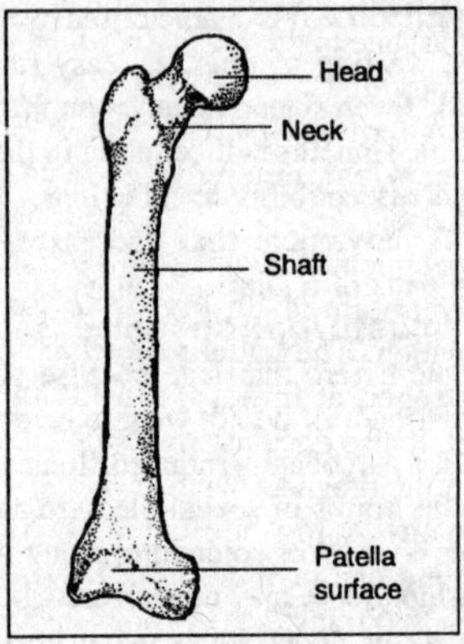

joint. Neck is a narrow point and vulnerable to fracture specially in old age. The shaft of femur is surrounded by powerful muscles.

Femur length A diagnostic parameter used in determining gestational age and skeletal dysplasia, whereby the femur is measured from the origin to the distal end of the shaft.

Fenestra Any window-like opening.

Fenestra ovalis Fenestra vestibuli

Fenestrated drape A drape with a round or slitlike opening in the center.

Fenestration Isolated area in which a root is denuded of bone when the marginal bone is intact.

Ferguson angle An angle measured on a lateral radiograph of the lumbar spine. It is formed between plane of superior margin of sacrum and horizontal line.

Ferguson's speculum It is a simple tubular speculum having no valves. It protects the wall of vagina when in use.

Fermentable Term applied to a substance that is capable of undergoing chemical change as a result of the influence of an enzyme; usually applied to substances that break down to an acid or an alcohol; applied to carbohydrate breakdown to form acid in the dental plaque.

Fermentation Energy-yielding anaerobic breakdown of a nutrient molecule, such as glucose, without net oxidation; yields lactate, ethanol, or some other simple product.

Fermentation balance The sum of the oxidized and the reduced compounds arising during a process of fermentation; this must equal the oxidation state of the substrate, which is calculated in arbitrary units.

Ferning A fern-like pattern seen microscopically when cervical mucus is viewed under the microscope.

The specimen is taken from the cervical area, usually obtained during a sterile speculum examination. The pattern confirms the presence of oestrogen at midcycle in the menstruating women. It also documents the rupture of amniotic fluid in the pregnant woman.

Ferredoxin A low molecular weight protein containing one or more iron-sulfur clusters that functions to transfer electrons from one enzyme system to another.

Ferritin One of the forms in which iron is stored in the body, an iron-protein complex.

Fertility The capability to reproduce; the ability to produce offspring. This can be expressed or measured as the number of live births produced by a group per unit of time.

Fertility awareness The development of familiarity with the bodily signs of impending ovulation and bodily signs after ovulation, which enables a woman to anticipate her fertile period and its ending.

Fertility, female It depends on normal ovulation and easy passage of egg into a fallopian tube towards the uterus. The process of fertility is

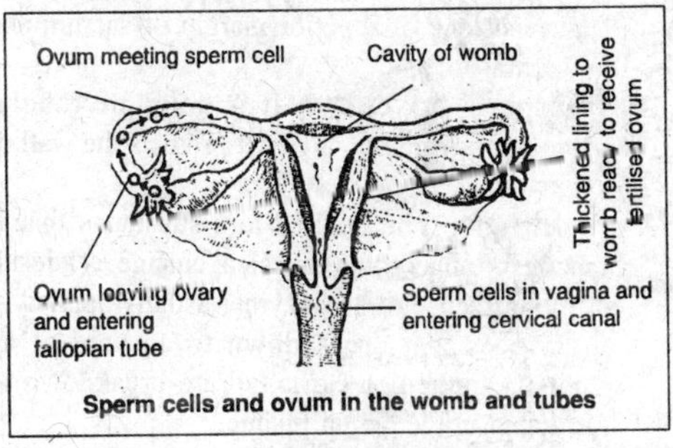

Sperm cells and ovum in the womb and tubes

dependent on gonadotropins, sex hormones, oestrogen and progesterone by the ovaries. Women become fertile at puberty and remain so until menopause.

Fertility, male Fertility of male depends on many factors such as healthy sperm in sufficient quantity, ability to erect and retain. One in 80,000 sperm ejaculated get entrance into vagina. Normal

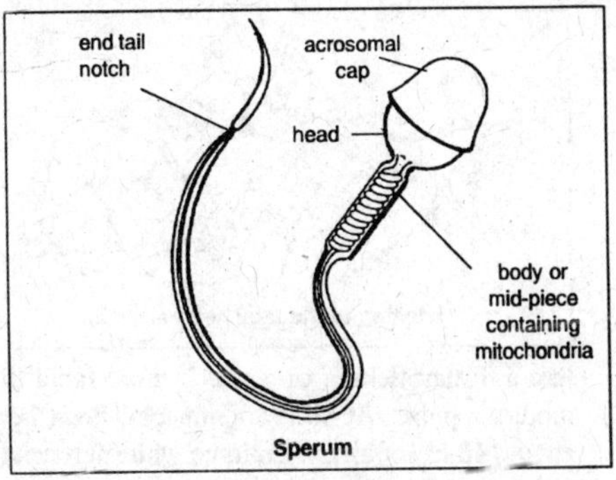

Sperum

fertility requires large number of sperms to be ejaculated to pass away the hostile environment of acidity of cervix. Men become fertile at the age of puberty and remain so till 70 years of age.

Fertilization Following fertilization and fusion cell division in the zygote does not begin upto 30 hours. Once the first division into two cells has occurred

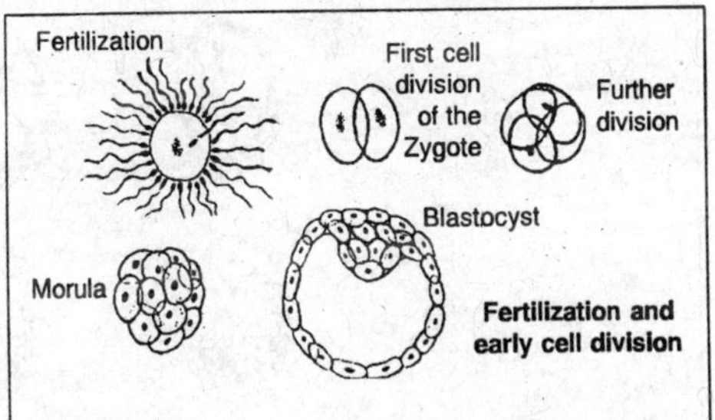

Fertilization and early cell division

further cell division follows rapidly. After 4 days one can identify an outer layer of cells, an inner mass of cells and a cavity containing clear fluid known as blastocyst.

Fertilization cone The microfilament-containing eruption on the egg's surface that assembles around the entering, successful sperm. There fertilization cone is responsible for the physical incorporation of the sperm into the egg cytoplasm in most nonmamalian systems.

FES Functional electrical stimulation.

Festoon Large roll of marginal gingiva, usually around the facial surface of a tooth.

Fetal heart The recognition of sounds of fetal heart is most conclusive of all clinical signs of pregnancy. The fetal heart sound sometimes can be heard by 24 weeks. At sixth month fetal heart sound is faint

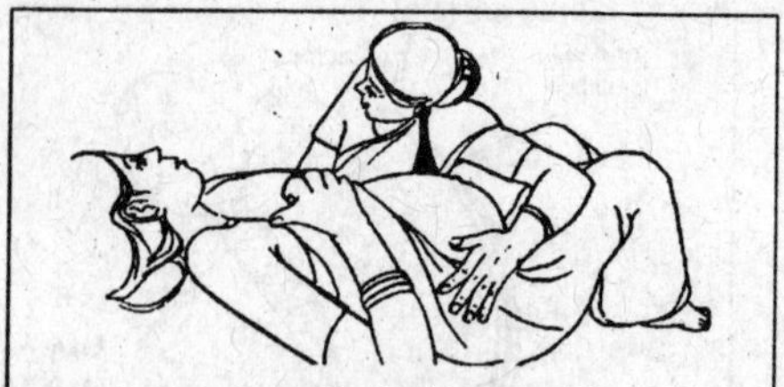

Listening to the fetal heart sounds

like a distant ticking of a watch more rapid than mother's pulse. At sixth month fetal heart beats about 140 to 160 times a minute while at term it is 120 to 140.

Fetal hydrops A large-for-date fetus may be the first indication of fetal hydrops with polyhydraminos. The presence of any two of following features allows a diagnosis of hydrops, fetal oedema, placental enlargement, polyhydraminos, ascites and pleural effusion.

Fetal lie Fetal lie is the relationship of the long axis of the fetus to the long axis of the mother. It can be detected by finding the two ends (poles) of the fetus. The head is usually harder and rounder than the large diffuse soft bottom of fetus. A line drawn between these two poles is the fetal axis.

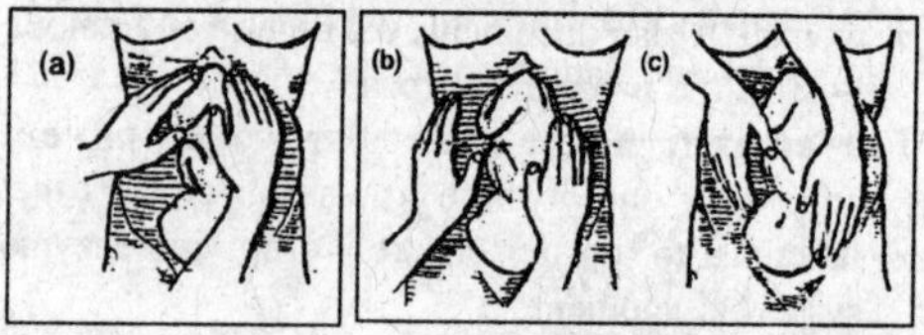

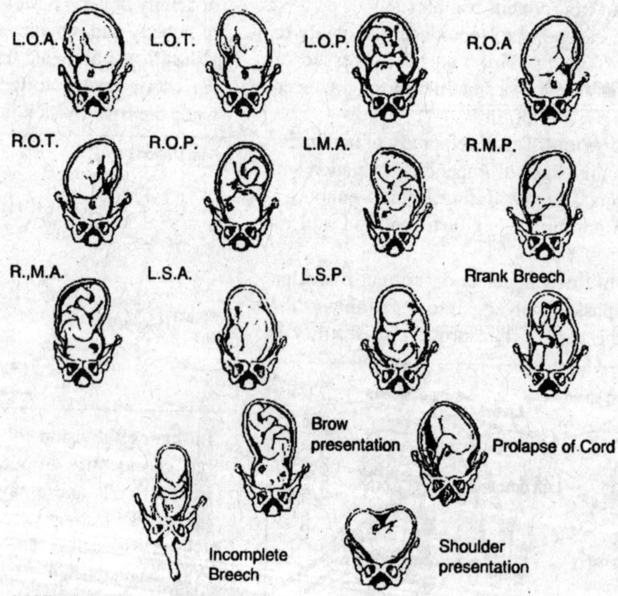

L.M.T.—Left mentum anterior
L.M.T.—Left mentum transverse
L.M.P.—Left mentum posterior
R.M.A.—Right mentum anterior
R.M.T.—Right mentum transverse
R.M.P.—Right mentum posterior
Breech presentations :
L.S.A.—Left sacrum anterior
L.S.T.—Left sacrum transverse
L.S.P.—Left sacrum posterior
R.S.A.—Right sacrum anterior
R.S.T.—Right sacrum transverse
R.S.P.—Right sacrum posterior
Transverse (shoulder) presentations :
L.Sc.A.—Left scapula anterior
L.Sc.P.—Left scapula posterior
R.Sc.A.—Right scapula anterior
R.Sc.P.—Right scapula posterior

Fetal alcohol effects Birth defects that may be attributed to maternal alcohol use but that do not manifest as the complete fetal alcohol syndrome.

Fetal alcohol syndrome A congenital anomaly resulting from maternal alcohol intake above 3 oz of absolute alcohol per day. It is characterised by typical craniofacial and limb defects, cardiovascular defects, intrauterine growth retardation (IUGR) and developmental delay. No safe alcohol limit has been determined. Alcohol consumption should totally be forbidden during pregnancy. Same is also true for drugs of abuse, drugs for recreation and smoking.

Fetal asphyxia Lack of oxygen is the most important and dangerous cause of depression of respiratory centre. Oxygen is brought to these respiratory centres by fetal blood. It will happen when uteroplacental circulation fails and when fetal head is subjected to prolonged compression during labour. It may be caused by premature detachment of placenta and placental insufficiency. Fetus has to make strenuous efforts to initiate pulmonary respiration prematurely while it is still *in utero*. In attempt, at the same time liquor amnii, mucus or meconium may be aspirated by fetus and even death may occur.

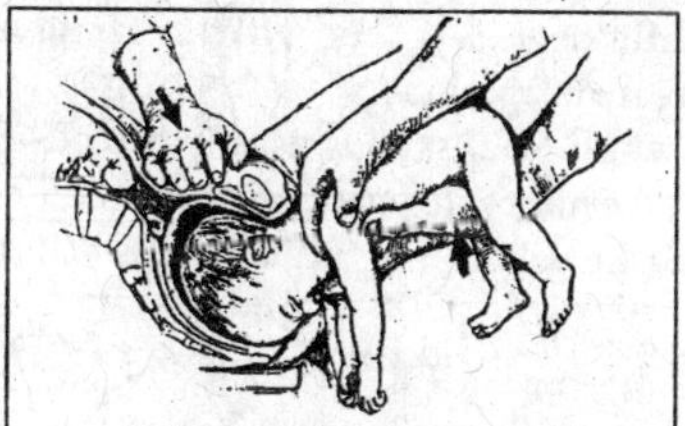

Delivery of after coming head

Fetal circulation Blood circulates differently in fetus than it does after birth. The fetus neither breathes nor eats. Fetus gets oxygen and nutrients from placenta and umbilical cord. Blood bypasses the lungs in the fetus. The oxygenated blood flows to the fetus along a vein in the umbilical cord then enters the right atrium after which, instead of flowing to the lungs it bypasses them. It does this bypassing into the left atrium through foramen ovale. The blood then passes to the left ventricle from where it is pumped into the upper parts. It then returns into right atrium and from there into right ventricle.

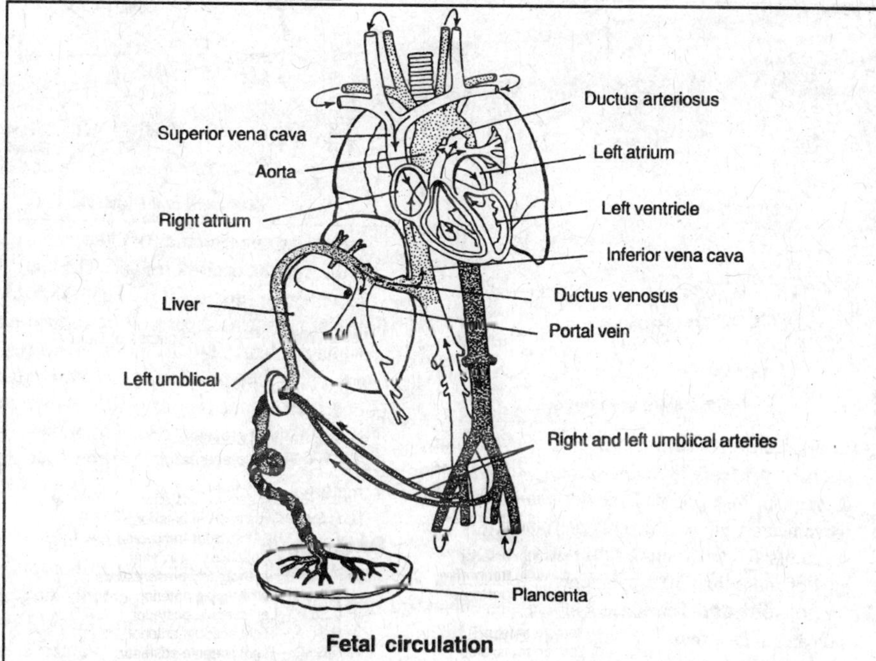

Fetal circulation

Fetal death Death of the fetus that occurs in the uterus prior to birth.

Fetal echocardiography A noninvasive technique used to identify structural cardiac defects and disturbances of cardiac rhythm.

Fetal excretion Fetal metabolism is mainly anabolic and excretion is not very great. Fetus is believed to pass urine contributing a small part of liquor amnii. The waste products urea, uric acid and salts pass through the placenta to the mother for excretion.

Fetal lung fluid fluid that fills that fetal lung; expanding the alveoli and promoting lung development.

Fetal membrane One of the extraembryonic membranes that usually participate in protection of the conceptus and/or the formation of placental structures that are sites of physiological exchange between conceptus and mother; these include the allantois, amnion, chorion, and yolk sac.

Fetal monitoring Auscultation of fetal heart sounds at frequent intervals, with regards to rate and regularity. Fetal echocardiography is of great help.

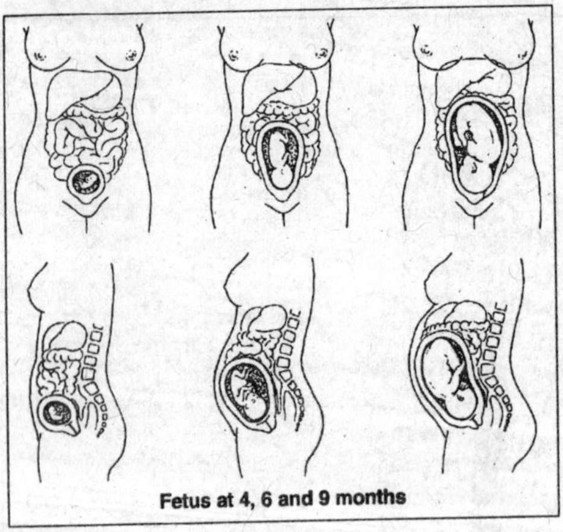

Fetus at 4, 6 and 9 months

Fetal movements count It is used to evaluate the status of the fetus at risk. Normally, fetus moves at frequent intervals and mother can count these movements well. Movements are counted in four segments for half-hour each, during the day. A total of more than 10 movements is reassuring.

Fetal personhood The concept of fetal personhood indicates that a fetus has legal and ethical rights outside of its mother's.

Fetal phase Period extending from the eighth to the thirty-ninth week of gestation; during this phase the term fetus is used.

Fetal position The direction that gives fetal landmark facing in the maternal pelvis.

Fetal scalp stimulation Variety of stimulators is a noninvasive method which shows a nonstress test acceleratory response in fetal heart pattern of a sleepy or otherwise non responsive baby.

Fetal size in diabetes Over sized fetus is a common complication. Weight of fetus may be more than 10 pounds. There will be round and cushingoid feature of face, an increased length proportionate to the weight. Oversized fetus is more seen in prediabetic women. The excess fetal insulin acts as a fetal growth factor causing increased deposition of fat.

Fetal skull Fetal skull is usually one of flexion so that submentobregmatic diameter (9.5 cm) will enter the pelvic brim. If the head is deflexed then

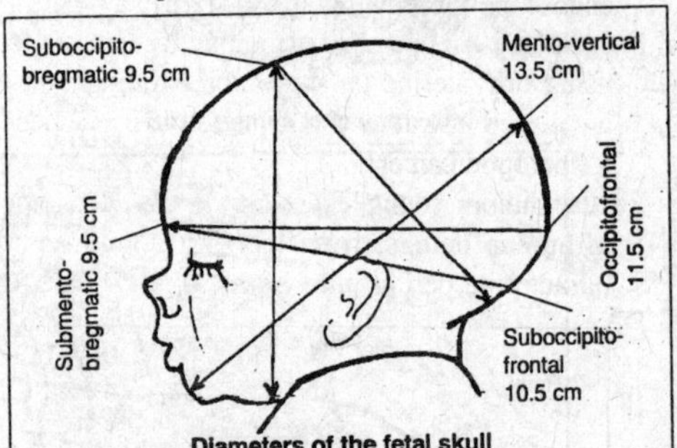

Diameters of the fetal skull

presenting diameter may be either submentofrontal (10.5 cm) or occipitofrontal (11.5 cm). In brow presentation, it is mentovertical (13.5 cm).

Fetal surgery An operation performed on a fetus while the fetus remains inside the uterus.

Fetal zone The unique large central compartment of the fetal adrenal cortex which secretes androgens and which regresses following birth.

Fetal-pelvic index A method that combines maternal X-ray pelvimetry with fetal sonography to predict fetal-pelvic disproportion.

Fetid breath Foul-smelling breath.

Fetishism It is a psychosexual disorder in which sexual gratification is repeatedly or exclusively achieved through fondling, kissing or licking inanimate objects such as women's bra, hair, undergarments, etc. Handling these objects is often accompained by sexual fantasies and masturbation.

Fetomaternal hemorrhage The transfer across the placenta of fetal red blood cells into the maternal circulation.

Fetor oris It is known as halitosis also. Bad breath may arise in any of areas, the lungs, breath passage, nose and mouth. Breath odour originating in lungs has smell of garlic and alcohol. Similarly there may be acetone breath in uncontrolled diabetes. Bronchiectasis and advanced malignancy also impart bad breath. Purulent sinusitis and atrophic rhinitis may also result it. In majority of cases bad breath originates in oral cavity. Ulcerative gingivitis, unfilled cavities, decomposed food remnants also give bad breath. Coated tongue and mouth breathing are source of foul breath.

Fetoscope 1. A head stethoscope designed especially for listening to fetal heart tones. 2. An endoscope for viewing a fetus.

Fetoscopy An operative technique for fetal surgery using tiny uterine puncture holes through which are placed instruments and a telescope attached to a fiberoptic camera.

Fetus Unborn young, especially in the later stages, in human beings, from the third month of the intrauterine period until birth.

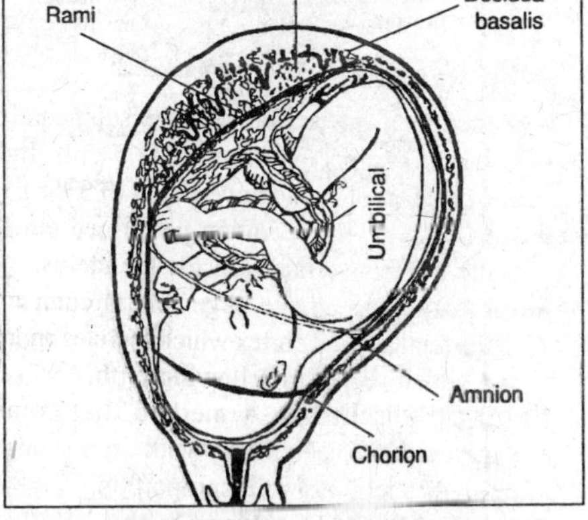

Fetus acardius Affected fetus is an amorphous mass. It may be an inherent development error and arises from interference with blood supply.

Fetus papyraceous In both monozygotic and dizygotic twins one fetus may overgrow more than the other fetus and deprive the other of its normal share of blood and nutrition. The second fetus dies due to compression between uterine wall and membranes of living child. Dead child is known as papyraceous.

Fever Pyrexia is defined as body temperature above 98.6°F. It is some time an indication of infection. It has different patterns in different diseases. In malaria, it may be with shivering followed by hot stage on alternate days. In typhoid evening rise of temperature, lower in morning but not normal at any time is seen. High fever in children may result in convulsions. Fever is an attempt to destroy the invading organism. Antipyretic drugs may be given to lower body temperature. These will relieve pain also.

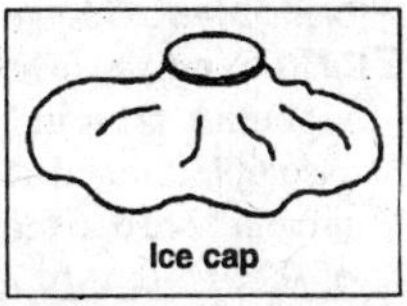

Ice cap

FHR Abbreviation for fetal heart rate.

Fiberoptics Transmission of light along a course of flexible material, plastic or glass. The intense light may be used to transilluminate teeth in diagnosing caries, to augment visualization of the operative field when incorporated in a handpiece, and to accelerate the initiator incorporated in visible (while) light-polymerized composites.

Fiber-reinforced polymer Glass, carbon aramid and ultrahigh-molecular-weight polyethylene have been used as a fiber reinforcing agents for removable and fixed prosthetic appliances.

Fibers Threadlike structures; for example, nerve fibers.

Fibre This is an indigestible component of plants some of which are fibrous. It includes certain types of polysaccharides, cellulose, gums and pectins. Lignin is also fibre. Humans do not contain any enzyme to digest these fibres. These are passed out as indigested and do not yield energy. These have capacity to bind water and adding bulk to faeces. Whole grains, root vegetables and fruits are good sources of fibre.

Fibre persistence A determination of the length of time that a foreign fiber remains on a recipient garment or fabric.

Fibre transfer Movement of a fiber or fibers from one textile material to another, usually through direct contact or through an intermediate contact.

Fibreoptic endoscopy One can inspect directly the oesophagus, the stomach, the duodenum and proximal small intestines. A colonscope allows direct inspection of colonic mucosa. Endoscopy is also valuable in the patient who is bleeding if the investigation is done within 24 to 48 hours.

Fibriae Fringe.

Fibrillation Munute skeletal muscle conractions resulting from denervation supersensitivity.

Fibrilloblast Odontoblast.

Fibrin Whitish, insoluble protein that forms the essential protein of a blood clot fibrinogen. Insoluble protein in clotted blood. A thread-like protein fibre derived from fibrinogen by the action of thrombin; forms a clot, that is, a network of fibres that traps blood cells, platelets, and fluid, which stops bleeding.

Fibrinase Plasmin.

Fibrinogen It is either formed in liver or controlled by it. When fibrinogen is removed from body replacing the blood by defibrinated blood, it is readily regenerated in a few hours if liver is intact. Fibrinogen has the property of clotting. Tissue injury and inflammation stimulate fibrinogen production.

Fibrinolysis Dissolution of fibrin by the enzymatic action of plasmin.

Fibrinolytic activity A measure of the ability of blood to dissolve a thrombus.

Fibrinolytic drugs These break down thrombus once formed. Warfarin and heparin are more effective in venous thrombus because it contains more fibrin while antiplatelet drugs are more effective in arterial thrombus.

Fibroadenoma It is a benign, fibrous tumour found commonly in breast. These are painless, firm, round lumps usually 0.5 to 2 inches in diameter. These are freely movable and not attached to skin. These generally develop in young women. Multiple fibroadenomas may develop in both breasts.

Fibroblast A flat, elongated cell associated with the formation of the fibro-collagenous network of the body, including tendons, aponeuroses, and supporting and binding tissues.

Fibroid It is a benign tumour of uterus. These are bundles of smooth muscles and connective tissue growing slowly within the uterine wall. These may be of different sizes and may protrude in uterine cavity. These develop between the age of 35 and 45. If fibroid is small it may not cause any symptoms. But if it grows and erodes uterine lining may cause heavy or prolonged bleeding. If twisted may cause severe pain. Distorting uterine cavity may cause infertility or miscarriage. Ultrasound is a good tool to examine it. Surgical removal is necessary if these become complicated. If no complications are there then no treatment is required.

Fibroid lung There is localised fibrosis in one or more areas often associated with bronchiectasis. Common cause is chronic pulmonary tuberculosis. Prominent symptom is shortness of breath may be at work or at rest. There is cough with change of position and sputum is copious and more purulent. Palpation confirms lack of movement and usually shows increased tactile and vocal fremitus. There is dull percussion over fibrotic area with unilateral fibrotic change.

Fibroids during pregnancy Uterine fibroids are found to complicate pregnancy depending on their size and location. All fibroids increase in size during pregnancy more due to oedema. Pregnancy in a submucus fibroid usually ends in abortion in first trimester due to distortion of cavity.

Fibrolysis The resolution or breakdown of abnormal fibrous tissue as in the creation of scar.

Fibroma Benign tumor composed primarily of fibrous connective tissue.

Fibromyalgia It is characterised by widespread pain with multiple tender points on examination. Patient will feel tiredness and nonrestorative sleep.

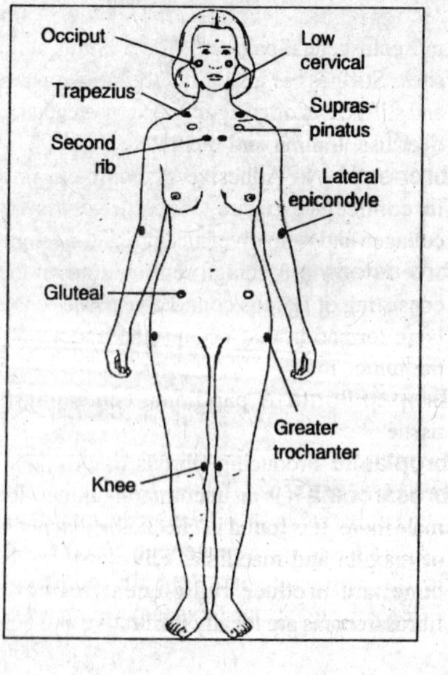

Patients feel unfreshed, stiffness, anxiety and depression. It can be extremely debilitating early morning.

Fibromyalgia pain pattern Typical pain is diffuse involving muscle groups in back and in upper and lower extremities bilaterally. Areas of subjective numbness are reported. Stabbing pain is often noted when trigger points coexist.

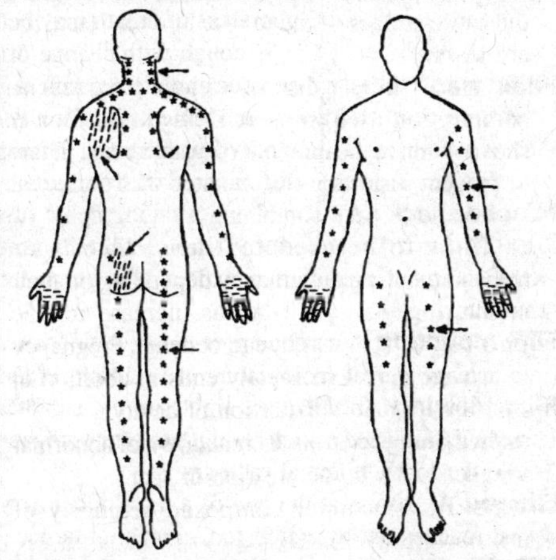

x Pain = Numbness /// Stabbing pain

Fibromyalgia syndrome It is a clinically recognizable condition with chronic musculoskeletal pain and tender points at multiple sites. Stiffness is also a bothering symptom. Pain and stiffness is often aggravated by weather factors, over use, trauma and mental stress.

Fibronectin An Adhesive glycoprotein important in connective tissue, where it cross links to collagen and is involved in aggregation of platelets.

Fibro-osteoma A benign central tumor of the jaws, consisting of fibrous connective tissue with foci of bone formation that occupy the major portion of the tumor mass.

Fibropapilloma A papilloma containing fibrous tissue.

Fibroplastic Producing fibrous tissue.

Fibrosarcoma It is an uncommon tumour. It affects male more. It is found in cheek, lip, and periosteum of maxilla and mandible. Fibrosarcoma destroys bone and produce radiolucent lesions. Most fibrosarcomas are locally infiltrative and persistent but they do not metastasise. The less common poorly differentiated fibrosarcomas metastasise widely and are fatal. Treatment includes wider excision.

Fibrosclerosis Fibrosis associated with sclerosis.

Fibrosis The reactive or preparative process in which fibrous tissue is formed.

Fibrositis It may cause pain and stiffness but inflammation is not proved on investigations. Tension and bad posture may cause the condition. If you sit in a cramped up position it may be caused.

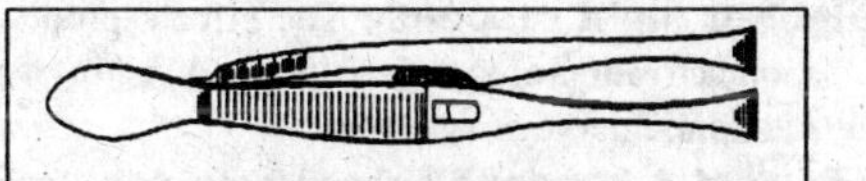

Fixation forceps

There is no restriction of movements. Pain killers, hot bath, analgesic anti-inflammatory massage relieves the pain and stiffness.

Fibroskeleton of the heart An intricate, malleable, three-dimensional continuum of dense and membraneous collagen forming the annuli of the principal valvular orifices.

Fibrous epulis It arises from the periosteum or from the periodontal membrane and forms a firm nodule at the junction of gum and tooth. Chronic dental sepsis is the predisposing factor. Histologically, it is a whorled fibroma and is composed of fusiform cells. It is more commonly found on the external aspect of gum, at the neck of canine or premolar tooth. It may be sessile or pedunculated. It is slowly growing. It is firm but not tender. The adjacent teeth are irregularly displaced and loosened. Draining lymph nodes are not enlarged. It has a tendency to recur after operation. Excision of the swelling is the choice of treatment.

Fibrous joint A type of articulation bound by fibrous connective tissue that allows little or no movement.

Fibrous proteins Insoluble proteins that serve as a protective or structural role; contain polypeptide chains that generally share a common secondary structure.

Fibrous tunic The superficial coat of the eyeball, made up of the posterior sclera and the anterior cornea.

Fibula The slender non-weight-bearing bone located on the lateral aspect of the leg.

Fick method Measuring the degree of deformity of hip flexion instance.

Fictive kin A concept from anthropology along the lines of chosen family but carrying the implication that the fictive kin is not "real."

Field potential The summed graded potentials of a number of neurons.

Field size The area and shape of a body portion to be irradiated.

Fifth lumbar root Fifth root syndrome includes unilateral limitation of straight leg raising, with increase in root pain on neck flexion. There may be cutaneous analgesia at outer leg.

Fight-or flight response The effects produced upon activation of the sympathetic division of the autonomic nervous system.

Figure of '8' bandage It is used for fracture clavicle and wrist joint. It begins with circular fixing turns above the wrist joint. The bandage is then passed obliquely down on the back of wrist and to the palm, round wrist at the base of fingers and then again to wrist back, over carpals, to the base of little finger and again round the wrist.

Figure-ground discrimination The ability to distinguish a figure from the background in which it is embedded.

Figure-ground relationships When one element of a stimulus stands out among the rest, that element is the figure and the remainder is background. An airplane is perceived against the sky or a song is heard in the context of talking.

Filarial fever It is periodic in nature. Onset is sudden with chill and rigor similar to malarial fever and fever of urinary tract infection. Temperature is often high 103 to 104 °F and may continue for several days. The temperature comes down by crisis and profuse sweating. There will be symptoms of toxaemia, i.e. tachycardia, flushed face, dry coated tongue, severe headache and loss of appetite. Simultaneously, there may be associated pain, swelling and tenderness of spermatic cord and scrotum. There is leucocytosis with increase of neutrophils.

Filariasis It is a disease caused by parasitic worm or larvae which are transmitted to man by insect bite. Blood sucking insects ingest the microfilariae while feeding on blood from infected people. Later on transmit them to others by biting. It may cause localised oedema. On repeated attacks, the lower limbs or scrotum become enlarged. Skin becomes thick, coarse and fissured. The diagnosis is done on microscopic examination of blood and lymph fluid. Three week course of hetrazan (Diethylcarbamazine) is effective.

File A surgical or a dental instrument with a finely serrated surface, for reducing surplus hard substance, such as bone or materials used in dental restorations, or for smoothing roughtened surfaces.

Filiform papillae Numerous small projections over the entire surface of the tongue in which taste buds are absent.

Filler wad Circular disc of various thickness and composition used in short shells to cushion the shot column at the moment of acceleration in order to prevent distortion due to inter-shot contact.

Film badge A pack containing a radiographic film or films to be used for the detection and measurement of radiation exposure in personnel monitoring.

Film mounting A cardboard or plastic holder used to arrange dental radiographs in anatomic order.

Film viewing An adequate light source, subdued room lighting and a magnifying glass are necessary in order to view dental radiograph.

Filopod A process at the end of a developing axon that reaches out to search for a potential target.

Filtrates Filtrates are the clean liquids obtained by passing a mixture containing a suspension through some type of filter system. The suspension is isolated as the residue.

Filtration The process whereby pressure produces a flow of fluid through a semipermeable membrane. Movement, resulting from a pressure difference, of a liquid through a filter, which prevents some or all of the substances in the liquid from passing.

Filtration membrane Site of blood filtration in nephrons of the kidneys, consisting of the endothelium and basement membrane of the glomerulus and the epithelium of the visceral layer of the glomerular (Bowman's) capsule.

Fimbria Fringe of white fibers along the edge of the hippocampus.

Fimbriae Hairlike proteinaceous appendages (100 to 1000 per cell) 2 to 8 nm in diameter, on the surface of bacteria. Often involved in adhesion to specific types of eukaryotic host cells.

Fimbriectomy The surgical removal of the end of the fallopain tube.

Fine motor skill The ability to use the small muscles of the body, esepcially the hand muscles, to perform tasks.

Fine-wire indwelling electrode Small diameter insulated wires inserted into the muscle belly by means of a hypodermic needle.

Finger adduction and abduction This test is often performed as a test of ulnar nerve function as the interossei are innervated by this nerve.

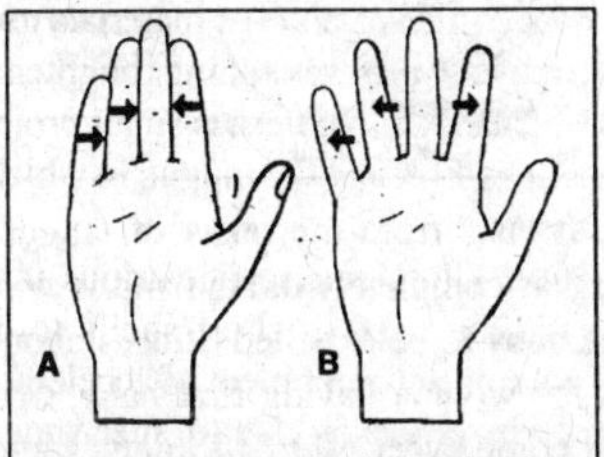

(A) Finger adduction (B) abduction

Finger agnosia The inability to identify the fingers on one's own hands or on the hands of the examiner, including difficulty in naming the fingers upon command, identifying which finger was touched.

Finger bandage Bandaging a finger is effectively done using a spiral and recurrent loop technique. In last narrow strip of adhesive is used.

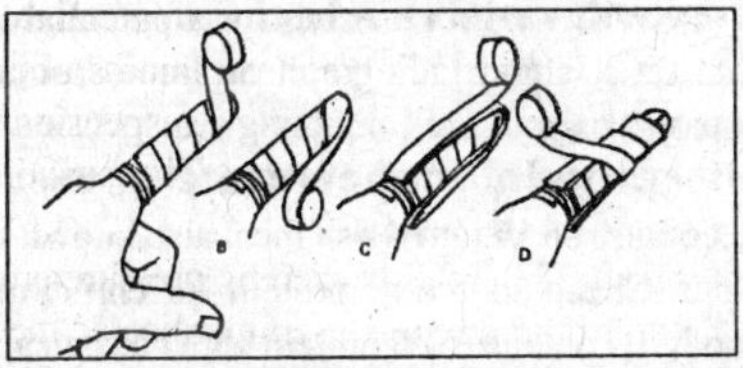

Finger Pad Kneading The basic circular kneading stroke is performed with the pads of one or more finger tips, using either hand or both. If the hands are placed opposite each other e.g., around the elbow region, then the fingers usually work in phase with each other.

Finger sweep Insertion of the index finger into the mouth along the inside of the cheek and deeply into the throat to the base of the tongue.

Fingernail artefact An artefact seen on dental radiographs when the film emulsion is damaged by the operator's fingernail during rough handling of the film; results in black crescent shaped marks.

Fingerprint artefact An aircraft seen on dental radiographs when the film is touched by fingers contaminated with fluoride or developer solution; results in black fingerprints on the film.

Fingerprint residue The chemical including proteins, lipids and water that are deposited on a surface from contact with the outer joint of a finger.

Fingerprints These are papillary ridges especially on the skin of terminal phalanges. The arrangement of these ridges is very specific and do not tally to each other. Chances are there that one in 6400 million may have similar pattern, hence thumb prints are used for identification marks. There are numerous sweat glands in the skin of palm and digits and their openings can be seen on papillary ridges.

Fingertipping First tactile experience between mother and newborn.

Finger-to-nose-test A test of cerebellar function.

Finish Degree of finish of a polished surface; the removal of excess restorative material from the margins and contours of a restoration; polishing the restoration.

Finishing Procedure by which roughness of a restoration is smoothed.

Finite Element Analysis In Implant dentistry, a computer assisted method in which a device and the bone or tissues with which it will be associated are theoretically modeled using geometric shapes (elements) in which each corner (node) of the shape (elements) in which each corner (node) of the shape can be analyzed for direction, magnitude, duration, and rate of force transfer along each axis.

Finkelstein's test It is useful in diagnosing de Quervain's disease. Patient is asked to fix the

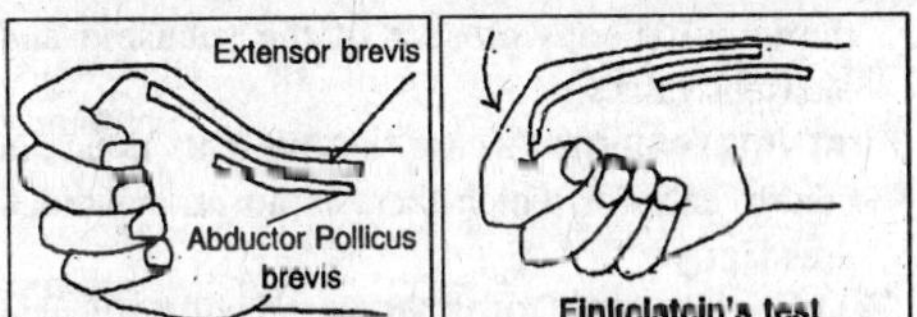

Finkelstein's test

thumb into the palm enclosing it in a fist. Then either active or passive ulnar deviation of wrist is executed. This motion results in moderate to severe pain.

Firbosis Abnormal formation of fibrous tissue.

Fire brigade In most of cities fire stations are there having many big vehicles, water tankers, cranes and well-trained people to control the fire. They are having specific fixed telephone number to be called upon in emergency.

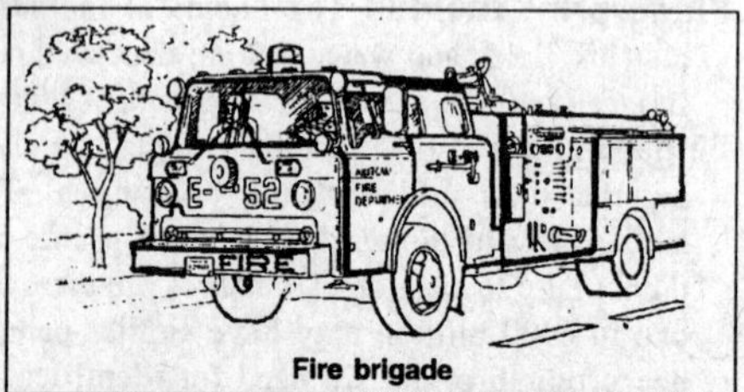

Fire brigade

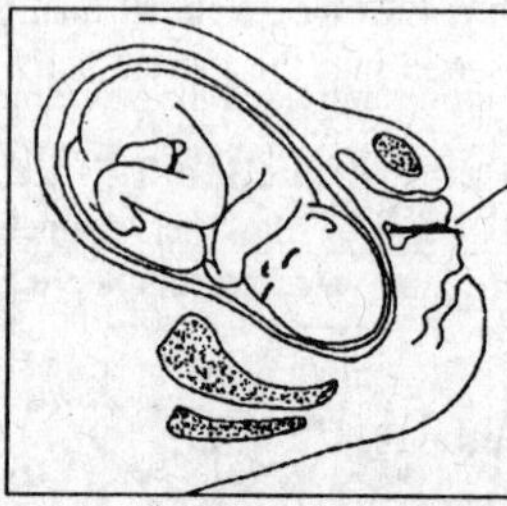

Fire plan Procedure followed if there is a fire.

Fire propagation The movement of a fire from the point of origin through to other places.

Fire seat The point of origin of a fire,

Fire triangle This is a simple geometric depiction of the three requirements for fire, that is, heat, oxygen and fuel. Without all of these components present, the triangle is incomplete and there will be no fire.

Firearm A device consisting of a barrel and associated firing mechanism which propels a projectile employing combustion of a powder fuel.

Firing pin The part of the firing mechanism that strikes the cartridge primer. This initiates the ignition process in the gun powder.

First aid kit It contains all items of emergency use stocked in a first aid box. It should be out of reach of children. Commercial first aid kits are available. It contains, dressing, antibiotic creams and certain known safe drugs. These items should be replaced off and on.

First heart sound The heart sound that results from the simultaneous closure of the tricuspid and bicuspid valves.

First impression A case that presents issues in controversy for which there is no prior judicial precdent.

First lumbar root Compression It will result pain in back radiating to region above trochanter and the groin.

First molars Primary and permanent teeth with four or five cusps and multiple roots.

First premolars Secondary teeth, also referred to as first bicuspids, located between the canines and first molars; usually have two cusps; replace the molars of the primary dentition.

First stage of labour This is the longest and hardest as it is the 'work' stage of labour and the time during which the cervix has to stretch and open. It lasts from the onset of labour until the cervix has completely dilated and is wide enough for the baby to be expelled. It lasts about 10 to 12 hours for woman having first baby. Contractions at first come every 10 to 15 minutes and lasts for 10 to 15 seconds. As labour progresses, contractions come closure. At the end of first stage they come every 2 to 3 minutes and lasts for 40 to 50 seconds.

First-degree atrioventricular block An impairment of the normal conduction between the atrial and the ventricles; characterized by a prolongation of the P-R interval.

First-intention healing Reparative process when wound edges are directly next to one another.

Fish mouth vertebra A biconcave vertebral body that on a lateral radiograph of spine specially in osteoporosis.

Fish protein concentrate Deodoused, decolourised, defatted fish meal also known as fish flour. Cheap source of protein for enrichment of foods. It contains 70% protein with biological value 75-80%.

Fission A mode of vegetative reproduction found in the yeast genus Schizosaccharomyces. Fission yeasts grow lengthwise and divide by forming a cell septum that separates mother cells into two equalized daughters.

Fissure A groove or narrow cleft that separates two parts, such as the cerebral hemisphere of the brain.

Fissure fracture A crack that penetrates the surface but does not go through a long way.

Fistula An abnormal opening between two internal structures or between an internal structure and the surface of the body.

Fitness The ability of an organism to pass on its genes to the next generation; the average reproductive success of a genotype in a particular environment, usually expressed relative to another genotype in that environment.

Fitness exercise Physical activity performed by healthy adults.

Five elements The chinese divided the world into five elements and every thing belongs to one or several of these five categories.

Fixed prosthodontics Phase of prosthodontics that deals with the replacement and/restoration of teeth by artificial substitutes that are not readily removable.

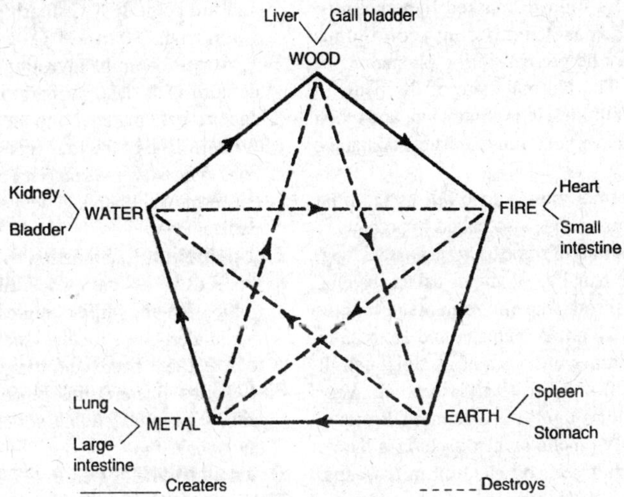

Five elements

Fix To make firm, stable and immovable.

Fixation The arrest of psychosocial development; may be considered pathologic, depending on the degree of intensity.

Fixation subluxation Lack of movement of a joint, caused by muscular spasm, a shortened ligament, or an intraarticular blocking.

Fixed appliance Orthodontic appliance that is cemented to the teeth or attached by means of an adhesive material.

Fixed cabinetry Nonmobile cabinetry found in the dental suite.

Fixed hip abduction An analogus manouevre is required to show or exclude fixed abduction.

Fixed macrophage Stationary phagocytic cell found in the liver, lungs, brain, spleen, lymph nodes, subcutaneous tissue, and red bone marrow.

Fixed nitrogen Chemically reduced or biologically converted nitrogen in a chemical form that can be assimilated readily by most microbes or plants.

Fixed partial denture A bridge replacing existing dentition that is permanently cemented to remaining teeth.

Fixed teeth The branch of prosthodontics concerned with the replacement and/or restoration of teeth by artificial substitutes that are not readily removable.

Fixed virus A laboratory strain that grows in tissue culture at a predictable rate, with predictable biological properties, and that will regularly kill inoculated animals within a predictable period.

Fixer cut-off An artefact on radiographs that results from a low level of fixer solution and represents an unfixed portion of the film; a straight, black border appears on the processed radiograph.

Fixer spots An artefact on radiographs caused by fixer solution coming in contact with the film before processing; light spots appear on the processed radiograph.

Fixing and suckling Infant is first made to feel the nipple. The nipple is then fixed and put into baby's mouth. Then with the baby's lips apart areola is made to contact the lips.

Fixture A type of root form implant.

Flaccid (hypotonicity) Paralysis of muscles in which there is an absence of reflexes in lower motor neuron disorders such as poliomyelitis.

Flaccid dysarthria Dysarthria associated with disorders of the lower motor neurons is characterized by mild to marked hypernasality, coupled with nasal emission; continuous breathiness may be present during phonation.

Flaccid Penis The Normal state of the penis in which the smooth muscle is contracied, and blood flow and intracavernous pressure are maintained at low levels.

Flaccidity Abnormal muscle tone felt as too little resistance to movement; also called hypotonus.

Flagella Motile strains of some bacteria possess long, thin, contractile hair-like filaments called flagella. These affect screw-like movements. Flagella measures 14 to 20 nm in diameter and 15 to 25 in length, several times of length of bacterial cell. It contains 1 to 20 or more flagella per cell. Very large number of flagella are seen in Proteus. Flagella can only function when bacteria is intact, Flagella are better seen by electron microscope. These are organs of locomotion.

Flagellar basal body The major structure of the flagellar motor, consisting of ring structures and a rod.

Flagellar pocket A depression in flagellates from which the flagellum emerges.

Flagellum A long hair-like motile process on the surface of a cell; usually only per cell, in contrast to cilia, which are short, motile, hair-like projections, with hundreds present on a single cell. Whip-like locomotor organelle similar to cilia except longer and there is usually one per cell; for example, spercells.

Flailing movements Thrashing about wildly.

Flange It is a part of denture base that extends from the cervical ends of teeth to the border of denture.

Flap surgery Incision and elevation of all or a portion of soft tissue in an area, completion of other procedures in conditions of good access and visibility, then repositioning and suturing of the soft tissue.

Flash back The feeling that one is re experiencing a traumatic event after it is over. Flash back may occur spontaneously or in response to sight, sound, smell and other sensation.

Flash point In frying oils the temperature at which the decomposition products can be ignited but will not support combustion. When they will support combustion this is a fire point. In case of cotton seed oil smoke point is 232° C, flash point 330°C and fire point 363° C. Flash point of different fat varies from 290 to 333°C.

Flasking Process of investing the cast and a wax denture in a flask preparatory to moulding the denture-base material into the form of the denture.

Flat bone One of the four types of bone; the frontal bone is an example of a flat bone. A bone that is in the form of a plate e.g. scapulae, ribs, pelvis and parietal bone.

Flat palpation Examination by finger pressure that proceeds across the muscle fibers at a right angle to their length, while compressing them against a firm underlying structure, such as bone. It is used to detect taut bands and trigger points.

Flat Sours Bacteria that render canned food sour without gas production. Ends of can are not swelled but remain flat.

Flatness of affect Dearth of emotional expression.

Flatogens Substances that cause gas production . Those identified include raffinose, stachyose and verbascose in a variety of beans.

Flatulence Production of gas in intestine hydrogen, CO_2 and methane caused by variety of foods onions, cabbage, gram, cauliflower.

Flatus Gas in the stomach or intestines; commonly used to denote expulsion of gas through the rectum.

Flatus tube This is a rubber tube thicker in diameter than Ryles tube. Passing a flatus tube into rectum may be required for relief of severe abdominal distension due to gas which may be arised postoperatively.

Flavedo The coloured outer peel layer of citrus fruits also called the epicarp or zest. It contains oil sacs and numerous yellow plastids. It is yellow in ripe fruits containing carotene and x-anthophyll.

Flavoprotein A conjugated protein containing a flacin pigment that is involved in electron transport within the mitochondria.

An enzyme containing a flavin nucleotide as a tightly bound prosthetic group. Proteins containing riboflavin derivatives.

Flavour enhancers These have little or no taste of their own but amplify the flavours. They exert synergetic and potentiation effect. Substances added to supplement, enhance or modify the original taste.

Flavour potentiator Substances that enhances the flavour of other substances. Without itself imparting any characteristic flavour of its own such as sugar, salt and vinegar.

Fleas These are blood sucking playing a role as intermediate hosts for helminth parasites. These

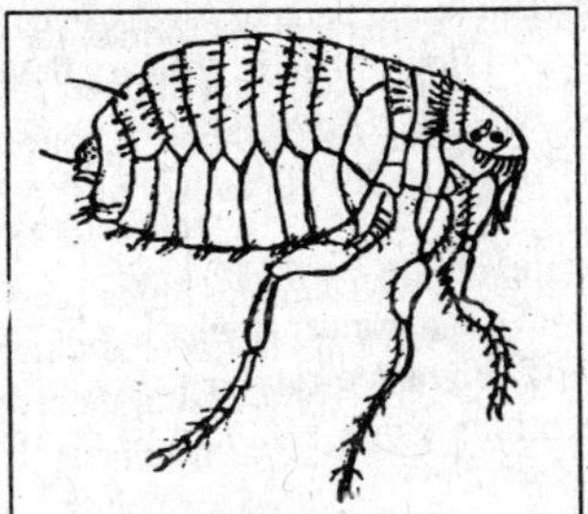

Flea—Female X-cheopis

are flattened laterally wingless and equiped with muscular hindlegs for jumping. A notorious organism transmitted by fleas is the bacillus Yersinia pestis causing bubonic plague.

Flexibility The ability to readily adapt to changes in position or alignment; may be expressed as normal, limited, or excessive.

Flexion The act of bending. In obstetrics, the process is the mechanism of labour referring to the bending

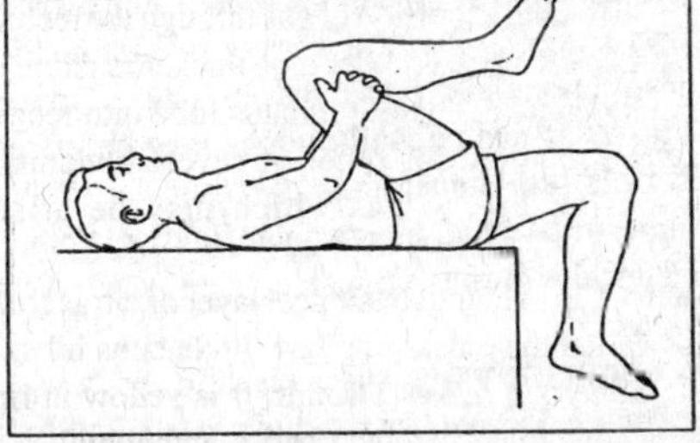

of the fetal head so that the chin is in contact with the chest, thus presenting the smallest anteroposterior diameter to the pelvis.

Flexion rotation fracture dislocation These result from flexion and rotation of lower dorsal or dorsolumbar region of spine. Fractures are unstable. Spinal canal is interrupted and posterior elements disrupted.

Flexor reflex It is a polysynaptic reflex requiring at least three neurons : (*i*) primary afferent neuron, (*ii*) interneuron in the dorsal horn, and (*iii*) alpha motor neuron supplying a flexor muscle. This is a protective mechanism. Peripheral receptors are free nerve endings. Suppose your hand is pricked by a needle, the limb flexes and withdraws from stimuli.

Flexor reticulum It is a strong fibrous band which lies on the anterior surface of wrist. It forms a tunnel on the front of wrist by virtue of curve. Several flexor tendons pass under it.

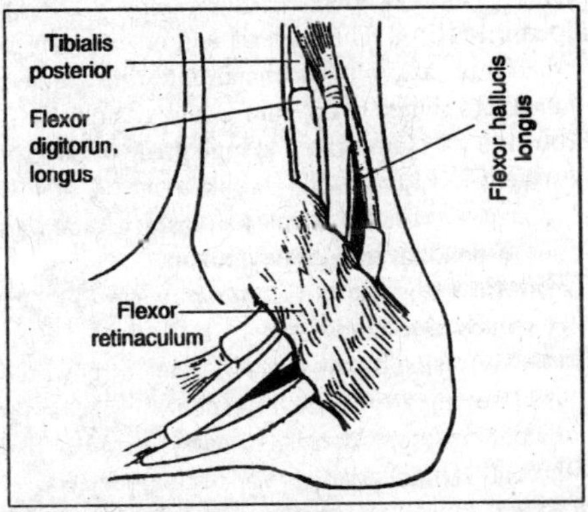

Flight path The path of the blood drop, it moves thorough space, from the impact site to the target.

Floatation time Time of floatation of dead body in drowning is ordinarily 24 hours after death in summer and 2 to 3 days in winter. Body floats sooner in shallow or saline water due to heavy specific gravity. Floatation is quicker in polluted water for quicker decomposition. Bodies of women due to higher fat floats earlier after drowning.

Floating ribs The eleventh and twelfth pairs of ribs, which are attached only to the thoracic vertebrae.

Floats Buoyanbt devices such as cork or inflated rubber tubes and rings used to support head, trunk or limbs of patient and to provide assistance or resistnace ot exercise.

Flocculus A part of the cerebellum that receives input from the vestibular receptors in middle ear.

Flooding Technique used to control the uncooperative patient to reduce anxieties.

Floor of the nasal cavity A bony wall formed by the palatal processes of the maxilla and the horizontal processes of the palatine bones; appears radiopaque.

Floppy infant In this child is having marked hypotonia of his muscles. Infant assumes a frog-like position. This menitests as decreased resistance to passive movement of limbs. Range of movement of peripheral joint is increased.

Floppy valve syndrome It is characterised by fibromyxomatous degeneration of valve leaflets resulting to aortic incompetence in men and mitral incompetence in women.

Flora The entire plant life of a geographic area; used to indicate the microorganisms that live together in a specific location.

Flora-intestinal The bacteria and other organisms that grow naturally in human intestine. Some of these are source of vitamin B and vitamin K.

Florence oil Name given to high grade of olive oil.

Florida (S. Fluouracil) Available as 1% and 5% cream and is used in actinic keratoses, genital warts not responding to podophylotoxin.

Floridation The use of fluorine in water to reduce incidence of tooth decay.

Floss Soft nylon or silk thread, waxed or unwaxed, used for cleaning the interdental spaces and dislodging loose debris, to carry a rubber dam through contact areas, or for testing contacts.

Flossing Floss can remove plaque in areas where toothbrush is inefficient. Draw an 18 to 24 inch length of unwaxed dental floss and twist the floss three times around the middle finger of the right hand and three times around middle finger of left

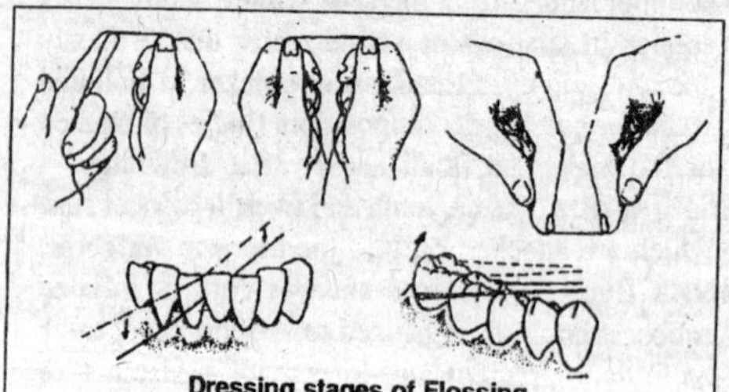

Dressing stages of Flossing

hand leaving a space of 1 to 4 inches between the hands. Thumbs and forefingers will guide the floss. Make the floss firm by stretching it. Press the flow against the tooth and carry it carefully under the free gingival margin of papilla. Once the floss is in sulcus wrap it firmly against the mesical tooth surface by applying pressure with both hands. Carry the floss apically. Then engaging any plaque move it incisally. Repeat the process. Unwaxed floss is efficient for plaque removal. Some persons may use floss carriers.

Flour enrichment Addition of certain vitamins and minerals to flour.

Flour high ratio Flour of very fine and more uniform particle size, treated with chlorine to reduce the gluten strength. Used for making cakes. one hundred fourty parts of sugar can be mixed to 100 parts of flour. while in ordinary flour only 70 parts of sugar can be mixed.

Flour strength A property of the flour proteins enabling the dough to retain gas during fermentation to give a 'bold' loaf.

Flow To move in a manner similar to a liquid stream.

Flow chart A graphic representation of sequence of operations using symbols to represent the operations.

Flow patter A change in the shape and direction of a bloodstain due to the influence of gravity or movement of the object.

Flow sheet Form of documentation that contains sections for recording frequently repeated assessment data.

Flowchart A diagram which shows the sequence of steps to be followed to solve a problem, often the expression of an algorithm in diagrammatic form.

Flowmeter Gauge used to regulate the number of liters of oxygen delivered to the patient.

Fluent aphasia A type of aphasia in which speech flows smoothly, with a variety of grammatical constructions and preserved melody of speech; paraphasias and circumlocutions may be present.

Fluid balance Homeostasis of fluids; the volumes of interstitial fluid, intracellular fluid, and plasma and total volume of water remain relatively constant.

Fluid compartments The areas in the body where the fluid is located; for example, interstitial fluid.

Fluid imbalance Condition in which the body's water is not in the proper volume or location in the body.

Fluid intelligence The form of intelligence that reflects speed of information processing, reasoning, and memory capacity rather than factual knowledge (crystallized intelligence); associated with Raymond Cattell.

Fluid volume deficit The state in which a person experiences vascular, cellular, or intracellular dehydration.

Fluid volume excess An alteration characterized by the abnormal retention of fluids and electrolytes in an isotonic fashion.

Fluorescein angiography The fluorescence can be observed directly by slit lamp or ophthalmoscope and can be photographed for permanent record. It is an alkaline dye of the sodium fluorescein. Its low molecular weight and high solubility in water allows rapid diffusion. For angiography, 5 cc of 10 % solution of dye is injected intravenously. It is mainly excreted in urine with a small amount in bile. Decreased fluorescence is seen in retinal vascular occlusion, atrophy of choriocapillaries, haemorrhages and abnormal tissue proliferation. Increased fluorescence is seen in vascular tumours. Leakage of dye can be seen in macular degeneration and central serous retinopathy.

Fluorescence The ability to absorb light at one wavelength and radiate part of it at another wave length. The property of a molecule that will absorb light and after a delay of less than one-millionth of a second remit light of a longer wavelength.

Fluorescent antibody An antibody conjugated to a fluorescent dye such as FITC.

Fluorescent microscope A microscope that uses an untraviolet light source to illuminate specimens that will fluoresce.

Fluoridation It is the addition of fluoride to the water supply as a means of reducing the incidence of dental caries. Fluoride is the natural content of water. Fluoride reduces the incidence of cavity. It acts by strengthening the mineral composition of the tooth enamel making it more resistant to acid attack. It reduces the ability of acid production of the organisms of plaque. Fluoride is most effective when ingested during formation of teeth. Water supply may naturally provide adequate amounts of fluoride. Ingestion of excess fluoride during tooth formation may lead to fluorosis, mottling of teeth that sometimes causes discolouration.

Fluoride Salt of hydrofluoric acid topically applied or added to the drinking water and dentifrices. Floride helps in the reduction of dental caries by combining with the hydroxyapatite of the hard tooth structure to form fluorapatite, which is more resistant to carious breakdown.

Fluoride gels and varnishes These are used to prevent formation of caries. Fluoride gel usually contains about 1.25% fluoride. It is present as sodium fluoride and hydrogen fluoride. The gel also contains small amount of phosphoric acid, a thickening agent and a colouring material.

Fluoride releasing agents Mouth rinses can be used at home. Fluoride is present as sodium fluoride, but dentifrice may contain stannous fluoride.

Fluorine Drinking water ranges in fuoride content between 0.05 and 14 parts per million, helps to protect teeth from decay. In larger amounts it causes chalky white patches to appear on surfaces of the teeth known as mottled enamel.

Fluorocil It is an anticancer drug used in cancer breast, bladder and intestine. In cream form it is used in basal cell carcinoma or when many tumours are there making surgery difficult. As side effects it may cause nausea, hair loss and impaired production of RBCs. After local application it may result in inflammation.

Fluorography It is a process where fluoroscopic image is photographed onto film using a lens camera (spot film camera). Generally, much higher dose rates are used for fluorography than for common fluoroscopy.

Fluorophore A molecule that will fluoresce when excited by light of a certain wavelength.

Fluoroscopy It the common name for production of real time images directly visible to eye during X-ray examination. Historically fluoroscopy was first done by WC Roentgen in 1985. Due to higher radiation dose lesser time should be used

Flutter A quick irregular motion.

FMRI Functional magnetic resonance imaging.

Foam bath The duckboard is covered to a depth of about 10 cm with hot water into which is put a

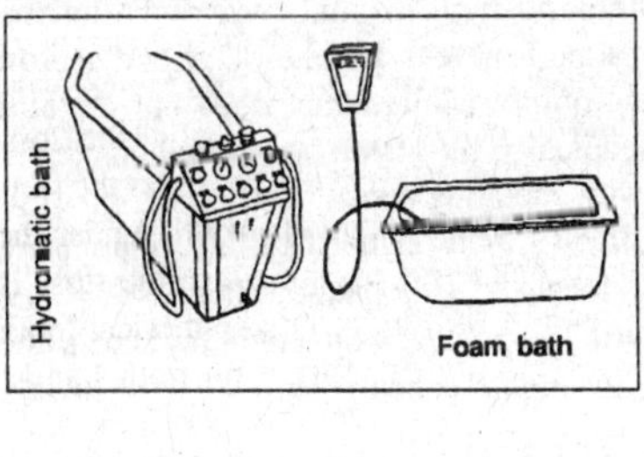

quantity of foam extract about 28 gm. Compressor is then started and continues to run until foam reaches almost the tip of bath. At this point, patient is slipped into a lying position. Head remains outside the foam. Crisp bubbles act as a very good insulation and prevent the heat from escaping. The normal length of time is 15 to 20 minutes.

Foam cells Cells that have accumulated or ingested material that dissolves during the tissue preparation, usually lipids.

Foam contraceptive A spermicidal preparation that is inserted vaginally prior to intercourse to prevent conception. Its effectiveness is enhanced when it is used with a diaphragm.

Focal The chief center of a morbid process, usually involving one area of the brain. Linear movement of the head leads to focal lesions at the site of impact or the opposite side of the brain.

Focal seizures These are seizures in which first clinical or EEG changes indicate activation of a group of neurons in part of cerebral hemisphere. Depending on area involved, partial seizure may be motor or sensory. Partial seizure with loss of unconsciousness is called a complex partial seizure. A seizure that arises in mesial part of one temporal lobe may produce perception of unpleasant and distorted smell. There may be complex visual hallucination. All partial seizure discharges can spread.

Focal biliary cirrhosis Damage to hepatic parenchymal cells as the result of bile duct obstruction.

Focal brain damage Localized injury to a specific part of the brain.

Focal infection Infection caused by bacteria or toxins carried in the blood from a distant lesion or focus.

Focal nodular hyperplasia of liver It is a reactive or hamartomatous lesion mostly found in children and women of child bearing age. It is mostly asymptomatic with normal liver function test. Calcification is absent. Haemorrhage and necrosis are uncommon. Malignancy does not develop. Microscopically, the lesion has central connective tissue with radiating septa.

Focal opacity A term used to describe a well-defined, localised radiopaque lesion.

Focal point The point at which light rays cross after passing through a concave lens.

Focal through In panoramic radiography, a three-dimensional curved zone or image layer in which structures are reasonably well defined; a patient must be positioned so that the dental arches are located within the focal through area.

Focus assessment Information that provides more details about specific problems.

Foetal distress It results from fetal hypoxia. It is suggested by slowing and irregularity of fetal heart and passage of meconium. Amnioscopy and sampling of scalp blood for estimation of pH helps.

Foetal surface placenta It is smooth shiny and white. Branches of umbilical vein and arteries can be seen radiating from the site of insertion. Surface is covered by amnion, underneath which chorion is closely applied.

Fog Darkening of the whole or part of a developed radiograph from sources other than the radiation of the primary beam to which the film was exposed.

Fogged film An artefact seen on dental radiographs when the film appears grey and lacks detail and contrast.

Fogging The production of fog.

Foil A very thin, flexible sheet of metal usually gold, platinum, or tin.

Fold A doubling back of tissue surface.

Foliate papillae Small indistinct papillae found on the folds of the posterior area of the sides of the tongue.

Folic acid It is a part of Vitamin B complex and responsible for production of RBC. Liver and raw vegetables are good source of it. During pregnancy it plays an important part in fetal growth. WHO has recommended the supplement of folic acid during pregnancy. Deficiency of it may result in megaloblastic anaemia.

Folk medicine Health practices unique to a particular group of people.

Follicle (dental) The sac that encloses the developing tooth before its eruption.

Follicles Specialized structures required for hair growth.

Follicle-stimulating hormone Hormone secreted by the anterior pituitary that initiates development of ova and stimulates the ovaries to secrete estrogens in females, and initiates sperm production in males.

Follicular Relating to or involving a follicle or the follicular phase.

Follicular phase The stage of the menstrual cycle during which the process of folliculogenesis is completed. The principal steroid hormone secreted in this phase and a mature follicle is ready for ovulation.

Folliculitis It is an infection of hair follicles produced by several microorganisms. Superficial folliculitis presents with tiny pustules around the coarse hair, surrounded by small erythematous zone, usually lesions form crusts and heal without scarring. Deep folliculitis gives rise to erythematous papules around coarse terminal hair. There are always deeper and larger abscesses communicating skin lesions. Lesions cause epilation and scarring. Management includes eradication of underlying infected foci. Mild cases can be treated with topical application of appropriate antibiotics. Resistent cases may be treated with fractional radiotherapy.

Follistatin A single-chain glycoprotein that acts as a binding protein for activin and neutralizes its diverse functions.

Fomite A term for an inanimate object that harbors pathogenic microorganisms and that may serve as a vehicle for transmission of infection.

Fondant Minute sugar crystals in a saturated sugar syrup. It is used as creamy filling in chocolates and biscuits and for decorating cakes.

Fondling It is, in general, caressing or handling in a loving way. Term is specially applied to the body caresses, including touching, and manipulating the sex organs for the purpose of sexual excitement.

Fones technique Toothbrushing technique in which the teeth are occluded, the brush is at a right angle to the teeth, the jaws parted, the palatal and lingual surfaces are brushed in an anteroposterior direction.

Fontanel A membranous-covered region on the skull of a fetus or baby where ossification has not yet occured; commonly called a soft spot.

Fontanelle It is a membrane covering gap between the bones of the skull. It is one of the two soft areas on a baby's scalp. At the birth the skull bones are not yet fully fused. Anterior fontanelle is diamond shaped about one inch across and usually closes by the age of one and half year. While posterior fontanelle is triangular area measuring about 0.25 inch and closes within two months of birth. A shunken fontanelle is a sign of dehydration. Early closure of fontanelles results in deformity called craniosynostosis.

Food Substances consumed orally to maintain life and growth.

Food additives There are many types of food additives : (*i*) those that preserve food and affects its keeping, (*ii*) those that affect texture, (*iii*) those that affect taste, and (*iv*) antifoaming agents. Antioxidant improves the keeping quality of food by preventing undesirable changes such as rancidity. Appearance and taste are improved by the use of colourings, sweeteners and flavourings. Artificial sweeteners such as saccharine and aspartum are commonly used.

Food energy Expressed in terms of calories per unit weight, food energy represents the energy available from the oxidation after deduction have been made for loses in digestion and incomplete oxidation.

Food fat Dietary triglycerides; consumed from food sources.

Food intolerance An adverse reaction to a food that does not involve the immune system.

Food liking The foods that we really like to eat.

Food poisoning It is suspected when many people of family or group or party become ill after eating the same food. It is of two types : infective and noninfective. The bacteria most commonly responsible for food poisoning is *Salmonella* which multiply rapidly. Poultry food harbour such bacteria. Other bacteria cause the formation of toxins that may be difficult to destroy even with thorough cooking. Such organisms are staphylococcal bacteria. Botulism is a rare, life threatening form of food poisoning caused by bacterial toxin. The symptoms of food poisoning develops within 30 minutes in case of chemical poisoning. In botulism there will be difficulty in speaking, visual disturbance, muscle paralysis and vomiting. Rehydration is very necessary.

Food preferences The foods we choose to eat when all foods are available at the same time and in the same quantity.

Food pyramid Guide for promoting the healthy intake of food.

Food technologist One who applies food science to preservation, processing preparation and packing or storage of food.

Food trolleys Serving desired and prescribed food to patient is the duty of nursing staff similar to medicine, and various types of food trolleys are available.

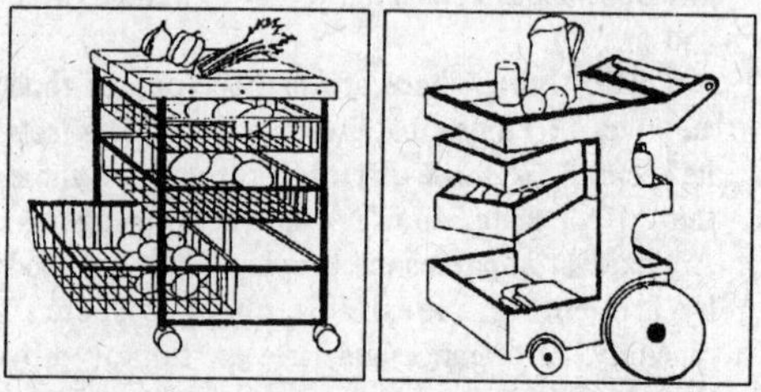

Foodborne Carried by food; resulting from the ingestion of a certain product in food.

Food-borne microbe A living organism less than 0.01 mm in diameter mainly bacteria, yeasts, and molds that can grow in foods and beverages and cause undersirable changes, food spoilage and foodborne diseases or desirable changes of food preservation and fermentation.

Foot It supports body weight and acts as a lever to propel the body forward. The stoutest bone of foot is calcaneum. Second prominent bone is talus. There are many bones which help in mobility of joint. Common deformities of foot are clubtoot flat foot and claw foot. Corns are small areas ot thickened skin on a toe usually caused by fitted shoes. Plantar warts appear on sole of skin. Gout is a metabolic disease affecting big toe mainly. Metatarsals are prone to fracture.

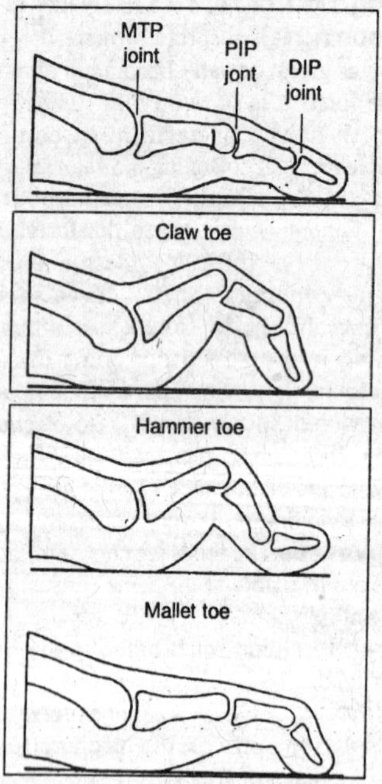

Foot control Device activated by the foot to operate dental handpieces.

Foot drop Permanent dysfunctional position caused by shortening of the calf muscles and lengthening of the opposing muscles on the anterior leg.

Foot print device An instrument that measures the pressure distribution between the human foot and the ground.

Foot pronation Foot pronation is the result of triplanar motion of the subtalar and midtarsal joints. It involves dorsiflexion, abduction, and eversion.

Foot supination Foot supination is the result of triplanar motion of the subtalar and midtarsal joints. It involves plantar flexion, adduction, and inversion.

Footboard Board placed perpendicular to the mattress, parallel to and touching the plantar surface of the client's feet and used to maintain dorsiflexion of the feed.

Footling breech A breech presentation in which one or both feet or the knees extend below the buttocks. It is also known as incomplete breech presentation.

Footprint Footprint confirms that a sole is arched anteroposteriorly and transversely and is best described as forming half a dome. The antero-posterior curve is most marked on the medial side and is called medial longitudinal arch consisting calcaneus behind and three metacarpals in front. The heads of metatarsals are regarded as the anterior end of arch. The lateral longitudinal arch

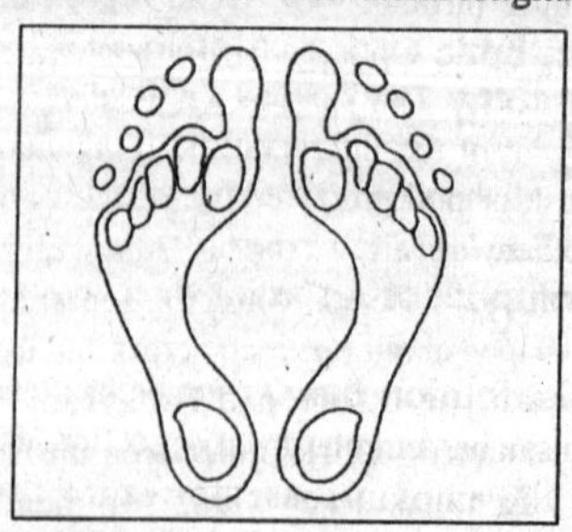

is much flatter than medial, lies along the lateral border of foot and is almost nonexistent. It is formed by calcaneus posteriorly and anteriorly by cuboid and lateral two metatarsals. An arched foot has the advantage of being resilient in response to varying forces. Segmentation of arch permits movements.

Footprint (tires) The shape and area of the portion of a tire in contact with the ground at a given inflation.

Footprinting A technique for identifying the nucleic acid sequence bound by a DNA or RNA-binding protein.

Foramen 1. Natural opening in a bone or other structure. 2. Natural opening in the root, usually at or near the apical end.

Foramen lacerum syndrome It is usually caused by congenital aneurysm of intradural portion of carotid artery. Clinically, there may be mental retardation, unilateral frontal or orbital headache, migraine and periorbital pain. Oculomotor palsy may cause ptosis and diplopia. There will be loss of light reflex.

Foramen magnum The large opening in the anterior and inferior part of the occipital bone, interconnecting the vertebral canal and cranial cavity.

Foramen ovale The valve of foramen ovale will be patent as the right atrial pressure exceeds the left atrial pressure. As pulmonary blood flow increases, the left atrial pressure will tend to rise and will exceed to right atrial pressure. The anatomical changes seen in adult will follow the functional closure of foramenovale. In the fetal heart, the oval opening in the interatrial septum with a valve that allows blood to flow from the right to left atrium but not in the opposite direction; becomes the fossa ovalis after birth.

Foramen, optic Optic canal, foramen.

Foraminotomy The surgical removal of a portion of the wall of the intervertebral foramen.

Force Push or pull produced by action of one body on another.

Force component A specific direction of applied force.

Force distribution bar On some plate/blade form implants, a bar, circular in cross section, extending along the implant base for more favorable distribution of forces.

Forced coughing Coughing that is purposely produced.

Forced expiratory technique Forceful exhalation techniques such as cough, huff, and active cycle breathing to clear the airways.

Forced vital capacity The largest volume of gas that can be forcefully exhaled from the lungs after a maximal inspiratory effort.

Forceps It is a tweezer-like instrument used for handling tissues during operation and dressing. These are of different types. Tissue forceps have fine teeth at the tip of each blade. Forceps used for

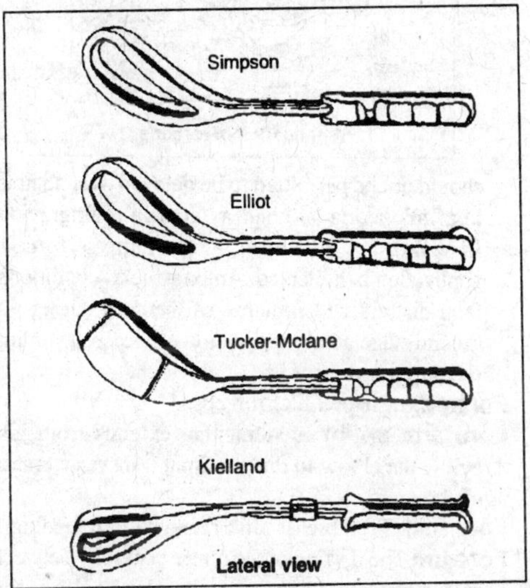

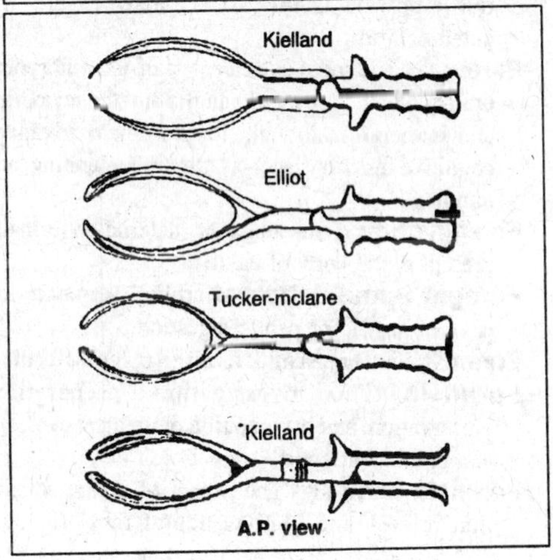

holding or removing wound dressings have scissor handles to make manipulation easier. Obstetric forceps has two wide, blunt blades designed to fit around the baby's head.

Forceps delivery Indications include delay in second stage of delivery. When the progress of descent of the head in vagina is absent or slow inspite of full dilatation of cervix. Second stage should not be permitted to be delayed over an hour in primigravida and half an hour in multigravida. In severe pre eclampsia and eclampsia forceps application is indicated. Amongst fetal conditions, fetal distress and prolapse of the cord during the second stage needs application of forceps avoiding pressure on the cord.

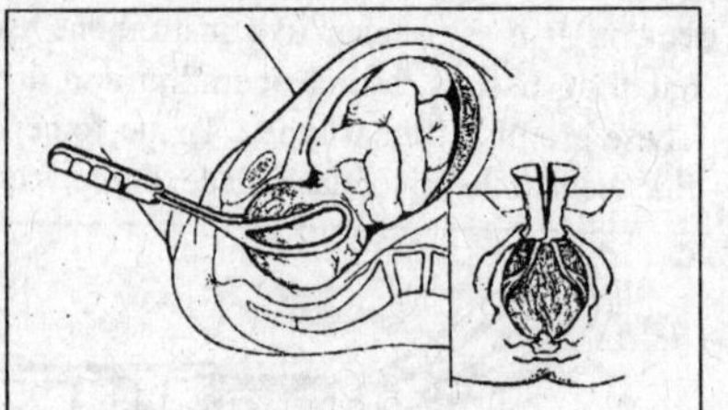

Application of forceps

Forcipate Shaped like forceps.

Fore arm splint A splint that extends from just below the elbow to the proximal transverse crease of the palm.

Fore milk First breast milk recieved in a feeding.

Forearm The portion of the upper extremity between the elbow and the wrist; also called the antebrachium.

Forebrain The most anterior part of the embryonic brain; contains the basal ganglia and the neocortex and is therefore thought to coordinate advanced cognitive functions such as thinking, planning, and language.

Foregin body A substance or material abnormally present in the body of cavity.

Foregut fermentation Microbial fermentation prior to gastric or peptic digestion.

Foremilk First breast milk received in breast feeding.

Forensic The investigation, preparation, preservation, and presentation of medical evidence and opinion in court.

Forensic dentistry The aspect of dental science that relates and applies dental facts to legal problems; encompasses dental identification malpractice litigation, legislation, peer review. and dental licensure.

Forensic engineering Forensic engineering is simply the application of engineering principles and knowledge to legal problems. It differs from forensic science primarily in the nature of the education, skills and experience brought to the analysis of the problem.

Forensic facial reconstruction Forensic facial reconstruction (FFR) is the term given to any system, which results in the construction of the soft tissues of the face over an unidentified skull, in an attempt to create a likeness of the original owner of the skull.

Forensic intelligence The collection and systematic exploitation of forensic science data and its integration into crime investigation and crime analysis.

Forensic medicine It is a branch of medicine which deals with criminal law, unnatural deaths and poisoning, etc. It includes to access the time of death, recognition of weapon and matching of blood, semen, hair and skin from victim. It has specific role to establish case of rape and poisoning.

Forensic psychiatry The application of psychiatric knowledge and practice in a forensic context.

Forensic psychology The application of psychological skills in the legal profession-for example, in jury selection, sanity determination, and assessing competency to stand trial.

Forensic psychophysiology A field of study combining theory and empirical knowledge from both psychology and physiology; generally it is used to refer to the detection and measurement of physiological events as they relate to behavioral changes.

Forensic urine drug testing Examination of urine to measure the presence and amounts of drugs or poisons for the purpose of determining their contribution to the cause of death or injury.

Foreshortening A radiographic error resulting from excessive vertical angulation; the teeth on the film appear shorter than their actual length.

Foreskin A loose-fitting retractable casing located over the glans of the penis; also known as the prepuce.

Forespore The cell compartment of a sporangium destined to become a spore.

Forewater rupture The forewaters are ruptured with the teeth of the amniotomy forceps. The method is adopted when the head has fitted well with good collection of forewaters. There is no risk of cord prolapse and there is no danger of injury to placenta as in high rupture of membranes.

Forgetting Absence of memory; specifically, the inability to recall, to recognise, or to relearn at an improved rate something to which the individual was exposed earlier.

Fork strap Prosthetic suspension and knee extension aid; consists of a fork-shaped elastic strap extending from the anterior portion of the below-knee prosthetic shank to a waist belt.

Form constancy The ability to perceive or to attend to subtle differences in form and shape. The perceptually impaired patient is likely to confuse objects of similar shape or to fail to recognize an object placed in an unusual position.

Formal operations The final stage of intellectual development, according to Jean Paget, beginning at approximately 11 years of age. The child or adult at this stage can imagine the possibilities in a given situation; reasoning can occur apart from concrete materials; hypotheses can be formed and tested in the abstract. Sometimes formal operations are simply referred to as abstract thinking.

Formaldehyde It is a pungent, irritant and colourless gas. Formaline is used to pressure the tissue to harden before they are examined. It is used as disinfectant also.

Formalin Formaldehyde is a colourless gas with a strong pungent smell. A 37 to 40% solution of formaldehyde in water is called formalin. The ingestion of 15 ml may be fatal. The inhalation of formaldehyde vapours causes severe irritation of eyes. Person may develop severe dyspnoea. Liquid ingestion causes burning pain in mouth, throat and abdomen. Ulceration occurs over the oropharynx. Face is flushed and pupils are small. Giddiness, unconsciousness and stertorous breathing could be a prominent feature. There may be severe metabolic acidosis, acute tubular necrosis and liver failure.

Formed element A cell, such as an erythrocyte or leucocyte, or cell fragments, such as a platelet, in blood.

Formic acid It is the simplest organic acid. This is found in ants and other insects and is part of irritant that produces itching.

Fornication It is a consensual heterosexual intercourse between two unmarried adults or juvenile. Fornication is sometimes confused with seduction and traditionally is illegal in most legal jurisdictions and is regarded as uncomplicated act of intercourse between unmarried persons of opposite sex. The act is private and consensual.

Fornix A recess around the cervix of the uterus where it protrudes into the vagina.

Fornix of the vagina The arched or vaulted surface of the vaginal mucous membrane onto the cervix uteri.

Forward Head Posture This posture involves flexion of the lower cervical spine in combination with extension of the upper cervical spine. It is often accompained by protracted scapulae and increased thoracic kyphosis.

Forward spatter Blood which travels in the same direction as the source of energy or force which caused the spatter.

Fossa A depression, usually more or less longitudinal in shape below the level of the surface or part such as a bone.

Fossa ovalis An ovoid depression above an to the left of the inferior vena cava orifice on the lower central portion of the septal wall of the right atrium.

Fossorial Having the behavior pattern of digging or burrowing; living in holes or burrows.

Fouid volume deficit An alteration characterized by the loss of fluids and electrolytes in an isotonic fashion.

Fouling A term for biodeterioration caused by the presence of living organisms, without significant structural damage to the material; in the case of microorganisms, it usually consists of aesthetic changes that create a generally unacceptable appearance.

Four tailed bandage It can be made from a strip of gauze or a roller bandage by splitting it at both ends. This bandage is convenient for making a loop or sling to retain small dressing on nose, chin and forehead.

Fourchette The posterior angle or commissure of the labia majora.

Four-dimensional ultrasound Acquisition of cardiac gated three-dimensional ultrasound data at several time points during cardiac cycle when these three-dimensional data sets are shown in a cine loop is referred as four-dimensional imaging.

Four-handed dentistry Technique of chairside operation in which four hands are kept busy working in the oral cavity simultaneously.

Fourth heart sound It is a low-pitched presystolic sound produced during late ventricular filling by contraction of atria. S_4 occurs when diminished ventricular compliance increases resistance to ventricular filling. It is heard in case of hypertension, aortic and pulmonary stenosis, coronary artery disease, acute myocardiopathy and mitral regurgitation

Fourth lumbar root compression Pain in inner quadrant of buttock, outer aspect of thigh and leg crossing over dorsum of foot, reaches the toe which often tingles.

Fourth stage of labour The recovery stage that begins with the delivery of the placenta and extends to the 1-4 hours post partum.

Fourth ventricle A cavity within the brain, between the cerebellum and the medulla oblongata and the pons, containing cerebrospinal fluid.

Fovea The region at the center of the retina that is specialized for high acuity; its receptive fields are at the center of the eye's visual field.

Fovea centralis A depression on the macula lutea of the eye, where only cones are located; the area of keenest vision.

Foveation Visual targeting so that the center of the scence is aligned with the fovea.

Fowler's position It is good for relief in breathlessness and for good drainage from abdomen and pelvic cavity postoperatively. It results in better blood circulation and preventing thrombosis.

It is as comfortable as half sitting position. Fowler's beds are available. The back of patient can be kept at a comfortable inclined position by mechanical adjustment. Otherwise also four pillows can be placed at the back of patient at comfortable inclination. Low blocks can be put at leg end to raise slightly to prevent slipping of patient downwards.

FPIA Fluorescent polarization immunoassay.

Fractal geometry The study of surfaces with a seemingly infinite area, such as the lining of the small intestine.

Fraction of inspired oxygen Portion of oxygen in relation to total inspired gas.

Fraction test meal Method of examining secretion of gastric juice of patients. Stomach contents are sampled at intervals.

Fractionation The administration of radiation in smaller doses over time rather than in a single large dose; minimizes tissue damage.

Fracture It is a break in periosteum of bone. If one side of periosteum is broken, it is known as greenstick fracture, when both periostea are broken it is known as fracture. Direct injury or fall may

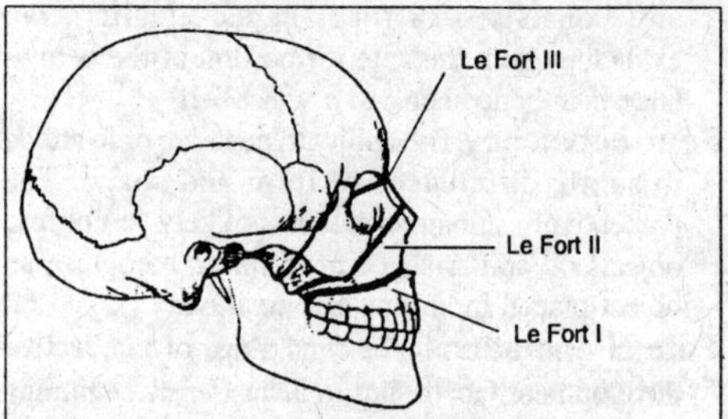

Fracture sites

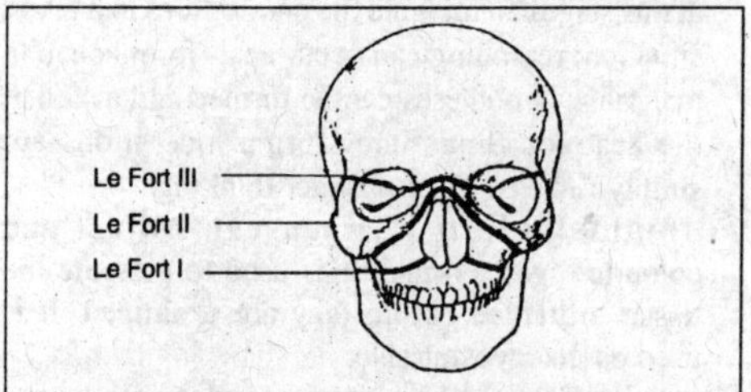

Sites of fracture of Maxilla

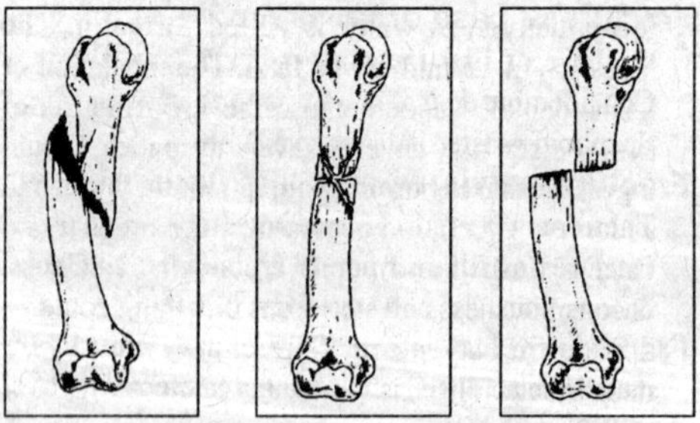

Different types of fractures

result it. Pain, swelling, deformity and presence of crepitation may be the symptoms. There may be loss of function and bleeding too if blood vessels have been injured. First aid includes not to try to force back a displaced bone yourself. Cover the open wound with a clean dressing. Move the patient as little as possible and apply splint. Do not give any fluid or food in case if operation is required.

Fracture dislocation A joint dislocation that is accompanied by a fracture of one or more bones that form the joint.

Fracture femur It is very common in old age and may be accompanied by marked concealed blood loss. Thomas splints suspend the thigh and Parson attachment applied to splint allows knee flexion.

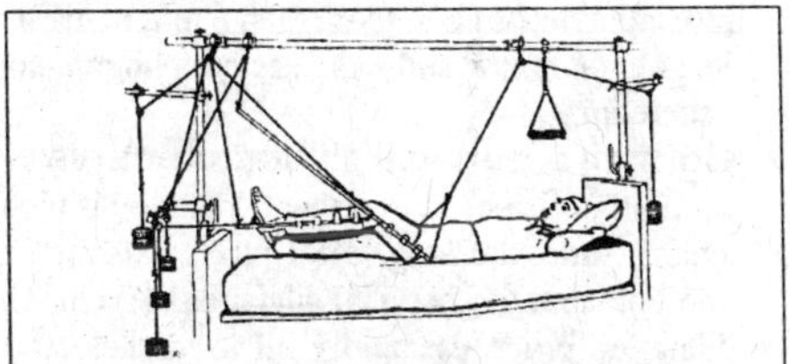

Thomas leg splint with Parson attachment

Fracture neck femur It is very common in old age. It may be through trochancter or through neck of femur.

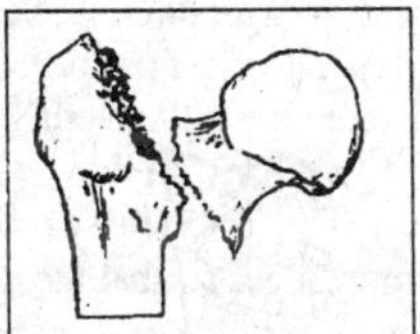

Hip fracture through trochanter of femer

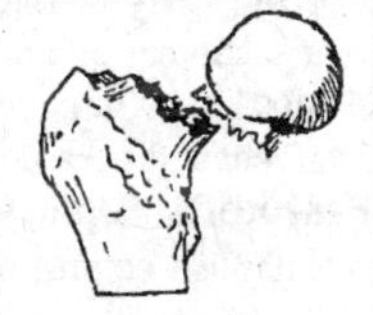

Hip fracture through neck of femur

Fracture of base of the first metacarpal Near the base of first metacarpal fracture is common. Considerable degree of angulation can be accepted. Scaphoid plaster is to be used.

Fracture pelvis without disruption of ring There may be muscle avulsion fractures, isolated fractures of ilium, fracture of ischium and pubis on one side.

Fracture rib Patient complains of pain while taking deep breath. There is local bony tenderness. There will be pain on anteroposterior compression on chest. Crepitus may be either felt or heard. X-ray for ribs will confirm it. Associated findings may be of surgical emphysema, pneumothorax, haemothorax and laceration of lung.

Fracture strength The degree of stress at which a material breaks.

Fracture toughness The ability of a material containing some type of flaw to resist propagation of a crack from the flaw; essentially resistance to fracture.

Fragile X-syndrome This is one of most important cause of mental retardation. Affected boys have long face, big ears, and big testes. Unstable region of DNA at this site can expand in successive generation.

Frame of reference A specific theoretical approach that is used to guide treatment activities.

Framework Skeletal portion of a prosthesis around which and to which are attached the remaining portions of the prosthesis to produce the finished restoration.

Franceschetti-Klein syndrome A hereditary and familial disorder characterised by hypoplasia of facial bones, palpebral antimongoloid fissure, malformation of ears, stretching of cheeks, buccal-auricular fistula, and skeletal deformities.

Franchise dentistry The practice of dentistry under the trade name, the rights of which has been purchased from another dentist or organization.

Frankfort plane The imaginary plane that intersects the orbital rim of the eye and the opening of the ear.

Frankia Symbiotic, nitrogen-fixing actinomycetes that form root nodules on diverse shrubs and trees which are not legumes.

Fraternal twins Twins that are the result of simultaneous fertilisation of two ova by two sperms. These twins may be of two different sexes and may have separate placenta.

Fraud Intentional perversion of truth for the purpose of inducing another, in reliance on it, to part with something valuable or to surrender a legal right; deliberate deception; deceit; trickery.

Fraudulent concealment Hiding or suppressing a material fact or circumstance that the part is legally or morally bound to disclose.

Freckle This condition starts as dark, pigmented, smooth but flat lesion, i.e. macule. It commonly appears on face and neck of elderly persons. The oral mucosa and conjunctiva can be involved. It is clinically a premelanomatous dermatosis but histologically, it is melanoma *in situ* with junctional changes but no dermal invasion. It has a tendency for steady centrifugal enlargement. There may be raised rough nodules showing malignant change. It is a benign disorder of abnormal pigmentation resulted from exposure to sunlight or to UV light. It may disappear in cointers. Lesions develop between 3 and 4 years and persist for years. Condition gives rise to multiple, small discrete, circular, grouped or confluent, tan red or light brownish evenly pigmented macules. Lesions are distributed symmetrically on exposed parts of body. Continued exposure to sunlight or to UV light makes the lesions of freckles to increase in number and to become darker. Surrounding skin becomes red and sore. Avoid further exposure to sunlight. Local application of keratolytic agent is effective.

Free association A technique designed to uncover unconcious feelings. Patient tells anything that comes into his mind. Neither the patient nor the therapist attempts to censor the throughts but the therapist listens and then interprets it.

Free energy The component of the total energy of a system that can do work at constant temperature and pressure.

Free floating hostility Behaviour characterised by hostile vocal inflection and fascial expression, ill temper, cynicism, sleeplessness, irritability and interpersonal conflict.

Free gingiva Gum tissue which is closest to teeth.

Free gingival junction Area where the free gingiva meets the sulcus area.

Free radical A molecule (monomer) containing an unpaired electron, making it very reactive toward other molecules.

Free-way space Distance between the occluding surfaces of the maxillary and mandibular teeth when the mandible is in its physiological rest position. This can be determined by calculating the difference between the rest vertical dimension and the occlusal vertical dimension.

Freeze concentration Concentration of a liquid by freezing out pure ice, leaving a more concentrated solution.

Freeze dry A process of rapidly freezing substance at an extremely low temperature and then dehydrating under vaccum. Moistre content is 3 to 10%.

Freeze drying It is a method in which material is frozen and subjected to high vaccum. The ice sublimes off as water vapour without melting. Freeze dried food is very porous. There is less loss of flavour.

Freeze-Dried Bone Allograft Bone harvested from donor cadavers, washed, ground to a selected particle size, immersed in ethanol, frozen in nitrogen, freeze-dried and ground to smaller particles ranging from 250 to 750 mm.

Frei test The test consists of intradermal injection of 0.1 ml of antigen prepared from chlamydial suspension. When the test is positive it produces red, indurated area of more than 6 mm in diameter in 24 to 48 hours, and indicates lymphogranuloma venereum.

Freidrman's cervical dilatation curve It is sigmoid in shape. The cervical dilatation is plotted against time. the long latent phase extends from onset of labor to a cervical dilatation of 3 cm. Then dilatation proceeds rapidly till it reaches 10 cm. This phase is active phase of dilatation. It has a phase of accelaration, a phase of maximum slope and a phase of deceleration.

Fremitus A vibration imparted to the hand resting on the chest or other part of the body.

Frenectomy 1. Excision of a frenum. 2. Surgical detachment and/or excision of a frenum from its attachment into the mucoperiosteal covering of the alveolar processes.

Frenkel's Exercises These exercises aim to extablish control of movement so that the patient is able and confident in his ability to carry out those activities whhich are essential for independence in everday life. The important points/essentials of Frenkel's exercise being :

Concentration of the attention.
Precision.
Repetition.

Frenulum A membranous structure that serves to anchor and limit the movement of a body part.

Frenulum linguae A sharp, thin ridge of tissue that arises in the midline from the base of the tongue and is attached to its undersurface for varying distances. Depending upon the distance of attachment, it restrains the movement of the tongue. Also called lingual frenum.

Frenum Fold of mucous membrane attaching the cheeks and lips to the mandibular and maxillary mucosa and limiting the motions of the lips and cheeks.

Frequency Number of complete cycles of a repetitive waveform in one second. Measured in Hertz (Hz).

Frequency bandwidth Frequency response of an amplifier, referring to the limits on the range of signal frequencies processed; for example, 10 to 1000 Hz.

Friable easily broken or crumbled.

Friction brake Device in a prosthetic knee unit that resists knee flexion during early stance phase, commonly a spring-loaded wedge that is forced into a groove upon transfer of body weight to the prosthesis.

Friction massage Deep circular massage to irritate or stimulate a muscle or increase its tonus and /or its arterial perfusion, or express swelling by moving the skin over the subcutaneous tissue.

Friction rub Dry grating sound heard during auscultation, caused by rubbing of tissue surfaces.

Friction sex It is a homosexual practice in which two male partners achieve sexual gratification by rubbing each other in a face to face position.

Friction skin The specialized configuration of ridged skin resembling corduroy, which appears only on the inner surfaces of the hands and the bottoms of the feet.

Friction Specific circular or transverse movements that do not glide on the skin and that are focused on the underlying tissue.

Frictional fit In implant dentistry, the state or retention of a plate/blade form or root form implant at the time of insertion that results from slight compression of the osteotomy walls by the implant body.

Friedman's ANOVA The nonparametric version of the repeated measures analysis of variance.

Friedman's test A modification of the Aschheim Zondek test for pregnancy, the urine of early pregnancy is injected in 4-ml doses intravenously twice daily for 2 days into an unmated mature rabbit. If, at the end of this time, the ovaries of the rabbit contain fresh corpora lutea or haemorrhagic corpora, the test is positive.

Frigi scanning Process of preserving food by controlled, heating sufficient to destroy vegetative form of microorganism.

Frigidity It is a female disorder of total unresponsiveness or various degrees of impairment of sexual response. Females having lack of interest in any sexual activity or sexual pleasure are called frigid. They may even have complete aversion to sexual relations.

Froin's syndrome It is characterised by greatly increased protein content in cerebrospinal fluid, spontaneous coagulation of cerebrospinal fluid immediately after withdrawal, and pleocytosis.

Froment's sign It is a sign of ulnar palsy. The patient grasps a piece of cardboard firmly with the thumb and index finger of each hand and pulls

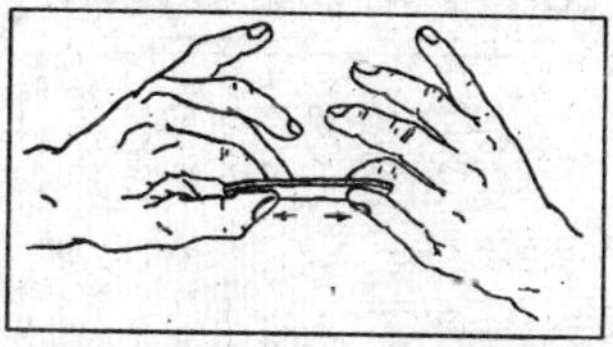

vigorously. If flexion of distal phalanx of thumb occurs, the test is positive and indicative of ulnar palsy.

Froments' paper sign Diagnostic test of ulnar nerve palsy. When the patient attempts to pinch of

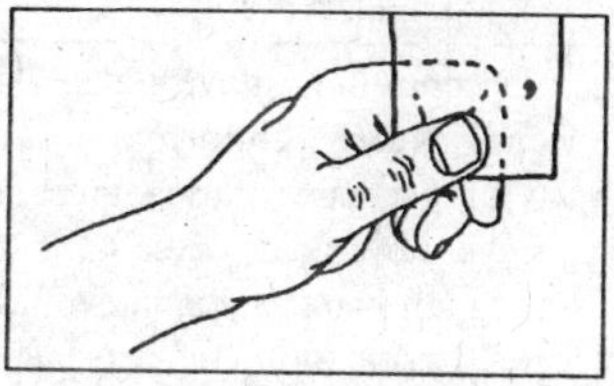

piece of paper forcefully between the thumb and index finger, increased flexion of the interphalangeal joint of thumb occurs.

Frontal bone Bone that forms the forehead.

Frontal eye area-8 It is largely extrapyramidal and concerned with voluntary eye movements. The stimulation of area number 8 causes conjugate deviation of eye and head to the opposite side.

Frontal leukotomy A surgical procedure in which nerve fibers to an from the frontal lobe are severed with a special knife called a leukotome (from the Greek leuko, meaning "white nerve fibers," and tome, meaning "a cutting").

Frontal lobe It observes voluntary and involuntary motor functions. It controls emotion, insight and personality and motor aspects of speech production. Brodmann's area 4 is related with movement. Area numbers 6 and 8 are also

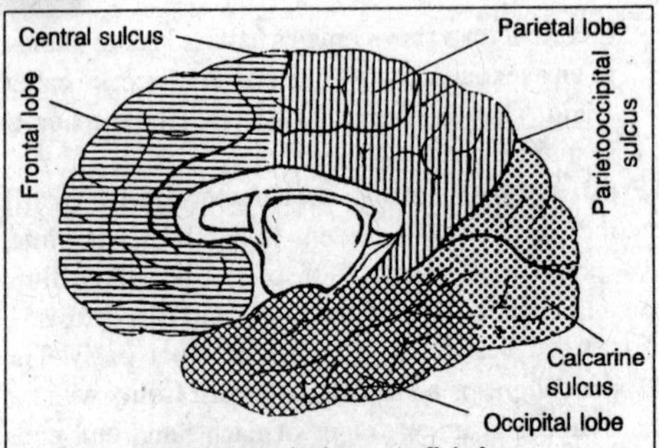

Cerebral hemisphere, medial view

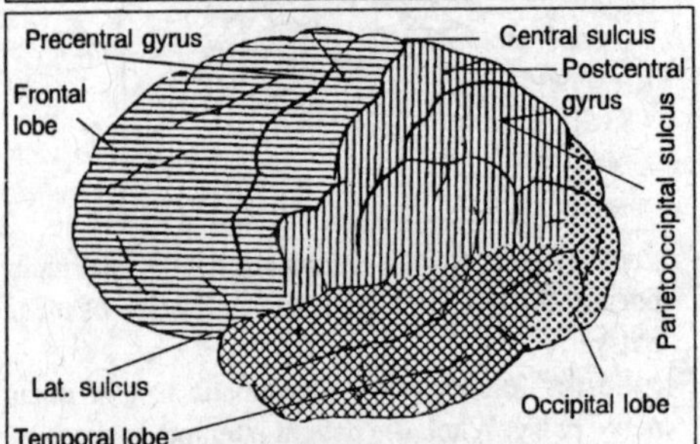

Lateral view

important in controlling movements. Damage to these areas causes abnormal involuntary movements and increased muscle tones. Area 8 is the area of eye movements. Area 44 is the motor speech area in left hemisphere, known as Broca's speech centre. Lesion of motor speech area causes motor dysphagia. On the inferior surface of frontal lobe lies area controlling higher functional centre.

Frontal lobe-lesions Frontal lobes are often contused in head injuries or may be compressed by slow growing meningiomas. Lack of social inhibitions may lead to urination or masturbation in public. Person becomes apathic and irritable. He or she may carry on doing one action when another is appropriate. Grasp, sucking and palmomental reflexes if present all suggest frontal lobe dysfunction. Jaw jerk may be increased. The pout reflex is elicited by gently tapping centrally just above the upper lip. If reflex is present lips come in kissing position. It is elicited by gently tapping the mandible when mouth is little open.

Frontal plane Vertical plane that passes through the body from the bead to the feet and is perpendicular to the sagittal plane.

Frontal sinusitis Inflammation in the frontal sinus.

Frontal sutures These lies between the two halves of frontal bone.

Frost bite It can affect any part of body below the temperature of 32°F. Specially toes, nose, ears and fingers are affected. So long only skin is affected recovery is possible but if blood vessels are also affected gangrene may follow and amputation may become necessary. Symptoms of frost bite includes pins and needle sensations followed by complete numbness. First skin looks white, cold and hard and later on it becomes red and swollen. Then blisters are formed and if skin becomes black it means skin has died. Lukewarm water can help and massage may not. Immediate attention of doctor is needed.

Frozen section It is a rapid technique for preparing biopsy section for microscopic examination. It is done during surgical procedures to know whether tissue is malignant or not. A small piece is removed by surgeon and after being frozen quickly in liquid nitrogen it is examined under microscope being cut in thin slides. Whole process hardly takes about 30 minutes.

Frozen shoulder It is stiffness and pain of shoulder making movements of the joint limited. It results due to inflammation and thickening of lining of capsule in which joint lies. Analgesics and anti-inflammatory drugs may be helpful. Sometimes cortisone has to be given. Exercises improve the stiffness.

Fructose Very sweet sugar ($C_6H_{12}O_6$) present in many fruits and honey and used as a preservative for foodstuffs and as an intravenous nutrient. Also called fruit sugar.

Fruits Edible portion of the reproductive body a plant which involves pulp. In fruits carbohydrate is in form of glucose and fructose. Sucrose may be found in fresh fruits. Sugar content varies from 6 to 20%, watermelon being the lowest and banana being highest.

Frusemide It acts on the thick portion of ascending limb of the loop of Henle. It is highly bound to plasma proteins. Half-life is 2 hours. It is highly successful for the relief of oedema. Taken orally it acts within hour and diuresis lasts for 6 hours. Given intravenous it acts within 30 minutes and can relieve acute pulmonary oedema. Oral dose is 20 to 120 mg by mouth per day.

Frustration Either a situational blocking or impending to behaviour toward a goal or the subjective feeling of being thwarted in attempting to reach a goal.

FSH Follicle Stimulating hormone; one of the two gonadotropic hormones secreted from the anterior pituitary. In females, FSH stimulates the development of the ovarian follicles; in males it stimulates the production of sperm in the seminiferous tubules.

Fugue Stress induced loss of memory in which the person looses personal identification and may assume a new one.

This is a state in which the patient wanders or carries on other apparently purposeful behaviour of perhaps hours or days without being able to remember what he was doing or why. It may result from alcohol intoxication, anxiety or suicidal depression.

Fugue state A flight from reality in which the individual develops amnesia, leaves his or her present situation, travels to a new location, and establishes a new identity.

Fulcrum Support upon which a lever rests when force is applied.

Full coverage crown Restoration that reproduces the entire surface anatomy of the clinical crown and fits over a prepared tooth.

Full liquid died A diet consisting of only liquids and foods that liquefy at body temperature.

Full penetration It is the maximum distance that an erect penis may enter into vagina. Depth of an average vagina is slightly less than 4 inches. For many couples full penetration is achieved when women is on top position.

Full-thickness burn Burn that destroys the epidermis and the dermis and sometimes the underlying tissue as well; sometimes called a third-degree burn.

Full-thickness flap Mucoperiosteal flap.

Fully functioning person A concept in the person-centred approach to personality, referring to an individual who shows trust in his or her experience and lives in a realistic fashion. The fully functioning person finds little incongruence between his or her experience and self-concept. This person is often characterised as engaging in self-actualisation tendency.

Fumes The products of explosion, which may contain toxic gases such as carbon monoxide and oxides of nitrogen.

Function of brain hemispheres Left hemisphere deals with speech, words, analysis, rational, logical, sequential, active, cognitive, somatic control. While right hemisphere deals with images, symbols, impulsion, creativity, intuitive, emotions, spirituality and automatic control.

Function of insulin It enables the liver and muscles to store glycogen from glucose and lowers the blood sugar level. It inhibits glucose formation from amino acids. It inhibits ketogenesis normally by keeping in check the ketogenic hormone.

Functional Without anatomical or organic problem. Also called physiological.

Functional disorder In this disorder it produces symptoms for which there is no apparent organic or structural cause. The term thus generally refers to symptoms caused by stress and anxiety.

Functional impotence It is a failure to achieve or maintain a penile erection because of circulatory or nervous disorder. Aging, depression, anxiety and use of excessive alcohol may result into it.

Functional amnesia An amnesia observed in adults of significant tune to an instigating tune usually stressful.

Functional areas of brain Brain has been divided in many areas according to the functional responsibility. Hence symptoms of CVA, injury or

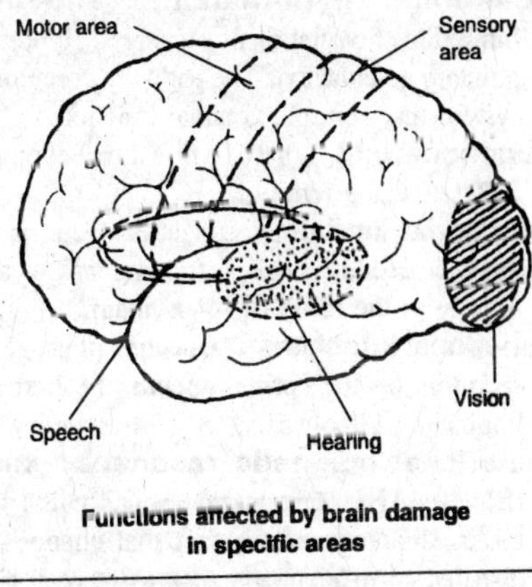

Functions affected by brain damage in specific areas

tumour depend upon the location and amount of brain damage involved.

Functional brace Brace that provides stability for a joint.

Functional capacity Ability or power to perform necessary activities.

Functional communication An individual's communicative effectiveness in everyday life; specifically, the ability to communicate needs, desires, and reactions.

Functional disease An ailment or problem involving body functions not caused by a structural defect or organic lesion.

Functional disorders Signs and symptoms for which no organic or physiological basis can be found.

Functional electrical stimulation Muscle rehabilitation by electrical stimulation at the motor point.

Functional fixedness An inability to think of novel uses for objects because of a fixation on their usual functions.

Functional food A food that provides health benefits beyond the nutrients it contains.

Functional genomics The study of gene function at the genome level.

Functional group The specific atom or group of atoms that confers a particular chemical property on a biomolecule.

Functional hypothalamic amenorrhoea Amenorrhoea associated with factors such as psychogenic stressors, excessive exercise or weight loss.

Functional hypothalamic anovulation Inhibition of ovulation due to stress. Hypothalamic pituitary gonadal axis The pathway of reproductive system that controls gonadal function.

Functional kin When fictive kin become fully integrated as a family.

Functional limitation Deviation from normal in the way an individual performs a task or activity, usually as the result of impairment.

Functional luteolysis The decline of progesterone secretion by the corpus luteum, the first sign of impending luteolysis.

Functional magnetic resonance imaging (FMRI) A type of magnetic resonance imaging that takes advantage of the fact that changes in the distribution of elements such as oxygen alter the magnetic properties of the brain. Because oxygen consumption varies with behavior, it is possible to map and measure changes that are produced by behavior.

Functional mobility The ability to move from one position or place to another.

Functional nursing Pattern in which each nurse on a unit is assigned specific tasks.

Functional occlusion 1. Occlusion in which attention is directed specifically to performance and is differentiated from structure and appearance. 2. Any tooth contacts made within the functional range of the opposing tooth surfaces. An occlusion that occurs during function.

Functional position Position that promotes continued use and mobility.

Functional residual capacity The sum of the expiratory reserve and residual volumes; it is the amount of air remaining in the lungs at the end of a normal tidal exhalation.

Functionalism A school of psychology which argued against the structuralists, that psychology should rather than with the nature of their conscious "structure", such as sensations, images, and feelings. Also called functional psychology.

Functionally illiterate Possessing minimal literacy skills.

Functioning of acupuncture It may close the 'gate' in the gate control theory of pain and central release of endorphins and possibly involvement of neurotransmitters. It may modulate the memory of pain.

Fundal grip Both hands are laid on the fundus of the uterus. By using the palmar surface of the full length of fingers held closed together. A breech feels like a mass.

Fundal height Fetus is just palpable above the symphysis pubis by the 12th week of pregnancy,

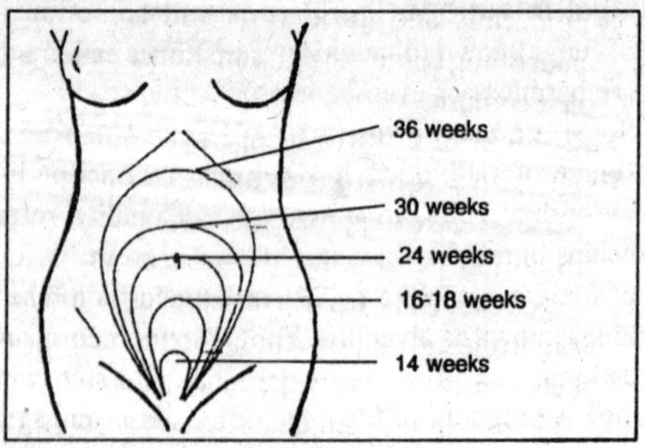

reaches approximately to the umbilicus by the 24th week and finally ceases to ascend at about 36 week. When the uterine fundus is about halt way from the symphysis pubis to the umbilicus; the gestation age is 16 weeks. Soon after the fetal movements may be felt. Uterine fundus grows 2 fingers every 2 weeks. The fundus of the uterus generally remains at the level of xiphisternum from 36th week.

Fundal massage It is done with hands and gentle massage stimulates the uterine muscles to contract. It restores normal tone and controls bleeding.

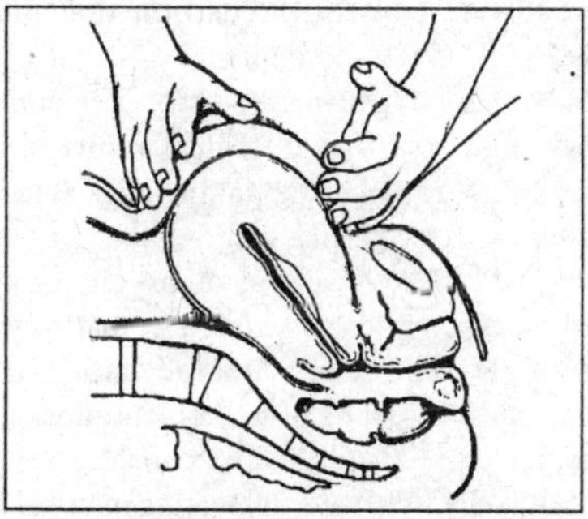

Fundamental attribution error Ascribing an individual's reactions to some internal condition or disposition when an explanation based on external factors seems more appropriate. When a person behaves in a dishonest fashion and this action is perceived as an enduring trait, attribution error may have occurred.

Fundus The bottom or base of anything; an anatomical term for any structure forming the bottom or case of an organ, or the part of a hollow organ farthest from its mouth.

Fungal Having to do with or belonging to the fungi.

Fungal infections There are more than one lakh of fungi known to medical science. Some of these are harmless or even beneficial to human beings. Some are used in baking and brewing, and are source of antibiotics. Yeast occurs as colonies of individual cells. In others cells divide to form chains of tubular filament. Inhaled spores of some of fungi can cause a persistent allergic reaction in lungs known as alveolitis. Fungal spores can cause asthma.

Fungi A kingdom of life forms that are eukaryotic, mycelial or yeast-like, heterotrophic, lacking in chlorophyll, sexually and/or asexually reproductive, and mostly aerobic.

Fungible Items that are so similar to one another that a consumer does not care if they are interchanged.

Fungicide A substance or agent used to kill fungi or to inhibit fungal growth.

Fungiform papilla A mushroom like elevation on the upper surface of the tongue appearing as a red dot; most contain taste buds.

Fungiform papillae Flattened, mushroom-shaped projections interspersed over the surface of the tongue in which taste buds are present.

Fungitoxic Extering a toxic effect on fungi.

Funic souffle A soft blowing sound, synchronous with the fetal heart sounds and supposed to be produced in the umbilical cord.

Funicular hernia Here the processus vaginalis is closed at its lower end so that sac of hernia is separate from the sac of tunica vaginalis. Testis lies below the hernia and can be felt separately from the contents of hernial sac. It is usually acquired but may be congenital.

Funiculus 'Small cord'.

Funnel pattern The pattern of burning, usually on a wall or other vertical structure, as a fire burns in an upward direction. The pattern is in the shape of a funnel opening upward.

Funtional sympathectomy Preganglionic sympathetic nerve section.

FUO Abbreviation for fever of unknown origin.

Furanose A simple sugar containing the five-membered furan ring.

Furcation Area or region lying between and at the base of two or more anatomically divided roots.

Furcation involvement Extension of periodontal disease into the area where the tooth roots separate.

Furious rabies The animal first becomes restless and apprehensive and may become apathetic. It then becomes hyperexcitable responding to minimal stimuli. Dog runs around snapping and biting without discrimination. There develops drooling of saliva due to inability to swallow. Vocal cords are affected and dog starts barking.

Furuncle A painful erythematous nodule caused by staphylococcus aureus and formed by localized inflammation of the dermis and subcutaneous tissue surrounding hair follicles.

Fusiform Tapering at both ends; spindle shaped.

Fusimotor Motor to intrafusal muscle fibers.

Fusion surgical The surgical formation of bony ankylosis.

Fusogen A chemical that induces the fusion of protoplasts, resulting in genetic recombination.

Fussol Systemic insecticide for treating fruits.

Fussy baby syndrome Condition in which the infant is easily upset due to bouts of ill temper; associated with infants who have sensory regulatory disorders.

F-Value Unit of measurement used to compare relative sterilizing effects of different procedures; equal to 1 minute of 121.1° C.

Fx Abbreviation for fractures.

G

"g" factor A hypothetical form of general intelligence, proposed by Charles Spearman, that can account for individual differences in human intelligence.

G protein A protein molecule usually imbedded in a cell's plasma membrane that plays an important role in getting a signal from a receptor (also in the plasma membrane) to the inside of the cell.

GABA Gamma aminobutyric acid; believed to function as an inhibitory neurotransmitter in the central nervous system.
The major neurotransmitter in the brain implicated in several psychiatric and neurologic conditions, most notably Huntington's disease.

GABA receptor A gamma-aminobutyric acid receptor on which sedatives, hypnotics and antianxiety drugs act.

Gaffelbitar Semipreserved herring product in which microbial growth is checked by addition of salt at a concentration of 10-12% and sometime by addition of benzoic acid.

Gag reflex Reflex contraction of the pharyngeal constrictors in response to stroking the oropharynx.

Gain Amplification of the reflected ultrasound waves. Echoes coming from deep tissues need more amplification than those coming from superficial tissues.

Gait There are many types of abnormal gait. *Paraparetic gait* is a walking pattern in which both legs are moved in a slow, stiff manner. Legs may tend to cross with each forward swing. It develops in cerebral palsy. *Steppage gait* is produced by weakness of ankle dorsiflexion. Because of foot drop, leg is to be lifted higher. If bilateral it is due to distal polyneuropathy and if unilateral it is due to L_5 radiculopathy. *Waddling gait* results from proximal lower limb weakness most often from myopathy. *Parkinson's gait* is characterised by a forward stoop with modest flexion at the hips and knees. The arms are flexed at elbows. Walking is initiated slowly by leaning forward and maintained with short rapid steps. *Cerebellar ataxic gait* is broad based gait disorder in which speed and length of stride varies regularly from step to step. *Hemiparetic gait* characterises spastic hemiparesis. Affected leg is flexed less than the normal during its forward swing and is more externally rotated. It is a common residual sign of stroke.

Gait Cycle The period between ipsilateral foot contacts (essentially two steps).

Galactosaemia In it physiological jaundice is exaggerated. Galactose phosphate accumulates in the blood in galactosaemia. This blocks the activity of enzyme phosphoglucomutase which helps in converting the glycogen into glucose. Diagnosis is suspected if a reducing substance is found in urine. There is an inability to metabolise galactose hence leads to high blood and tissue galactose level and galactosuria. Classic glactosaemia is due to glucose1 phosphate uridyestransferase deficiency, an autosomal recessive disease. Symptoms may be cataract, cirrhosis and mental retardation. Hydration of lens and precipitation of protein occurs due to dulcitol, a derivative of galactose. Within weeks of birth child may develop diarrhoea, vomiting, progressive hepatomegaly and jaundice. Galactokinase deficiency also produces galactosaemia and cataract during infancy.

Galactose Simple sugar $CH_2OH\ (CHOH)_4\ CHO$ (Commonly occurring in lactose).

Galeazzi fracture This results on the outstretched hand with forearm in pronation. There is fracture

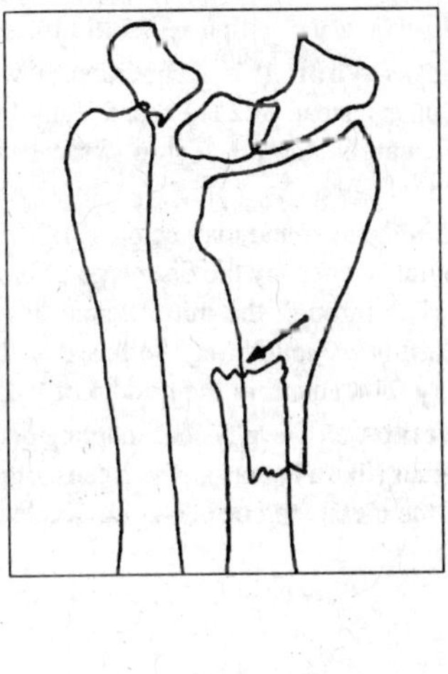

of distal third of radius with associated dislocation of distal radioulnar joint. Ulna is dislocated dorsally and medially.

Galen vein Great cerebral vein.

Galenic Pertaining to the ancient system of medicine taught and practiced by Galen.

Galenicals Crude drugs, infusion and tincture preparations from medicinal plants.

Gall bladder It is a pear-shaped organ situated underneath the liver to which it is attached by fibrous tissue.

Bile produced in liver reaches gall bladder through cystic duct. Within gall bladder it is stored and concentrated.

When food passes from stomach to duodenum, secretin and cholecystokinin cause the gall bladder to contract and expel its content of bile into duodenum where bile emulsifies fats.

Gall bladder cancer Chronic cholecystitis with stone may lead to malignancy. The cancer may cause tenderness in right upper abdomen. But sometimes it may be symptomless. Ultrasound can diagnose it. Surgical removal in early stage is feasible.

Gall stones These are round or oval smooth or faceted lumps of solid material. Only 20 per cent of gall stones cause symptoms. When impacted in bile duct they cause biliary colic. Indigestion is made worse by food containing fats. These may result in cholecystitis. Silent stones can be left alone. When symptoms are severe, cholecystectomy can be done.

Gallates Salts and esters of gallic acid.

Gallon Imperial gallon is 4.546 litres.

Gallop rhythm It is a condition in which 3 heart sounds instead of 2 are heard. Pathological causes are bundle branch lesion. First heart sound is reduplicated.

Third heart sound may be present in early stage of mitral stenosis by the discharge of blood from left auricle through the mitral valve in mid diastole. Third heart sound may be heard at the apex as a very faint sound in the middle of diastole.

Galvanic cell The physical coupling of two different metals (like a battery), which causes the least noble of the metals to corrode at an accelerated rate.

Galvanic skin response (GSR) Lowered resistance of the skin to passage of an electrical current following emotional and other forms of stimulation. Recorded with the psycho-galvanometer.

The change in the electrical resistance of the skin in response to diverse stimuli; an easily measured variable widely used in experimental studies.

Galvanism Direct current created by a battery. An electromotive force of 500 mV may exist in the mouth.

Gamete a haploid sex cell; either an egg cell or a sperm cell.

Gamete intrafallopian transfer (GIFT) A procedure in which aspirated secondary occytes are combined with a solution containing sperm outside the body, and the mixture is then immediately inserted into the uterine (Fallopian) tubes.

Gametogamy Sexual reproduction by fusion of gametes to produce a zygote.

Gametogenesis Development and maturation of sperm and ova.

Gamma (g) motor neuron Fusimotor neuron supplying the intrafusal muscle fibers of a muscle spindle.

Gamma camera Imaging device used in nuclear scanning. It was first used in 1960. Principle of it may be used in position-emission tomography (PET) camera too using six crystals in hexagonal configuration.

Gamma counting It is the process by which the intensity of a flux of gamma-rays is measured or imaged. Gamma-rays interacts with matter through photoelectric absorption.

Gamma globulin These have been demonstrated in saliva as other proteins. Certain gamma globulins known as immuno globulins possess antibody activity.

Saliva also contains several coagulation factors (VIII, IX, X, PTA and Hageman factor) that hasten blood coagulation and tend to protect wounds from invasion by microorganisms.

Gamma knife A stereotactic radio surgery device that allows well defined, deep seated brain tumors less than 3 cm in diameter to be treated in a single session under local anaesthesia using the overlapping of narrow collimated beams from 201 cobalt 60 sources.

Gamma-ray Electromagnetic wave of high energy emanating from a nucleus rather than from the electronic shell of an atom.

Gamontogamy Sexual reproduction by the pairing of parent cells and exchange of gametes, usually resulting in cross fertilization.

Ganglion It is a cystic swelling that develops as a result of mucoid degeneration of connective tissue of the joint capsule usually at back of wrist and dorsum of foot. It is a rounded firm and elastic swelling, of the size of bigger pea nut. It contains a jelly-like substance under tension system.

Ganglion, dorsal nerve root Enlargement of the dorsal root of the spinal nerve located at or just medial to the junction of the ventral and dorsal spinal roots. It contains the cell bodies of the afferent neurons, including visceral afferents, entering the spinal cord by the dorsal root.

Ganglion, sympathetic chain A connected series of sympathetic ganglia located anterolateral to either side of the vertebral column from the upper cervical region to the coccyx. At the coccyx the left and right chains are joined, forming the ganglion impar. The superior cervical, middle cervical, and stellate ganglia are located within the sympathetic chain ganglia.

Ganglioneuroma These are benign tumours of the sympathetic chains or the adrenal medulla. Common location is mediastinum but 20% are found in adrenal also. These are well encapsulated small tumours consisting of ganglia cells and nerve fibres. These are found incidentally.

Gangliosides Sphingolipids, containing complex oligosaccharides as head groups; especially common in nervous tissue.

Gangrene It is a death of tissue due to loss of blood supply. Pain is felt in dying tissues but once they become dead become numb. The affected skin and underlying tissue turns black. Bacterial infection may develop giving a typical smell. In *dry gangrene* there is no bacterial infection. This does not spread to other tissues and is caused by arteriosclerosis and diabetes mellitus. *Wet gangrene* develops when wound becomes infected by bacteria. Treatment includes to improve circulation. Antibiotics may be given to prevent wet gangrene. If wet gangrene develops amputation is the only solution.

Gänsslen syndrome It is an autosomal dominant disorder. Clinical features include haemolytic anaemia, splenomegaly, deformities of external ear, hypogenitalism and retinal haemorrhage. X-ray will show frontal and parietal prominence, oxycephaly and polydactly. Dental deformities are noted.

Gap junction Small channels that allow materials to pass from one cell to an adjacent cell; provides a means of intercellular communication.

Garden's femoral neck fracture It is an intracapsular fracture. It may be complete or partial. There may be rupture of ligaments with or without dislocation.

Gardener's syndrome It is a hereditary disturbance. Osteomas of maxilla, mandible and other facial bones are associated with polyps of large intestine, odontomas and epidermal cyst of skin. After about 15 years of onset many of polyps in large bowel develop adenocarcinoma.

Gardner wells Tongs It is hard, rigid device applied to the sides of skull for traction.

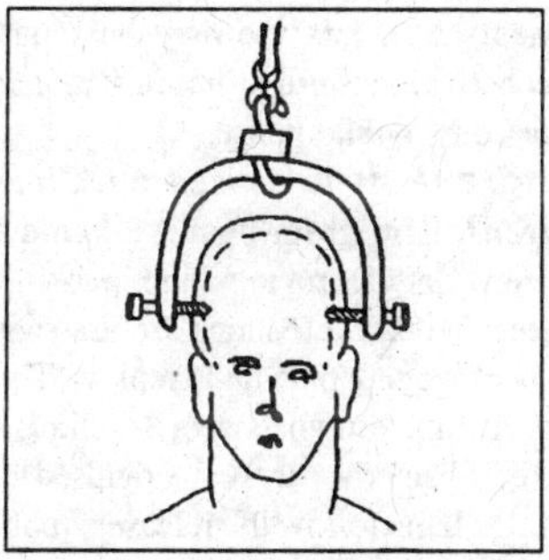

Gardner's femoral neck fracture Stage I is an incomplete fracture, stage II complete but

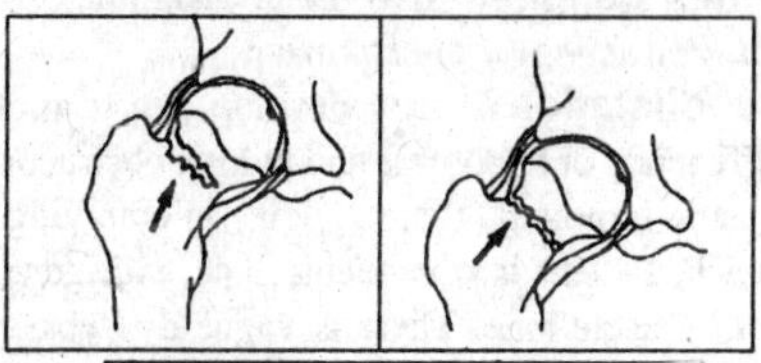

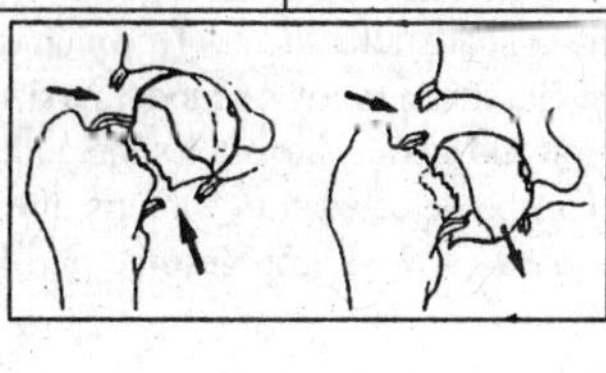

undisplaced fracture, stage III complete and partially displaced fracture while stage IV completely displaced fracture.

Gargle It is a liquid preparation to wash and freshen the mouth. Liquid may contain saline, black tea, antiseptic and local anaesthetic. Antiseptic gargles are helpful in sore throat.

Garlic Bulb of allium sativum with pungent adour.

Garre's disease In some patients with osteomyelitis there is significant growth of new bone tissue underneath the periosteum. This type of proliferative or sclerosing reaction in bone is known as Garre's osteomyelitis. The mandible is involved more frequently than the maxilla and commonly occurs in children. There is an inflammatory lesion within jaw. Microscopic sections show elevation of periosteum and new bone formation. Treatment of Garre's disease consists of removal of cause.

Gartner's duct Longitudinal duct of epoophoron, remains of mesonephric duct in female.

Gas chromatography Procedure whereby components of a mixture may be separated by partition between a solid or liquid stationary phase and a gaseous mobile phase.

Gas gangrene It is caused by *Clostridium perfringens*. The gram-positive spore bearing bacilli are widely found in nature, particularly soil and faeces. Wound infections are associated with severe local wound, pain and crepitus. The wound presents a thin, brown, sweet smelling exudate from which bacteria can be recognised on Gram staining. Oedema follow the release of collagenase and hyaluronidase. Prophylaxis in patients at risk should always be considered.

Gasserian ganglion Trigeminal ganglion.

Gastric Pertaining to the stomach.

Gastric dilatation It may develop due to motor insufficiency or hypotonia and pyloric obstruction. In gastric hypotonia there is delay in emptying of stomach. Patient is of asthenic type with general loss of muscle tone. There is vague dyspepsia or discomfort usually after meals. True pain is absent. Prolonged lassitude follows a moderate sized meal. Depression and anxiety are often superadded. Food residue can be detected 6 to 8 hours after meals. The disease is always troublesome and liable to relapse.

Gastric emptying Control of gastric emptying is essential to maintain the reservoir function of stomach by allowing adequate mixing of gastric content and formation of chyme. Emptying of stomach depends on osmolarity of meal, pH of meal, physical state of meal, i.e. solid and liquid phase. Liquids are handled primarily by the fundus and proximal part of body of stomach. A satiety hormonal system probably exists, slowing emptying and reproducing a central sensation of satiety the most likely hormone being CCK/PZ (cholecystokinin/pancreozymin) Gastric emptying method has been studied by dye dilution method.

Gastric erosion It is the break in continuity in the innermost layer of the membrane that lines the stomach. It occurs in some cases of gastritis. Break beyond this layer is known as gastric ulcer. Ingestion of alcohol, iron tablets, aspirin may cause it. It may be asymptomatic although erosions may bleed. It may cause haematemesis or melena. Gastric erosions heal completely in a few days with antacid drugs and ranitidine.

Gastric glands Glands in the mucosa of the stomach composed of cells that empty their secretions into narrow channels called gastric pits. Types of cell are chief cells (secrete pepsinogen), parietal cells (secrete hydrochloric acid and intrinsic factor), mucous surface and mucous neck cells (secrete mucus), and G cells (secrete gastrin).

Gastric intrinsic factor A glycoprotein secreted by the stomach that is needed for the absorption of vitamin B_{12}.

Gastric juice It is the most acid secretion of body. Acidity of it is due to HCl. The strength of HCl secreted by glands is about 0.55%, pH 0.9. Total chloride is 0.165 N. Mucus of stomach helps to neutralise HCl. Gastric juice contains about 0.55% solids of which a little over 0.4% is organic. This organic portion includes enzyme pepsin, gastric lipase and renin.

Gastric lavage It is done by nursing staff and is not a sterile procedure. It can be done one hourly to rest the gastrointestinal tract as in paralytic ileus or after operation over stomach or duodenum. Nasal tube can be kept for 24 hours while tube through mouth may be removed after procedure is over. It is commonly done to remove poisonous material and to remove irritable material in paralytic ileus. It helps in relieving nausea and vomiting. In case of poisoning aspirated fluid is to be kept for analysis. It is the preferred method of emptying the stomach and should follow the instillation of one dose of activated charcoal. It is most effective if it is done within one hour of ingestion of poison. In case of ingestion of phenothiazines, tricyclic antidepressants, antihistamines can be recovered after several hours of ingestion. To prevent aspiration and to reduce entry of lavage fluid into duodenum, place the patient in left lateral position. About 200 ml of tap water may be used for lavage. In young children isotonic saline may be used.

Gastric reflux Reverse flow of gastric contents.

Gastric residual Volume of liquid remaining in the stomach.

Gastric secretion There are five components of gastric secretion : hydrochloric acid, pepsinogen, bicarbonate, mucus and intrinsic factor. Control of secretion of acid by parietal cells is mediated by hormonal and neural factors. Division into three classic phases of stimulation are cephalic, gastric and intestinal phase hormonally.

Gastric test meal This is done to analyse gastric acidity to rule out ulcer or carcinoma of stomach. Patient is kept 12 hours fasting before the procedure starts in the morning. Nothing is given

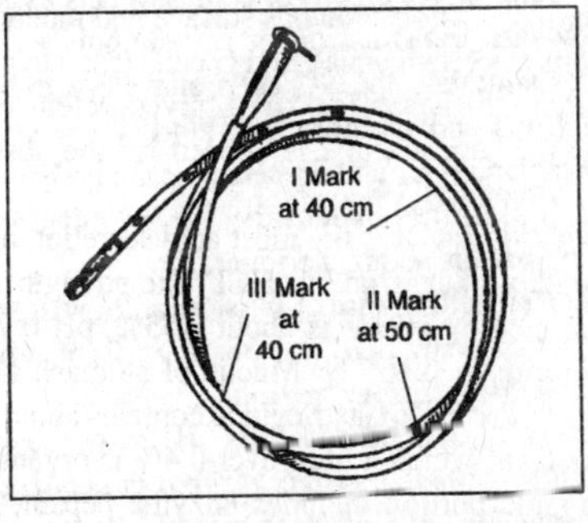

orally too. Then insert the Ryles tube with glycerine in nostril. Patient should swallow the tube. Attach the 20 cc syringe to the tube end and withdraw the content of stomach. Remove all content and label this specimen as fasting specimen. Then give 100 cc of 7% alcohol or half a *chapati* as gruel. After half an hour collect again stomach content and label as first specimen. Similarly collect 4 samples after every 30 minutes are to be taken.

Gastric ulcer Many gastric ulcers may be asymptomatic. These are deep, penetrating beyond the mucosa of the stomach. Almost all benign gastric ulcers are found immediately distal to the junction of antral mucosa and acid secreting mucosa. Benign gastric ulcers are rare in fundus of stomach. Gastric emptying is delayed in gastric ulcer. Clinical features include epigastric pain. Nausea and vomiting may occur without obstruction. Weight loss may occur. These tend to heal but then recur often in same location. Haemorrhage is a common complication. Pain increases by taking food. Ulcers larger than 3 cm in diameter are likely to be malignant. Endoscopic visualisation of ulcer shows definition of its size, location and biopsy gives its histological characteristic.

Gastrin It is an acid stimulating substance isolated by Edkins in 1905. It is produced primarily in G-cells but also in duodenum and pancreas. Microvilli in G cell surface are pH sensitive and this is one of the mechanism of gastrin release. Acid and pepsin release are activated by gastrin. It increases motility of antrum, relaxation of the pylorus and contraction of lower oesophageal sphincter. It inhibits sodium and water absorption in small intestine and stimulates pancreatic secretion. Level of gastrin is increased in atrophic gastritis, pyloric stenosis, phaeochromocytoma and vagotomy.

Gastrinoma Almost all of these are in pancreatic non-beta cell islets. These are smaller than 1 cm and may be multiple. Most are slow growing but malignant. Metastases occur in duodenum. These develop duodenal ulceration with diarrhoea. These may be multiple and may be at unusual site. These may cause watery diarrhoea due to inhibition of salt and water absorption in small intestine but additional factors are the large volume of gastric secretion to be absorbed and intestinal hurry which limits absorption. The steatorrhoea is partly due to inactivation of pancreatic lipase by low pH consequent upon the high acid secretion. Endoscopy shows hypertrophied gastric folds. A basal serum gastrin of greater than 1000 pg/ml is virtually diagnostic.

Gastritis It is the inflammation of gastric mucous membrane. *Acute gastritis* may be caused by aspirin, alcohol, butazolidine, etc. Clinical features include nausea, vomiting, haematemesis and melena. There may be epigastric distress. Bland liquid diet with antacids are useful. H_2 blockers may also be given.

Chronic gastritis may be associated with pernicious anaemia, gastric ulcer, alcohol, tobacco and spicy diet. Gastric mucosal folds are enlarged. Clinical features include anorexia, nausea, vomiting particularly in the morning. There is upper abdominal discomfort. Gastric acid secretions will be found low by augmented histamine test. Mucus is present in all samples in abundance. Gastroscopy will show absence of mucous folds and visible submucosal veins.

Gastro intestinal tract obstruction Most common causes are intussception, volvulus and hernia.

Gastrocolic reflex Increased peristaltic activity.

Gastrodermis In Hydra, the inner epithelium of the body wall that surrounds the gastrovascular cavity.

Gastroenteritis It is the inflammation of stomach and intestine caused by virus, bacteria and other organisms. Symptoms include nausea, vomiting, cramps and diarrhoea. It develops suddenly and continues for 3 to 4 days.

Oral rehydration and antibiotics help. In severe cases where shock and collapse occur hospitalisation is necessary. Patients are to be given IV fluids. Recovery usually is complete without any complication.

Gastroenterology The medical specialty that deals with the structure, function, diagnosis, and treatment of diseases of the stomach and intestines.

Gastroesophageal reflux The return of gastric contents into the esophagus that results in a severe burnning sensation under the sternum.

Gastroesophageal sphincter A ring of smooth muscle around the opening of he stomach at the lower end of the esophagus that acts as a valve to allow food to enter the stomach but prevents stomach contents from moving back into the esophagus.

Gastrointestinal tract Technically only the stomach and intestines. Often used as a synonym for digestive tract, which extends from the mouth to the anus.

Gastroparesis Paralysis of the stomach caused by vagal autonomic neuropathy; causes delayed gastric emptying.

Gastroschisis An abdominal wall defect at the base of the umbilical stalk.

Gastroscopy It is the examination of lining of oesophagus, stomach and first part of duodenum with the help of oesophagogastroduodenoscope. It is used to investigate symptoms such as severe pain and bleeding. It may be used to monitor therapeutic effects. Attachments at the end of instrument helps physician to take biopsy. Procedure is done using a local anaesthesia being sprayed. Whole procedure takes about 20 to 30 minutes.

Gastrostomy Creation of an artificial opening into the stomach through the abdominal wall, used for feeding purposes.

Gastrostomy feeding tube Long, hollow, glexible tube inserted into the stomach through a stab wound in the upper left abdominal quadrant.

Gastrostomy tube, G-Tube Transabdominal tube located in the stomach.

Gate control theory of pain It correlates physiological and pathological data. It is postulated that both large and small fibres act on target cells. Some substantia gelatinosa (SG) cells have an inhibiting effect on target cells and acts as a gate to onward transmission of pain impulses. Large fibres stimulate the SG cells and close the gate. Emotions and memory can modify the system. Prostaglandin E_1 and E_2 sensitise the body to pain and histamine especially in infection and inflammation acting peripherally.

Gating Controlling ease of passage of impulses from one set of neurons to another, e.g., from primary to secondary sensory neurons.

Gaucher's disease This is a disease of reticuloendothelial system, a lipid is deposited in the reticular cells of liver, spleen, lymph nodes and bone marrow. It can occur at any age. Skin shows brown pigmentation. Oral lesions are rare. Because of replacement of marrow and thrombocytopenia, there is gingival bleeding. Under microscope there is presence of large foam cells with striations called Gaucher's cells.

Gaucher's syndrome It is a deficiency of an enzyme glucosidase as a result of which breakdown of flucocerebrosides is reduced. It affects children with weakness, fatigue and progressive dementia. There develops hepatosplenomegaly. Neurological manifestation predominates with hypotonia, dyspnoea, nausea and cranial nerve involvement. There is abnormal modelling of long bones, pathological fractures and compression of vertebral body.

Gauge Diameter

Gavage Feeding through a tube passed into stomach through the oesophagus.

Gavage feeding Forced feeding, as through a tube into the stomach.

Gay These are male or female homosexual persons. The term is favoured by homosexuals themselves. Gay liberation is a social movement in which homosexuals of both sexes assert their right to their own sexual orientation. They want that homosexuality be recognised as a normal variation of gender in human relationship.

Gaze avoidance The tendency to avert one's eyes in order to avoid eye to eye contact with another.

Gel A solution or colloidal suspension that has set to a jelly.

Gelatin Water soluble protein prepared from collagen by boiling with water or from bones.

Gelatin sugar Glycine.

Gelation The conversion of a solution into a gel.

Gender The way in which different sexes behave. Femininity encompasses long hair, makeup, and soft speech; masculinity includes athletic prowess, aggressiveness, and never wearing dresses. Femininity is usually associated with females and masculinity with males. However none of these behaviors is biologically driven; there is no gene in women telling them to curl their hair. Females and males in practice combine many masculine and feminine traits in their daily lives.

Gender identity Confidence in one's self as male or female. It is influenced by the extent to which an individual adopts a typical sex role, but individuals with a high degree of gender identity do not necessarily follow social stereotypes.

Gender marker A protein or DNA determinant that differs beween males and female individuals.

Gender role Everything one says and does to indicate to others or the self the degree to which one is male or female or ambivalent. It includes but is not restricted to sexual arousal and response. Gender role is the public expression of gender identity.

Gene Every human cell holds within its nucleus more than 50,000 different genes. These influence the functioning of all organs. Genes also influence IQ, mental talents and behaviour. The physical material of inheritance DNA is an extremely long, chain-like structure. Gene correspondences to a small section of DNA within a chromosome.

Gene bank There is a collection of large number of diverse genotypes of species. A genotype once lost will not be available to scientists for future evolutionary activities. In gene bank large number of genotypes of a species and its wild relatives all over world are preserved under artificial environmental condition.

Gene disruption The physical disruption of the integrity of a gene by insertion mutagenesis or by deletion, usually of an internal segment of the gene. Gene disruptions are commony constructed by recombinant DNA methods to study gene function.

Gene expression Transcription and, in the case of proteins, translation to yield the product of a gene; a gene is expressed when its biological product is present and active.

Gene flow The transfer of DNA that results from matings between individuals belonging to different populations.

Gene fusion Genetic manipulation to fuse two genes together. Transcriptional fusions are done in such a way that expression of the first gene could be monitored by the phenotype of the second. Translational fusions lead to the in-frame fusion of two coding sequences.

Gene linkage Refers to the fact that all the closely located genes of a given chromosomes are inherited together.

Gene splicing The enzymatic attachment of one gene, or part of a gene, to another.

Gene transfer Any of various methods used for carrying new or altered genes into cells.

General acceptance Accepted among the preponderance of practitioners with an an area of expert endeavor.

General adaptation syndrome Collective physiological processes that occur in response to a stressor.

General anesthetic Irregular, reversible depression of the cells of the higher centers of the central nervous system that makes the patient unconscious and insensible to pain.

General intelligence The term by Spearman—as his concept G—to represent an alleged general ability or capacity which expresses itself through many specific abilities, such as social, mathematical, and mechanical skills.

General practioner A doctor working in primary care in the community. He is the first point of contact for medical cases of all kinds.

Generalised anxiety disorder Chronic, persistent and excessive feelings of anxiety and worry.

Generalised neurofibromatosis It is a multiple neurofibromatosis with numerous malformations. There are lesions in skin, oral cavity, GIT, and bones. Skin may show brown pigmented spots. In the oral cavity, lesions occur in soft tissues and/or jaws. Tongue is commonly affected. If neurofibromas are deep, tongue looks enlarged. If superficial, it appears fissured. It may occur within periodontal membrane and may lead to migration of teeth. Jaw shows radiolucencies.

Generalized transduction The transfer of random fragments of chromosomal DNA from one cell to another cell via a bacteriophage.

Generativity versus stagnation The next-to-last stage in Erikson's psychosocial stages. The issue here is the expansion of one's interest and include the concerns of the next generation, called generativity, versus an exclusive concern with one's own well-being, referred to as stagnation. Generativity is not exclusively a biological concept; it concerns the success of the whole of humanity.

Generator potential The graded depolarization that results in a change in the resting membrane potential in a receptor (specialized neuronal ending); may trigger a nerve action potential (nerve impulse) if depolarization reaches threshold.

Generic Relating to or descriptive of an entire group or class.

Generic drugs Drugs called by their approved and pharmacological names and not by proprietary names. For example, paracetamol is generic name and proprietary name is Crocin.

Generic name Chemical name of drug that is not protected by a manufacture's trademark.

Genes It is estimated that there are over 70,000 genes distributed on human chromosome and that each gene is the DNA code for a specific protein.

Genetic anomaly A marked deviation from the expected standard as a result of an inherited defect.

Genetic code The linear sequence of bases in DNA that ultimately determines the sequence of the amino acids into proteins.

Genetic conditions Disorders that occur as a result of abnormal or absent genes.

Genetic counselling A process in which individuals or families are given information that is needed to understand a hereditary disorder. Advice is being given by genetic specialist to the parents who have chances of having children with congenital defects. It requires exhaustive investigations.

Genetic drift Changes in gene frequency caused by the random sampling of genes during transmission across generations rather than by natural selection.

Genetic engineering Genetic engineering has been used for producing some human hormones, i.e. insulin and growth hormone. The main technique for mass production by genetic engineering is called DNA technology. DNA is the substance in cells that consists of strings of genes controlling the manufacture of different proteins. The types of cells or organism suitable to such genetic alteration are *E. coli* and various yeasts.

Genetic linkage An association of genes in inheritance due to their localization on the same chromosome or other nucleic acid molecule.

Genetic nomenclature The designation of genes according to an abbreviated letter code that is italicized, for example fabH and plsB. The corresponding protein products of these genes are abbreviated as FabH and PlsB.

Genetic recombination The formation of new combinations of genes, as by crossing-over between homologous chromosomes.

Genetic sex Sex determined at conception by union of two X-chromosomes or an X and Y chromosome. It is known as chromosomal sex also.

Genetic sex determination A mechanism of sex determination present in the majority of vertebrates, in which sex is determined by the genetic constitution of individuals.

Genetic traits These are characteristics from parents. It depends whether the genes are dominant over any recessive ones. Genetic traits may predispose to blue eyes, blonde hair, etc.

Genetic transcription The process by which RNA is produced with a sequence of nucleotide bases that is complementary to a region of DNA.

Genetic translation The process by which proteins are produced with amino acid sequences specified by the sequence of codons in messenger RNA.

Genetics It is the study of heredity. Heredity depends on genes. A multitude of paired genes make up paired chromosomes present as strands of DNA.

Development of body depends how specific genes or combination of genes are paired with the corresponding genes from the other parent whether one is dominant or recessive. Some congenital disorders may be inherited through the presence or absence of specific genes.

Genial tubercles Tiny bumps of bone in the anterior region of the mandible that serve as attachment sites for the genioglossus and geniohyoid muscles; appear radiopaque.

Genicular Pertaining to the knee.

Geniculate Knee-form, meaning bent.

Geniculostriate system A system consisting of projections from the retina to the lateral geniculate nucleus to the visual cortex.

Genital herpes A sexually transmitted diseased caused by type 2 herpes simplex virus.

Genital stage The stage at which, according to Freudian theory, full maturity has been attained; in the genital stage, the individual has achieved mature relations with the opposite sex.

Genital tubercle The embryonic primordium of the phallus. Seen in both males and females, it enlarges in the male to from the penis. In the female significant growth does not occur and it forms the clitoris.

Genital warts Several types of viruses may be involved. It gives rise to moist, soft, pink, pedunculated papillomatous or vegetating growth on any mucocutaneous surface such as coronal sulcus, cervix in females and in rectum and perianal region in both. No treatment is satisfactory.

Genitalia The reproductive organ.

Genitourinary tuberculosis Organism reaches the urinary tract via blood stream from a primary focus elsewhere. Common complaint will be urinary frequency and dysuria. Other symptoms

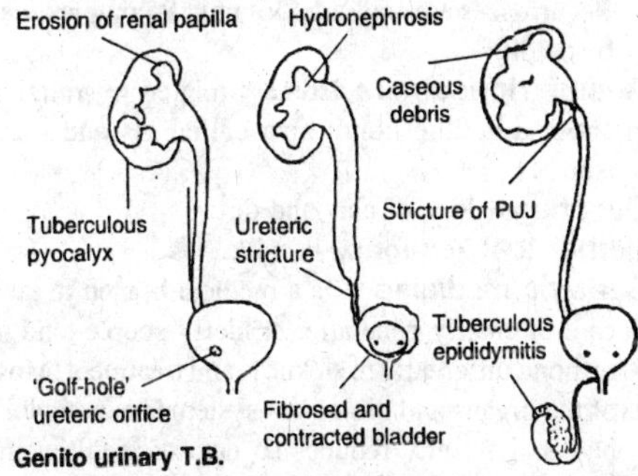

Genito urinary T.B.

include loin pain, haematuria, and nonspecific symptoms such as lethargy, malaise and anorexia. Chemotherapy is the mainstay of treatment. But it may lead to accelerated fibrosis and in rapid restricturing of one or both ureters.

Genome The genetic makeup of cells and viruses. It represents the total number of chromosomes which is the diploid number in somatic cells and the haploid number in gametes.

Genomics Relating to or involving the genome. The study of genome, or all of the genes of an organism.

Genotype The total set of genes present at the time of conception, producing the genetic constitution.

Genotyping It is a genetic constitution. Genotyping of father is indicated where RH negative mother gives birth to a child suffering from hemolytic disease. It helps in determining whether father is homozygos or heterozygos

Gentian violet It is a purple coloured dye to make bacteria visible under microscope. Being antiseptic it is used to treat burns, boils and carbuncles, and fungal infections. In oral thrush also it was used widely.

Genu Meaning a bend.

Genuineness In the person-centred approach to therapy, the capacity of a counsellor to express his or her thoughts or attitudes openly at any given moment in the therapeutic process.

Geographic tongue It shows one or more irregular areas of desquamation on tongue. These may be due to allergy because it is more common in asthma and allergic rhinitis patients. Emotional state is often associated. The spots are bald and filiform papillae are absent. These heal but other areas develop nearby. Lesions do not respond to treatment and may disappear drastically. Recurrences are common. Vitamin B complex may be helpful.

Geometric isomers Isomers related by rotation about a double bond; also called cis and trans isomers.

Geophagia Pica of clay and dirt.

Gerber test Test for fat in milk.

Geriatric medicine It is a medical branch to take care of elderly generation. Elderly people tend to respond differently to sickness and treatment. Most of the organs and biological systems become dull, physical activity reduces so energy requirement becomes lesser. Doses of drugs are to be regulated accordingly. Population of elderly persons is increasing daily so in future separate physicians will be required to look after their interest.

Germ The part of cereal that grows and produces new plants.

Germ cell cycle Asexual reproduction in digenea during which progeny arise through differentiation of germinal cells passed from one generation to the next.

Germ line The arrangement of the genetic material as transmitted through the gametes.

Germ wheat The embryo or sprouting portion of wheat comprising 2.5% of seed. It contains 64% of thiamine, 26% or riboflavin, 21% of pyridoxine.

German measles Oral lesions known as Koplik's spots do not consist of vesicles. They consist of a few or cluster of white or yellow pinpoint papules on an inflamed, red background on buccal mucosa but German measles is not associated with Koplik's spots. Oral lesions when present consist of erythema of mucosa or a few macules in posterior part of mouth.

Germfree Free of all known microoganisms, though not necessarily free of virus for all species.

Germicide Anything that destroys bacteria; applied especially to chemical agents that kill disease germs, but not necessarily bacterial spores; applied to both living tissue and inanimate objects.

Germinal center Discrete areas within lymph node and spleen where B cell maturation and memory development occur.

Germinal disc A 2-3 mm region of the surface of the avian oocyte that contains the female pronucleus, cellular organelles, and the only continuous oolemma with microvilli.

Germinal epithelium A layer or bed of germ cells in the ovary that divide mitotically and give rise to primary oocytes.

Germinal vesicle The diploid nucleus of the oocyte.

Germination When a single tooth germ splits or attempts to split to form two or partially separated crowns the process is called germination. There is usually a single root canal.

Germogen The germinal area of the ovary.

Gerodontics That branch of dentistry which treats all problems peculiar to the oral cavity in old age and the aging population. Also called geriatric dentistry.

Gerogogy Techniques that enhance learning among older adults.

Geronotic Refers to working with the elderly.

Gerontology The study of an old age.

Gerota's Fascia Renal fascia.

Gestalt psychology The school of psychology which disparages the partist approach to experience and behaviour and argues for emphasis upon wholes, which, Gestalt psychologists say, are more than the sum of as opposed to trial and error; in perception, it stresses primitive organisations, such as figure-ground relationships and the phiphenomenon, which appear to be independent of past experience. The word "gestalt" is often translated as configuration or form and the school is sometimes referred to as configurationalist, i.e. as emphasising configurations rather than their constituent parts.

Gestalt therapy A form of psychotherapy, initiated by Fritz Perls, that emphasizes awareness of the present and employs an active therapist-client relationship.

Gestation The period of development from fertilization to birth.

Gestational age The age of the product of conception between fertilisation and birth.

Gestational diabetes Diabetes initially diagnosed during pregnancy, due to glucose intolerance.

Gestational diabetes mellitus A form of diabetes occurring during pregnancy, most commonly after the twentieth week of gestation.

Gestational hypertension A relatively benign condition of elevated BP during pregnancy without signs of proteinuria and edema.

Gestational surrogate A woman who carries the embryo of an infertile couple and relinquishes the child after birth.

Gestures The way patient touches the body while explaining a problem. These movements may indicate whether the problem is a muscle problem, a joint problem, or a visceral problem.

Geyser sign While doing shoulder arthrogram leakage of dye outline glenohumeral joint in subdeltoid bursa due to rotator cuff tear.

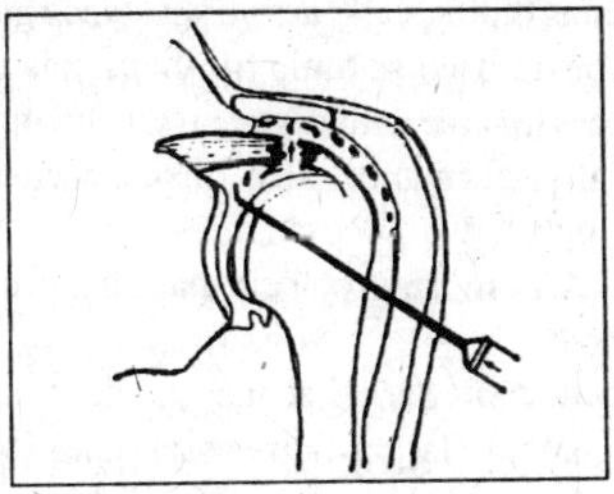

Ghee Clarified butter fat made by heating, and separating the water. It is made from milk of cow, buffalo, goat or sheep.

Ghost image An artefact on dental radiographs produced when an area of increased density is penetrated twice by the X-ray beam; appears radiopaque.

Gianotti-Crosti syndrome The syndrome is characterised by papular eruptions on the extremities and face generally associated with gastro-intestinal or respiratory symptoms, and mild fever.

Giant cell arteritis It is also known as cranial arteritis or temporal arteritis. It is a disease of elders with temporal headache and tenderness. Temporal artery pulsation reduces and person even may become blind due to involvement of ophthalmic artery. Biopsy shows giant cell infiltration. Treatment is with 40 to 60 mg of prednisolone till symptoms are controlled.

Giant cell granuloma It is seen in patient under 20 years of age mostly in females. Mandible is more commonly involved. Lesion is usually expansile. Regional teeth may migrate. X-ray shows a single cystic area or a soap bubble appearance. It contains multiple nucleated giant cells with numerous small vessels. Local curettage is the treatment of choice.

Giant cell tumour Initial complaint is of localised pain and swelling accentuated by trauma. Histological picture is of richly vascular tissue consisting of plumb spindle cells and numerous giant cells with 50 to 100 nuclei. X-ray shows soap bubble appearance. Penetration of thinned cortex with tumour leads to soft tissue mass.

Giant motor unit A motor unit potential with a peak to peak amplitude and duration much greater than normal ranges. Often seen following collateral sprouting with regeneration of peripheral nerves.

Giardiasis It is the infection caused by *Giardia lamblia*. The disease is spread by contaminated food and water. 75 per cent infected children do not show any symptom. After 3 to 4 days child may have attack of diarrhoea with gas formation. Child may develop foul smelling faeces which is greasy. There may be abdominal pain and cramps. Microscopic study gives diagnosis. Metronidazole or quinacrine helps in relieving symptoms.

Gibson murmur A rumbling murmur continuously heard without interruption in both systole and diastole, and is found in patent ductus arteriosus.

Gifted persons With special talents also individuals with an IQ of 130 or above, such as Terman's gifted children, in the upper 2 per cent of the general population.

Gigantism Growth hormone produced by eosinophilic cells promotes the growth of cartilage and connective tissue. It stimulates growth of skull and skeleton. If an adenoma of eosinophilic cells, occurs before the cessation of normal growth period, gigantism will be the result. There is an enlargement of maxilla and mandible, a marked increase in vertical dimension, early eruption of teeth and an enlarged tongue. There may be hypercementosis.

Giganto A combining form meaning huge.

Gilles de la Tourette syndrome It is characterised by gradually worsening of habit spasms consisting of brief, purposeless, semivoluntary or involuntary contraction of muscles.

Gimbernat's ligament : Lacunar ligament.

Gin Spirit containing 31% of alcohol.

Ginger Rhizome of Zingiber officinale used as favouring spice.

Gingiva The fleshy covering over the mandible and maxilla through which the teeth protrude within the mouth; also called the gum.

Gingival abrasion The attrition of gingival tissue by harsh irritants, faulty tooth brushing and coarse foods.

Gingival clefts A cleft of marginal gingiva. It may be caused by faulty tooth brushing.

Gingival dehydration The dying of gingival tissue leading to a lowered tissue resistance resulting in gingival inflammation. It is seen in mouth breathing.

Gingival flap plastic surgery In implant dentistry, the surgical procedure by which gingival flaps are reduced in thickness, trimmed, or otherwise recontoured in preparation for suturing to promote long-term health and improve prosthodontic retention and esthetics.

Gingival graft Excision and moving of a piece of gingiva or thick mucosa from one area to another.

Gingival index A scale in which a score is assigned based on observed gingival conditions around teeth or implants, particularly pocket depth, mobility, and propensity of fluid transfer inducing bleeding.

Gingival lichen planus Lesions are usually atrophic and gingiva appears shiny, inflamed and smooth. Striae are uncommon. It involves limited segments. Tooth brushing becomes difficult.

Gingival margin The soft tissue of gums next to the tooth.

Gingival receptor site A site in attached gingival tissue of the maxillary crest or lingual incline prepared to receive an intra-mucosal insert.

Gingival retracting clamp Rubber dam clamp that provides retraction of the gingival tissue.

Gingival sulcus Space between the free gingiva and the tooth.

Gingivectomy The surgical removal of diseased gingiva to eliminate periodontal pockets.

Gingivectomy knife Instrument, with specially designed blades used to incise gingival tissue.

Gingivitis Inflammation of the gingiva; usually a result of poor oral hygiene and an accumulation of bacterial plaque on the teeth.

Gingivobuccoaxial Pertaining to or formed by the gingival, buccal, and axial walls of the cavity preparation of a tooth.

Gingivolabial Pertaining to the gingivae and lips.

Gingivoplasty The surgical contouring of the gingival tissue to produce the physiologic architectual form necessary for the maintenance of tissue health and integrity. Grit the size of abrasive particles determined by the number of particles which, end to end, equal one inch; fine, stony, hard particles used for grinding. Plastic surgery of the gingiva to shape it to physiologic contour.

Gingivoglossitis Inflammation of the gingivae and tongue.

Gingivolabial Pertaining to the gingivae and lips.

Ginseng It is a root of two plants of same family. It contains biologically active substance ginsenoside. It is being used as tonic for thousands of years. It appears to have antifatigue effect and may increase sexual performance. Side effects include oedema and high BP.

Girdle A bony ring or belt that attaches a limb to the body.

Glabrous skin Skin that does not have hair follicles but contains larger numbes of sensory receptors than do other skin areas.

Gland A single cell or a multicellular structure that secretes substances into the blood, a cavity, or onto a surface.

Glanders It is an acute and often fatal, condition causing ulceration and necrosis of nasal mucosa and septum and occasional skin ulcers. It is caused by gram-negative, small rod, *Pseudomonas malleian* infection of horses and donkeys. The condition gives rise to abscess on the skin which spreads along the lymphatics and invades the blood stream and produces metastatic abscesses in lungs and bones. There may develop cellulitis, necrosis, abscess and thrombosis with septic embolism.

Glandilemma The capsule or outer envelope of a gland.

Glands, swollen Lymphadenopathy develops due to enlargement and infection of glands, specially children. When the physician examines the patients he should try to palpate glands. Soft, flat submandibular nodes lesser then 1 cm are often palpable in healthy children and healthy adults may have palpable inguinal nodes up to 2 cm. Symptoms such as sore throat, cough, fever, night sweats, weight loss, chronic cough or pain in nodes need examination of glands. Localised or regional adenopathy implies involvement of single anatomic area. Occipital adenopathy often reflects an infection of scalp and preauricular adenopathy accompanies conjunctival infections. The chief malignant causes include metastatic cancer from head and neck, breast, lung and thyroid primaries. Enlargement of supraclavicular and scalenus nodes is always abnormal. Axillary lymph node enlargement is due to injuries or localised infection. Inguinal lymphadenopathy is usually secondary to infection. Tenderness is found when capsule is stretched during rapid enlargement secondary to inflammation. Leukaemia may produce rapid enlargement and pain in nodes. Nodes involved by lymphoma tend to be large, discrete, firm, mobile and non-tender. Nodes containing metastatic cancer are often hard, nontender and fixed. Tuberculosis may result in matted cervical lymphadenopathy. Enlarged intra-abdominal or peritoneal lymph glands are generally malignant.

Glandular epithelium Cells that are specialized for secreting activity.

Glandular fever It is particularly common in young adults. It causes sore throat with reddening of fauces and tonsils and enlargement of lymphatic glands. Spleen is enlarged. On palate multiple petechiae may occur. After 1 to 2 weeks of malaise and fever the throat becomes sore. This infection is seen in young adults. There is generalised lymphadenopathy. Incubation period is 5 to 15 days. There will be droplet infection caused by herpes virus. There will be low-grade fever, weakness and myalgia. Throat will be sore with splenomegaly. Transient macular or maculopapular or petechial rash will be seen over palate. There will be lymphocytosis and agglutination test will be positive by 4th week. A titre above 1:128 is considered significant.

Glans The distal end of the shaft of the penis.

Glans penis The slightly enlarged region at the distal end of the penis.

Glare The more the eye is dark adapted, the easier it will be dazzled by glare. Physiological glare decreases visual performance. It decreases the differential threshold for brightness, the potential capability for resolution and the speed with which an object of a certain brightness can be recognised. Lower half of retina is apparently less sensitive to glare than the upper. Glare sensitivity may increase with age.

Glaserian fissure Petrotympanic fissure.

Glass ionomer A dental material composed of an acidic polymer liquid and a fluoride-containing aluminosilicate glass. used as a restorative material, base, liner, and cement.

Glass ionomers These are used in liners, bases, sealants, restorative and luting cements. These are composed of acidic polymer liquid mixed with silicate glass powder containing calcium, aluminium and fluorine. These minimize the formation of secondary caries.

Glass state A highly viscous liquid that appears to be solid. Biopesticides dried in the presence of various carbohydrates can be stabilized when encapsulated in the glass state formed by the carbohydrate.

Glass transition temperature A characteristic temperature for certain types of materials, such as glasses and polymers, at which material physically transforms from a hard, glassy state to a soft, moldable state.

Glaucoma In it pressure of eye fluid is very high. A minimal pressure is required to maintain the shape of eyeball. If pressure is very high it may press blood vessels and nerve fibres causing loss

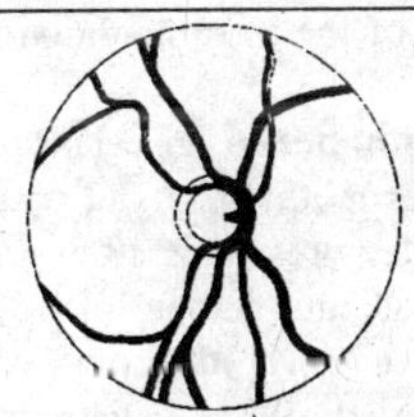

Retinal changes in glaucoma

of vision. *Open angle glaucoma* rarely develops below the age of 40. It is due to gradual blockage of outflow of aqueous humour over a period of years. It may run in families. In *close angle glaucoma*, there is sudden obstruction to the outflow of aqueous humour and pressure rises suddenly. *Congenital glaucoma* is due to a structural abnormality in the drainage angles of eye. Repeated tonometry and visual field testing should be done. Drugs have to be taken life long. Surgery includes peripheral iridectomy.

Glaucomatous optic atrophy Most important finding is the cupping of disc. The cup is deep and reaches up to the margin of optic disc. The vessels bend sharply at margin. There is a parallax between the vessels on retina and vessels at the bottom of the cup. In case of glaucomatous optic atrophy there shall be an increased intraocular pressure while it is normal in anterior ischaemic optic neuropathy.

GLBT "Gay, Lesbian, Bisexual, and Transgendered".

Glenoid fossa A concave, depressed area of the temporal bone on which the mandibular condyle rests; appears radiolucent.

Glia Supporting cells of nervous tissue; also called neuroglia.

Gliadin A plant protein fraction of wheat gluten.

Gliding Movement in which the joint surfaces are flat or only slightly curved and one articulating surface slides on the other.

Gliding joint A synovial joint having articulating surfaces that are usually flat, permitting only side-to-side and back-and forth movements, as between carpal bones, tarsal bones, and the scapula and clavicle.

Gliding motility Spontaneous movement on solid surfaces in the absence of flagella.

Glioblast A progenitor cell that gives rise to different types of glial cells.

Glioma One of the most common types of brain tumors.

Glioma of optic nerve Visual disturbance, squint, proptosis, exophthalmos and optic atrophy are presenting features. It is slow growing. It is a primary ectodermal tumour of optic nerve. Glial tumours are derived from astrocytes and oligodendroglial cells of optic nerve. Glioma is a non-neoplastic and self-limiting tumour of the optic nerve with good prognosis. It develops below the age of 10 years.

Gliosis Scarring produced by astrocytes.

Glisson's capsule Perivascular fibrous capsule of liver.

Global aphasia Severe aphasia characterized by marked impairments of the production and comprehension of language; all sensory modalities may be impaired. The individual may be unable to use any expressive speech and may use some gestures or pantomime instead.

Global burden of disease The collective impact of disease on all nations of the modern world.

Globalization In public health, the phenomenon that the processes of food importation, international trade, travel, tourism, etc., significantly affect the ability of a sovereign state to protect the health of its citizenary.

Globin A hemoprotein that reacts with dioxygen, generally reversibly and without reduction of the released oxygen.

Globose Globose nucleu of the cerebellum.

Globular leukocytes Migratory cells of the tracheobronchial epithelia, possibly derived from mast cells; postulated to play a role in the immunological process.

Globular proteins Soluble proteins with a globular shape.

Globulin A type of plasma protein that incudes antibodies.

Globus Usually refers to the globus pallidus in the cerebral white matter.

Globus pallidus One of the nuclei of the basal ganglia, the globus pallidus plays a role in motor control.

Glomerular capsule The double -walled proximal portion of a renal tubule that encloses the glomerulus of a nephron; also called Bowman's capsule.

Glomerular filtrate The fluid produced when blood is filtered by the filtration membrane in the glomeruli of the kidneys.

Glomerular filtration rate (GFR) The total volume of fluid that enters all the glomerular (Bowman's) capsules of the kidneys in 1 min; about 125 mL/min.

Glomerular ultrafiltrate Fluid filtered through the glomerular capillaries into the glomerular capsule of the kidney tubules.

Glomerulonephritis It is the inflammation of glomeruli. Generally both kidneys are affected. It hampers the removal of waste products, salt and water from blood stream.

Mild form of glomerulonephritis does not produce any symptom. There may be some puffiness below eyes. In advance cases there may be high blood pressure and dull ache in loins. Urine may contain RBCs and albumin. At last kidney failure may result.

Glomerulus Mass of capillary loops at the beginning of each nephron, nearly surrounded by Bowman's capsule. A coiled tuft of capillaries surrounded by the glomerular capsule. It filters urine from the blood.

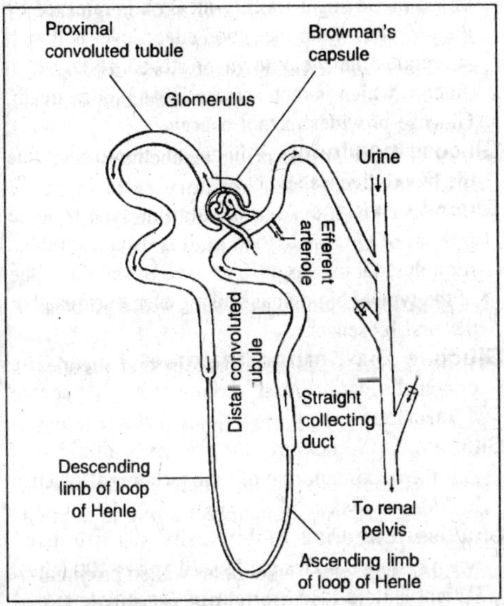

Glomus tumour A benign, extremely painful tumour of modified smooth muscle cells arising from glomus body. Grossly tumours are less than 1 cm in diameter and may be pinpoint. Histologically they consist of branching vascular channels separated by stroma.

Glossitis Inflammation of the tongue.

Glossodynia It refers to pain an unpleasant sensation of itching in tongue. Cause may be nutritional deficiency, anaemia, xerostomia and postmenopausal syndrome. Burning mouth is seen in postmenopausal syndrome. Symptom is mostly accompanied with psychogenic factor.

Glossograph An apparatus for recording tongue movements.

Glossology The sum of knowledge regarding the tongue.

Glossomantia Prognosis based on the appearance of the tongue.

Glossoncus A swelling of the tongue.

Glossopathy A disease of the tongue.

Glossopexy Lip-tongue adhesion.

Glossopharyngeal Sensory distribution of the glossopharyngeal nerve and to its motor supply to stylopharyngeus.

Glossopharyngeal air space An air space on a panoramic film that appears as a radiolucency posterior to the tongue and oral cavity.

Glossopharyngeal nerve block It can be used for the evaluation of atypical facial pain, the treatment of glossopharyngeal neuralgia and the treatment of intractable plain caused by pharyngeal cancer. Refractory hiccups have also been treated successfully. It also helps in manipulations as endoscopy or laryngoscopy.

Glossopharyngeal neuralgia It is the severe pain in the posterior part of tongue and pharynx. It occurs in older people and is unilateral. Its cause is unknown. It is a rare condition associated with paroxysmal pain. Pain is less intense than trigeminal neuralgia. Location and trigger zone of pain sensation follows distribution of nerve specially pharynx, posterior tongue, ear and infraauricular area. Pain starts by chewing, talking and swallowing, all of which stimulate mucosa of pharynx. It is mostly due to intra or extracranial tumours. Treatment includes carbamazepine and baclofen.

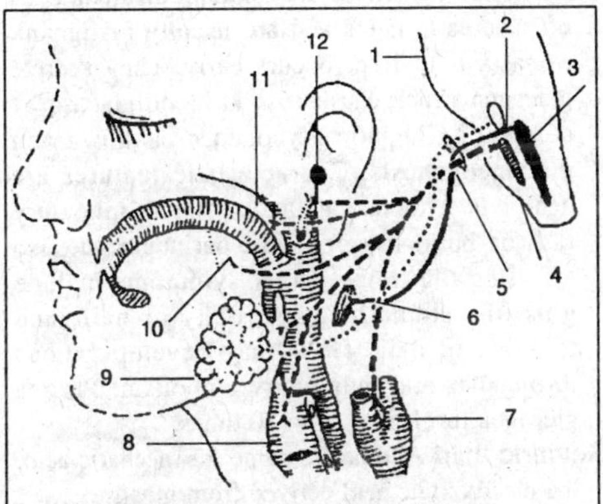

Distribution of the glossopharyngeal nerve

1. pons
2. inferior salivary nucleus
3. nucleus ambiguous
4. solitary nucleus
5. jugular foramen
6. stylopharyngeus muscle
7. carotid sinus
8. larynx
9. parotid gland
10. posterior 1/3rd of tongue (taste and sensory)
11. soft palate
12. middle ear

Glossoplasty Plastic surgery of the tongue.

Glossoptosis Retraction or downward displacement of the tongue.

Glossotrichia Hairy tongue.

Glottis The vocal apparatus of the larynx, consisting of the true vocal folds and the opening between them.

Glotz syndrome It is also known as focal dermal hypoplasia syndrome. It is a familial disorder usually lethal in character. Exact cause is not known. At birth skin shows irregular linear streaks of telangiectasis. One can notice atrophy and pigmentation over trunk and limbs.

Glucagon It is the hormone produced and secreted by pancreas to raise the level of glucose in blood. It promotes the reabsorption of glucose from the tissue cells. Too little glucagon may result in very low level of blood sugar level. Its effect is opposite of insulin.

Glucagonoma These are tumours of alpha cells of pancreatic islets and are usually malignant. Metastasis to liver occurs early. They secrete glucagon which causes rise in blood glucose by stimulating hepatic glycogen breakdown and gluconeogenesis. Characteristic features are necrolytic erthematous and vesicular migratory rash on buttocks, groin and perineum but also affecting the limbs. Other symptoms include glossitis, stomatitis, dystrophy of nails and thinning of hair. There may develop venous thrombosis and pulmonary embolism. Plasma glucagon level rises 10 to 20 times.

Glucaric acid Alternative name for saccharic acid, the dicarboxylic acid derived from glucose.

Glucide Name occasionally used for saccharine.

Glucocorticoid Hormones from the adrenal cortex capable of increasing the rate at which lipids are broken down to fatty acids and proteins are broken down to amino acids; elevates blood glucose levels, and acts as an anti-inflammatory substance.

Glucogenic amino acids Amino acids with carbon chains that can be metabolically converted into glucose or glycogen via gluconeogenesis.

Glucometer Instrument that measures the amount of glucose in capillary blood.

Gluconeogenesis The formation of glucose from noncarbohydrate molecules, such as amino acids and lactic acid.

Glucose It is the body's chief source of energy for cell metabolism. In normal human beings blood glucose level is maintained between 60 and 110 mg per cent. It is maintained by the level of insulin. Insulin is released by pancreas in response to raised blood sugar level. Glucagon is released by the pancreas when the blood sugar level is low. It stimulates the breakdown of stored glycogen to glucose which is then released into blood stream. Glucose provides instant energy.

Glucose monitoring A diagnostic test to detemine the blood glucose level.

Glucose oxidase An enzyme that catalyzes the process of glucose oxidation. It is usually suitable for industrial use because of its high stability. One of the typical biological sensing elements; used in the first biosensor.

Glucose Six-Carbon (hexose) sugar The principal sugar in blood, serving as a major source of metabolic energy.

Glucose Tm It measures the efficiency of kidneys. It is the maximum rate of reabsorption of glucose by kidney tubules.

Glucose tolerance test Usually this is ordered when fasting blood sugar level is above 120 mg%. Patient should take 300 gm of carbohydrate and 80 gm of protein. No food should be given for 12 hours of taking sample in morning. Blood and urine are to be tested simultaneously. In morning 3 ml blood is collected in oxalate tube and labelled. Then 75 gm of glucose powder is given in half a glass of water. At intervals of 30 minutes 3 ml blood is collected and properly labelled as 1st, 2nd, 3rd, 4th and 5th sample.

Glucosides Complexes of substances with glucose.

Glucostatic theory The theory that the level of blood sugar affects cells in hypothalamus of the brain to arouse eating behaviour when blood sugar is low.

Glulathione peroxidase Selenium enzyme which prevents oxidation and destroys free radicals. It depends on selenium supply fo optimal activity.

Glutamate An amino acid whcih stimulates the CNS. It is usually used in chinese food. It is harmful in large quantities.

Glutamate analogue A drug that acts like glutamate on glutamate receptors.

Gluteal Of or near the buttocks.

Gluteal injection A frequently used site for intramuscular injections in the gluteal region. Large sciatic nerve travelling through the area

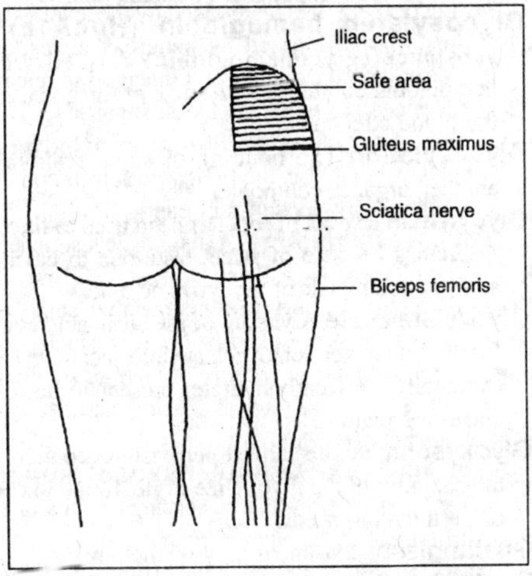

remains in danger of being punctured with the needle. To avoid the nerve, injection is given in the upper lateral quadrant of buttock into belly of gluteus medius supply.

Gluteal region This region is limited above by the iliac crest. In males it forms a watershed between gluteal muscles and muscles of back. In females fat of this region is continuous with the fat of lumbar region so that iliac crest is not a prominent feature. Three main gluteal muscles are there: gluteus maximus, gluteus medius and minimus.

Gluten The protein complex in wheat which gives dough the viscid property that holds gas when it rises. A mixture of two proteins, gliadin and glutenin found in many cereals and grains.

Gluten free foods Formulated without any wheat or rye in case of coeliac disease.

Gluten-induced enteropathy It is an important cause of malabsorption in childhood. Proximal part of small intestine is involved. Villi in jejunum are flattened. Chronic recurrent diarrhoea with large pale bulky frothy stools starting from the time of weaning is the most characteristic feature. Illness is accentuated with worsening of loose motions, vomiting and severe diarrhoea. Physical growth is retarded in children. Anaemia and vitamin deficiency are associated.

Gluteus maximus Major extensor of the thigh and also supports the torso in an erect position.

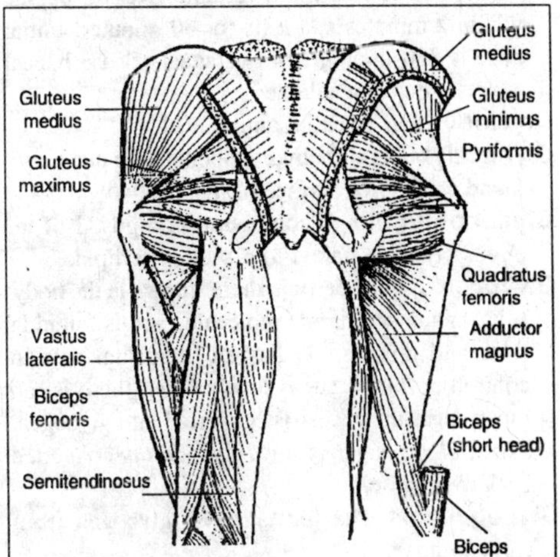

Muscles of gluteal region

Gluteus medius syndrome Pain from gluteus medius syndrome is in the low back in the distribution of L4. Pain is more when walking uphill.

Glycemia Presence of glucose in blood.

Glycemic threshold The blood glucose concentration at which a specific event is triggered during development of hypoglycemia i.e. onset of symptoms.

Glycerin It is a colourless liquid made out of glycerol. It has a high water content, evaporates slowly and is absorbed easily. It softens the skin making it shining. It is put in ear to soften the wax. It is a constituent of cough syrups. It relieves constipation also.

Glycerin suppository This is a evacuant suppository used for starting defaecation reflex. This is available in two forms, adult and child. It acts as hygroscopic agent slowly causing evacuation by withdrawing fluid from tissue.

Glycerol A three-carbon carbohydrate which combines with fatty acids to form triglycerides (neutral fat).

Glyceryl trinitrate Half-life is 3 minute. It is an oily preparation. It is the drug of choice in the treatment of an attack of angina pectoris. The tablets should be chewed and dissolved under the tongue or placed in the buccal sulcus where absorption is rapid and reliable. Action begins within 2 minutes and lasts for 30 minutes. Initial dose is 300 microgram. Sustained release buccal tablets are also available.

Glycine A non essential amino acid.

Glycocalyx The carbohydrate-containing outer coat found on the free surface of most cells.

Glycoconjugate A compound composed of an oligosaccharide linked to a protein or lipid.

Glycogen It is the carbohydrate storage in the body. It has many saccharide molecules and is found in liver and muscles. It has an important role in controlling blood sugar level. When there is too much sugar the excess is converted into glycogen. When blood sugar is low, glycogen is converted back to glucose.

Glycogenesis The formation of glycogen from carbohydrates.

Glycogenolysis The hydrolysis of glycogen to glucose 1-phosphate, which can be converted to glucose 6-phosphate, which then may be oxidized via glycolysis or (in the liver)converted to free glucose.

Glycolysis The metabolic pathway that converts glucose to lactic acid; forms small amounts of ATP in the absence of oxygen. Anaerobic process during which one glucose molecule is converted to two pyruvic acid molecules; a net of two ATP molecules is produced during glycolysis.

Glycolytic pathways General central pathways for the metabolism of sugars for production of energy and precursors for biosynthesis.

Glycoprotein An organic molecule composed of a protein and a carbohydrate.

Glycosome A membrane-bound, microbody-like organelle, peculiar to the hemoflagellates, that contains enzymes essential for glycolysis.

Glycosuria It is the presence of sugar in urine. Generally glucose is filtered through kidney. The filtered fluid passes down many tubules where all except unwanted products are reabsorbed. Glucose is being reabsorbed. If tubules have been damaged or there is hyperglycaemia sugar may be noted in urine. But blood glucose level is normal.

Glycosyl transferase An enzyme catalyzing the transfer of a sugar residue, generally from its activated nucleotide sugar derivative, to an acceptor molecule.

Glycosylase An enzyme that hydrolyzes N-glycosyl bonds linking purines and pyrimidines to carbohydrate components of nucleic acids.

Glycosylated hemoglobin (HgbA1c) A substance (glycohemoglobin) formed when hemoglobin combines with some of the glucose in the blood stream.

Glycosylation The bonding of sugar residue to another organic compound.

Glycyrrhzia Extract of root has been used to flavour medicines because of sweet taste due to calcium and potassium salt of glycyrrhizic acid.

Glyoxylate cycle A variant of the citric acid cycle, for the net conversion of acetate into succinate and, eventually, new carbohydrate; present in bacteria and some plant cells.

Glyoxysome A specialized peroxisome containing the enzymes of the glyoxylate cycle; found in cells of germinating seeds.

Gnathoplasty Plastic surgery of the jaw.

Gnotobiotic Indicating the presence of well defined microbial forms.

Goal Expected or desired outcome.

Goal-directed behaviour A sequence of events presumed to underlie motivation; need, drive, incentive, and reward, Need refers to a biochemical imbalance or deficit, giving rise to a drive, which is directed by some incentive in the environment, and therefore the organism's goal is to attain the incentive, resulting in reward.

Goals Desired outcomes.

Goblet cell A goblet-shaped single cell gland that secretes mucus; present in epithelium of airways and intestines.

Goitre There is an enlargement of thyroid gland seen as swelling of neck. The thyroid gland may enlarge during puberty or after taking birth control tablets. Main cause of goitre is lack of iodine in diet. Excessive production of thyroid hormone leads to thyrotoxicosis. It results in increased appetite, warm, dry skin, weight loss, tremor or insomnia. A goitre can be caused by taking antithyroid drugs for overactivity of thyroid gland. Large swelling may press on the oesophagus or the trachea making breathing difficult.

Gold foil It has been used in restoration of both anterior and posterior teeth. Pure gold is soft malleable metal with excellent resistance to tarnish and erosion. It has a thermal expansion coefficient similar to tooth structure. But it lacks aesthetics. It is available in thin gold foil of 25 mm.

Gold standard A term for the best available approximation of the truth, generally indicating a test method currently accepted as reasonably, but not necessarily 100% accurate.

Golden berry Gooseberry.

Golgi An organelle in the cytoplasm of cells consisting of four to six flattened sacs (cisterns), stacked on one another, with expanded areas at their ends; functions in processing, sorting, packaging, and delivering proteins and lipids to the plasma membrane, lysosomes, and secretory vesicles.

Golgi apparatus It is a reticular structure of viscous consistency, embedded in cytoplasm at one pole of cell or near the nucleus. It is concerned with metabolism in the cell and bring about the combination of fatty acid and glycerol. It is composed of protein and lipid substance. Vitamin C and enzymes are absorbed on to it. Named after Camillo Golgi, Italian histologist and Nobel laureate, 1843-1926; stacks of flattened sacks, formed by membranes, that collect, modify, package, and distribute proteins and lipids.

Golgi body A membrane in neurons that provides a membrane covering for proteins manufactured by the cell.

Golgi cell This is an interneuron. Its dendrite ramifies in the molecular layer where these are synaptically contacted by parallel fibres of granule cells. Its axon does not leave the cerebellar cortex but breaks up into many collateral branches and form cerebellar synaptic glomerulus.

Golgi organ This is found in tendon close to its point of attachment to the muscle. The tendon bundles split into smaller fasciculi. The structure enclosed in a fibrous capsule continuous with the areolar tissue covering the bundles of tendon. These are tension receptors.

Golgi tendon organ a sensory receptor found near the junction of tendons and muscles.

Golgi tendon receptors Sensors that are responsible for proprioception.

Gomphosis A fibrous joint in which a cone-shaped peg fits into a socket.

Gonad Reproductive gland that produces gametes and sex hormones. Female gonads are ovaries while male gonads are testes.

Gonadal sex The sex of an individual determined by the presence of either testes or ovaries as gonads, or in the case of a true hermaphrodite, the presence of gonads of both sexes.

Gonadotropic Stimulating the gonads.

Gonadotropic hormone Anterior pituitary hormone affecting the gonads.

Gonadotropins Hormones from embryonic sex glands.

Goniometer It is a protactor with a movable arm. The arm can move in a complete circle. In pre and

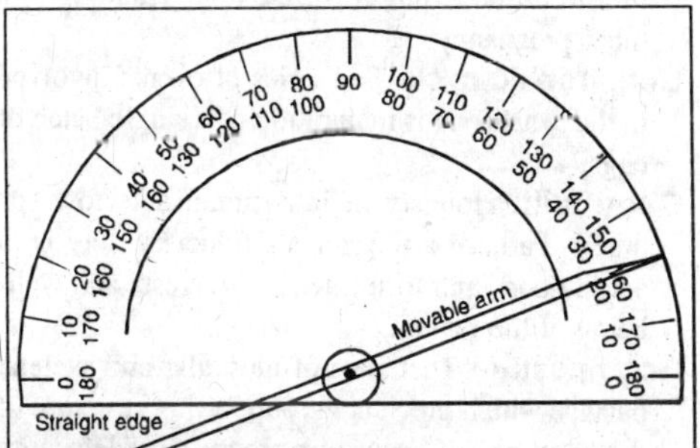

Goniometer

post-operative physical therapy it is important to measure individual joint with much greater accuracy. It helps in knowing improvement after therapy.

Goniometry It is the use of instrument for measuring the range of motion in body joints. Initial range of motion measurements provide a basis for developing a treatment plan and repeated

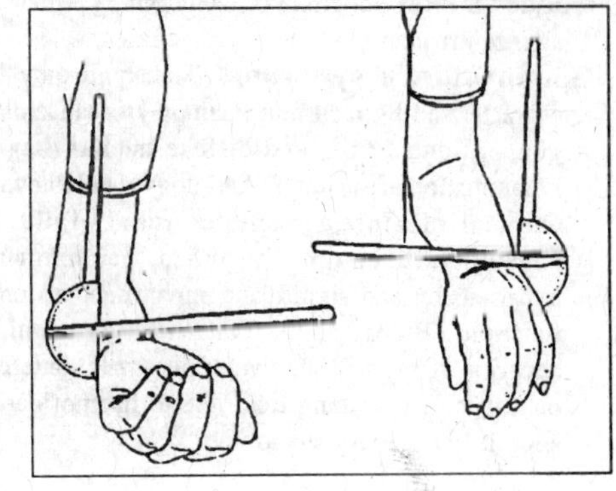

measurement throughout the course of rehabilitation help determine whether improvement has been made and goal achieved. Joint range of motion can be measured with excellent reliability.

Gonopore In some invertebrates, a ciliated, discrete invagination of the epidermis where the eggs and sperm are released.

Gonorrheal conjunctivitis Severe form of conjunctivitis caused by gonococci.

Gonorrhoeal salpingitis An infection of the fallopian tube caused by the *Neisseria gonorrhoeae* bacteria. It may cause narrowing of the fallopian tube, which may subsequently prevent the passage of a fertilised ovum down the tube, resulting in a tubal pregnancy.

Gonotrophic cycle The series of events involved in the synchronous maturation of a single batch of eggs.

Good faith Honesty in intentional acts towards others. Parts of a physician's fiduciary duty is to act in good faith to further the interests and well-being of the patient.

Good posture That state of muscular and skeletal balance which protects the supporting structure of the body against injury or progressive deformity irrespective of the attitude (erect, lying, squatting, stooping etc.) in which these structures are working or resting.

It involves using energy in the most efficient manner, because each body movement begins and ends with the posture.

Good samaritan laws Legal immunity for passerby who provide emergency first aid to accident victims.

Goodell's sign Softening of the cervix, a probable sign of pregnancy.

Goodpasture's syndrome The syndrome is characterised by recurrent haemoptysis, anaemia, glomerulonephritis, and diffuse haemorrhagic inflammation of the lungs. Aetiology is not known. Clinical features include renal failure, haemoptysis, cough, dyspnoea, haematuria, hypertension and significant impairment of lung functions. Biopsy shows concentric glomerulonephritis. X-ray will show multiple small scattered opacities all over lung field due to haemosiderin deposit like miliary shadows.

Gooping Gooping is an extra heavy deposit of ink which often occurs following a sharp curve written with a ball-point pen. Document examiners use this characteristic to assist in determining the direction of ball-point pen ink strokes.

Gorlin goltz syndrome Characteristic facies with frontal and parietal bossing with broad nasal root. There will be multiple keratocysts of jaw with bifid ribs and abnormally shaped sellaturcica.

Gossypoe Yellow toxic pigment found in 2-4% dry weight in some varieties of cotton seed.

Gossypol A derivative of cottonseed oil that has male contraceptive actions by suppressing sperm production and affecting sperm structure and mobility.

Gottron's sign It indicates the presence of scaly patches over the dorsum of the proximal interphalangeal and metacarpophalangeal joints as seen in polymyositis and dermatomyositis.

Gout It is a metabolic disorder causing arthritis. An acute attack affects a single joint specially the big toe but it may affect other joints also. Affected joint is red, swollen and extremely tender. It may be confused with cellulitis. Pain becomes severe within 24 to 36 hours. First attack generally involves one joint and lasts for a few days.

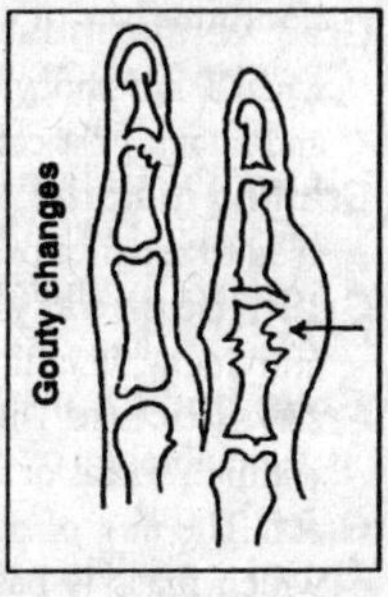

Most have second attack within 6 months. Treatment includes nonsteroidal anti-inflammatory drugs (NSAIDs).

Gouty tophi These are hard, non-tender, freely movable, subcutaneous nodules of urate deposits occurring in the periarticular fibrous tissue, cartilage of external ear, or kidney. These are pathognomonic of gout.

Gower's sign A diagnostic marker in muscular dystrophy and congenital myopathies that reflects hip extensors and trunk weakness.

Graafian follicle A mature ovum in its sac.

Graded exercise test (GXT) The observation and recording of an individuals cardiopulmonary responses during gradually increasing exercise challenges to determine the body's capacity to adapt to physical work.

Gradient A slope or difference between two levels; for example, blood pressure gradient: a difference between the blood pressure in two different vessels

Grading of heart disease

Grade I - Female has no symptoms and can take all physical activities.

Grade II - Anymore exertion will result in fatigue and dyspnea

Grade III - Patient is comfortable at rest but becomes dyspnoeic when attempting physical work.

Grade IV - Patient is breathless at rest and is in cardiac failure.

Graffian follicles or vesicles Small spherical bodies in the ovaries, each containing an ovum.

Graft failure Failure of transplanted tissue to function in the recipient.

Graft surveillance A procedure to measure flow through a surgically repaired bypass graft to assess for restenosis.

Graft versus host reaction Reaction occurring when T lymphocytes presents in a graft recognize and attack host cells.

Grafting material A substance, natural or synthetic, used to repair a tissue defect or deficiency.

Grain boundary The boundaries separating individual metallic grains (crystals).

Grain structure The orientation of grains or crystals within a metal or other substance.

Gram The unit of measure in the metric system on which mass is based (approximately 454 grams equals one pound).

Gram molecular weight The weight in grams of a compound that is numerically equal to its molecular weight, the weight of 1 mole.

Gram staining Process of adding a dye to a microscopic specimen.

Grand mal Epileptic seizure that is seen as generalized involuntary muscular contraction and cessation of respiration with tonic and clonic spasms of the muscles.

Grandiosity Exaggerated belief or claims of one's importance or identity, often manifested by delusions of great wealth, power, or fame. See also bipolar disorder and mania.

Granular leukocytes Leukocytes with granules in the cytoplasm, on the basis of the staining properties of the granules, these cells are classified as neutrophils, eosinophils, or basophils.

Granulation The formation of very small, rounded connective tissue projections that form on healing surfaces.

Granulation tissue Soft, pink, fleshy projection of tissue that forms during the healing process in a wound not healing by primary intention.

Granule cell These are the only excitatory cell in the cerebellar cortex. In man there are about 7 million granule cells per cubic millimetre of cerebellar cortex. All fibre endings terminate upon the dendrite of these cells. Each dendrite ends in a claw-like terminal which takes part in formation of a cerebellar synaptic glomerulus.

Granulocyte Leucocyte named according to the appearance, in stained preparations, of large cytoplasmic granules; neutrophils, basophils, and eosinophils.

Granuloma A circumscribed mass or nodule consisting mainly of histiocyte.

Granulomatosis Any condition characterized by the formation of nodular inflammatory lesions.

Granulomatous angitis It affects segments of arterioles or venules. Disorder may occur in association with lymphoma and with varicella infection. Headache is prominent with ischaemic events. CSF may contain many lymphocytes and ESR is elevated.

Granulomatous epulis It consists of mass of granulation tissue which forms around a carious tooth or at the site of chronic irritation by a denture. This is a false epulis. It is rapidly growing and soft swelling is bright red in colour. Overlying mucous membrane is granular and persistently ulcerated. It bleeds on touch or during brushing. There is an offensive smell of infection. Draining lymph nodes are enlarged and tender. Treatment includes scraping of granulation tissue, extraction of carious tooth and maintenance of oral hygiene.

Granulomatous peritonitis A granulomatous peritonitis may occur in Crohn's disease and may mimic tuberculosis very closely. It is also rarely seen in sarcoidosis and schistosomiasis. Starch granules are seen in fluid obtained from the peritoneal cavity and there are peritoneal nodules. Histologically epithelioid and giant cells are prominent and starch granules are characteristic. Non-steroidal analgesics or cortiosteroids hasten recovery.

Granulomatous uveitis It occurs due to invasion of eye by living organism. The inflammation tends to be insidious in onset and chronic in nature with minimal reaction of tissue. Such inflammation is characterised by dense nodular infiltration of the tissue.

Granulomatuous aortitis Inflammatory nodule in the aorta.

Granulosa cell A female somatic cell type of epithelial origin in the ovarian follicle that surrounds the oocyte and provides the required micro environment for its maturation.

Granulosis A type of enveloped, double-stranded DNA virus reported only from insects of the order Lepidoptera moths, butterflies that replicate initially in the nucleus and later in the cytoplasm of infected cells, virions are occluded individually in small occulsion bodies called granules.

Granzymes Serine esterases present in the granules of cytotoxic T lymphocytes and NK cells. They induce apoptosis in the target cell which they enter through perforin channels inserted into the target cell membrane by the cytotoxic lymphocyte.

Graph A visual representation of the results of research, in some quantified form.

Grapheme A written syllable.

Graphology Also called grapho-analysis; the attempt to discern personallity traits from examination of a subject's handwriting.

Graphomotor Pertaining to movements involved in writing.

Grasp reflex The reflex present at birth in an infant's hands and feet causing the fingers and toes to curl around an object touching them.

Grass tetany Magnesium deficiency in cattle.

Grattage The process of rubbing, brushing, or scrapping the surface of a slowly healing ulcer or wound to stimulate healing.

Graves' disease A hyperthyroid condition believed to be caused by excessive stimulation of the rate, high metabolic rate, and other symptoms of hyperthyroidism.

Graves' ophthalmopathy Most patients with thyrotoxicosis have some eye signs when seen with lid retraction, proptosis and gritty soreness affecting the eyes. There is damage to external ocular muscles. These become infiltrated by lymphocytes and oedematous. Pathology remains obscure. It may become worse or may thyrotoxicosis brought under control. Choice of treatment is immunosuppression with prednisolone.

Gravid Pregnant

Gravid uterus Pregnancy increases weight of uterus 40 to 60 gm to 1.1/2 to 2 pounds at term. Non-pregnant uterus is pear shaped. At the end of 12 weeks it is nearly globular in shape about 9 to 10 inches in diameter and fills the pelvic cavity and in primi gravida is felt just above pubes. In multipara it is higher. At the end of 16 weeks it becomes pyriform. Average height of fundus above pubes at term is about 12 to 14 inches.

Gravida A pregnant woman.

Gravitation force line During relaxed standing it acts through the center of mass.The line lies in the median plane and runs anterior to the throacic vertebra, through the body of S_2 vertebra, behind the hip joint and in front of knee and ankle.

Gravitational Forces 1) Gravitational moment is defined as torque that is produced by the force of gravity acting on the body, 2) When the line of gravity falls anterior to the joint axis, the resulting torque causes motion of the proximal segment in an anterior direction, 3) when the line of gravity falls posterior to the joint axis, the resulting torque causes motion of the proximal segment in a posterior directions.

Gravity A physical force that draws all matter toward the earth's center; in varying degrees, a force that is resisted by all human's upward motions.

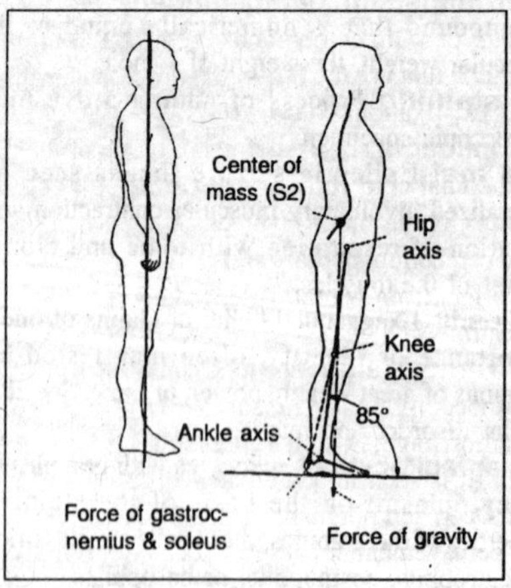

Gravity Assisted Traction With this type of traction, the patient is placed in a position that favours distraction.

Gravity line A vertical line through the center of gravity; a line analogous to the intersection of the midsagittal and midcoronal planes.

Gray matter Those areas of the nervous system composed predominantly of cell bodies, leading to a gray appearance.

Great cardiac vein Vein that runs from the apex of the heart to the base of the ventricles in the anterior interventricular sulcus, before turning to the left in the coronarysulcus to reach the back of the heart.

Greater omentum A double layered peritoneal membrane that originates on the greater curvature of the stomach. It hangs inferiorly like an apron over the contents of the abdominal cavity.

Greater vestibular glands A pair of glands on either side of the vaginal orifice that open by a duct into the space between the hymen and the labia minora.

Great-person theory The view, not generally held in psychology, that the leader of a specific group is an all around capable individual, likely to be the leader of any group of which he is a member. This view is based on the uncertain premise that leadership involves a single dimension, general leadership ability. Current psychological research suggests instead that different groups require different, specific characteristics in a successful leader.

Green nonsulfur photosynthetic bacteria A group of filamentous anoxygenic photosynthetic bacteria that use the 3-hydroxypropionate pathway of CO_2 fixation.

Grey matter It consists of nerve tissue of the brain and spinal cord forming the cortex.

Cortex is the outer layer of cerebral hemisphere and cerebellum in brain and medulla of spinal cord. It differs from white matter having less of myelin sheath.

Grey Turner's sign The flanks may be discoloured from ecchymoses in cases of intraperitoneal haemorrhage, which represents Grey Turner's sign. It is seen in acute pancreatitis.

Grief Deep and poignant distress caused by or as if by bereavement, a cause of such suffering.

Grief response Psychological and physical phenomena experienced by those who are grieving.

Grief work Activities involved in grieving.

Grieving Process of feeling acute sorrow over a loss.

Grill To cook by radiant heat.

Grip Power grip places the tool handle across the supports of index-little finger arch and then clamps

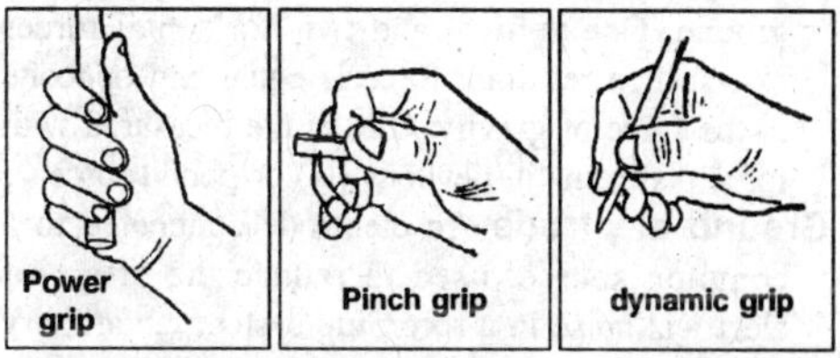

between these two points with the support of thumb. Lateral pinch grip and tip grip uses only the index-thumb arch support in a centripetal motion. The dynamic tripod grip uses index thumb arch to hold the tool.

Grip size Optimal grip circumference should equal the distance from the proximal palmar crease to the tip of ring finger.

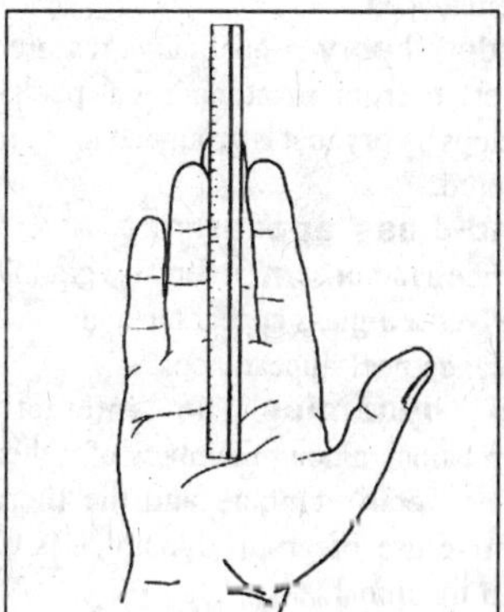

Grist Cereal for grinding.

Grit Degree of roughness based on size and shape of abrasive particle. Larger sizes and irregular shapes are rougher.

Gravida Pregnant women.

Groin The depression between the thigh and the trunk; the inguinal region.

Gross anatomy The branch of anatomy that deals with structures that can be studied without using a microscope. Also called macroscopic anatomy.

Gross motor coordination The use of large muscle groups for controlled movement.

Gross pathology The description of changes in the tissue and organs of the body resulting from disease that is visible to the naked eye.

Ground (Floor) Reaction Forces (G.R.Fs) are the forces that react to the body's weight on the ground. One vertical and two horizontal forces exists; then resultant force is equal and opposite to the force of gravity. G.R.Fs are measured with force platforms in newtons (N) or pound force.

Ground electrode An electrode connected to a common source, used to reduce the effect of electrical noise in a recording system; an arbitary zero potential reference point.

Ground itch A localized irritation and rash caused by penetrating larvae of hookworms and accompanying bacteria.

Ground state The normal, stable form of an atom or molecule; as distinct from the excited state.

Ground substance The amorpous gel-like material in which connective tissue cells and fibers are embedded.

Grounded theory A qualitative research approach that starts from an atheoretical perspective and develops theory that is grounded in the information gathered.

Ground-glass appearance A term used to describe a radiopacity; refers to a granular, pebbled or pulverised-glass appearance; also referred to as an orange-peel appearance.

Group dynamics The interactions and interrelations among members of a therapy group and between members and the therapist. The effective use of group dynamics is essential in group treatment.

Group marriage It is a non-legal social arrangements in which three or more adults live together as a family and engage in sexual relationship with one another. Group marriage is an extension of swinging or open marriage. It may be seen as extension of open marriage.

Group practice The combined practice of 3-4 professionals who share office, space, equipment, expenses and income.

Group sex It is sexual activity by a group of people in the same place and at the same time. It usually involves exchange of partners and observing each other. A group may include both homo and heterosexuals.

Group therapy It is a form of therapy in which two or group of persons talk and discuss their problem in presence of a treating doctor. It is more effective in case of drug addition and alcoholism.

Growth An increase in side due to an increase in (1) the number of cells, (2) the size of existing cells as internal components increasing size, or (3) the size of intercellular substances.

Growth cone The conical tip of a growing axon.

Growth factor Generally, any compound that facilitates or that is required for cell division or whole animal growth; specifically, certain polypeptides that bind to target cell membrane receptors and promote cell division and various other cellular functions.

Growth hormone A hormone secreted by the anterior pituitary that stimulates growth of the skeleton and soft tissues during the growing years and that influences the metabolism of protein, carbohydrate, and fat throughout life.

Growth medium An aqueous solution containing all the nutrients necessary for microbial growth.

Growth of hair Hair in scalp grows for 2 to 5 years. Rate of growth is 0.33 mm/day. Variations in the hair growth and duration of hair growth cycle account for individual differences in uncut hair length. While hair growth is underway the cells of hair root are absorbing nutrients. As it grows, root of hair is firmly attached to the matrix of the follicle.

At the end of growth cycle, the follicles become inactive and hair is termed as club hair. The follicle gets smaller and over the time connection between hair matrix and root of club hair breaks down. When another growth cycle begins, the follicle produces a new hair and old hair gets pushed toward the surface.

Growth optimum The particular state of a variable environmental factor e.g., temperature or salinity at which an organism grows fastest.

Growth plate fracture In children damage to growth plate may result in growth arrest. This may be partial or complete. Salter and Harris classified it into 5 types.

Growth spurts Brief periods of a rapid increase in growth rate.

Guaiac test Diagnostic test to detect blood in the stool.

Guanine One of the bases in a DNA (deoxyribonucleic acid) strand that binds to a base (cystosine) in another strand to form double-stranded DNA.

Guardian A person appointed by the court to protect the interests of a ward: a minor or legal incompetent. The guardian has the rights of a parent for minors. A guardian may have full powers over an incompetent, or the court may limit the guardian's powers to a specific task such as managing the finances of the incompetent. A guardian has a right to full informed consent before making medical decisions for a ward.

Guardianship In most jurisdictions, in the context of mental illness, a person under guardianship by reason of mental illness is under the total control of another person or persons and in the status of a ward with respect to both his body (as in consenting to surgery) and fiscal or contractual affairs.

Guillain-Barre syndrome It may lead to death from progressive paralysis of the ventilatory muscles within 48 hours. Symptoms like flu illness precede before polyneuropathy by about 2 weeks. The cellular infiltrate is associated with segmental demyelination. Sometimes the pathological process appears to be confined to spinal roots and on occasions to nerves. After prodromal illness, patients complain of painful rubbery legs.Pace of weakness may advance to quadriparesis and ventilating insufficiency within 48 hours. Maximum deficit reaches within 3 weeks. Sensory disturbances include numbness and feeling of tingling. Ataxia may be prominent. The autonomic nervous system is also affected. Urinary retention may occur. More important are cardiac irregularities and bradycardias. Corticosteroids help but mortality rate is higher.

Guilt Emotion resulting from doing what one conceives of as wrong, thereby violating superego precepts; results in feelings of worthlessness and at times the need for punishment.

Gumma A rubbery tumor like lesion associated with tertiary syphilis.

Gummatous ulcer of leg Duration is short. It occurs classically on outer side of leg commonly above knee. There is history of sexual exposure, ulcer is typically of punched-out appearance with clear-cut vertical edge and wash leather slough on the floor. Ulcer may be round. Ulcer is painless and may be multiple. There is no varicosity.

Gums Substances that can disperse in water to form a viscous mucilaginous mass.

Gustatory Pertaining to the sense of taste.

Gustatory cell Cells of taste.

Gutta percha Non reactive filling material used to fill root canal.

Gynandromorph The individual mosaic for male and female tissues.

Gynecoid pelvis This is a typical normal and functionally perfect pelvis in women. The brim is slightly oval transversely and anterio-posteriorly it is well rounded. Brim may present picture of circle. The AP diameter of brim is 11.2 cm and maximum transverse diameter is 13.2 cm. The sacrosciatic notches are wide.

Gynecological age Number of years past onset of menarche.

Gynecology The branch of medicine dealing with the study and treatment of disorders of the female reproductive system.

Gypsum Plaster of Paris; material used for casts as it becomes hard and rigid.

Gyrase An enzyme that introduces supercoiling into the DNA duplex in an ATP-dependent reaction.

Gyrate Having or characterized by a ring or spiral shape.

Gyrus A groove in brain matter, usually a groove found in the neocortex or cerebellum.

Gyrus, fusiform Medial occipito-temporal gyrus, hippocampal, Parahippocampal gyrus.

H

H1 receptors Located in vascular, respiratory and gastrointestinal smooth muscle; targeted for blockade by antihistamines.

Hease's rule A method for calculating the length of an embryo or fetus. During the first 5 months, the number of months should be squared to approximate the length in centimetres (e.g. second month of pregnancy, the fetus is about 4 cm in length). After the fifth month, the number of months should be multiplied by 5.

Habenula It is made up of two nuclei concerned with basic emotions and olfaction. It receives its afferents from medial olfactory area on the medial surface of frontal lobe, lateral preoptic area, anterior thalamic nucleus and corpus striatum. It sends its efferents to the hypothalamus and the reticular formation of the brainstem.

Habilitation Application of measures that will assist a person in obtaining a state of health, efficiency, and independent action; make over in an improved form.

Habit The tendency toward an act or an act that has become a repeated performance, relatively fixed and consistant.

Habitat A location where a given organism occurs, especially a usual or characteristic location for this organism.

Habitual abortion It refers to the occurrence of 3 or more consecutive spontaneous abortions.

Habitual cheek biting It occurs as an unconscious nervous habit. Rough tooth surfaces may also result. Plastic occlusal night guards may be necessary. More severe cheek biting is common with uncontrolled tongue thrusting or chewing and in neuromuscular disorder.

Habituation A sensory processing ability that allow a child to inhibit irrelevant stimuli, when exposed to numerous repetitions of the same stimulus, the intensity of the response diminishes and often the child stops responding altogether. Decrease in responsiveness upon repeatitive exposure to stimulus.

Hackenbroch sign In claw foot a shortened distance between lateral malleolus and achilles tendon.

Hacking A type of *tapotement* that alternately strikes the surface of the body with quick, snapping movements. Originally the term hacking was used for person with outstanding programming skills. Today the term hacking refers to persons that unlawfully penetrate computer systems and networks.

Haemangioma It is a tumour like malformation of blood vessels.

• Capillary and cavernous haemangiomas may be seen at any age. These present as elevated, partly elevated or submerged circumscribed, reddish lesion of varying size. The most common site is tongue and cheek. There may be interference in speech and mastication. Haemangiomas are benign and seldom ever become malignant. Superficial lesions can be removed surgically or fibrosis may be induced by sclerosing solution.

• Juvenile haemangioma of infancy occurs most frequently in parotid and submaxillary glands or on lip. The involved site is diffusely enlarged and tumour is not red or bluish but appears as a firm mass of normal mucosal colour. It grows slowly. The salivary gland lobules may be completely replaced by blood vessels and only the presence of a few ducts identify the tissue as a salivary gland. Lip musculature is replaced and infiltrated by some blood vessels and endothelial buds. It has a better chance of spontaneous regression.

Haemarthrosis It is bleeding in a joint space. It results due to severe damage to a joint which results in torn capsule, torn ligament or fracture itself. Haemophilia can also result in haemarthrosis. Swelling just after injury causes joint to swell. If swelling occurs after 12 to 24 hours of injury it is due to synovitis. It may cause joint to be fixed in a stiff position. Ice packs reduce the swelling. Analgesic anti-inflammatory drugs relieve the pain. Sometimes aspiration is being done. Repeated haemarthrosis may damage the surface of joint and may result in osteoarthritis.

Haematocolpos It develops in an adolesent girl in which menstrual blood accumulates inside the vagina due to hymen not being perforated. Girls develop intermittent and colicky abdominal pain. Menstruation has not yet set although secondary sex characters have started appearing. Vagina gets progressively distended with blood and on separation a bulging bluish membrane can be recognised. Treatment is surgical.

Haematocrit The percentage of total blood volume composed of erythrocytes. Formerly, it meant the procedure used to determine this number; now it is the result of that determination.

Haematoma A blood clot formed from blood that has been released by trauma or pathology and that accumulates within a tissue.

Haematuria There is blood in urine. Blood may or may not be visible. Urine may be reddish or of smoky appearance. Kidney stone, cystitis, urethritis often cause haematuria.

Bleeding disorders, or glomerulonephritis lead to it. Urine examination will confirm the diagnosis and ultrasound, CT scan will help in locating the defect.

Haemochromatosis It is a disturbance of iron metabolism in which ferritin and hemosiderin are deposited in the body tissues leading to fibrosis of involved organs. It is characterised by cirrhosis of liver, cardiac failure, diabetes and skin pigmentation. Skin becomes bronzed and oral mucous membrane is pigmented. Pigmentation of skin takes place due to melanin and haemosiderin in connective tissue.

Haemocytoblast Single population of cells that differentiate to give rise to the formed elements of blood.

Haemodialysis It is a temporary extracorporeal circulation which is established usually from artery to vein in the arm. In it, a semipermeable membrane separates blood from dialysis fluid and the poison passes passively from the blood (where it is present in high concentration). It is effective for salicylates and isopropranol poisoning.

Haemoglobin The protein colouring matter of the red blood cells, conveys oxygen to the tissues; occurs as oxyhaemoglobin in arterial blood and reduced haemoglobin in venous blood.

There are 350 million haemoglobin molecules in the average blood cell and each can carry four molecules of oxygen. It is a large molecule made in bone marrow from two components haem and globin. Defects in haemoglobin production may be genetic or acquired.

Haemoglobin deficiency Haemoglobin deficiency leads to anaemia. Anaemia results in pallor of mucous membrane, skin, muscle and fatty change in heart and liver. There may develop atrophy of oral and GIT membrane. There may be haemorrhages in oral mucosa.

Haemoglobin percentage Normally it is 14-18 grams per 100 cc of blood. At birth it is 23 grams per 100 cc. This falls to above 10.5 grams by the end of 3rd month. It then gradually rises and at the end of first year reaches to about 12.5 grams per 100 cc of blood.

Haemoglobinopathy A disorder of the blood resulting from a genetically caused altered molecular structure of haemoglobin.

Haemolysin It is a specific substance present in serum. Due to presence of this substance the serum hemolyses the red cells. Its haemolytic activity is destroyed when serum is heated to 55°C.

Haemolysis There develops abnormal degeneration of RBCs into their component parts which releases haemoglobin into blood plasma. It may be caused by abnormal types of haemoglobin, malaria, blood group incompatibility and certain poisons. It results in anaemia, jaundice and high temperature with chills.

Haemolytic anaemias In it, there is destruction of erythrocytes.

- Thalassaemia is characterised by anaemia, yellow colouration of skin, splenomegaly, fever and malaise. Head is enlarged and radiograph shows thickening of diploe and 'hair on end' appearance, Oral manifestations are protrusion of upper anterior teeth. Jaw shows osteoporosis with peculiar coarsening of trabeculae.
- Sickle cell anaemia is characterised by distorted erythrocyte. Oral mucosa becomes pale. Jaw shows osteoporosis and coarse trabecular pattern. These are prominent between apices of teeth and inferior border of mandible. Trabeculae between roots of teeth may be arranged in step ladder fashion. There may be pain in mandible and lip paraesthesia.

Haemolytic disease, newborn Destruction of erythrocytes in the fetus or newborn caused by antibodies produced in the Rh-negative mother acting on the Rh-positive blood of the fetus or newborn.

Haemolytic uraemic syndrome It is manifested by acute renal insufficiency with haemolytic anaemia and thrombocytopenia. Underlying mechanism is microangiopathy affecting glomerular capillaries. Passage of red cells and platelets from injured walls results in damage. In late stage severe anaemia, purpura, sensorial disturbance and oliguria are main features. Hypertension, oedema and circulatory congestion are often present. Urine examination shows haematuria, protein urea and casts. Blood urea values are elevated.

Haemophilia Deficiency of thromboplastin precursor as well as accessory factors leads to haemorrhagic disorder of varying severity. Lack of antihaemophilic globulin factor VIII produces classical haemophilia or hemophilia A. Lack of plasma thromboplastin component leads to haemophilia B. Lack of factor XI produces mild or pseudohaemophilia. The oral manifestation of all these disorders is spontaneous bleeding. Even after minor trauma there may develop persistent bleeding. *Haemophilia-A* is a hereditary disorder of coagulation of blood due to deficiency of antihaemophilic globulin in blood resulting in haemorrhagic disorder. It is inherited as a sex-linked recessive character.

Disease manifests in infancy. Bleeding follows trauma. Characteristic feature of bleeding is not profuseness but its persistence. It may persist for weeks, cutaneous haemorrhage is rare although bruise may occur after slight knock. Recurrent haemorrhage in joints is a disabling symptom. There may be repeated small haemorrhages in joints. *Haemophilia-B* is due to deficiency of factor IX. The clinical picture simulates haemophilia-A. Here bleeding occurs usually after trauma and deep-seated bleeding in muscles, joints and viscera. Bleeding time is normal but coagulation time is prolonged. PTT is also prolonged. Level of factor IX is low.

Haemophilus influenzae It generally develops between 3 months and 4 years and are nearly always associated with septicaemia. Onset is gradual with nasopharyngeal infection. Child has moderate fever, dyspnoea, grunting respiration and retraction of lower intercostal spaces. Course is subacute and prolonged.

Haemorrhagic cyst These are blood-filled cys containing echoes that may form a fluid leve Severe pain develops when the bleeding into cy takes place.

Haemorrhagic diathesis A predisposition abnormal bleeding.

Haemorrhagic disorder The mechanism of bloc coagulation may be expressed in three steps.

- Platelets+calcium+thromboplastin precursor thromboplastin.
- Prothrombin+thromboplastin+ accessory factor thrombin.
- Fibrinogen + thrombin—fibrin. Disturbance blood coagulation may occur any where i platelets, plasma proteins, vitamin K, calcium any other factor described. There develops a overall picture of spontaneous bleeding around th teeth and prolonged bleeding after even minc surgical procedures.

Haemorrhagic otitis media It is a definite oti media seen in influenza epidemics and may be see with bulbous eruptions of membrane. Culture c discharge when not sterile reveals a haemolyti *Streptococcus*. There may be severe earache an early mastoid tenderness. It is managed as a simpl otitis media.

Haemorrhoids Internal piles arise from interna haemorrhoidal venous plexus and external pile from the external plexus. Constipation an straining at stool aggravate piles as does pelvi venous congestion and pelvic filling in pregnancy Blood flow is obstructed by increased pressur between the faecal mass and the anal sphincters Venous congestion occurs and plexus become engorged by inflow from arterial supply Haemorrhoidal enlargement occurs and surfac epithelium may show squamous metaplasia Symptomatic classification is—first degree onl bleeding, while in second degree there will b prolapse but being reducible. In third degree pile prolapse is not reducible.

Haemostat An instrument or other agent used t arrest the escape or flow of blood.

Haemothorax It is rare. Signs and symptoms wi be like hydropneumothorax. Person becomes pal and shocked due to haemorrhage. One may aspirate practically pure blood. Blood remain fluid for several days. Fracture rib or perforatin wound may cause it or tuberculosis may result in it.

Hair The root of each hair is embedded in a tiny pit in the skin called a hair follicle. During the growing phase of a hair the root is firmly enclosed by live tissue called a bulb which supplies the hair with keratin. From the fourth month, the fetus is covered with downy hair which is shed during ninth month. After birth till puberty, vellus hair which is fine, short and colourless covers most of the body. The third type of terminal hair is thicker, longer and pigmented grows on the scalp. the eyebrows and eyelashes. Hair colour is determined by amount of pigment called melanin in hair shaft. Melanin is produced by melanocyte. Red melanin is responsible for red hair and black for other colours.

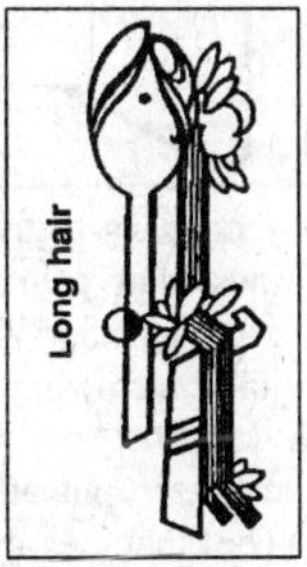

In old age, cortex of each hair becomes transparent resulting hair white. The degree of curliness of a hair depends on the shape of its follicle.

Hair cell Cell of the inner ear containing hair-like processes (microvilli) that respond to bending of the hair by depolarising. Specialized receptor nerve endings for detecting sensations, such as in the spiral organ.

Hair changes in pregnancy Mild degree of hirsutism are common during pregnancy. Face is frequently affected. Abdominal hair growth is less common. Hirsutism may result from placental androgen production as well as elevated levels of cortisol. There is a loss of scalp hair 2-4 months after delivery.

Hair colour Variation in hair colour reflects differences in structure and variations in pigments produced by melanocytes at papilla. These characteristics are genetically determined but condition of hair can be influenced by hormonal or environmental factors. As pigment production decreases with age, the hair lightens towards grey. White hair results from the combination of lack of pigment and presence of air-bubbles in medulla of hair shaft.

Hair content Keratin is the chief constituent. Human hair contains 15.6 to 21.2% of cystine and is differentiated from all other animal hair or wool. Hair has the highest sulphur content. Hair contains 12 to 15% water, 3 to 5% lipids and 1 to 1.5% ash. Blonde, brown and black colour is due to varying amounts of melanin. Bright red human hair contains a pigment with high content of iron, grey is due to absence of pigments and white by an increased proportion of calcium carbonate and phosphate.

Hair follicle A small tube where hair growth occurs. A hair follicle is a complete pocket in the skin formed by a downgrowth of the epidermis, which directly surrounds the hair root.

Hair papilla A small, cap-shaped cluster of cells located at the base of the follicle where hair growth begins.

Hair removal For cosmetic purpose hair is removed from different parts of body. Shaving removes hair at skin level and is suitable for face, leg, armpit and pubic hair. Shaving is quick on the face but the hair grows back. Depilatory cream dissolve the hair just below the skin surface creating a smoother effect than shaving. Plucking with tweezers is suitable for small areas. Permanent removal of hair requires electrolysis in which electric current is used to destroy the growing part of hair. Nowadays hair transplantation is feasible.

Hair skin Skin that contains hair follicles, in contrast with glabrous skin, which does not.

Hairy cell leukaemia It is a rare form of chronic B-cell leukaemia in which tumour cells have fine, hair-like projections. Lymphadenopathy is rare. Leucocytosis is present in 25 % of patients but hairy cells are present in peripheral blood. Average survival is 4 years.

Hairy root A tumorous plant disease provoked by Agro-bacterium rhizogenes.

Hakim's syndrome It is also called occult hydrocephalus. Condition results from subarachnoid haemorrhage, head injury, meningitis and vertebral anomalies. It is a condition of communicating hydrocephalus in which ventricular dilatation occurs due to obstruction of brainstem or cerebral hemisphere. Clinically there will be mental retardation and downward displacement of eyes. CT shows enlarged ventricles.

Half disease Acute paroxysmal myoglobinuria suffered by fisherman.

Half-life The time in which half the atoms of a particular radioactive substance disintegrate to another nuclear form, varrying from millionths of a second to billions of years.
This is the time taken for the activity of its substance to reduce to half. Actually it is used for the level of radiation by a radioactive substance to decay, to half of its original retain. The term half-life is used for medicines to retain its half potency in blood.

Halfway house A specialised residence for patients who do not require full hospitalisation but who need an intermediate degree of care before returning to independent community living.

Halibut liver oil One of the richest natural source of vitamin A & D. Contains 5 mg vitamin A and 8 mg vitamin D per 100 gm.

Hallucination A sensory perception in the absence of an actual external stimulus. May occur in any of the senses.

Hallucinogenic A term applied to drugs which commonly produce hallucinations.

Hallucinosis A condition in which the patient hallucinates in a state of clear consciousness.

Hallus Great toe.

Hallux rigidus It is a painful condition affecting metatarso-phalangeal joint of great toe and is characterised by restriction of motion. It is usually

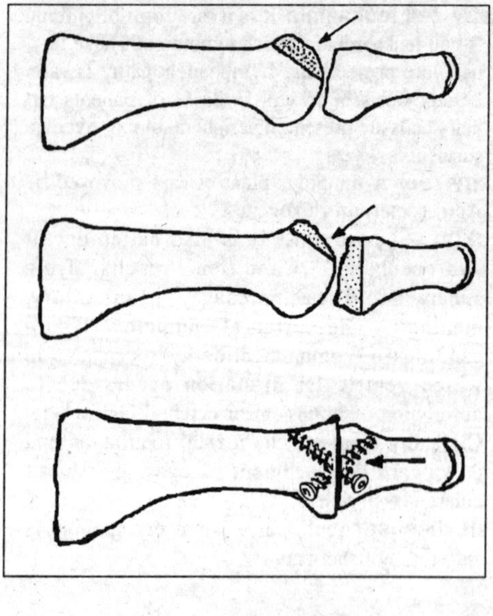

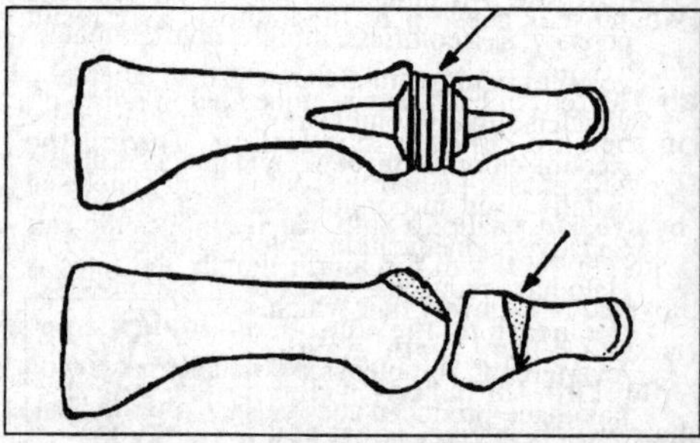

secondary to traumatic osteoarthritis. Gradually increasing pain and stiffness are common. Passive motion of dorsiflexion is painful. X-ray will show joint narrowing and spur formation.

Hallux valgus The great toe is abducted at the metatarsophalangeal joint. Condition is bilateral. The other toes are crowded together and the second toe may be hammer toe. Short and pointed shoes with high heels are the usual cause. It is commonly seen in patients with a wide variety of disorders such as lax ligaments, weak muscles and abnormal bone anatomy. Angle between first and second metatarsal should normally be 3 to 9°. Angles more than 10° or more are described as having metatarsus primus varus deformity. In an attempt to compensate for medial angulation the hallux deviates laterally. Normally this deviation is 10°, beyond it is hallux valgus.

Hallux varus It is a deformity usually seen in children in which medial angulation of great toe occurs at the metatarsophalangeal joint. It is usually congenital and associated with other foot deformities. Mild cases in children may respond to passive stretching exercises and proper shoe wear. In severe cases surgical correction is needed.

Halo effect The tendency to make a biased judgment based on irrelevant information. A student who is highly capable athletically and academically may erroneously judged by an instructor as capable socially. In the halo effect, the teacher's judgement of social skills is influenced by knowledge of the student's academic and athletic prowess.

Halophile Literally, salt-lover; an organism that grows optimally at high salt concentrations.

Halophilic Pertaining to or characterized by an affinity for salt; applied to microorganisms which require a high concentration of salt for optimal growth.

Halothane An inhalation anesthetic of moderate potency; as a colorless, mobile, nonflammable (but volatile) liquid with a characteristic ethereal odor, which is slightly soluble in water and miscible with alcohol, chloroform, ether, and oils. In oral surgery, usually used in conjunction with nitrous oxide. Sedative premedication prolongs the recovery time. Halothane reduces the flow of saliva and sensitizes the heart to the action of epinephrine and levarterenol. Hypotension is usually present during halothane-produced anesthesia. Contraindicated in patients with liver and biliary tract disease. Trademark: Fluothane.

Ham's test A diagnostic test for paroxysmal nocturnal haemoglobinuria and acute haemolytic anaemia in which haemolysis of the patient's red

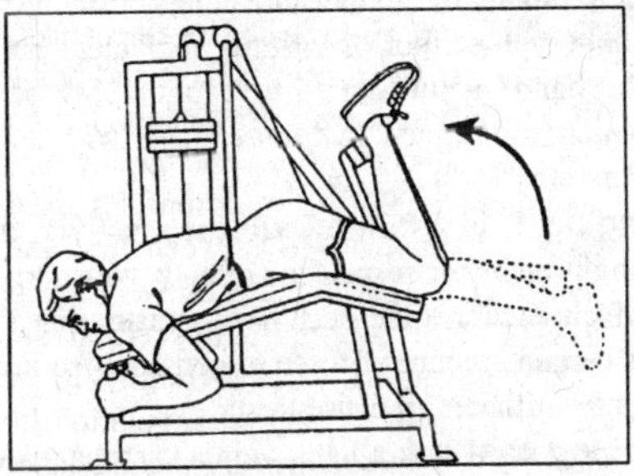

blood cells occurs in acidified normal human serum.

Hamartomas It is an excessive amount of normal tissue seen in its usual location. This tumour like mass is hamartoma. When it occurs in abnormal location it is known as choristoma. Mostly these are located on dorsum of tongue or lip. These are circumscribed, slow growing masses consisting of salivary glands, cartilage, nerves and fats. In oral cavity tongue is mostly involved. Some of these may undergo malignant degeneration.

Hamman-Rich syndrome Interstitial fibrosis of the lung, leading to severe right ventricular failure and cor pulmonale.

Hammer toe This deformity is often associated with hallux valgus. It affects the second toe, along with third and fourth. There is hyper-extension at the metacarpophalangeal joint, hyperflexion at first interphalangeal joint and hyperextension at terminal joint. Generally corn develops over first interphalangeal joint.

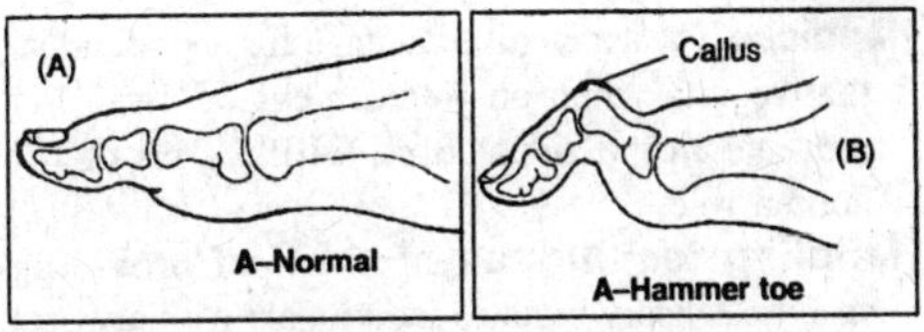

Hammock ligament The slinglike meshwork of periimplant collagenous fibers contiguous with the outer layer of the periosteum that sheathes a subperiosteal implant in the periosteal mode of tissue integration.

Hamstring curl The leg pad on exerciser is adjusted just above the Achilles tendon. The athlete lies on the bench with knees on the surface of the pad and aligned with the axis of the pivot arm, lifts the weight by bending both knees, pauses, lowers the weight to the starting position in a slow and controlled manner and repeats.

Hamstring insufficiency Muscle is not long enough to be stretched over each joint individually. If you flex your hip with your knee exterded you cannot complete the range.

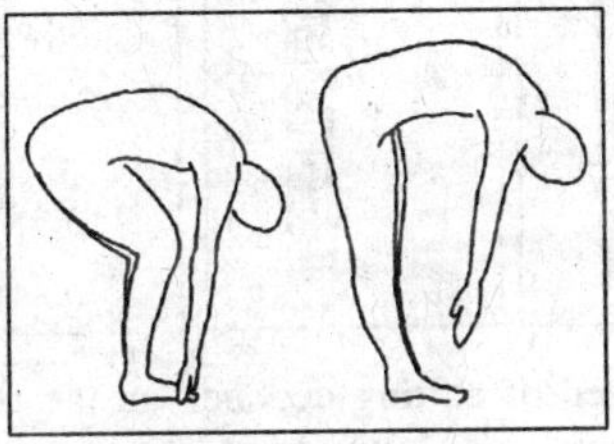

Hamstring muscle One of the three major muscles of the posterior thigh. Powerful flexors of the hip made up of the semimembranosus, semitendinosus, and biceps femoris muscles.

Hand It is the most flexible and useful part of the body. It is composed of wrist, palm and fingers. Movements of hand is achieved by small bones and tendons.

These tendons are covered in synovial sheath having lubricating fluid avoiding friction. Hand is most susceptible to burn, cuts, bites and fracture. Rheumatoid arthritis involves it. Damage to muscles may result in Volkmann's contracture.

Hand hygiene It is the single most effective method of reducing cross infection. The purpose of hand washing is to remove dirt, organic material and transient microorganisms.

Handicap The social disadvantage for an individual that results when an impairment or disability prevents an individual from fulfilling his or her normal role.

Handling techniques Methods of providing specific sensory input to indiviudals with atypical muscle tone, posture, and movement.

Hand-over-mouth Method of behavior managemnet in pediatric dentistry.

Handpiece Instrument used to hold rotary instruments in the dental engine or condensing points in mechanical condensing units. It is connected by an arm, cable, belt, or tube to the source of power (motor, air, water). Tooth cavities are cut with burs fitted in handpieces.

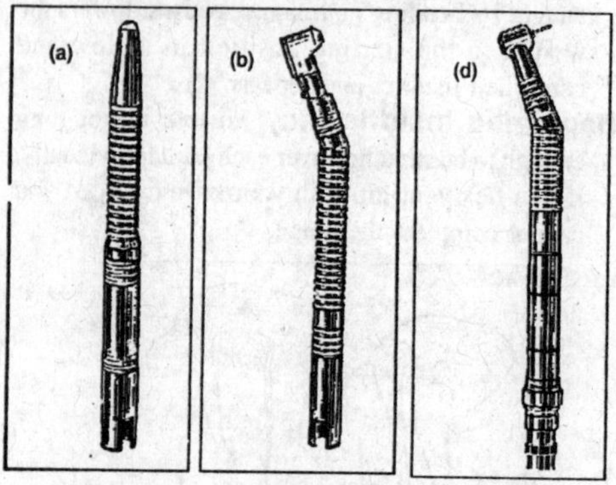

The speed of cutting depends on the type of handpiece used. Low speed handpieces upto 4000 revolutions a minute are driven by a miniature compressed air or electric motor at the base of handpiece. A contraangle handpiece is used most often as it provides access to every tooth. For easily accessible teeth and laboratory work, a straight handpiece is used. Air turbine handpieces run at very high speed of 400,000 revolutions a minute.

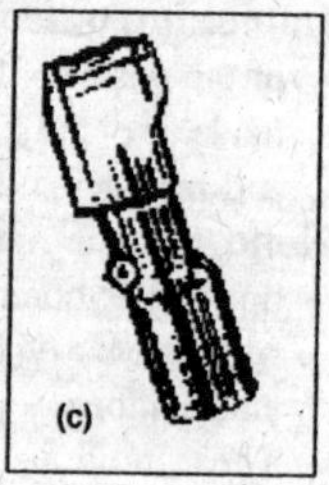

Hand-Schüller Christian disease It develops in first decade of life. Skull is commonly affected. There may be papular rashes or petechial eruptions, skin, ulceration and necrosis of oral mucosa. There is enlargement of liver, lymph nodes and spleen. There may be triad of :

(*i*) bone lesions,

(*ii*) exophthalmos displacing eyeball outward, and

(*iii*) diabetes insipidus. This syndrome basically consist of proliferation of histiocyte cells in bone marrows, spleen, liver, lymph glands and lungs. This is a chronic form of histiocytosis. Children below 5 years are commonly affected. Malaise, anorexia, fever and irritability develop. One will notice hepatosplenomegaly, exophthalmos, diabetes insipidus, and otitis media. Skull shows lytic lesions.

Hand washing It is very necessary to wash hand with soap and plenty of water after food and passing stools.

Handwriting The formation of letters, characters or symbols, by human movement, usually using some type of tool or writing implement held by the hand, according to a recognizable pattern which is designed to communicate with another person.

Hanging It is a form of violent asphyxial death produced by the suspension of body with a ligature which encircles the neck with constricting force. A certain amount of force to constrict the neck is quite sufficient to cause death.

Hanging cast It is a light weight cast that extends from the upper arm to the hand.

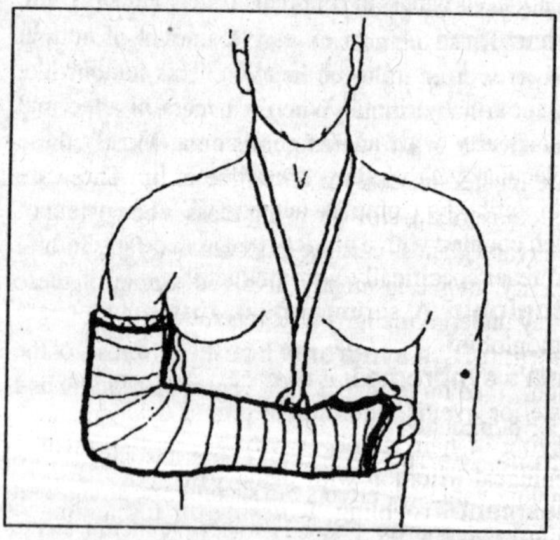

Hangman's fracture This is a fracture through the pedicle and lamina of axis with instability between axis and third cervical vertebra. It may be caused by road traffic accident.

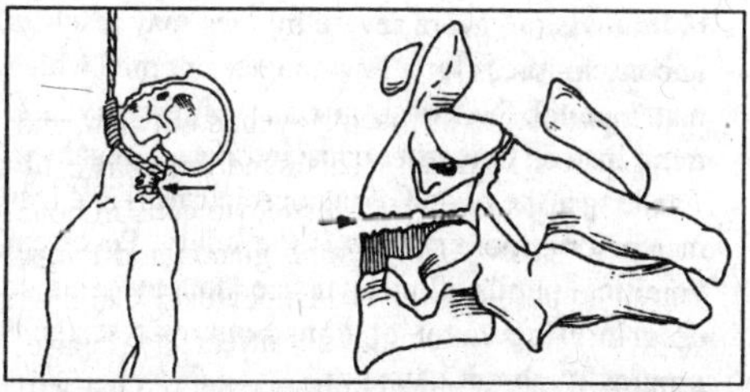

Hangnail It is an extraneous strand of skin tissue which has become partly detached between the fold of skin at the side of the nail. It should be cut.

Hangover It is the unpleasant effect in the early morning experienced on waking up after indulgence in alcohol. Person feels headache, nausea, vomiting, vertigo and depression. Brandy and wine having high concentrations of congeners produce bad hangover. Some think it may be due to dehydration caused by diuretic effect of alcohol. Same central hervous depressant drugs like antihistamines also cause of.

Hanulus A small book-like projection of bone that extends from the medial pterygoid plate of the sphenoid bone; appears radiopaque.

Haploid A cell that has one of each chromosome type and therefore half the number of chromosomes present in most other body cells; only the gametes (sperm and ova) are haploid.

Hapsis The perceptual ability to discriminate objects on the basis of touch.

Haptens These are not antigenic by their own right and are thus unable to stimulate antibody production by themselves. But these can react specifically with antibodies. These are of low molecular weight compounds which do not react with antibody. Complex haptens are those which when coupled with a carrier will produce antibody and react specifically with this antibody.

Haptoglobin A serum protein that scavenges hemoglobin.

Harada's syndrome It is characterised by bilateral posterior uveitis, choroiditis, retinal detachment, greying of hair, alopecia, vitiligo, and signs of meningeal irritation with pleocytosis.

Harassment Troubling, worrying, or tormenting another person with repeated questions, comments, or attacks. Sexual harassment is particularly common in females, especially at crowded places, workplaces and academic institutions.

Hard corn A cone shaped hyperkerototic skin lesion that occurs where there is irritation between the skin and outside source.

Hard of hearing Whose hearing power is impaired.

Hard palate Hard palate is formed by horizontal plates of maxillae and horizontal plates of palatine

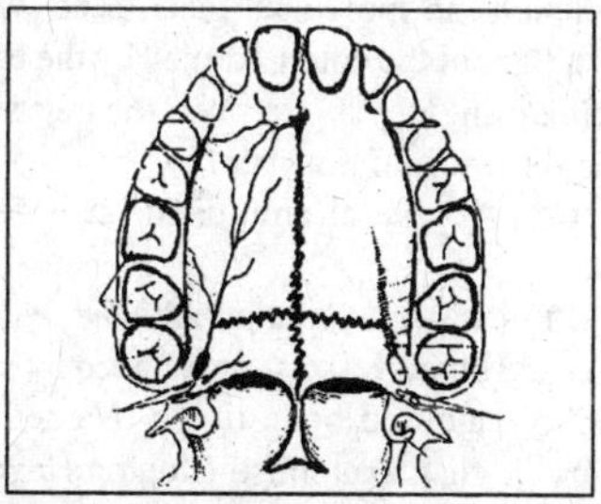

bones. Anteriorly there is an incisive fossa into which open four small foramina that transmit nasopalatine nerves and vessels.

Hard plate The bony partition between the oral and nasal catities, formed by the maxillae and palatine bones and lined by mucous membrane.

Hard water Water that contains high amounts of minerals such as calcium and magnesium.

Hardiness A composite of three dimensions labelled control, commitment and challenge.

Hardness It is the ability of a material is resist forces of indentation. It is often equated with being resistant to wear and abrasion.

Hardy-Weinberg Law The state, for a genetic locus in a population, in which the alleles making up the genotypes are in random proportions.

Harrington system A method used for internal instrumentation of the spine. It is used for correction of scoliosis.

Harris splint Expandable splint that supports the thigh in skeletal traction.

Harrison's groove A transverse depression at the level of the diaphragm running round the front of the chest, causing flaring of the lower ribs. It is seen in rickets.

Hartnup syndrome It is characterised by aminoaciduria, pellagra-like skin rash, and cerebellar ataxia.

Hasner, fold Lacrimal fold.

Hasse's rule A method for calculating the length of an embryo or fetus. During the first 5 months the number of months should be squarred up to approximate the length in cms. After fifth month the number of months should be multiplied by 5.

Hassle Minor life events whose effects divorce in a day or two.

Hassles scales An instrument measuring the irritating and frustrating demands of everyday transactions an individual feels faced with.

Haustra Sacs of the colon, formed by the teniae coli, which are slightly shorter than the gut; so that the gut is thrown into pouches.

Haustrum A general antomical term denoting a recess.

Haversian canal A canal in bone tissue containing nerves and blood vessels; surrounded by concentric layers of calcified bone tissue. Named for 17th century English anatomist, Clopton Havers; canal containing blood vessels, nerves and loose connective tissue and running parallel to the long axis of the bone.

Haversian system A single haversian canal, with its contents, and the associated lamellae and osteocytes surrounding it.

Hay fever A seasonal type of allergic rhinitis caused by pollen; it is characterized by itching and tearing of the eyes, swelling of the nasal mucosa, attacks of sneezing and often by asthma.

Hayem-Widal syndrome The syndrome is characterised by anaemia, jaundice, slight splenomegaly, urobilinuria, and increased fragility of red blood cells.

Hazardous waste Any material or substance that poses a significant threat to human health or environment, requiring special handling, processing, or disposal.

HBV Viral form of hepatitis B that is transmitted in contaminated serum in blood transfusions or by the use of contaminated needles and instruments.

Head The superior part of a human, cephalic to the neck. Also the superior or proximal part of a structure.

Head injury It occurs generally due to accident, fall, sports injuries or bullet wounds. It may damage the scalp or brain in any combination. It is not necessary that with every skull fracture brain will be damaged. While on the other hand in closed injury without external injury brain may be damaged. Head injury may cause oedema. In concussion there may be confusion, dizziness and blurred vision. More severe injuries may result in unconsciousness for a few minutes or coma which may be fatal. Postconcussive loss of memory lasts more than an hour after consciousness is regained. The longer the period of unconsciousness and loss of memory, more serious is the injury. Persistent vomiting, pupils of unequal size, double vision or deteriorating level of consciousness suggest progressive brain damage.

Head mirror It consists of a concave mirror with viewing aperture in centre and attached to an adjustable head belt. Focal length of mirror is 8"

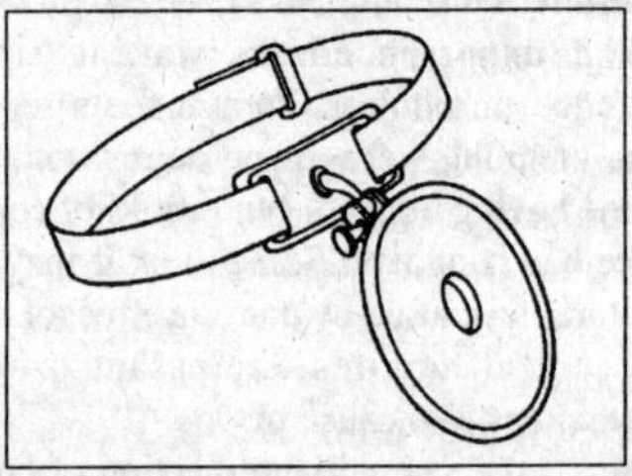

and diameter is 4". Mirror is worn by surgeon and light source is Bull's lamp. Surgeon views through aperture in mirror. It is most commonly used in ENT examinations.

Head of the rib The end of the rib that articulates with the vertebrae.

Head start Program that provides comprehensive developmental services for low-in-come, pre-school children, ages 3 to 5, as well as social services for their families. Education, social and emotional development, physical and mental health, and nutrition are all components.

Head, Intramucosal Insert Theretentive portion of the intra-mucosal insert that seats within the gingival receptor site.

Headache The main cause of headache is fatigue and tension. Other causes include refrective error and hypertension. In *ophthalmic headache* there will be pain around eye which increases at the end of day. In glaucoma severe local pain with hardening of eyes may be present. In *muscle contraction* headache one feels occipital pain with stiffness which increases by neck movement. In hypertension pain is on both sides–either at front or at the back of head—is bursting or throbbing. Headache due to brain tumour generally occussin patients above the age of 50. Pain may aggravate by bending, coughing, sneezing or on exertion. Headache is more in the morning. l In sinusitis pain

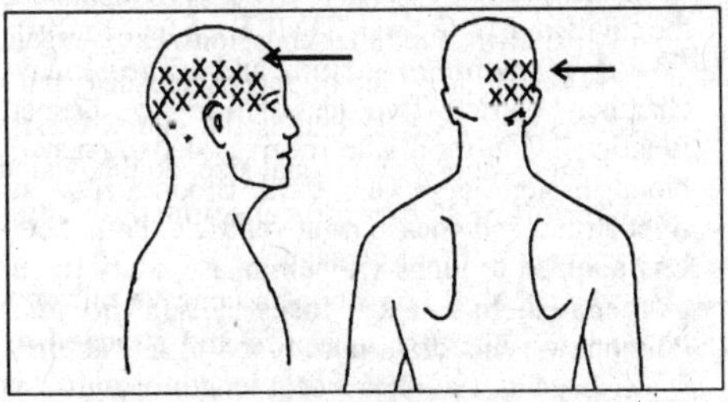

is in affected area. Bending forward or blowing nose will develop pain. It is the pain felt to be in head. It may be caused due to refractive error, high blood pressure, severe fatigue, anaemia and brain tumour. In usual case of headache pain killer helps.

Headgear Orthodontic apparatus encircling the head or neck and providing attachment for an intraoral appliance in use of extraoral anchorage.

Head-righting reflex A reflex, engaging the static labyrinth and medial vestibulospinal tract, designed to keep the head upright.

Headspace The volume above a liquid containing the vapors of the liquid. By analyzing this vapor, information concerning the liquid can be obtained.

Healing The restoration of structure and function to injured or diseased tissue.

Healing of cortical bone In normal cortical bone healing takes about three months in 5 stages.

Healing ridge Induration of collagen deposits beneath the skin extending to about 1 cm on each side of the wound.

Healing, bone fracture On fracture there will be a formation of haematoma between the ends of bones. Then there will be development of acute inflammation and accumulation of macrophages. It takes about 5 days. Then develops growth of granulation tissue and new blood vessels. In about 3 weeks, large number of osteoblasts develop, which secrete nonlamellar osteoid which is quickly turned into lamellar osteoid and calcified forming callus. In months shaping of new bone is done by osteoclasts which remove excessive callus and open up a medullary canal in the callus.

Healing, wound When cut surfaces are proximated or closely sutured the wound heals without scarring. The first step in repair is the formation of clot which helps to hold the parts together. Since the cut area is the site of inflammation it is oedematous and contains leucocytes and macrophages. In 3 to 4 days the clot is slowly replaced by tissue consisting of blood vessels and young fibroblasts. The epithelium grows across the wound and healing is almost completed.

Health State of complete physical, mental, and social well-being, not merely the absence of disease.

Health belief model Before seeking preventive measures, people generally must believe that the disease at issue is serious, if acquired; that they or their children are personally at rick for the disease; that the preventive measure is effective in warding off the disease; and that therre are no serious risks or barriers involved in obtaining the preventive measure.

Health care Practitioner An individual who directly provides health care services. In India, private hospitals cater 80% of heath requirements.

Health care provider An individual or an institution who provides health care services. In India Private Hospitals cater 80% of the health requirements.

Health maintenance organizations Prepaid group practives consisting of a legal and fiscal entity that does the contracting and financial transactions and seeks to control the costs of medical care; a group of physicians that provides the outpatient and inpatient medical care; and an associated hospital or hospitals.

Health patterns The daily activities and behaviors families and their members perform to promote and protect optimal physical, mental, and social well-being, not merely to ensure the absence of disease and incapacitation.

Health promotion Activities that improve or maintain the well-being of people.

Health psychology The use of psychological principles and findings in health-related issues. These issues can include prevention, treatment, education, and any other measures directed to physical and mental health.

Health related life style A collective pattern of health promoting or health damaging behaviour.

Health risk assessments Use of questionnaires or computer programs to elicit and evaluate information concerning individuals in a clinical or industrial medical practice.

Healthplan employer data and information set A national data set of information about the performance of selected services by each managed care organization. HEDIS emphasizes data on preventive services.

Healthy carriers These are individuals harbouring pathogenic organisms in their system but himself not showing any clinical manifestation of disease and are capable of disseminating a causative organism to other person. These persons constitute an unsuspected and dangerous source of infection.

Healthy worker effect Because people with jobs must be in reasonably good health to remain employed, their risk of death and illness is lower than that of the population as a whole. A carrier that insures a group of workers will benefit from this effect.

Hearing aids It is an appliance which converts sound waves into electrical impulses, amplifies these impulses and reconverts them into sound waves. Microphone has a diaphragm able to set into vibrating motion to the sound waves. The movement of diaphragm raises electric current by magnetic induction which is passed through the amplifier. The receiver built into ear piece receives the amplified electric impulses and reconverts them to sound.

Aids other than electrical such as speaking tubes and trumpets have a very limited use. The efficiency of a hearing aid depends mainly upon the qualities of amplifier and the fit of earmould into the ear. The amplifier should amplify speech sounds without distortion.

Heart It is an efficient muscular pump. In one minute it contracts about 70 to 80 times and in life span more than 2.2 billion times. A thick septum divides the cavity into right and left half. Each half consists of upper chambers–atrium and larger lower chamber–ventricle. Two sides of heart have distinct functions. The right side receives deoxygenated blood through large vena cava. Blood arrives at right atrium and goes to right ventricle. From here it is pumped to lungs via pulmonary artery to be oxygenated. In lungs it loses carbon dioxide. Pulmonary veins drain pure blood to left atrium.

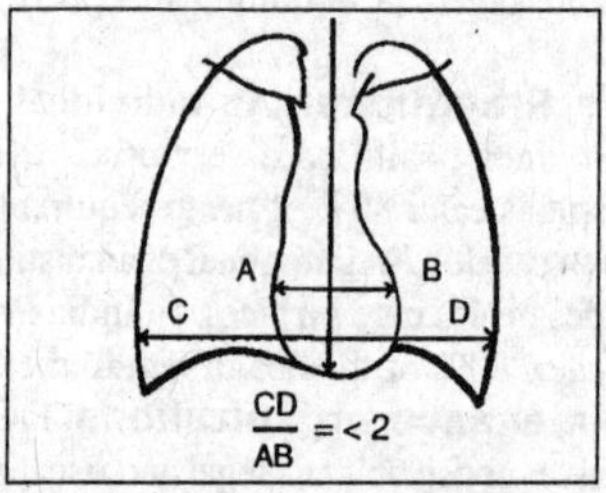

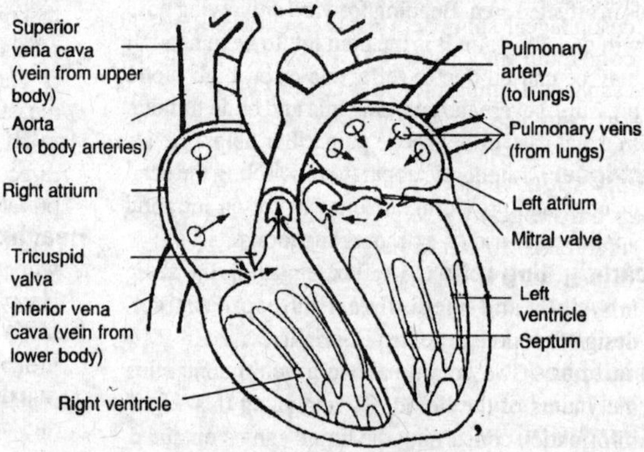

The heart showing the four chambers

From here it goes to left ventricle to be pushed to body.

Heart and lung machine It is the machine which takes over the function of respiration and blood circulation for a patient who is temporarily unable to manage either. Tubes inserted into the patient's venae cavae draw venous blood out of body. Machine simultaneously feeds a constant supply of oxygenated blood into a major artery. It is used in cardiac surgery. Russians use hypothermia in controlled conditions instead of this machine with good results.

Heart block Improper formation of sinoatrial impulse and its propagation through the junctional tissues of heart is known as heart block. It may be SA block, AV block, bundle branch block or arborisation or Purkinje block. It leads to dizziness, stroke or fainting attacks. It may be caused by coronary heart disease, myocarditis, overdose of digitalis drug. The rate of ventricle beat is slower than normal and in complete heart block the rate does not increase after exercise. Pulse becomes lesser than 50 per minute. Mild block does not require treatment. In severe case pace maker is fitted.

Heart burn It is the burning pain in epigastrium and may be caused by overeating, spicy prickles, and alcohol consumption. This pain is generally mistaken for heart attack. Antacids and anticholinergic drugs are helpful.

Heart burn in pregnancy It is a common complaint of pregnancy due to relaxation of oesophageal sphincter. Overeating of spicy food contribute may to it. Liquid antacids coat the esophageal lining more effectively.

Heart rate The number of complete cardiac cycles (heart beats) per minute.

Heart sugar Inositol.

Heart transplant It is a complex form of surgery undertaken to replace a patient's diseased heart either with a healthy one from donor or a mechanical one. Cross matching has to be done. It was first performed by Cristian Bernard in 1962. In India, it was performed by Dr. Venu Gopal of All India Institute of Medical Sciences, New Delhi.

Heartburn A burning sensation felt in the esophagus; caused by acid influx into stomach.

Heart-lung transplantation Removal of a patient's heart and two lungs, which are then replaced with donor heart and lungs.

Heat exhaustion It is caused by overexposure to heat, when person is not accustomed to work in hot environment. Insufficient water intake and diminished consumption of salt precipitate it. Symptoms include faintness, fatigue, headache, restlessness and heat cramps. Skin is pale and clammy. Breathing is shallow and fast. Pulse is rapid and weak. Glucose saline intravenous drip and antipyretics help the patient. Patient should be shifted to cooler place and whole body sponging will relieve the fever.

Heat resistance Capacity to withstand temperatures higher than 37°C without significant loss of functions.

Heat shock gene A gene inducible by heat shock or any other stressor.

Heat shock proteins Proteins induced by heat shock and related stress.

Heat shock response A rapid change in gene expression that occurs when there is a temperature shift to an elevated temperature.

Heat stroke It is a life threatening condition. In some cases exposure to direct heat may raise the body temperature to 106°F.
Constipation, dehydration humid hot weather and drinking too much alcohol are contributory factors. Person feels fatigue, weakness and profuse sweating. Skin becomes hot and dry. Without treatment person may loose consciousness and die. Treatment includes lowering the temperature and maintaining of fluid balance.

Heave A lift or thrust felt during palpation of the heart.

Heavy pressure Compressive force that extends to the bone under the tissue.

Hebb synapse A synapse that can change with use so that learning takes place.

Heberden's nodes These are cartilaginous and bony outgrowths at the sides of the terminal interphalangeal joints, usually accompanied by some deformity. These are seen in osteoarthritis.

Hedonic Associated with the seeking of pleasure and the avoidance of pain.

Heel pad Cushioning or protective material placed in the heel seat of a shoe.

Heel pain syndrome It is the most common cause of inferior heel pain in runners. Pain is more while rising up in the morning and bearing weight on the heel after sitting for a long time. Pain and

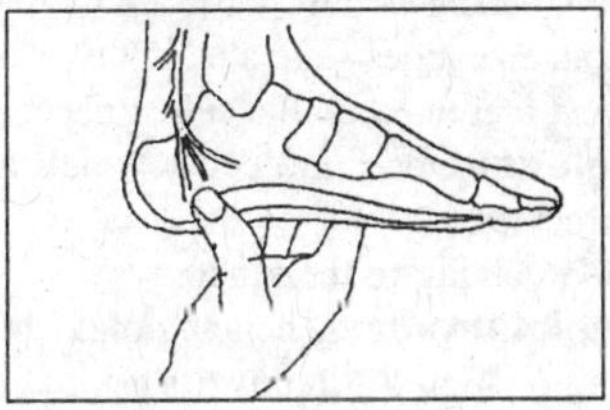

stiffness typically improve with activity, after prolonged activity the pain returns. Maximum amount of pain is felt on the medial aspect of calcaneus at the insertion of plantar fascia.

Heel Toe gait Walking in which the heel strikes the ground first and the toes are the last part of foot to leave the ground at the end of stance phase.

Heel-to-knee-test A test of cerebellar function.

Hegar's sign It can be recognised between 6th and 10 weeks of pregnancy. At this time fundus and upper part of body are enlarged by presence of ovum and lower uterine segment is soft and empty.

Hegar's sign depends upon this difference of consistency. Lower segment is soft and collapsed as to be impalpable, and fundus and cervix appear to be separate entities. Two fingers are placed in anterior vaginal fornix which appear almost to meet the fingers of the other hand pressing backwards and downwards suprapubically with the fundus above and cervix below their level of contact. This is a positive sign. Markedly softening and compressibility of lower segment of the uterus which gives rise to easy flexibility at the junction of the body of the uterus and cervix. The sign is present by the 6th week of pregnancy.

Heimlich maneuver Emergency procedure to dislodge food or other obstruction from the trachea, thereby preventing asphyxiation.

Helical CT scanner It is the CT system in which continuous X-ray tube rotation using slip ring technology is used. Term is equal to spiral CT scanner. In helical scanning the data acquisition is 100 % and no time is lost. It is more helpful in CT angiography and multiphase abdominal imaging.

Helium dilution method One of the most commonly used methods for the measurement of static lung volumes.

Helper T cells T cells that help B cells respond to antigen, or activate macrophages to become microbicidal; generally, these are CD4 T cells that recognize peptides generated in the vesicles of the cell and presented on the cell surface.

Hemaglutinin Any molecule which aglutinates erythrocytes.

Hemal Pertaining to the blood.

Hemangiofibroma A hemangioma characterized by proliferation of fibrous tissues.

Hemangioma A benign proliferation of vascular endothelium that creates a mass resembling neoplastic tissue. It is usually asymptomatic.

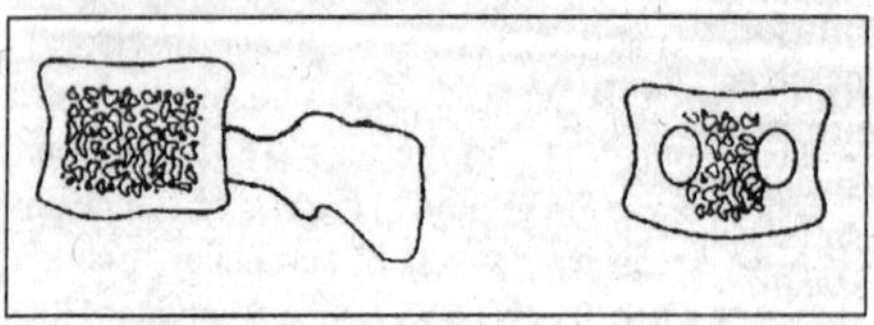

Hematemesis Vomiting of blood.

Hematinic An agent that increases the hemoglobin level and number of RBCs.

Hematocrit The ratio of packed red blood cells to total blood volume in a centrifuged sample of blood, expressed as a percentage.

Hematology The study of blood cells.

Hematopoiesis The formation and development of blood cells in bone marrow.

Hematosis Oxygenation or aeration of venous blood in lungs.

Hematuria and hypertension Pathological findings include neutrophils and macrophages. There will be increased number of endothelial cells.

Heme A iron containing metal ion, customarily iron in the Fell state, chelated in a tetraphyrrole ring.

Heme iron Iron which is bound to protoporphyrin in hemoglobin and myoglobin. Absorption of heme iron is not affected by phosphate or phytic acid or by vitamin C.

Hemianopia Caused by a lesion of the geniculocalcarine pathway or primary visual cortex.

Hemianopsia Inability to see half the field of vision in one or both eyes.

Hemibalism Involunatry, 'throwing' monements of arm and/or leg on one side, associated with damage to the subthalamic nucleus.

Hemicrania It is a form of recurrent paroxysmal headache often confined to one side of head starting in adulthood. It is a disturbance of carotid and vertebrobasilar system. Initially, there is vasoconstriction which leads to cortical and brainstem ischaemia resulting in aura. This is soon followed by vasodilation. Before actual headache starts there is rise of serum 5-hydroxy trytamine level. Anxiety, overwork, emotional upsets, hypertension and premenstrual tension may precipitate it. Actual attack of aura starts after waking from sleep. It may be in a form of visual disturbance, coloured lights, ocular pain, lacrimation and photophobia. Sometimes, tingling and numbness of face may be seen. After aura passes of headache starts. This may be uni or bilateral. Pain gradully increases in intensity having a throbbing or expansile character. The side affected is constant on each attack.

Hemidiaphragm One of the two domes of the diaphragm. Co-ordination is necessary to maintain adequate performance.

Hemiparesis Muscular weakness of one half of the body.

Hemiplegia It is a paralysis of one side of body. There is difficulty in swallowing, loss of use of extremities and bowel and bladder incontinence. There are two types of aphasia. Expressive aphasia is an inability to select words to communicate by speaking and writing.

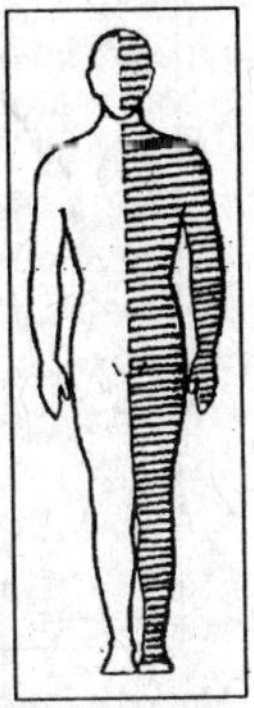

Hemiplegic Pertaining to or affected with hemiplegia.

Hemisacralization There is fusion of 5th lumbar vertebrae to the first segment of sacrum on only one side.

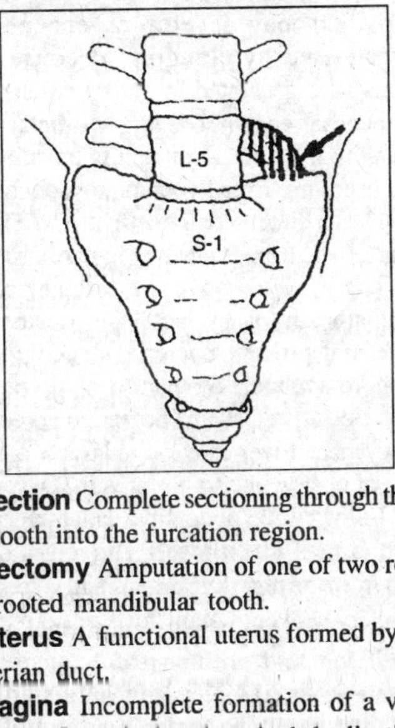

Hemisection Complete sectioning through the crown of a tooth into the furcation region.

Hemisectomy Amputation of one of two roots of a two-rooted mandibular tooth.

Hemiuterus A functional uterus formed by a single Mulerian duct.

Hemivagina Incomplete formation of a vagina in the case of cervical and vaginal duplication.

Hemivertebra A congenital anomaly of spine caused by the incomplete development of one side of vertebra.

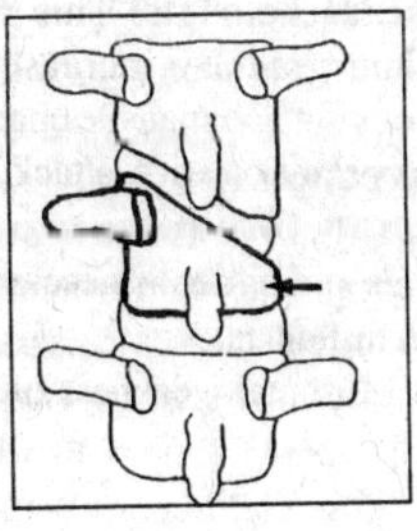

Hemochromatosis A genetic disorder causing excessive dietary iron absorption.

Hemocoel The body cavity of insects within which the hemolymph, or blood circulates freely.

Hemocomcertration The concentration of red blood cells in ome area.

Hemodialysis A procedure to remove impurities or wastes from the blood, used in treating renal insufficiency, by shunting the blood from the body through a machine for diffusion and ultrafiltration and then returning it to the patient's circulation.

Hemodilution The dilution of the blood.

Hemodynamic stability Stable heart rate and blood pressure.

Hemodynamics The study of movements of the blood and of the forces concerned therein.

Hemodynamics of placenta About 500-700 ml blood is flowed through placenta each minute Any reduction may interfere with nutritional transfer mechanism of placenta. Infants born being dysmature have reduced chances of survical.

Hemolymph The circulating fluid or blood of insects, which is pumped by a dorsal tubular heart and circulates freely in the body cavity, or hemocoel; it serves to transport nutrients, immunity factor, and hormones but not oxygen; several types of hemocytes, but no erythrocytes, are present.

Hemolysis An antibody that causes hemolysis of RBCS.

Hemolytic disease of the newborn A hemolytic anemia of a newborn child that results from the destruction of the infant's erythrocytes (red blood cells) by antibodies produced by the mother; usually the antibodies are due to an Rh blood type incompatibility.

Hemolytic uremic syndrome A trail of renal failure, thrombocytopenia, and hemolytic anemia frequently associated with Shiga toxin-producing E. coli.

Hemopexin A serum protein that strongly binds heme.

Hemophilic pseudotumor A progressive cystic swelling produced by recurrent hemorrhaging into soft tissue. Infections and trauma can also produce swelling in these cases.

Hemophore A secreted bacterial protein that shuttles environmental heme to the bacterial surface.

Hemopoiesis The production of red blood cells.

Hemopoietein Erythroproietin

Hemopoietic tissue Specialized connective tissue that is responsible for the formation of blood cells and lymphatic system cells; found in red bone marrow, spleen, tonsils and lymph nodes.

Hemorrhage-postpartum It is bleeding from genital tract after labour. Blood loss measuring 570 ml or more from genital tract within 24 hours of delivery is called primary postpartum hemorrhage. Bleeding after 24 hours is known as secondary PPH. It is a major cause of maternal death.

Hemorrhagic colitis Bloody-diarrhea caused by enterohemorrhagic Escherichia coli.

Hemorrhagic fever An infection manifested by acute onset of fever and hemorrhagic signs; typical of many zoonotic viruses.

Hemosiderosis Large amount of hemosierin are deposited especially in liver and spleen. It may result due to excessive break down of RBCs. It is treated by repeated removal of the blood in controlled manner or by heating the primary cause. At times spleen removal in necessary.

Hemostasis The arrest or checking of bleeding through natural process or through the use of artificial means.

Hemostat Instrument used to compress or treat bleeding vessels to arrest hemorrhage.

Hemovac drain A type of closed drain system.

Hemovae A proprietary name for a closed wound, suction drainage device.

Henle's ligament Part of conjoint tendon.

Hensen's duct Ductus runiens.

HEPA A high-efficiency particulate filter that can remove bacteria and some virus from air.

Heparin An anticoagulant given to slow the conversion of prothrombin to thrombin, thus reducing the risk of blood clot formation; also found naturally inbasophils and most cells.

Heparin lock An intravenous needle connected to a small "well" that allows for the intermittent injection of medication without the need for repeated venipuncture.

Heparinnized The use of an antithrombin factor to prevent intravasculat clotting.

Hepatic Pertaining to the liver.

Hepatic colic flexure The bend between the ascending colon and the tranverse colon.

Hepatic duct Tubules that drain bile from the liver and merge with the cystic duct from the gallbladder to form the common bile duct.

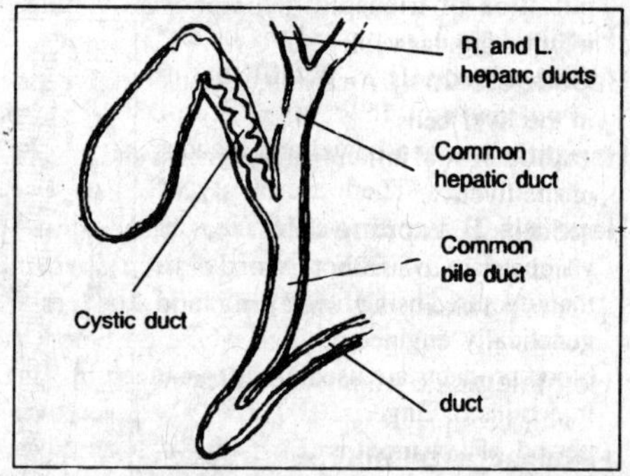

Hepatic encephalopathy In fulminant acute liver failure due to viral hepatitis secondary to cirrhosis the patient may develop an encephalopathy characterised by clouding of consciousness. Ammonia is generated in gut by colonic bacteria and mucosal enzymes acting on dietary protein. In healthy liver this ammonia is transformed into urea. In failing liver hyperammonaemia develops which has a direct sedative effect. The EEG shows characteristic triphasic waves in paroxysmal bursts and runs of delta waves. Treatment of hepatic encephalopathy is by lactulose. Restrict protein intake and prevent bacterial decomposition of protein to ammonia by the use of ciprofloxacin.

Hepatic oedema Oedema begins and predominates in abdomen. Liver may be enlarged if not other cause of obstruction to portal vein. Dyspnoea will have followed the abdominal enlargement.

Hepatic portal circulation The return of venous blood from the digestive organs and spleen through a capillary network within the liver before draining into the heart.

Hepatic portal system Blood flow through the veins that begin as capillary beds in the small intestine, spleen, pancreas, and stomach and carry blood to the liver, where they end as a capillary bed.

Hepatic portal vein The vein that carries blood from the intestines, stomach, spleen, and pancreas to the liver.

Hepatic pulsation Systolic pulsation of liver can be detected in case of severe tricuspid incompetence. Finer adjustment of pressure will allow him to feel and see pulsation superimposed on respiratory movements. These pulsations are systolic and coincident with the typical single pulsation of tricuspid incompetence visible in internal jugular vein.

Hepatic steatosis An accumulation of triglycerides in the liver cells.

Hepatitis A viral inflammatory process and infection of the liver.

Hepatitis B vaccine Two types of hepatitis B-vaccines are available : plasma derived where it is manufactured using blood and blood products, and genetically engineered, and where no blood and blood products are used in the manufacture. Three injections of Engerix 'B' have to be given over a period of six months. First dose—at an elected date. Second dose—One month after first dose. Third dose—Six months after first dose.

Hepatitis, viral It is an inflammation of liver by virus. Common viruses are Hepatitis A and Hepatitis B.

- Hepatitis A is thought to spread by virus from infected person's faeces, food and drinking water.
- Hepatitis B is spread through blood transfusions, blood products and infected needles. Nowadays it is more prevalent in male homosexuals. It is more serious having bad prognosis. In many cases virus persists for years and may lead to chronic form. Symptoms include loss of appetite, fatigue and jaundice. Diagnosis is made by identification of virus.

Hepatocellular carcinoma A cancer originating in the liver, probably from neoplastic transformation of hepatocytes.

Hepatocyte A major cell type of the liver, comprising ~70% of liver cells; a specific target of infection by viruses that cause hepatitis.

Hepatomegaly Enlargement of the liver.

Hepatopancreatic ampulla A small, elevanted area within the duodenum where the combined pancreatic and common bile duct empties; also called the ampulla of vater.

Hepatotoxic Potentially destructive to liver cells. Many drugs like paracetamol, carbon tetrachloride, and rifampicin etc.

Hepatotropic Having a special affinity for or exerting a specific effect upon the liver.

Hepatoxicity A toxic condition of the liver.

Herbal medicine A system of medicine based upon the healing properties of medicinal plants for the promotion and maintenance of helath of treatment of physical, physiological and spiritual concomittents of disease.

Herbal therapy The use of plant material is as old as civilisation with every known culture. Herbalism is known as art of simpling. Herbs were known as

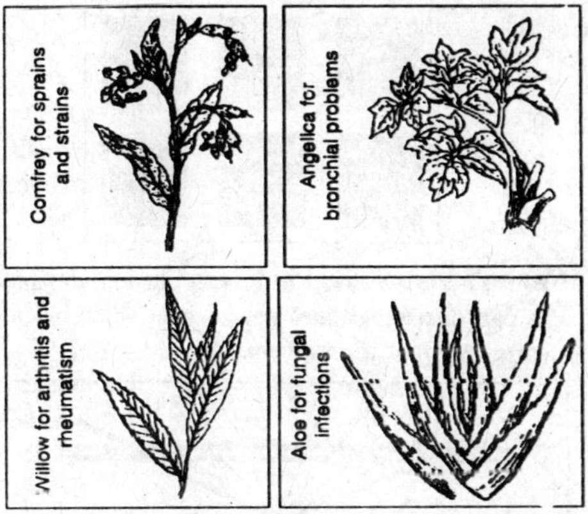

simples because one herb can cure many different conditions. These herbs work biochemically in the body and taken in moderate doses for long enough, these biochemical responses become automatic even after one stops taking the herbs.

Herbert screw Double ended threaded screw with different pitches. It allows compression of fracture fragment.

Herbicide A substance or agent used to kill plants, especially weeds.

Herbs Not clearly distinguished from spices, except that they usually refer to the whole of soft stemmed aromatic plant while spice is only part of plant.

Hereditability estimate A mathematical estimate of magnitue of the importance of genetic factors in a condition or disease.

Heredity That which is passed on from parents to offspring biologically through the genes. Dependent upon the genes. The inheritance of resemblance, physical qualities, or diseases from a familial predecessor; the passage of characteristics from one generation to its progeny by genetic linkage.

Hering Hermann grid This grid consist of black blocks separated by white broadlines, vertically horizontally. The patient sees a dark shadow at the intersections of white bonds. It is seen due to lateral inhibition and does not occur for the fixed point.

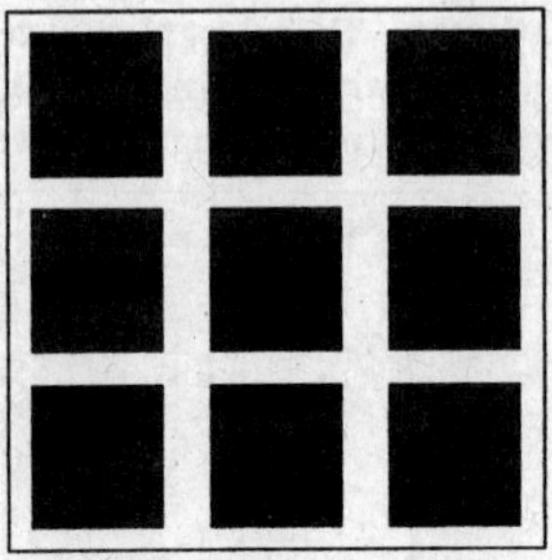

Hering's visual illusion It is an illusion. In which a pair of parallel lines appear bent when placing diagonal lines across them.

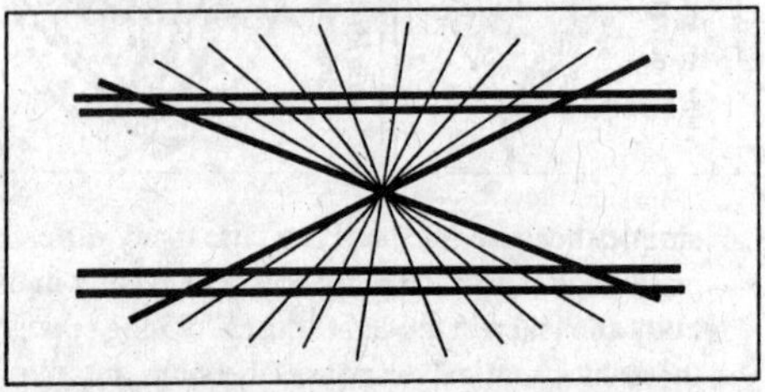

Hering-Breuer reflex A reflex in which distension of the lungs stimulates stretch receptors, which in turn act to inhibit further distension of the lungs.

Heritability The proportion of the variation among individuals in a phenotype that is attributable to differences in genotype and not to environmental effects.

Hermaphrodite An animal possessing gonads of both male and female type, often at the same time.

Hermaphroditism A congenital condition of ambiguity of reproductive structures so that the sex of the individual is not clearly defined as exclusively male or female. The condition is named for Hermes and Aphrodite, the Greek god and goddess of love.

Herniated nucleus pulposus There may be disc protrusion, nuclear material may protrude into spinal canal or there may be sequestration of nuclear material.

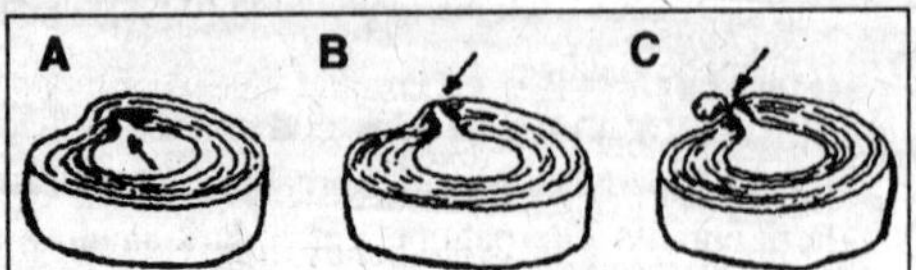

A - disc protrusion
B - nucleus protruding in spinal canal
C - sequestration

Herpangina Main symptoms include sore throat, odynophagia, high fever, headache, malaise and loss of appetite. It affects the younger age group. Tonsils become slightly red and swollen. Disease runs a brief course. Infective virus is coxsackievirus-A.

Herpes auricularis There develops uncomfortable, hot, stiff feeling in the ear becoming a dull ache punctured by sharp pain. Preherpetic pain is very severe and interfere with sleep. Meatus or tympanic membrane may present a red, swollen, erysipeloid appearance or 3rd day. Malaise, pyrexia and swelling of lymphatics are there. Vesicles may appear on concha, lobule and tragus. In a few days the vesicles desiccate. Disturbance of sensation may present.

Herpes genitalis Herpes simplex type 2 is the most common virus encountered in vulval disease. Infection is acquired in early adult life with commencement of sexual activity. Virus may remain dormant during recurrences. Antibodies persist indefinitely. It may be primary or secondary infection. The incubation period of primary is 2 to 7 days. Prodromal symptoms include, tingling, itching and paraesthesia. Vesicles rapidly erode leaving behind painful ulcer. Dysuria and retention of urine may be present. Inguinal lymph glands are enlarged. Treatment is symptomatic.

Herpes labialis Changes follow a consistent course with prodromal paresthesia or burning sensation, then erythema at the site of attack. Vesicles form after 1-2 hours in clusters along the mucocutaneous junction of lips. Vesciles enlarge, coalesce and weep. After 2-3 days they rupture leaving a crust. Then new vesicles appear.

Herpes simplex Infection caused by the herpes simplex virus.

Herpes simplex encephalitis It is a DNA virus with two related antigenic subtypes I and II. Type I affects nongenital areas while type II affects urogenital tract and skin below waist. Clinical features include fever and altered consciousness as initial signs, but focal hemisphere sign such as hemiparesis often follows. Seizures may develop. CSF contains high number of lymphocytes and sugar becomes low. Electroencephalography shows local slowing over one or both temporal lobes. Acyclovir may be given IV in a dose of 10 mg/kg delivered over 1 hour every 8 hours for 10 days. Prognosis depends on level of consciousness.

Herpes virus These have an icosahedral composed of 162 capsomers. Surrounding the particle is a loose lipoprotein envelop giving the overall diameter of 150 nm. Herpes virus remains latent, localised to certain sensory nerve ganglia. Virus produces vesicular lesions of the skin, especially face, lips and nose. Man is the only natural host and the sources of infection are saliva. Lesions are very painful but are mostly self-limiting. The most common manifestations are vesicular pharyngitis, tonsillitis and gingivostomatitis. Disease may be reactivated.

Herring bone pattern An artefact on a radiograph caused by a film being placed backward in the oral cavity; the pattern embossed in the lead foil appears on the radiograph, resulting in a lighter image.

Hertz It is a unit in which temporal frequency is measured. It defines the number of sinusoidal oscillations per second and is measured in Sec^{-1} As the frequencies of electromagnetic waves are usually very high, the terms kHz (kilohertz 10^3 Hz) MHz (megahertz=10^6Hz) GHz (gigahertz= 10^9 Hz) are often used. Unit of frequency representing cycles per seconds.

Herxheimer reaction The reaction may be both generalised and local, and may include general malaise, headache, pains in the limbs, sweating, rigors, fever, intensification of local lesions, skin rash and sore throat, and may occur after the first administration of any potent treponemacidal agents. It is seen in syphilis, and also in other spirochaetal infections such as relapsing fever.

Heschl's gyrus The primary auditory cortex found in the temporal lobes.

Hesperidine A vitamin from the bioflavonoid group.

Hess test A test for capillary fragility in scurvy.

Hesselback's ligament Inter-foveolar ligament.

Hesselback's torcular of Confluence of the cranial venous sinuses

Heterochromatin A condensed, inactive form of chromatin.

Heterochromic uveitis There are 3 main features of it, i.e. iris heterochromia, keratic precipitates and cataract. On examination one will find iris stromal atrophy, diffusely scattered small white keratic precipitates and mild aqueous flare.Fundus remains normal.

It affects young people. The loss of vision is due to cataract and glaucoma. Patient responds to steroids well.

Heterocrine Secreting more than one kind of matter.

Heteroduplex DNA Duplex DNA in which the two strands have different genetic origins. A heteroduplex may contain mismatched bases.

Heteroecious Describing a parasitic life cycle with a seasonal alternation between primary and secondary hosts.

Heterogeneity Dissimilarity in the genotypical structure of individuals originating through sexual reproduction.

Heterogonic Describing a life cycle in which free-living generations may alternate periodically with parasitic generations.

Heterogony The alternation of generations between asexual and sexual phases.

Heterograft A heterologous graft in which the tissue is obtained from another species.

Heteroinfection Infection from outside the body; exogenous infection.

Heterokaryon Genetically dissimilar nuclei found in a common cytoplasm, as in certain fungal cells.

Heterologous Derived from a different source or species; not native to the host.

Heterophil antibody test In this test demonstration of heterophil antibody is done by agglutination of the patient's serum with sheep red blood cells. The test is positive in infectious mononucleosis.

Heterophoria It is a condition in which eye shows duration when the fusion is broken.

It is a condition of imperfect balance of eye due to weak fusion. Heterophoria can be elicited only by dissociation tests. To check it requires a conscious effort.

Heteropolysaccharide A polysaccharide containing more than one type of sugar.

Heterosexism Prejudice against people who are not heterosexual or straight.

Heterosexuality The fact of experiencing sexual and/or romantic attraction to individuals of the opposite sex to oneself. Homosexuality is having sexual attachment with ones own sex.

Heterotopic transplantation The donor heart is anastomosed to the native heart without removal of the native heart.

Heterotroph Literally, feeder on others; an organism dependent upon organic material from an external source to provide carbon for growth; contrasted with autotrophs that can utilize inorganic materials for this purpose. Thus, heterotrophic.

Heterotrophy The fact of being a heterotroph; obtaining carbon from some external organic source.

Heterozygous Having two different allelic genes specifying the same genetically determined component.

Hexachlorophene It is a diphenol. In concentration of 1 to 3% it has been incorporated into soaps and combined with detergents used for preoperative hand scrubs of surgical team and postoperative patient's skin. It is long retained on skin from where it can be recovered even after 48 hours. Its bactericidal benefit is attributed to the bactericidal film left over the skin. It is the most universal of antibacterial agent.

Hexaflora A stable, six-member microflora often introduced to normalize, specific anomalies of germfree animals such as the enlarged cecum. The most often consist of Lactobacillus brevis, Streptococcus fecalis, Staphylococcus epidermidis, Bacteroides fragilis, vulgatus, Enterobacter aerogenes, and a Fusibacterium.

Hexose A simple sugar with a backbone containing six carbon atoms.

Hiatus An opening or fissure; a foramen.

Hiatus hernia and pregnancy Hiatal hernia is more frequent during pregnancy and there is higher incidence in multiparous mothers. Symptoms are heart burn, epigastric discomfort, vomiting and occasional hematemesis. The second stage of labour of patients with known hiatus hernia should by shortened by doing low forcep delivery.

Hibbard maneuver It involves application of pressure with the flattened hand against the fetal head posteriorly and upward and displace the anterior shoulder from behind of symphysis.

Hibbs spinal fusion A surgical technique fusion of lumbar spine.

Hibs angle It is an angle between the talus and the first metatarsal used as a measurement of cavus.

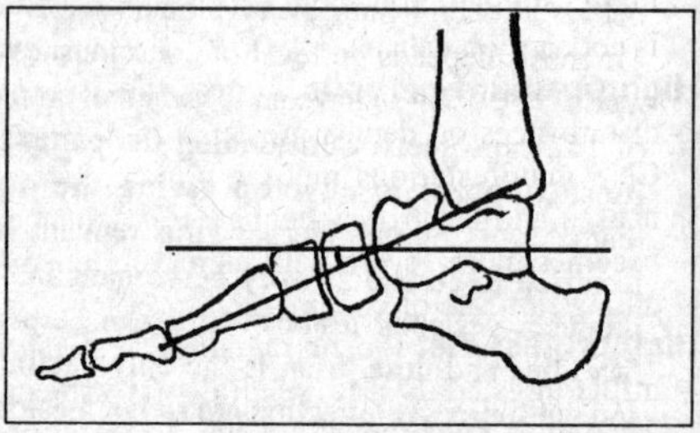

Hiccup This is a state of intermittent spasm of diaphragm accompanied by sudden closure of glottis. It may be caused by stimulation of sensory nerve endings of phrenic which are connected with the coeliac and other intra-abdominal autonomic plexus. The vagus may also act as part of afferent arc of reflex. Through these pathways hiccup may arise from impulses in any abdominal viscus. Alcoholic intoxication, uraemia and encephalitis may result it.

Hickey-Hare test According to this test intravenous infusion of hypertonic saline does not induce antidiuresis in the patients with diabetes insipidus.

Hidden transfer Technique commonly used to transfer the anesthetic syringe out of the view of the patient.

Hierachy of needs Pyramid of needs, described by Dr. Abraham H. Maslow, that motivate behavior; physiologic, safety, social, ego and self-actualization.

Hierarchy A system that organizes things into successive ranks or grades.

High concentration syntocin drip Increasingly high concentration of syntocin 5% glucose drip is effective in terminating missed abortion. Water intoxication and convulsions may develop.

High density cholesterol HDL has a different and apparently beneficial role. It carries cholesterol away from cells back to liver and promotes its excretion from body. HDL removes cholesterol from artery walls too Regular exercise increases HDL while obesity lowers it.

High Fowler's position Placement of a client in a semisitting position by raising the head of the bed up more than 4560 degrees.

High impact resistant acrylic It has a much higher impact strength. It is more expensive material and is not easily breakable.

High pressure nervous syndrome Behavioral disturbances on depths greater than 150 meters. CNS manifestations include tremor, dizziness, nausea and electro enchephalogram changes. It becomes more severe with increasing depth and during fast rate of compression.

High protein diet Protein rich diets are meat, fish, milk, eggs, dals and specially soyabean. In vegetables mushrooms contain 40 to 50 gm of protein per 100 gm. Dals contain 22 to 26 gm/100 gm and groundnut 20 gm%. Meat contains 18 to 20 gm %.

High-density lipoprotein (HDL) One of the major classes of lipoproteins, containing about 50% protein and much smaller concentrations of phospholipids than either VLDL or LDL; has a flotation fraction density between 1.063 and 1.21.

Highet's scale A method of grading muscle stength based on scale of 0 to 5.

High-output congestive heart failure Heart failure resulting from a volume overload.

High-quality protein A food containing the best balance and assortment of essential and nonessential amino acids for protein synthesis homocysteine.

Hill reaction The evolution of oxygen and the photo reduction of an artificial electron acceptor by a chloroplast preparation in the absence of carbon dioxide.

Hilton's methods–buccal abscess An incision should be parallel to the alveolar ridge and at least 1.3 cm in length. The closed blades of a pair of sinus forceps are thrust into the abscess and then

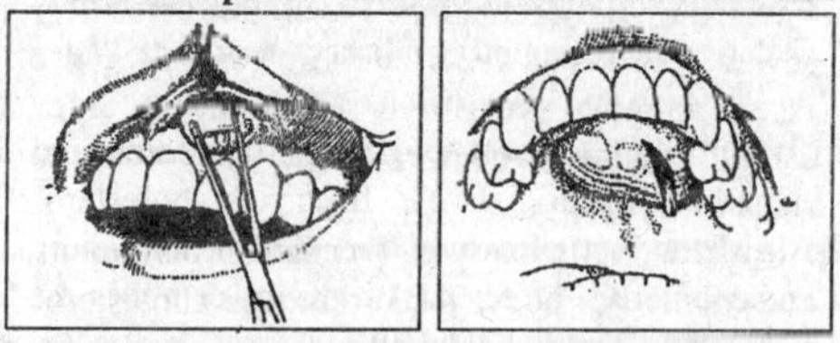

opened liberating the pus. This method of opening an abscess ensures that no blood vessels or nerve is damaged and is known as Hilton's method. This method is commonly used to drain abscesses.

Hilum Part of an organ where the nerves and vessels enter and leave.

Hilus An area, depression, or pit where blood vessels and nerves enter or leave an organ. Also called a hilum.

Hind brain It is a rear lower part of brain. It consists of bulbar area of brainstem, medulla oblongata and cerebellum.

Hind foot Posterior portion of foot consisting talus and calcaneus.

Hind milk Breast milk recieved at the end of a feeding. It contains higher fat.

Hind water rupture Hind water is ruptured with the introduction of 'S' shaped catheter.

Hindbrain The embryonic part of the brain that contains the brainstem and cerebellum; thought to coordinate movements and support movements of walking and posture.

Hinge joint A type of synovial articulation characterized by a convex surface of one bone fitting into a concave surface of another such that movement is confined to one plane, as in the knee or interphalangeal joint.

Hinged solid ankle-foot orthosis Plastic orthosis with similar trimlines that has a transverse separation to provide sagittal plane motion.

Hip The joint connecting the legs of the trunk.

Hip extension test Patient is aligned in neutral position, raises the nontest limb. Examiner maintains trunk and limb alignment in neutral position and if knee or ankle or both are unstable, manual support is provided by assistant.

Hip replacement Hip joint is the joint between hip bone and head of femur. If fractured or severe osteoarthritis causing crippling, hip replacement may be done. In it head of femur is replaced by metallic one. Patients become fit to walk.

Hip spica The use of hip spica with the hip internally rotated may help to alleviate some of the pain experienced with daily activity. Lateral movements and abduction with external rotation should be avoided until symptoms subside.

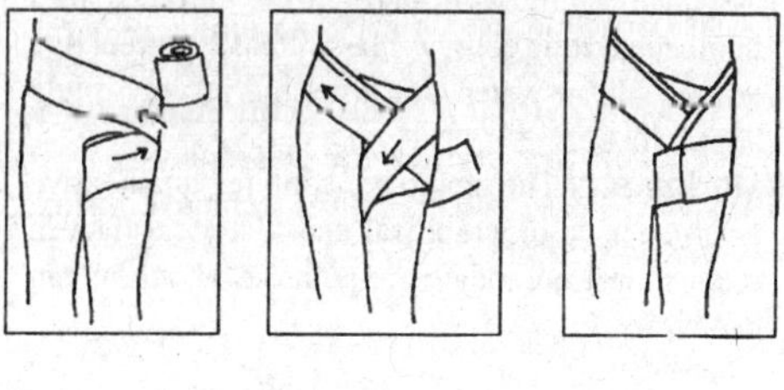

Hippocampal formation A general term referring to the hippocampus and a number of associated structures and pathways.

Hippocampus A brain structure with implications for remembering and forgetting. The term is based on the Latin word for seahorse, which is curved, like this structure. Injuries to this area of the brain have resulted in various forms of amnesia.

Hirsutism It is an excessive hairiness specially in women. Additional hair are coarse. Certain conditions in which level of male hormones are high such as polycystic ovary syndrome, congenital adrenal hyperplasia.
Consumption of cortisone for long period may also result in hirsutism. Hair can be bleached and removed by different ways.

His, bundle Atrioventricular bundle.

Histamine A compound secreted by tissue mast cells and other connective tissue cells that stimulates vasodilation and increases capillary permeability. It is responsible for many of the symptoms of inflammation and allergy.

Histaminergic system Widespread hestaminergic innervatio of cerebral cortex by the tuberoinfundibular nucleus of hypothalamus.

Histidine An aminoacid essential for growth and repair of human tissue.

Histochemistry Pertaining to the composition of the tissues.

Histocompatibility It is the degree of matching between the tissues of patient and donor. Tissues have at least 20 antigens to reject the tissue so maximum matching is required to avoid rejection.

Histogenesis Formation of tissues from primary germ layers of embryo.

Histograph A bar graph. It is a graphic representation of frequency distribution.

Histology Microscopic study of the sturcture and function of tissues.

Histones The family of five basic proteins that associate tightly with DNA in the chromosomes of all eukaryotic cells. A class of basic protein that are soluble in water and insoluble in very dilute ammonia.

Historiometry The method of applying quantitative techniques to biographical and historical data in order to test nomothetic hypotheses about human behavior.

History Information from the client about past and present medical conditions and patterns of symptoms.

HIV dementia Most common neurological syndrome of HIV infection is AIDS dementia complex, impairment of cognitive function and memory and later motor disturbance. Dementia is produced by primary neuronal loss and inflammatory encephalopathy. Early symptoms are loss of concentration, loss of memory and interest in environment. Person may develop agitation, inappropriate behaviour and hallucinations. Depression of consciousness and seizures are uncommon. Towards the end many patients develop ataxic spastic para-or tetraparesis and become mute and incontinent. Lumbar puncture in HIV encephalopathy usually shows a moderate pleocytosis. Electroencephalography (EEG) shows moderate degree of slowing. MRI shows areas of increased signal in the central white matter in T_2 weighted image.

HIV oral melanosis Such patients undergo progressive hyperpigmentation of skin, nails and mucous membranes. Aetiology remains undermined. Buccal mucosa is the most frequently affected site but gingiva, palate and tongue may be involved. Microscopically, it is characterised by basilar melanin pigment.

HLA Abbrevaition for human leukocyte antigens.

Hodgkin's disease It involves lymphoid tissue in the lymph node. It starts as a painless enlargement of lymph nodes. As disease progresses various viscera may be involved. Half of patients present with adenopathy in neck or supraclavicular area. Nodes involved tend to be centripetal or axial. Patient develops low grade fever with night sweats. Fever may be fluctuating. Fever can persist for several weeks followed by afebrile intervals. There is unexplained weight loss. Person develops fatigue, malaise and weakness. It responds to radiation therapy.

Hodgkin's lymphadenoma Generally young adolescents are affected. All groups of nodes are involved sooner or later. Cervical group is affected first. Several nodes are simultaneously affected. Mass becomes rubbery and elastic. The individual nodes remain discrete with little tendency of matting and softening of suppuration. Spleen and liver are enlarged with secondary anaemia.

Hoe Scaler that resembles a garden hoe.

Hoffas fat pad The infrapatellar fat pad of knee.

Hoist Hoist is an overhead gantry with winch and chain used for loading a large pool.

Holism An approach to the study of the individual in totality, rather than as an aggregate of separate physiologic, psychologic, and social characteristics.

Holistic, holism Viewing something as a unified whole, i.e. the whole person.

Homan's sign It is manifested by pain at the calf or back of the knee occurring due to forcible dorsiflexion of the ankle with the knee extended of during straight leg raising. It is seen in venous thrombosis.

Home care The provision of equipment and services to the patient in home for the purpose of restoring and maintenance of health at maximal level.

Home care agency A agency that contracts with nurses and practitioners to provide home-based services.

Home traction Any type of traction used by a patient and his family outside the hospital.

Homelessness A state of losing one's possessions, doubling up with relatives during hard times, or simply having no home.

Homeostasis The compensatory mechanism by which a constant physical or chemical state is maintained. Physiologically exemplified by sweating and other processes which maintain a constant body temperature, psychological homeostasis may be illustrated by maintaining one's self-respect through such compensatory devices as rationalising and blaming others.

Homeostatic mechanism A system that maintains a constant environment enabling body cells to function effectively.

Homocysteine Elevated levels of this vitamin/hormone compound increase the risk for coronary artery disease; low levels of folate and vitamin B6 are related to increased circulating homocysteine. Now a days, increase in levels have been correlated with thrombosis or other disorders of blood coagulation.

Homocystinuria It is an autosomal recessive trait due to deficiency of cystathionine-beta synthetase leading to defective homocystine metabolism and formation of excessive homocystine. The manifestations are ectopia lentis, mental retardation, bony abnormalities and osteoporosis. Thrombi occur in artery as well as vein resulting in infarction of brain, lung and heart. Long bones become thin developing pathological fracture.

Homodimer A molecule composed of two identical subunits.

Homoeopathy It is based on the fact that disorder can be treated by tiny doses of drug which in large doses itself produces symptoms of disorder. Homeopathic drugs are diluted with water and milk sugar.

Homofermentative Describing or referring to microorganisms that produce lactic acid as the sole product of carbohydrate metabolism.

Homogeneity The state or quality of being homogenous.

Homogeneous Composed of similar elements or ingredients.

Homogonic Describing a lifestyle that is consistently either parasitic or free living.

Homologous Very similar or the same, as in form, structure, position, appearance, etc. or having a shared common ancestry with another.

Homologous chromosomes Two chromosomes that belong to a pair.

Homologous recombination A process by which two nearly identical genetic elements are brought together for the purpose of combining them or separating them.

Homology The fact of being homologous; having a common or corresponding origin structure, organization, etc.

Homonymous (a) Matching motor neurons (ch. 8); (b) matching parts of the binocular visual field.

Homonymous hemianopia Blindness of an entire left or right visual field.

Homonymous hemianopsia Blindness in the outer half of the visual field of one eye and the inner half of the visual field of the other eye, producing an inability to receive information from either the right or the left half of the visual environment.

Homophobia A general term for various forms of prejudice and discrimination against homosexuals.

Homosexual This term was invented at the beginning of the twentieth century by psychoanalysts studying people who found themselves attracted to their own sex. Because of the term's use as a disease category, it is generally not used within the communities to which it refers.

Homosexual behavior Sexual actions with some one of same sex.

Homosexual panic An acute and severe attack of anxiety based on unconscious conflicts involving gender identity.

Homosexual pattern There are three types of homosexuality: (i) an active role in which the individual functions sexually as a male (performing), (ii) a passive role in which person plays a female role in which person plays a female role (receiving), and (iii) mixed active and passive roles.

Homosexuality The sexual interactions, behavioral or in fantasy with persons of one's same sex even in conditions of available and willing opposite sex partners.

Homosexuals It is a sexual act between two males. Homosexuality was well accepted in ancient Rome and a few Roman emperors were known to engage in homosexual behaviour. Most pairs engage in foreplay activities such as hugging, kissing and petting. Among male homosexuals fellatio and mutual masturbation are the most common methods of inducing orgasm.

Homotherm Any animal, including mammals and birds, that tends to maintain a constant body temperature; also referred to as warm blooded.

Homovanillic acid (HVA) A principal metabolite of dopamine, a catecholamine found in the brain and other organs.

Homozygos Having two identical alleles for a genetic trait.

Homozygos Having two identical alleles.

Homunculus The representation of the human body in the sensory or motor cortex; also any topographical representation of the body by a neural area.

Honey A sweet, sticky liquid made by honeybee from nectar of plants. Bees suck the nectar from flowers and store it in their honey sacs where it undergoes certain changes. Later on bees deposit the liquid in honeycombs where due to certain changes it becomes honey. Honey is predigested sweetner.

Honeymoon cystitis It is an inflammation of the bladder found among women who have just been married or who engage in frequent and regular intercourse for the first time. Condition is painful during micturition and often caused by vaginal dryness.

Hook grip It involves second through fifth fingers flexed around an object in a look manner.

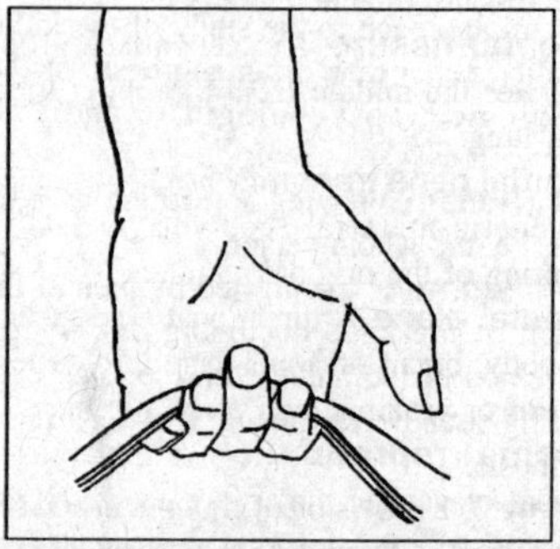

Hookworm Adults of two species of hookworms, Ancylostoma duodenale and Nector americans cause infection resulting in anemia.

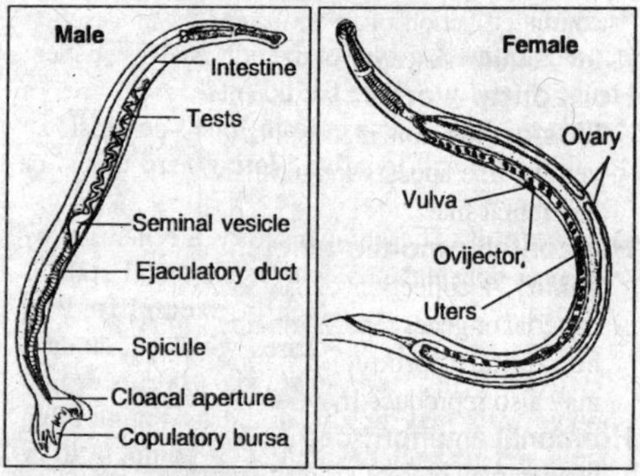

Hope Reflects a positive congnitive set that people have about their future out come in life.

Hops The dried flowers of the female Humulus lupulus plant that contribute flavor and antibacterial compounds to beer.

Hordeolum internum It is a suppurative inflammation of the meibomian gland. It occurs due to secondary infection of chalazion. symptoms are more than of stye because gland involved is larger and embedded in a thick layer of fibrous tissue. There is an acute pain and tenderness with swelling of lid.

On examination there is large and hard tender nodule in lid. Abscess usually points on conjunctival side. Pus appears as a yellow spot shining through conjunctiva. Once abscess has formed then there is only treatment of evacuation.

Horizontal angulation The angulation of the position indicating device (cone) in a horizontal (side-to-side) direction.

Horizontal fissure The secondary groove that separates the middle from the upper lobe of the right lung.

Horizontal gene transmission The reappearance of genetic material received by HGT in the offspring of the original recipient.

Horizontal plane A directional plane that divides the body, organ or appendage into superior and inferior or proximal and distal portions.

Horizontal reproduction An increase in the amount of genetic material e.g., DNA, genes, or sets of genes e.g., viruses and plasmids by transfer between organisms rather than through organismal reproduction.

Horizontal resistance Resistance conferred by the combined action of several genes; can vary from low to high susceptibility.

Horizontal vertical visual illusion Illusion in which the vertical line appears longer than horizontal line.

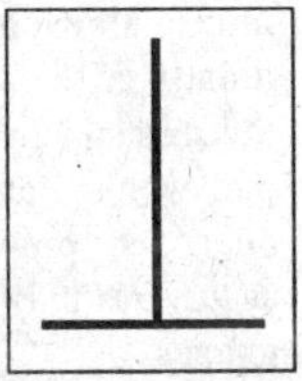

Horizontally mobile element (HME) A collection of genetic material or genes reproducing by horizontal reproduction, that may also reproduce by vertical reproduction.

Hormonal amenorrhoea Affected premenopausal woman may present with amenorrhoea. Pregnancy tests may give false positive results due to cross reactions with other pituitary hormones.

Hormonal sex The sex of an individual determined by the preponderance of either oestrogen (female) or testosterone (male) sex hormones.

Hormone Substance secreted by endocrine tissues into the blood that acts on a target tissue to produce a specific response. These are glandular secretion that stimulates one or more specific organs in the body to fulfil their function. Important hormones are growth hormones, sex hormones and thyroid hormones.

Hormone implant Small capsules of progestin inserted subcutaneously to provide contraception.

Hormone receptor A protein in, on the surface of, target cells that binds a specific hormone and initiates the cellular response.

Horn An area of gray matter (anterior, lateral, or posterior) in the spinal cord.

Horner's muscle Pars lacriminalis of orbicularis oculi.

Horner's syndrome In this syndrome paralysis of the cervical sympathetic ganglia produces enophthalmos, ptosis, miosis, facial hemiatrophy, and absence of sweating on the ipsilateral side of the face and neck.

Horse back riders knee A common term for posterior dislocation of tibular head in proximal tibiofibular joint.

Hortnet freezing test The test for adulteration of milk with water by measuring the depression of freezing point. Normal range is 0.53 to 0.55°C.

Hospice An alternative to traditional medical care of dying person giving highest priority to pain and other symptoms to be relieved.

Hospital An institution that provides medical care.

Hospital dust It is a potent source of disease. Hospital dust contains sand particles coming inside by foot wear or blown in by wind, scales from skin, dried infected matter like pus and other debris of wound, dried throat and nasal secretions, particles of dried excreta and food particles.

Various types of virulent organism particles may be found in dust. Dust can spread disease either by direct contact with wound, eyes, throat and inhalation of lungs.

Host Generally, any living organism that provides the site where another organism of a different species resides and obtains nutrition or an organism in which a pathogen can replicate and potentially cause disease or an organism or cell culture in which a virus or group of viruses may replicate.

Host defence system A complex system that enables the organism to defend itself from tissue injury.

Host range The number and nature of organisms in which is given virus or group of viruses replicate, or the particular group of species in which genes transferred from another particular organism can replicate.

Host Site In bone augmentation, the site into or onto which a graft or transplant material is placed.

Host specificity The extent to which a parasite can exist in more than one host species.

Host, definitive The host in which a parasite attains sexual maturity.

Host, intermediate The host in which a parasite undergoes developmental changes but does not yet reach sexual maturity.

Host, parasitic The host in which a parasite resides without further development; a transfer host.

Host, reservoir A host, usually non-human, in which a parasite lives and remains a source of infection but usually produces no symptoms.

Hostile aggression Aggressive behavior, that is associated with anger and is intended to harm another.

Hostility An attitudinal disposition of antagonism toward another person or social system.

Hot application Local and general application of heat to the body is useful for relieving the stasis of blood and to increase absorption of inflammatory products. It relieves stiffness of muscle and muscle pain. It increases blood circulation and thereby to improve nutrition to the part.

Hot bath 36.5°C-40°C. Chronic arthritic patient, muscle tightness, fatigue, strain.

Hot compress This is an improvised method of application of heat to a part of body where water bottle is not applicable or in folds when hot water bottle cannot be put. Folded thick guage or compressed cotton is brought to source of heat. Check its tolerable limit and apply over the desired part of the patient. Make sure that patient is not having paralysis, numbness or loss of sensation or poor circulation which are absolute contraindications for application of heat.

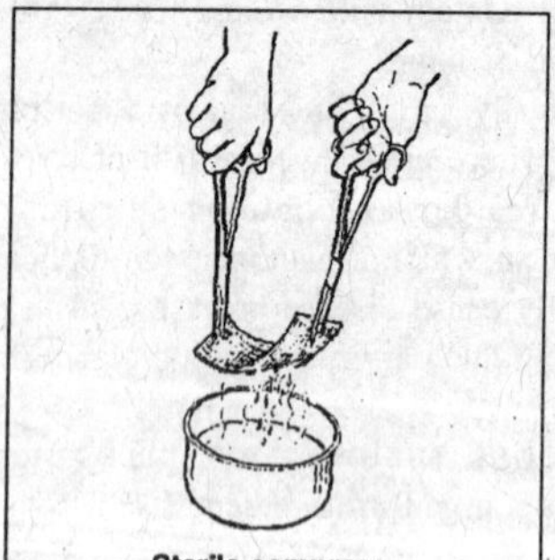

Sterile compress

Hot compresses and packs Pack is usually applied to an extensive body area and consists of warm, moist flannel while a compression normally applied to a limited body area and consists of warm, moist, gauge dressing. Material can be wrung with forceps so that it does not drip on the patient. Generally, it is done for 15 to 20 minutes.

Hot flushes A brief, subjective sensation of intense heat mainly of the upper body; associated in the human female with a decline in circulating estrogen levels during or after menopause. These are heat waves over face and whole body developing at the time of menopause but also during emotional upset. Hot flushes are reddish in colour.

Hot pack Any device which provides superficial heat therapy to a body part.

Hot spot imaging It depends on the accumulation of radio-labelled tracers in area of damaged myocardium. Bone scanning agents such as ^{99m}Tc-pyrophosphate accumulate at these sites probably secondary to membrane breakdown and microcalcifications. Images become positive mostly after 12 to 24 hours of an attack of myocardial infarction and remain positive for about one week. Patients with ongoing myocardial necrosis, post MI and those who develop aneurysms may show persistently positive infarct images.

Hot water bag, ice bag cleaning These are to be cleaned with soap water and rinse properly. Never use boiling water and hang it upside down to drain water. Fill some air to keep separate the opposing inner walls. Place stopper before storing. In infectious ward dip it in 1:40 solution of carbolic acid for 4 hours before cleaning with soap water. Hot water bottle is filled with hot water at 50° to 55°C. For general warmth of body and sometime to provide extra comfort to needy patient in extreme cold climate, a hot water bottle can be put inside the quilt.

Hot water bottle It is used to relieve pain of the part of the body, to relieve distension of abdomen and congestion. It relieves retention of urine and provide warmth to the body.

House staff Physician and other health care professional who are still under training.

Houston's valves or folds Transverse rectal folds.

Hoyer lift Mechanical device that uses a canvas sling to easily lift dependent clients for transferring.

HPLC High pressure liquid chromatography.

HPTLC High performance thin layer chromatography.

HTST High temperature short time treatment, defined as sterilization by heat ranging from a few seconds to 6 minutes. Usually applied to flow sterilization in which, the process time is less than about 1 minute.

Hubbbard tank It is a large container made of metal in shape of a keyhole or modified figure of 8.

Huber needle Special needle with a deflected point designed to prevent damae to the silicone septum of implanted infusion ports.

Hue The term used in the munsell color system to describe the dominant color of an object (i.e.,red, yellow, blue).

Huffing Inhaling toxic substances by breathing them through the nose; seen in substance-related disorders.

Human chorionic gonadotrophin (HCG) A hormone secreted by the placenta that prolongs the life of the corpus luteum. It is excreted in the mother's urine and makes possible the standard tests for pregnancy.

Human factors psychology A speciality in which the psychologist is concerned with the design of tools, machines, and systems of all types best suited for human use. The field began largely with development of tools and equipment to include the design of administrative systems and organisations. Formerly called engineering and human factors engineering.

Human immunodeficiency virus The retrovirus that causes acquired immunodeficiency syndrome (AIDS).

Human menopausal gonadotrophin (HMG) A hormone excreted in the urine of postmenopausal women that has the property of stimulating growth and maturity of ovarian follicles.

Human physiology It is the science that deals with a consideration of the activities of man and the manner in which the individual parts of human body carry out the process of life.

Human placenta lactogen Hormone secreted by placenta influencing somatic growth and maturity of ovarian follicles.

Humanistic viewpoint The study of personality which focuses upon human uniqueness, especially the differences, between human beings and other species. Human complexity, subjectivity, and capacity for growth are stressed. This viewpoint stands largely in opposition to behaviourism and psychoanalysis.

Humectant A substance that prevents loss of moistre.

Humerus The second longest bone in the body; the long bone of the arm.

Humerus triangular space A triangular anatomic space in the upper posterior arm through which, brachial artery and radial nerve leaves the area.

Humoral Circulating or found in the blood or another fluid of the body.

Humoral immunity The form of acquired immunity in which antibody molecules are secreted in response to antigenic stimulation as opposed to cell mediated immunity; also called antibody-mediated immunity.

Humphrey, ligament Anterior meniscofemoral ligament.

Humus The organic fraction of soil, characteristically black-brown in color; organic by-products consisting of microbial cell walls and other resistant molecules formed from free-radical reactions of sugars, aminoacids, and products of lignin decomposition.

Hunger A physiological need for food.

Hunt syndrome Patient develops sharp, stabbing pain which may be continuous or paroxysmal. Pain is radiating to roof of the palate and deep into the ear and face. There may be abnormal taste sensations with facial paralysis.

Hunter syndrome It is a X-linked recessive disorder involving abnormality in mucopoly-saccharide or glycoprotein metabolism. Clinically there will be various degrees of mental retardation, corneal clouding and skeletal changes. Progressive retinal degeneration is noted along with optic atrophy and loss of vision.

X-ray will show microcephaly and 'J'-shaped sella along with hook-shaped vertebral bodies and ilium bones are widely flared. CT may show optic atrophy.

Hunter's canal Adductor canal.

Hunting season A period of time during which a specified species can be legally hunted within a specified area.

Huntington's disease It is an autosomal dominantly inherited disorder that usually begins in middle life; characterised by involuntary choreic movements and dementia. Illness generally starts with psychological features, inability to concentrate and loss of social skills.

An impression of restlessness and fidgeting may be initially seen. It may become difficult to catch a knife and fork. Mean duration of illness from onset to death is about 13 to 15 years. MRI may show atrophy of caudate nuclei with enlargement of frontal horn.

Hurdles technology In the temperature control of microbial acitivity, a calculated use of combinations of different preservation factors or techniques in order to acheive multi-target, mild but reliable preservation effects.

Hurler's disease (gargoylism) A hereditary disorder caused by an enzyme deficiency. It is the characterised by gargoyl-like features of the head (depressed bridge of the nose, large prominent tongue, and widely spaced teeth), dwarf structure, short neck, broad short hands, severe mental retardation, blindness, deafness, and cardiovascular defects.

Hurler's syndrome The syndrome includes severe abnormality in skeletal development with dwarfism, kyphosis, deformed limbs, corneal clouding, deafness, mental retardation, and hepatosplenomegaly. It is also known as gargoylism. Syndrome is also a disorder of mucopolysacchrides.

Clinical features include prominent eyes, puffy lids, heavy brows, large tongue, hydrocephalus, widely spread teeth, mental retardation and deafness. X-ray will show oxycephally and enlarged sella with cardiovascular anomalies.

Husk This is the outer woody cellulose covering. In wheat it is loosely attached and removed during threshing, in rice it is firmly attached.

Hutchinson teeth A pathognomonic sign of congenital syphilis represented by the presence of oval-shaped notch on the permanent central incisors.

Hutchinsons fracture A fracture of radial styloid.

HVE system High-velocity evacuation system used to remove oral fluids and debris.

Hyalin A translucent substance, one of the products of amyloid degeneration.

Hyaline cartilage A cartilage with a homogeneous matrix. It is the most common type, occurring at the articular ends of bones, in the trachea, and within the nose. Most of the bones in the body are formed from hyaline cartilage.

Hyaline membrane An eosinophilic membrane lining the alveolar ducts of infants suffering from respiratory distress syndrome.

Hyaline membrane disease (HMD) A disease of premature infants characterised by the formation of a translucent membrane in the respiratory passages and the incapacity of the lungs to expand adequately. Also known as respiratory distress syndrome (RDS).

Hyalinization Conversion to a substance resembling glass.

Hyaluranidase An enzyme that catalyzes the hydrolysis of hyaluronic acid.

Hyaluronic acid A viscous, amorphous extracellular material that binds cells together, lubricates joints, and maintains the shape of the eyeballs.

Hybrid composite These give durability with esthetics. This contains a mixture of small and microscopic particles making up 70 to 80% of total weight. Most common are minifills. Their largest particles are 1 to 2 mm. Hybrids with larger particles are known as mid fills. Larger particles have greater amount of fillers and higher strength.

Hybridization The mating of two genetically distinct individuals.

Hybridoma Fused or hybrid cells that continue to produce the same antibody as the original lymphocyte.

Hydatid cyst of kidney It becomes difficult to differentiate from other cysts unless it opens into pelvis of kidney. The passage of vesicle may cause renal colic. The cyst may be suspected when it has thrill on palpation along with eosinophilia and history of hydatid cyst elsewhere. Prognosis is not grave. Treatment is surgical.

Hydatid liver It depends on the presence of liver of parasite *Echinococcus granulosus*. Enlargement of liver may be smooth, globular and elastic and sometimes fluctuating. Right chest may be bulged outwards with dullness in axilla. Pain is absent unless tumour is near surface. When liver capsule is involved it may produce pain. No constitutional symptoms appear. Rupture of cyst may produce shock.

Hydatidiform mole When the chorionic villi are converted into a mass of vesicles, the condition is termed hydatidiform mole. Hyperactivity of trophoblastic layer is the essential feature. Uterus is filled with a mass of clear vesciles of varying size. Uterine bleeding is the commonest feature. The bleeding varies from mere spotting to frank bleeding. There may develop abdominal pain due to uterus growth.

Hydraminos There is excess of liquor amnii. Quantity of liquor becomes greater than 2000 ml. The may be over production of liquor or diminished disposle of it. Causes include, abnormal fetuses, multiple pregnancy and diabetes mellitus. There develops abdominal enlargement with pain and discomfort. Complaints are dysponea and orthopnoea. Hyperemesis gravidorum may be precursor. Odema of lower extremities and labia may be present. In acute hydraminos abdomen is tense, tender and disproportionately large.

This may be the resuslt of deficit absorption and excessive production. Uterus is disproportionately large and its contour more globular. Fluid thrill may be obtained in all directions. Signs of pregnancy will be found. A large ovarian cyst may be found with pregnancy. During labour hydraminos causes more risk of malpresentations, prolapse of cord, uterine inertia, APH and PPH. There may be respiratory distress to fetus.

Hydraminos in diabetes It occurs practically in all diabetic pregnancies.

The volume of liquor does not show any relationship with its glucose content.

Hydranencephaly This condition involves absence of cerebrum There is an intact cranial vault, meninges and posterior fossa. The cranium is normal sized or enlarged and is fluid filled. The entire cerebrum consists with CSF density and normal ventricles are not visualised. There are intact, posterior fossa, thalamus and basal ganglion.

Hydraulic couch It is made of heavy steel with adjustable head end to examine a patient in comfortable situation.

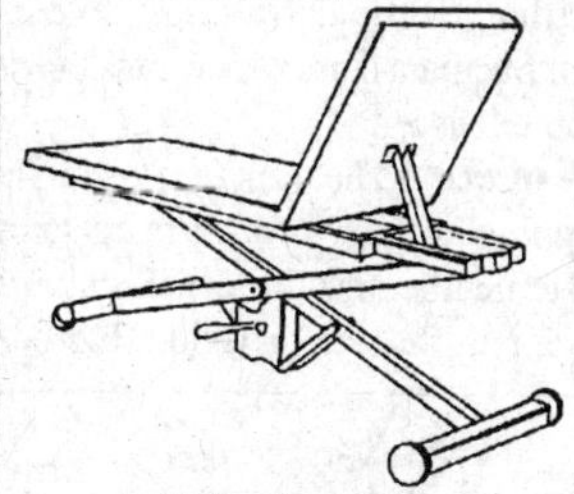

Hydraulic couch

Hydraulic effect In implant dentistry, the shock-absorbing quality that results from the movement of fluid within interstitial spaces or anastomosing blood or lymph vessels of the tissue around a functioning osteopreserved or periosteal integrated implant.

Hydraulic lift It consists of an upright pillar mounted outside and it one end of pool. The outer sleeve is mobile and has projecting arms, onto which fits a chair or stretcher.

Hydroarthrosis The accumulation of excessive synovial fluid in a joint.

Hydrocele In it tunica vaginalis becomes irritated and an effusion of fluid occurs into the cavity between the parietal and visceral layers. Normally 2 to 3 ml of fluid is present in it but if larger amount accumulates in tunica vaginalis it is known as hydrocele. Fluid is of amber colour. It is odourless,

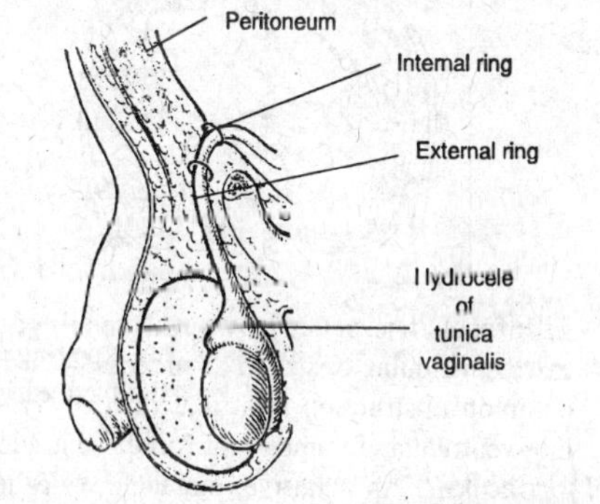

natural in reaction and its specific gravity varies from 1010 to 1.025. It contains albumin and occasionally cholesterin. It may be caused by acute inflammation of testes, trauma or neoplasm. Wall of hydrocele is usually thin. Sac may be multilocular. Clinical findings reveal smooth nontender, fluctuant mass which translucents it, may be congenital also.

Hydrocele of cord The testicle is readily palpated. When tapping of the hydrocele is contemplated, it is well to remember that the testicle and epididymis lie posterior to the sac or fluid. Hydroceles as a

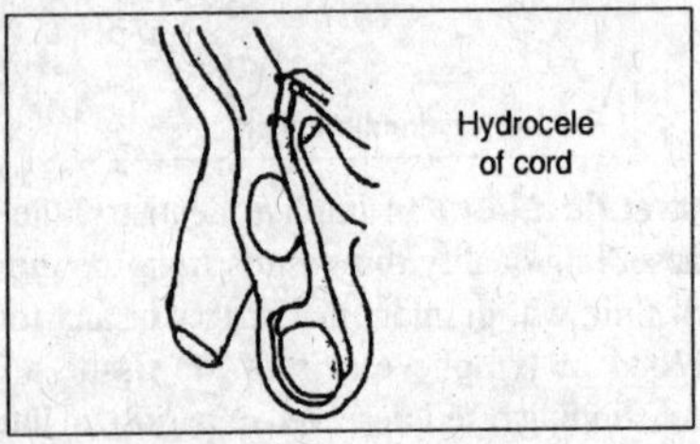

rule are painless, but occasionally may produce a dragging sensation when the mass reaches such proportion as to be embarrassing or inconvenient to the patient.

Simple hydrocele must be differentiated from scrotal hernia which produces an impulse on coughing. The mass can be palpated.

Hydrocephalus It is a pathophysiological condition due to imbalance of CSF production compared to reabsorptive capacity. It results in ventricular enlargement that is not caused by brain atrophy.

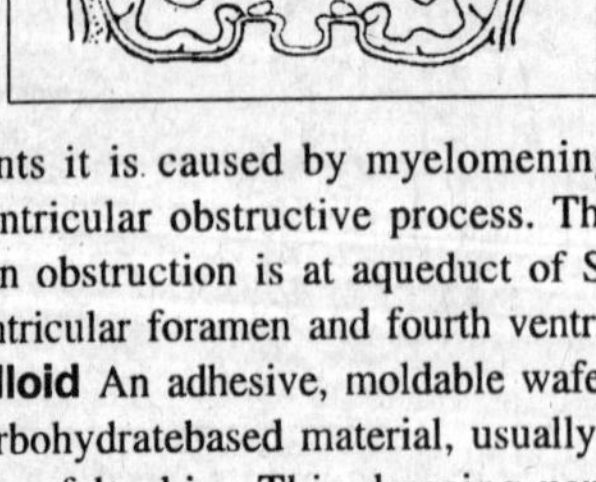

In infants it is caused by myelomeningocele, extraventricular obstructive process. The most common obstruction is at aqueduct of Sylvius, intraventricular foramen and fourth ventricle.

Hydrocolloid An adhesive, moldable wafer made of a carbohydratebased material, usually with a waterproof backing.This dressing usually is impermeable to oxygen, and water.

Hydrocortisone Major corticosteroids are produced and secreted by adrenal glands. Hydrocortisone assists in metabolism of carbohydrates, fats and proteins and body's reaction to stress. It helps in severe allergy, asthma, eczema and inflammation.

Hydrodynamic injection An injection mode used in capillary electrophoresis in which the sample is injected inside the capillary by hydrostatic pressure, gravity or syringe.

It is opposed to electrokinetic injection, in which the sample is introduced by application of an electric field.

Hydrodynamic theory A theory explaining the etiology of pulpal sensitivity, based on fluid flow through the dentinal tubules.

Hydrogel A waterbased, nonadherent, polymerbased dressing that has some absorptive properties.

Hydrogen bond A bond between the positively charged hydrogen of a polar molecule and the negatively charged region of another polar molecule.

Hydrogen ion Found in water and water solutions; produces an acidic solution; H^-.

Hydrogen sulphide It is a colourless gas with an odour of rotten eggs. It is formed during the decomposition process of organic substances containing sulphur. It is formed in sewers. A concentration of 0.18% is immediately fatal when inhaled in pure form. Otherwise it causes irritation to eyes, nose, throat and respiratory passages. This is followed by dizziness, headache and cyanosis. It can lead to pulmonary oedema. If inhaled in very diluted form it gives rise to sleepiness and may lead to death.

Hydrogenase An enzyme capable of redox activation of molecular hydrogen.

Hydrogenation Breaking a bouble bond on a fatty acid carbon chain and saturating it with hydrogen.

Hydrogenosomes Cytoplasmic organelles present in anaerobic protozoa and fungi, containing enzymes that produce hydrogen from the oxidation of reduced cofactors.

Hydrolectomy When hydrocele is large hydrolectomy may be indicated. A site is chosen on the anterior superior scrotal wall between the larger vessels and a wheal is made, using local anaesthetic to permit passage of a 17 to 18 guage needle into the sac to drain fluid content. All fluid should not be taken out at fast.

Hydrolysis Reaction or association of a chemical substance with water molecules.

Hydropathy index A scale that expresses the relative hydrophobic and hydrophilic tendencies of a chemical group.

Hydropericardium Abnormal accumulation of fluid in the pericardial cavity.

Hydroperoxidase An enzyme whose major function is the decomposition of peroxides that is involved in the oxidation of Hg.

Hydrophilic Refers to a substance that binds weakly to polar water molecules also known as water soluble.

Hydrophobic Literally, water-fearing; describing molecules or regions of molecules that cannot form hydrogen bonds or other polar interaction with water.

Hydrophobic effect The tendency of hydrophobic regions of molecules to avoid contact with water.

Hydrophobin A small cysteine rich protein found associated with the aerial hyphae of filamentous fungi.

Hydropic Involving an abnormal collection of fluid.

Hydropneumothorax It is caused mostly due to TB focus in lung. A small quantity of fluid first

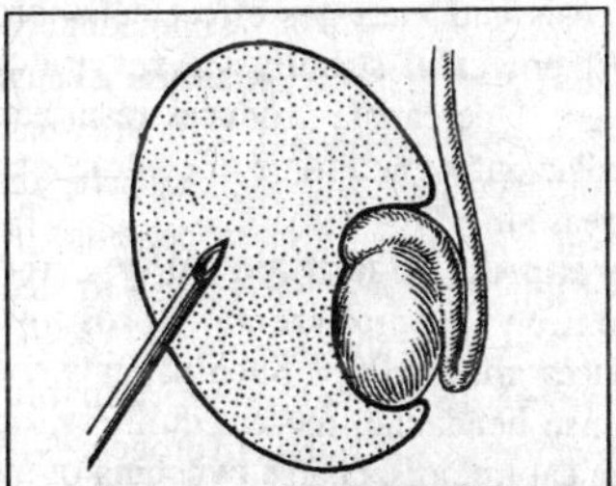

Aspiration of hydrocele fluid

fills the costophrenic angle and later fills lower half of chest. the fluid moving with the position of patient. Upper level of fluid is always horizontal unlike the level of pleural effusion.

Hydrostatic bed Water bed

Hydrostatic pressure The force of a fluid pushing against some surface.

Hydrotherapy It was first used by Greeks in the time of Hippocrates (460-375 BC) who treated diseases with hot and cold water, diet and rest. Later on Romans used baths for recreational and curative purposes. It the body is immersed to waist level, the weight relief is 50% of body weight. Pain due to weight bearing can be relieved by

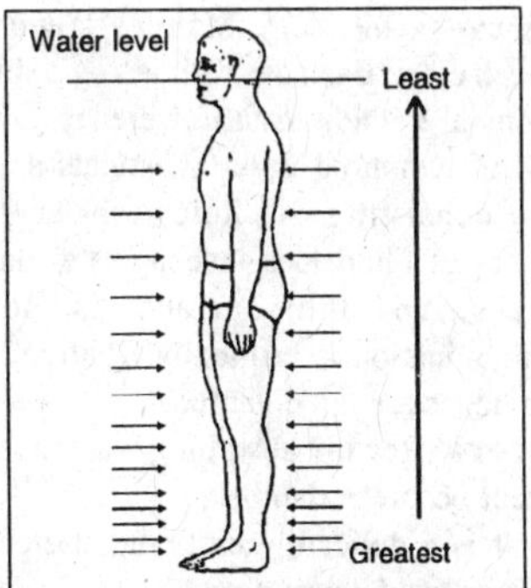

Water pressure

hydrotherapy. Hydrostatic pressure is greater in deeper water and less near surface. Temperature of water is maintained at 35°C to 36°C.

Hydrothorax It is a chronic collection of serous fluid in pleural cavity. Onset is usually gradual and as hydrothorax a secondary condition. Dyspnoea is usually present and its degree depends on large amount of fluid present. If there is no inflammation then there will be no pain, pleural rub or pyrexia. The most common cause is combination of right and left sided heart.

Hydroxide ion Found in water and water solution; produces an acidic solution; H^-.

Hydroxyapatite A mineral or ceramic composing much of bone and teeth that contains calcium and phosphorus; a synthetic (artificial) forms is used as an implant material

Hydroxyl radical A very strong, reactive, cell destroying radical, formed from the reaction of a super oxide radical with hydrogen peroxide.

Hyesthesiae Abnormal burning or pain sensation.

Hygiene The science that deals with the preservation of health.

Hygoformic Device used to isolate the mandibular teeth and remove fluids from the oral cavity.

Hygroma cystic It is a collection of lymphatic sacs containing clear colourless lymph. It is a congenital malformation affecting the lymphatic channels and arise from the congenital lymph sacs which are precursors of adult lymphatic channels. It appears very early and may be found at birth or within first few years of life. It is multilocular and multilobular. Cysts are filled with clear lymph. Larger cysts are situated at periphery and the smaller cysts at the centre. Many cysts communicate with each other. Each cyst is lined by a single layer of columnar epithelium and covered externally with a shell of lymphoid tissue. Contents are clear or watery consisting of cholesterol crystals and lymphocytes. Fluid does not coagulate. Fluctuations are positive and surface is lobulated. Transillumination is brilliantly positive. Regional lymph nodes are not enlarged.

Hygroscopic Readily absorbing water as and when table salt becomes damp.

Hymen It is a delicate membrane stretching over the entrance of vagina and partially closing it. Some women have large hole in hymen and some

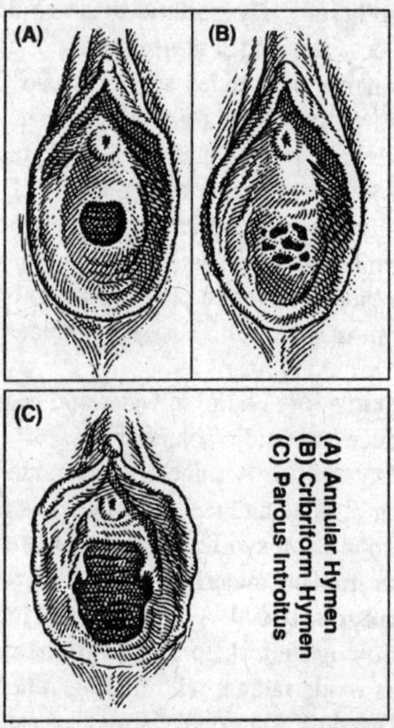

(A) Annular Hymen
(B) Cribriform Hymen
(C) Parous Introitus

do not have any. Previously its presence was thought to be a sign of virginity but it could be torn during play, games, cycling, swimming, etc.

Hyoid bone A horseshoe-shaped bone located at the base of the tongue just below the thyroid cartilage; appears radiopaque. It supports the back of tongue protecting epiglottis. It is kept in position with the help of muscles and ligaments.

Hyper Beyond excessive.

Hyper thermophilic. Organism with an optimal temperature for growth of 80ºC or higher.

Hyperactive airways Excessive activity of the bronchioles; increased bronchoconstriction.

Hyperacusis Increased perception of hearing. It occurs in a condition called otosclerosis.

Hyperaemia An increase in the flow of blood through a region of the body.

Hyperalgesia An increased response to a stimulus that is normally painful.

Hyperalimentation The administration of nutrients beyond the normal minimum requirement.

Hyperathia Increased reaction to stimuli, especially when repetitive; increased threshold to stimuli.

Hyperbaric oxygen Oxygen fas present at greater than atmospheric pressure.

Hypercalcemia High blood levels of calcium.

Hypercaloric More than one kcalorie per ml.

Hypercapnia Ill-effects are due to CO_2 excess. It may result due to gross impairment of venilation due to respiratory obstruction, profound necrosis or relaxants. Severe bilateral lung disease and hyperpyrexia may also result it. Mild hypercapnia up to $PaCO_2$ 10.5 Kpa commonly causes dysrhythmia during anaesthesia. At the level of $PaCO_2$ rises towards 25 KPa, narcosis deepens into coma. Effects of hypercapnia result in increased cerebral volume and fluid pressure, progressive narcosis and inert gas effect. CO_2 provides the most powerful stimulus to respiratory centre. Severe hypercapnia produces respiratory failure. Cardiac output and force of contraction of heart is increased.

Hypercapnic encephalopathy Carbon dioxide retention in emphysema, fibrosing alveolitis reduces arterial PO_2. Such patients complains of intense headache, mental dullness, drowsiness, frequent tremors, coarse twitching of muscles and papilloedema. During carbon dioxide narcosis EEG shows bilateral synchronous slow activity. Such patients need immediate ventilatory assistance with intermittent positive pressure respiration. Acidosis is to be corrected by bicarbonate administration.

Hypercementosis An excess deposition of cementum on root surfaces; appears radiopaque.

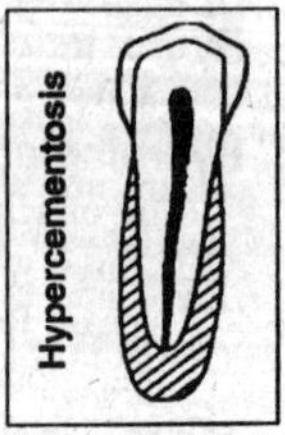

Hypercementosis

Hypercholestrolemia Total blood cholesterol levels over 200 mg/dl.

Hypercortisolemia Excessively high concentration of adrenal corticosteroids in plasma.

Hyperechoic Tissues creating brighter echoes than adjacent tissues, i.e. bone, fat.

Hyperemesis gravidarum The morning sickness of pregnancy may become more severe and instead of abating it becomes more and more persistent. Vòmiting begins to occur independently of food being taken. Every thing swallowed is being rejected. Vomiting soon leads to carbohydrate starvation and glycogen depletion. Tongue may become furred. Sleeplessness and muscular twitchings also develop. Severe epigastric pain is complained of. If pregnancy continues disease may pass into toxaemic phase characterised by scanty urine, containing albumin, blood and casts. Pulse becomes faster.

Hyperemia Congestion; increased and excessive amount of blood in a tissue. The hyperemia may be active or passive.

Hyperesthesia An elevation of threashold for touch stimulation.

Hyperextension Movement of a body part beyond its normal resting extended position.

Hyperflexia An abnormally increased or exaggerated action of reflexes.

Hyperglycemia Elevated blood glucose levels (>120mg/dl).

Hypergonadotropic hypogonadism A condition characterised by elevated gonadotrophins due to ovarian failure and diminished ovarian hormone secretion.

Hyperhidrosis It represents exessive sweating which develops due to varieties of psychological elements. It may develop even after consumption of hot and spicy food. It may be an accompaniment of several endocrine dysfunction such as hyperthyroidism and wasting diseases. Localised hyperhidrosis may be due to hereditary, excessive intake of tea/alcohol and even flat foot. Localised hyperhidrosis may cause offensive sweating due to decomposition of sweat and cellular debris by bacteria or fungus. It may be due to prolonged use of nylon socks and tight shoes. Use of various chemicals can cause sweating black blue or red.

Hyperhidrosis states Disorders associated with involuntary movements.

Hyperinflated Distended beyond the normal extent.

Hyperkalaemic periodic paralysis This is inherited through an autosomal recessive gene, now mapped to chromosome 17q. Paralytic episodes tend to occur in early life and is of shorter duration usually less than one hour. The serum level of potassium rises during the period of paralysis as potassium leaks from muscle fibres into circulation. Myotonia may be seen in periocular muscles during an attack.

Hyperkeratosis Abnormal increase in the thickness of the keratin layer (stratum corneum) of the epithelium. Benign hyperkeratosis is one of the most common white lesions of the oral mucous membrane.

Hyperkinesis Excessive motility; excessive muscular activity.

Hyperkinetic pulse This pulse is large and bounding. It indicates rapid ejection of blood from left ventricle and is usually associated with decreased peripheral resistance. It occurs in states of hyperdynamic circulation like fever, exercise, thyrotoxicosis, patent ductus arteriosus (PDA), aortic regurgitation, ventricular septal defect (VSD) and complete heart block.

Hyperkinetic states Disorders associated with involuntary movements.

Hyperkinetic symptom A symptom of brain damage that involves involuntary excessive movements.

Hyperkyphosis A kyphosis of greater than normal range.

Hyperlipidemic Excess lipids in the blood.

Hyperlordosis A lordosis of greater than normal range.

Hyperlucent lung syndrome A variant of panacinar (panlobular) emphysema.

Hypermagnesemia Refers to solutions with sodium concentrations greater than 147 mEq/L.

Hypermenorrhoea Prolonged bleeding at regular intervals (1 and 2 are sometimes used interchangeably).

Hypermetabolism An increase in BMR above expected levels based on age, sex, and body size.

Hypermetropic eye In hypermetropia the eyeball is short thereby the retina is placed forward than its normal position at 24 mm behind the cornea. In hypermetropic eye the parallel rays coming from a distant object does not come to focus. Focus forms behind the retina. The far point in hypermetropic eye is virtually behind the eyeball. So hypermetropic cannot see distant or near objects clearly. Hypermetropia is treated by providing requisite convergence to the rays before they enter the eye by prescribing convex lens.

Hypermobile joint Overflexible link in a series of articulated bodies.

Hypernasal speech There is production of speech sounds with predominantly resonance due to velopharyngeal incompetence. It may be due to congenitally soft palate or psychogenic.

Hypernatremia An abnormally high concentration of sodium ions in the plasma.

Hyperopia A refractive disorder in which rays of light are brought to a focus behind the retina as a result of the eyeball being too short; also called farsightedness.

Hyperosmolality An increase in the osmotic concentration of a solution.

Hyperosmolar Abnormally increased osmolarity.

Hyperosmotic Relating to or causing an increase in osmotic pressure or osmolality.

Hyperostosis The presence of excessive growth of bone.

Hyperpathia A painful syndrome characterised by over reaction and after sensation to a stimulus. In it stimulus that would be felt in a healthy person as no more than mildly unpleasant is perceived to have burning quality of unusual intensity. It is found in patients with partial lesions of peripheral nerves and in thalamic lesions.

Hyperphagia A disorder in which an animal overeats, leading to significant weight gain.

Hyperpigmentation Unusual darkening of the skin.

Hyperplasia It constitutes an increase in the number of cells in an organ. It is usually accompanied by hypertrophy. Hyperplasia can occur only with cells capable of synthesising DNA. Nerve, cardiac and skeletal muscle cells have little or no capacity for hyperplastic growth and so muscle cells undergo almost pure hypertrophy. Hyperplasia may be physiological or pathological.

Hyperpolarization An increase in the electrical charge across a membrane, usually due to the inward flow of chloride ions or the outward flow of potassium ions.

Hyperprolactinemia Elevation of the serum or plasma prolactin concentration above the normal range.

Hyperpyrexia Above 40°C.

Hyperreactivity An increase in the sensitivity of the airway walls to stimuli.

Hyperreflexia Exaggerated tendon reflexes; associated with upper motor neuron disease.

Hypersecretion Too much of a substance is being secreted.

Hypersensitivity Some form of immune reaction instead of providing exumptions or safety to affected individual can produce severe and sometimes fatal results. These are known as hypersensitivity reactions. It is acute and delayed type.

Hypersensitivity pneumonitis Pulmonary inflammation resulting from an allergic response to an inspired antigen.

Hypersexuality It is an excessive, insatiable need for sexual activity often associated with inability to achieve complete gratification. This condition may arise to cover one's impotence or frigidity.

Hypertension Abnormal elevation of systolic and/or diastolic arterial pressure. Systolic hypertension is generally related to emotional stress, sclerosis of the aorta and large arteries, or aortic insufficiency. Diastolic hypertension may be due to obscure causes renal disease, or endocrine disorders.

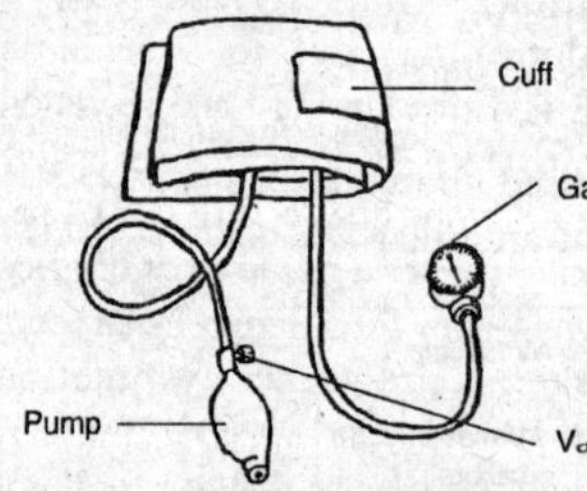

Blood pressure cuff

Level of blood pressure depends on physical activity, stress, age and on certain diseases. It is labelled if in younger age group it rises above 140/90 mm Hg at rest. *Essential hypertension* is that when no obvious cause is known for high BP. When *high BP* is due to kidney or other diseases usual complications of constant high BP may be retinopathy, heart failure and kidney damage.

Hypersomnolence A condition of drowsiness approaching coma.

Hypertensive encephalopathy It is an acute event usually associated with severe hypertension in a previously normotensive patient. Person may be suffering from glomerulonephritis or toxaemia of pregnancy. Clinical features include headache, seizures, visual disturbances, or confusion. There may be focal neurological signs in limbs. Fundus may show retinal oedema, retinal haemorrhage and exudates. There may be cerebral oedema.

Hypertensive haemorrhage There are four common sites of hypertensive intracerebral haemorrhage : putamen and adjacent internal capsule, thalamus, pons and cerebellum. Once bleeding stops recurrence is unusual. The surrounding brain oedema is very conspicuous. Unlike thrombosis which occurs during sleep, haemorrhage occurs when patient is active and awake. Onset is usually sudden with bursting headache, vomiting and dizziness. In putaminal haemorrhage, there develops contralateral hemiphagia with conjugate deviation of eyes. If haematoma is large bilateral motor palsy, irregular respiration and dilated fixed pupils may ensue. Pontine haemorrhage produces deep coma, pinpoint reactive pupils, quadriplegia, hyperthermia and rigidity. Cerebellar haemorrhage presents with gait ataxia, vomiting and occipital headache.

Hypertensive retinopathy Ophthalmoscopic findings are due to vasoconstriction and leakage from vessels. Vasoconstriction manifests as generalised arteriolar attenuation. The presence of focal arteriolar attenuation is a sure sign of

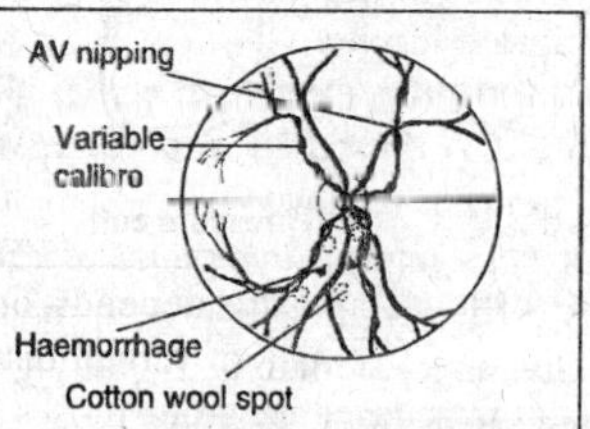

Hypertensive retinopathy

raised blood pressure. Leakage of vessel leads to haemorrhage. In grade I, there is generalised arteriolar attenuation of small branches. In grade II, there is an increased generalised arteriolar attenuation with focal arteriolar attenuation. While in grade III, there is generalised and focal arteriolar attenuation with haemorrhages, cotton-wool spots and hard exudates. In grade IV, there is hard exudate and swelling of optic disc.

Hyperthermophile Literally, heat-lover; an organism having an optimal temperature for growth of 80°C or higher.

Hyperthermophilic Relating to or describing organisms that grow optimally at temperatures above 80°C.

Hypertonia A state of increased muscle tension, rigidity or spasm.

Hypertonic A solution containing a higher level of salt (NaCl) than is found in a living red blood cell (above 0.9% NaCI).

Hypertonic labour dysfunction Ineffective labour characterized by erratic and poorly co-ordinated contractions. Uterine resting tone is higher than normal.

Hypertonic solution One that has a higher molecular concentration than another with which it is compared; of greater concentration than isotonic.

Hypertrichosis Excessive growth of hair on the body.

Hypertriglyceridemia A condition in which the triglyceride concentration in the blood is greater than normal.

Hypertrophic Pertaining to enlargement of an organ due to increase in size.

Hypertrophic bone union Exuberant bone reaction with hypertrophy and sclerosis of bone ends. Abundant callus is formed.

Hypertrophic cardiomyopathy It is uncommon in children. There is asymmetrical hypertrophy of the ventricular septum. Patients present with exertional dyspnoea, anginal type of chest pain, palpitation and syncope or a murmur. Sudden death can occur. Pulse has a sharp upstroke with a bisferience character. Apex beat is forcible. Second sound may split. Ejection systolic murmur develops. ECG shows hypertrophy of left ventricle.

Hypertrophic emphysema It is a common disease of lung occurring in later middle life. It develops gradual shortening of breath. Face is congested with appearance of polycythemia. Chest becomes barrel shaped and ribs are raised. Expiration phase becomes longer.

Hypertrophic scar It is a type of scar characterised by hypertrophy or proliferation of mature fibroblast or fibrous tissue without any proliferation of blood vessels. It is caused by some extra stimulus to fibrous formation during healing such as excessive tension of infection.

Scar is raised above the surface. Surface becomes glossy. There is no claw-like process and no sign of increased vascularity. There is no itching and it does not spread. It may regress gradually after six months. It does not recur after excision if the causative factors are eliminated. It does not involve normal skin.

Hypertrophic tuberculous enteritis Here dose and virulence of organism is less and resistance of host is more. So the net result is formation of granulation tissue.

Clinical features include pain in right iliac fossa, anorexia, vomiting, diarrhoea, wasting and evening rise of temperature are less marked. Visible peristalsis are present typically of ladder pattern type. A fixed mass may be palpable at right iliac fossa. Barium meal studies may show a filling defect.

Hypertrophy It is an increase in the number of organ cells, size of cells and with such change an increase in size of organ. It is caused by increased functional demand or specific hormonal stimulation such as uterine hypertrophy during pregnancy. Actual number of cells remains the same. After long-term exercise muscles hypertrophy.

Hyperventilation It is deliberately breathing fast without undergoing any exertion. Thus person consumes large quantity of oxygen. Abnormally low CO_2 may also cause unconsciousness.

Hyperviscosity syndrome The syndrome consists of fatigue, weakness, skin and mucosal bleeding, neurological involvement, and visual disturbances from increased viscosity of the blood.

Hypervitaminosis Condition caused by excess amounts of vitamins; usually associated with the use of vitamin supplements.

Hypha The thread-like tubular cell that constitutes the basic growth unit of filamentous fungi.

Hyphomycetes A grouping of asexually reproducing fungi in which the asexual spores are produced on loose, cottony hyphae.

Hyphopodium In certain fungi, an attachment and infection structure that develops from short hyphal branches.

Hypnagogic Referring to the semiconscious state immediately preceding sleep; may include hallucinations, which are of no pathologic significance.

Hypnagoic hallucinations These are not dreams but half awake sensory errors with fragments of waking imagery incorporated into near dreams, which can be summoned and on occasion dispersed at will.

Hypnosis An artificially induced state of extreme suggestibility in which the patient is insensible to outside impressions. It is a state of extreme suggestibility induced by one person. Person undergoes in a state of sleep and obeys the other person. It is useful in case to relieve pain.

Hypnotic Any agent that induces sleep. Although sedatives and narcotics in sufficient dosage may produce sleep as an incidental effect, the term hypnotic is appropriately reserved for drugs employed primarily to produce sleep.

Hypnotic induction A series of suggestion that focus attention and bring about the transition from an ordinary waking experience to hypnosis.

Hypnotic susceptibility A subject's measured level of responsiveness to hypnotic suggestions on standardized scales.

Hypnozoite The dormant stage of *Plasmodium vivax* and *Plasmodium ovale* in hepatocytes of the human host. A resting life stage of certain parasites.

Hypoadaptive A failure in a occurrence of expected or anticipated results.

Hypoalbuminemia Decreased serum albumin.

Hypoalgesia A decreased response to a stimulus that is normally painful.

Hypoarousal It refers to symptoms of PTS disorder such as difficulty in sleeping or concentration, irritability, angry outbursts, hyper vigilance and an exaggerated startle response.

Hypobiosis A lag phase at some stage of development in the life cycle of a nematode.

Hypocalcification Deficiency in the mineral content of a calcified tissue, for example in the enamel, results from disturbance in the maturation phase during development; may be due to systemic, local, or hereditary factors.

Hypocapnia Reduction of CO2 in body which is the result of hyperventilation.

Hypochondriasis It is an abnormal condition of the nervous system which has features common to both melancholia and some of neurosis. Patient suffers from prolonged emotional disturbance. Male hypochondrias appear to be excessively worried most frequently about their sexual functions and fear impotence. Treatment is difficult.

Hypochromic Decrease in colour due to decrease in hemoglobin content of RBCs as an iron deficiency.

Hypodermic injection These are used very often. The drug is deposited in the tissues just beneath the skin, generally on the outer aspect of the arm or thigh. From 0.5 to 2 ml (cc) may be given in this

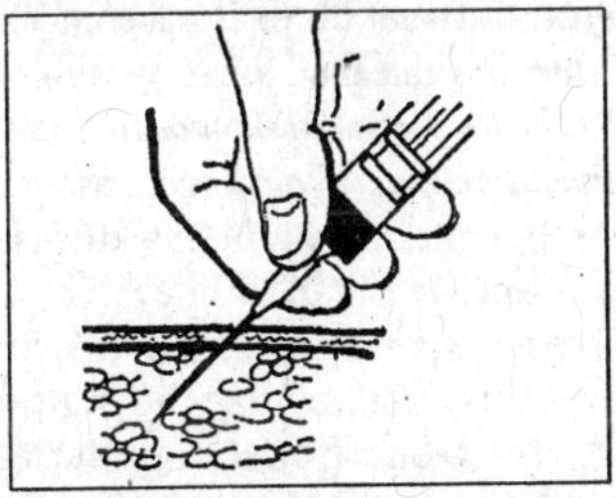

way, and the drug will become effective in about 15 to 20 minutes.

Hypodermis The loose, ordinary (areolar) tissue just under the skin and superficial to the muscles; also called subcutaneous tissue or superficial fascia.

Hypodermoclysis Large amounts of isotonic solutions can be given by hypodermoclysis. The administration set for this procedure consists of two

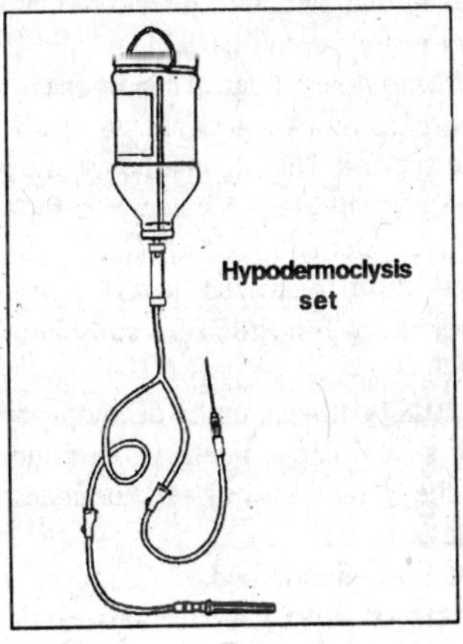

outlet tubes in an inverted "Y" formation. The amount of fluid in the subcutaneous tissues at each of two injection sites can be regulated by clamping the tubing.

Hypodermolysis It is a subcutaneous administration of saline when intravenous route is not available. It is given in thighs. Hyaluronidase is a spreadig factor which helps in absorption of injected fluid in subcutaneous and intramuscular tissues. It is a mucolytic agent. This system is used in infiltration anaesthesia. It is used in burns and infants.

Hypodontia Condition of congenitally missing teeth; partial anodontia.

Hypodontia, Book's syndrome It is characterised by premature whitening of hair, hyperhidrosis of palms and soles and aphasia of the premolars and third molar. It is inherited as an autosomal dominant trait.

Hypoechoic Tissues that create dimmer echoes than adjacent tissues, i.e. lymph nodes and fluid.

Hypofunction A condition of being subjected to force that is below the minimum physiologic limits for health.

Hypogammaglobulinemia A less than normal amount of the gamma fraction of serum globulin.

Hypoglycaemia It is an abnormally low level of glucose in the blood. Generally, insulin dependent patients suffer from it. Hypoglycaemia can also occur if a diabetic misses a meal, fails to eat enough or excercises too much. Person develops sweating, weakness, hunger, dizziness, confusion and even double vision. Person becomes aggressive and movements become uncoordinated like that of alcoholic. Such person should keep a card in their pocket mentioning 'patient of diabetes' and a small packet of glucose. Condition existing when the concentration of blood sugar is 40 mg/100 ml or less. Symptoms may not occur even when the concentratoni is considerably less. Hypoglycemia may occur in the fasting state and following the injection of insulin.

Hypogonadotropism A hormonal state characterized by low circulating concentrations of the pituitary gonadotropins.

Hypokalaemic periodic paralysis It begins in adolescence. Episodes of paralysis occurs on waking after a heavy carbohydrate meal and after exercise. Leg muscles are predominantly affected.

Cranial muscles are spared. Paralysis usually lasts for several hours. During an attack the serum potassium falls to 2.5 mmol/L or less. Several attacks may be shortened by the use of oral potassium salts. Attacks may be prevented or reduced of severity. Episodes of paralysis become less frequent in middle age.

Hypokalemia An abnormally low concentration of potassium ions in the circulating blood.

Hypokinetic gait This type of gait is characterised by slow nonfluid positioning of legs with few or no associated movements and with stiff posture.

Hypokinetic symptom A symptom of brain damage that involves a paucity of movement.

Hypomagnesemia Refers to solutions with magnesium concerntations less than 1.5 mEq/L.

Hypomania A psychopathologic state and abnormality of mood falling somewhere between normal euphoria and mania.

It is characterised by unrealistic optimism, pressure of speech and activity, and a decreased need for sleep. Some people show increased creativity during hypomanic states, while others show poor judgement, irritability, and irascibility.

Hypomenorrhoea Decrease in amount and duration of menses.

Hyponatraemia Patient may develop stupor, seizures and coma with serum sodium concentration of less than 110 to 115 mmol. This situation arises in patients within appropriate secretion of antidiuretic hormone (ADH) such as in bronchial carcinoma. Some patients with severe hyponatraemia develop central pontine demyelinating lesions. An abnormally low concentration of sodium ions in the circulating blood.

Hyponychium A thickened, supportive layer of stratum corneumk at the distal end of a digit under the free edge of the nail.

Hypophagia Eating less than usual.

Hypopharyngeal abscess It is more laterally situated than retropharyngeal abscess and produces more severe symptoms. Pyriform sinus is effaced. There is unilateral oedema of laryngeal inlet with or without involvement of protuberant. Foreign body injuries are the most common cause.

Hypophosphatemia A less than normal concentration of alkaline phosphatase in the blood: hypophosphatasia.

Hypophysis Endocrine gland attached to the hypothalamus by the infundibulum; the pituitary gland.

Hypoplasia Defective or incomplete development; enamel hypoplasia results when the enamel matrix formation is disturbed.

Hypoplastic small-for-date babies Growth retardation usually occurs in early part of pregnancy due to intrauterine infections, genetic defects and chromosomal aberrations. The number of body cells is reduced. The prognosis as regards postnatal physical growth and mental development is poor. Baby is smaller in all parameters.

Hypopyon corneal ulcer It is a corneal ulcer with pus in anterior chamber. Many pyogenic organisms like *Staphylococcus, Streptococcus* may be a cause but *Pseudomonas pyocyanea* is most virulent. Toxins liberated bacteria can diffuse through corneal lamellae and ulcer in eye.

Diffused toxins are irritant to iris causing iridocyclitis. There may be outpouring of leucocytes from dilated capillaries of iris. Leucocytes settle at the bottom of anterior chamber to form a hypopyon. Hypopyon is sterile because it develops due to toxins.

There will be severe pain in eye and marked photophobia. Person develops redness of eye with lid swelling and discharge from eye. There will be greyish white and yellowish disc near the centre of the cornea. The edges of an ulcer are well marked in one particular direction. Cornea starts looking lustreless and hazy.

Hyporeflexia A neurological condition characterzed by weakened reflex reactions.

Hyporheic zone The ecotone between a steambed and the groundwater, characterized by a mixture of surface water and groundwater.

Hyposalivation Decreased flow of saliva.

Hyposecretion Too little of a substance is being secreted.

Hyposexuality It is an under-development or total lack of sexual drive, interest of activity. It may result due to low level of sex hormones or some brain lesions.

Hyposite Low energy food.

Hypostasis of lung It is a serous exudation into

and around air vesicles. It is known as hypostatic pneumonia also. It is never a primary condition. The onset is insidious and considerable amount of dyspnoea is present. There is frothy mucous expectoration. Percussion note is dull, expansion and air entry at bases is diminished.

Hypotension It is better known as low blood pressure. When systolic pressure comes to 60 to 90 mm of Hg and blood supply to brain is reduced.

Hypothalamic dysfunction An abnormal function of the hypothalamus.

Hypothalamic hormones Hormones produced by the hypothalamus. These include antidiuretic hormone and oxytocin, which are secreted by the posterior pituitary, and both releasing and inhibiting hormones that regulate the secretions of the anterior pituitary.

Hypothalamic pituitary gonadal axis The pathway of reproductive system that controls gonadal function.

Hypothalamic-pituitary portal system Series of blood vessels that carries blood from the area of the hypothalamus to the anterior pituitary; originates from capillary beds in the hypothalamus and terminates as a capillary bed in the anterior pituitary.

Hypothalamo-hypophyseal tract The tract of nerve fibers (axons) that transports antidiuretic hormone and oxytocin from the hypothalamus to the posterior pituitary.

Hypothalamus Functions of hypothalamus include maintenance of body temperature and body's water balance. It helps in sexual development and reproductive functions. It is involved in emotional responses. It controls food intake. It plays an important role in metabolic functions and emotional reactions working intimately with hypophysis and is under control of telencephalon. Hypothalamus plays a part in evoking attack and defence reaction of individual and the development and maintenance of sexual functions. Subthalamic nucleus represents the principal motor coordinating centre. Its destruction leads to uncontrollable movements, choreic in type and violent in character.

Hypothermia It is a method used to lower the metabolism of body as a whole and to reduce the dangers from hypoxia and the cellular damage resulting from regional occlusion of the circulation of brain, heart, liver and legs. It has also been used to treat hyperpyrexia, during and after operation and to treat shock. Dysrhythmia occurs at temperature below 30°C. Measurement of human cerebral oxygen consumption indicates that at 30°C it is only 39 %. The oxygen dissociation curve is shifted to left so that liberation of oxygen to tissues is hindered. Acidosis is developed due to respiratory insufficiency. Rapid change of pH may cause cardiac iregularities. Consciousness is usually lost between 28°C and 30°C. With each fall of 1°C the metabolism is reduced 6 to 7%. Functions of liver and kidneys are depressed. Utilisation of glucose is decreased.

Hypothermia therapy Techniques used to reduce elecated body temperature.

Hypothesis A tentative explanation, an unconfirmed interpretation of a condition or event. In lay terms, a guess.

Hypothetical average-work curve A hypothetical curve showing the productivity of an average worker in an industrial setting. Productivity starts low, increases during an initial warm-up period, then reaches a plateau, and afterwards declines in a work decrement, presumably because the worker is tired or bored. At the end of the work period there may be another sharp increase in activity, called the end spurt, suggesting that the worker is motivated to complete the job.

Hypothetical situation Assumed or proved fact and circumstances so as to constitute a specific situation.

Hypothyroid myopathy It is characterised by muscle pain, stiffness and cramps. Muscles show pseudomyotonia—a prolonged contraction after percussion without continuing electrical discharge, occasionally hypothyroidism is accompanied by an inflammatory myopathy.

Hypothyroidism It leads to insufficient synthesis of thyroid hormone. Cretinism may manifest at birth. The symptoms include short stature, coarse features, protruding tongue, broad flat nose, dry skin and sparse hair. There is impaired mental development and delayed dentition. In older child there is delayed puberty. Adults develop fatigue, lethargy, cold intolerance, stiffness and cramping of muscles. Intellectual and motor activity becomes slow and weight increases. Hair becomes dry. Face becomes dull and expressionless. Tongue becomes large.

Hypotonic A solution containing a lower level of salt (NaCI) than is found in a living red blood cell (below 0.9% NacI)

Hypotonic babies These are markedly depressed with weak Moro reflex and poor subcutaneous movements. They suck poorly. Seizure may develop after birth.

Hypotonic labour dysfunction Ineffective labour characterised by the weak, infrequent and brief but coordinated uterine contraction. Uterine resting tone is normal.

Hypotonic solution One that has a lesser molecular concentration than another to which it is compared of less concentration than isotonic.

Hypotonic uterine dysfunction An abnormality in the functioning of the uterus to propel the fetus through the birth canal in which contractions decrease in strength and the tone of the uterine muscles is less than usual.

Hypotonic uterine inertia -Uterine contractions are weak, inadequate and of short duration. Dilalation of cervix is slow but polarity of stomach is normal. Patient does not suffer from any discomfort.

Hypovirulence The fact of having low virulence.

Hypovirulent Describing a pathogen with low virulence; e.g. fungi that are reduced in virulence because of infection with a transmissible virus, and may therefore be used for bilogical control of the pathogen.

Hypovitaminosis Condition of having too few vitamin molecules in the body for normal function.

Hypovolemia Decreased volume of circulating blood.

Hypovolemic thirst Thirst produced by a reduction in the amount of extracellular fluid.

Hypoxemia A condition in which arterial oxygenation is below normal.

Hypoxia Abnormally low concentration of oxygen in the blood or tissue fluids.

Hypoxic-ischaemic encephalopathy Selective necrosis of neurons of deeper cerebral cortical layers is the hallmark of hypoxic injury to the perinatal brain. Hypertonic infants are generally hyperalert. These have extensor posture, brisk stretch reflexes and strong Moro reflex with low threshold.

Hysdiadochokinesia Impaired ability to perform rapdi alternating movements.

Hysmetria Impaired ability to judge the distance or range of a movement.

Hysterectomy Surgical removal of the uterus.

Hysteresis The ability of viscous solutions to recover instantaneously to initial viscosity values after removal of shear stress forces.

Hysteria Patients are egocentric. The hysterical reaction is a manifestation of childish need for any organic disease. When rigidity is present it is proportional to the force used to overcome it. Person may mimic very close to organic disease but is never complete. Flaccid hysterical palsies are common than rigidity. All kinds of bizarre hysterical gaits are met with. The muscles react normally to electrical stimulation. Hysterical tremors and tics vary in degree and are increased by attention. Hysterical tremors may closely simulate the tremor of paralysis agitans. In hysterical aphonia the patient whispers but can phonate normally on coughing. In mutism there may be complete abolition of speech. Sensory loss affects only cutaneous sensibility and is usually complete. Hysterical blindness is often sudden in onset and may be complete. In hysterical deafness patient can be awakened from sleep if called by name but when awakened he or she cannot hear.

Hysterical amnesia Loss of memory for a specific period associated with trauma.

Hysterical behaviour It is a form of neuritis which is characterised by physical and behavioural symptoms. shallow and emotional relationship. Hysteria is of two types : in conversion hysteria mental aspects of repression are converted into behavioural symptoms such as paralysis or inability to speak whereas in dissociate type person is having multiple personalities. Psychiatric treatment helps.

Hysterical fit These never occur between definite hours of day as do epileptic fits. These never occur during sleep. Fits develop only in presence of onlookers. Incontinence of urine neither occurs nor tongue biting results. The eyes are scewed up and hands clenched. Every movement is purposeful. Patients specially females may develop outbursts of laughing or crying.

Hysterosalpingectomy Surgical removal of the uterus and one or both fallopian tubes.

Hysterosalpingography A x-ray procedure in which dye is passed through the fallopian tubes to test for tubal blockage.

Hysterosalpingoophorectomy Surgical removal of one or both ovaries and fallopian tubes alongwith the uterus.

Hysteroscope A viewing instrument for examination of the cervix and interior of the uterus.

Hysteroscopy Endoscopy of the uterine cavity.

Hysterotomy A miniature caesarean section, wherein the incision of uterus is made either transabdominally or vaginally to remove products of conception.

Hysterotrachelorrhaphy Surgical repair of a lacerated cervix uteri.

Hz Abbreviation of hertz.

Hzv Abbreviation of herpes zoster virus.

I

Iatrogenic Resulting from the activity of the clinician; applied to complications induced in the patient by the clinician.

Iatrogenic diabetes Diabetes caused by administration of certain drugs, such as corticosteroids certain diuretics, and birth control pills.

Iatrogenic disease and injuries Diseases an injuries generated during the process of treatment.

Ice cap This is a local dry application of cold. As the ice is kept in a rubber cap, the effect of cold persists without soiling or wetting the skin. It is used to control bleeding, to reduce swelling, to relieve headache, to relieve local pain and prevent cerebral congestion.

Ice creams A frozen confection made from fat, milk, solids and sugars.

Ice packs Cold causes blood vessels to contract and reducing blood flow. Ice is applied to skin to relieve pain. After injuries it is used to minimise swelling, bruising and further tissue damage. Ice is applied to skin surface being wrapped in a wet cloth.

Ice water enema This is given in case of hyperpyrexia when by routine procedure of cooling down becomes uneffective. It is given very slowly or by drop method. The temperature of cold water is maintained at 15°C. About 300 to 600 CC of cold water can be given to cool the body.

Iceberg phenomenon The earliest identified cases of a new disease are often fatal or severe however, as more becomes known about the disease, less severe cases and asymptomatinc cases are usually discovered.

Icon A visual image, based on residual stimulation in the sensory system after the original stimulus has disappeared. The icon is in the sensory register, and it forms the initial basis of later memory.

Iconic memory Brief sensory memory for vision. Id: The part of the psyche that contains the instincts and is directed solely by pleasure seeking; it is the most primitive part of the psyche and was thought by Freud to fuel the ego and superego.

Icterus neonatorum The jaundice of a newborn.

ICU Nurse She should be perfectly trained in handling equipment like oxygen cylinder, artificial respirator and incubator, etc. She should be trained in CPR and cardiac massage. She should be active, smart confident in profession, and co-operative. Politeness will be her virtue.

Id In Freudian theory, the part of the personality that is the unconscious source of unstructured desires and drives.

Ideal alignment The alignment used as a standard when evaluating posture.

Idealisation A mental mechanism, operating consciously or un-consciously, in which one overestimates an admired aspect or attribute of another.

Ideas of reference Incorrect inter-pretation of casual incidents and external events as having direct reference to oneself. May reach sufficient intensity to constitute delusions.

Ideational apraxia An inability to perform a purposeful motor act, either automatically or upon command; an inability to retain the idea of the task and to formulate the necessary motor patterns. The patient no longer understands the overall concept of the act.

Identification A defence mechanism, operating unconsciously, by which a person patterns himself after some other person. Identification plays a major role in the development of one's personality and specifically of the superego. To be differentiated from imitation or role modelling, which is a conscious process.

Identification marks Generally two identification marks on exposed part of the body are noted down, mostly on face, forehead and arms. These include scar, mole and tattoo marks. These marks are more or less permanent and generally are not destroyable.

Identity The aggregate of characteristics by which an individual is recognized by himself and others.

Identity crisis A loss of the sense of the sameness and historical continuity of one's self and inability to accept or adopt the role one perceives as being expected by society; often expressed by isolation, withdrawal, extremism, rebelliousness, and negativity, and typically triggered by a combination of sudden increase in the strength of instinctual drives in a milieu of rapid social evolution and technologic change.

Ideological immunisation In persuasion, the technique of providing resistance to later counter arguments by exposing the audience to them in small doses. Speaker A may attempt to immunise his audience against the rhetoric of speaker B by describing B's assets and also emphasising his limitations before speaker B has an opportunity to address that same audience.

Ideological code Words and beliefs that seek to guide how members of society perceive the world.

Ideology A belief or value system.

Ideomotor apraxia An inability to perform a task upon command and to imitate gestures, even though the patient understands the concept of the task and is able to carry out habitual tasks automatically.

Idiocy It is an obsolete term for mental retardation. IQ is less than 20 and mental age of a person is of only 2 years.

Idioglossia Imperfect articulation with utterance of meaningless vocal sounds.

Idiographic Pertaining to a particular case in a particular time and context; the opposite of nomothetic.

Idiographic measures No standardised but devised to assess the problems specific to an individual.

Idiopathic Of the nature of an idiopathy; self-originated; of unknown causation; essential.

Idiopathic congestive cardiomyopathy A myocardial dysfunction that has no discernible cause.

Idiopathic illness One whose cause is unexplained.

Idiopathic osteolysis Heritable condition in which there is dissolution of bone with predictable debilitating and disfiguring consequences.

Idiopathic polymyositis Onset is acute with fever, muscle pain, oedema and tenderness of limbs. Being acute, myoglobinuria results. Serum lelvel of phosphocreatine kinase is raised. Symptoms develop over weeks and months. Weakness is greater than the degree of atrophy. Tendon reflexes are preserved. There may be dysphagia and non-erosive arthritis.

Idiopathic steatorrhea Fat malabsorption as a result of unknown causes.

Idiosyncrasy Any tendency, characteristic, peculiar to an individual.

Idiosyncratic reaction It is defined as those ADRS which cannot be explained by any pharmacologic or biochemical mechanism. It is neither an overdose nor an allergic reaction. There may be depression following administration of stimulant. Being unpre-dictable treatment is symptomatic only.

Idiot A person with gross mental retardation who nonetheless is capable of performing certain remarkable feats in sharply circumscribed intellectual areas, such as calendar calculation or puzzle-solving.

Idiotope An epitope made up of amino acids within the variable region of an antibody or T cell receptor which reacts with an anti-idiotope.

Idiotype network A regulatory network based on interactions of idiotpes and anti-idiotypes present on antibodies and T cell receptors.

Idnetity confusion Subjective feelings of uncertainity, puzzlement or conflict.

IgA nephropathy It is a major cause of recurrent glomerular haematuria. Under microscope one notices mesangial proliferation and IgA deposition. Defects in regulation of IgA synthesis, secretion or clearance may be the cause.

The haematuria lasts for several days and then subsides only to recur after a few months. In old age, resulting in hypertension may poor prognosis.

Ignition temperature The minimum temperature required to initiate the self-sustaining chemical process referred to as fire or burning.

Ileocaecal junction The junction of the ileum of the small intestine and the caecum of the large intestine.

Ileocecal valve The sphincterlike structure between the end of the small intestine and the beginning of the large intestine.

Ileostomy The removal of the entire colon and rectum; surgical formation of an opening of the ileum onto the surface of the abdomen through which, fecal matter is emptied.

Ileum It is the narrowest, final part of small intestine. It is the part between jejunum and large intestine.

It contains millions of villi which increases surface area to absorb. It may develop Crohn's disease, celiac sprue and lymphoma.

Ileus Dilated loops of bowel that do not show any evidence of peristalsis. Ileus is associated with many abdominal problems, pancreatitis, sickle cell crisis, prolonged bowel obstruction.

Iliac crest The thickened and expanded superior border of ilium.

Iliac crest block It blocks the ilioinguinal, iliohypogastric and lower 2/3 intercostal nerves providing anesthesia of lower ipsilateral abdomen.

Iliopsoas A flexor of the thigh and an important stabilizing muscle for posture.

Iliotibial tractitis This is the fascial insertion of tensor fascia lata as it passes over the bony expansion of lateral femoral condyle at the knee. There is local pain and hydrocortisone injection gives local relief.

Ilium One of the three separate bones that forms the os coxa.

Illegitimate child Child becomes illegitimate or bastered if it can be proved that the husband could not possibly be the father of child. It may be under circumstances when father has not attained the age of puberty. When father did not have sexual access to his wife when the child was born. It has the importance in case of inheritance, disputed paternity and affiliation cases.

Illiterate Unable to read or write.

Illness What the patient experiencs when he or she is sick.

Illness behavior The recognition and assessment of body symptoms along with seeking and following of medical advice.

Illness patterns The processes and phases of illness that families go through to manage a disease and the medical treatments that becomes a part of their daily lives. Families usually respond differently to acute, chronic, and life-threatening phases of illness.

Illusion A perception considered as mistaken because it does not agree with objective measurement of the physical form or pattern, which is regarded as more fundamental.

Image contrast In microscopy, the ability to distinguish various components of the structure of the object by different intensity levels in the image.

Image intensifier A device used to convert X-rays that have passed through the object or patient into image which can be recorded with a television camera or photographic camera. It was introduced in 1950's.

Imagery It refers to the experiencing of vivid mental images which lack the immediacy or substantiality of perception and which are under the conscious control of will. Iidotic imagery, the capacity to experience a vivid memory of visual scene is normal in children. One may see black clouds hanging over them or hearing something inside to do something.

Imaging Creating a picture.

Imago A term used by Jung for an unconscious mental image, usually idealised, of an important person in one's early history.

Imbecility It is an obsolete term of mental retardation. Intellectual capacity of a person is 3 to 6 years and IQ between 20 and 50.

Imbrication Th1e surgical technique of suturing tissues in ovelapping layers.

Imitation The performance of behaviors that were learned by observing the actions of others.

Immature cataract As long as there is any clear lens substance between the pupillary margin of iris and the opacity in lens, the iris throws a shadow upon the grey opacity of the lens.

Presence of iris shadow is a sure sign of an immature cataract. Vision is reduced. At this stage visual acuity is low, pupils appear grey white and iris shadow is present. There is no red glow on plane mirror examination and on ophthalmoscope. Only treatment is removal.

Immediate denture Complete or removable partial denture constructed for insertion immediately following the removal of natural teeth.

Immediate hypersensitivity Hypersensitivity (allergy) mediated by antibodies of the IgE class that results in the release of histamine and related compounds from tissue cells.

Immediate postoperative prosthesis Application of a temporary prosthesis immediately following amputation; usually consists of a plaster of Paris socket, pylon, and foot.

Immediate recall The ability to remember information that has been stored for a few seconds.

Immersion bath The body, or any part of it except the head, may be immersed in water of different temperatures for different purposes.

Immersion foot A circulatory disturbance similar to trench foot.

Immigration The movement of individuals toward a certain site; specifically, movement toward a breeding site in advance of reproductive activity.

Immobility Pertaining to the inability of a body part or limb to e moved.

Immobilized cell A cell attached to a solid support over which substrate is passed and is converted into product.

Immobilizer Commercial splint made from cloth and foam.

Immounocompromised A state of defective of failed immuno response that makes a person more likely to acquire an infection.

Immune complex Complex of antibody bound to antigen which may also contain complement components.

Immune deficiency syndrome Oral lesions are common. Kaposi's sarcoma syndrome develops in palate. It appears as a bluish discolou-ration of mucosa which may be mistaken for a bruise. Moniliasis is a very common opportunistic oral infection.

Immune response The capacity of a vertebrate to generate antibodies to an antigen, a macromolecule foreign to the organism.

Immune suppression Medical treatment interventions that results in dampening of immune survilence mechanism.

Immune suppressive therapy It is done to control immune responses in patients with certain conditions, i.e, cancer or auto immune disease.

Immune system The body's internal defence against foreign substances such as bacteria/ parasite.

Immunity It is a resistance offered by an individual to infection by microorganisms or injury by their products is called immunity. This resistance may be of all degrees from almost complete susceptibility to complete unsusceptibility.

Immunization The process in which an organism becomes immune; e.g., by means of injection of a specific antigen foreign to the organism to promote the formation of antibodies.

Immunoassay Any of a number of laboratory or clinical techniques that employ the specific binding between an antigen and its homologous antibody in order to identify and quantify a substance in a sample.

Immunobiology That branch of biology dealing with immunologic effect.

Immunocompetence The ability or capacity to develop an immune response i.e. antibody production and/or cell-mediated immunity following antigenic challenge. Thus, immunocompetent.

Immunocytes Cells of immune system.

Immunodeficiency A deficiency of the immune system, which may be long-term (as in AIDS) or may be transient lasting for a short period following some types of infections or the administration of chemotherapy for certain types of cancer.

Immunodominant epitope The major antigenic determinant of a particular antigen in its native state, stimulating the strongest antigen-specific immune response of the immunized animal.

Immunogen Any substance which elicits an immune response. Whilst all immunogens are antigens, but all antigens are not immunogens.

Immunogenicity The capacity to elicit adaptive immunity.

Immunoglobulin (IgG) This is a major immunoglobulin component of serum making 75% of antibody present in normal adult human serum. The IgG is bivalent having two combining sites per molecule. It allows two antigenic molecules forming a complex. It passes in the placenta and gives passive protection to fetus against many infectious agents for up to six months of age.

Immunoglobulin A (IgA) It constitutes about 10 % of immunoglo-bulins in human serum. It is found in seromucous secretions such as saliva, tears, colostrum, bronchial mucus, intestinal and urinary tract secretions. On mucous surfaces, it forms an antibody paste, and plays important role in local immunity against respiratory and intestinal pathogens. It is fully responsible for local immunity.

Immunoglobulin E (IgE) These are responsible for severe, acute and occasionally fatal response. It is present in serum in very low quantity. IgE would appear more harmful than beneficial for many individuals who are allergic or hypersensitive to certain substances. It is heat sensitive and is labile at 56°C for about 4 hours. These are abundant in mucosa of respiratory and intestinal tracts.

Immunoglobulin M (IgM) Being a pentamer, IgM has increased capacity for antigen combining and thus is extremely efficient in agglutination lytic reactions. About 80 % is intravascular in distribution. IgM antibodies are short lived. Hence their demonstration in the serum indicates recent infection. A single molecule of IgM can bring about immune haemolysis whereas 1000 IgM molecules are required for the same effect. Septicaemia is often associated with deficiency of IgM.

Immunological memory Active immunity is associated with immunological memory which implies that the immune system is able to retain the memory of a prior antigenic exposure for long periods and produce a secondary type of response when it meets with same antigen again.

Immunosuppressant An agent capable of suppressing immune responses.

Immunosuppressive Any agent that prevents or interferes with the development of a immunologic response.

Immunosurveillance The concept that the immune system recognizes and attacks maligant cells that produce antigens nor recognized as "self". This function is believed to be cell mediated rather than humoral.

Impact pattern Bloodstain pattern created when blood receives a blow or force resulting in the random dispersion of smaller drops of blood.

Impact site That point where force encounters a source of blood.

Impaction Presence of large or hard fecal mass in the rectum or colon.

Impaction tooth It is a failure to emerge fully or part from gum because of mechanical impediment. It may be embedded in bone or soft tissue. Impaction is caused by overcrowding where little space is left for eruption. *Impacted upper canines* are not removed but are put in order with the help of orthodontic appliance. *Impacted wisdom tooth* is very common and cause trouble unless they partially penetrate the gums. Plaque bacteria and food debris then may collect between teeth and gum and become inflamed. Warm saline gargles and analgesics do help.

Impaired fecundity Difficulty or danger in achieving or carrying a pregnancy to term.

Impaired immunity A defect in host defense; a lack of immune response.

Impairment Any loss or abnormality of anatomic, physiologic, or psychologic structure or function; a direct and natural consequence of pathology or insult.

Impedance Resistance to flow of an alternating current in an electrical circuit dependent on currents frequency.

Impetigo It is a highly contagious infection due to bacteria in children. It causes skin rash which forms yellow crusts on face and limbs. Antibiotics help the patient.

Impinge To press or encroach upon; to come into close contact; an obstructing lesion causing pressure on a nerve.

Impingement An encroachment on the space occupied by soft tissue, such as nerve or muscle. In this test, impingement refers to nerve irritation from pressure or friction associated with muscles.

Implant A metallic or ceramic device that is placed on or within the jaw to provide a stable support for a dental prosthesis.

Implant dentistry Dental treatment associated with the use of dental implants. ,

Implant, dental A prosthetic device of biocompatible material placed within or against the mandibular or maxillary bone.

Implantation The placement within body tissues of a foreign substance, for example metal or plastic, for restoration by mechanical means. In dentistry, a foreign material placed into or onto the jaw bone to support a crown, partial or complete denture.

Implantation bleeding During process of imbedding of the ovum, the blastocyst erodes the endometrium and may cause source amount of bleeding in some cases. This may be mistaken as a normal menstruation.

Implantation dermoid It arises from the in driven epithelium beneath the skin following a trauma particularly a puncture injury. Commonly involved sites are pulp or tips of fingers, palms or soles. It may be painful and tender. It contains white greasy material which is desquamated epithelium cells with mucoid degeneration.

It is spherical smooth swelling, usually 0.2 to 1 cm in diameter. Cyst feels tense and hard. Overlying skin is scarred. Infection may develop in it and cosmetically it looks ugly. Cyst on sole may cause limping. Complete excision is convenient.

Implantology Surgical insertion of material and devices into, onto and about the jaws.

Implement To put into action.

Implementation It involves carrying out or putting into effect the care plan developed during the planning phase.

Implicit memory Memory in which subjects can demonstrate knowledge or skin but cannot explicitly retrieve the information.

Implied contract A contract not evidenced by explicit agreement of parties but inferred by the law, act and circumstances surrounding the transections.

Implosion therapy A therapy in which the patient imagines his or her feared situation, plus elements from psychodynamic theory that the therapist thinks are related to the fear, until fear decreases.

Impotence Inability to maintain an erection.

Impregnation The act of becoming pregnant.

Impression A negative replica of a dental structure, usually a prepared tooth, used in the fabrication of a dental restoration or prosthesis; the impression material may be rubbery or hard and rigid.

Impression mercaptan An impression made of mercaptan, a rubber base elastic material.

Impression waxes These are used for taking edentulous impressions. These waxes must be deformable at oral temperatures to record the detail of oral tissues.

Imprinting A term in ethology referring to a process similar to rapid learning or behavioural patterning that occurs at critical points in very early stages of animal development. The extent to which imprinting occurs in human development has not been established.

Impulse A psychic striving usually refers to an instinctual urge. This is a sudden and irresistable force compelling a person to the conscious performance of some action without any motive or fore thought. A specific desire or urge to perform a particular action on some occasion.

Impulsive A tendency to obey internal drives, without regard for acceptance by others or pressure from society.

Impulsivity Reduced ability to resist an impulse or temptation to perform some action. These are directed for obtaining immediate gratification without regard for delayed consequences of the behaviour.

In situ In its original or normal place or natural position.

In vitro Refers to the glass laboratory container where a mature ovum is fertilized by a sperm. Literally, in glass; describing studies carried out in the test tube, or, more broadly, in any setting outside the living organism.

In vitro fertilization (IVF) Embryos are generated outside the body and transferred at least two of them after successful fertilization with sperm.

In vivo In life; describing studies carried out in the living organism.

Inactivated vaccine Vaccine that contains killed micro organism.

Inactivation gate The chemical e.g., neurotransmitter or electrical e.g., membrane potential action that closes an ion channel after it has been opened.

Inanition Exhaustion and wasting due to complete lack of or non assimilation of food.

Inapparent infection The presence of infection in a host without recognizable clinical signs or symptoms. It can only be identified through laboratory tests.

Inborn error-phenyl ketonuria There is a failure of hydroxylation of phenylaline metabolism. High blood level of phenylaline is chiefly responsible for progressive mental deterioration. Deficiency of tryosine is there.

Melanin synthesis is inhibited and infants become of light colour. The baby has a 'mousy odour' Repetitive finger movements, restlessness, clumsy gaits and major epileptic fits are seen in childhood. A low phenylaline diet in the form of protein hydrolysate prevents mental retardation.

Inborn immunity Immunity to disease that is inherited.

Inborn motives Motivation which is part of the organism's biological inheritance, such as the need for food, drink, rest and so forth. Also called primary motivation.

Inbred strain A set of animals that is produced by at least 20 consecutive generations of sisters and brothers or parent and offspring mating. These are fully homozygos.

Inbreeding Matings between genetically related individuals.

Incendiary communication Communication characterized by bringing up old unresolved issues, to reach a solution, yelling and screaming at other family members, and walking away from conflicts without much resolution.

Incentive A reward attached to a desired goal; used in rehabilitation and department management.

Incentive salience Refers to cues that, after having been associated with drug use, become sought out.

Incentive spirometer A flow or volume-dependent device that is used to facilitate slow, deep, sustained inspiratory efforts in patients who might otherwise be disposed to breath shallowly.

Incentive spirometry Lung expansion technique designed to encourage deep breathing to reduce atelectasis.

Incest Incest is any form of overt sexual contact including fondling, masturbation or intercourse between persons related to each other by either blood or marriage. Practically all societies consider incest to be taboo for religious reactions and because of belief that deformed offspring would result from the sexual union of blood relatives. Incest creates sexual rivalries and jealousy within family.

It is the sexual relationship between blood relations such as between father and daughter, brother and sister, niece and nephew or cousins. Social taboos or laws against incest exist in every society but the degree of relationship may differ.

Incidence A measure of the rate of new cases of a disease; the number of people in a given population developing a specified disease or becoming infected within a specified period of time.

Incidence density The frequency (density) of new events per person-time. Incidence density is expecially useful in studying the frequency rates of diseases or events that occur more than once for an individual, such as otits media, colds, or hospital admissions.

Incidence density measures Measures of the frequency of adverse health events that are used, for example, to determine the optimal timing for administration of new vaccine and the duration of the immunity produced.

Incidence rate The number of incident cases over a defined study period, divided by the population at risk at the midpoint of that study period.

Incident report Written account of an unusual event involving a client, employee, or visitor that has the potential for being injurious.

Incidental additives Substances that inadvertently contaminate processed foods.

Incipient Beginning to exist; coming into existence.

Incisal Relating to the cutting edge of the anterior teeth, incisors, or canines.

Incise Cut into

Incision Incision should be made with a firm pressure upon a sharp scalpel through the skin.

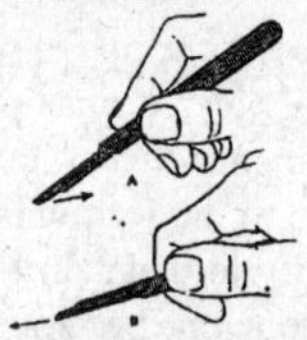

(A) correct and
(B) incorrect use of scalpel

Scalpel should be used as pen and not as a plough and soft tissues should be cut at right angles to the surface of underlying bone if any.

Incisive canal A passage way through bone that extends from the superior foramina of the incisive canal to the incisive foramen; appears radiolucent.

Incisive foramen An opening or hole in bone located at the midline of the anterior portion of the hard palate directly posterior to the maxillary central incisors; appears radiolucent.

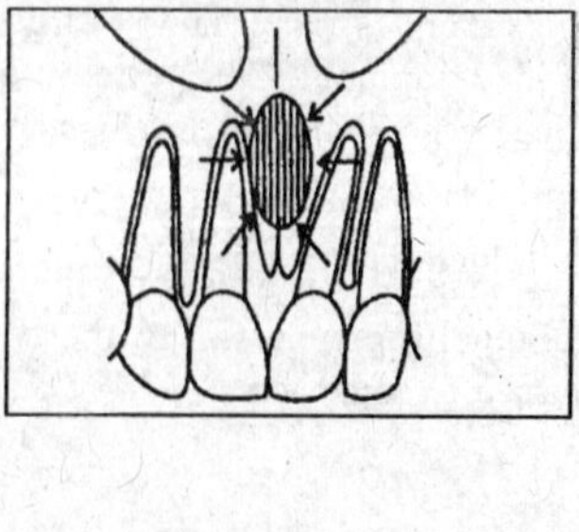

Incisive papilla The elevation of soft tissue covering the foramen of the incisive or nasopalatine canal.

Incisors These are 8 in number and are chisel-shaped cutting teeth located anteriorly between the canines. Purpose is to bite.

Incitant An inciting or causative agent, as one that causes infectious diseases or induces an allergic reaction.

Inclination angle Angle formed by the incident of the longitudinal axis of the neck with that of shaft.

Inclinometer A wide range of joint motion measure instruments based on the principle of gravity are called Inclinometer. It may be a circular scale to the centre of which is attached a weighted pointer at one end so that it remains vertical while the scale rotates around it (Pendulum Goniometer). It may also be a calibrated instrument with a starting Zero position that indicated by a fluid level (Bubble goinnometer).

Inclusion conjunctivitis It is a common cause of ophthalmia neonatorum. The causative organism is *Chlamydia trachomatis*. Characteristic inclusion bodies are found on bacteriological examination. The primary source is subclinical venereal disease producing mild urethritis in males and cervicitis in females. It is transmitted from mother to newborn and in adults transmitted from genitals by fingers and through water of swimming pools.

Incompatible blood groups RH incompatibility only infrequently may lead to late recurrent abortion, still births and erthroblastosis.

Incompatible transfusion All patients receiving blood transfusion should be carefully watched during first 15 minutes of transfusion. Conscious person may feel fullness of head, tingling of limbs, precordial pain, lumbar pain, dyspnoea, and circulatory collapse. Under anaesthesia one can note hypotension, tachycardia, general oozing from wound and may be in 5% cases jaundice and oliguria may develop.

Incompetent cervical os A mechanical defect in the cervix, which causes late habitual abortion or preterm labour.

Incompetent cervix A mechanical defect in the cervix, which causes the cervical os to dilate prematurely during the midtrimester of pregnancy resulting in late habitual recurrent abortion or preterm labor.

Incompetent valve A leaky valve; usually refers to a leaky valve in the heart that allows blood to flow through it when it is closed.

Incomplete abortion In it some portion of placenta or of embryo has been retained in uterus. Continuance of bleeding with absence of expected involution of uterus are chief signs.

Incomplete inevitable abortion It means that some products of conception are still retained within the uterus. The uterus does not appreciably diminish in size and bleeding continues. Patient may have pain or no pain.

Incomplete lesion Some preservation of sensory or motor function below the level of the lesion.

Incomplete proteins Those that contain some, but not all, of the essential amino acids.

Incontinence Involuntary voiding of urine/feces.

Incontinence urine It is uncontrolable, involuntary urination due to injury or disease of urinary system. It is very common in females after child birth. In *urge incontinence* an urgent desire to urinate is accompanied by inability to control the bladder. Sometimes even sudden change of posture may result it. *Total incontinence* refers to a complete lack of bladder control. In this sphincter does not work. *Overflow incontinence* occurs in chronic retention. Person becomes unable to empty bladder fully. It may be due to obstruction of enlarged prostate. Incontinence may be caused by bladder stones, prolapse of uterus or mental impairment. Pelvic floor exercises may help to restore sphincter function. In irritable bladder, anticholinergic drugs are helpful.

Incontinentia pigmenti It is autosomal dominant trait causing patchy hyperpigmentation. It develops within first few weeks of life and lesion shows deposition of melanin. It presents with crops of inflammatory papules, vesicles occurring mostly on trunk. There is no distinctive pattern.

Incorporation A primitive defence mechanism, operating unconsciously, in which the psychic representation of a person, or parts of the person, is figuratively ingested.

Incretory Pertaining to internal secertion; endocrine.

Incubation The behavior pattern of sitting on eggs to provide the correct environment for embryo development; also, the provision of a comparable artificial environment for eggs to hatch.

Incubator A container in which controlled environmental conditions e.g., temperature , pressure, gas composition may be maintained.
An apparatus for maintaining a premature infant in an environment of proper temperature and humidity.

Incus The anvil, the middle ear bone that is shaped like an anvil.

Indecent assault This is an offence committed on a female with intent or knowledge to outrage her modesty. This is usually sexually motivated and obviously done without her consent. It may include kissing any part of female, pressing female'sbreasts or private parts. Even doctor should examine female patient with her consent and in presence of a female attendant.

Indemnity A contractual agreement in which one party agrees to reimburse an other for loses of a particular type. Many insurance policies have indemnity clauses that allow them to recover paid to an insured who later recovers damages in court for the same injury.

Independent The condition of a study or clinical trial being conducted by investigators who are disinterested in the potential success or failure of the experimental protocol.

Independent 't' test A parametric test of differences between two independent samples.

Independent variable A factor that is suspected in influencing the ourcome of an analytical study.

Index Scoring system in which a number describes a designated oral condition; for example, oral hygiene, periodontal disease, caries.

Index case In a disease outbreak, the first affected individuals to be identified.

Index of nutritive quality It refers to the ratio of nutrients to energy in a food. INQ more than 1 is useful.

Indian childhood cirrhosis It develops around the first year of life. There is progressive distension of abdomen, marked irritability, unexplained irregular low-grade pyrexia, a firm hepatomegaly with sharp margin. Spleen may enlarge with ascites and jaundice. Prognosis is poor.

Indian sitting A means of sitting in which the legs are bent and crossed over each other.

Indication A therapeutic application that promotes health or assists in a healing process. A strong reason for believing that a particular remedy or course of treatment is appropriate.

Indicator A microorganism that on detection gives a quantitative representation of a group of organisms, often of contamination or pathogens in foods or drinking water or a target organism sensitive to bacteriocin.

Indictment A formal written accusation of crime brought by the prosecuting attorney against a person charged with criminal conduct.

Indigenous Native or natural in a given site or region; not exotic.

Indigenous flora Microorganisms that consitute the normal or resident flora of a system, especially those that colonize animals or humans without causing known disease.

Indigenous societies Societies that are native to a particular locality in which people speak a distinctive language and have a dinstinctive heritage and are technically less complex.

Indigestion It may be caused by eating too quickly and of fatty food. Symptoms include bloated feeling around diaphragm, belching and regurgitation of liquid contents. There may develop heart burn and flatulence. Later on symptoms similar to peptic ulcer may develop. Antacids and ranitidine group of drugs help.

Indirect calorimetry The rate of metabolism and heat production is calculated from the oxygen intake. By determining either the oxygen consumed or CO_2 exhaled in a given number of minutes the caloric expenditure can be calculated.

Indirect causality One factor influences one or more other factors that are, in turn, directly causal.

Indirect contact Method of transmitting infection or disease without coming into direct contact with the source of the containant.

Indirect development A life cycle that includes a larval stage and metamorphosis.

Indirect hernia Hernia is a protrusion of abdominal viscera through a weakened portion of abdominal wall. It can be congenital or acquired. Indirect hernia occurs in men below 30. A weakness around deep inguinal ring allows sac to protrude through the ring into inguinal canal and occasionally extends into scrotum.
Diect hernias result from weakness in an area of fascia, bounded by rectus abdominis muscle, the

inguinal ligament and epigastric vessels. Occurs in elderly person.

Indirect impairments The sequelae or secondary complications occurring in systems other than the system affected by the original pathology or insult; the clinical manifestations of expanding multisystem dysfunction.

Indirect inguinal hernia The hernia enters the inguinal canal through the deep inguinal ring lateral to the inferior gastric artery. It is usually congenital due to persistence of patent processus vaginalis. It appears at or soon after birth. Acquired variety may develop at any age.

Indirect laryngoscopy Hoarseness and other laryngeal symptoms may be an early sign of malignancy. Any hoarseness persisting for 2 weeks mandates laryngeal examination. In many cases indirect laryngoscopy coupled with history will lead to diagnosis of persisting hoarseness, upper respiratory obstruction, stridor, haemoptysis and dysphagia. In case of acute epiglottiditis it should not be done.

Indirect ophthalmoscopy The eye is made highly myopic by placing a strong convex lens in front of the eye, so that a real inverted image of the fundus

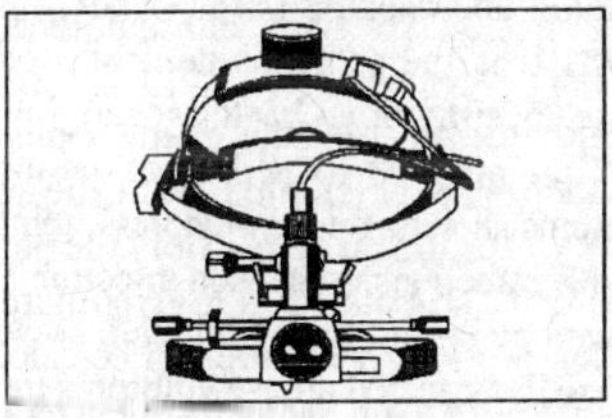

is formed between the observer and the convex lens. The image is magnified five times with a lens of 13 dioptres. The weaker the lens the large is the size of the image formed.

Indirect pulp cap A cement or calcium hydroxide material placed over a deep suspected caries or possible exposure in order to "cap"and protect the pulp.

Indirect vision Use of a dental mouth mirror to provide vision of the treatment site.

Individual development The expected changes in each family member associated with growth and development.

Individual psychology A system of psychiatric theory, research, and therapy developed by Alfred Adler which stresses compensation and overcompensation for inferiority feelings.

Individual supply Single container of drugs with several days' worth of doses.

Individuation The time provided for each family member to be alone to develop a sense of self and spirituality.

Indole, skatole Simple offensive smelling proteins produced by bacterial degradation of those proteins usually present in the body.

Indomethacin It is highly effective anti-inflammatory analgesic and antipyretic agent. Absorption from gut is rapid and complete. Half-life is 4 hour. It is used to relieve moderate to severe pain and the inflammation of rheumatoid disease, acute musculoskeletal disorders, gout and during postoperative period. The oral dose is 50 to 200 mg daily in divided doses. Suppository of 100 mg at night is effective for relief of morning stiffness. Main side effects are gastric irritation with ulcer formation. It may cause salt and fluid retention. Headache is common. Vomiting, dizziness and ataxia occur.

Induced abortion An abortion that is produced artificially and intentionally.

Induced enzyme An enzyme that is produced by an organism in response to the presence of its substrate or a related substance.

Induced movement A false perception involving illusory motion; attributing movement to a stationary stimulus. Without an adequate reference point, it may appear that your subway car is moving and the adjacent car is at a standstill, but when you notice the edge of the stationary ticket booth, you discover that the reverse is true.

Inducer A signal molecule that , when bound to a regulatory protein, produces an increase in the expression of a given gene.

Inductance cardiography It is to determine changes in intrathoracic volumes used for estimating cardiac output.

Induction An increase in the expression of a gene in response to a change in the activity of a regulatory protein.

Induction of labor Artificial initiation of labour.

Induction period It is the lag period during which the fat shows stability to oxidation because of its contents of antioxidants. After this induction period there is sudden and large consumption oxygen and fat becomes rancid.

Inductive reasoning Reasoning that proceeds from the specific (i.e., from data) to the general (i.e., to formulas or conclusions).

Induration A area of the skin that feels hard.

Industrial psychology A speciality in which the psychologist works in an industrial setting and is generally concerned with such problems as employee recruitment and selection, employee training, job analysis, and techniques for improving work efficiency.

Industry versus inferiority The fourth stage of Erikson's psychosocial stages and the last childhood stage. The issue here is the development of feelings of accomplishment in the child. If the child is presented with tasks appropriate for his or her ability, a sense of industry, rather than inferiority, should develop. The key in this outcome is the presentation of tasks appropriate to the child's ability.

Indwelling catheter Catheter designed to remain stable as it runs through the urethra.

Inefficacy Feeling of incompetence and lack of achievement in work.

Inelastic The quality of not being elastic; a rigid, nonflexible material.

Inert Without intrinsic active properties; no inherent power of action, motion, or resistance.

Inert gas nacrosis Loss of consciousness caused by inhalation of high partial pressures of inert gases i.e. argon and nitrogen.

Inertia Property that makes a body resist a change in motion.

Inevitable abortion Free and pronounced bleeding with severe uterine cramps are characteristics. It usually follows threatened abortion. Open external OS is seen. Membranes may remain intact and may be seen to bulge through dilating internal OS. If internal OS can be closed, pregnancy can be continued.

Infancy From birth to about 18 months of age.

Infancy period First year of life.

Infant death The death of a live-born child before that child's first birthday.

Infant feeding The baby is offered 15 to 30 ml of 5% glucose four hours after birth. After 6 hours newborn is allowed breast feeding. Baby gets colostrum which protects the child from certain infections.

Infant mortality rate The number of death's of all children under a year per 1000 live births

Infant respiratory distress syndrome Leading cause of death in premature babies, due to a lack of surfactant in the alveolar air sacs.

Infantile colic Infants below three months of age often have paroxysms of sudden crying followed by flushing of face, distension of abdomen and drawing up of lower limbs on the abdomen. It is relieved when faeces or flatus is passed. It may be caused by aerophagy, hunger and overfeeding.

Infantile eczema It usually starts within first 3 months of birth specially in boys. There is severe itching. There is bilaterally symmetrically distributed papulovesicular lesions on cheeks and extremities. Secondary infection may develop.

Infantile strabismus Strabismus which develops in first year of life.

Infantilism There develops mental retardation and retention of childhood characteristic in adult hood.

Infarct Area of necrosis resulting from a sudden insufficiency of arterial blood supply.

Infarction Cessation of blood flow by thrombus formation and causing tissue death.

Infection It is the establishment of a colony of a disease causing virus/ bacteria/ fungi in the body. Infection may be localised or general. Toxic symptoms such as fever, weakness, joint aches are systemic infections. Localised infection is generally followed by inflammation which increases flow of blood to the infected area. Symptoms include pain, redness and swelling. There may or may not be pus formation. Invasion of the body by pathogenic microorganisms and the body's response to the microorganisms and their toxic products; transfer of disease from one part to another or one person to another.

Infection control The use of medical and surgical asepsis and standard precautions to prevent or control the spread of microorganisms.

Infection control precautions Physical measures designed to curtail the spread of infectious diseases.

Infection of finger spaces An abscess in the finger pulp is known as felon. A localised subcutaneous abscess over phalanges is not much painful. Still it has to be opened up. While an

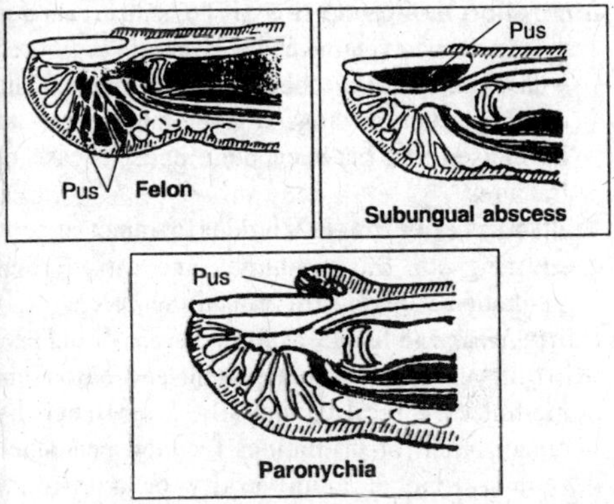

abscess under nailfold is known as paronchyia, is to be treated by incising and freeing up the nail fold. Sometimes proximal portion of nail is to be removed.

Infection thread A plant-derived tube through which rhizobia move down the root hair, or between cells in the root cortex.

Infectious agent Any bacterium, virus, protozoan, prion, or other such form that can cause infection or disease in a human, animal, or other host.

Infectious disease Diseases spread from one person to another.

Infectious dose The number of microbes needed to cause symptoms.

Infectious mononucleosis It is caused by Herpes like virus. Incubation period is 7 weeks. Disease lasts for about a week. Patient develops fatigue, sore throat, malaise, headache and elevation of temperature. Cervical lymph glands enlarge. Oral lesions include gingivostomatitis, gingival bleeding and multiple pin point petechiae at the junction of hard and soft palate. A heterophil antibody test is diagnostic.

Infectious parotitis It is highly infectious and is commonly known as mumps. It occurs in children and affects parotid gland. Gonads, pancreas and breast may also be involved. Incubation period is 2 to 3 weeks.

Person develops fever, malaise and pain in parotid area. Patient complains of bad taste. Disease regresses in 2 weeks. Under microscope one notices degenerative changes in epithelium of ducts, a few areas of acinar atrophy and presence of polymorphonuclear leucocyte.

Infectious waste Any material capable of producing an infectious disease; a subset of medical waste.

Infectiousness The state or quality of being infectious.

Infectiousness of an organism A measue that is caluclated as the proportion of exposed persons who become infected, although it is also influenced by the conditinos of exposure and the immune status of the exposed person.

Inference The act of drawing a conclusion or making a deduction.

Inferior Down, or lower, with reference to the anatomical position.

Inferior alveolar canal A canal that traverses the ramus and body of the mandible between the mandibular and metal foramina, transmitting the inferior alveolar vessels and nerve.

Inferior alveolar nerve Inferior alveolar nerve and vessels as combined are in a true osseous canal in the ramus of the mandible. There may be multiple branches.

Inferior colliculus A structure on the dorsal surface of the midbrain; used in auditory processing.

Inferior nasal conchae Water-thin curved plates of bone that extend from the lateral walls of the nasal cavity and appear radiopaque.

Inferior pulmonary vein The vein returning blood from right or left lower lobes of the lungs to the left atrium.

Inferior vena cava The blood vessel that receives blood from the lower limbs and the greater part of the pelvic and abdominal organs; it begins at the level of the fifth lumbar vertebra on the right side, pierces the diaphragm at the level of the eight thoracic vertebra, and empties into the back part of the right atrium of the heart.

Inferiority complex It is a set of strong emotive feelings and ideas of lack of confidence.

Infertility It is an inability to conceive. It depends on production of healthy sperms by man and healthy eggs by woman. There should not be any mechanical obstruction of passage of sperm from reaching to ova. Then fertilised egg must be able to implant. *Male infertility* may be due to azoospermia or oligospermia. In some cases sperms even may be malformed. Orchitis or hypogonadism may cause it. Certain men may not be able to deliver normal healthy sperm in vagina due to impotency. *Female infertility* is caused due to failure of production of ova. It may be due to hormonal imbalance, tumour or ovarian cyst. Blocked fallopian tube may be due to inflammation of fallopian tubes. Fibroids and endometriosis may hamper plantation of fertilised ova. Chromosomal abnormality and allergy to her partner's sperms may result in infertility. As regards azoospermia nothing much can be done and artificial insemination by donor can only be the choice. If the sperm count is low artificial insemination by husband can be useful. In case of female infertility failure to ovulate requires ovarian stimulation with clomiphene. Microsurgery can repair damaged fallopian tubes. If cervical mucus is hostile husband's semen can be pushed by syringe directly into cervix.

Infiltrated When solution is deposited in tissue outside the vein.

Infiltration Escape of intravenous fluid into the tissue.

Infiltration analgesia It is to abolish the pain due to surgical intervention and to ease pain associated with trauma and injection of irritant drugs. The direct injection of drugs is given into the area to be incised and between bone ends in case of fractures.

Infiltration anesthesia It is done for minor surgery, suturing etc. Subcutaneous and intradermal infiltration is performed around the lesion.

Infirm Weak and feeble, as from disease or old age.

Infirmary A short-term inpatient and outpatient medial care facility, usually established by organizations or institutions for their personnel, such as one at a university or a military establishment.

Inflammation Symptoms of inflammation include redness, swelling, heat and pain. When body tissues are damaged mast cells release a chemical called histamine. Histamine increases blood flow to damaged tissue resulting in redness and heat. Capillaries start leaking blood which results in swelling. The pain or inflammation is the

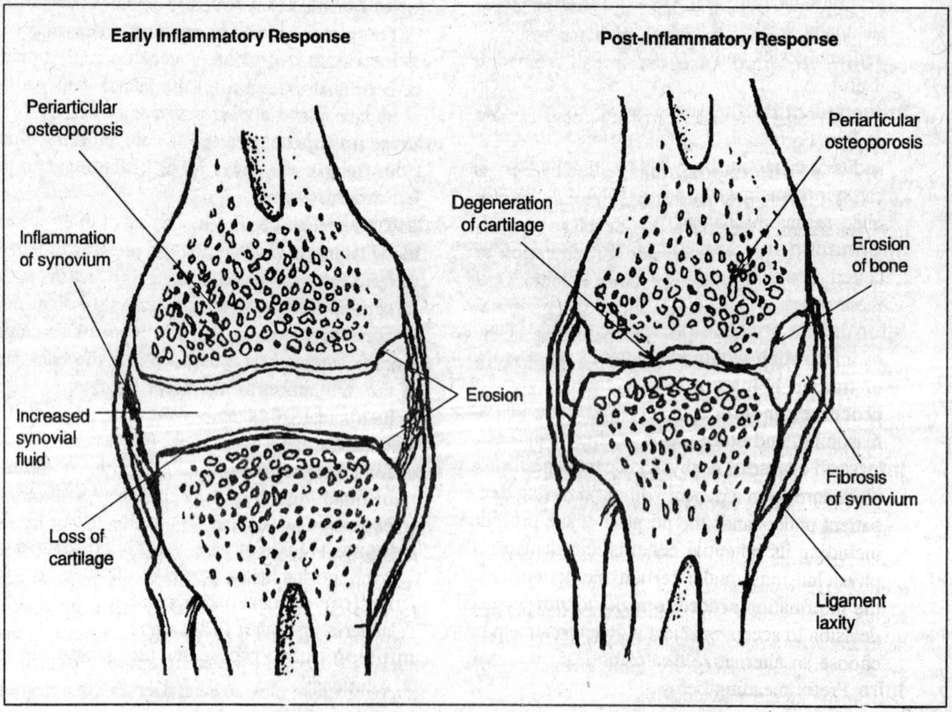

stimulation of nerve endings. This way we notice that inflammation is an essential part of body's response to injury or infection.

Inflammatory response Complex sequence of events involving chemicals and immune system cells that results in the isolation and destruction of foreign substances such as bacteria; symptoms include redness, heat, swelling, pain, and disturbance of function.

Inflatable penile proshtesis An artificial device placed into the corpora to achieve girth and rigidity for the treatment of impotence.

Inflatable splint Immobilizing device that becomes rigid when filled with air.

Influenza Commonly known as flu is the viral infection of respiratory tract. It results in headache, backache, muscle ache and severe weakness. Epidemics do occur in winter.

There are 3 types of virus A, B and C. A and B viruses cause chill fever, headache, muscular ache, loss of appetite and fatigue. Virus A causes mild disease similar to common cold. Symptoms generally clear up in 7 to 10 days. Cough persists for many weeks. There is no specific treatment and analgesics and high doses of vitamin C are useful.

Influenzal otitis There develops severe excruciating otalgia. Formation of blood, blisters in the external auditory canal on the tympanic membrane. Inner ear symptoms may occur. Paracentesis releases a pink, serous discharge.

Information It is formed by condensed chromatin coiled into spiral filaments (chromatids) joined more or less in the center by the centromere.

Information processing The storing and handling of information within a system, as in a computer or human being. In human beings, the chief processes include perceiving, remembering, reasoning, and other forms of thinking.

Informed consent A physician cannot perform any procedure upon a patient without ensuring that the patient understands the purpose of the procedure, including its potential benefits and dangers. The physician must make certain the patient has all the information needed to make a knowledgeable decision to accept or reject a given treatment or to choose an alternative treatment.

Infra Prefix meaning below.

Infrabony pocket Pocket with base below the level of the alveolar crest.

Infranculear lesion Lesion of the trunk of a cranial nerve.

Infranuclear lesion Lesion of the trunk of a cranial nerve.

Infraorbital foramen A hole or opening in bone found inferior to the border of the orbit; appears radiolucent.

Infrared lamp It is a red coloured electrical lamp which remits infrared rays. These are invisible rays of spectrum used for therapeutic purpose on patients for production of heat in tissue. Length of

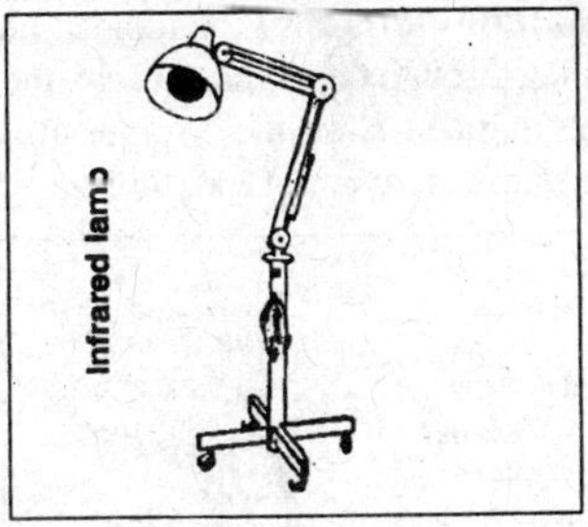

heat penetration is about 3 mm It is used to relieve muscle spasm and pain. It is used for promoting healing of bed sores, to dry casts and to relieve muscle stiffness and backache.

Infrared thermometers For use in ear measuring the temperature of tympanic membrane quickly.

Infrared treatment Infrared rays are radiant heat. These reach their peak output 30 seconds after switching on. Radiant heat lamps have a built-in reflector system which projects the waves from the lamp in a more or less parallel beam resulting in fairly evenly dispersed heating. It is applied for sprains/strains and contusions. Heat often has a soothing effect. It produces hyperaemia, relief of pain and tissue relaxation.

Infundibulum Funnel-shaped structure or passage, for example the infundibulum that attaches the pituitary to the hypothalamus; funnel-like expansion of the uterine tube near the ovary.

Infusate Volume of parenteral fluid infused a client over an established period of time.

Infusion A suspension resulting from boiling material in water; for example, tea.

Infusion pump Device that uses pressure to infuse solutions.

Ingestion The process of taking food or liquid into the body by way of the oral cavity.

Ingestive behaviour The action of taking food or fluid into the body as nourishment.

Ingrowing toe nail Ingrowing toe nail of big toe develops due to encasing sweaty feet in tight shoes. There may be family history. Many patients have wide, fleshy nail folds and thin nail plates. Wedge resection of nail is advised.

Inguinal Pertaining to the groin region.

Inguinal canal The passageway through which a testis passes as it descends from the abdominopelvic cavity to the scrotum.

Inguinoscrotal hernia It is an indirect hernial sac protruding through the inguinal canal, the external inguinal ring and down the scrotum. It is seen as a mass within scrotum. There will be a palpable

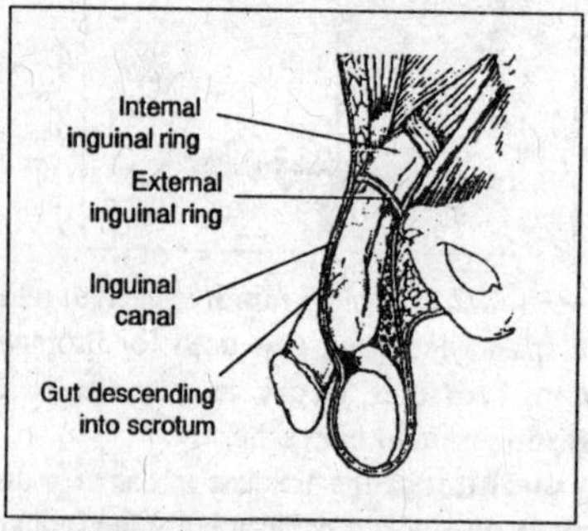

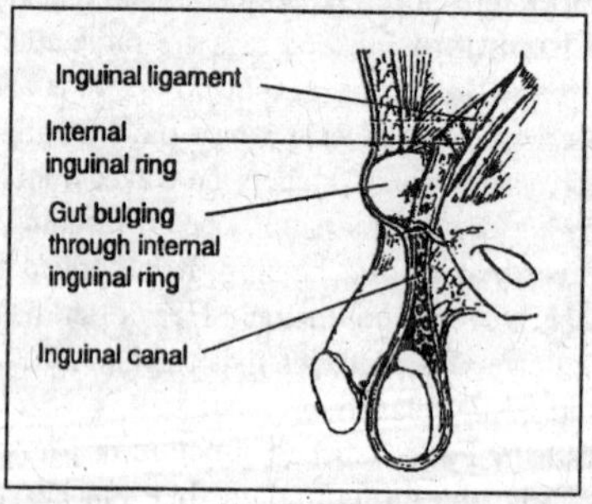

thickening along the entire course of spermatic cord. Hernia may consist of omentum or bowel or both. Auscultation over scrotum should reveal bowel sound. Transillumination may be possible. Herniation being strangulated is an emergency.

Inhalant abuse Volatile substance abuse.

Inhalant route Drug administration into the lower airways.

Inhalation It is the breathing in part of process of respiration. In it lowering of diaphragm takes place. Rib cage is drawn upwards and outwards.

Inhalation therapy Respiratory treatments that provide a mixture of oxygen, humidification, and aerosolized medication.

Inhaler Hand-held device for delivering medication to the respiratory passages.

Inhaling drugs A few drugs which are volatile are administered by inhalation to produce its effect. Examples are ether, tincture benzoin, tincture chloroform, etc. Ether and chloroform are anaesthetic drugs used by anaesthetist. Tincture benzoin inhalation is advised by ENT specialists for nursing care.

Inherited immunity Inborn immunity.

Inhibin A polypeptide hormone secreted by the testes that is believed to specifically exert negative feedback inhibition of FSH secretion from the anterior pituitary.

Inhibited gait Act of walking is slowed. Feet are pushed forward with evident difficulty often scraping audibly along the floor.

Inhibiting agents These inhibit the action of enzymes. Salts of mercury, silver and gold are especially potent in this respect. Certain preservatives such as chloroform, glycerol and thymol may inhibit some. Aldehydes destroy enzymes. An inactivated enzyme can often be reactivated by removing the inhibiting substance.

Inhibiting hormone Hormone produced by the hypothalamus that slows the release of anterior pituitary hormones.

Inhibition It is a conscious or unconscious wish to avoid taking a specific action because something unpleasant or immoral may happen. Behavioural evidence of an unconscious defence against forbidden instinctual drives; may interfere with or restrict specific activities.

Inhibitor Any agent that restrains or retards physiological, chemical, or enzymatic action.

Initial phase of treatment Conservative, nonsurgical actions taken as a first step toward elimination of periodontal disease.

Initial Swing Begins at toe off and continues untill maximal knee flexion occurs.

Initiation factor A protein factor that promotes the correct association of ribosomes with mRNA;

required for the initiation step of protein biosynthesis.

Initiative Willingness to try.

Initiative versus guilt The third stage of Erikson's psychosocial stages. The crisis here concerns the child's willingness to accept a given task. If the child's effort is supported, rather than the outcome, then initiative should be developed. If the child is unsuccessful and the parent blames the child for wasting materials, wasting time, or making a mess, then the child's initiative is reduced, and guilt is a likely outcome. This stage has implications for the next one, which concerns the development of real skills, rather than the imaginary play associated with initiative versus guilt.

Injection Act of forcing a liquid into the body by means of a syringe.

Injection molded polymers These are usually made of nylon or polycarbonate. Material is supplied as a gel in the form of patty which is to be heated and injected into a mold.

Injunction A court order preventing a person or entity from performing a certain act. A preliminary injunction is temporary and awarded prior to a trial on the merits of the case. A permanent injunction is awarded after the trial and is a final order.

Injury Damage or impairements resulting from an accidental or intentionally inflicted trauma.

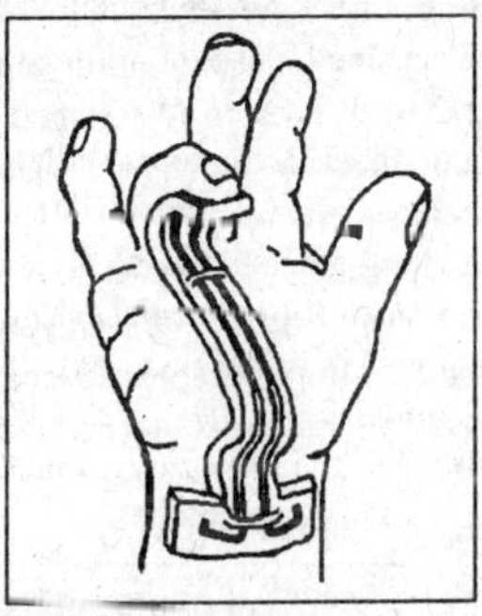

Injury severity score It is at trauma scale used to grade severity of multiple injuries based on abbreviated injury scale.

Injury to brachial plexus A high velocity impact of tip of shoulder with the road or a distraction between head and shoulder will tear the upper part of plexus. Lower part may be torn by forcible abduction of arm. The roots are often avulsed from cord. The tear lies proximal to the dorsal root ganglion and there is no possibility of regeneration of central axon. Upper plexus injuries involve the muscles innervated by the fifth and sixth cervical roots. Lower plexus injuries are characterised by involvement of finger flexors and small muscles of hand innervated by C_8,T_1.

Injury to ureter Risk of injury to ureters are enhanced in complicated vaginal deliveries associated with lateral uterine ruptures. Hematoma of lateral vaginal fornices and broad ligament may compress the lower ureter. Caesarian hysterectomy is associated with hazard of ureteral injury.

Injury to urethra It may develop due to compression necrosis of posterior urethra in difficult forcep application, symphysiotomy operation or fractured pelvis. Urethral injury may be asymtomatic. Urethral damage at the vesicourethral junction results in fistula with incontinence of urine.

Inlay A dental restoration made from metal, ceramic or composite that is cemented within the crown of a tooth and does not include a replacement of any cusps.

Inlet The upper limit of the pelvic cavity (brim).

Inlet of pelvis The space within the brim of pelvis.

InLoco Parent is Literally, in the place of the parents.

Innate Inborn; hereditary.

Innate immunity Immune system response that is the same upon each exposure to an antigen; there is no ability to remember a previous exposure to a specific antigen.

Innate intelligence The inborn capacity of an organism to heal itself and adapt to the dynamics of the external and internal environment; roughly synonymous with vis medicatrix naturae.

Inner cell mass Group of cells at one end of the blastocyst from which the embryo develops.

Inner liner An airtight rubber liner, forming the inside surface of tubeless tires.

Innervation The distribution of nerve fibres that end in association with a particular structure, region or organ.

Innervation ratio The number of muscle fibres per motor nerve fibre.

Innominate It consist of 3 parts pubis, ilium and ischium. They fuse together in the walls of acetabulum. Two pubic bones meet anteriorly to form pubic symphysis.

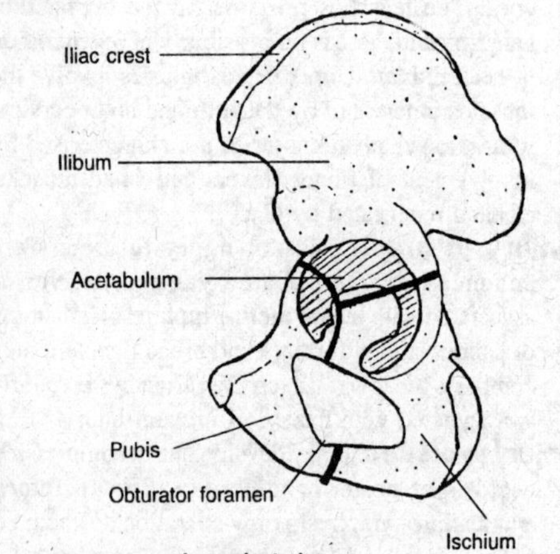

Innominate bone

Inoculation Introduction of microorganisms or some substance into living tissues or culture media; introduction of a disease agent into a healthy individual to induce immunity.

Inoculum The causative agent that is introduced into the body.

Inorganic Molecules that do not contain carbon atoms; originally defined as molecules that came from nonliving sources; the original definition is no longer valid, because carbon dioxide produced by living organisms is considered an inorganic molecule.

Inorganic nutrients Mineral elements are sometimes called inorganic nutrients.

Inotrope An agent that influences the contractility of muscular tissue.

Inotrophy The characteristic contractile state of muscular tissue.

Inotropic Influencing the contractility of muscular tissue.

Inotropic drugs Drugs which increase myocardial coutractility increasing cardiac output.

Inotropism The strength of cardiac muscle contraction.

Inpatient surgery Operative procedures performed on patients who are admitted to the hospital and are expected to remain for a period of time.

Inquest It is a form of court presided over by a coroner with or without of jury. It declares publicly the exact cause of death.

Insall-salvati ratio The ratio of patellar tendon length to the height of patella. The value is normally 1.03 ± 20%.

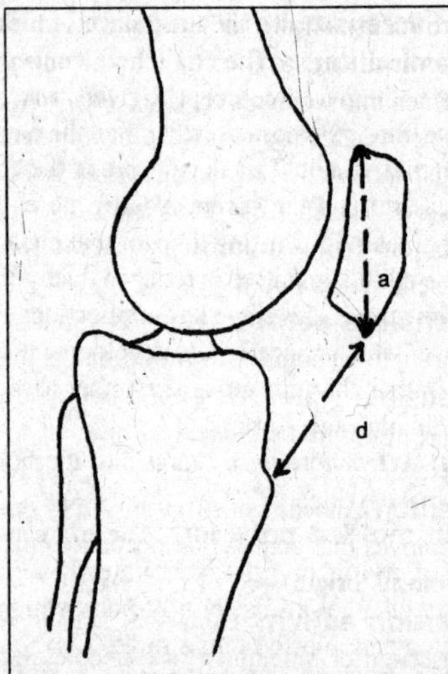

Insall-salvati ratio d/a

Insanity It is a condition of mental illness or instability in a person that he cannot be allowed to drive or handle firing arm and cannot be held legally responsible for his adverse actions.

Insect stings Bees, hornets and yellow jackets are able to sting. Insect venom contains inflammatory substance causing local pain, redness and swelling for about 2 to 3 days. In rare cases it may cause anaphylactic shock. Symptoms include severe itchy rash, dizziness, facial and throat swelling. As treatment stung area should be washed with soap and water and cold compression is applied. Antihistamine and analgesic anti-inflammatory drugs are given.

Insects Body is divided into 3, head, thorax and abdomen, lacking appendages.

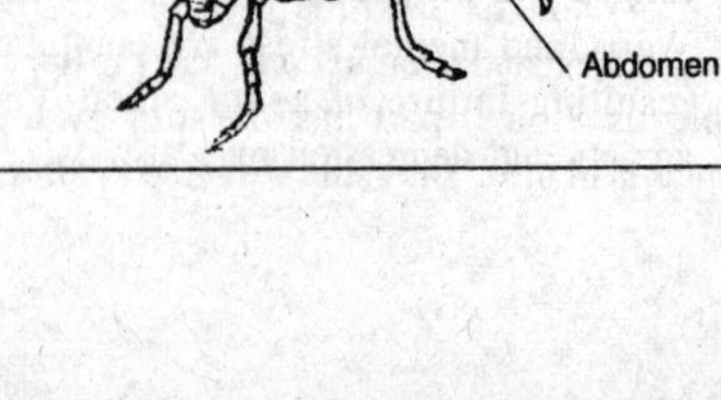

Insemination It is the ejaculation by a man of semen into woman's vagina for the purpose of becoming father. In case of non-feasiblity it can be introduced artificially known as artificial insemination.

Insemination, artificial It is an introduction of semen into woman's cervical canal so that she may conceive. It is done in case of impotent or sterile husband. Artificial insemination husband is the use of semen from husband only, while using semen from unknown person is artificial insemination donor.

Insensible perspiration Water lost invisibly through evaporation from the lungs and skin.

Insensible water loss Unmeasurable amount of pure water loss per day. It is normally 1200 mL at rest.

Insertion Attachment of a muscle to the bone that it moves that contraction occurs (as distinguished from its origin).

Insertion activity Electrical activity caused by insertion or movement of a needle electrode in a muscle. Can be described as normal, reduced, increased, or prolonged.

Insertion mutation A mutation caused by insertion of one or more extra bases, or a mutagen, between two successive bases in DNA.

Insertion sequence Specific base sequences at either end of a transposable segment of DNA.

Insertional inactivation The insertion of foreign DNA into a functional gene, causing its loss of function, or inactivation.

Insertional mutagenesis Intoduction of an in-frame addition of one or more codons, resulting in altered local or global properties of the proetin. Used to disrupt and thereby identify gene functions.

Insidious Coming on gradually or almost imperceptibly; as in a disease, the onset of which is gradual, with a more serious effect than is apparent.

Insoluble dietary fibers Dietary fibers that do not dissolve in fluids.

Insomnia It is an insufficient and troubled sleep. Many persons complain of increased day time fatigue and irritability.

Worry and mental stress are common cause in resulting failure of sound sleep. People with anxiety and depression may also cause difficulty in getting sound sleep. Withdrawal syndrome from hypnotic drugs may cause weeks of insomnia. Sleeping drugs should be taken on medical prescription only.

Inspection A physical examination skill involving the examiner's looking at external and internal body parts for physical characteristics.

Inspiration Moving air into the lungs; same as inhalation, opposite of exhalation or expiration.

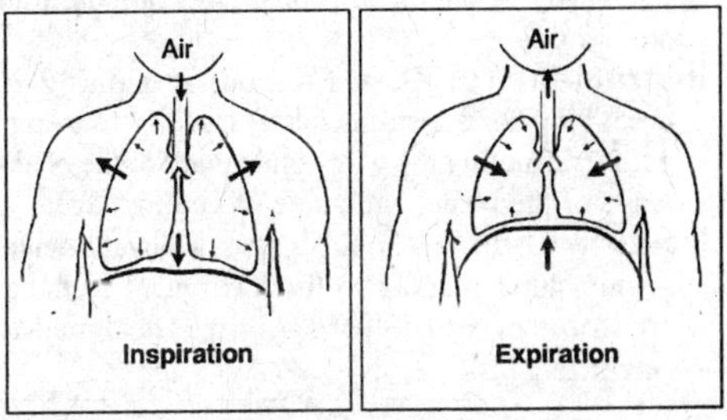

Inspiratory : expiratory ratio Ratio of inspiratory time; expiratory time. Usually it is 1:2.

Inspiratory capacity The total amount of air that can be inspired after a tidal exhalation. Inspiratory reserve volume plus residual volume equals inspiratory capacity.

Inspiratory center One of the two most important controls centers located in the medulla; the other is the expiratory center.

Inspiratory muscle The muscles that increase the size of the thorax, including the diaphragm and external intercostals, and allow air to rush into the lungs.

Inspiratory reserve volume The additional volume of air that can be taken into the lungs beyonds the normal tidal inhalation.

Instability index In congenital dislocation of hip, a measurement of the inherent tendency to dislocate.

Instant foods Dried foods that reconstitute rapidly when water is added.

Instillation of drugs The drugs applied to eyes, ears and nose comes under this group. The application of eyedrops, eardrops and nasal drops gives relief locally.

Instinct An inborn drive. The primary human instincts include self-preservation, sexuality, and—according to some proponents—aggression, the ego instincts, and hero or social instincts. Freud also postulated a death instinct. A descriptive term for a complex, unlearned adaptive response; an unlearned pattern or reflexes appearing in all members of species. If the adjustment were learned, the behaviour pattern would be called a habit.

Instrument exchange Method of transferring instruments between the dental assistant and operator; a method of reducing unnecessary movement at chairside to decrease fatigue, time and motion.

Instrument formula Method of naming of describing hand instruments. A three or four-digit number denoting the width and length of the blade, angle of the blade, and angle of cutting edge.

Instrument number Number assigned by the dental manufacturer relating to the instrument formula.

Instrumental behaviors Actions designed to complete a task.

Instrumental conditioning Conditioning in which the response is instrumental in achieving some end, such as obtaining food or escaping punishment. Often used as synonym for operant conditioning, but some psychologists make distinctions in the usages of these two terms.

Instrumentation Use of any tool, appliance, or apparatus; work performed with instruments.

Insula 'Island' of cereral cortex covered by the opercula.

Insulator A material that has a low thermal and electrical conductivity and, therefore, can be used to protect a sensitive structure from electric current or temperature changes.

Insulin It is the hormone produced by pancreas. It depends on the level of blood glucose. Increased blood glucose level stimulates the pancreas to produce sufficient insulin to neutralise it. Insulin

Sites of insulin injection

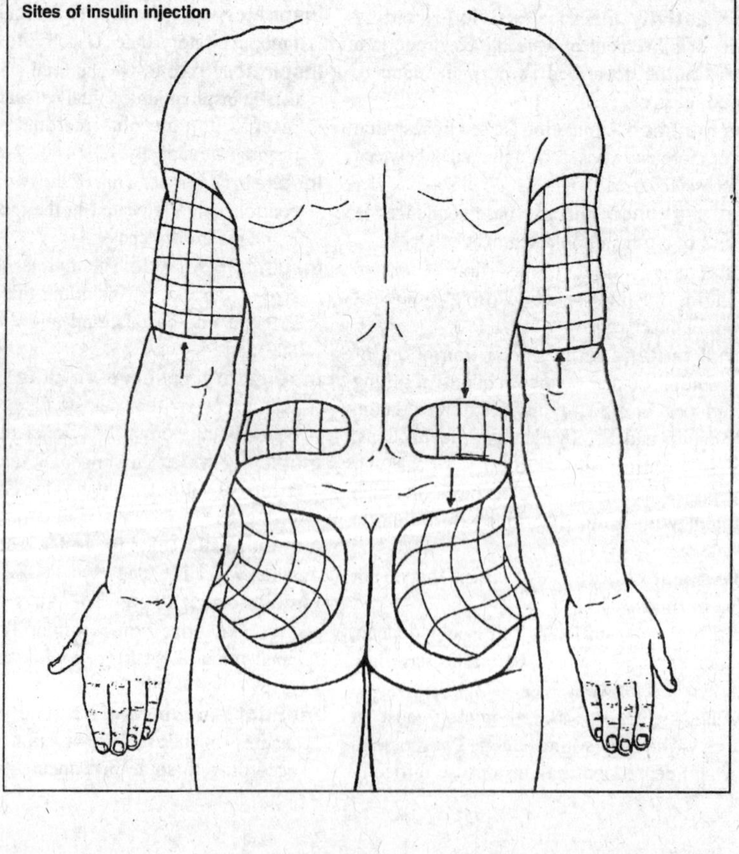

promotes absorption of blood glucose in liver and muscle cells. Diabetes mellitus develops when pancreas produces little or no insulin leaving glucose unutilised. In such cases oral hypoglycaemic drugs are given. If it fails then insulin has to be injected. Insulin may be injected before meals to act on increased blood glucose. Dose is to be regulated when there are variations in diet, exercise and during illness. High dose of insulin may cause hypoglycaemia.

Insulin and pregnancy Insulin therapy in diabetic pregnancy needs careful consideration of the course of diabetes in first half of pregnancy. In first half of pregnancy dose of insulin is reduced to 2/3rd. While in second half dose of insulin is increased by 70%.

Insulin intoxication Therapeutic dose of insulin with an inadequate diet is a common cause of hypoglycaemia. Excessive dose of insulin produces hypoglycaemia of varying durations depending upon the formulation used. After 1 to 8 hours of injections hypoglycaemia develops due to catecholamine release. These include tremors, shivering, tachycardia, palpitation, pallor and anxiety. Later patient develops lethargy and confusion.

Insulin resistance A glucose sparing mechanism that allows for an abundant supply of glucose for fetal use.

Insulin resistance syndrome A constellation of physiological and metabolic abnormalities.

Insulin shock therapy Injection of insulin in sufficient quantity to produce a coma, for which the patient recovers through administration of glucose. Used in treating certain psychotic conditions.

Insulin syringe These are small, narrow and accurately marked to able to push the desired dose of insulin.

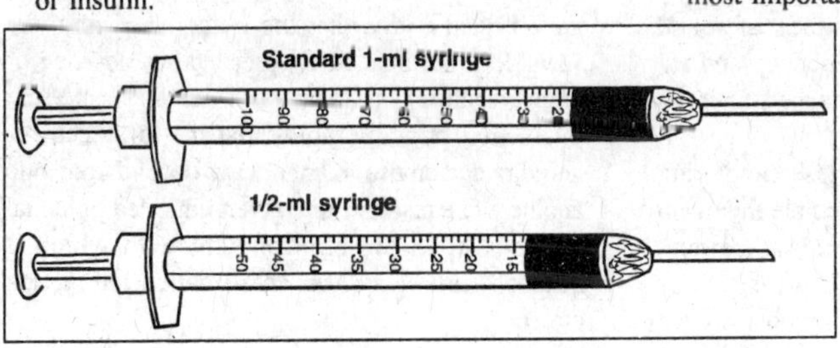

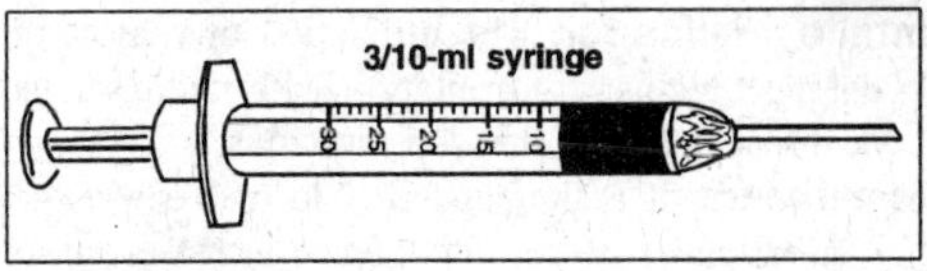

Insulinase An enzyme that accelerates insulin degradation.

Insulinklike growth factor (IGF) Small protein, produced by the liver and other tissues in response to stimulation by human growth hormones (hGH), that mediates most of effects of human growth hormone.

Intake and output Record of a patient's fluid intake and fluid loss over a 24 hour period.

Integrated approaches Combined methods of various forms of massage and bodywork styles.

Integrated model The result of combined concepts for several theories to formulate or provide direction for interventions when working with families.

Integration The useful organisation and incorporation of both new and old data, experience, and emotional capacities into the personality. Also refers to the organisation and amalgamation of functions at various levels of psychosexual development.

Integrity versus despair The last of Erikson's eight psychosocial stages. In this crisis, an elderly person attempts to find meaning in his or her memories. Integrity refers to integration, especially emotional integration; a person who finds meaning in past experiences is said to have achieved integrity, rather than despair.

Integument Skin and its appendages; hair, nails, and sweat and sebaceous glands.

Integumentary Relating to the covering of a body or body part.

Integumentary system The skin; the largest and most important organ in the body.

Inteligibility The degree of clarity with which one's utterances are understood by the average listener; influenced by articulation, rate, fluency, vocal quality, and intensity.

Intellectual health Use of intellectual abilities to learn and to adopt to changes in one's environment.

Intellectualisation The utilisation of reasoning defence against confrontation with unconscious conflicts and their stressful emotions.

Intelligence It is the capability to understand the concept and analyse. Intelligence increases up to the age of 6 years, then it stabilises. Intelligence quotient (IQ) as measured by intelligence tests continues to increase up to about 26 years of age. Most of the intelligence is inherited but social background and upbringing also affect it. Majority of persons have IQ between 80 and 120. IQ above 140 groups a person as most intelligent.

Intelligence A. Hebb's term for innate intellectual potential, which is highly heritable. This form of intelligence cannot be measured directly.

Intelligence B. Hebb's term for our observed intelligence, which is influenced by experience as well as other factors, such as disease, injury, or exposure to environmental toxins, especially during development. This intelligence is measured by intelligence tests.

Intelligence quotient (IQ) A numerical rating determined through psychologic testing that indicates the approximate relationship of a person's mental age (MA) to chronologic age (CA).

Intelligence test Generally, any method for measuring mental ability. There are group and individual tests of intelligence; the latter are likely to include nonverbal and verbal items. The chief individual tests are the Stanford-Binet Intelligence Scale and the Wechsler Scales.

Intelligibility enchancement Any method used to compensate the degradation of a speech signal due to different types of noise.

Intensifying factor The ratio of exposure time without an intensifying screen to that when a screen is used other conditions being the same.

Intensity The quantitative as contrasted with the qualitative aspect of stimulation or experience. For example, the magnitude or amplitude of sound wave as distinguished from its frequency and the brightness of a colour as distinguished from its hue.

Intensive care It is the process of close monitoring of patient which caters for an immediate treatment and to take care of fast deteriorating patient. Doctors and nurses posted in ICU are specially trained and alert professionally. It is most needed for patients who are on artificial ventilation, unconscious patients of ascending paralysis and myocardial infarction.

Intensive care unit (ICU) It is a ward having limited number of beds where seriously ill patients are kept. Extra specialised treatment, nursing care and other facilities are made available which are not available in general ward. It provides medical or surgical care in case of life-saving emergencies. A case of poisoning with deteriorating condition, heart patient, cerebrovascular accident patients and patients of major surgery are kept in ICU.

Intention tremor Tremor appearing during performance of purposive movements; associated with cerebellar disease.

Intentional The law punishes intentional acts more severely than negligent acts. A physician who negligently fails to obtain an informed consent may be used only if an injured patient can established that he or she would have refused the surgery had he or she been given sufficient information. A physician who intentionally deceives a patient about surgery can be sued for battery even if the surgery is a success.

Intentional food additives Substances purposely added to food products during manufacturing.

Intentional infliction of mental distress A cause of action for intentionally causing emotional suffering. The defendant must intend to cause the suffering, the defendant's conduct must be outrageous, and the suffering must be more than just the ordinary distress of daily living.

Intentional tort Lawsuit in which a plaintiff charges that the defendant committed a deliberately aggressive act.

Inter pedicular distance In AP X-Ray distance between two pedicles in millimeter.

Interaction principle The concept of reciprocal influences between or among two or move variables; the idea that the outcome of any one variable is influenced by presence or absence of other variables. In the nature-nurture issue, the interaction principle holds that the influences of heredity and environment always depend upon one another. The result of any given inherited potential depends upon the environment with which it interacts and *vice versa*. Also called interaction effect.

Interactive effect When the influence of one variable depends on another variable. The influences are not independent of one another; they combine to produce an outcome which is not predictable on the basis of each factor separately. Food A may be mildly nutritious; when consumed together, these foods may be more nutritious than the sum of their independent nutritive value.

Interalveolar septum The tissue between two adjacent alveoli; comprises the alveolar epithelium, the capillary epithelium, and the interstitial space.

Interatrial septum The wall separating the right and left atria.

Intercalated disc Connection between cardiac muscle cells; important in co-ordinating the contractions of cardiac muscle cells; contains gap junctions which allow action potentials to pass from one cardiac muscle cell to adjacent cardiac muscle cells. Cross striations and unique dark bands that are found in cardiac muscle fibers.

Intercellular substance The matrix or material between cells that largely determines tissue types.

Interceptive orthodontics It is an extension of preventive orthodontics that may include minor local tooth movement in an otherwise normally developing dentition.

Intercompetition massage Massage provided during an athletic event.

Intercondylar Between the condyles, in humerus and femur.

Intercostal Between the ribs.

Intercostal muscle The respiratory muscles located between the ribs.

Intercostal nerve block Used for pre and post operative analgesia and in fracture rib.

Intercurrent Occurring during the course of an existing process.

Interdental Situation between the proximal surfaces of adjacent teeth.

Interdental aids Devices used to mechanically remove certain dental deposits from tooth surfaces.

Interdental papilla Part of the gingivae filling the interproximal spaces between adacent teeth, consisting partly of free and partly of attached gingivae.

Interdependence The mutual dependence of two or more persons on one another.

Interdigital neuroma Compression and shearing forces at the bifurcation of neurovascular bundle between the metatarsal heads can lead in the formation of a benign tumour of fibrous tissue

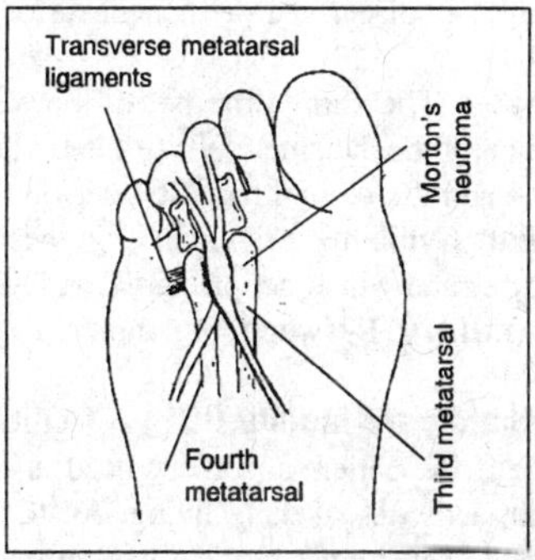

called Morton's neuroma. Pinching and squeezing occur in the hypermobile foot. Chief complaint is that of burning or electric shock sensation in the forefoot that radiates into toes. Lesion is usually located between the third and fourth metatarsals.

Interdisciplinary team A team consisting of two or more disciplines of professions that are considered distinct.

Interface, Implant The surface of an endosteal or subperiosteal implant in contract with its investing tissues.

Interface, Tissue The border to the tissues in contact with the dental implant.

Interferon It is a protein, moderately stable and changes to pH (2-10). It is non-toxic and poorly antigenic if at all. Interferon is inactivated by proteolytic enzyme such as trypsin and pepsin but not by lipase. It is non-dialysable. Interferon does not interfere with antibody formation. Non virulent or poorly adopted viruses are better interferon inducers than are virulent strains. Togaviruses and vesicular stomatitis virus are efficient interferon inducers. Three principal types of protein (alpha, beta, gamma) naturally produced by virus-infected host cells; induce uninfected host cells to synthesize antiviral proteins that inhibit intracellular viral replication.

Interim denture Dental prosthesis to be used for a short interval for reasons of esthetics, mastication, occlusal support, convenience, or to condition the patient to the acceptance of an artificial substitute for missing natural teeth until more definitive prosthetic therapy can be provided.

Interim dressing Material placed in a tooth or on oral tissues to provide protection and function until healing takes place or a permanent restoration is placed.

Interkinesis The short time period between the formation of the daughter cells of the first meiotic division and the second meiotic division.

Interleukin Cytokines principally synthesized by leukocytes and which act primarily on leucocyte.

Intermaxillary Between the maxilla and the mandible.

Intermediate care facility (ICF) A facility that is suitable if the patient's primary need is for help with the activities of daily living. An ICF is not required to have registered (skilled) nurse on duty at all tiems.

Intermediate cells May be undifferentiated forms of ciliated or secretory cells in the tracheal epithelium.

Intermediate fetal death Delivery of dead fetus between 20 and 28 seeks of gestration.

Intermediate hospital A medium to large community hospital that has a considerable amount of the latest technology but less research and investigational activity than a tertiary medical center.

Intermediate host The host in which a parasite having an indirect life-history pattern underoges development but would not normally attain sexual maturity.

Intermediate plateau A flat section in a performance curve, indicating no further improvement, attributable to a motivational failure, fatigue, or even the refinement of skills, Later there is further progress, as indicated by a rise in the curve.

Intermenstrual bleeding Any bleeding or spotting between menses.

Intermittent fever Temperatures alternate between pyrexia and normal or subnormal temperatures within a 24-hours period; an intermittent fever with fluctuations between high and low temperatures is termed a hectic fever.

Intermittent acute porphyria There will be severe burning or colicky pain, vomiting or constipation suggesting as acute abdominal emergency but surgery is not to be done. There is no abdominal rigidity or rebound tenderness. No leucocytosis develops and urine darkens on standing. Infection precipitates the attacks. Neurological symptoms include delirium, convulsions and coma.

Intermittent claudication It is manifested by dull ache or sharp constricting pain with spasticity and cramping of the involved muscles, particularly those of lower extremity, during activity but is relieved by rest. It is seen in peripheral atherosclerotic disease, thromboangiitis obliterans, and arterial hypertension.

Intermittent feeding Gradual instillation of liquid nourishment four to six times a day

Intermittent fever Intermittent fever is called when body temperature remains elevated but falls to normal or subnormal level once or more in 24 hours as seen in certain malaria and septicaemia.

Intermittent infusion Parenteral administration of medication over a relatively short period.

Intermittent mandatory ventilation A mode of mechanical ventilatory assistance; the mandatory preset ventilator breath is delivered at a preset regardless of the phase of the patient's breathing efforts.

Intermittent Mechanical Traction It involves a mechanical device that alternatively applies and release the traction for brief intervals, usually from 15-60 seconds.

Intermittent positive pressure breathing (IPPB) Assisted ventilation of the lungs with a mechanical apparatus; primarily used for patients who are able to breathe spontaneously but have an inadequate depth of respiration.

Intermittent pulse Pulse that occasionally skips a beat.

Intermittent reinforcement Any schedule of reinforcement in which less than 100 per cent of the organism's correct responses are reinforced; noncontinuous reinforcement.

Intermittent venous access device Sealed chamber that provides a means for administering intravenous medications or solutions on a periodic basis.

Internal Toward the center, away from the surface of the body.

Internal ballotment It is the most useful sign felt per vagina between 16th-28th week pregnancy

PLATE-1

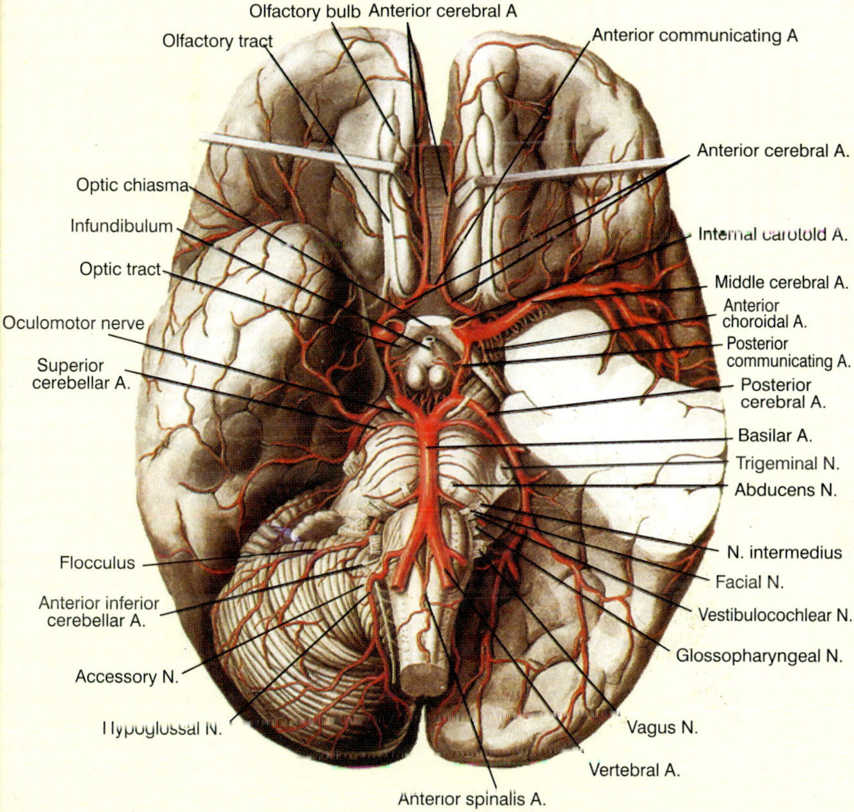

BRAIN

PLATE-2

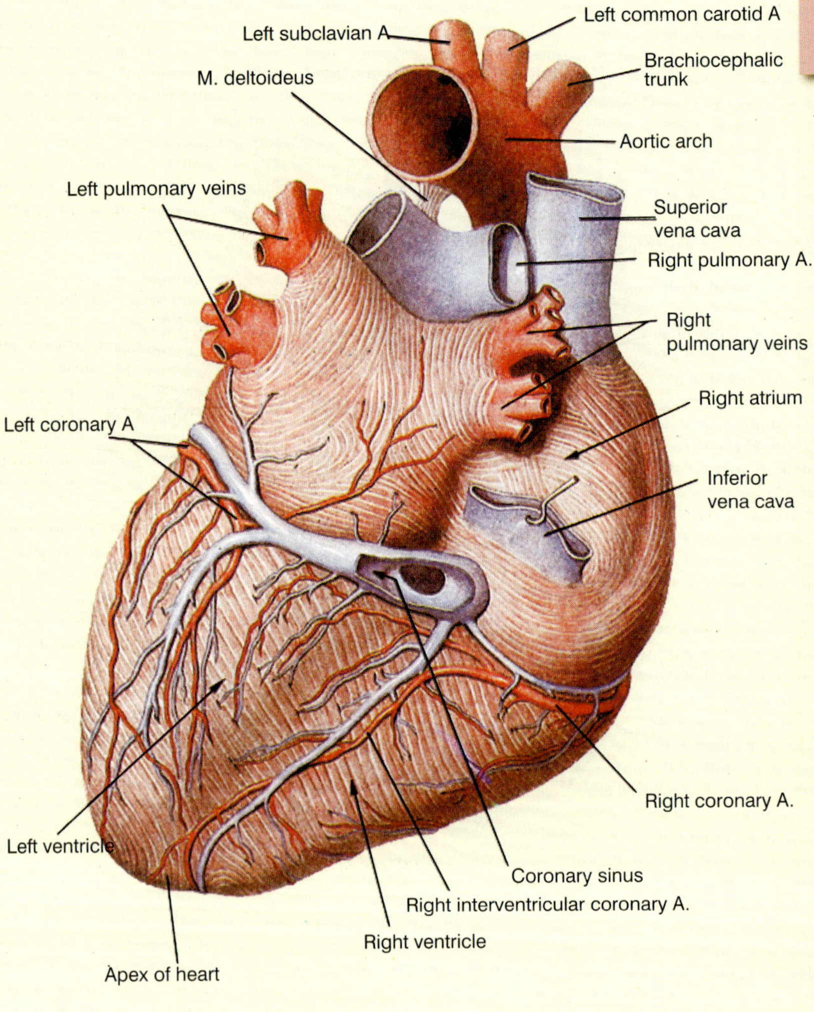

HEART VESSELS

PLATE-3

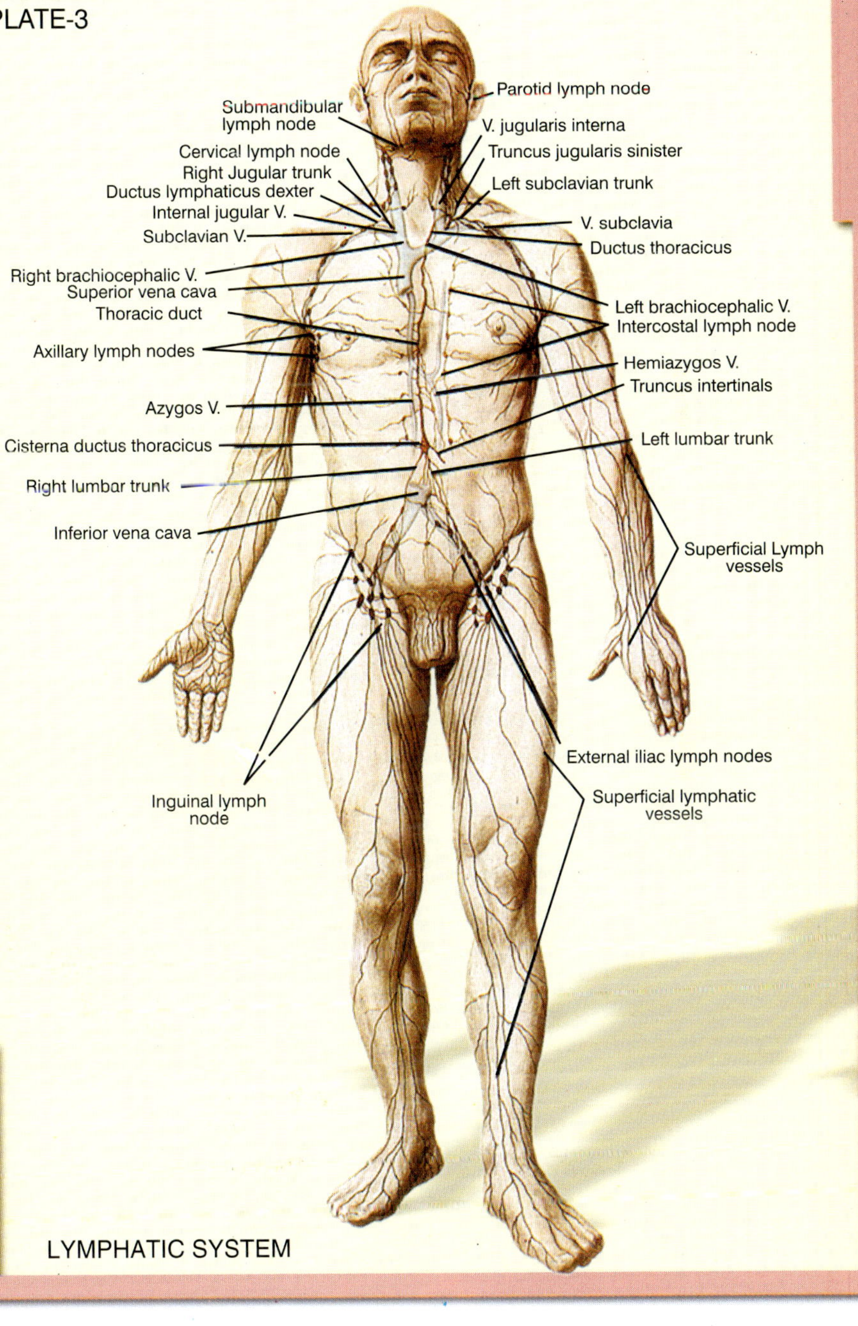

LYMPHATIC SYSTEM

PLATE-4

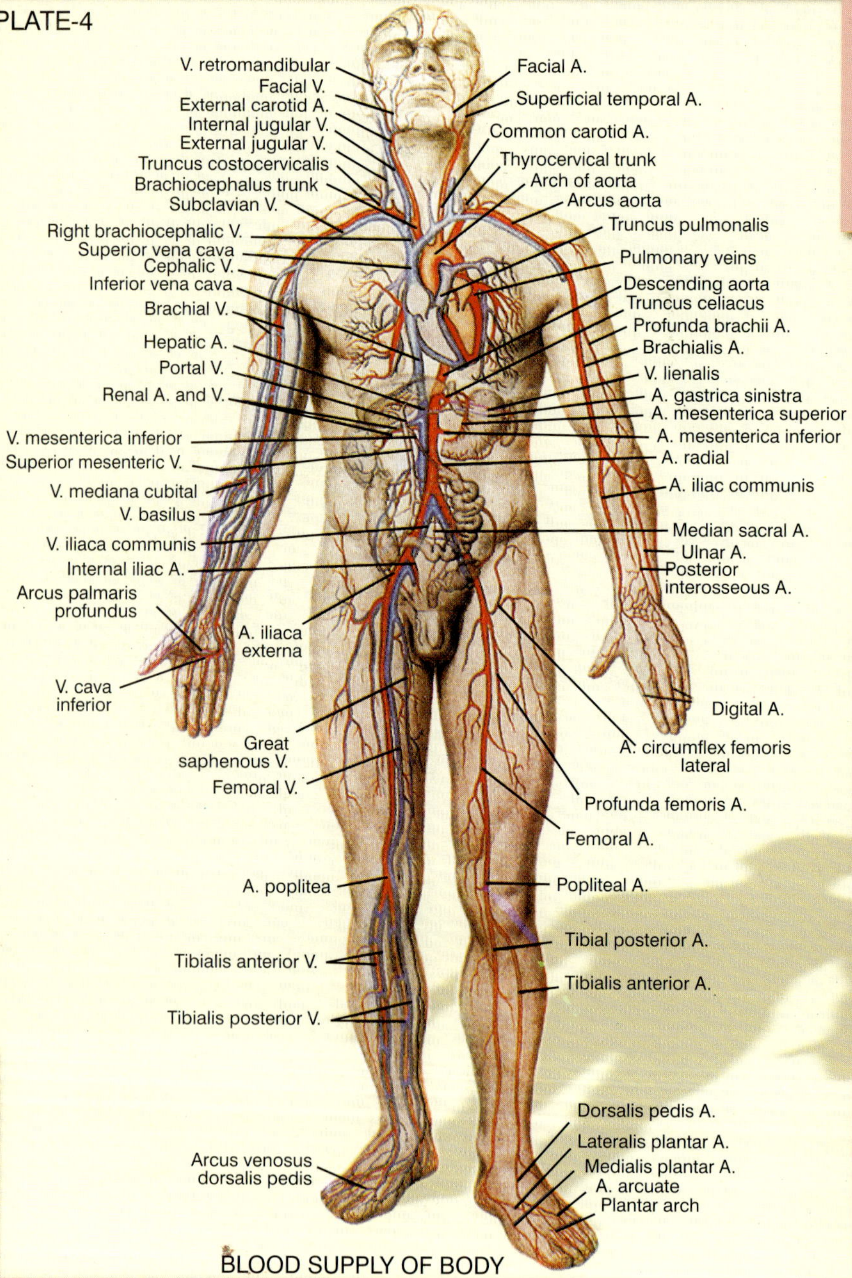

BLOOD SUPPLY OF BODY

PLATE-5

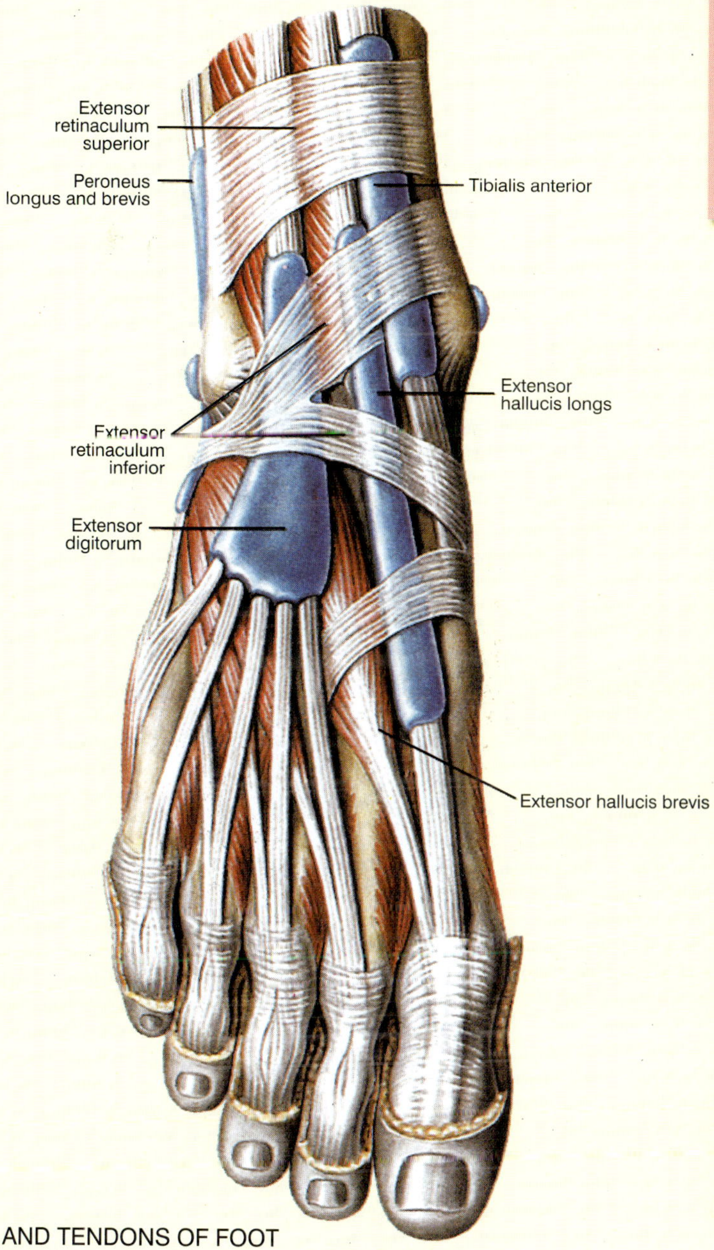

MUSCLES AND TENDONS OF FOOT

PLATE-6

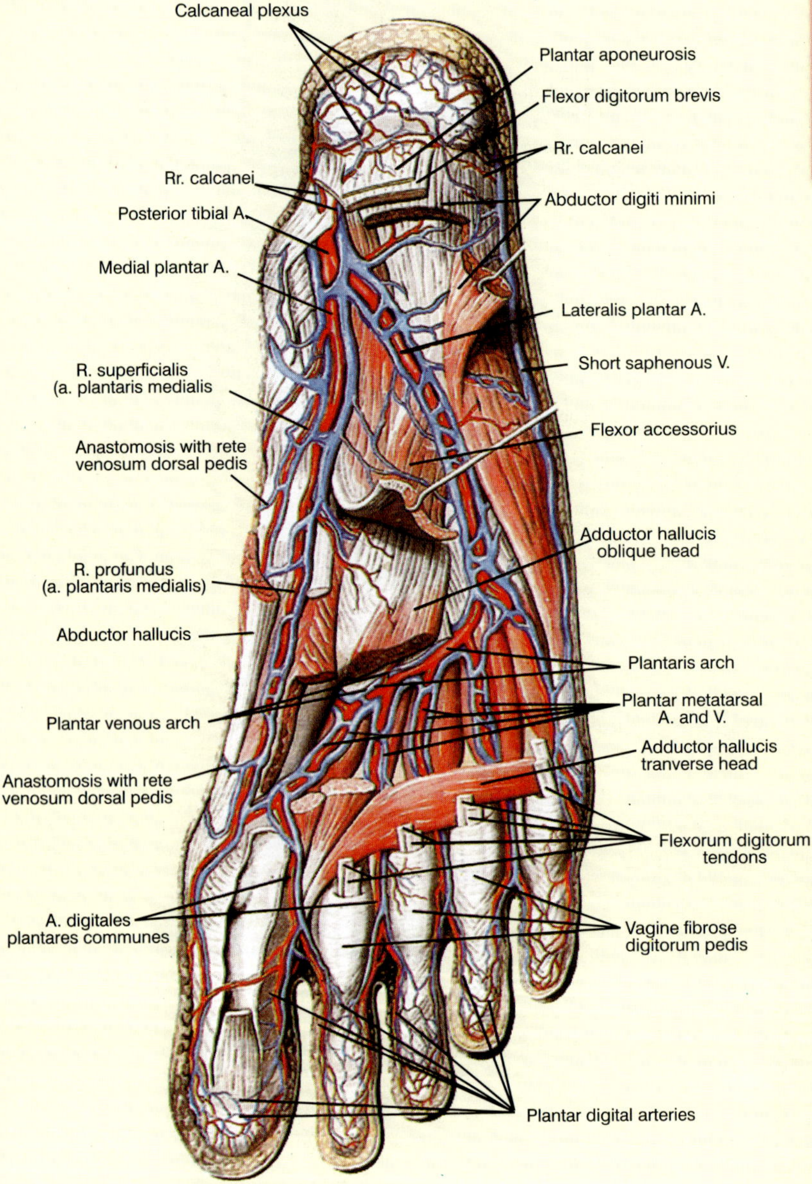

BLOOD VESSELS OF FOOT

PLATE-7

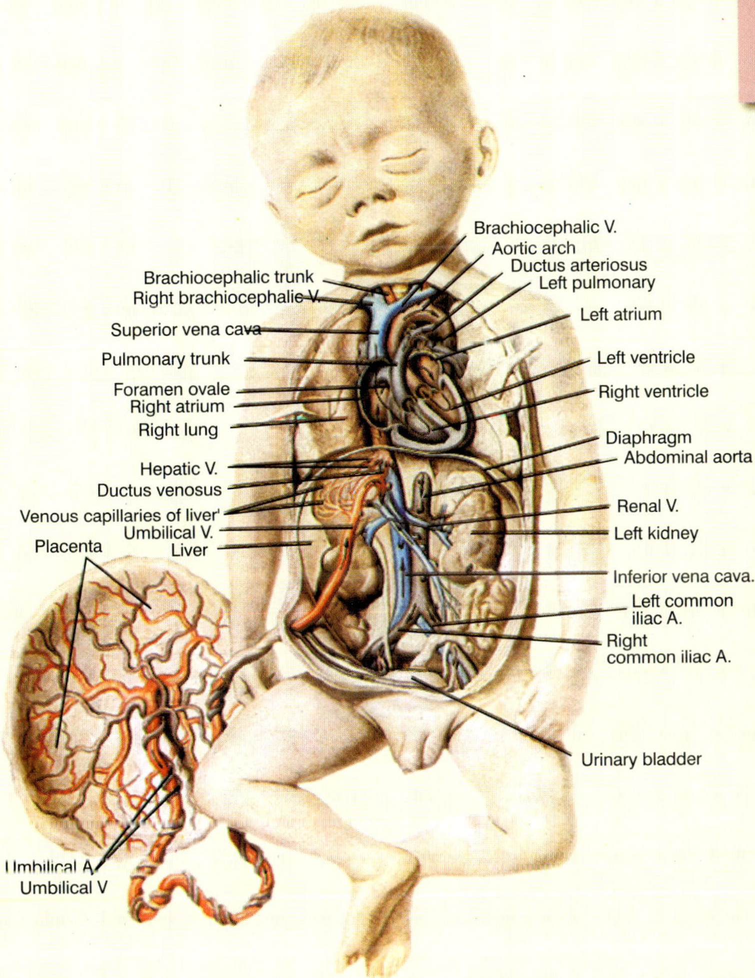

FETAL VESSELS

PLATE-8

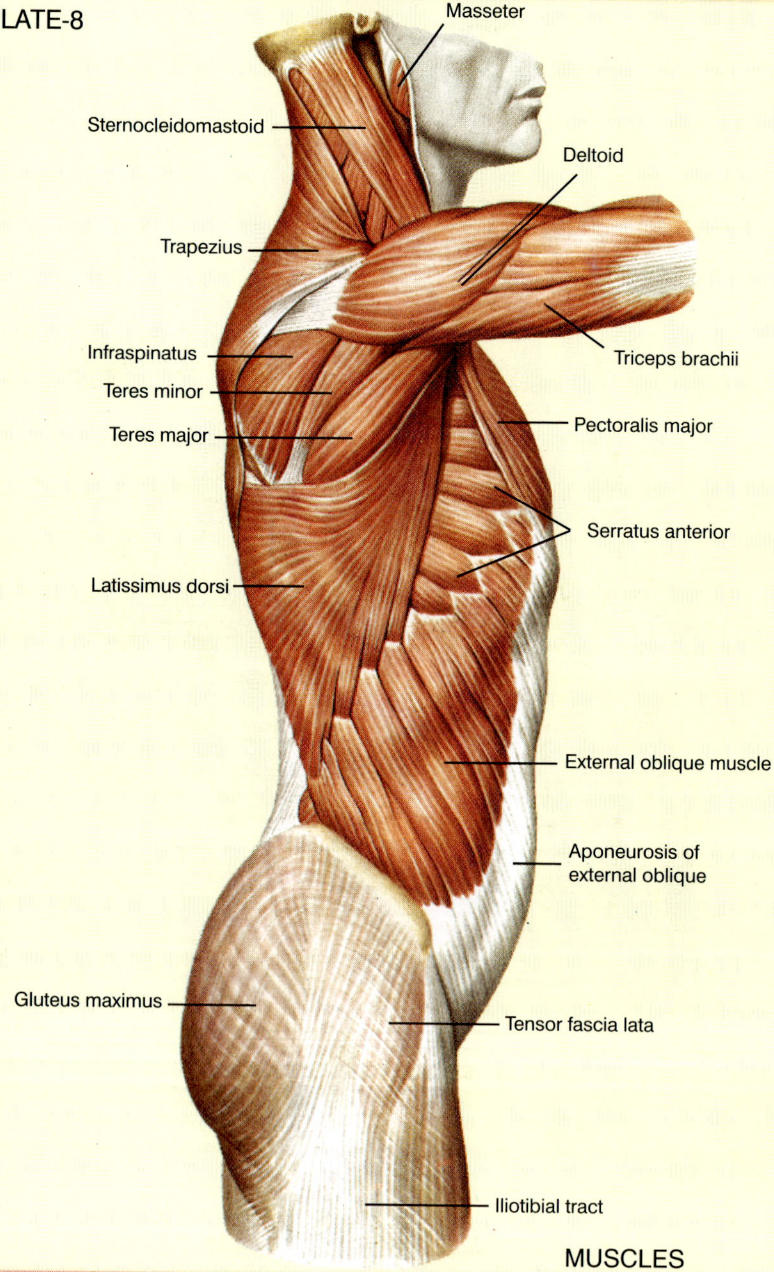

MUSCLES

PLATE-9

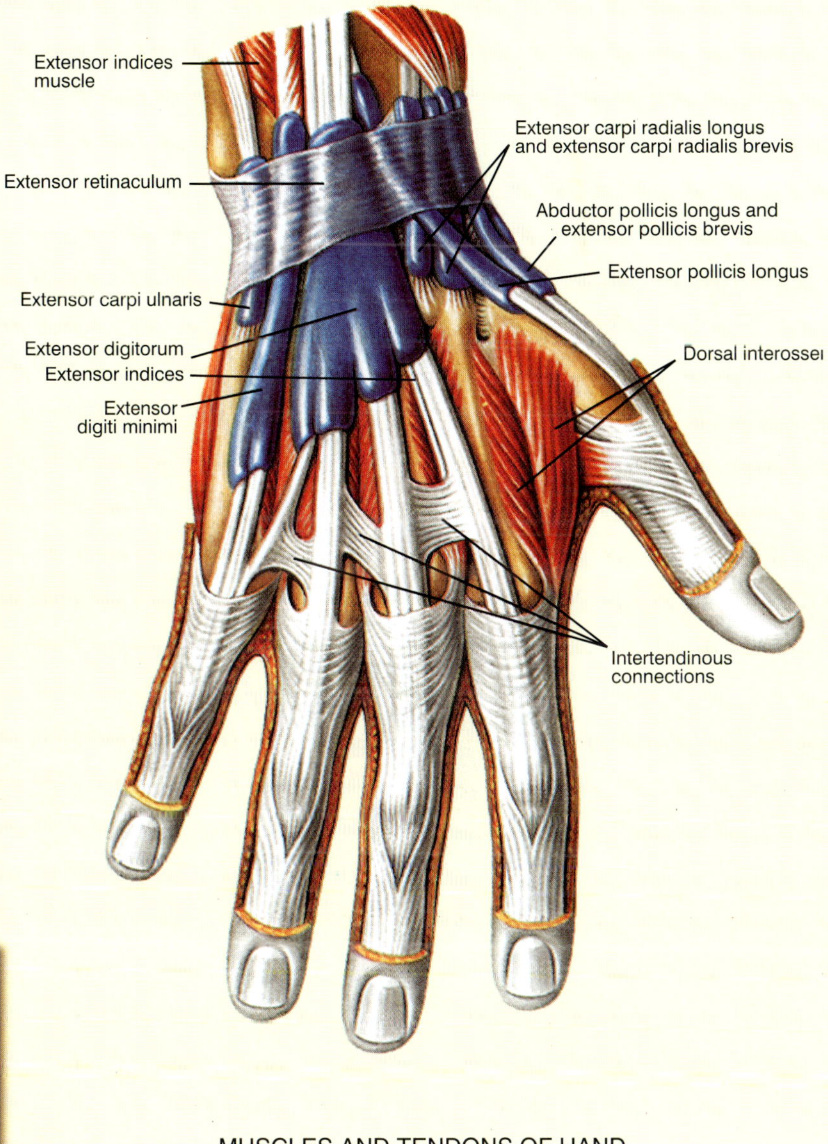

MUSCLES AND TENDONS OF HAND

PLATE-10

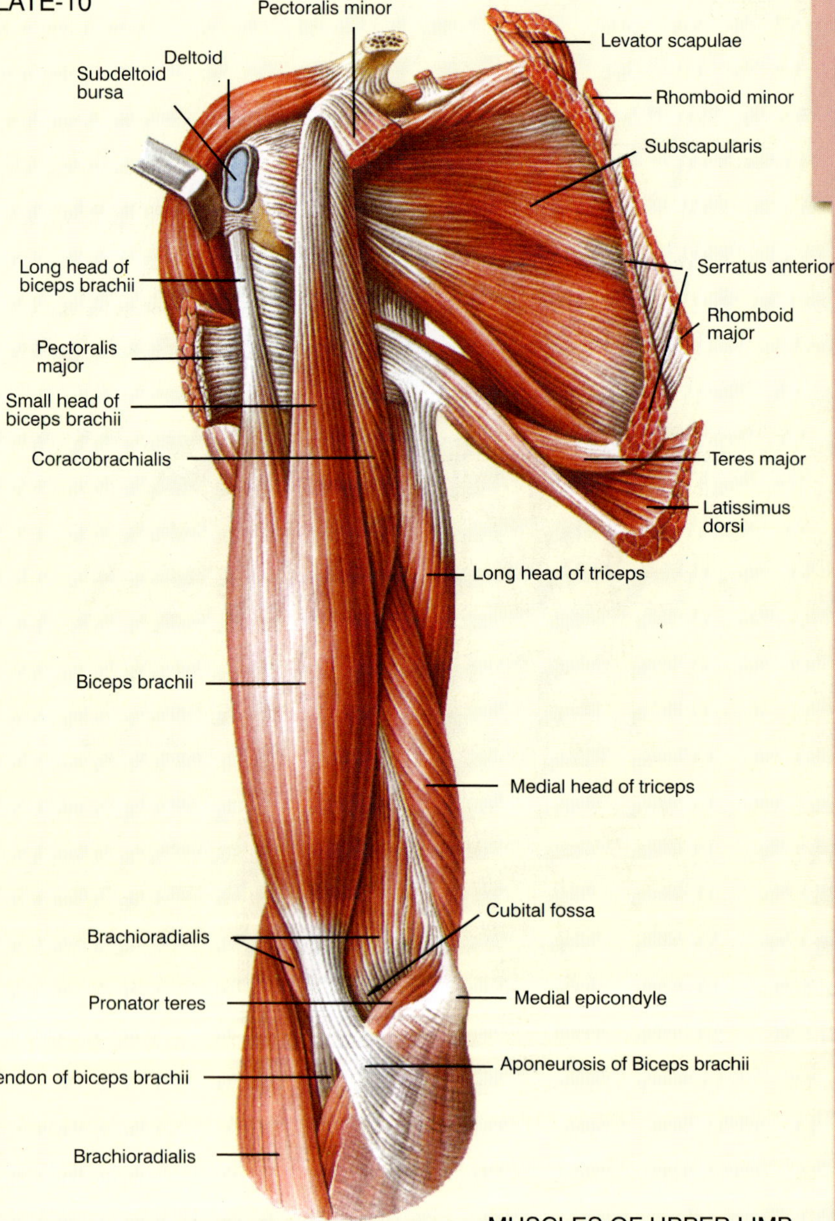

MUSCLES OF UPPER LIMB

PLATE-11

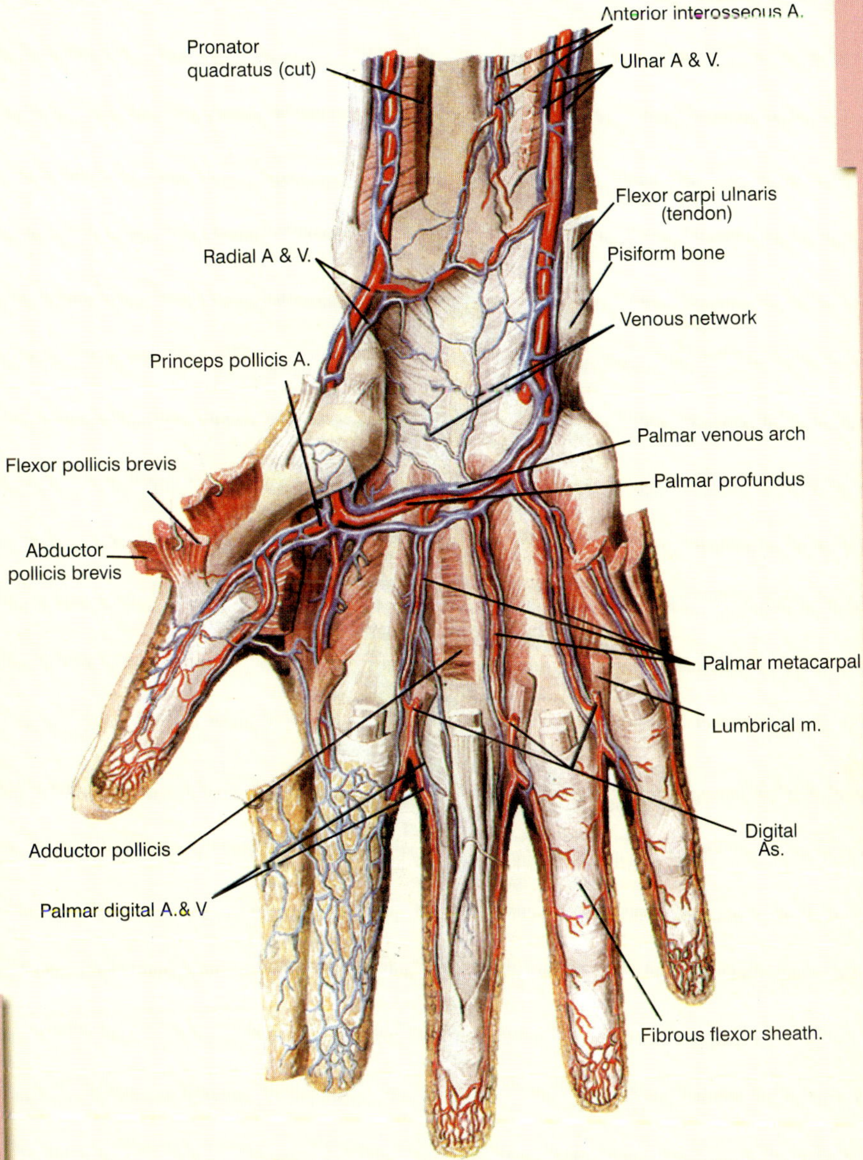

ANATOMY OF HAND

PLATE-12

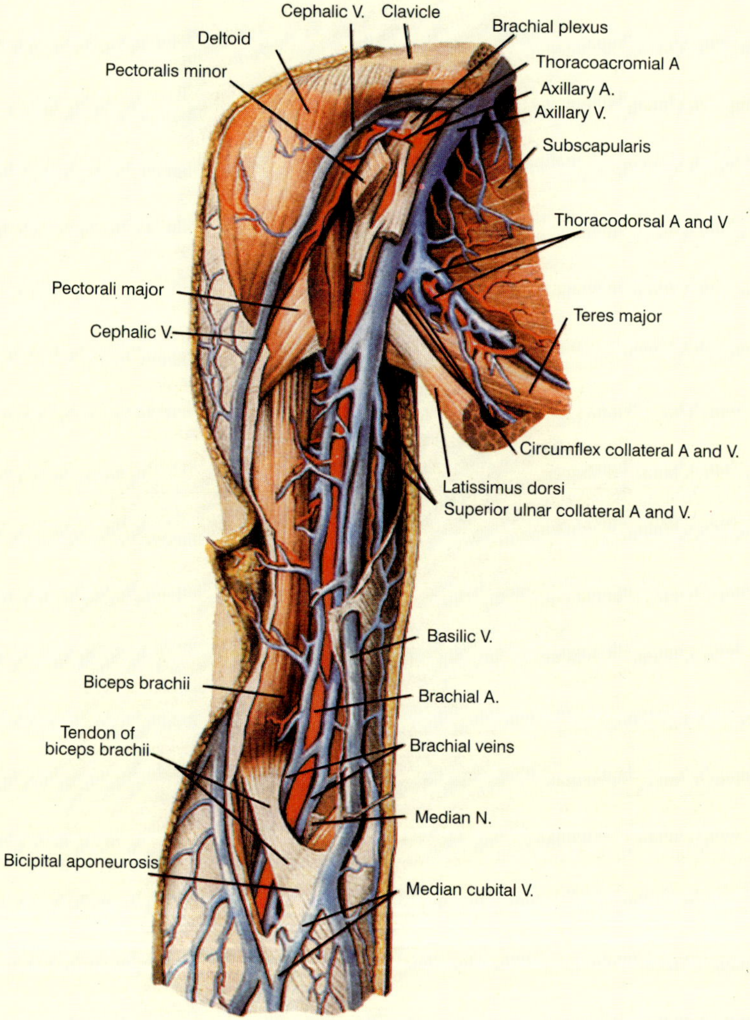

MUSCLES AND BLOOD SUPPLY OF UPPER ARM

PLATE-13

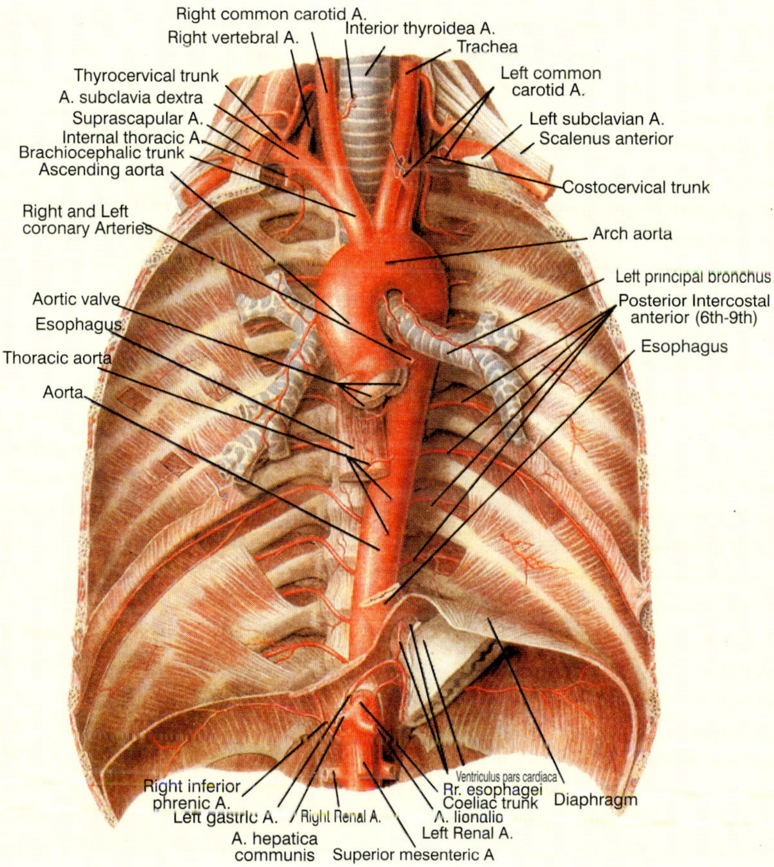

BLOOD VESSELS CHEST

PLATE-14

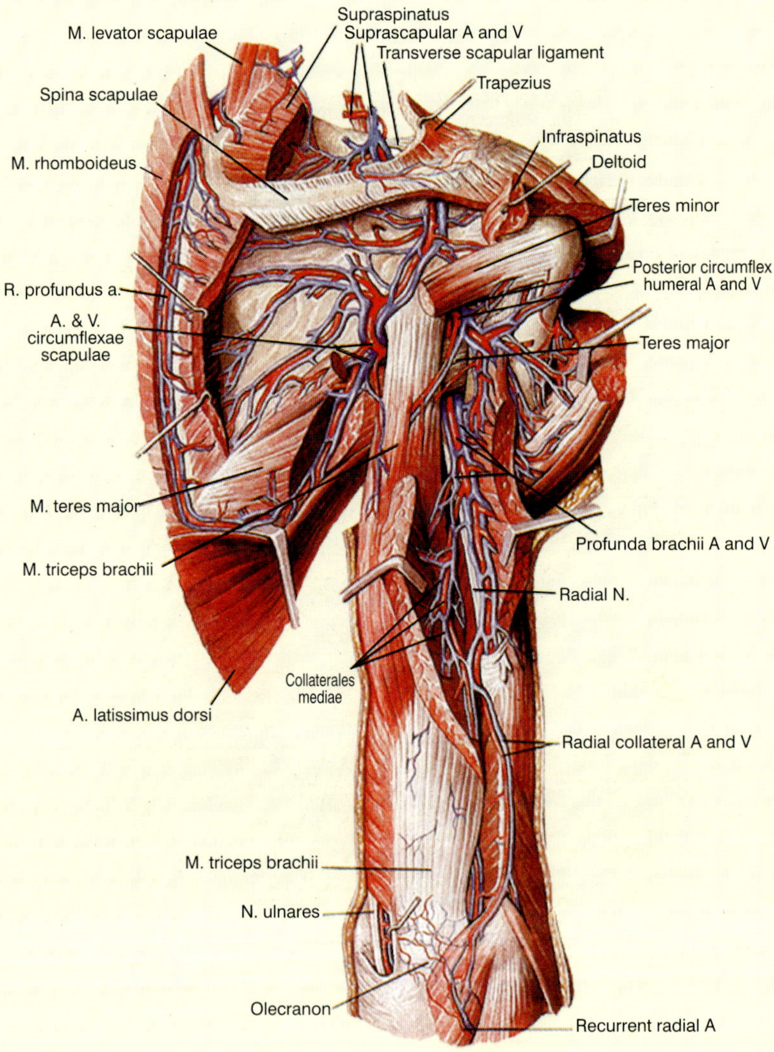

BLOOD VESSELS UPPER ARM

PLATE-15

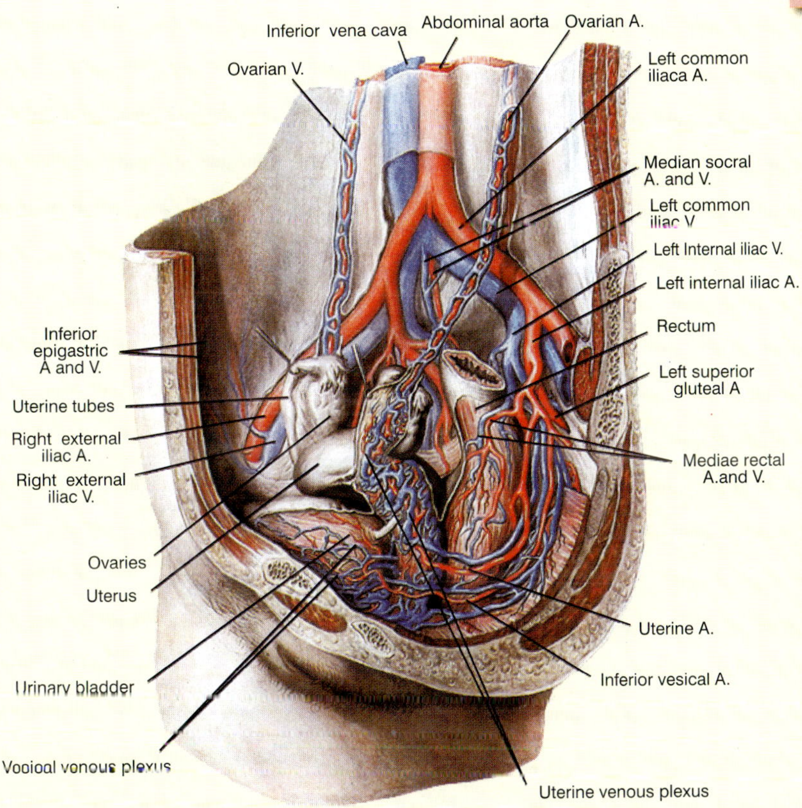

BLOOD VESSELS IN PELVIS

PLATE-16

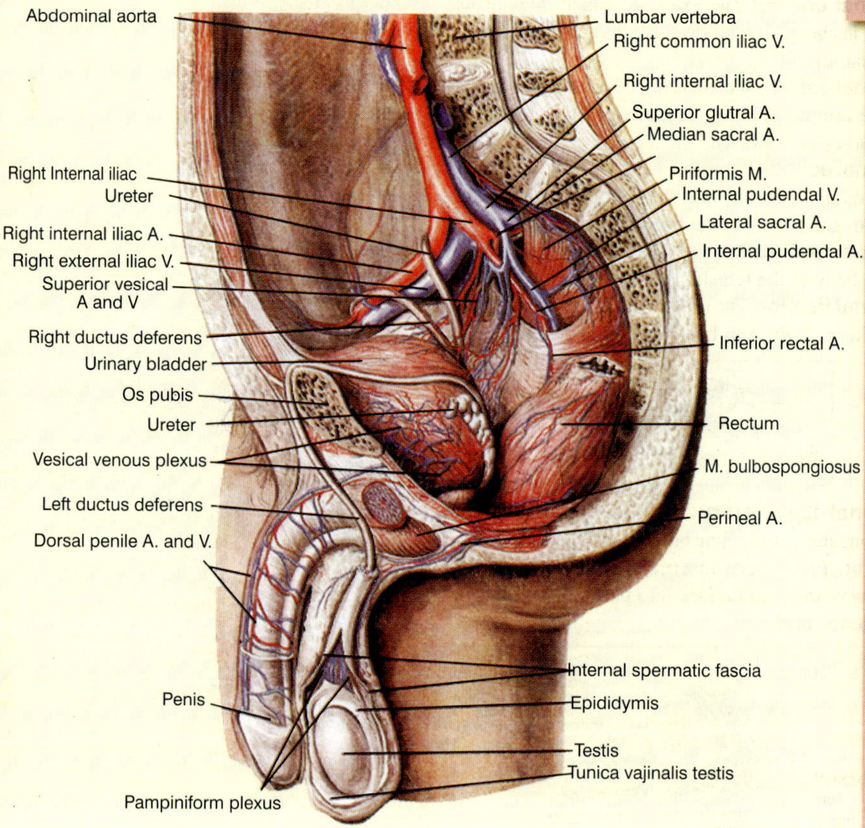

PELVIS VERTICAL SECTION

when a sharp tap at the cervix causes fetus to float upwards in the amniotic cavity. When the fetus sinks back the vaginal fingers can feel the rebound of the fetus.

Internal clock A neural structure, such as the suprachiasmatic nucleus, that determines the time at which a behavior will occur.

Internal control The extent to which individuals are in charge of their own actions and the outcome of an activity.

Internal ear The inner ear or labyrinth, lying inside the temporal bone, containing the organs of hearing and balance.

Internal echoes Ultrasound reflections from tissues of different density within an organ. It may arise from gall stones or debris within abscess.

Internal fertilization Fertilization occurring within the body of the female.

Internal fixation The use of metallic or other device to keep the broken bone parts in alignment.

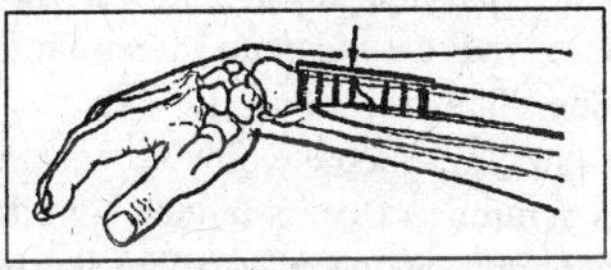

Internal iliac artery The common iliac artery bifurcates at the pelvic brim opposite the sacroiliac joint. From here internal iliac artery passes downwards and divides into posterior and longer anterior division.

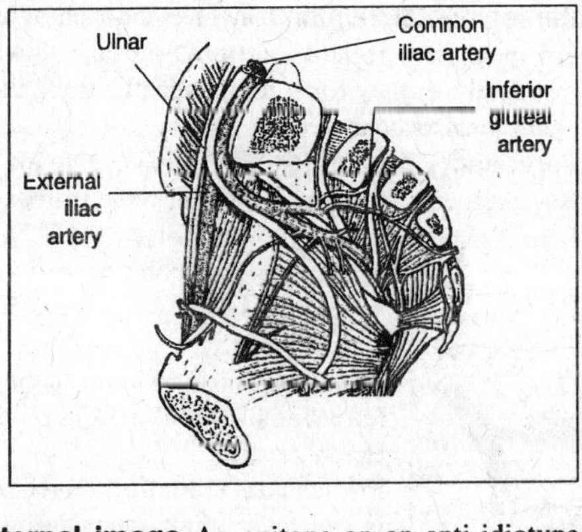

Internal image An epitope on an anti-idiotype which binds in a way that structurally and functionally mimics the antigen.

Internal nervous system A functional division of the nervous system that controls the body's internal organs; also called the autonomic nervous system

Internal oblique The middle layer of the anterolateral abdominal walls.

Internal oblique ridge A linear prominence of bone located on the internal surface of the mandible that extends downward and forward from the ramus; appears radiopaque.

Internal os The length, dilatation and texture of cervix before the onset of labour is extremely variable. It may be long and undilated. A ripe cervix at the time of term is soft, effaced slightly and patulous. At labour cervix is shortened and the canal opens at both ends, the internal os being wider than external. Dilatation of internal os is of necessacity where head of fetus is to be engaged.

Internal podalic version Operation is performed under anesthesia by introducing a hand into the uterus through a well dilated cervix grasping and pulling down a leg and displacing a head towards the fundus.

Internal receptor The space within the coronal portion of a conventional root form implant body into which components are fastened.

Internal resorption A regressive alteration of tooth structure that occurs within the crown or root of a tooth; appears as a radiolucency.

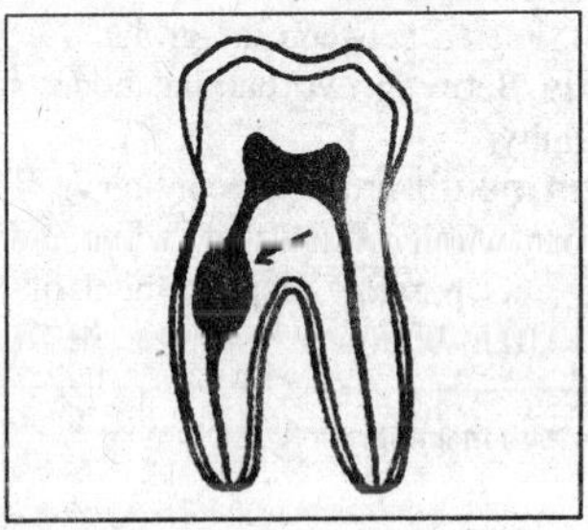

Internal respiration The exchange of respiratory gases between blood and body cells.

Internal rotation The process in the delivery of a baby in which the fetal head is rotated so that it enters the pelvis in the transverse position and exists in the anteroposterior position.

Internal validity Concerns whether the independent variable is the probable cause of changes in the dependent variable. Is is present when the results of a study are true and meaningful for the participants.

Internarial Situated between the nostrils.

International units Used as a measure of comparative potency of vitamin.

Internet Network of computers linked via telephone and other communication lines spinning the world.

Interneuron A neuron interposed between a sensory neuron and a motor neuron; thus, in mammals, interneurons constitute most of the neurons of the brain.

Interneuron nerves That conduct impulses from sensory neurons of motor neurons.

Internodal atrioventricular tracts or bundles Specialized conduction pathways between the sinoatrial and atrioventricular nodes.

Internuncial 'Messenger between'. Refers to small connecting neurons.

Interobserever variability A measure of disagreement betweenor among different observers.

Interocclusal Between the occlusal surface of maxillary and mandibular tooth.

Interocclusal clearance The difference in the height of face when mandible is at rest and when teeth are in occlusion.

Interoceptors Sensory receptors that respond to changes in the internal environment (as opposed to exteroceptors).

Interorbital Situated between the orbits.

Interosseous Between two parallel bones in the same extremity.

Interosseous membrane It is a continuous fibrous joint between whole of shaft of radius and ulna which prevents parallel displacement of these bones. Overstrain of arm may rupture its fibres.

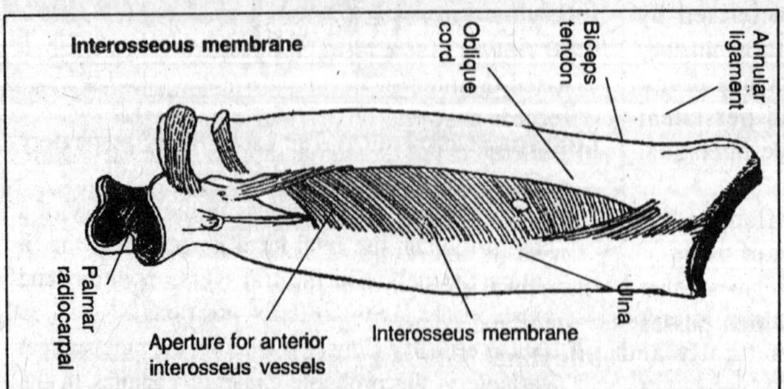

Interoversion Inward concentration on oneself and one's body.

Interpalpebral Between the eyelids.

Interparoxysmal Occurring between paroxysms.

Interphalangeal osteoarthritis There is loss of joint space due to attrition of cartilage, osteosclerosis of juxta-articular bone, bone cyst and osteophytes capped with cartilage known as Heberden's nodes.

Interphase The phase immediately before the visible stages of cell division when the DNA of each chromosome replicates itself.

Interpleural analgesia Injection of local anaesthetic agent into pleural cavity for thoracic surgery and rib fractures.

Interpolated To occur, or be inserted, between other things.

Interpretation The process by which the therapist brings the patient to an understanding of a particular aspect of his or her problems or behaviour. In psychoanalysis, the search for some symbolic or indirect meaning in certain thoughts or actions, The most popular form is dream interpretation, in which the obvious content of the dream is scrutinised for its hidden significance.

Interracial Families or people of more than one race.

Interrupted amorphous periosteal reaction It is discontinuous and appears irregular. It is a reaction to a localised process. Healing fracture is a common cause. There may be thickening of cortex.

Intersegmental traction It involves the application of mechnical rollers that move up and down vertically as they track longitudinally along the paraspinal structures.

Intersensory perception Perception arising from the contribution of more than one sensory modality, such as perceptions commonly arise from several sensory processes simultaneously.

Intersex An individual having both female and male sexual characteristics.

Intersexual selection A process in which variation in reporduction of members of one sex occurs because of behavioral, physiological, or morphological inter-action with members of the opposite sex.

Intersexuality gender Ambiguity; the intermingling in one individual, to various degrees, of both female and male sexual characteristics may result from a disturbance in sex determination during embryonic development.

Interspecific Involving two different species.

Interstitial Between and around cells.

Interstitial cell Small specialized cells in the testes that secrete the male sex hormone, testosterone. Cell between the seminiferous tubules of the testes; secretes testosterone; also called cell of Leydig.

Interstitial cell-stimulating hormone (ICSH) A term sometime used to refer to luteinising hormone in males. Hormone of the anterior pituitary that stimulates the secretion of testosterone in the testes.

Interstitial fibrosis The laying down the fibrous tissue in the interstitial tissues between normal structure.

Interstitial fluid Fluid in the tissue space between and around cells.

Interstitial keratitis It is an inflammation affecting the stroma of cornea without primary involvement of epithelium and endothelium. It is associated with congenital syphilis and tuberculosis. To begin with there is slight ciliary congestion. It is marked in florid stage of disease. Pain, lacrimation and blepharospasm are common symptoms and person is not able to open eyes. Vision is reduced to hand movements. There is always iridocyclitis and keratic precipitates seen. Do not expect much improvement after one and half years.

Interstitial nephritis It refers to renal morphological abnormality chracterised by infiltration of interstitial tissue with inflammatory cells. Common causative agents include drugs, bacterial infection, radiation and persistent hypokalaemia. Late features include interstitial fibrosis and tubular atrophy.

Interstitial pneumonitis An inflammation involving the spaces within an organ or tissue.

Interstitial pregnancy An ectopic pregnancy that develops in that portion of tube which passes through the uterine wall.

Intertrigo It results due to moisture, warmth and friction. Diabetes also predisposes it. Condition shows marceration of superficial epidermis. It gives rise to localised erythematous patches and plaques on groins and skin flexures, where opposition of folds of skin prevent evaporation of moisture. Patient complains of itching, stinging and burning. There may also be fissures, erosions and exudations. There may be weeping glazed appearance. Treatment includes in keeping the pant clean and dry.

Intertrochanteric fracture A fracture expending between the trochanters.

Interval of fertility Those days during the menstrual cycle during which a woman can conceive, determined by considering the life span of both ova and sperm and the cyclic variability. It ranges from about 7 to 15 days in duration.

Interval minilaparotomy A sterilisation technique in which a small incision is made below the pubic hair line for tubal ligation.

Interval scale Has the real-number system properties of order and distance, but lacks a meaningful origin.

Interval training A method of organizing an exercise routine into periods of activity with warm-up, peak, and cool-down periods.

Intervening variables Intermediary factors involved in indirect causality.

Intervention The active process of treatment.

Interventricular foramen The opening that separates the interventricular septum from the endocardial cushions.

Interventricular septum The septum that develops from the ventricular apex, growing toward the fused dorsal and ventral endocardial cushions, and separating the ventricle into left and right halves.

Interview survey A type of cross-sectional survey.

Interviewer assessement Process in which the assessor interviews or questions a subject and records answers.

Intestinal crypt A simple tubular digestive gland opening into the surface of the intestinal mucosa that secretes digestive enzymes; also called the crypt of lieberkuhn.

Intestinal decompression Removal of gas and intestinal contents.

Intestinal flatulence It may be due to fermentation of carbohydrate specially in colon. Anything which causes congestion of intestinal veins will delay the absorption of intestinal gases and gives rise to distension and flatulence. There is sense of fullness with discomfort. Eructance and passing flatus may be useful.

Intestinal glands Tubular glands in the mucous membrane of the small intestine.

Intestinal juice It is secreted abundantly from duodenal mucosa and in smaller amount along the jejunum and ileum. It is similar to pancreatic juice. The chief difference between pancreatic and intestinal juice is of enzymes. pH is about 7.7. Enzymes include pepsin, lactase, maltase, sucrase, lipase, phosphatase, amylase and protease.

Intestinal lymphangiectasia This refers to distension of lymphatics in villi. It is presumed to be due to obstruction or rise in pressure. This gives rise to severe loss of proteins and also lymphocytes in lumen. It may be congenital or acquired. Predominant symptom is browny oedema of legs due to low plasma albumin. In congenital case due to abnormalities of peripheral lymphatics there may be gross asymmetry. Sometimes there is ascites which may be chylous. Diarrhoea occurs in some patients. Unexplained abdominal pain occurs in some patients. Pyogenic infection also occurs.

Intestinal obstruction Common causes of intestinal obstruction are intussuception, volvulus and hernia.

A. Intussuception

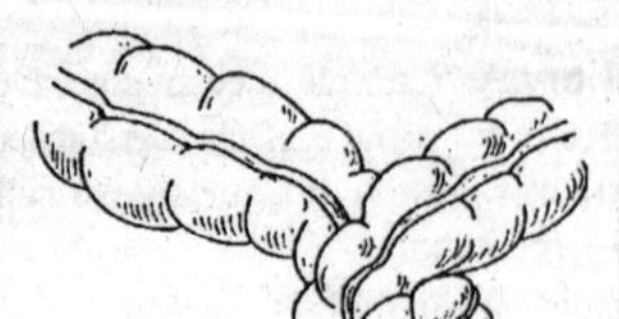

B. Volvulus

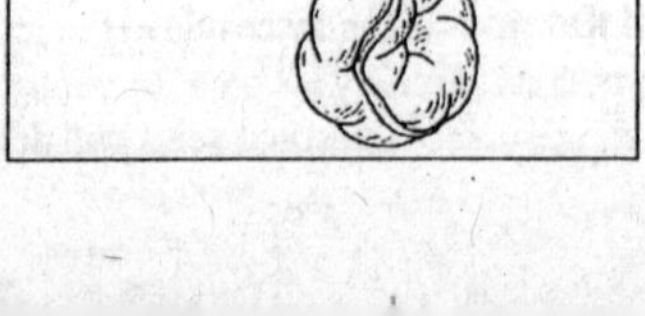

C. Hernia

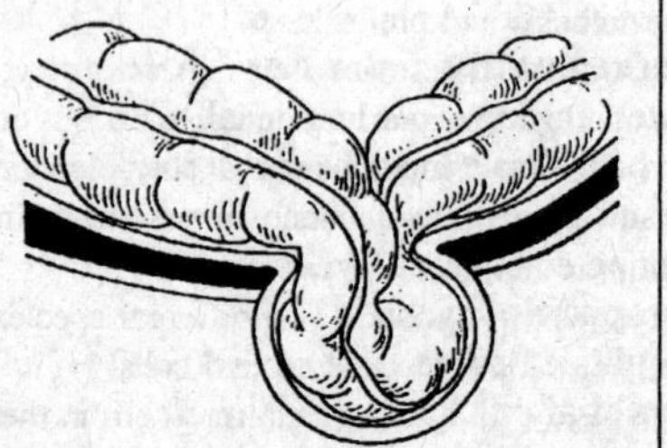

Intestinal pseudo-obstruction This is a syndrome with clinical features to suggest intestinal obstruction but with no mechanical cause. By definition radiology does not show any mechanical obstruction and disordered motility is seen. This is a complication of other illness, for example pneumonia, acute pancreatitis and heart failure. There may be episodes of constipation.

Intima The innermost coat of a blood vessel also called the tunic intima.

Intimacy It is a close, trusting personal relationship between two people who are completely at home with each other and feel free to express their innermost feelings. Intimacy is a basic ingredient of marriage and satisfying relationship. Although it is possible for people to be sexually involved without being intimate.

Intimacy versus isolation The sixth stage and first adult stage in Erikson's psychosocial scheme. The crisis here lies in attaining a close personal relationship with someone else, usually a person of the opposite sex. If this crisis is adequately resolved, then the individual, with this personal support, will progress to the achievement of other goals. The commitment to someone else requires relinquishing personal goals to some degree and true intimacy is presumed to be impossible without first resolving the prior crisis of personal identity.

Intimate space Distance within 6 inches.

Intoductory phase Period of getting acquainted.

Intolerance Any adverse reaction ranging from lactose intolerance to inborn errors of metabolism.

Intoxication The state of being poisoned by a drug or other toxic substance resulting in a mental and/ or emotional change in the individual.

Intra Intralaminar nucleus of thalamus.

Intra arterial Directly within artery or vein.

Intra cranial birth injury It is the commonest cause of neonatal death and morbidity. Subdural hemorrhage, sub arachnoid hemorrhage, intraventricular hemorrhage contribute to the fatal case. Anoxia produces venous congestion and thrombosis and predisposes to brain damage.

Intra ocular pressure Normal pressure is 10-15 m.m. Hg increased in glaucoma.

Intra uterine blood transfusion It is indicated in severely affected fetus, where intra uterine fetal death is apprehended and where there is a history of still birth Group 'O' RH negative packed red cells are injected into the peritoneal cavity of the fetus prior to 32 weeks. 80 to 100 ml is injected.

Intraabdominal pressure Amount of tension within the abdominal cavity.

Intra-abdominal spesis A disease process in humans that occurs following spillage of colonic contents within the periotneal cavity.

Intra-amniotic injection This procedure is indicated in obstetric practice for therapeutic abortion. Before 16 weeks of pregnancy amniotic sac is punctured through vaginal route by 10 cm special tap needle in anterior vaginal fornix. After 16 weeks the amniotic sac is punctured through abdominal route. Usually 50% glucose or 20% saline is injected to amniotic sac after removing 200 ml of amniotic fluid. To detect bladder puncture, the bladder is filled with 15-20 ml of methylene blue by catheterisation.

Intra-amniotic injection with glucose Mid line of sub umbilical skin area is infiltrated with 0.5 percent or one percent xylocaine. A medium bore spinal needle is inserted transabdominally into amniotic cavity and clear fluid is withdrawn. About 150-200 ml of 25 percent glucose or 20% saline is injected into the amniotic sac. Fatal complications include cerebral hemorrhage in accidental injection of hypertonic saline into blood stream

Intra-aortic balloon counterpulsation A means of assisting ventricular ejection by reducing aortic pressure just before and during ventricular systole with an intra-aortic balloon pump activated by an automatic mechanism triggered by the ECG.

Intra-aortic balloon pump A pump connected to a balloon catheter that is inserted into the descending aorta to provide temporary cardiac assistance by means of counterpulsation.

Intra-articular injection This is a local administration of drug into joint cavity. Here the drug acts locally and not by absorption to blood stream. Usually hydrocortisone injections are given

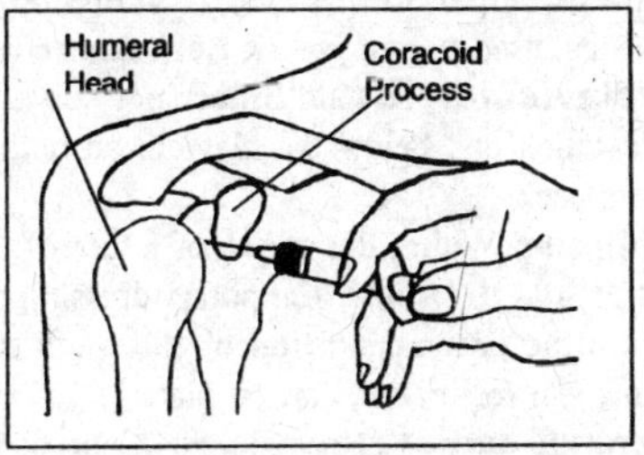

in orthopaedic practice. Great aseptic precaution is to be taken. Usually big joints like shoulder, knee and ankle are given intra-articular injections.

Intrabronchial tumours These produce paroxysmal progressive dyspnoea with wheezing and eventual stridor. With a slow growing tumour the stenosis may remain clinically silent for sometimes. Some may produce haemoptysis, weight loss and pain chest.

Intracapsular forceps The purpose of this forceps is to hold the anterior capsule of the lens during

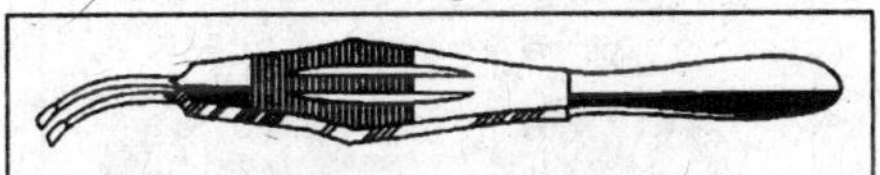

Intracapsular forceps

delivery of the lens for intracapsular cataract surgery. Most surgeons either use cryo of an aspiration irrigation unit for cataract surgery.

Intracapsular fracture A fracture occuring within capsule.

Intracardiac injection It is given during cardiac arrest or to revive a failing heart during terminal stage. Usually coramine, micoren and adrenaline 1:100 are given intracardially. These are given in very emergency without even following strict sterilisation process. The site of precardiac region in second and third intercostal space in midclavicular line. Needle is inserted at 90° angle perpendicular to chest.

Intracavitary Within a body cavity.

Intracellular Refers to the inside of the cell.

Intracellular fluid The fluid within the cells composed of water plus concertrations of potassium and phosphates.

Intracerebral hematoma Extravascualr blood mass located with the brain tissue.

Intraclass correlation coefficient (ICC) A family of correlation, correlation coefficients that allows comparison of two or more repeated measres; used to analyze measurement reliability.

Intraclavicular fossa Small pocket area or indentation just below the clavicle on both sides of the neck.

Intracoronal Within the crown of a tooth.

Intracoronal dressing Temporary dressing placed within the coronal portion of the tooth until a permanent restoration can be placed.

Intracranial content Normally 50-70 mL of blood, 50-120 mL CSF and 1.5 kg of brain tissue.

Intracranial haemorrhage Bleeding within the cranium. When it occurs in a newborn as a result of a long labour or difficult delivery, it is extremely

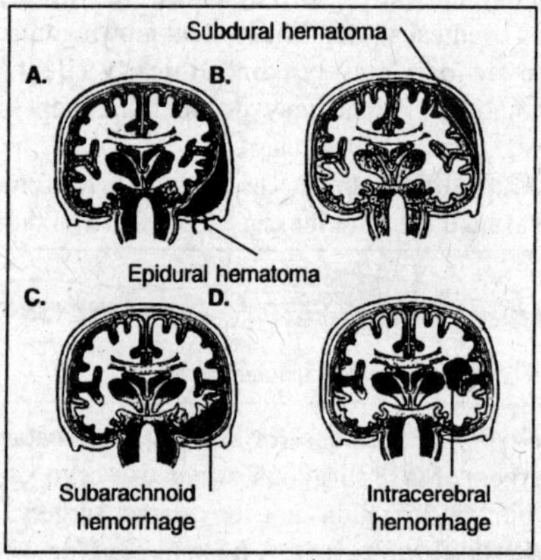

grave. Also called subdural haematoma. It includes, epidural hematoma, subdural hemetoma, subarachnoid hemorrhage and intracerebral hemorrhage.

Intracranial pressure Pressure exerted by CSF in the frontal horns of lateral ventricles of brain. Normally it is 7-17mm Hg.

Intracranial sarcoidosis There will be cranial nerve palsies of facial and abducens and hydrocephalus caused by CSF obstruction. Clinical findings are caused by basilar meningitis. Sarcoid granulomas do not calcify.

Intractable pain Pain unresponsive to methods of pain management.

Intradermal Into the dermis.

Intradermal injection There is difference between intradermal injection and hypodermal or subcutaneous injection. Intradermal means into the skin while hypodermal means below skin. Usually

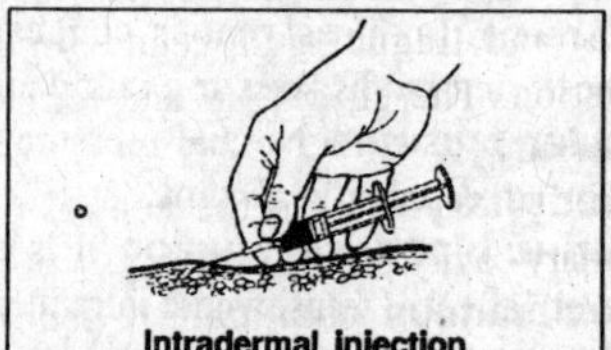

Intradermal injection

intradermal injections are given for diagnostic purpose for testing the reaction on the skin. By a thin needle it is injected into depth of skin such as tuberculin test, Schick test and sensitivity test of penicillin, tetanus, etc.

Intradermal naevus This type usually appears as an elevated, dome-shaped, soft, smooth or warty lesion. It is of skin colour to light brown in colour. It is known as hairy mole due to the presence of hair. Lesion can develop anywhere except soles, palms or genitalia. These are mostly common on face. Microscopically, the overlying epidermis appears normal. The dermal naevus cells are usually arranged in characteristic alveolar ribbons. The cells often becomes spindle shaped. The cells have lost the typical features of clear cells and some of them may coalesce to form giant cells. It never changes to malignancy.

Intraductal papilloma The papillary growth within a duct usually is a lactiferous duct. There is serous or bloody nipple discharge or a small subareolar tumour.

Intrafusal fibers Modified muscle fibers that are encapsulated to form muscle spindle organs, which are muscle stretch receptors.

Intraligamentary injection Some patients specially children, find an inferior dental block injection unpleasant due to numb tongue and lip

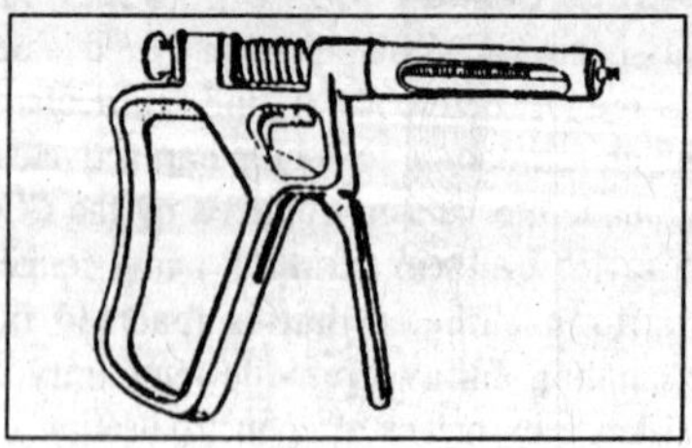

it produces. An alternative for these is an injection directly down the gingival crevice into the periodontal ligament on the mesical sides of tooth. It immediately anaesthetises the tooth and its buccal and lingual gum ready for filling or extraction. The cheek, lip and tongue remain unaffected.

Intramedullary Within the central portion or medullary cavity of bone.

Intramembranous ossification Bone formation within connective tissue membranes.

Intramuocsal Inserts Mushroom-shaped devices fastened to the tissue surface of a maxillary removable partial or total denture that fit within prepared gingival receptor sites for increased retention and stability of the denture.

Intramural plexus A nerve plexus within the walls of the gastrointestinal tract; involved in local and autonomic control of digestion.

Intramuscular (IM) Into the muscle.

Intramuscular injection Drugs more than 2 CC or irritating drugs which cause irritation over skin are given through muscular route. If site of buttock is used upper and outer quadrant is used while in arm insertion of deltoid muscle is the site. Use friction to clean site with cotton swab moistened

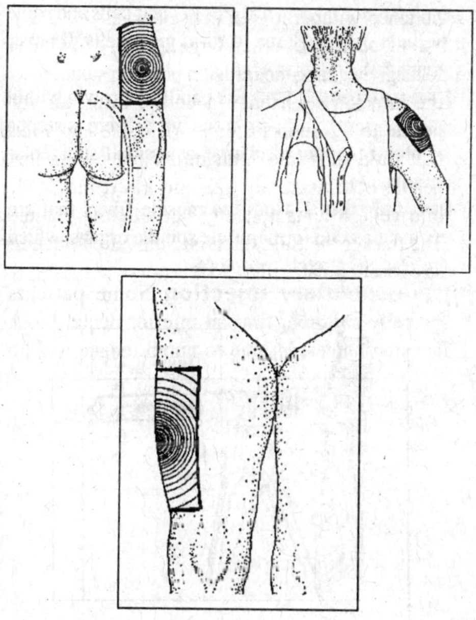

with spirit. Remove any air-bubble in the syringe by holding the syringe with needle pointing upwards and pushing in the plunger. Stretch the skin by grasping the area and use the other hand to hold the needle at 90° angle and pierce the skin firmly. Before injecting the drug pull back the plunger to make sure that the needle has not entered into blood vessel.

Intraocular fluid The composition of aqueous humour is very similar to that of CSF without cells. The most characteristic of gel-like vitreous humour is that it contains a mucoprotein (0.02%) and another unidentified protein (0.02%) not found in aqueous humour, otherwise the composition of two humours is very similar.

Intraocular lens It was Harold Ridley a British ophthalmologist who placed first intraocular lense (IOL) in capsular bag in 1949. Results were encouraging but due to many complications came

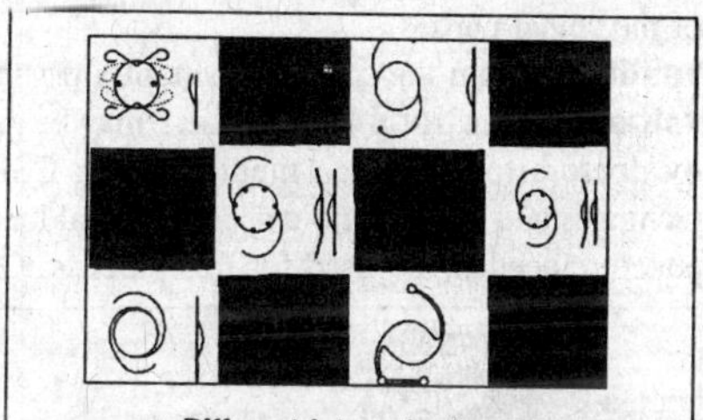

Different Introcular lenses

the era of anterior chamber lens. It also caused corneal oedema and pillous keratopathy. Then came the iris clip lens. It gave new direction for various present day contact lens.

Intraoperative period Time during which the patient undergoes surgery.

Intraoral Inside the mouth.

Intraoral examination Examination of all intraoral structures.

Intraoral radiograph Radiography of teeth and facial bones by placing films within the oral cavity and directing X-Rays at various angles.

Intraovserver variability A measure of inconsistency in repeated assessments by a single observer.

Intrapartum A term referring to the time interval during the birth process

Intraperitoneal injection Peritoneum is a thin paper-like membrane which covers the abdominal organs. Peritoneum provides a good surface area for absorption of drugs in liquid form to blood stream. Proper antiseptic precaution is to be taken. Antirabies vaccine is given intraperitoneally. During intraperitoneal dialysis also injections are given intraperitoneally. Needle is kept at 30° angle, then pierced.

Intrapleural Pertaining to, or affecting, the potential space between the parietal and visceral pleurae.

Intrapulmonic Pertaining to, or affecting, the spaces within the lungs.

Intrarater reliability The consistency with which one rater assigns scores to a single set of responses on two or more occasions.

Intraspecific Within a single species.

Intraspinal Within spinal canal.

Intraspinal analgesia Method of relieving pain by instilling a narcotic or local anesthetic via a catheter into the subarachnoid or epidural space of the spinal cord.

Intrastitial Within the cells or fibers of a tissue.

Intrathecal injections Usually these may be given by doctors to introduce medication in CSF to meninges and subarachnoid space. Special lumbar puncture needles are used for this purpose. Great

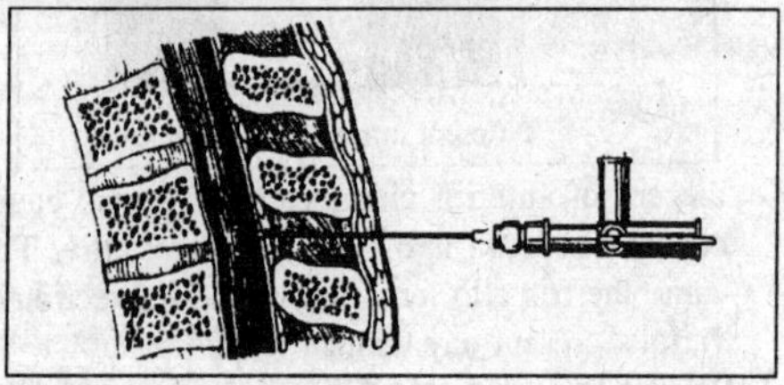

sterilisation care is taken to handle as there is possibility of introducing bacteria to meninges or brain. Streptomycin and penicillin are not given. Certain sera is given intrathecally usually in meningitis. The route is preferred for quick action.

Intrauterine Within the uterus.

Intrauterine device A mechanical device inserted into uterus to prevent pregnancy.

Intrauterine fetal death The mother ceases to feel fetal movements. Uterus is small for date and uterus cease to grow. Fetal heart sounds are not audible. Doppler studies are helpful. Oestriol excretion is markedly reduced. Some patients with retained dead fetus may develop easy brusing and bleeding.

Intra-uterine fetal death of diabetic mother The still birth rate of diabetic mothers is 3 to 4 times more. Cause of fetal death is due to placental insufficiency secondary to endarteritis.

Intrauterine growth standards Graphic charts that are used to compare a newborn's weight (in grams) and gestational age with population averages.

Intrauterine packing It is now not recommended It may be occasionally necessary if vaginal bleeding continues after evacuation and curettage is risky. It is forbidden in shock state because it may aggravate.

Intrauterine resuscitation In case of severely abnormal fetal heart rate during preparing for caesarian section a small bolus dose of beta adrenergic drug or magnesium sulphate can be given to inhibit uterine activity.

Intravasation The entrance or injecting of foreign matter into a vein.

Intravascular Within a vessel.

Intravascular fluid Watery plasma, or serum, portion of blood.

Intravenous (IV) Within a vein or veins.

Intravenous conscious sedation Anesthetic procedure in which anesthesia or analgesia is obtained without loss of consciousness.

Intravenous drip When large quantity of fluid is to be given, hang the infusion bottle in stand. Insert the infusion set needle in bottle. Insert air vent needle to the rubber stopper of bottle and watch that fluid runs into infusion rubber tubing upto needle is to make air free and insert the needle into vein. Maintain steady rate of flow of fluid. The thicker the fluid the lesser the rate. Watch for any reaction carefully.

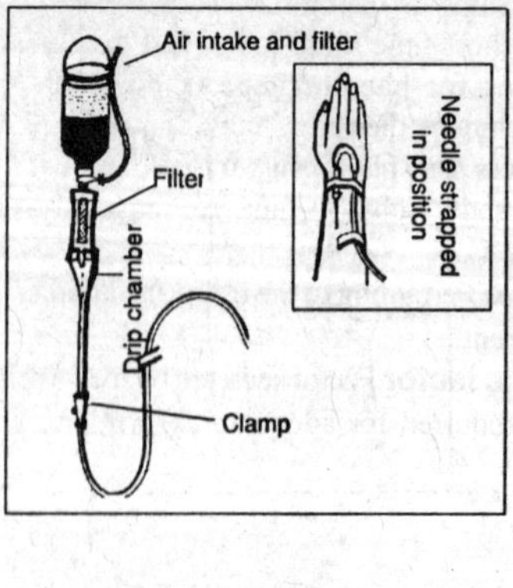

Intravenous fluids Solutions infused into a patients's vein.

Intravenous injection It is given when very quick action is required like cardiac stimulants, respiratory stimulants and antispasmodics. It is used to avoid local irritation and when large quantity is to be given. It is a route for general anaesthesia. Usual site is large vein at cubital fossa, the next site is visible vein at dorsum of foot or hand. When due to severe dehydration in burn or haemorrhage cubital veins are not available, femoral vein or veins at inner side of ankle is tried. Needle is inserted at an angle of 30° or above, when needle pierces the vein, blood comes out in syringe then push the drug slowly.

Intraventricular hemorrhage Bleeding into ventricles of brain.

Intraventricular injection This is to introduce medication to ventricle of brain, not of heart. The administration may be required either for therapeutic or diagnostic purpose. Usually neurosurgeon performs such procedures. Great aseptic care is to be taken.

Intravital Occurring during life.

Intravitreal haemorrhage The common causes of intravitreal haemorrhage are trauma, vitreous traction, retinal tear, posterior vitreous detachment and retinal vein occlusion. A massive haemorrhage in the vitreous tends to diffuse anteriorly and centrally causing marked loss of visual acuity. On ophthalmoscopy there is no red reflex from pupil. A slit-lamp biomicroscopy shows haemorrhage debris in the anterior vitreous and on posterior lens capsule. A haemorrhage in healthy vitreous shows finger-like projections in vitreous from the bleeding site. It resolves slowly while haemorrhage in a degenerated vitreous resolves early. Patient complains of seeing red vision to begin with and in a short time there is marked loss of vision. If causes for haemorrhage is posterior vitreous detachment then they may complain of vitreous floaters and photopsia. A slit-lamp examination may show debris behind the lens and in anterior vitreous.

Intrinsic Pertaining to the essential nature of a thing; inherent.

Intrinsic factor Factor secreted by the gastric glands and required for adequate absorption of vitamin B_{12}.

Intrinsic incubation In the vertebrate animal, the time from infection of the animal until viremia occurs at a level sufficient to infect an arthropod.

Intrinsic muscle Muscle located within the structure on which it acts.

Intrinsic parameters A term for naturally occurring attributes of foods which may influence food spoilage, preservation and fermentation: pH, oxidation/reduction potential, moisture contents, antimicrobial agents, and biological structures.

Introitus It is the orifice of the body cavity such as the sensitive entrance to vagina which is ordinarily relaxed and may tighten during intercourse.

Introjection A defence mechanism, operating unconsciously, whereby loved or hated external objects are symbolically absorbed within oneself. The contract of projection. May serve as a defence against conscious recognition of intolerable hostile impulses. For example, in severe depression; the individual may unconsciously direct unacceptable hatredness or aggression toward himself. Related to the more primitive fantasy of oral incorporation.

Intromittent organ A term for the male copulatory organ; e.g., in reptiles.

Introns Intervening sequences in the coding portions of genes that are transcribed into RNA and are removed during RNA splicing.

Introspection The self-report of one's own sensations, perceptions, experiences, and thoughts; analyses of and reports on the content of one's own conscious experiences.

Introversion The turning outside in, more or less completely, of an organ.

Intrusion In orthodontic therapy, a technique of depressing a tooth back into the occlusal plane or an effort to prevent its eruption or elongation during the correction of an excessive overbite.

Intubated The condition of having a hollow cylindrical device inserted through the nose or mouth into the trachea.

Intubation The insertion of a hollow cylindrical device through the nose or mouth into the trachea.

Intuition Knowing something by using subconscious information.

Inulin A polysaccharide of fructose, produced by certain plants, that is filtered by the human kidneys but neither reabsorbed no secreted. The clearance rate of injected insulin is thus used to measure the glomerular filtration rate.

Inunction Medication incorporated into an agent such as an ointment, oil, lotion, or cream.

Invasin An adhesin that can mediate bacterial invasion into host eukaryotic cells.

Invasion of privacy Wrongful intrusion into one's private activites such as to cause humiliation or mental suffering.

Invasive Referring to procedures that involve puncture, incision, or insertion of a foreign object into the body.

Invasive procedures Procedures that require entry into the body.

Inventory Itemwise compilation of materials on hand.

Inversion A combination of supination and forefoot adduction; talipes varus. Inversion is more free in plantar flexion than in dorsiflexion.

Inversion of the uterus The state of the womb being turned inside out associated with a placenta that has fundal implantation. It is a condition in which uterus literally turns inside out partly or completely. In incomplete degree the fundus does not come out through the cervix while in complete whole fundus has passed entirely completely through center.

Invert sugar Mixture of glucose and fructose produced by hydrolysis of sucrose.

Invertase Enzyme that splits sucrose into invert sugars glucose & fructose.

Inverted 'Y' A radiographic landmark that represents the intersection of the maxillary sinus and the nasal cavity; appears radiopaque.

Inverted nipple A nipple that recedes rather than becoming erect.

Inverted-U theory (Yerkes-Dodson law) There is an optimal level of arousal for performance; too much or too little arousal can cause marked deterioration in performance.

Investment oven Device used to heat an invested mould to eliminate a wax pattern and expand a mould during the burnout procedure.

Invitro fertilization A system of impregnation in which ova are extracted from a woman, fertilized in a test tube, and implanted in the uterus.

Involuntary muscle Smooth muscles that are not under conscious control and are found in organs such as the stomach and small intestine.

Involution It is the process by which uterus regains its gravid state. Immediately after parturition uterus is 8x4½ inches. Thickness of body is 1½ inches while at the end of puerperium it becomes 3x2x1 inch thick. The involution is produced by the process of autolysis.

Involutional melancholia A term formerly used to describe an agitated depression in a person of climacteric age. Currently, such patients are not distinguished from depressed patients of other age groups.

Involutional of decidua Within 2 or 3 days following labour, the decidua becomes differentiated into 2 layers.

The superficial becomes necrotic and cast off in lochia. Process of regeneration is fairly rapid except at placental site.

Iodine fuming Application of iodine vapor to develop latent fingerprints on various items. Prints are visible as light brown images.

Iodine uptake The function of thyroid gland is better understood by its capacity to concentrate iodine, 10000 times more than other tissues. Patient is given a tracer quantity of radioactive iodine and uptake is directly measured by Geiger Muller counter 24 hours after the dose imbibed. In healthy uptake iodine uptake is 20 to 40%. An uptake of 55% or more indicates hyperthyroidism and uptake of 20% or less indicates hypothyroidism.

Iodine value Measure of degree of unsaturation of a fat by the extent of uptake of iodine. (Grams iodine per 100 grams of fat).

Iodism Acute or chronic intoxication due to ingestion or absorption of iodides.

Iodoxin A substance in the retina which plays a role in visual adaptation. It makes the eye less sensitive to light, thus enhancing vision under conditions of intense illumination.

When you awaken in the middle of the night and turn on the light, at first you cannot see, but partly due to the influence of iodoxin, you gradually adjust to the increased illumination.

Ion Atom or group of atoms carrying a charge of electricity because of a loss or gain of one or more electrons.

Ion Channel An integral membrane protein that provides for the regulated transport of a specific ion, or ions, across a membrane.

Ion pump A specialized cellular component that moves ions from an area of low concentration to an area of high concentration.

Ionic bond A strong primary chemical bond characterized by the donation of an electron form one atom to another to make both atoms stable.

Ionisation Process in which ion pairs are created. The ionisation energy is the energy required to remove the outermost electron from an atom thereby creating a positively charged ion. Ionisation radiation is able to produce ions via photoelectric effect. When a salt such as sodium chloride is put into solution. The NaCL splits into positively charged Na ions and negatively charge CL ions.

Ionophore One of a class of antibiotics that alter ruminal fermentation end-products.

Ionotropic receptor A receptor that has two parts: a binding site for a neurotransmitter and a pore that regulates ion flow.

Ions Substances that carry either a positive or negative electrical charge.

Iontophoresis Use of electric current to aid penetration of drug into tissues. It is suitable for drugs of low molecular weight.

IP Abbreviation for interphalangeal.

Ipsilateral Pertaining to, situated on, or affecting the same side.

IPSP Inhibitory postsynaptic potential; hyperpolarization of the postsynaptic membrane in response to a particular neurotransmitter chemical, which makes it more difficult for the postsynaptic cell to attain a threshold level of depolarization required to produce action potentials. It is responsible for postsynaptic inhibition.

Iradiation A procedure by which food is exposed to radiation, destroying microorganisms, insect growth, and parasites that could spoil food or cause illness.

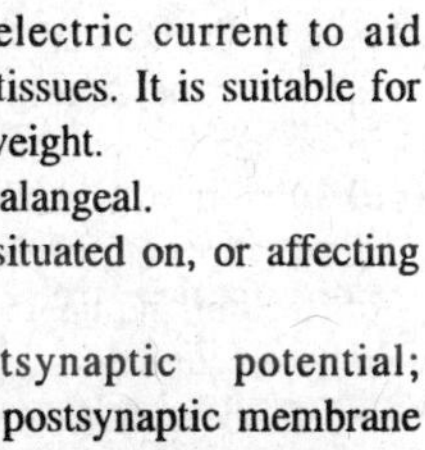

Iris It is a coloured circular diaphragm with an aperture in the centre the pupil. The iris divides the posterior surface of cornea and anterior surface of lens into 2 parts : anterior chamber and posterior chamber. The colour of iris depends on the pigment in the stromal cells of the iris. There is a collarette which demarcates the iris into two portions : the papillary and ciliary zone which differs in colour.

Iris cysts These may occur spontaneously in the stroma or in the pigment epithelium. These are lined by several layers of epithelium. These transilluminates easily. Cysts with or without stalk may lie freely in the anterior chamber or in the vitreous.

Iris forceps It is used to hold the iris and bring it out of the section to perform an iridectomy or an

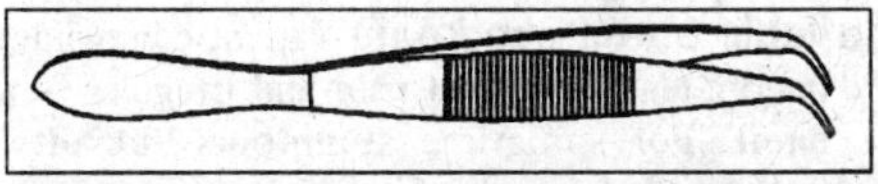

iridotomy. The iridectomy can be peripheral or complete. It is required in all cases of cataract and glaucoma.

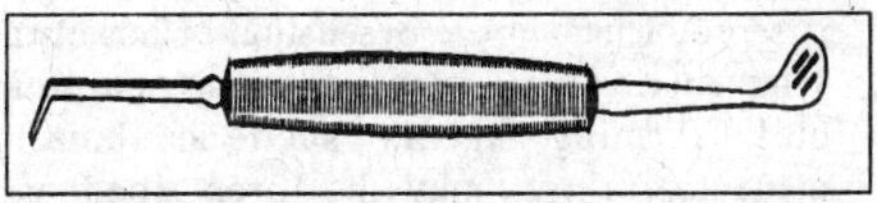

Iris repositor It is used to replace the iris in the eye after an iridectomy. It helps to free the iris from the lips of the section. It helps to make the pupil circular, after reposing the iris.

Iron absorption study 0.2 MBq ^{59}Fe is given orally as ferrous citrate with 100 mg of ascorbic acid and iron as carrier. The patient should fast overnight and for a further 4 hours should take no oral iron for a week before and after test. Normal absorption 10 to 35% is variable estimated by stool collection or by whole body counting after 2 weeks. The amount in the blood at 10 days with normal haemopoiesis represents about 70% of absorbed activity.

Iron lung A large, relatively airtight chamber into which a patient is placed with head exposed for mechanical ventilation; used during polio epidemic in 1950s, but rarely used today.

Irregular emphysema Atypical emphysema.

Irregular pulse Pulse that varies in both force and rate.

Irregular, expansile Terms used to describe a radiopacity that often represents a malignant condition.

Irreversible contracture A contracture that cannot be released by treatment because elastic tissue has been replaced by inelastic tissue.

Irrigate To flush with a fluid, usually with a slow, steady pressure on a syringe plunger. Done to cleanse a wound or clear tubing.

Irrigation The flushing or washing out of anything with water or other liquid for the purpose of making it moist, diluting another substance present, or cleaning the area.

Irritability of uterus Some women are so excitable that with the least fright and excitement they may abort. The irritability is believed to increase in subsequent pregnancy.

Irritable bowel syndrome Patient complains of intermittent abdominal pain and irregular bowel habit. For sometime symptoms subside or disappear but again surface up. Basic abnormality is disturbance of involuntary muscle movement. Anxiety also plays its role. The symptoms include intermittent cramp-like pain in abdomen. There is sense of incomplete evacuation of bowels and symptoms increase after food. As part of treatment bulk forming agents such as bran or methylcellulose may be prescribed with antispasmodics and antidiarrhoeals.

Irritable hip It is known as transient synovitis. It is diagnosed by exclusion from septic arthritis. Generally the child between the age of 4 and 8 years presents with pain of variable severity in hip. There may be a history of minor trauma or viral infection. There will be minor restriction of movements. X-ray and blood picture may be normal except a slight rise in ESR. Management is bed rest.

Ischaemia It means insufficient supply of blood to a specific organ or tissue which may be due to atherosclerosis or as a result of injury. Ischaemia refers to lack of oxygen due to inadequate perfusion which results from an imbalance of oxygen supply and demand. Coronary blood flow can also be limited by arterial thrombi, spasm and emboli. Person needs medical help for chest discomfort, heaviness, squeezing, or chocking. Rarely there may be a frank pain. Patient can pinpoint the location of pain. Episodes of angina are typically caused by exertion, emotion, anger, fright and fear. Rest brings relief. Patients are advised to keep nitroglycerine tablets in his pocket.

Ischaemic encephalopathy Cerebral anoxia results from prolonged hypotension or respiratory failure, cardiac arrest, myocardial pump failure, shock and suffocation are the principal causative factors. Mild degree of anoxia causes inattentiveness, impaired judgement and incoordination. Anoxia persisting beyond 3 to 5 minutes inflicts permanent CNS damage. The features of global brain death are dilated fixed pupils, and absence of brainstem reflexes. Some patients even when fully recovered may develop apathy, confusion and some of them may have progressive neurologic deterioration resulting in death.

Ischemic stroke A deficiency of blood to the brain caused by an occlusion of an artery from a thrombus or embolism.

Ischiadic Sciatic.

Ischial containment socket Above-knee socket that covers the ischial tuberosity and is relatively narrow in width.

Ischium The posterior and inferior bone of the pelvis, distinct and separate in the fetus and the infant, or the corresponding part of the hip bone in the adult.

Ischium and pubic rami fracture with disruption of pelvic ring These include fracture of ischium and pubic rami on each side, on both sides, fracture with separation of pubic symphysis etc. In these external fixature is required.

Ishihara test It is a method for detecting colour blindness. It involves seeing a series of cards on which there are dots of many sizes and colours of different shades and tones. Certain plates may not be recognised by those who are colour blind.

Islets of Langerhans Areas of pancreas from which the insulin is secreted.

Iso- Isocortex, uniformly containing six layers of neurons.

Iso immunization The sensitized maternal red cells are stimulated in second pregnancy to produce antibody against RH antigen to destroy this antigen. This antibody production once initiated is permanent. This is different from antibody formation against bacerial antigen which is temporary.

The maternal RH antibody reaching to fetal circulation causes hemolysis. Sensitization of mother is likely to be cumulative. It may result in jaundice and anemia.

Iso-A Ret-20 Vitamin A derivative is highly effective therapy for serious and debilitating cystic acne.

Isobestic point Point at which two substances absorb a certain wave length of light to the same extent.

Isoelectric focusing An electrophoretic method for separating macromolecules on the basis of their isoelectric pH.

Isoenzymes Enzymes that are very similar in catalytic properties but can be differentiated by variations in their physical properties.

Isofrequency stripes Bands of primary auditory cortex responding to particular tonal frequencies.

Isograft A tissue transplant from one individual to another genetically identical .

Isoimmunisation This occurs when there is blood group incompatibility between the baby and the mother.

When fetal blood crosses the placenta into the mothers circulation in labour IgG type antibodies are formed crossing placenta. In the fetus these produce haemolysis of fetal RBCs.

Isokinetic dynamometer An exercise device that controls the velocity of a limb movement, keeping it at a constant rate while offering accommodating resistance through the range of motion.

Isokinetic exercise Exercise using a constant speed of movement of the body part.

Isolation A mechanism of defence operating unconsciously central to obsessive–compulsive phenomena in which the effect attached to an idea is rendered unconscious, leaving the conscious idea colourless and emotionally neutral. Most of the hospitals are having special wards where contagious and infected patients are kept separately. Patients of chickenpox, etc. are kept in it.

Isoleucine An essential amino acid rarely limiting in foods.

Isomerases Enzymes that catalyze the transformation of compounds into their positional isomers.

Isomerism Existence of two or more ions or compounds that have same atomic composition but different structural arrangements often with different properties.

Isomers Organic compounds having the same empirical formula. The same number of atoms but different structural formulas and therefore different physical and chemical properties.

Isometric Maintaining, or pertaiing to the same measure of length; of equal dimensions.

Isometric contraction Muscle contraction in which the muscle shortens in length and maintains approximately the same amount of tension throughout the shortening process.

Isometric exercise Contraction of a muscle that is not accompanied by movement of joints that would normally be moved by that muscle's action.

Isoprene The hydrocarbon 2-methyl-1,3-butadine, a recurring structural unit of the terpenoid biomolecules.

Isoreceptors Eukaryotic cell membrane components which contain identical receptor determinants recognized by a bacterial adhesin.

Isothermal Isothermic; having the same temperature.

Isotonic Having a uniform tonicity or tension. Solution that causes cells to neither shrink nor swell. Of the same tension or pressure. Normal saline is the commonly available isotonic solution.

Isotonic contraction Contraction in which the tension remains the same; occurs when a constant load is moved through the range of motions possible at a joint.

Isotonic exercise An active exercise in which there is muscle contraction and movement of joint through an arc of motion against a constant resistance. Dynamic, musclestrengthening exercises that cause muscle contraction and change in muscle length e.g., walking or aerobics.

Isotonic solution A solution having the same total solute concentration, osmolality, and osmotic pressure as the solution with which it is compared; a solution with the same solute concentration and osmotic pressure as plasma.

Isotope It is a form of chemical element in which the atomic nuclei have the same number of protons but a different number of neutrons. Radioactive isotopes emit alpha, beta or gamma particles. Certain radioctive isotopes may be artificially created by bombarding elements with neutrons.

Isotype An antibody constant region structure present in all normal individuals, i.e. antibody class or subclass.

Isovolumic contraction The action of the ventricular muscle fibers in early systole, when they initially increase their tension without shortening and thus without an associated alteration of ventricular volume.

Isovolumic relaxation The Phase immediately following aortic valve closure and continuing until the mitral valve opens when ventricular pressure falls below atrial pressure.

Isozymes Multiple forms of an enzyme that catalyze the same reaction but differ from each other in their amino acid sequence, substrate affinity, Vmax, and/or regulatory properties; also called isoenzymes.

Isthmus A narrow neck or portion of tissue connecting two structures.

I-type receptors Stretch receptors in the interstitium of the lung.

IUGR Abbreviation for intrauterine growth retardation.

Ivory bones Very dense bones due to osteopetrosis and osteoblastic lesions.

J

Jackscrew It is a threaded device used in appliances for separation or approximation of teeth or jaw segment.

Jackson's tracheostomy tube It consists of 3 parts : inner tube, outer tube and obturator. The obturator has a provision to lock itself.

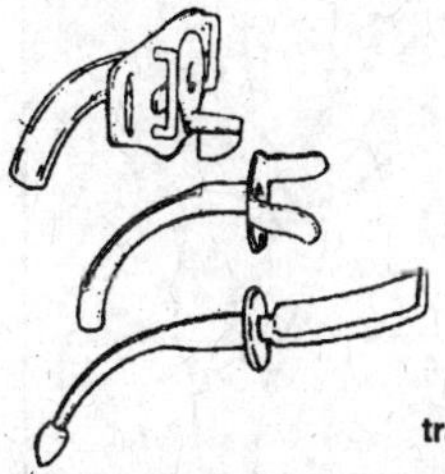

Jackson's tracheostomy tube

Jacksonian epilepsy Form of epilepsy that includes spasms seen in one area of the body or group of muscles.

Jackson pratt drain A closed drain system.

Jacquemier's sign It is the darkening of vaginal mucosa due to pelvic congestion. Sign appears at 8 week of pregnancy. It may occur in pelvic cellulitis or retroversion of uterus.

Jaeger chart Visual assessment tool with small print.

Jaggery Coarse dark sugar made from sap of coconut palm or raw sugar cane juice.

Jam Fruit preserve set to a gel by reaction between acid pectin and added sugar.

Jamais vu 'Never seen'. Epileptic aura where a familiar scene appears novel.

James lange theory A theory based on the work of W. James that emotions result from afferent feed back from the periphery to the brain.

Jargon aphasia Jumbled speech asociated with a lesion of wernicke's area.

Jaundice It is yellowing of skin and sclera of eye. Bilirubin is formed from haemoglobin when old red cells are broken down by spleen. Pigment is absorbed from the blood by liver, where it is excreted in bile. Jaundice may be due to many causes. In *hepatocellular jaundice* due to acute hepatitis, bilirubin builds up in the blood. Transfer from liver cells of bile is prevented. In *obstructive jaundice,* bile is prevented from flowing out of liver because of disorders causing blockage or bile ducts. In *haemolytic jaundice* the amount of bilirubin produced is too great to be processed by liver. Obstructive jaundice is usually accompanied by pale faeces and dark urine. While in haemolytic jaundice both urine and faeces colour are normal. In hepatocellular jaundice, the faeces are normal but the urine may be dark.

Jaundice in pregnancy Jaundice is yellow colouration of skin, sclera and other tissues as a result of increased serum bilirubin above 0.8 mg%. When serum bilirubin exceeds 2 mg/100 ml visible staining of tissue appears.

Jaw thrust manoeuvre The first priority in resuscitation of unconscious patient is airway. It should be opened by neck extension. If there is no suspected cervical injury, the mandible is to be displaced forward. It helps to alleviate obstruction caused by tongue prolapse and hypotonia of pharyngeal musculature.

Jaw winking syndrome In this syndrome chewing causes increasing width of the eyelids, and sometimes rhythmic elevation of upper eyelid when the mouth is open and ptosis, when the mouth is closed.

Jaw, giant cell granuloma It is a tumour or tumour like growth of jaw and may involve gingiva. Mandible is involved more. Lesion is asymptomatic. It is usually expansile. Regional teeth may migrate and covering mucosa is intact. X-ray shows a single cystic area or a soap bubble like deformity. It consists of numerous multinucleated giant cells dispersed throughout specimen. But soap-bubble appearance is not very specific and develops in ameloblastoma too. Local curettage is the treatment of choice. Prognosis is excellent.

Jaw, osteogenic sarcoma The lesion more commonly afflicts male and mandible is involved more commonly. The tumour is initially seen as rapidly growing swelling associated with vague pain and paraesthesia. There is a history of bone trauma and tooth extraction. Tooth may be loose.

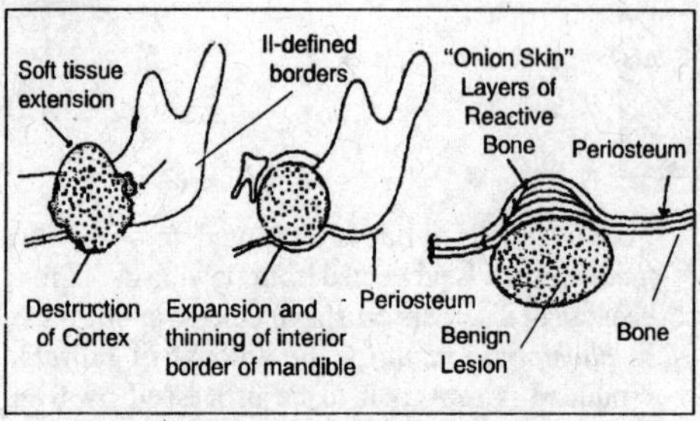

Slow migration and root absorption is seen. Spontaneous pathologic fracture may occur. X-ray shows radiopacity in which bone trabeculae radiate from periphery of lesion producing a sun ray appearance. In some cases widening of periodontal space is an earliest radiographic finding. It is an osteogenic sarcoma which is most malignant. It meta-stasises widely and has a poor prognosis. For jaw lesions, a radical resection with or without chemotherapy and radiation is the gold standard.

Jaw-thrust maneuver Alternative method for opening the airway.

J-chain A molecule which forms part of the structure of pentameric IgM and dimeric IgA.

Jejunostomy A hollow tube inserted into the jejunum through the abdominal wall for administration of liquefied foods.

Jejunostomy tube; J-tube; transabdominal tube that leads to the jejunum of the small intestine.

Jejunum That portion of the small intestine which extends from the duodenum to the ileum.

Jelly A soft substance which is coherent, tremulous, and more or less translucent; generally, a colloidal semisolid mass.

Jendrassik maneuver Method used to facilitate eliciting the deep tendon reflexes of the lower extremities; the patient hooks together the fingers of the hands and attempts to pull them apart. While the pressure is maintained, the reflex is tested. It is believed due to increase in resterent discharge from central nervous system.

Jerk The sudden contracture of a muscle.

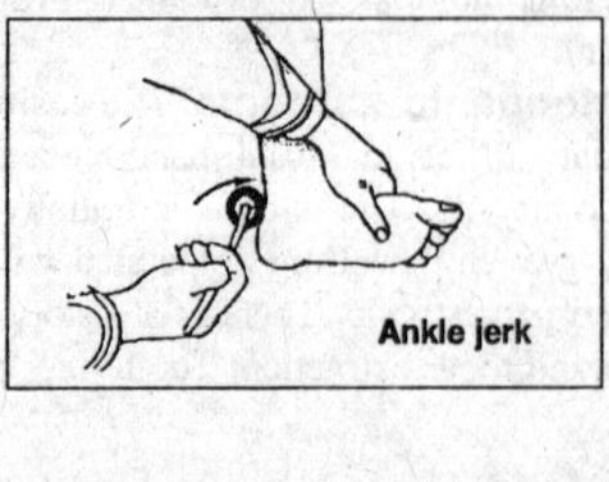
Ankle jerk

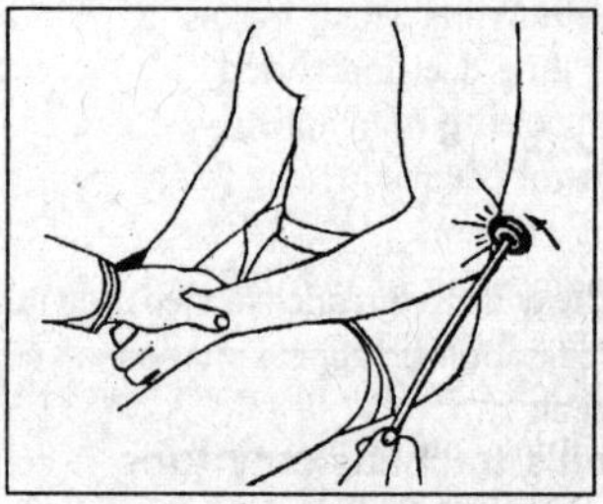
Elbow jerk

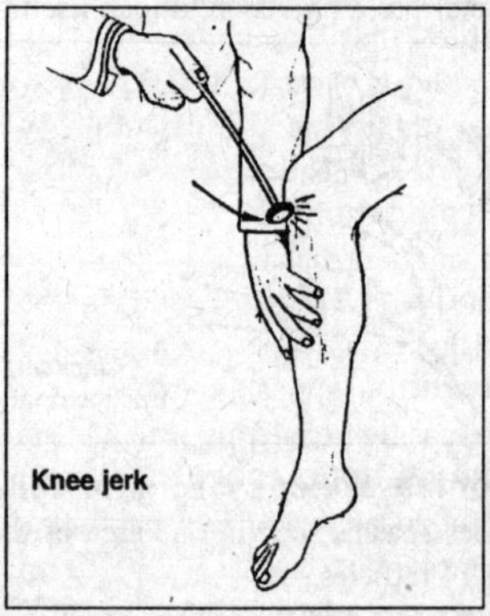
Knee jerk

Jet gun tuberculin test It is done when tuberculin test is done on massive scale because it is painless and rapid way to test. The testing material is driven

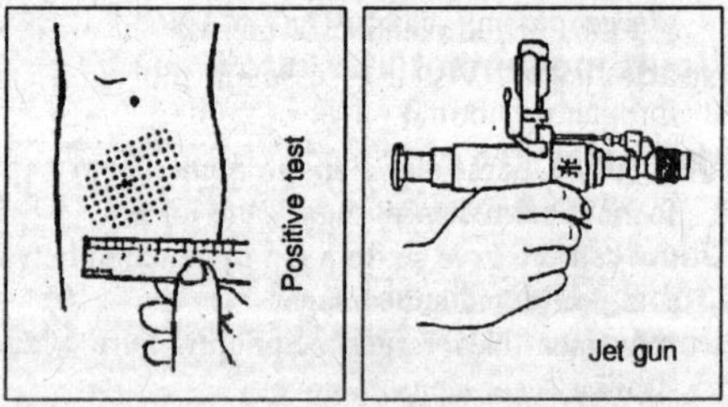

intradermally by high pressure without a needle. The gun delivers O.I ml 5 IU of PPD tuberculin. A positive reaction is 10+ mm for tuberculosis.

Jet lag Emotional and physical changes experienced when arriving in a different time zone.

Jet lag syndrome The malaise experienced by the majority of travellers during the days following a flight across time zones. The symptoms include day time fatigue, difficulites initiating and maintaining sleep, deterioration of mood and G.I.T. disorders.

Job A regular activity performed for payment.

Job stain Work which makes heavy demands but offers little decision latitude for the worker.

Jobst stocking A compressive elastic stocking used to control edematous conditions such as phlebitic edema or burns.

Joint A meeting of two bones for the purpose of allowing movement.

Joint block Iujection of anaesthetic block out pain from joint, and which may be used to confirm source of back pain.

Joint distributin graph A plot of two continuous veriables that can be used to visualize the relationship between the two variables (if on exists) and to determine the direction (positive or negative)and linearity of such a relationship.

Joint dysfunction Joint mechanics showing area disturbances of function.

Joint end-feel The sensation felt when a normal joint is taken to its physiological limit.

Joint fusion A surgical procedure that fixes a joint in one position rendering it immovable.

Joint kinesthetic receptor A proprioceptive receptor located in a joint, stimulated by joint movement.

Joint knee Knee contains two joints the tibiofemoral with its associated collateral ligaments, cruciate ligaments and menisci. Second is patellar femoral joint which obtains stability from large patellar tendon passing anteriorly over patella.

Joint movement The movement of the joint through its normal range of motion.

Joint play The small amount of joint motion that occurs at the end range and is not under voluntary control.

Joint sense The sense of direction of passive movement of a joint affected in posterior column disease.

Joint stiffness 'Active joint stiffness is the element of resistance to movement introduced by autogenetic inhibition and designed to prevent oscillation 'Passive' joint stiffness is progressive resistance to passive movement caused by intramuscular collagen accumulation following an upper motor neuron lesion.

Jones fracture A fracture of proximal diaphyseal portion of fifth metatarsal.

Jorgensen Technique of sedation In it, 30-300 mg pentobarbitone, pethidine up to 25 mg and hyoscine 0.3 mg IV to allow dental surgery is used.

Joule Unit of energy 4.184J = 1 calorie. Junket- Precipitated protein of milk. It is a unit of energy. One joule equals to the work done by a force of one Newton acting through one metre.

JRA Juvenile rheumatoid arthritis.

J-shaped episiotomy First part of incision is like the median episiotomy and after extending 2 cm in the middle line the incision is diverted towards 8'O clock. Such repair is difficult and the repaired area gets puckered.

Judgment The court's official decision in a legal case. The judgement in a case establishes what damages, if any, must be paid, and the legal responsibilities of all the parties in the lawsuit.

Judicial electrocution In some states of USA death penality is carried out in the electric chair. Victim is strapped to a wooden chair and one electrode is put on the shaven scalp and other on right lower leg and current is passed for 1 minute. Same current is passed again for one minute.

Jugular bulb catheterization It is done to allow access to the blood draining brain and providing information about cerebral metabolism.

Jugular foramen syndrome Constellation of symptoms and signs associated with injury to the glossopharyngeal, vagus, and accessory nerves related to the jugular foramen.

Jugular venous distension Stretching or overfilling of the jugular vein.

Jugular venous pressure It is done by noting the height in centimeters of visible pulsations in the jugular veins above the sternal angle patient reclining at 450. Venous pulsations normally are not seen.

Jump sign General pain response of a patient, who winces, may cry out, and withdraws in response to pressure applied on a trigger point.

Junction A place of coming together Labial-Near lips.

Junctional naevus These are usually macular lesions that are smooth, flat or slightly raised 1 mm to 1 cm in diameter. These are usually hairless, light brown to dark brown in colour often darken at centre than at periphery. Most pigmented naevi on the soles, palms, digits or genitals are of junctional type. Microscopically, there is proliferation of melanocytes at the epidermodermal junction with varying amounts of melanin. These cells are potentially unstable and may become malignant.

Junctional rhythm The rhythm of the heart when the atrioventricular node initiates the depolarization wave; nodal rhythm; atrioventricular junctional rhythm.

Junctional tachycardia A junctional rhythm in which the heart rate exceeds 100 beats per minute.

Jurisdiction Jurisdiction over the subject matter of a claim is the power of a court to hear the case and bind the parties. There are monetary, geographic and political limits on jurisdiction.

Just right challenge Therapy that challenges an individual to achieve by using acitivities that are not too hard to too easy.

Juvenile melanoma It is a type of compound naevus, growing in young children. The most common site of involvement is face. Microscopically, cells are spindle shaped and there may be presence of mitoses which can lead to the diagnosis of malignancy. Lesion is entirely benign though it shows junctional component. Like the compound naevus, it has a tendency to become completely intradermal.

Juvenile pause A period of slow growth without sexual maturation, between age 2 years and the onset of puberty, accompanied by low gonadotropin levels.

Juvenile periodontics Peridontics characterized by severe pocketing and loss of bone, specially in anterior and first molar region.

Juxta A combining from meaning near, in the vicinity.

Juxta-articular nodule These are firm fibrous nodules near the joints, usually the large joints of the extremities, often symmetrically arranged and not attached to the skin or deeper structures. These are seen in yaws, pinta, occasionally in endemic syphilis, and rarely in acquired syphilis.

Juxta-epiphyseal fracture These are usually salter type II fractures. The distal fragment includes a flake of metaphysis as well as growth plate and epiphysis.

Juxtaglomerular In close proximity to a renal glomerulus.

Juxtaglomerular apparatus (JGA) Consists of the macula densa (cells of the distal convoluted tubule adjacent to the afferent and efferent ateriole) and juxtaglomerular cells (modified cells of the afferent and sometimes efferent arteriole) : secretes renin when blood pressure starts to fall.

K

KAFO Abbreviation for Knee Ankle Foot Orthoses.

Kala-azar A disease, also known as visceral leishmaniasis and dumdum fever, caused by *Leishmania donavani.* It is prevalent in costal areas of India.

Kanner's syndrome The syndrome is identified by infantile psychosis presenting with strict loneliness, preferences for same thing and practice, differences in intellectual performances, and speech and language disorder.

Kaolin A fine white clay; used in pharmacy in ointments and for coating pills.

Kaplan's Cardinal line A topographic guide to the deep structures of the hand.

Kaplan mier method of life table analysis The most commonly used approach to survival analysis in medicine. The Kaplan-Meier method is different form the actuarial method in that the occurrence of each death defines the end of one observation period and the beginning of the next. Therefore, with this method, the duration of observation periods for which survival is determined varies throughout.

Kaposi's sarcoma With the spread of AIDS, the clinical aspects of Kaposi's sarcoma have changed dramatically. Lesions are much more generalised and disseminated and 50 per cent of AIDS patients show oral lesions. Oral lesions are flat or raised. These are non-tender, pigmented and reddish purple bruise or a vascular growth. Microscopic studies show spindle cells, some of which show mitosis, atypical vascular channels and haemosiderin.

Kappa A reliability coefficient designed for use with nominal data; corrects agreement percentages to account for chance agreements.

Kappa test A measure of the extent to which agreement between two of correlation test observers improves on chance agreement.

Kardex Quick reference for current information about the patient and the patient's care.

Karell diet For patients with severe cardiac failure. It is a low calorie of fluid diet consisting 800 mL of milk in four feeds.

Karyogenesis The development of the nucleus of a cell.

Karyokinesis (mitosis) The prime purpose of this type of division is to ensure the normal somatic number of chromosomes in each daughter cell by the equal division of nucleus and initiates cell division.

Karyotype The chromosome make-up of the nucleus of a human cell; also, the photomicrograph of chromosomes arranged in an organised way.

Katharometer It is used for gas analysis following separation e.g. by gas chromatography.

Kawasaki's disease A polymorphous erythematous febrile disease of unknown origin; characterized by a desquamation of fingers and toes and a furrowing depression of the nails; mucocutaneous lymph node syndrome.

Kayser-Fleischer ring In hepato-lenticular degeneration (Wilson's disease), a rare congenital familial condition, faulty metabolism causes deposition of copper in the posterior surface of the cornea. This produces greenish-brown pigmentation of the cornea, known as Kayser-Fleischer ring. It occurs due to deficiency of ceruloplasmin.

Kegel exercises Alternate contracting and relaxing of the pelvic muscles. These movements strengthen the pubococcygeal muscle, which surrounds the meatus and vagina. The tightening and relaxing of the pubococcygeal muscle. It aids in toning the vagina, strengthening the perineum, preventing haemorrhoids, and controlling stress incontinence of urine.

Kehr's Sign Symptoms of pain referred to shoulder.

Keloid It is a clinical condition characterised by proliferation of immature fibroblast, collagen fibrils and immature blood vessels on the top of scar caused by a pin prick, burn or incision. Keloid is usually associated with itching, oozing and blanching. Causative factors may inlcude familial diathesis and tuberculosis. Majority of cells proliferate in claw-like processes to the surrounding tissue hence the name keloid. Some keloids are nonprogressive. Swelling is raised from the surface, and surface of the swelling is lobulated and firm to feel. Claw-like processes extend beyond the original scar both in length and breadth. It is bluish and pinkish in colour. Patient complains of itching. It becomes tender and there may be oozing of serosanguineous fluid. It is a raised, hard, irregularly shaped scar on the skin. There will be itching too. It develops due to defective healing process. Keloid can occur anywhere in the body. These may be unsightly. Local injections of corticosteroid drugs directly into keloid reduce itching and may cause shrinkage.

Kelvin unit Unit of temperature K is minus 273 degrees centigrade.

Kempner diet It is a rice diet low in salt comprising rice, fruit, fruit juices, sugarnd vitamins containing about 2000 KCal.

Kendall rank corelation test A nonparametric significanhce test of correlation used for ordinal data.

Kennedy classification A method of classifying partially edentulous conditions and partial dentures based on location of edentulous spaces in relation to remaining teeth.

Kepalins Phosphatides similar to lecithins but composed of glycerol, fatty acid and ethanolamine.

Keratin A protein material formed as a transformation product of the cellular proteins of the flat cells on the surface of the epithelium; form of protective adaptation to function. It is a fibrous protein a main content of outer most layer of skin, nails and hair. It is a tough substance that is resistant to damage.

Keratinisation Process of formation of a horny protective layer on the surface of stratified squamous epithelium of certain body surfaces including the epidermis and masticatory oral mucosa. Production of keratin and changes in the structure and shape of epithelial cells as they move to the skin surface.

Keratinocyte The most numerous of the epidermal cells; produces keratin.

Keratitis It is the inflammation of cornea. True keratitis is rare. Symptoms include eye pain, excessive watering and photophobia. Treatment with antibiotics is useful.

Keratitis disciformis It is caused by viral infection affecting lid margin. It is characterised by appearances of central grey disc in middle layers of stroma which is dense in central part. On slit-lamp examination, there is thickening of cornea and fold in Descemet's membrane. The cornea becomes insensitive. There is no ulceration. There is mild irritation which lasts for months. Vision is markedly reduced. Topical steroids help.

Keratoacanthoma It is a rapidly growing pseudocarcinomatous hyperplasia. It gives rise to small pimple on the part of body exposed to sunlight. The pimple grows very rapidly over a period of 10 to 12 weeks to 1 to 2 cm in diameter, even if left untreated tumour undergoes spontaneous resolution having atrophic scar.

Keratoconjunctivitis Inflammation of the cornea and conjunctiva, the delicate membrane lining the eyelids and covering the eyeball. It is the disorder of cornea associated with conjunctivitis. Epidemics develop due to viral infection. It is highly infectious. It is severe with redness, swelling or destruction of surface layer of conjunctiva having whitish membrane. Tiny opaque spots may remain for months in cornea. There is no specific treatment.

Keratoglobus It is a hemispherical protrusion of whole cornea occurring bilaterally as a congenital anomaly. It is a familial and hereditary condition. In it cornea is clear and there is no rise of intraocular pressure. Anterior chamber angle is clear and there is not cupping of disc on fundus examination.

Keratomalacia It is a condition in which there is necrosis of cornea and cornea seems to melt away within a few hours. It develops due to marked deficiency of vitamin A . On examination conjunctiva looks dry, lustreless with xerotic spots. Cornea looks dull, insensitive, hazy with necrosis. Soon the whole cornea gets necrosed and melts away. There is no inflammatory reaction in the eyes. In late stage it is difficult to save the eye.

Keratome The purpose of keratome is to make a small incision at the limbus for surgery. The incision can be enlarged by use of corneal scissors which are again universal or right and left.

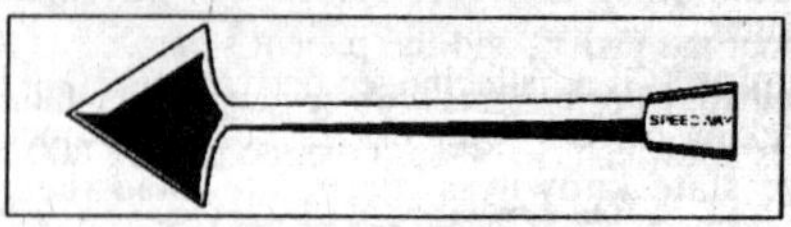

Keratometer Two types of keratometers used in practice are Javal-Schiotzmodel and Limbe model.

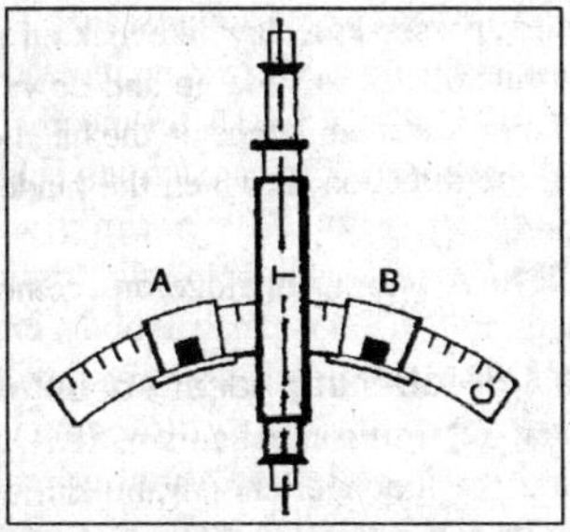

Javal-Schiotz model kerato-meter consists of two illuminated wires AB fixed on a rotatable circular arc-C and a viewing telescope T.

Keratosis follicularis It is rare, chronic, intractable disorder and begins in early life. Histopathologically it shows large epidermal cleft with free lying acantholytic cells and irregular proliferation of epidermal cells. Condition presents with small follicular and intrafollicular, keratotic, brown red papules which may become confluent to form plaques covered with brown or black crusts. Lips may be crusted, fissured and swollen, scalp is covered with greasy crusts.

Nails are brittle. Palms and soles show horny patchy thickening.During summer condition becomes worse. Lesions cause intense itching and bleed easily. No effective thereapy of disease is available.

Kernicterus It is a brain jaundice. Basal ganglion are coloured yellow. If infant survives then may develop convulsions, lethargy, spasticity and muscular incoordination.

Kernig's sign When a patient lies flat with one lower extremity and the other thigh is flexed at a right angle and then holding the ankle an attempt is made to extend the leg at the knee, the patient complains of pain or the examiner meets with a sharp passive resistance. This is Kernig's sign. It is seen in cases of meningeal irritation and low back pain. The test is, however, unreliable in infants.

Ketamine It is a hallucinogen derivative, acting by blocking NMDA receptors. It produces a trance-like state known as dissociate anaesthesia. Anaesthesia persists for 15 minutes after a single intravenous injection. It does not produce hypotension. Disadvantage is that it does not produce any muscular relaxation. It tends to raise heart rate, intracranial and intra orbital pressure. It should always be preceded by premedication with atropine to reduce salivary secretions. 5-10 mg/kg by deep IM injection produces surgical anaesthesia in 3-5 minutes and may last up to 25 minutes. Through IV route 1 to 2 mg/kg by slow injection over a period of 60 seconds. 2 mg/kg produces surgical anaesthesia within 1-2 minutes and may last up to 5 to 10 minutes. Return to consciousness is gradual. It should not be given in moderate to severe hypertension, cardiac failure and in pregnancy.

Ketch up Spicy sauce mostly made of tomato.

Ketoacidosis A condition of abnormally low blood pH (acidity) caused by presence of an abnormally large number of ketone bodies or "keto acids" that are produced when fats are converted to forms of glucose to be used for cellular respiration; often occurs in diabetes mellitus, when it is more specifically called diabetic ketoacidosis (see also acidosis).

Ketogenesis The formation of ketone bodies from fatty acids and some amino acids.

Ketone bodies Substances produced primarily during excessive trighlyceride catabolism, such as acetone, acetoacetic acid, and beta-hydroxybutyric acid. Breakdown products of fatty acid catabolism.

Ketones Normally urine does not contain hydroxybutyric acid, acetoacetic acid and acetone. These appear in starvation and uncontrolled diabetes mellitus. Ketones enter urine readily at low blood plasma concentration. Rothera's test is sensitive to acetoacetic acid

Ketonuria Acetone bodies in the urine.

Ketose A simple monosaccharide in which the carboxyl group is a ketone.

Ketosis It is a condition in which there is an abnormal quantity of ketone products of normal metabolic breakdown of fats in the tissues of body. Ketones are normally further broken down to be excreted and may be noted in urine in diabetes mellitus.

Keyes technique Use of salt, baking soda, and hydrogen peroxide to prevent or control periodontal disease.

Kg Abbrebiation for kilogram.

Kidney There are two kidneys in body. Kidney is responsible for filtering the blood and excreting waste products. Size of kidney is 4 to 5 inches long and about 6 ounces in weight. Renal arteries supplying blood to kidneys arise from aorta. Each

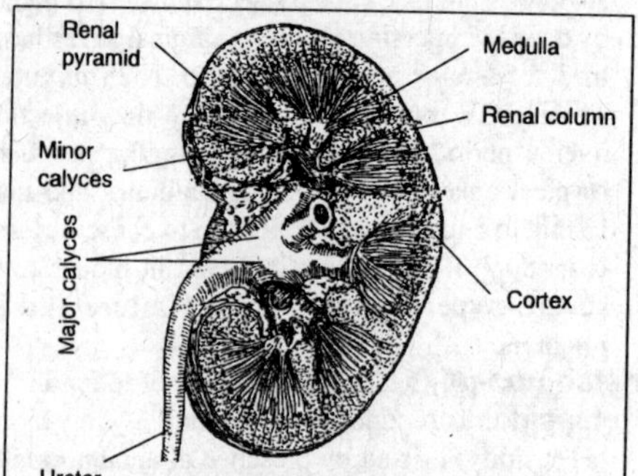

Coronal section

kidney contains about 1 million glomeruli which pass the filtered blood through long tubules into medulla. The glomeruli and tubules make up nephrons. Nephrons are the functioning unit of kidney. As person becomes old these number of units are diminished. Kidneys also control acid-base balance. Kidney produces several hormones including erythropoietin. When blood pressure falls kidney produces enzyme renin.

Kidney cyst These are non-malignant. Above the age of 60 many develop these cysts without reason. These do not produce any symptoms. But when becomes very big may cause pressure. Multiple

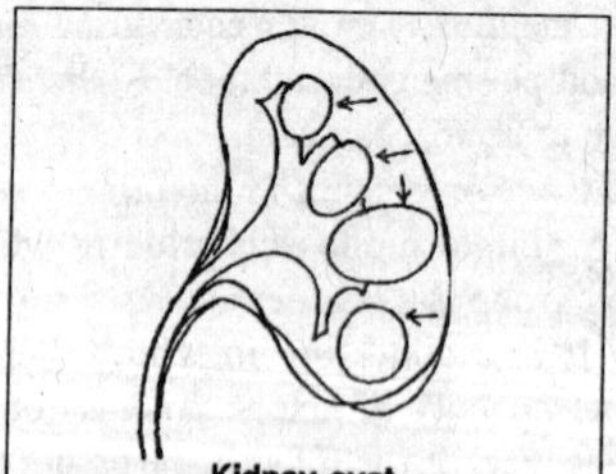
Kidney cyst

cysts may develop in both kidneys. Treatment is generally not needed and aspiration in selected cases may help.

Kielland's forceps This special device of rotation-extraction forceps is named after kielland (1916) It possesses a cephalic curve and a very shallow pelvic curve. The concavity of the pelvic curve is directed towards the child's occiput. The instrument possesses a claw like lock on the shank and permits blades to slide up and down on each other. There are small knobs on the handles which point in the direction in which the blades should be turned.

Kilian's line A prominent ridge on promontary of sacrum.

Killiani's self-retaining nasal speculum It has got a self-retaining mechanism. It is used for retracting the mucoperichondrium during septal surgery. Its self-retaining quality is better.

Kilocalorie 1000 calories. The amount of heat required to raise the temperature of 1000 g of water 1°C from 14°C to 15°C; the unit used to express the energy content of foods and to measure metabolic rate.

Kilovoltage In X-ray machines, the potential difference between the anode and cathode of an X-ray tube.

Kinases Enzymes that catalyze the phosphorylation of certain molecules by ATP.

Kindling Progressively increasing group response of hippocampal neurons to a repetitive stimulus of uniform strength.

Kinesics Body Language.

Kinesiology The study of movement as it relates to physiological processes, physical principles, and anatomy of the body.

Kinesthesia Sense by which muscular motion, weight, position, etc. are perceived.

Kinesthetic Related to the ability to perceive the existence or direction of weight or movement.

Kinetic Chain Exercises In mechanical engineering, a closed kinematic system is where both ends of a linked chain are fixed, so that movement of one of the rigid linked segmetns cause predictable movement of other segments. By this definition only isometrics are true closed chain exercises, but the defination has broadend to include dynamic exercises wherever the hand or foot meets resistance, such as in squats, leg press, trepups, push ups or chin ups. An open kinetic chain exists when the peripheral joint of an extremity can still move freely and resistance is applied more proximally, as in leg extension or leg curls. In practical terms, closed chain exercises

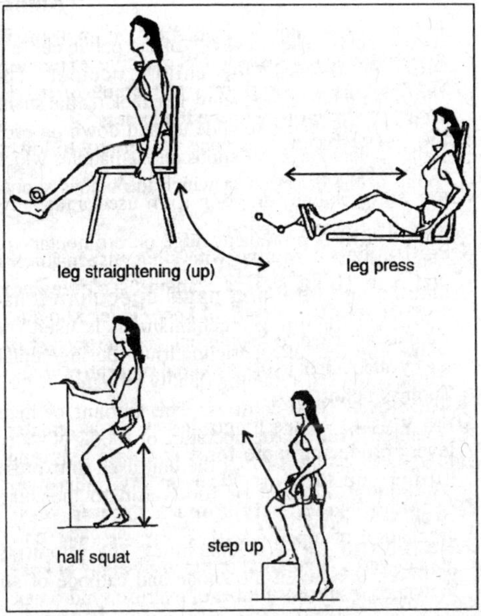

usually involve movement while weight bearing through the limb. In open chain exercises, the limb may move against resistance but does not bear weight of the body (non-weight bearing).

Kinetic information This information can also be descriptive and includes the joint centers as well as joint angles. Video based information can be collected.

Kinetics Body of knowledge that deals with the effects of forces that produce or modify body motion.

Kinins A family of polypeptides released during inflammatory responses and which increase vascular permeability and smooth muscle contraction.

Kink Band or twist.

Kitol An inactive form of vitamin A.

Kleine-Levin syndrome Periodic episodes of hypersomnia; first appears in adolescence, usually in boys, and is accompanied by bulimia.

Kleptomania It is a strong, unavoi-dable desire to steal. Objects stolen may not be of any value or desirable. It is a mental aberration and is associated with depression

Klinefelter's syndrome There is male hypogonadism associated with two or more X-chromosomes and at least one Y-chromosome. It is a leading cause of male infertility. There will be minimal or no mental retardation with failure of male secondary sexual characteristics. Testis will atrophy with hyperplasia of Leydig cells. Plasma FSH and oestrogens will be elevated with lowering of testosterone.

Klippel-Trenaunary syndrome It consists of congenital angiomatosis of an extremity which is larger, longer and hotter than the other, and there may be ulceration and gangrene of the affected limb.

Kluge's sign There develops vulval varicosities appearing in ten weeks of pregnancy.

Kluver-Bucy syndrome Constellation of personality changes following anterior temporal lobectomy.

Kneading Kneading is a manipulation in which the muscles and subcutaneous tissues are alternately compressed and released. The movement takes place in a circular motion.

Knee This is the joint between the femur, tibia and fibula. Patella lies over the joint frontally. There are two triangular cartilage called meniscus covering the surface of tibia and femur. It is a modified hinge joint. Joint is partly surrounded by a fibrous capsule lined with synovial membrane. Synovial membrane secretes a lubricating fluid which allows the cartilage to move freely. Severe damage to joint such as sports injury may result in blood collection in joint. It may result in synovitis.

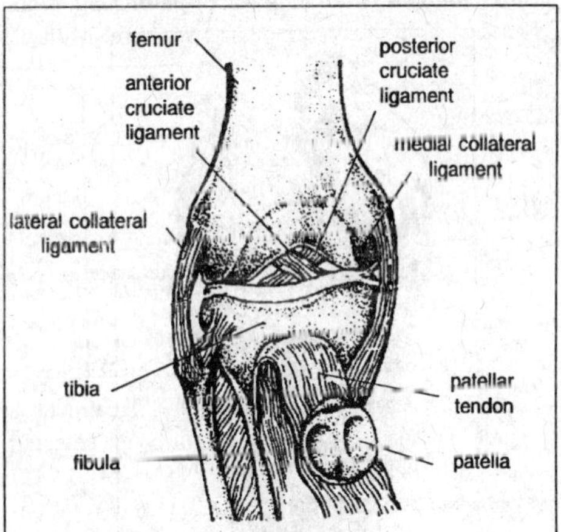

Joint knee

Knee joint is involved in osteoarthritis and rheumatoid arthritis. In old age fracture of femur disrupts the movement of joint. Nowadays surgical procedures can replace knee joint with an artificial substitute.

Knee aspiration To determine that what kind of fluid it is blood, synovial fluid or pus it is necessary to perform a needle aspiration. Blood implies that some intra-articular structure has been ruptured.

Knee exercise Mechanical apparatus for passive exerceses of the knee joint.

Knee extension exerciser Patients back and knees are aligned with the axis of the pivot arm. The leg pad is adjusted to just above the ankle.

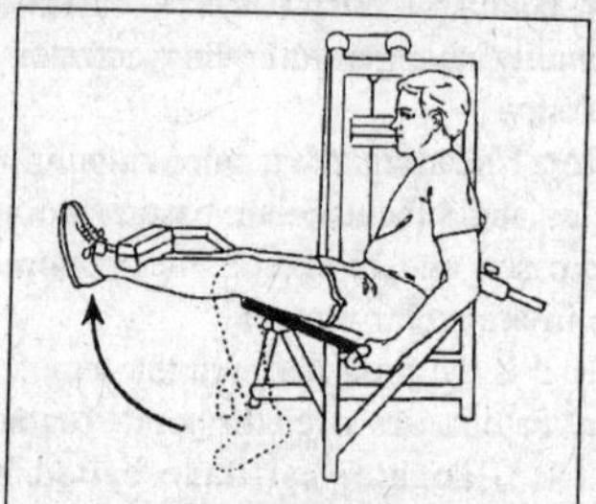

Knee extension

The athlete lifts the weight by straightening both knees, pauses, lowers the weight to the starting position in slow controlled manner and repeats the process.

Knee joint line It is easily palpable edge of the tibial plateau. Patient with effusion and pain

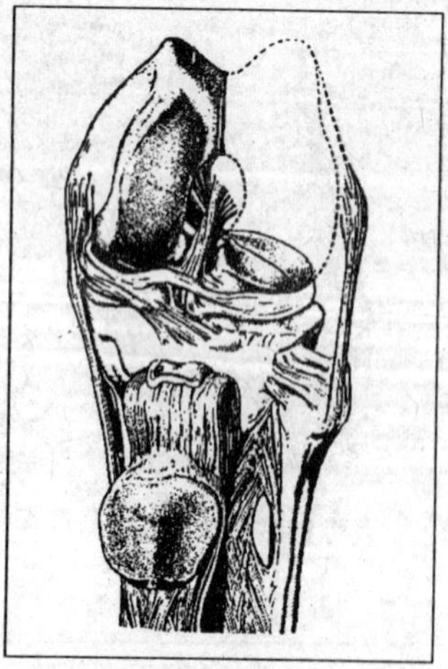

follows a sport injury. Tenderness on joint line is associated with loss of full passive extension suggesting meniscus injury. Osteoarthritis is common cause of joint line tenderness.

Knee nerve block It is done for surgery to lower leg and foot.

Knee sling Support in sling form used under the knee for Russell traction.

Knee traction It is used with sling suspension so that 3 to 10 kg weight transmit a downward pressure over the dorsum of knee. Three kilogram weights are used to counterbalance the weight of leg by attachment to the proximal ring and reversed Thomas splint.

Knee valgus Men's longer bones act as greater levers producing more force in sports requiring hitting and kicking. Women have narrower shoulder, wider pelvis and a greater varus angulation of hip and valgus of their knee. The greater varus angulation of hip and valgus of knee in women results in number of overuse syndromes. Because of their wider pelvis and shorter lower extremities, women have lower centre of gravity which gives dinstinct advantage in gymnastics.

Knee-ankle-foot orthoses Main function is to reduce the stress within leg and stabilise the knee in the sagittal and coronal plane. It is useful in cases of delayed union of lower limb fractures, to limit range of motion at knee, valgus/varus instability due to arthritis. These can be made of traditional leather and metal cons-truction or moulded plastic.

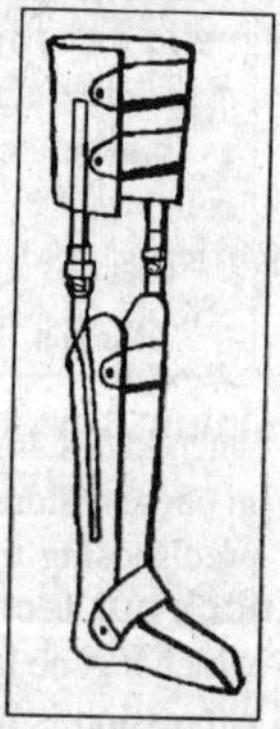

Knee-chest position This is used for gynaecological purpose, like examination of vagina and rectum and for first aid treatment of cord prolapse and retroverted uterus. Patient lies with breast downwards facing down on bed. Knees

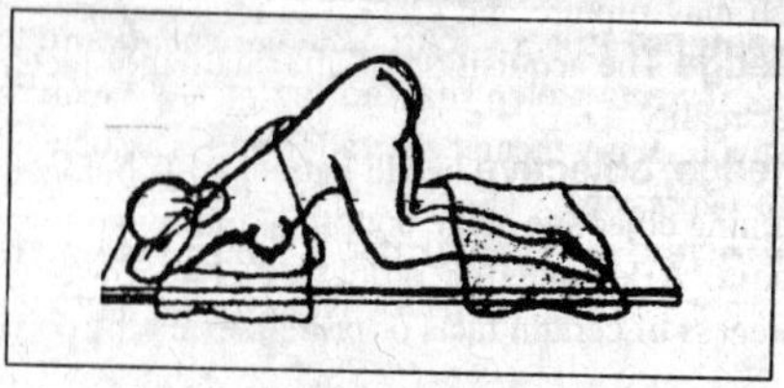

and thighs are flexed with buttocks high up in air. Thighs remain at right angle to bed. Hands are flexed. Small pillow can be given under chest.

Kneel position A posture in which both knees are bent and the hips are in neutral position.

Knife A cutting instrument, an instrument used to remove or smooth the rough margin of a metallic restoration, such as gold foil, or tissue in a surgical procedure.

Knight spinal brace This is a rigid lumbar orthosis that is very useful in treating chronic low back pain when more support is required. It is also used in treatment of disc disease and spondylolisthesis.

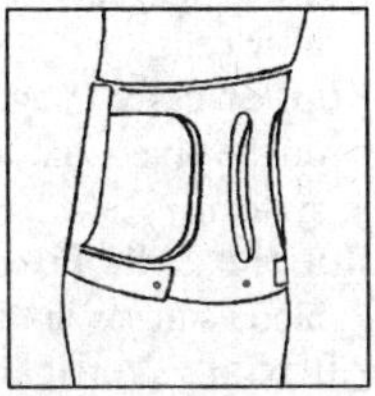

Knight spinal orthosis Lumbosacral flexion, extension, lateral control orthosis.

Knock-knee In this deviation the lower legs bow outwards with the result that ankles ae forced apart when knees are touching. It is a postural deviation in obese children. It creates poor alignment of knee predisposing to strain and injury.

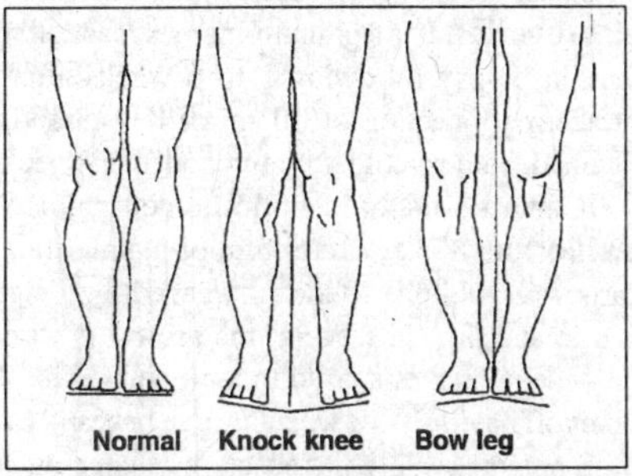

Knock-out technology A method in genetics in which a gene is deleted from a chromosome or its expression is blocked.

Knots of cord True knots are commonly encountered. False knots occur due to varices which may rupture and can cause fetal death.

Knowledge The acquisition of information of facts about reality.

Knowledge, objective In edu-cational psychology, a learning objective at the bottom of the congnitive domain. A knowledge objective concerns the awareness of certain facts or principles on the part of the learner. No analysis, application, synthesis, or other use of this knowledge is expected.

Knuckle It refers to the dorsum of metacarpophalangeal joint prominence when the hand is clinched.

Knuckle bender brace In it rubber bands create tension on a spring wire brace that can be positioned to overcome extension or flexure

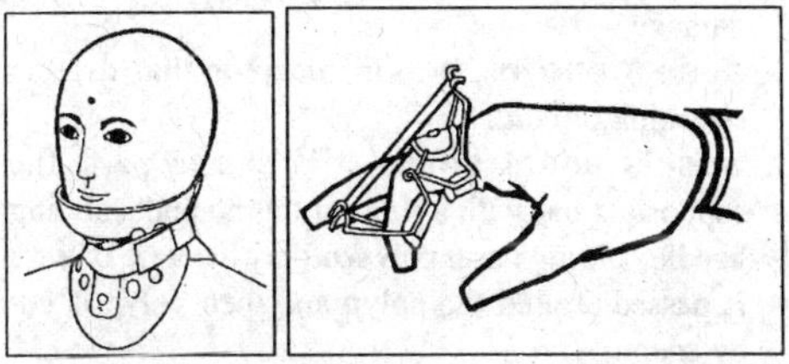

contracture of PIP joints. It is used once infection has largely subsided and is applied for 20 minutes at the interval of 4 to 5 hours.

Knuckle Kneading For small areas when greater depth is required, the dorsal surface of the middle or proximal phalanges may be used. Significant pressure can be generated with the closed fist, applying the same basic circular motion.

Kocher maneover A technique for the reduction of anterior dislocated humeral head into glenoid.

Kock's lymphadenitis Usually one group of cervical lymph nodes is infected, most frequently the upper jugular group of nodes is affected. The organism is tubercle bacilli. There are 3 stages of infective process. In first stage, the lymph nodes become enlarged and slightly tender but remain discrete. In second stage, the lymph node becomes matted with perilymphа-denitis. While in third stage, caseating material liquefies and breaks through the capsules of lymph nodes to form cold abscess. In the beginning abscess remains deep, later fascia is eroded at one point and pus tracks into superficial space.

Koebner's phenomenon It is a reaction in which any injury can produce at the site of trauma a typical lesion in such condition as psoriasis, lichen planus, lichen nitidus, infective eczematoid dermatitis, and verruca plana.

Kohlers disease An avascular necrosis or osteochondrosis of tarsal navicular bone.

Kohn'a pores Interalveolar foramina.

Korotkoff's sounds Sounds heard over an artery when pressure over it is reduced during the determination of blood pressure by the auscultatory method.

Krabbe disease Characteristic globoid cells are present in white matter of brain. The onset of symptoms is before the age of 6 months. Disease is usually fatal. Child may develop irritability, hypertonicity, blindness, deafness and neurological damage.

Krause's end blub Skin receptor that detects sensation of cold.

Krause's nasal snare It is of two parts the supporting bar with a ring for thumb and a sliding handle. During nasal polypectomy the loop of wire is passed around the polyp and then polyp is cut by snare.

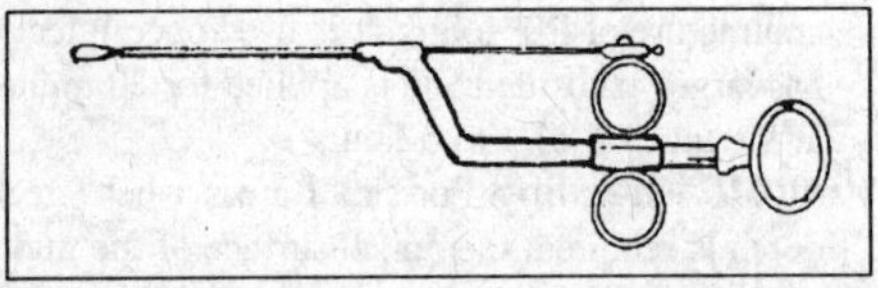

Krebs cycle A series of biochemical reactions that occurs in the matrix of mitochondria in which electrons are transferred to coenzymes and carbon dioxide is formed. The electrons carried by the coenzymes then enter the electron transport chain, which generates a large quantity of ATP. Also called the citric acid cycle.

Kresis test For oxidative rancidity of fats.

Krukenberg's spindle It is a spindle in which pigment derived from the uveal tract is deposited on the endothelium of cornea in a shape of vertical spindle. It is usually seen in the aged and mostly is myopics and females. It is acquired in nature and pigment is derived from uvea. A case with Krukenberg's spindle must be watched for granuloma, diabetes and myopia.

Kruskal-wallis one-way ANOVA A nonparametric significance test used to compare three or more groups of ordinal data. It is analogous to the one-way ANOVA used for three or more groups of continuous data.

Kruskal-Wallis test The nonparametric version of the one-way analysis of variance.

KUB Abbreviation for kidney, ureters and bladder.

Kulchitsky's cells The rarest type of bronchial epithelial cell; Kulchitsky's cells are neurosecretory cells believed to play a role in the regulation of lobular growth.

Kupffer Cell macrophage found in spaces between liver cells.

Kupffer cells Phagocytic cells lining the sinusoids of the liver that are part of the body immuity system.

Kuppfer cells Fixed tissue macrophages lining the blood sinuses in the liver.

Kurtosis Vertical distortion of a frequency distribution.

Kussmaul breathing When the respiration is slow and deep, with normal breathing capacity and the occurrence of dyspnoea is rare, it is known as Kussmaul breathing. It is seen in diabetic acidosis.

Kveim reaction It is a granulo-matous reaction seen on skin biopsy following 3 to 6 weeks after an intradermal injection of 0.1 ml of Kveim antigen obtained from sarcoidal lymph nodes or spleen. It is a diagnostic aid for identification of sarcoidosis.

Kwashiorkor It is a severe form of malnutrition. It starts when child is suddenly weaned onto a poor calorie and protein diet. In this growth is stunted but oedema makes a child to look puffy. The skin flakes off having a raw weeping area beneath. Liver often enlarges and child loses resistence against severe infection. High calorie+high protein diet with sufficient vitamins and zinc helps the child.

Kyphosis It is the excessive backward curvature of spine resulting in lump or a more gradually rounded back. It may result from osteoporosis, fracture of vertebra or tuberculosis. Treatment is to be done of causing factor.

Kyphotic posturing Excessive convex curvature of the thoracic spine as viewed laterally.

L

L.T.T. cleanser It is a creamy lotion containing emulsifiers. It eliminates grime, excessive sebum, dead cells and applied make up. This tends to open the pores allowing the sweat glands to release waste.

L4 root syndrome Pain radiates over the ventral aspect of thigh to the knee, and can radiate further on the anteromedial aspect of leg to the lateral medial ankle, and even of the medial aspect of the big toe. In this syndrome, positive femoral nerve syndrome is marked. There is weakness of quadriceps and of the hip flexors. The patellar reflex is weakened or absent. There is hypoaesthesia mainly on the anterior aspect of the L_4 dermatome owing to weakness of the knee extensors.

L_5 root syndrome Pain radiates on the lateral aspect of thigh and leg to the lateral ankle to the big toe and to the second and third toes. There is weakness of foot and toe extensors. Patient may not walk on his or her heels and there is a drop foot. Hypoaesthesia is found in L_5 dermatome.

Labbe, vein inferior Anastomotic vein of cerebrum.

Labeling Labeling theory suggests that we give people labels as woman, black, Latino, cop, addict to categorize them and so know how to interact with them. If someone is simply a woman, she loses the complexity of her humanity.

Labia The nominative pleural of labium. Lips or liplike structures.

Labia majora One of two rounded folds of skin surrounding the labia minora and vestibule. "Large lips" of the vulva.

Labia minora "Small lips" of the vulva. One of two narrow longitudinal folds of mucous membrane enclosed by the labia majora; anteriorly they unite to form the prepuce.

Labial bar A major connector that is located labial to the dental arch and that joins bilateral parts of a mandibular removable partial denture.

Labial frenulum A longitudinal fold of mucous membrane that attaches the lips of the gum along the midline of both the upper and lower lip.

Lability It is an exaggerated changeability of mood and marked activity to outside events. Emotions are poorly sustained and sadness or tears may quickly change to gaiety and laughter when gloomy topics are changed to cheerful humorous ones. Lability is a striking feature of hysterical personality. It is the most common kind of emotional change in dementia when it is known as emotional incontinence.

Labiomental groove Horizontal depression which separates the lower lip from chin.

Labioversion Displacement of a tooth labially from the line of occlusion

Labor The process that results in the birth of the baby.

Laboratory Information Management Systems A computer system to track and manage the flow of evidence, laboratory processes and resultant data.

Laboratory requisition/prescription Directions given to a laboratory technician by a licensed dentist for the construction of a dental prosthesis.

Laboratory test Procedure that involves the examination of body fluids or specimens.

Labour pain during 1st stage During first stage of labour pains are short lasting, mild and separated at intervals of ten to twenty minutes. There will be mild discomfort in upper sacral regions and lower abdomen during uterine contraction. With the progress of labour pains become frequent, stronger and longer. With more lasting uterine contractions the head becomes engaged if it has not so far.

Labour pains These are intermittent contractions recognisable on palpation occurring in the wall of gravid uterus. Patient may become even semiconscious but these do not produce any ill-effect on ovum. At term, these become labour pains. This transformation is gradual, vague transient abdominal pain. At first they are slight lasting for half a minute separated by inervals of 15 to 30 minutes. They change in frequency, severity and duration.

Labrum A general anatomical term for an edge, brim, or lip. Lamellar Pertaining to or resembling lamellae.

Labrum, glenoid Acetabular labrum.

Labyrinth Bony labyrinth consists of three semicircular canals, posteriorly, vestibule in the middle and snail-like cochlea anteriorly. Bony

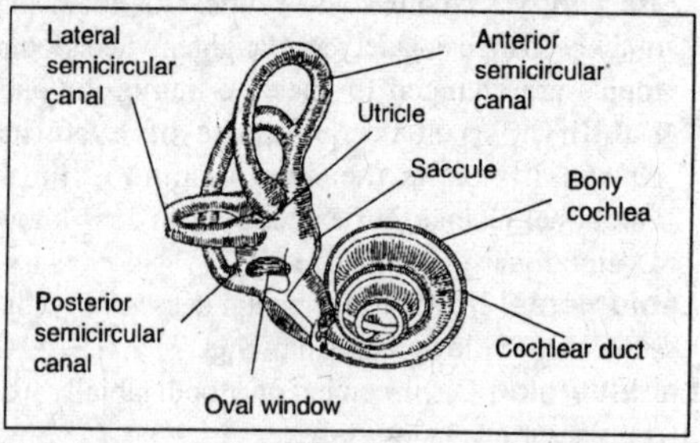

labyrinth is hollow and contains perilymph. Suspended from the bone by delicate filamentous strands is the membranous labyrinth. This is a complex of tubes and sacs containing endolymph and subdivided into three semicircular canals.

Laceration A wound produced by tearing or irregular cutting.

Lacertus fibrosus Bicipital aponeurosis.

Laches A defense in which the defendant claims that the plaintiff waited so long in brining the complaint that it would be unjust to allow the case to go to trial. The laches defense is important in claims that have no clear statute of limitations.

Lachman's test It is considered to be the most sensitive test for anterior cruciate ligament (ACL) injury. It is performed with the patient positioned supine and the therapist supporting the affected knee between terminal extension and 20° of flexion. The distal femur is stabilised by one of the examiner's hands while proximal tibia is translated forward by other hand. A normal knee exhibits either minimal anterior movement of tibia. An indefinite or soft end point is a positive Lachman test indicating ACL injury.

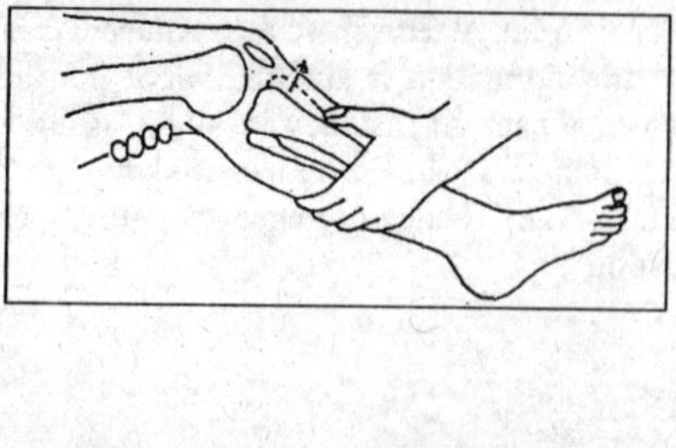

Lack of arousal A female sexual dysfunction formerly called frigidity. It involves failure to respond adequately with congestion and lubrication–even with appropriate sexual stimulation.

Lack of personal accomplishment A decline in one's feelings of competence and successful achievements in one's work with people.

Lacrimal Relating to tear or tear production.

Lacrimal bone Small fragile bone of the face found in the anterior portion of the medial wall of the orbit.

Lacrimal canal A duct, one on each eyelid, beginning at the punctum at the medial margin of any eyelid and conveying tears medially into the lacrimal sac.

Lacrimal canaliculus A drainage duct for tears, located at the medical corner of an eyelid. It conveys the tears medially into the nasolacrimal sac.

Lacrimal dissector It is used to dissect the tissue around the lacrimal sac. It is very useful during the sac surgery.

Lacrimal gland Secretory cells, located at the superior anterolateral portion of each orbit, that secrete tears into excretory ducts that open onto the surface of the conjunctiva.

Lacrimal papilla A small elevation at the inner canthus of each eyelid containing a punctum lacrimale.

Lacrimal probes These are used for probing of the nasolacrimal duct.

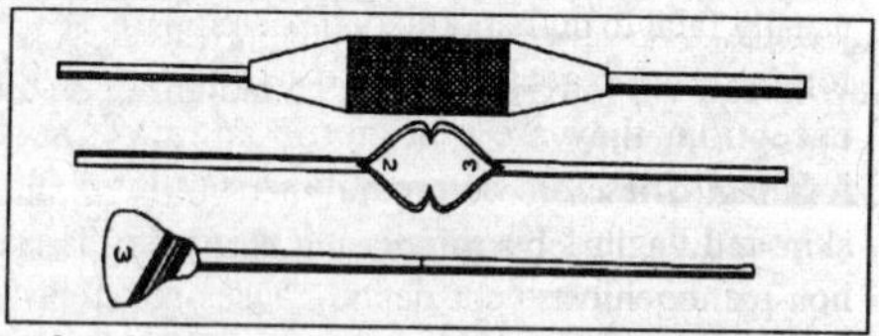

Lacrimal retractor This is used to retract the skin after giving an incision in the lacrimal sac area for lacrimal surgery. It helps the surgeon to provide a good field and also acts as haemostat.

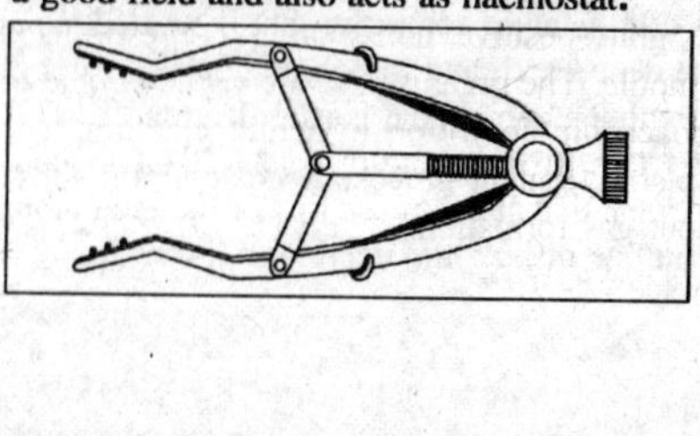

Lacrimation It is an active process of excessive secretion of tear fluid. Although lacrimal drainage system is functioning normally yet it is not able to drain the excessive secretion of tear fluid. It may occur in inflammation or ulceration of cornea, irritation of conjunctiva and uveitis. Emotional factors may also results in it.

Lactate A salt or an ester of lactic acid.

Lactation In mammals, the production and secretion of milk from the mammary glands, or the period following parturition when this process occurs.

Lactational anestrus The absence of ovulatory estrous cycles during lactation.

Lacteal A lymphatic vessel located in each villus of the intestine; serves to absorb fat materials from the chyme passing through the small intestine.

Lactic acid The acid produced by fermentation of milk, sugar and responsible for the flavour of sour milk and precipitation of casein curd in cottage cheese.

Lactic acid bacteria A diverse group of bacteria, composed chiefly of genera that produce lactic acid as the primary metabolic endproduct from the fermentation of carbohydrates; members of the genera lactococcus, lactobacillus, pediococcus, and entercococcus.

Lactic acidosis Metabolic acidosis accompanied by plasma lactate levels.

Lactiferous duct The duct that drains the grapelike cluster of milk-secreting glands in the breast.

Lactobacillus The *Lactobacill*us produces considerable amount of lactic acid from simpler carbohydrates and withstand a degree of acidity, usually fatal to non-sporulating bacteria. These are long, slender gram-positive bacilli and with exception, they are non-motile and non-spore forming. These are commonly present in mouth, skin and vagina. Essentially, these organisms are non-pathogenic except dental causes and febrile disease.

Lactobacillus acidophilus These are able to flourish in a highly acid medium at pH 4. These occur in faeces, saliva and milk. These are basically large, gram-positive, non-sporing, non-capsulated and motile. The organisms grow under aerobic or microaerobic condition in acidic medium. The organisms ferment glucose, lactose and maltose without gas formation.

Lactochrome Pigment in milk.

Lactoferrin A glycoprotein present in the mucosal secretions and phagocytic cells of vertebrates that binds and transport iron.

Lactogen A factor that stimulates milk production; specifically, one of the lactogenic hormones.

Lactones These are oxygen containing heterocyclic compounds.

Lacto-ovo-vegetarian One whose diet is composed of vegetables, fruit, milk and eggs but no flesh food.

Lactose The carbohydrate found in milk, which is composed of a molecule of glucose and galactose. It is the primary osmotic determinant of milk.

Lactose intolerance A disorder resulting in the inability to digest lactose because of an enzyme, lactase, deficiency. Symptoms include bloating, intestinal gas, nausea, diarrhea, and cramps.

Lactovegetarian dietary pattern A food plan consisting of only plant foods and dairy products.

Lacuna A small space, cavity or depression; a space in bone matrix or cartilage in which an osteocyte or chondrocyte is located; cavity containing maternal blood in the placenta.

Lacunar It is known as cerebral atherosclerosis or multi-infarct dementia. Mental symptoms are always present. Impairment of memory of recent incidences may take place. Lack of grasp and storage of facts exist. Headache, vertigo attacks, giddiness and convulsious may take place. There may develop homolateral cerebellar ataxia. Brain infarctions are 0.9 to 1.5 mm diameter and iregularly distributed.

Lacunar infarct Brain infarct in the form of a lacuna, associated with hypertension.

Ladin sign Elastic area offering decreased resistance to palpation located just above corporocervical junction.

Laevulose Alternate name for fructose.

Ladin sign Elastic area offering decreased resistance to palpation located just above corporocervical junction.

Lag glycosuria It is a condition where blood sugar rises rapidly after a meal to a value above renal threshold. The fasting value is normal and blood sugar returns to normal at usual rate. It happens due to delay in action of insulin.

Lag phenomenon Difference between active and passive range of motion.

Lagophthalmos It is a condition of incomplete closure of palpebral aperture when an attempt is made to close the eyes. It may be caused by congenital deformity of lids and ectropion of lower lid. Proptosis, absence of reflex blinking is extreme in all patients. On examination there is conjunctival congestion in lower bulbar fornix. Lower part of cornea shows erosions of opacities. There is constant epiphora.

Lamaze method of delivery The most widely used prepared childbirth method in the United States. It uses an individualised approach with classes for both parents in the anatomy and neuromuscular activity of the reproductive system, breathing techniques in labour, and exercises. Sometimes other subjects such as nutrition, hygiene, and child care are taught. Also called psychoprophylactic method of prepared childbirth.

Lambdoid suture Area that denotes the union of the occipital and the parietal bones of the skull.

Lambert's canals Collateral interalveolar ducts.

Lamella A concentric ring of matrix surrounding the central canal in an osteon of mature bone tissue.

Lamellar ichthyosis The clinical manifestations are at birth. It begins with diffuse erythema and scaling which also involves the flexor areas of body such as subcubital and popliteal fossae. Most of body shows large and coarse scales. Skin loses its elasticity and shining with fine wrinkles. During puberty only a little improvement is seen. In ichthyosis congenita baby may born with severe hyperkeratosis as if encased in a thick sheet cover. Even feeding becomes difficult. So it becomes fatal.

Lamellated corpuscle Oval-shaped pressure receptor located in subcutaneous tissue and consisting of concentric layers of connective tissue wrapped around a sensory nerve fiber. Also called a Pacinian corpuscle.

Lamina A layer; a portion of the vertebra which extends from the transverse process to the spinous process.

A thin plate of bone that extends superiorly from the body of a vertebra to form both sides of the arch of a vertebra.

Lamina dura Dense cortical bone lining the alveolus as it appears on a radiograph; white line between the dark periodontal ligament space and light gray trabecular alveolar bone on a radiograph.

Lamina papyracea Orbital lamina of ethmoid bone.

Lamina propria The connective tissue layer of a mucous membrane.

Laminar or streamline flow In this type of movement, all molecules are moving parallel to each other and paths do not cross.

Laminaria A genus of seaweeds. Also, a small stick of hygroscopic material that absorbs moisture rapidly and expands. It is used to begin initial dilation of the cervix prior to abortion.

Laminaria tent It is a stick sike wooden material. It is derived from sea wood which absorbs water very easily. It swells enormously. At one end thread is attached for making it convenient to pull out. It is used for cervical dilatation. One laminaria tent introducer pushes it into cervix.

These are made from compressed seaweed root, 6 to 7 cm in length and 0.2 to 0.6 cm in diameter available in a presterilized disposable set and may be used prior to curettage to avoid cervical tear. Inserted 18 to 24 hours before D & C. The laminaria tent usually dilates the cervix to No 9 or No 10. Hegar dilator.

Laminate Restoration made by forming a thin sheet or layer of dental material, such as porcelain to form a restoration; commonly used in anterior teeth for esthetic purposes.

Laminotomy Removal of only part of the lamina to reach to disc.

Laminectomy The surgical removal of posterior boney arches of one or more vertebra.

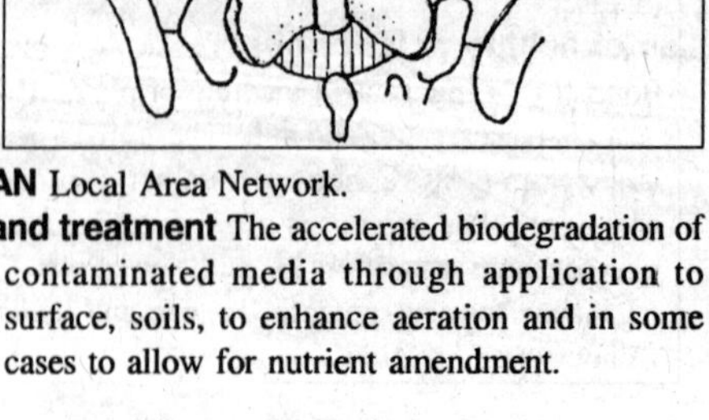

LAN Local Area Network.

Land treatment The accelerated biodegradation of contaminated media through application to surface, soils, to enhance aeration and in some cases to allow for nutrient amendment.

Landolt ring A test object for measuring visual acuity consisting of incomplete ring resembling the letter C.

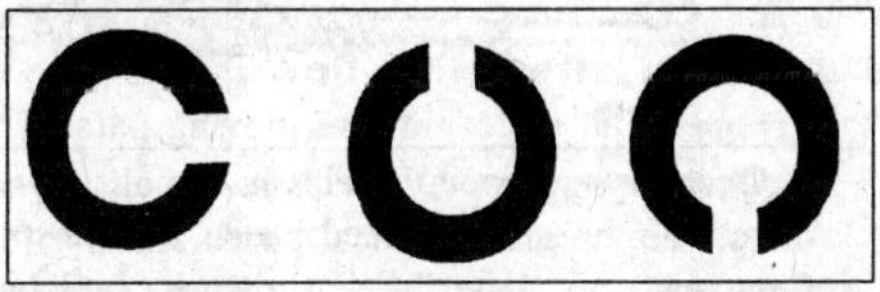

Langer' lines Cleavage lines of skin. These are the lines visible in skin representing the aligned formation of connective tissue beneath. The best examples are creases of palms and hands.

Langerhands cell Epidermal dendritic cell that functions as an antigen-presenting cell (APC) during an immune response.

Language analyser Also known as a language-acquisition device, it is speculated to lie at the basis of the child's ability to learn language. A condition of our biological inheritance, it enables children to acquire language in the very earliest years of life.

Language habits Learning the names for things; acquiring the use of words. The emphasis here is upon vocabulary development, the use of the basic sounds, and the simple constructions in a given language.

Language rules In language learning, the understanding of syntax and sentence construction. Understanding the complexities of a given language, making proper sentence constructions and grammatical transformations.

Lanugo The fine, downy hair found on nearly all parts of the fetus's body except the palms of the hands and the soles of the feet.

Laparoscope Specialized optical viewing tube.

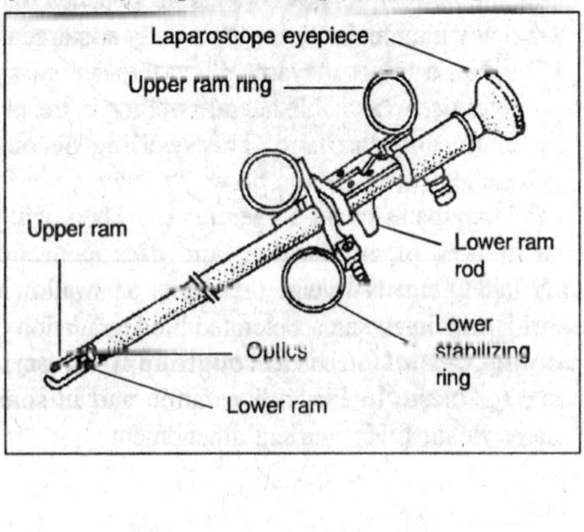

Laparoscopy It is the insertion of a scope about 10 mm into peritoneal cavity through 2 cm subumbilical incision to allow visualisation of

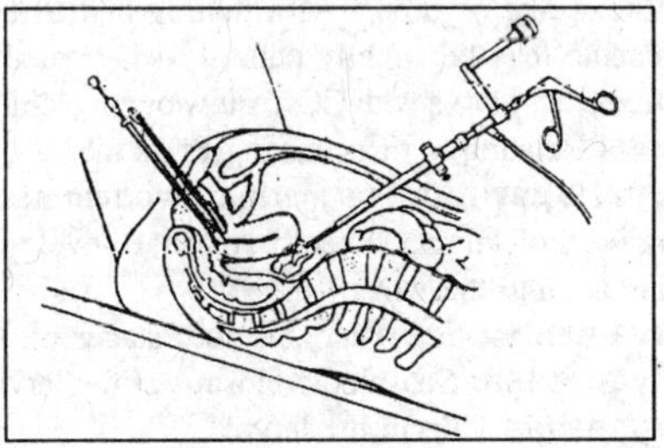

pelvic structures. Indications are diagnostic but it is also possible to do minor operation as tubal sterilisation/ovarian biopsy and dilatation and curettage (D & C).

Laprotomy A large incision through the abdominal wall, made to operate on or view the abdominal contents.

Larazèpam It is used for insomnia, epilepsy and sedation. Half life is about 12 hours. It produces more amnesia.

Lard The fat rendered from fresh, clean, sound fatty tissues of hogs at the time of slaughter. It is used as an ingredient of margarine and cooking fats. It contains high concentration of saturated fatty acids.

Large for gestational age (LGA) Pertaining to an neonate weighing above the 90th percentile for the gestational age. LGA infants are immature but overgrown and are typical of diabetic mothers.

Large for gestational age infant An infant whose size is above 90th percentile for gestational age.

Large intestine The portion of the gastrointestinal tract extending from the ileum of the small intestine to the anus, divided structurally into the cecum, colon, rectum, and anal canal.

Larsen syndrome It is an autosomal dominant condition in milder form and recessive in severe form. Clinical features include short stature, multiple joint dislocation, specially knee and hip joint. Face will be flat with cleft palate and foot deformities.

Larson's joint A congenital disorder of multiple dislocations of joints.

Larva migrans It is caused by migration of parasitic larva in epidermis. It commonly affects those walking bare footed or working bare handed on contaminated soil. It presents with papule at the site of inoculation followed by slightly raised thread-like erythema with itching and irritation. Papule may be slightly painful. It is treated with freezing of larva with CO_2, snow or ethyl chloride.

Larval Relating to or occurring as larvae.

Larval spawning In marine invertebrates, the release of larvae, or embryos that develop into larvae, into the water.

Larva-nematodes There are four stages of larva.

Larygospasm Spasmodic closure of the larynx.

Laryngalgia Pain in the larynx.

Laryngeal of or pertaining to the larynx.

Laryngeal carcinoma Most warning signs are, hoarseness, habitual throat clearing, cough, haemoptysis, dyspnoea and dysphagia. Metastasis to lymph nodes may develop.

Laryngeal cellulitis Symptoms are rapidly progressive. Severe pain radiates to ear, dysphagia, hoarseness, stridor, fever and severe systemic illness. Laryngoscopy shows swelling, redness and possible fistula formation. Bacterial infection is the cause.

Laryngeal forceps It is a long handled, curved forceps with a clubbed beak. The beak or tip of

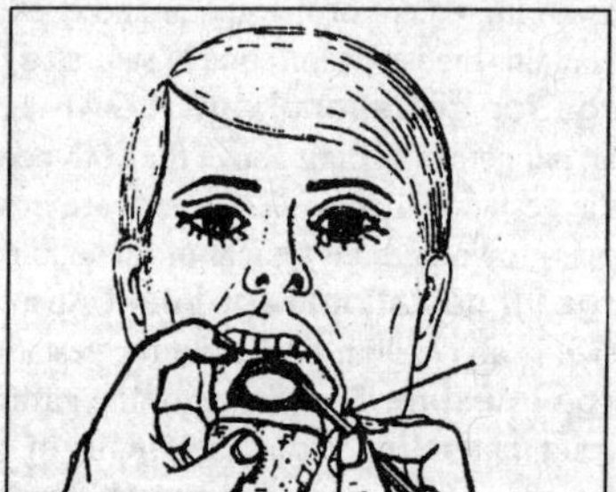

forceps may be cupped with sharp margins. It is best used to get biopsy from larynx and base of tongue and to remove foreign body from larynx.

Laryngeal mask airway It is a device supporting and maintaining airway without tracheal intubation.

Laryngeal mirror It is a small circular mirror of approximately 1" diameter mounted at the tip of long slender metal staff at an angle. It is used for

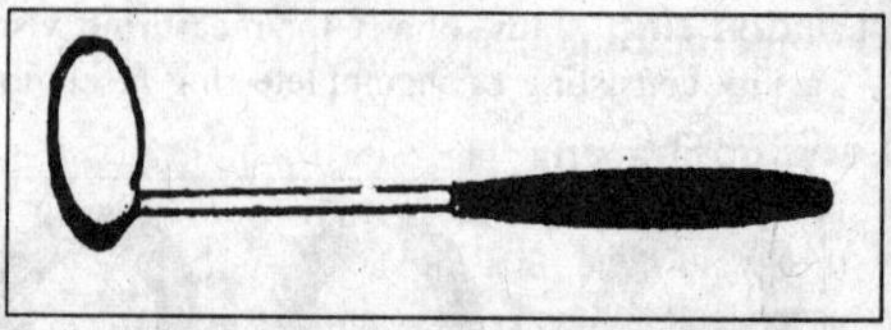

indirect laryngoscopy. It helps in visualising base of tongue, epiglottis, vocal cords and pyriform fossa, well.

Laryngeal oedema Oedematous swelling in the larynx may be circumscribed or diffuse. The symptoms depend on location, extent and rate of development. There will develop hoarseness to aphonia, occasional dyspnoea, pressure sensation, frequent throat clearing and cough. There is no pain. Laryngoscopy shows a glassy oedema or general swelling of epiglottis. Inflammation is the cause.

Laryngeal syphilis Secondary syphilis produces syphilitic eruptions in the larynx. Tertiary cases are marked by endolaryngeal gummata. Dark red swellings are succeeded by ulcers. Ulcers are punched out in shape. Pain and dysfunction may be absent for sometime. There will develop oral fetor.

Laryngitis Inflammation of the mucous membrane lining the larynx.

Laryngitis sicca Person develops habitual throat clearing, accompanied by a dry, barking cough. There will be variable hoarseness. Stridor may be present. Vocal cords become narrow, reddened and may be covered by crusts. Dyspnoea occurs.

Laryngocele It is a diverticulum containing air, formed due to herniation of laryngeal mucosa through the thyrohyoid membrane. It is mostly unilateral. It simulates cervical air pouches found in many mammals. These are mostly acquired and found in trumpet players. When the sac enlarges it gives rise to a visible lateral swelling in the neck over thyroid cartilage. The swelling becomes prominent when person blows. It is baggy in feel and may be resonant on percussion. There will be a history of appearance and disappearance. Swelling moves up with the larynx on swallowing which is diagnostic.

Laryngocentesis Surgical puncture of the larynx.

Laryngomalacia Flaccidity of the epiglottis and aryeiglottic folds.

Laryngopharyngeal Pertaining to the larynx and pharynx.

Laryngopharynx The inferior portion of the pharynx, extending downward from the level of the hyoid bone, that divides posteriorly into the esophagus and anteriorly into the larynx.

Laryngopyocele A suppurative form of laryngocele.

Laryngorrhagia Hemorrhage from the larynx.

Laryngoscope Instrument used to perform laryngoscsopy. It may be flexible or rigid.

Laryngotracheal diverticulum The pouch that develops from the laryngotracheal groove as a precursor of the laryngotracheal tube.

Laryngotracheal groove The depression in the posterior wall of the pharynx from which the lower larynx and the trachea, bronchi, and lungs eventually develop.

Larynx It is a organ of voice, the sphincter between the pharynx and trachea. It extends from root of tongue to trachea. It is opposite the 3rd, 4th, 5th, and 6th cervical vertebrae. Average length is 44 mm in males and 36 mm in females. Transverse diameter is 43 mm, its AP diameter averages 36 mm. It is covered by depressor muscles of the hyoid bone by the thyroid gland and cricothyroid muscles. Cavity of larynx extends from superior laryngeal aperture to the lower border of cricoid cartilage. The entrance of larynx is wider in front than behind and slopes downwards and backwards. The vestibule of the larynx is the superior part of the cavity and extends from aryepiglottis fold to vestibular fold.

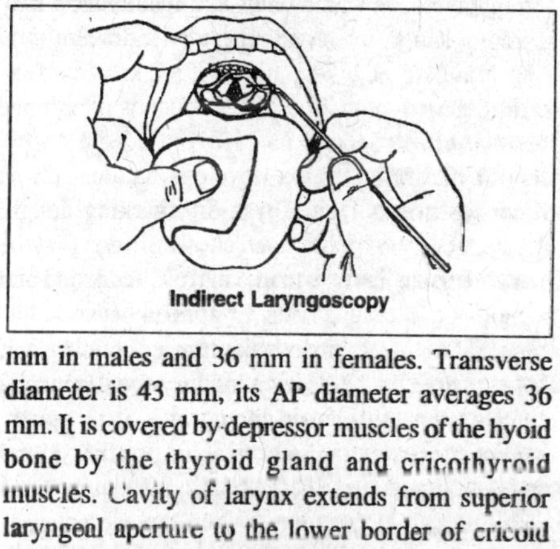

Indirect Laryngoscopy

Vestibular folds are false cords. The vocal cords stretch from thyroid cartilage anteriorly to the arytenoid cartilage of the corresponding side posteriorly. Space between cords is glottis. Glottis is the narrowest part and measures about 2.5 cm. Nerve supply is from vagus. The sensory supply from the larynx ascends in the internal and recurrent laryngeal nerve.

Laseque's sign Patient lies supine with hip flexed. An attempt of dorsiflexion of the ankle then produces muscle spasm and pain in the posterior thigh. It is seen in the cases of irritation of sciatic nerve or lumbar nerve root.

Laser It is the device that amplifies light into a very concentrated beam. It can be used as a scalpel and its heat used to cauterise and seal minor blood vessels. For retinal surgery it is being used. As a wider beam it is used to destroy precancerous mass.

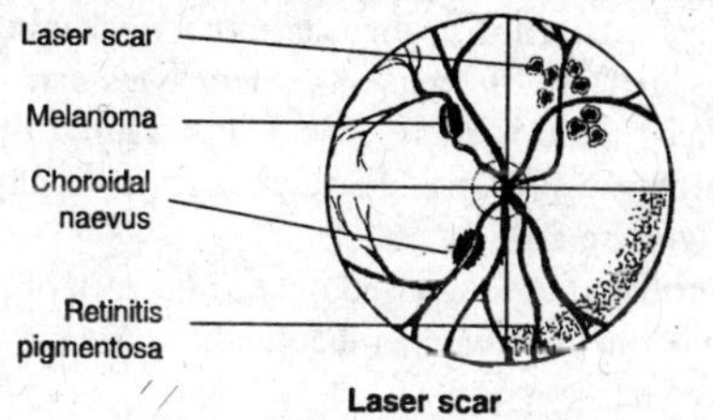

Laser scar

Laser angioplasty It is a method to open vascular occlusions and narrowings exploiting the theoretical possibility of achieving plaque ablation by a laser beam transported along a glass fibre.

Laser argon Laser with ionised argon gas as the active medium which limits a blue green light beam with a wave length of 514 nm. It is used to do iridectomy.

Laser camera It is a device in which digital data from an imaginary modality are encoded by variations in the intensity of a laser beam which is scanned line by line over the film. The variable laser intensity thus exposes the film to the desired grey scale or the desired degree of colours in a laser camera.

Last rites A religious rite performed by a clergyman to the individual just prior to death.

Latch on Attachment of infant to the brain.

Late blight The disease of potatoes caused by Phytopthora infestants that led to the disastrous Irish Potato Famine of the mid-19th century. The term also applies to infection of P.infestans on tomatoes.

Late deceleration Increasing of the fetal heart rate after the onset of a uterine contraction.

Late fetal death The death of a product of condeption after 28 weeks of gestation by before birth.

Late look bias Bias that occurs when mild, slowly progressive cases of a disease are preferentially detected in a survey because patients with this form of the disease live longer and can be interviewed, whereas more severe cases result in death and go undetected by the survey.

Lateal canal stenosis It follows a disc prolapse as a result of organisation and fibrosis of sequestrated disc material with thickening and ossification of ligaments osteophytes narrow the canal. Pain is more severe than caused by disc prolapse sitting is also uncomfortable physical signs are few.

Latency stage A period of apparent lack of sexual interests. In Freudian theory, the stage before the genital period.

Latent Concealed, not apparent, potential.

Latent content The hidden (unconscious) meaning of thoughts or actions, especially in dreams or fantasies. In dreams, it is expressed in disorted, disguised, condensed, and symbolic form.

Latent fingerprint technique Any method employed to visualize, invisible fingerprints on various surfaces.

Latent heat Energy required solely to change are state of a substance without changing its temperature.

Latent infection The virus persist in the quiscent form most of the time with very little viral replicative activity. A symptomless or inapparent infection that is chronic and in which a certain host-parasite relationship is established.

Latent motivation A chronic or ongoing desire that may not be active for a particular moment such as desire for money or sex.

Latent phase of delivery This starts at the onset of contractions and is completed when cervix reaches 3 cm of dilatation. In primigravida, it takes about 8 hours and lasts an average of 6 hours.

Latent virus A virus which has entered into a non-replicative mode of existence in a cell but, which allow limited viral genome replication without full expression of virus functions and production of mature infectious virus particles.

Lateral Position either to the right or the left of the midsagittal plane.

Lateral basal segmental bronchus The portion of the tracheobroncheal tree arising from the right or left lower lobe bronchus that is distributed to the lateral basal segment.

Lateral corticospinal tract In the lateral spinal cord, a pathway that carries information instructing movement.

Lateral episiotomy The incision starts 1 cm away from the centre of the fourchette but it may result in free bleeding. Levator ani muscles may be torned and bartholin's glands and ducts are injured.

Lateral frenum Folds of tissue connecting cheeks to tooth structures.

Lateral grip By this grip the lie of the fetus and situation of the back of fetus are determined.

Lateral horn The small, lateral extension of spinal cord grey matter; located only in spinal cord regions T_1-L_2 and S_2-S_4; containing preganglionic autonomic nerve cell bodies.

Lateral hypothalamus Region of the hypothalamus in which damage impairs eating and drinking and in which animals will in tracranially self-stimulate at a very high rate also known as eating center.

Lateral incisor Second incisior tooth distal to the central incisor.

Lateral listhesis Lateral translatory excursion of the vertebral body.

Lateral medullary syndrome Characteristic symptoms and signs following thrombosis of the certebral of posterior inferior cerebellar artery.

Lateral meniscus The knee meniscus in the lateral compartment. It is more circular in form than the medial meniscus.

Lateral oblique position Variation of a side-lying position.

Lateral or external rotation Turning the anterior surface of the extremity away from the midline of the body.

Lateral position This can be left lateral or right lateral position. This is used for giving back care, enemas, colonic irrigation, for gynaeçological examination and rectal examination. Patient lies on his or her right/left with legs flexed. Upper leg is flexed more than lower leg. In this position there is less chance of chest infection or pressure sores.

Lateral pterygoid plate A wing-shaped bony projection of the sphenoid bone located distal to the maxillary tuberosity region; appears radiopaque.

Lateral stenosis Nerve root compression as it exits the neural framen.

Lateral surface The outer side.

Lateral thoracotomy A surgical incision into the lateral chest wall.

Lateral ventricles It is a cavity in brain hemispheres which has its anterior horn in frontal lobe, sends posterior horn towards occipital lobe and inferior horn in temporal lobe. These dont communicate with other side.

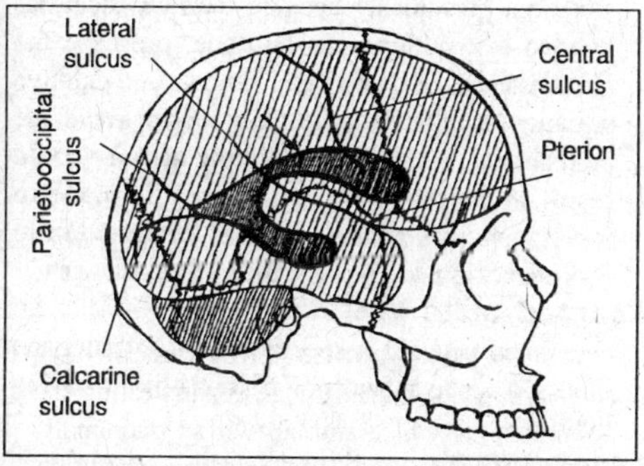

Lateralization A process whereby functions become located primarily on one side of the brain.

Laterally condensed cold gutta parcha It is an extension of single cone whcih fits accurately in the apical 2 or 3 m.m. with this an attempt is made to obturate the unfilled space around primary gutta percha with additional secondary points. These are condensed without heat.

Latex A colorless or milky sap that exudes from wounds of some plants, such as milkweed.

Latex sensitivity Allergic response to the proteins in latex.

Latex-safe environment Room stocked with latex-free equipment and wiped clean of glove powder.

Lathyrogens Spastic paralysis of legs is caused by lathyrus sativum.

Laticifers Cells or a series of cells forming ducts containing latex and occurring in some vascular plants.

Latissimus dorsi An extensor of the upper arm.

Lattice degeneration Lattice degeneration of retina is directly related to retinal detachment. Lattice is not an age-related phenomenon and is seen in young myopes above minus three dioptres. Lattice degeneration appears as spindle-shaped, sharply demarcated areas which are circumferentially oriented. These lattice areas may form 2 or 3 rows. Lattice is generally bilateral and seen more commonly in superior temporal quadrant of fundus. The vitreous over the lesion is synchytic with firm attachment at borders. A retinal hole in lattice remains quiet. Detachment progresses slowly.

Laurence-Moon-Biedl syndrome An autosomal recessive disorder usually characterised by hypogonadism, obesity, mental defects, polydactylism, and perhaps retinitis pigmentosa, optic nerve atrophy, strabismus, and nystagmus.

Lauric acid A saturated fatty acids. One of the long chain fatty acids.

Lavage The irrigation or washing out of an organ or cavity.

Law A scientific statement that is true uniformly for a whole class of natural occurrences.

Laws Rules of conduct established and enforced by the government of a society.

Law of Bell and Magendie Named after its cofounders, this law states that the dorsal roots of the spinal cord are sensory and the ventral roots are motor.

Law of gases The kinetic theory of gases postulates that molecules of a gas in space are constantly moving and bumping each other and into walls of enclosing space. This bumping gives rise to pressure or tension of gas in space. The greater the number of molecules the greater will be tension. Temperature increases movement and so increases tension.

Laxative Substances that accelerates intestinal movements.

Lay Non professional.

Layette The complete outfit of clothing for a newborn.

LDH Licensed Dental Hygienist.

Lead hand It is a simple and effective hand shaped device made of malleable type lead. During surgery it positions the hand of patient.

Lead intoxication It occurs both in organic and inorganic form. Ten per cent consumed lead is being absorbed by an adult. Majority of lead poisoning occur after the absorption of inorganic lead and needs extended periods of absorption to achieve levels to cause symptoms. First sign of inorganic lead toxicity is anaemia. It results in fatigue, irritability, anorexia and paleness. GIT symptoms include abdominal pain, intermittent vomiting and constipation. Lead colic is more common. Lead encephalopathy develops after excessive chronic exposure. It usually occurs at blood lead levels of more than 100 mg/ml. Lead encephalopathy is characterised by vomiting, irritability clumsiness and loss of recently acquired developmental skill. Person develops ataxia and jerky movements. If untreated, stupor, coma, convulsions and death may follow. Lead line occurs in gums and around anal margin.

Lead pipe rigidity Uniform resistance to passive joint movement; characteristic of parkinson's disease.

Lead poisoning It causes excessive salivation, metallic taste, swelling of the salivary gland and a dark line along a gingival margin. Under microscope one finds that lead line consist of a granular pigment in the perivascular area of basement membrane. This pigment is lead sulphide. There will be GIT disturbances, neuritis and convulsive seizures.

Lead rubber It is a combination of lead and rubber used for shielding in areas where flexibility as well as protective shielding is required. The lead can be used as a linning in the rubber material.

Lead rubber gloves Gloves worn when handling radioactive material. Lead can be combined with other materials such as rubber to enable them to be flexible enough to be worn whilst maintaining its protective value.

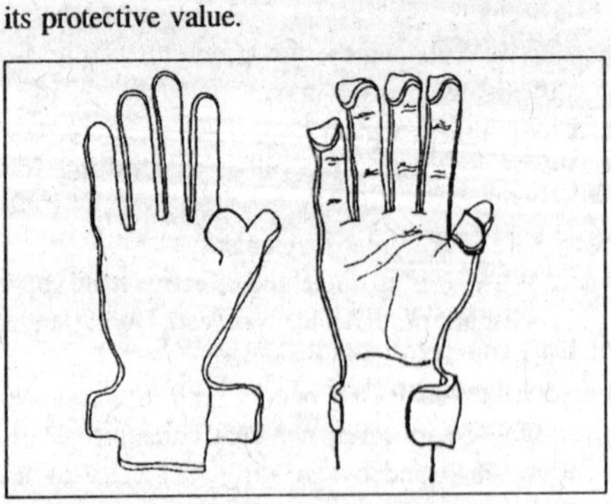

Lead-time bias Bias that occurs when screening detects disease earlier in its natural history than would otherwise have happened, so that the time from diagonsis to death is lengthened. Having additional lead time does not necessarily alter the natural history of the disease and therefore may not indicate longer life.

Leafy vegtables Their less digestible carbohydrates provide an abundance of roughage. Although proteins content is low but is of higher quality.

Learned helplessness Inactivity is an aversive situation, presumably because the individual has learned that nothing can be done to escape the circumstances. Experimental animals in a punitive situation eventually take no steps to avoid the punishment, even when a simple activity could result in its removal. An analogy is made to individuals in a ghetto, some of whom seem to make no effort to alleviate their circumstances.

Learned taste aversion Acquisition of an associated between a specific taste (or odor) and illness; leads to an aversion of food objects having that taste.

Learned tolerance Experience in performing a behavior under the influence of a drug results in improved performance of the behavior when subsequently under the influence of the drug.

Learning A more or less permanent modification of an individuals's behaviour which results from previous activity, special training, or observation.

Learning disability A syndrome affecting school age children of normal or above normal intelligence characterised by specific difficulties in learning to read (dyslexia), write (dysgraphia), and calculate (dyscalculia). The disorder is believed to be related to slow developmental progression of perceptual motor skills.

Learning disorders Academic skill disorders; developmental arithmetic disorder (dyscalculia); writing disorder (dysgraphia); and reading disorder (dyslexia).

Learning objective An outcome that the learner is expected to achieve at the end of a given unit of instruction, sometimes called an instructional objective, especially from the teacher's viewpoint. Learning objectives can be established at different levels of difficulty and in three domains : the cognitive domain, usually concerned with verbal learning; the motor domain, usually concerned with physical skills; and the affective domain, involving attitudes, feelings, and values. Commonly, learning objectives involve more than one domain.

Learning set An understanding of how a problem can be solved with a rule that can be applied in many different situations.

Learning theory The body of theory that exists in experimental psychology that attempts to account for how animal and human behaviour change takes place.

Leaven Yeast.

Lebers Optic atrophy, vernal conjunctivitis and Down's syndrome. Patient complains of gradual loss of vision, photophobia and monocular diplopia. Visual acuity is markedly reduced with distorted vision. Retinoscopy reveals a scissors shadow. Refraction shows a high degree of irregular myopic astigmatism.

Leboyer method of delivery A method of delivery based on theories of a French obstetrician, Frederick Leboyer. The method avoids harsh, sudden sensory stimulation of the newborn by providing him a quiet, dimly lit delivery room and warm bath to make birth less of a traumatic event.

Lecithin Freshly prepared lecithin is a pale yellow waxy solid which is crystalline. On exposure to air and light oxygen is readily absorbed and colour darkens. Fresh lecithin in contact with water swells up.

Lectins A family of proteins, mostly of plant origin, which bind specific sugars on glycoproteins and glycolipids. Some lectins are also mitogenic e.g. PHA, conA.

Lectovegetarian Vegetarian whose diet includes milk.

LeFort fracture It is a vertical avulsion fracture of anterior medial aspect of distal fibula.

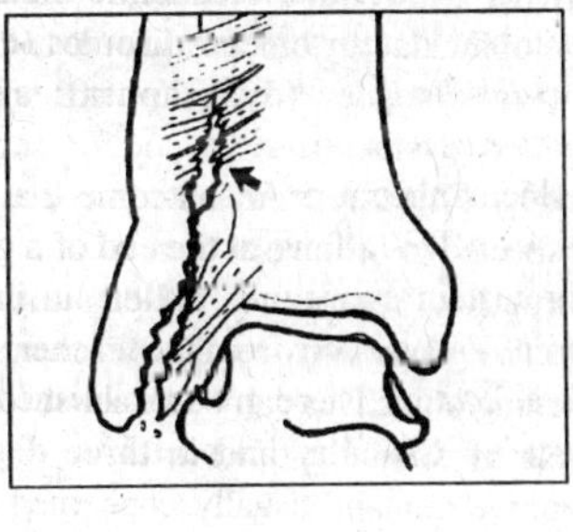

Left atrioventricular orifice The opening leading from the left atrium into the left ventricle.

Left bronchus It is narrower but longer than right. Length before dividing into upper and lower lobe bronchi is 5 cm. Aorta arches over it and it enters the left lung opposite 6th thoracic vertebra. It leaves the treachea at angle of 45° from vertical.

Left bundle branches The left crus of the atrioventricular (His) bundle of specialized myocytes that ramifies in the subendocardium of the left ventricle; part of the specialized conduction system of the heart.

Left common carotid artery Arises from the highest part of the arch of the aorta to the left of the brachiocephalic trunk.

Left coronary artery Originates in the left posterior aortic sinus, passing between the pulmonary trunk and the left auricle, as it proceeds to the atrioventricular sulcus, where it typically divides into two branches; The anterior interventricular ramus and the circumflex ramus; usually supplies almost all of the left ventricle and atrium and most of the interventricular septum.

Left coronary plexus Primarily and extension of the left half of the deep part of the cardiac plexus, although it does receive some fibers from the right half; it follows the distribution of the left coronary artery, supplying the left atrium and ventricle.

Left fibrous trigone The part of the fibroskeletion of the heart that is located between the left side of the left annulus of the mitral valve and the aortic annulus.

Left handedness One in 21 persons may be left handed. There is dominance of right cerebral hemisphere.

Left inferior pulmonary vein The vein that returns blood from the lower lobe of the left lung to the left atrium.

Left lateral view Refers to the preferred view for a lateral radiograph of the chest; taken with the left side of the chest against the film cassette.

Left margin of the heart The left border of the heart, descending obliquely (convex toward the left) from the left auricle to the cardiac apex; formed mainly by the left ventricle, separates the sternocostal and the left surfaces of the heart.

Left marginal artery A large ventricular branch of the circumflex artery, occurring gin about 90% of cases.

Left marginal vein One of the larger tributaries to the great cardiac vein; delivers blood from the left ventricle.

Left occipito anterior (LOA) The denominator 'occiput' points towards the left ileopectinal eminence and the sagittal suture lies in the right oblique diameter of pelvic brim.

Left occiptio lateral (LOL) The occipit points towards the left side of the pelvic brim midway between ileo pectineal eminence and left sacroiliac joints and the sagittal suture is in the transverse diameter of the brain.

Left pulmonary artery The left branch of the pulmonary artery distributed to the left lung; runs in front of the descending aorta and the left primary bronchus to the root of the lung.

Left subclavian artery The last branch from the arch of the aorta.

Left surface of the heart The surface of the heart, consisting almost entirely of the left ventricle, that faces upward, back and toward the left; it is convex and widest above, narrowing toward the cardiac apex.

Left ventricular enddiastolic pressure The pressure in the left ventricle at the end of the diastolic phase of the cardiac cycle.

Left ventricular failure It is the failure of left ventricle to propel blood forwards resulting in accumulation of blood in pulmonary circulation, characterised by paroxysmal nocturnal dyspnoea, gallop rhythm, pulsus alterans and basal crepitation.

Dyspnoea to start occurs on exertion and then may occur even at rest. Dyspnoea at rest may be paroxysmal and often nocturnal. At midnight patient suddenly gets up in bed or rushes to window and feels suffocated. During early stage patient coughs up and bring out lot of cough which is frothy. There may be cold clammy sweat often drenching the garments due to excessive catecholamine secretion. Central type of cyanosis is present. Pulse is high.

Leg The portion of the lower extremity between the knee and ankle.

Leg press This exercise is done on weight machine exerciser. The feet are placed shoulder width apart. The athletes lift the weight with both legs are almost straight without locking the knees, pauses, lower the weight to the starting position in a slow and controlled manner and repeats.

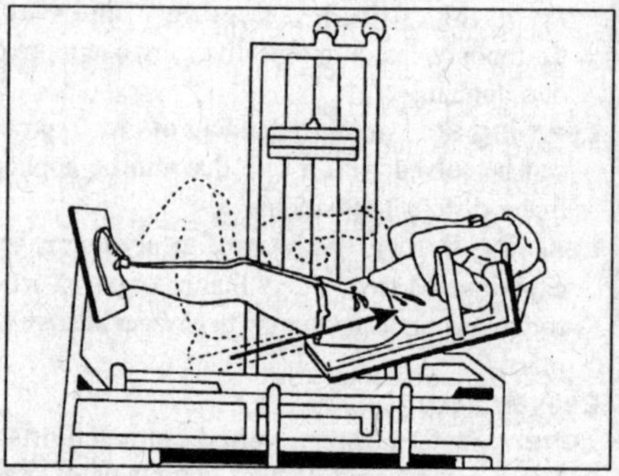

Legal psychology A speciality concerned with the application of psychological knowledge to legal issues. Specialists in this field sometimes testify on the ways in which the basic psychological processes, such as perception and motivation, may influence recall and other behaviours. Sometimes the concern is with the uses and abuses of psychological testing; psychiatric issues and the plea of insanity also are important concerns. Sometimes called forensic psychology.

Leger card Accounting form for keeping track of debits, expenditures, credits and charges.

Legitimate tools Instruments that are in accordance with established and accepted standards for a profession or discipline.

Legumin Globulin protein in pea, bean and lentil.

Leih Chueh Located 1.5 to 2.0 cm proximal to the transverse crease just above the styloid process of radius supplied by branches or radial nerve. This site is indicated for headache and neck pain. Needle is inserted obliquely and upward to 0.5 cm.

Leishman-Donovan body Leishman-Donovan (LD) bodies are non-flagellated form of protozoa, *Leishmania donovanosis*, and are seen in kala-azar. It is intracytoplasmic, small, oval or round unicellular body with one tiny and another little larger nuclear bodies, occurring in the reticuloendothelial cells and macrophages.

Leminiscus It is a longitudinal bundle of fibres in the brainstem conveying sensory impulses from different part of body to the different centres in cerebral cortex. There are two such longitudinal bundles—a mesial and a lateral.

Lengthening The process in which the muscle assumes a normal resting length by means of the neuromuscular mechanism.

Lens It is a transparent biconvex lens with a capsule. It lies between iris and vitreous. It has two surfaces, two poles and equator. The curvature of anterior surface is about 10 mm while that of posterior surface is 6 mm. It is suspended by suspensory ligaments to the ciliary body. Lens matter is plastic one while the lens capsule is elastic. It helps the lens to change its curvature in the act of accommodation. Anterior surface is lined by epithelium while posterior surface is not. The lens derives its nutrition from aqueous humour.

Lens bifocal A lens which is having two portions of different focal powers. Upper portion is larger and used for distance vision while lower one is smaller and used for near vision.

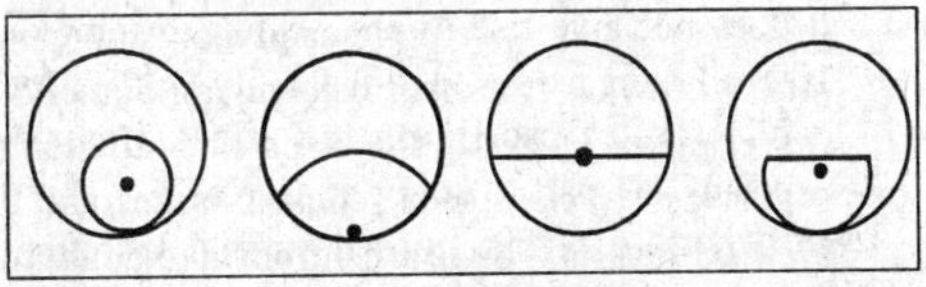

Lens measure It is an instrument for determining the radius of curvature of spherical or cylindrical surface based on measuring the sq of curve.

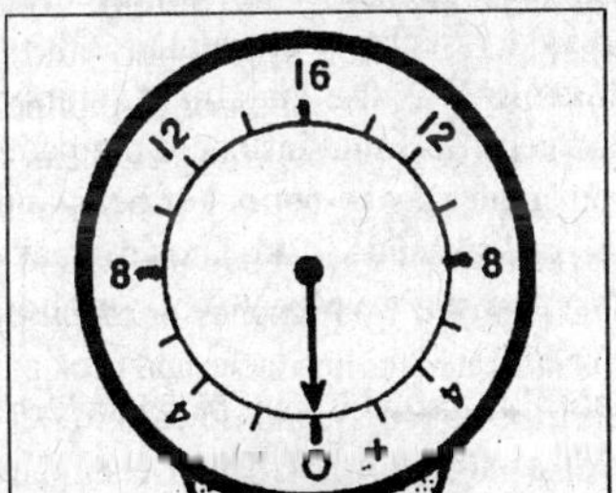

Lens orthoscopic A lens corrected for peripheral aberrations.

Lentavirus A retrovirus such as HIV that primarily infects immune cells and can induce AIDS.

Lenthyosis vulgaris It is the most common variety. In it lesion generally appears in first year of life. Lesions present with fine scales affecting extensor surfaces of limbs and trunks. It appears on antecubital and popliteal fossa and other flexor areas. Hyperkeratosis causes exaggerated creases and thickening of palms and soles. At puberty it improves but may persist for life.

Lentic Describing still or standing waters, as in a lake or pond.

Lentiform Lens-shaped nucleus, part of the corpus striatum (caudate and lentiform nuclei).

Lentigo maligna melanoma It is least common and least malignant. It generally occurs on face after the age of 60. It can develop on any exposed part of body. It starts as irregularly pigmented, brown macule which grows slowly over a period of 10 to 15 years. Malignant change is recognised by thickening and development of discrete nodule. Malignant change may grow up to 5 cm become and irregular in outline.

Lentils Seeds of many varieties of lens esculenta fall into same group as peas and beans.

Lentula A flexible spiral wire instrument used in hand piece to apply past like filling material in root canal.

Leopolds manueuvres It is an obstetrical palpation of four manueuvres of left occipito anterior lie.

Leopord's method Four maneuvers for diagnosing the fetal position.

Lepido A combining form meaning flake or scale.

Lepromin skin test Intradermal injection of boiled extract of lepromatous tissue produces, in cases of positive action, nodule at the site of inoculation. The test is, however, non-specific but in known cases of leprosy a positive test indicates tuberculoid leprosy and a negative test lepromatous leprosy.

Leptomeninges 'thin membranes' comprising the arachnoid and pia mater.

Leptospirosis *Leptospira interrogans* is excreted in urine of wild and domestic animals most often rodents. Organisms enter through scratched skin and enters in nervous system within 2 to 3 days. Organisms disappear from the CSF before active meningitis begins. Uveitis may occur with meningitis. Occasionally ascending polyneuropathy may occur.

Leriche's syndrome There is atheromatous occlusion of abdominal aorta and iliac arteries. The atheroma extends upwards but stops at origin of renal arteries. Clinical features include intermittent claudication of buttock, thigh and calf muscle. Femoral pulse is absent.

Lesbian Equivalent to "homosexual," lesbian is a preferred term for women whose sexual objects of choice are other women.

Lesbianism Lesbian relationship reveals a facet of loving in which a woman shares her joy and fulfilment with another woman. A lesbian is a woman who sexually loves another woman only.

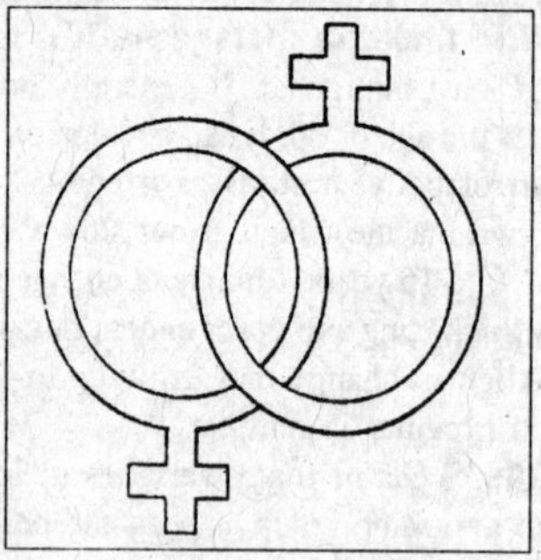

She is not in any way biologically different from other woman, still it is a taboo. Lesbians practise mutual masturbation and cunnilingus. Use of an artificial penis is not very frequent. They practice long periods of foreplay and caressing in general.

Leschke's syndrome The syndrome is characterised by hyperglycaemia, numerous brownish macules on the skin, and general weakness.

Lesion Pathologic disturbance of a tissue resulting in the loss of continuity, enlargement, or function.

Lesser omentum A peritoneal fold of tissue extending from the lasser curvature of the stomach to the liver.

Let-down reflex The activation of a process by which contractions of the myoepithelial cells in a mother's breast propel milk along the duct into the lactiferous sinuses. Also called *milk ejection reflex*.

Lethal mutation A mutation that inactivates a biological function essential to the life of the cell or organism.

Lethality In pathology, a measure of the potency of a disease, defined as the percentage of people who die of a disease among the total of people sickened by that disease.

Lethargy Condition of drowsiness or sleepiness.

Lethologica Temporary inability to remember a proper noun or name.

Leucite It is an important content of porcelain. It is a crystalline potassium-aluminium silicate mineral. It strengthens, toughens and raises the thermal expansion coefficient of normal porcelain.

Leucocin One of water soluble proteins of wheat flour.

Leucocyte White blood corpuscle; a formed element of the blood consisting of a colourless mass of protoplasm, having amoeboid movements and involved in the destruction of disease producing microorganisms.

Leucocytosis An increase in leukocytes in blood.

Leucoderma It is a loosely applied terminology to express depigmented skin lesions. The condition presents with varying and irregular sized and shaped, sharply demarcated, completely depigmented patches surrounded by normal or hyperpigmented skin. Lesions may coalese to form large patches or may involve whole skin surface. It does not give rise to any scaling. Ammoidine 10 to 40 mg is given once daily orally, local application of psorlin on the affected part and exposing the part to sunlight may help.

Leucorrhoea In this, normal vaginal secretion is increased in amount. Discharge is not purulent. The increase in normal vaginal secretion develops during puberty, and during ovulation. During pregnancy discharge simply increases due to increased vascularity of uterus.

Leukaemia It is the malignant tumour of white blood cells. In some instances the patient's white blood count may be normal or below normal. The cause of leukaemia is not known. Leukaemias are classified as myelocytic, lymphocytic and monocytic.

Leukaemia, acute It may begin suddenly and run a rapid course in a few weeks or months. To start there may be aleukaemic phase but later on blood count becomes very high. Blood contains myeloblast or lymphoblasts. Oral lesions are most common and constant finding in acute leukaemia. Enlargement, bleeding and necrosis of gingiva and bleeding around teeth are seen. There may be necrosis of oral mucosa. Tooth extraction is followed by profuse bleeding.

Leukaemia, chronic It may extend up to many years. Acute exacerbation and death may occur at any time. Enlargement of spleen and lymph node may be the first sign. *Chronic myelocytic* shows great increase in granular leucocytes in blood. Many immature cells are present and total count may reach 500,000 per cubic millimetre. Platelet counts may increase but red cells diminish in number. *Chronic lymphocytic* leukaemia is characterised by white cell count than myelocytic type. Count is lesser than 100,000 per cubic mm of which mostly are lymphocytes. Lymph nodes are enlarged. *Chronic monocytic* leukaemia in which immature cells appear in between monocytes and myeloblasts. Oral symptoms are usually present and consist of gingival hyperplasia. There is a dense infiltration of the connective tissue by immature cells of the lymphoid or monocytic series. Usually acute myelogenous leukaemias arise in bone marrow and disseminate in various organs and tissues of body.

Leukocyte White blood cells.

Leukocytosis Increased production of white blood cells.

Leukoderma An acquired type of localized loss of melanin pigmentation of the skin.

Leukopenia Reduction of the number of leukocytes in the blood.

Leukoplakia A white patch on a mucous membrane that will not rub off.

Leukoplakia of vulva The most common white lesion of vulva is lichen sclerosis. It affects prepubertal and post menopausal women but can coexist with pregnancy.

Leukopoiesis The formation and development of leukocytes.

Leukotriens End product of arachidonate metabolism. It plays a key role in inflammation like allergic reactions.

Levator ani muscle It supports pelvic viscera and is supplied by pudendal nerve.

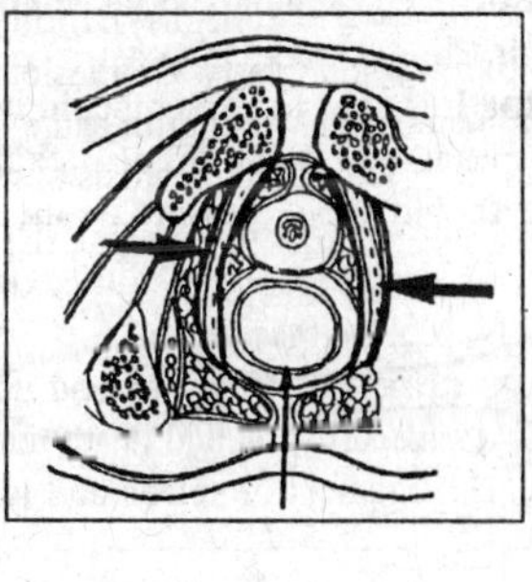

Levator scapulae It raises scapulae.

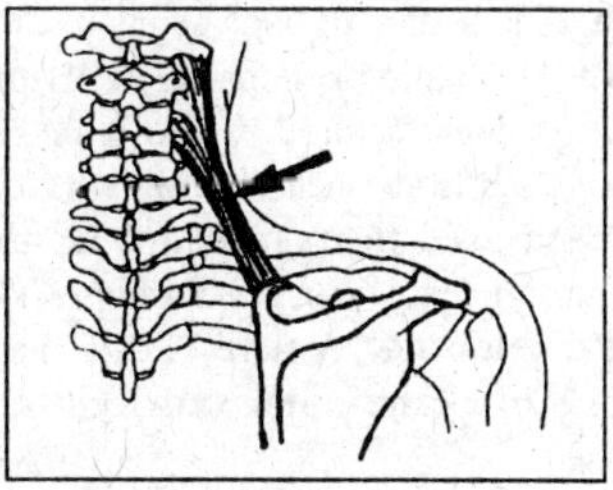

Level of severity The relative degree of involvement or disability.

Level of support The relative degree of asistance required by an individual who is disabled.

Level or arousal The amount of alertness and attention needed for an activity; must be at the optimum level for learning to take place.

Levell's levels Three levels of preventive health care (primary, secondary, and tertiary levels based on the premise that all of the activities of physicians and other health professionals have the goal of prevention. What is to be prevented depends on teh stage of health or disease in the individual receiving preventive care.

Levels of amputation Upper extremity amputation stumps are classified by level of amputation using different terminology. Above-elbow stumps are measured from the tip of acromion to the lateral epicondyle. Below-elbow measurement is made from the medial epicondyle to the end of ulna.

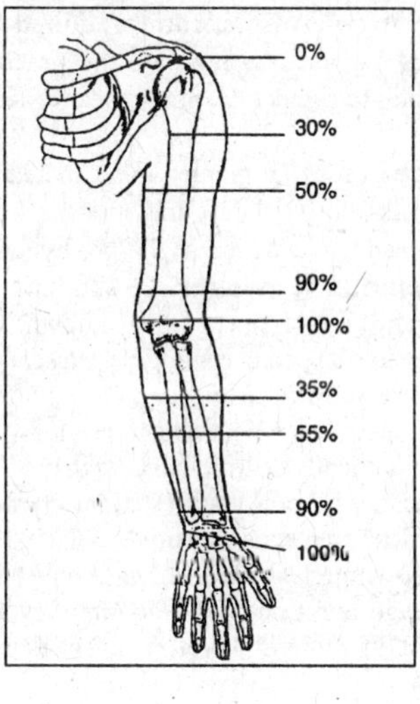

Lever A rigid bar moving about a fixed joint, Distance between joint centers of body segments.

Levodopa Also called L-dopa (el DOH-pah), this chemical is manufactured by the brain cells and then converted to the neurotransmitter dopamine; it has been used to treat disorders involving dopamine deficiencies such as Parkinson's disease.

Levorotatory isomer A stereoisomer that rotates the plane of plane-polarized light counter-clockwise.

Lexicon The vocabulary or list of all the words in a language.

Leydig Cell of Leydig.

Lhermitte's sign A sensation like an electric shock running down the spinal cord and legs and produced by flexing the neck.

Liability State of being bound by law or justice to do something or to make something good; legal responsibility.

Liability insurance Contract between a person or corporation and a company who is willling to provide legal services and financial assistance when the policyholder is involved in a malpractice lawsuit.

Liable Responsible.

Libel Defamation by written or printed materials, including pictures.

Libel Damaging Statement that is written and read by others.

Libido The desire to have sex.

Licence A type of credential required by law; licenses are used to regulate the practice of a profession to protect the public health, safety, and welfare.

Licensure Credential granted to a candidate by the state after the candidate has met the necessary requirements to practice in the profession.

Lichen planus It involves the skin and mucous membrane. Exact cause is not known. On skin lichen planus appears as multiple red scaly lesions which are pruritic. Most common sites are the flexor aspects of wrists and lower legs. Lesions are symmetrically distributed. Less than 50 per cent of patients with oral manifestations show dermal lesions. Lichen planus constitutes about 90 per cent of whole white lesions of the oral mucosa. It has an average duration of 45 months. Seventy five per cent of lesions develop in cheek mucosa. Mucosal lesions appear as minute white papules forming a reticular, annular or plaque pattern. Slender white lesions in form of lines radiate from the papules are typical feature. Lesions are asymptomatic. Patient may complain of burning sensation. Lesion may spontaneously disappear in a few months. Microscopic sections show thickening of keratin layer, formation of 'raw tooth' ridges in the epithelium, oedema of basal layer of epithelium. Lichen planus does not require any surgery. Lesions that are rapid in onset disappears promptly. Besides the usual form of lichen planus bullous or vesicular, erosive, atrophic and hypertrophic forms are recognised but are rare. In all these varieties white lines are seen on the periphery of vesicle, in the erosion area, in the area of atrophy and in area of hypertrophy, respectively. The bullous or vesicular form is usually seen on lateral or ventral surface of tongue. Erosive form is usually developed on cheek and tongue. Hypertrophic form is accompanied by thick, white plaques.

Lichen ruber planus Lesion may present as milky white dots that cannot be wiped away or they may be arranged in a reticular, annular or spider web pattern. Buccal mucosa is commonly affected. It is considered a potentially precancerous lesion.

Lichen simplex chronicus In it person feel intense irritation due to varieties of emotional stress. Histologically there is thickening of epidermis, acanthosis with hyperkeratosis, oedema and perivascular infiltration. It presents with severely itchy, thickly arranged, fat papules or dry lichenified patches with well-demarcated borders on back and side of neck. Lesions tend to persist for a long time and show an exaggeration on emotional stress. Repeated scratching may lead to bacterial infection.

Lichenification Thickening and hardening of skin resulting in chronic scratching.

Lid retractor It is used to retract the lid in cases of blepharospasm and in children to examine the eyes. One should avoid pressure on the eye as in

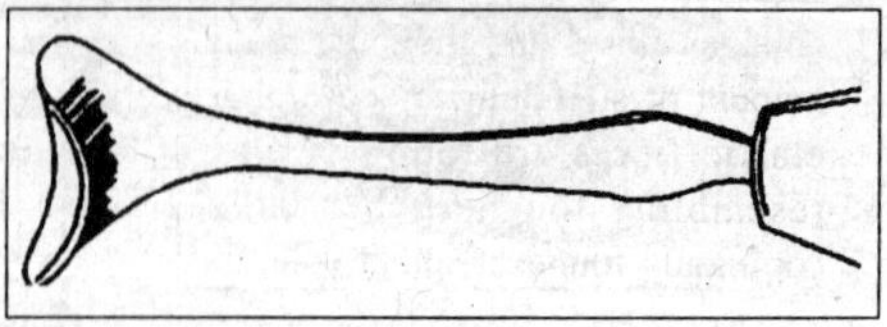

cases of ulcer threatening to perforate, the pressure may cause perforation. Various types are available.

Lie of fetus It is the long axis of fetus to the long axis of uterus.

Life cycle The sum of successive stages in the growth and development of an organism that occur between the appearance and reappearance of the same stage e.g., spore of the organism.

Life cycle events The events that typically occur during an individual's life.

Life event A discreate event or change in course of person's life.

Life expectancy These are number of years somebody might be expected to live. It is calculated on average statistics related to age, sex and location, environment and other relevant factors. Traditionally, defined as the average number of years of life remaining at a given age.

Life instinct In psychoanalysis, one of the two basic forces of the id. An inborn tendency towards survival, including the sex impulse, as well as the intake of food and drink, seeking of protection, and sleep. Its consequence is the maintenance of life in the organism and also in the species as a whole.

Life table analysis A statistical analysis of survival in which roportionate survival is assessed repeatedly over the intervals of observation. This shows the pattern of mortality, as well as the overall rates of death and survival.

Lifespan The number of years of a person's life.

Lifestyle A pattern of behaviors.

Life-threatening illness pattern The family's responses to caring and preparing for the death of a member at the end of life, as well as the grieving, mourning, and healing after the death.

Ligament Teres An intracapsular ligament of hip that arise from margins of acetabular notch.

Ligaments These resemble tendons but they extend from one bone to another. Ligaments often contain significant numbers of elastic fibres as well as collagen fibres and they can tolerate a moderate amount of stretching. Even higher proportion of elastic fibres are found in elastic ligaments resembling tough rubber bands. These are commonly found in spinal column.

Ligamentum arteriosum The remains of the ductus arteriosus of the fetus; between the left pulmonary artery and the arch of the aorta.

Ligamentum teres The remains of the umbilical vein of the fetus.

Ligamentum teres of femur Ligament of the head of the femur.

Ligamentum venosum The remains of the ductus venosus of the fetus.

Ligand A chemical substance that binds to a specific receptor. A small molecule that binds specifically to a larger one; for example, a hormone is the ligand for its specific protein receptor.

Ligase An enzyme that covalently joins strands of DNA.

Ligate To tie or bind with a ligature or suture.

Ligation The binding or tying of a vessel with a substance such as string or catgut. Tubal ligation is the sterilisation of a woman by surgically interrupting her fallopian tubes to prevent ova from being transported to the uterus and to prevent sperm from fertilising the ovum. The method may involve ligation, crushing, burning, coagulating, or embedding the ends of the tubes.

Ligature tie Wire or threadlike substance used to tie a tooth to an orthodontic appliance.

Light The electromagnetic radiation having a velocity of about 3×10^{10} cm (186, 284 miles) per second, and the vibration in space being at right angles to the direction of transmission.

Frequently construed as limited to the range of wavelength between 3900 and 7700 angstroms, which provides the stimulus for the subjective sensation of sight, but sometimes considered as including part of the ultraviolet and infrared ranges as well.

Light adaptation Decreasing visual sensitivity when a person remains in a condition of bright light, such as the glare of sunlight upon a sandy beach or the water.

Light dermatoses Skin area exposed to the sun will show pigmentation, atrophy, telangiectasia, ulcers and malignant tumours. Nodules, ulcers, atrophic areas, desiccation and squamous cell carcinoma may appear at limbus.

Light leak The accidental exposure of film to white light; exposed area appears black.

Light reactions The reactions of photosynthesis that require light and cannot occur in the dark; also known as the light-dependent reactions.

Light-curing The process of applying light energy to a resin-based material containing specific light-sensitive initiators that cause polymerization of the resin.

Lightening It differs only in degrees from electric current. A flash of lightening is due to passage from a thunder cloud to the earth of a direct current of enormous potential. Along the track much energy is liberated which is converted into heat. Immediate death occurs due to syncope or paralysis of CNS. Delayed death is due to complications of burns.

Ligneous conjunctivitis It is characterised by white grey yellow membranous deposits on conjunctiva which can be several mm thick. It may be attached by peduncle to the underlying tissue. It is difficult to tear off. Deposits may occur in both eyes.

There is rarely a tumourous or granulomatous proliferation.

Lignin A highly stable polymer of mostly methoxylated phenylpropanoic residues, synthesized as part of the cell wall of vascular plants; the second most abundant organic polymer on earth after cellulose.

Lignocaine hydrochloride It is the most commonly used local analgesic. It is very stable and is not decomposed by boiling, acid or alkalies. Solutions of 0.25 to 0.5% for infiltration with adrenaline 1 to 250,000 ; 4% for topical analgesia in surgery of throat, larynx and pharynx. For nerve block 1.5 to 2 % with adrenaline and for extradural block 1.2 to 2 % with adrenaline.

It is neither a vasodilator nor does it interfere with vasoconstrictive action of adrenaline. It has a cerebral effect causing drowsiness and amnesia.

Likelihood ratio negative The ratio of the falsenegative error rate of a test to the specificity of the test.

Likelihood ratio positive The ratio of he sensitivity of a test to the false-positive error rate of the test.

Limb An extremity, arm or leg.

Limb Length Discrepancy : (LLD) is a measurable difference in overall length of the two legs. This difference can be true, apparent and of functional nature.

Limb lengthening Any procedure that results in increased length of extremity.

Limbic Forming or occupying a limbus; i.e., a border.

Limbic cortex Cortical regions within the limbic system; includes both the cingulate cortex and the cortex adjacent to the hippocampus.

Limbic system An area in the brain associated with the control of emotion, eating, drinking and sexual activity.

For functional reasons, the limbic system is also called visceral brain or emotional brain. Its main functions involve emotional expression like pleasure, excitement, anger, fear and discomfort.

Limbus The cornea is set into sclera like a watch glass so that sclera overlaps the cornea all around in the periphery.

The junction of these two tissues : the cornea and sclera is known as limbus. There is minute arcade of blood vessels about 1 mm broad at the limbus. The cornea gets its nutrition partly from the diffusion of tissue fluid from these perilimbal capillaries.

Limbus marginalis The line of demarcation between the muscular septum and a thin, rounded, collagenous area immediately below the right and posterior cusps of the aortic valve.

Limen nasi The upper limit of the lower nasal cartilage.

Limit Restriction.

Limiting amino acid The essential amino acid or amino acids that incomplete proteins lack.

Limits of stability The maximum angle from vertical that can be tolerated without a loss of balance; normally 12 degrees in an anteroposterior direction and 16 degrees in a mediolateral direction.

LIMP Refers to an abnormal gait pattern due to pain, weakness or deformity of the Neuromusculo-skeletal system. Dysambulation is another term used for the limp.

Line A term for a family of animals derived from a founder animal and possessing the same germline modification.

Line angle Angle formed by the junction of two walls along a line; designated by combining the names of the walls forming the angle.

Line of gravity It passes behind hip joint but in front of knee and ankle joint. It maintains the balance of body.

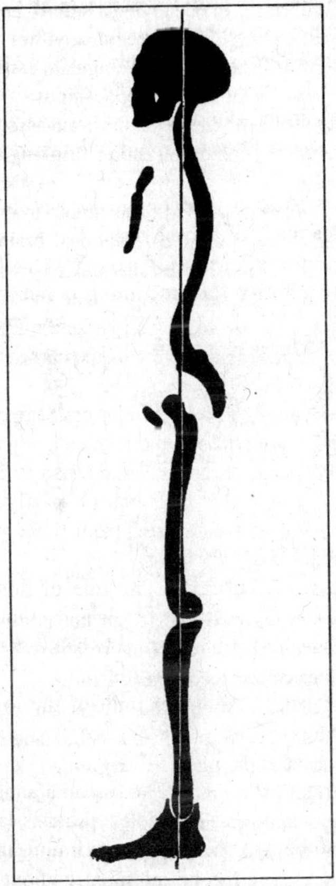

Linea alba White line in the centre of the abdomen where muscles of the abdominal wall insert. A vertical fibrous band extending down the anterior medial portion of the abdominal wall.

Linea semicircularis Arcuate line of sheath of rectus abdominis.

Linea terminalis The oblique ridge on the inner surface of the ilium, continued on the pubis, which separates the tube from the false pelvis. Formerly called the *iliopectineal line*.

Linear causation One event causes another but the second does not affect the first event.

Linear polymer A polymer with no chemical bonds between individual molecular chains.

Linear salpingostomy Incision along the length of fallopian tube to remove an ectopic pregnancy and pressure the tube.

Liner It is applied in a thin sheet to seal the dentin on the floor and walls of the cavity from influx of bacteria.

Liner regression analysis A statistical test of the strength of the linear relatinoship between one independent and one dependent variable, both of which must be continuous.

Lingua alba Tongue, white hairy.

Lingual bar A major connector that is located lingual to the dental arch and that joins bilateral parts of a mandibular removable partial denture.

Lingual foramen An opening or hole in bone located on the internal surface of the mandible near the midline; it is surrounded by the genital tubercles and appears radiolucent.

Lingual frenum Fold of tissue that connects tongue to floor of mouth.

Lingual groove Vertical groove located on the middle of lingual surface of maxillary molar teeth.

Lingual nerve The lingual nerve may be hidden beneath or in the mucosa lateral to the location of a mandibular third molar near the crest. More than one branch of nerve may be present.

Lingual tonsillitis Inflammation localised to the lingual tonsil at the base of tongue. Symptoms include swelling, redness, yellow deposits and severe pain.

Lingula A small tongueshaped projection of bone seen adjacent to the mandibular foramen; appears radiopaque.

Lingula frenulum A longitutinal fold of mucous membrane that attaches the tongue to the floor of the oral cavity.

Liniment Lotion for topical application on the skin surface, usually to relieve muscular sprain. Many liniments contain alcohol.

Link Distance between joint centers of body segments.

Linkage blindness Impossibility to reveal link within information caused by a physical or logical barrier that prevents data to be compared.

Linoleic acid An essential polyunsaturated fatty acid with the first duble bond located at the sixth carbon atom from the omega end.

Lip biting An oral habit in which either lip is placed between the teeth or forcible teeth to the lips.

Lipase An enzyme that breaks down lipids.

Lipemia The presence in the blood of excessive amounts of fats.

Lipid A small water-insoluble biomolecule generally containing fatty acids, sterols, or isoprenoid compounds. An acylated and phosphorylated di- or monosaccharide that forms the hydrophobic part of lipopolysaccharide.

Lipid bilayer Arrangement of phospholipid, glycolipid, and cholesterol molecules in two parallel sheets in which the hydrophilic "heads" face outward and the hydrophobic "tails" face inward; found in cellular membranes.

Lipid emulsion A soybean oil.

Lipid peroxidation Rancidification of fats due to free radicals and inflammation.

Lipidosis A disorder of cellular lipid metabolism that involves abnormal accumulation of lipid. The lipidoses include Tay-Sachs disease, Niemann-Pick disease and Gaucher's disease.

Lipoatrophy Breakdown of subcutaneous fat at the site of repeated insulin injection.

Lipofuscin Brown age pigment which arises from the influence of oxygen free radicals and promotes ageing.

Lipogenesis Anabolism (synthesis) of lipids; triglycerides, phospholipids, cholesterol, and prostaglandin synthesis.

Lipogenesis The formation of fat or triglycerides.

Lipogenic substances Substances such as insulin that stimulates the production of fat.

Lipohypertrophy Buildup of subcutaneous fat at insulin injection sites.

Lipoic acid Essential growth facture for various microorganism.

Lipolysis The breakdown of triglycerides to release fatty acids.

Lipoma A usually benign growth of breast tissue, typically composed of mature fat cells.

Lipomatosis An abnormal, localized, or tumorlike accumulation of fat in the tissues.

Lipopenia Deficiency of lipids in the body.

Lipophilic Affinity for fatty substances.

Lipophyalinosis A condition characterized by fat and hyaline degeneration.

Lipoprotein A lipid-protein aggregate that serves to carry water-insoluble lipids in the blood. The protein component alone is an apolipoprotein. One of a class of proteins carrying at their amino terminus a cysteine to which glycerol is linked that has its hydroxyl groups substituted by fatty acids. Particles circulating in the blood that contain triglycerides, phospholipids and proteins.

Lipoprotein lipase An enzyme that regulates fat uptake.

Lippe's loop It is a commonly used intrauterine device made of polyethylene. The woman should be below 40 years of age. Wearer has little responsibility for preventing conception once

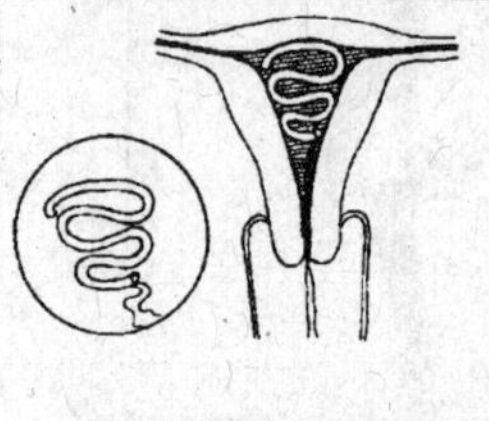

Lippe's loop in uterus

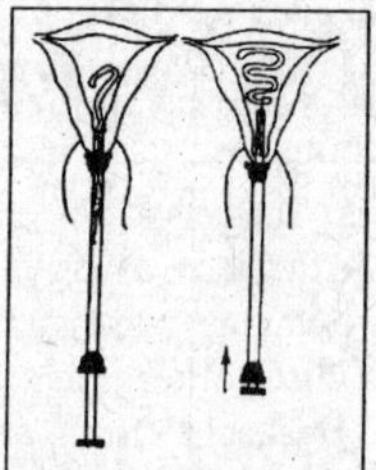

Lippe's loop insertion

device is inserted and it can be removed when pregnancy is desired. But it cannot be used in presence of gynaecological disorder.

Lipproteinse Combination of fats and proteins.

Lips These become pallor in anaemia and cyanosed in case of right sided heart failure. Dry lips are due to climatic conditions and in gastroenteritis. Dry cracked lips are seen in nervous people and in dry winters. Swelling of lips may be due to injury, urticaria or angioneurotic oedema. In exfoliative cheilitis there is persistent vesiculation and crusting of lips. Scars left by syphilitic fissures are white.

Liquid diet It is for easy digestion, specially when there is difficulty for mastication or in semiconscious or unconscious patients, liquid diets are prescribed. Following food items, tea, coffee, milk, soup, sagoo water, fruit juice, Horlicks or Complan may be given.

Liquid oxygen unit Device that converts cooled liquid oxygen to a gas by passing it through heated coils.

Liquid-phase extraction Extraction of drugs or poisons using solvents from an aqueous matrix.

Lisfranc fracture It occurs after a fall from height or down a flight of stairs. The lisfranc ligament between the first cuneiform bone and base of second metatarsal bone is disrupted or avulsed.

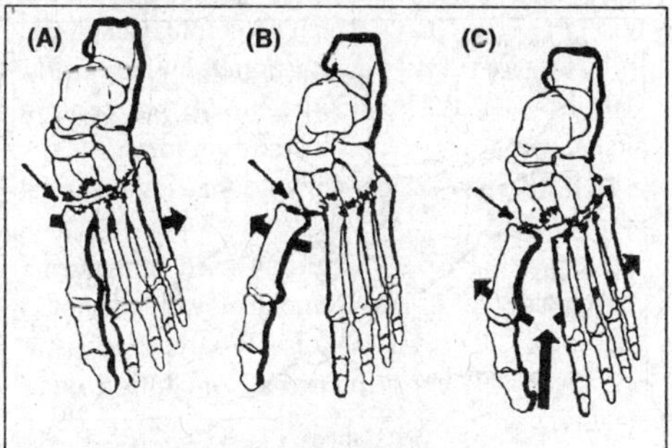

Lisfranc tarsometatarsal dislocations : (A) homolateral; (B) isolated; (C) divergent

List Tendency of lean to one side.

Listeria monocytogenes This is the most common cause of bacterial meningitis in patients with other causes of immunosuppression. Headache, fever and confusion predominate in listeria infections and clinical evidence of meningeal inflammatioin may be slight. Organism can be easily cultured. Ampicillin IV in a dose of 12 gm/day is treatment of choice.

Literacy Ability to read and write.

Literature search The scrutiny of research reports and other writings in a given area, providing a background for an investigation, the development of a test, or a related procedure. In test construction of the test, the aim is to make use of currently existing information and technique.

Lithium poisoning It is used in patients with manic depressive psychosis. Intoxication may result in prolonged therapy. In case of acute ingestion features may develop after 16 hours only. Prodromal phase of lithium intoxication lasts for several days and be manifested by a combination of vomiting, diarrhoea, drowsiness, coarse muscle tremors, muscle twitching, lethargy and slurred speech. Severe toxicity presents with tremors, confusion, restlessness, extrapyramidal signs, muscle fasciculations, neuromuscular irritability, hyperreflexia, clonus, stiffness, grunting, stupor and coma. There will be severe memory loss. Other features include hyperalgesia, acute generalised polyneuropathy and flaccid quadriplegia.

Lithocholic acid One of the bile acids that form bile salt in conjunction with glycine.

Lithoplaxy It is a time honoured method of taking out bladder stone. The crushing instrument lithotrite is introduced into bladder via urethra and

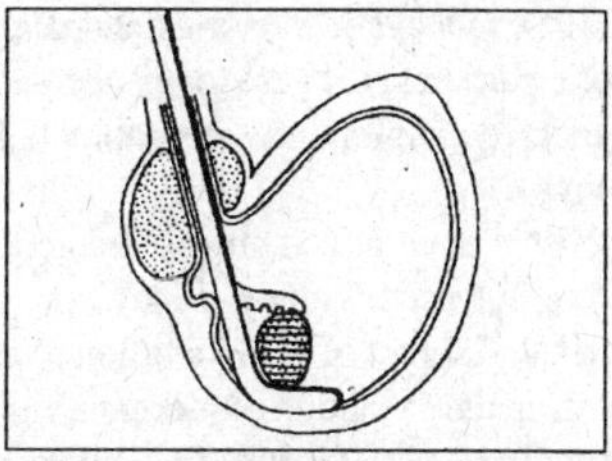

rotated with its jaw open until stone can be gripped in the jaws. Once gripped the stone is crushed enough to be washed out of bladder via a cystoscope.

Lithotomy position This position is used for gynaecological purpose for adequate exposure of pelvis and vagina. For rectal operation also this

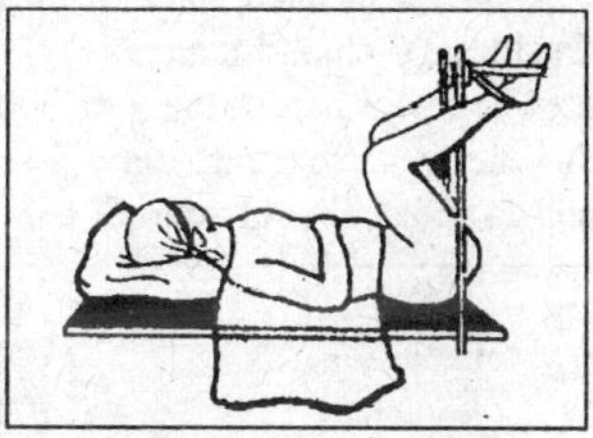

position is used. Patient lies flat facing upwards. But the legs are held or fixed in position by lifting from table and hanged on the special table.

Lithotripsy Extracorporeal shock-wave lithotripsy (ESWL) is now established way of taking out gall

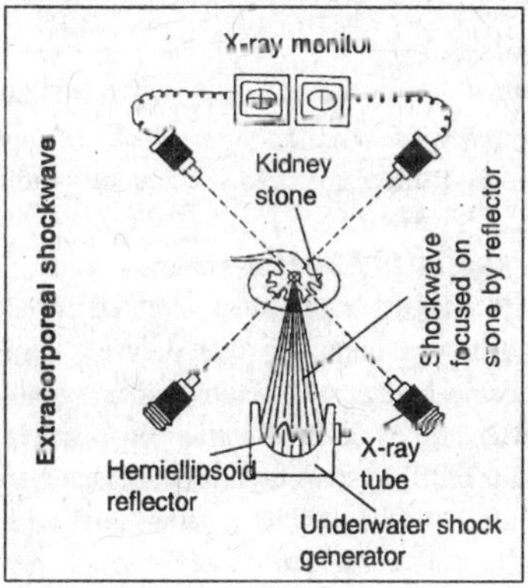

stones. Indications of lithotripsy are that gall stone volume should be less than half the volume of gall bladder and should not exceed 3 ´ 3 cm in diameter. Stone should be primarily of cholesterol but gall bladder must be functioning well. Common bile duct (CBD) and cystic duct must be patent to drain out stone particles. Larger stones need endoscopic retrograde cholangiopancreatography (ERCP) and basketing.

Lithotriptor A specialized ultrasound generator that is used to pulverize kidney stones.

Lithotrophy The fact of being a lithotroph; deriving energy from the oxidation of inorganic compounds.

Litigation Trial of a dispute in a court of law or other legal forum to determine factual and legal issues, rights, and duties between the parties.

Litten's phenomenon According to this phenomenon the line of diaphragmatic insertion estimated externally on the chest is lowered during inspiration and elevated during expiration. This movement is absent in pneumonia of lower lobe, pleural effusion and emphysema.

Little's area The lower part of the nose is supplied by branches derived from maxillary artery. The internal and external carotid sources anastomose

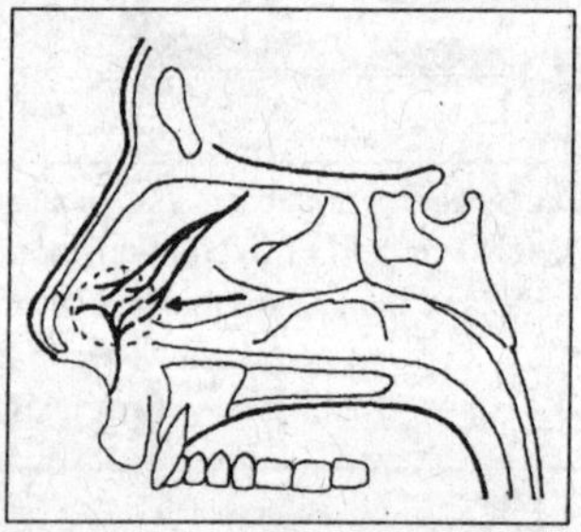

freely in the nose. An aggregation of poorly supported vessels on the anterior part of septum is known as. Little's area and is frequently the source of nasal bleeding.

Littre, glands of Urethral glands.

Live attenuated vaccines Created by altering infectious organisms so that they are no longer pathogenic butare still viable and antigentic.

Live birth This is defined as that birth where there are signs of life such as breathing, presence of heart beat, after the conceptus is completely expelled from the mother irrespective of the age of gestation.

Livedo A discolored spot or patch on the skin, commonly due to passive congestion.

Liver It is the largest organ in the body and weighs about 1.5 kg. It lies under diaphragm mainly in

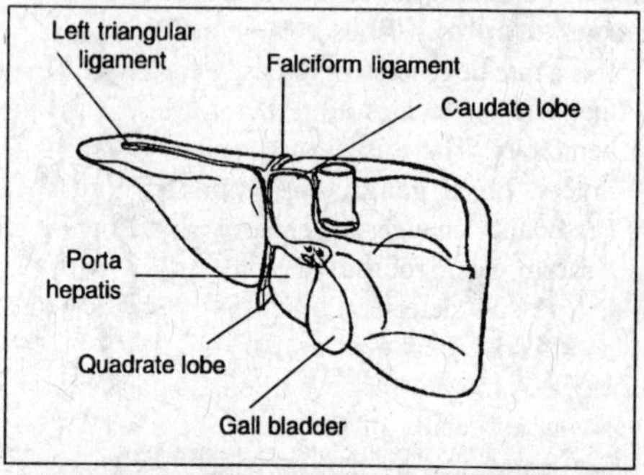

right hypochondrium. It is wedge shaped having rounded diaphragmatic and visceral surface. Its upper border lies anteriorly at the level of 5th or 6th intercostal space.

Liver biopsy It is done in chronic liver disease and malignancy. The patient lies on his or her back at near the right hand edge of the bed. Right arm is supported above his head to provide clear access

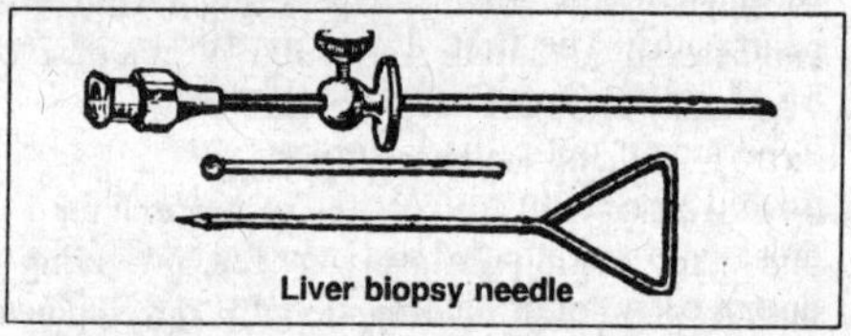

to the right intercostal space. Needle is introduced in mid or anterior axillary line among 8th, 9th and 10th rib. Before liver biopsy blood group, haemoglobin, bleeding and clotting time should be done and for 24 hours patient should rest on bed.

Liver glycogenolysis Chemical process by which liver glycogen is converted to glucose.

Lividity The quality of being livid; discoloration, as of dependent parts, by the gravitation of the blood.

Living will A legal document stating what medical treatment a patient chooses to omit or refuse in the event that he or she is terminally ill and is unable to make those decisions for himself or herself.

Living wills A legal document that outlines the patient's wishes for refusing or discontinuing lifesaving medical treatment if the patient becomes incompetent.

Loading dose Larger dose of a drug administered initially or when pain is intense.

Lobar Pertaining to, or affecting a lobe.

Lobar atrophy It is also known as Pick's disease. It is a rare degenerative disease of presenile period that affects females more than males. It is often hereditary. There is diffuse neuron loss in outer layers. Basal ganglia are commonly affected. Personality changes, orientation and attention are first to be affected than retentive memory. Progressive deterioration is the rule and there is no effective treatment available.

Lobe 1. A more or less well-defined portion of any organ; especially of the brain and glands. Lobes are demarcated by fissures, sulci, and connective tissue, and by their shape. A part of a tooth formed by any one of the separate points of the beginning of calcification.

Lobectomy A severe form of psychosurgery, no longer in use, which involved removal of a portion of the frontal lobe of the brain.

Lober's optic atrophy There develops acute or subacute loss of vision in young man due to optic neuropathy. The first change is enlargement of blind spot. Optic fundus shows a swollen hyperaemic optic disc, tortuous arterioles and dilated vessels in retina near disc. Virtually all those who are affected are men but their sperms do not carry mitochondria. Lober's subjects have been shown to be deficient in enzyme thiosulphate sulphur transferase.

Lobes of prostate This is an accessory genital gland, the secretion or which add bulk to semen. It is cone shaped. It has a posterior, an anterior and two inferolateral surfaces. The posterior surface of gland is directly related to the rectum

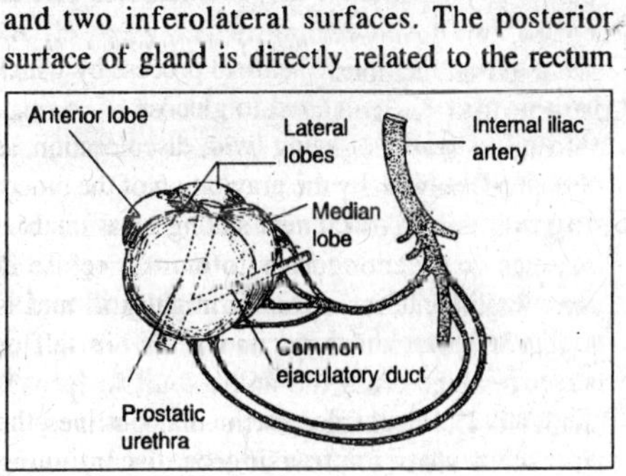

and can be palpated during rectal examination. The gland surrounds the prostatic urethra and is divisible into four lobes. The median lobe lies between the urethra in front and two common ejaculatory ducts behind. On either side of median lobe are the two lateral lobes which extend backwards forming the posterior surface of the gland.

Lobotomy An operation which involves cutting some nerve fibres that connect the frontal lobes with the thalamus in order to relieve psychotic symptoms, now largely replaced by chemotherapy.

Lobstein's syndrome The syndrome consists of laxity of the ligaments, fragility of the bones, osteosclerosis, fineness of hair, defective dental enamel, and blue sclera.

Lobular bronchiole The bronchiole that enters the secondary lobules of the lung; each lobular bronchiole gives off about six terminal bronchioles.

Lobule A small lobe; specifically, such a structure of the breast.

Local Restricted to one spot or area; not generalized.

Local anaesthetics Useful substance must be water soluble, sterilised by heat and should have a rapid onset of effect. Local anaesthetics prevent the propagation of the nerve impulse. By injection or

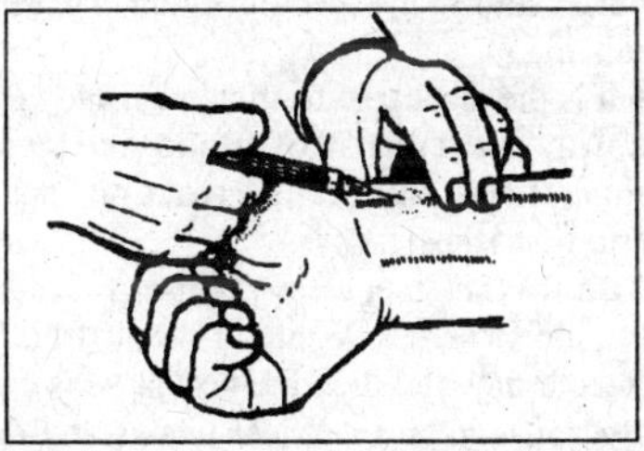

infiltration it is effective within five minutes and has a useful duration of 1 to 1.5 hours. Absorption from mucous membrane on topical application varies according to compound. Well-absorbed surface anaesthetics are cocaine, lignocaine and prilocaine. Local anaesthesia is generally used when loss of consciousness is neither necessary nor desirable.

Local application of drugs Drugs can be applied on skin or mucous membrane. For local application dress in the semisolid preparations can be spread on to the skin. It can be applied by rubbing or massage of antiseptic ointment. Creams and powders are applied without rubbing. Throat paints, gentian violet or boroglycerine paints are applied over mucous membrane.

Local community hospital Hospital that provides services such as rutine diagnosis, treatment, and surgery but lacks the personnel and facilities for complex procedures.

Local Immersion This method involves placing part in a container of iced water-a mixture of water flaked ice, Varying the amount of ice used can control temperature.

Local inflammation Inflammation confined to a specific area of the body; symptoms include redness, heat, swelling, pain, and loss of function.

Local lesion A symptom found in a plant leaf inoculated with a virus, caused by the death of, or changes in, cells around the original point of entry; lesion localised to one part of body.

Local norms The compilation of test results for a given community or group of subjects, constituting only a subgroup of a larger population. A high school may develop local norms for a test which is administered on a national basis. In this way, the students may be judged against other from their same community.

Local therapy Treatment that is used to remove or kill cancer cells in the specific region, e.g., surgery or radiation.

Lochia It is the discharge from uterus following the childbirth and consist of blood and necrotic decidua. It has an alkaline reaction in which bacteria flourishes easily.

Lochia alba Whitish or clear vaginal discharge that follows lochia serosa. White in colour from ninth to fifteenth day and then the discharge is creamy in colour. It contains cervical mucus and debris. Persistent red colour indicates that some products of conception are retained. In such cases severe post partum hemorrhage may result. Lochia is sterile.

Lochia rubra Red in colour persist for three days mainly contains blood, shreds of decidual and fragments of vernix. Meconium may also be present.

Lochia serosa Pink in colour between fourth to 8th day. It contains less blood but more serum. Leucocytes and bacteria are present.

Locked twins Mostly primigravidas are victims. Two forms of locking occurs, chin to chin interlocking or both heads in collision at the brim.

Locked-in syndrome Patient is conscious but has great difficulty in expressing it. Usual cause is large infarct in anterior part of pons. There develops total disconnection of lower cranial nerves. Only cortical pathway to cranial nerves III and IV are spared to make vertical eye movements. All other muscles are paralysed. Within a few weeks either partial degree of recovery of motor function occurs or patient dies.

Locking It describes intermittent blocking of some part of normal range of joint movement. It is due to interposition of something between articulating surface and is seen in meniscal lesions in knee. There becomes inability to extend the joint fully. Loose bodies in knee may produce a similar picture if they get between the articulating surfaces.

Lockjaw Same as Tatanus.

Locomotion Moving from place to place. An infant progresses from relatively small movements to crawling, walking, running, and so forth.

Locomotor ataxia It is also known as tabes dorsalis similar to tertiary syphilis affecting sensory and motor nerves. There will be sharp pain anywhere from wrist down. There will be gradual loss of voluntary co-ordination, bladder incontinence and blurring of eyesight.

Locus ceruleus A small area in the brainstem that is considered to be a key brain centre for anxiety and fear.

Locus of control The perception of one's ability to control life events and experiences.

Loeffler's syndrome Larvae of many intestinal parasites enter the portal circulation, liver and then they pass through the hepatic vein and inferior vena cava into heart and lungs. In lungs larvae penetrate into capillaries. There are fleeting patchy pulmonary infiltration. Clinical features include cough, low fever, feeling of being unwell and scattered crepitations.

Logrank test A signigicance test used to compare the rates of survival as determined by kaplanmeier life table analysis.

Long muscles of anterior leg There are four long muscles on anterior surface of lower leg. These are, tibialis anterior, extensor digitorum longus, extensor hallucis longus and peroneus tertius. Their tendons cross the ankle joint in front of malleoli. These all are dorsiflexors of ankle joint.

Long term depression A long lasting stable

reduction in the size of post synaptic response.

Long term potentiation A long lasting stable increase in the size of post synaptic response.

Long term satiety Satiety that results mainly from a substantial excess of body fat.

Long tract signs Signs indicative of damage to major sensory and motor pathways, especially in relation to brainstem vascular lesions.

Longitudinal Pertaining of long axis of a structure or part.

Longitudinal arch Two arches, the medial and lateral, that extend lengthwise.

Longitudinal arch of foot The anteroposterior arch

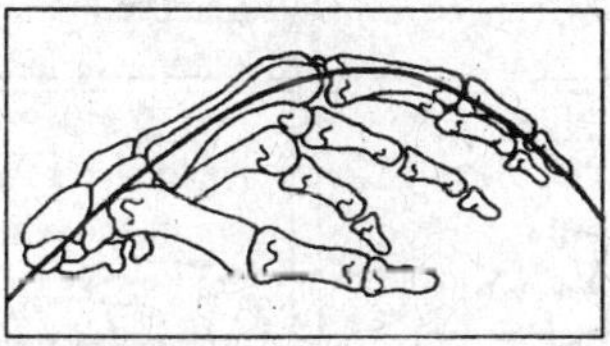

of foot formed by tarsal and metatarsal bones.

Longitudinal axis It is vertical extending in a cranial

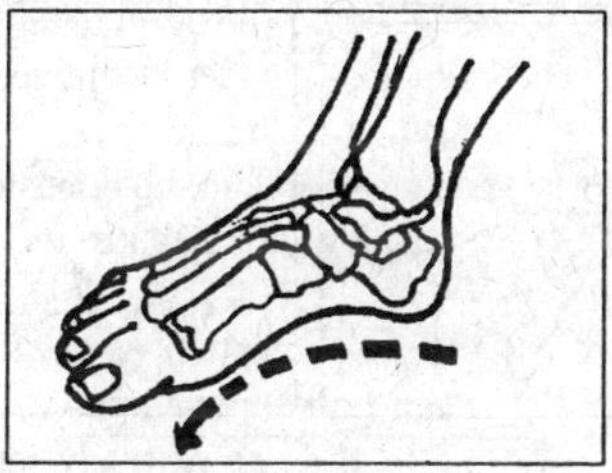

caudal direction. The movements of medial and lateral rotation and abduction and adduction at shoulder take place about this axis.

Longitudinal ecologic studies Use of ongoing surveillance or frequent cross-sectional studies to measure trends in disease rates over year in a defined population.

Longitudinal method A developmental study which follows the same individuals from early to later age levels. Contrasted with crosssectional studies. In which different groups represent each age level.

Longitudinal plane Invisible vertical line that dissects the body, object, or organ.

Longitudinal section A cut made through the long axis of an organ.

Longitudinal study A technique where research is carried out over a period of time so that changes in individuals can be observed. It is particularly used in development research so that the effects of independent variables on developmental outcomes can be observed.

Long-term memory (LTM) Retention which has been established for long periods, presumably involving a consolidation of the memory trace.

Loop diuretic One of a group of agents that enhances the exertion of urine; acts by inhibiting sodium and chloride reabsorption not only in the proximal and distal tubules but also in Henel's loop. High doses of loop diuretics cause an inhibition of enzyme activity which interfere with electrolyte transport in the cochlea. There may be bilateral high tone hearing loss within a few days. Hearing loss and tinnitus are reversible with immediate withdrawal of drug.

Loop of Henle U-shaped part of the nephron extending from the proximal to the distal convoluted tubule and consisting of descending and ascending limbs; many of the loops of Henle extend into the renal pyramids.

Loops (fingerprints) Loops consist of at least one ridge entering the pattern area from one side, recurving and exiting on the same side of entry, and one point of delta.

Loose bodies These may arise from synovial fluid. Fibrinous loose bodies resulting from haemorrhagic or inflammatory effusion. From synovial membrane numerous cartilaginous loose bodies develop within villous synovial processes. There may be detached osteophytes in case of osteoarthritis.

Loose tooth A loosened tooth may be partially displaced, intruded, extruded or avulsed. When tooth has been displaced outwards or laterally try to place the tooth back in normal position. The damaged tooth is splinted to surrounding tooth for 2 to 3 weeks. Any attempt to move the teeth

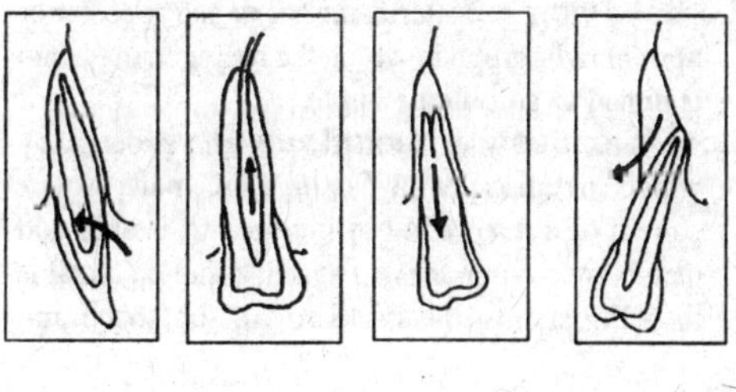

vigorously may result in permanent loss of it.

Loosening of associations A disturbance of thinking in which ideas shift from one subject to another in an oblique or unrelated manner. The speaker is unaware of the disturbance. When loosening of associations is severe, speech may be incoherent.

Lophodont Having molar teeth with crested occlusal ridges.

Lorain-Levy syndrome The syndrome is manifested by retention of infantile characteristics, lack of sexual development, absence of pubic hair, and low urinary 17-ketosteroids.

Lordosis Accentuation of thoracic curve is called kyphosis. Lateral curvature of spine is known as scoliosis. The lateral deformity is coupled with rotational deformity. Abnormal exaggeration of lumbar curve or lordosis is often associated with weakened muscles and forward pelvic tilt.

Causes of lordosis include congenital spinal

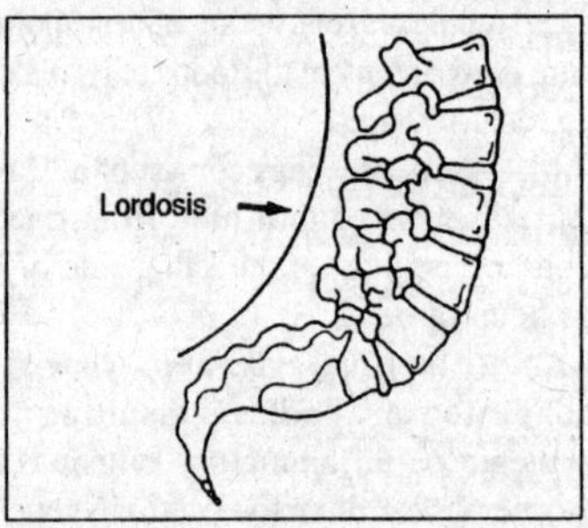

deformity, weakness of abdominal muscles, poor postural habits and over training in sports. Because lordosis places added compressive stress on the posterior element of spine low backache is the symptom.

Lordotic Posture Lordotic posture combines an increase in the lumbosacral angle with an increase in lumber lordosis, anterior pelvic tilt, and hip flexion.

Lordotic view A posterioanterior or anteroposterior upright radiograph in which the roetngen ray beam is aimed at an oblique angle.

Lost wax casting technique The process by which metallic dental castings are made a wax pattern of a restoration in invested in a mold and then burned out to leave a space; a molten metal is then thrust into the mold to fill the space and produce a metallic restoration on cooling.

Lotic Having to do with swiftly flowing waters, as in a stream or river.

Louisiana ankle wrap About 100 inches webbed bandage is used. Patient sits on table holding the ankle at 90 degrees. The wrap may even be applied over stocking. Steps one and two secure the wrap.

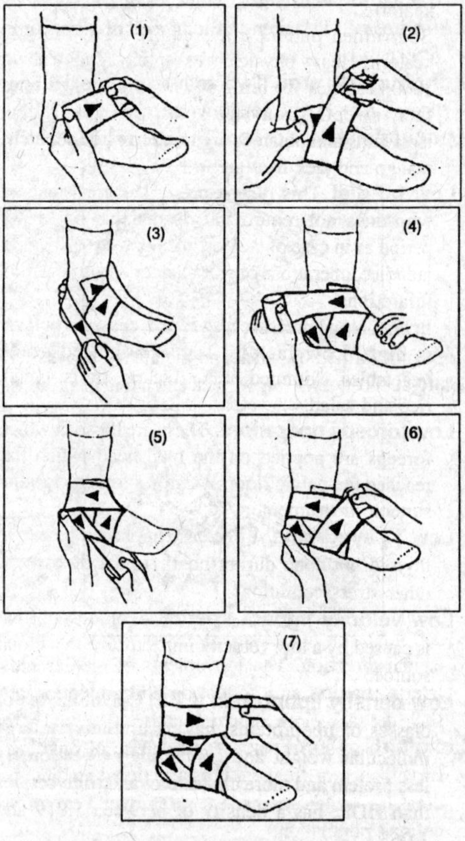

Steps three, four and five are the lateral and medial heel tracks that prevent eversion and inversion respectively. Steps six and seven are done as shown in figure to prevent needless ankle injury.

Lovastatin It is an effective drug which lowers the blood cholesterol by inhibiting the production of cholesterol in liver.

Love play It includes the entire gamut of erotic activities ranging from teasing, fondling to various ways of expressing tenderness and affection which may lead more or less to direct gratification.

Low birth weight Weighing less than 5.5 lbs (2500g) at birth.

Low calorie diet Calorie requirement of a person varies depending on age, type of work, sex, climate, etc. An average sedentary worker requires 1800 to 2400 kcalories. Moderate worker requires 4000 kcalorie.

Bed-ridden patient may require 1400 to 1800 kcalorie. Heavy physical worker may require about 3900 kcalories. To bring down number of calories fats, sweets, nonvegetarian fat rich foods, icecreams and potatoes are to be reduced. Banana, mango and jack fruit are to be avoided.

Low fat diet This diet is prescribed for a patient who does not require fat during that particular period as in case of steatorrhoea or fatty diarrhoea, jaundice, operations of gall bladder and myocardial infarctions.

In high blood pressure also where cholesterol level is high. Low fat diet includes boiled green vegetables, skimmed milk, chicken, fruits, bread, rice and salad.

Low forceps operations These are those in which forceps are applied on the fetal head which has reached the pelvic floor. Wrigley's forceps is quite suitable instrument.

Low T_3 syndrome A decrease in plasma bioactive thyroid hormone during nonthyroidal illness and other stress conditions.

Low velocity impact spatter A bloodstain that is caused by a low velocity impact/force to a blood source.

Low-density lipoprotein (LDL) One of the major classes of lipoproteins, having a relatively large molecular weight and containing proportionally less protein and more cholesterol and triglycerides than HDL; has a density of between 1.019 and 1.063.

Low-energy phosphate compound A phosphorylated compound with a relatively small standard free energy of hydrolysis.

Lower esophageal sphincter Lower 2-5 cm. portion of lower esophagus of increased intra luminal pressure extending above and below diaphragm.

Lower extremity A lower appendage, including the hip, thigh, knee, leg, and foot.

Lower lobe bronchus The portion of the trancheobronchial tree that gives off the segmental and subsegmental bronchi of the lower lobe of the lung.

Lower vertebrates A collective term for reptiles, amphibians, and fish (cartilaginous and bony); i.e, vertebrates other than mammals and birds.

Low-grade lymphomas This includes three tumours, small lymphocytic lymphoma, follicle predominantly small clear cell lymphoma and follicular mixed lymphoma.

Lowman plinth It is made of stainless steel and tapers in width to allow free leg movement in prone position; It is long enough to support the body while leaving the legs free.

Low-output congestive heart failure The description most frequently associated with heart failure; the result of a low cardiac output at rest or during exertion.

LTD Long-term (prolonged) depression of neuronal responsivity following conditioning stimuli.

Lubricant An oily liquid applied to moving parts of a mechanism in order to reduce friction, heat, or wear, or to surfaces in close contact to prevent them from adhering to one another.

Lucid dream Dream in which the dreamer is aware that he is dreaming.

Lucid interval Lucid interval means temporary return to mental health. This is a period occurring in course of a mental disease during which there is complete loss of symptoms of insanity. Lucid interval occurs commonly in connection with mania and melancholia. An insane can make a valid will during the lucid period.

Luciferin Literally, light bearing; the generic name for a substrate that is oxidized to give light in a bioluminescent reaction, identified as a flavin in bacteria and a tetrapyrrole in dinoflagellates.

Lumbagosciatica syndrome The syndrome includes low back pain, limitation of back motion, pain and tenderness of paravertebral muscles, radiation of pain down to the posterior aspect of the thigh and calf to the outer border of the foot, paraesthesia and later numbness over the distribution of the nerve root.

Lumbar Lower back between the ribs and pelvis.

Lumbar canal stenosis Both the anteroposterior and transverse diameter vary in person to person. The available cross-sectional area in those with massive pedicles may be only just sufficient for the passage of cauda equina. A relatively minor posterolateral disc protrusion or central bulge of annulus ligament will compromise the roots. It is known as lumbar canal stenosi person may develop recurrent back pain and sciatica.

Lumbar disc herniation The herniations are most often postero-lateral, as the posterior longitudinal ligament reinforces the intervertebral disc

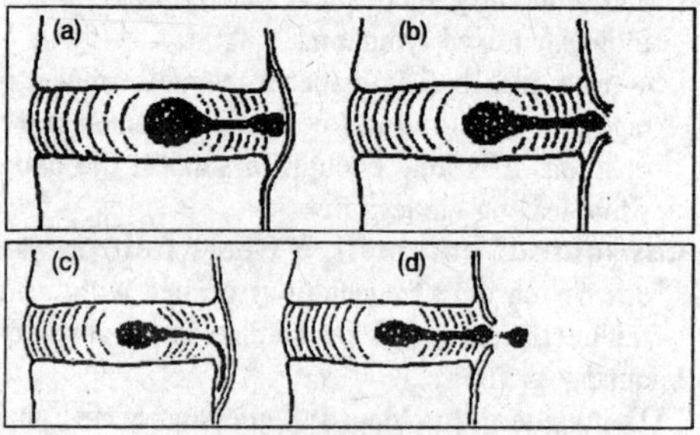

(a) without rupture of post ligament
(b) with rupture of post ligament
(c) Disk extrusion beneath p. ligament
(d) Sequestrated fragment

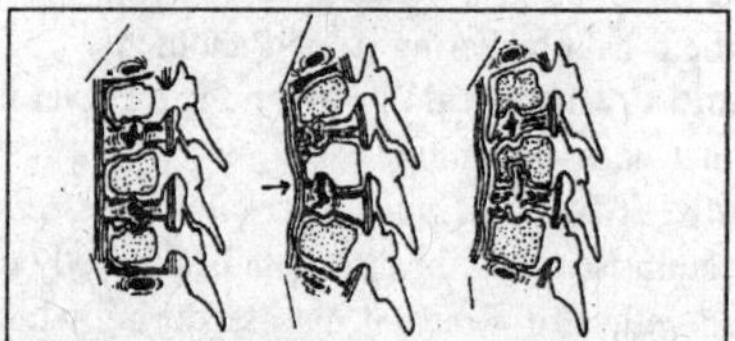

Different stages of Sheurmann's disease

posteriorly. Some heriations remain ligamentous but others break through this ligament. In younger age group Sheurman's disease develops.

Lumbar disc herniation pain There is a history of recurrent episodic low back pain Disc herniation at L5/S1 will result in pain radiating down the back of thigh, outer side of lower leg and outer side of foot to fifth toe. In case of L4/L5 disc herniation pain radiates from lower back down the posterolateral part of thight, lower leg and front of foot to big toe. With L2L3 root lesions pain radiates down the front of the thigh. Disc prolapse pain is aggravated by sitting, lifting and coughing, sneezing, laughing and straining to defecate.

Lumbar epidural analgesia Local anesthetic is injected into epidural space.

Lumbar hernia It is of two types, primary and secondary. It may take place following an operation upon an infected kidney or drainage of lumbar abscess. It may occur after local paralysis of anterolateral abdominal muscles, e.g. due to poliomyelitis also known as phantom hernia. The hernia protrudes through the lumbar triangle of Petit. Patient will develop swelling in lumbar region just above the iliac crest. Swelling is soft and cough impulse is present on lying and on applying pressure hernia reduces.

Lumbar puncture It is the process of insertion of a long lumbar puncture needle into the spinal canal in subarachnoid space in order to obtain a specimen of CSF. It helps in introducing drugs in meningitis.

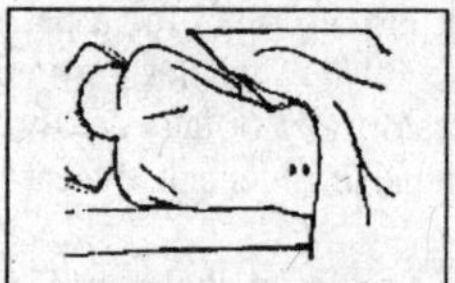

Lateral decubitus position

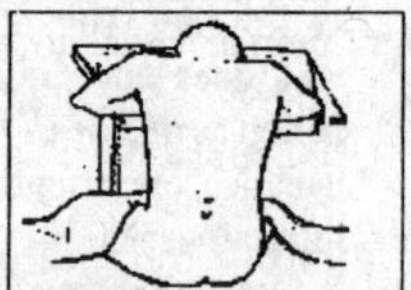

Sitting position for L.P.

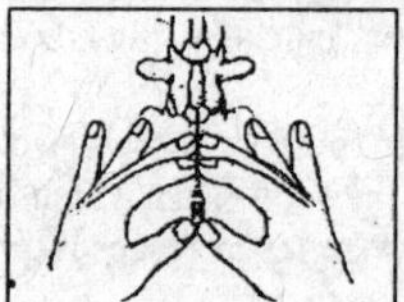

Inserting L.P. needle in subarachnoid space

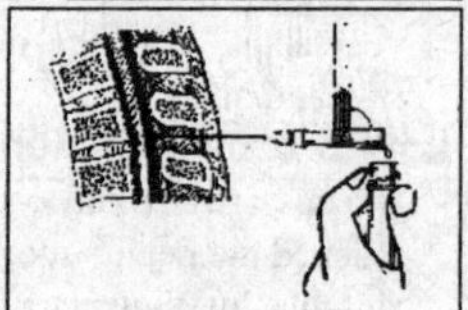

Collect cerebrospinal fluid

It reduces intracranial pressure. It is used for spinal anaesthesia. Usual position of patient is left lateral with patient's chin and knee as close as possible and his or her back along the edge of the bed. Doctor punctures in 3rd and 4th lumbar space. Collect the CSF fluid and later on seal with tincture benzoin.

Lumbar spondylosis, degenerative Prolapsed intervertebral disc occurs in younger age. It is due to rupture of annular ligament. There is extrusion of soft disc material from the nuclear pulposus. In old age water content of disc decreases and herniation of soft disc material is much less. Radicular lesions in middle-aged people are largely due to hypertrophic degenerative changes in facetal joint with subsequent compression. Generally disc protrusion takes place in L_4-L_5 level compressing fifth lumbar root. Pain is characterised by sciatica, pain in buttock and down the back of thigh. There

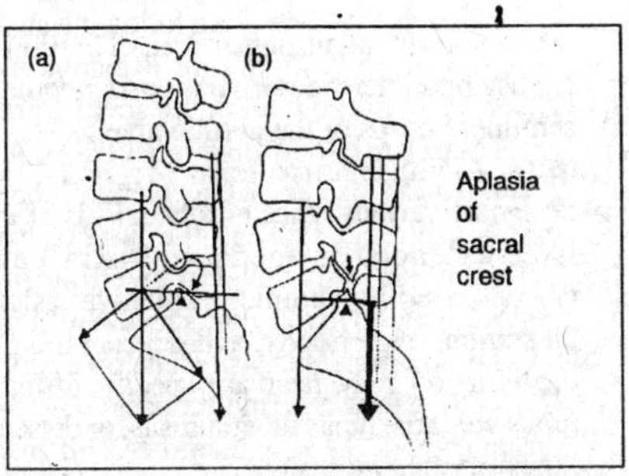

may be tingling along outer side of foot in S_1 involvement L_5 lesions are characterised by some degree of foot drop. In L_4 lesions foot drop is prominent due to weakness of tibialis anterior. In L_2 and L_3 lesions pain radiates down from the thigh, qurdriceps may be weak and knee jerk is depressed.

Lumbar sympathetic block The blocking of neuropathways of pain by injecting a local anaesthetic at L_2. It abolishes pain in the uterus only.

Lumbar traction in bed Bed rest is often prescribed

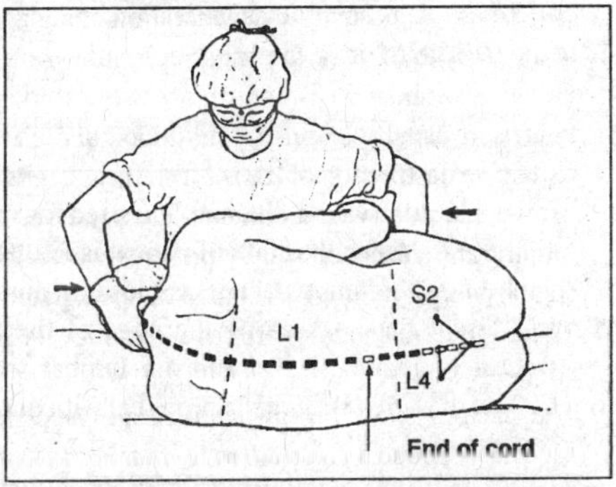

for treatment of acute lumbar pain and sciatica. Additional continuous traction in bed is tolerated poorly and patient compliance is low. Automotor frame is useful.

Lumbosacral angle Inclination of the superior

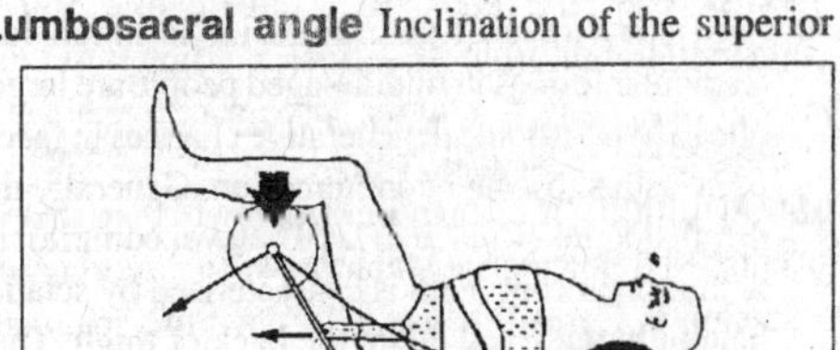

surface of the first sacral vertebra to the horizontal. Usually measured from standing lateral x-ray films. Last segment of spine is sacrum. In adult this

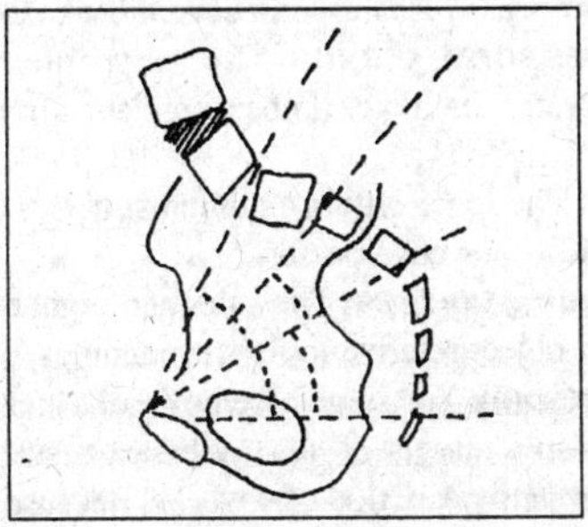

consists of one fused mass which normally is inclined at 30° to 45° to the horizontal.

Lumbosacral chair back brace It is a leather or plastic brace. A pelvic band is located between the iliac crest and the greater trochanter. Firm abdominal compression is applied. This brace is

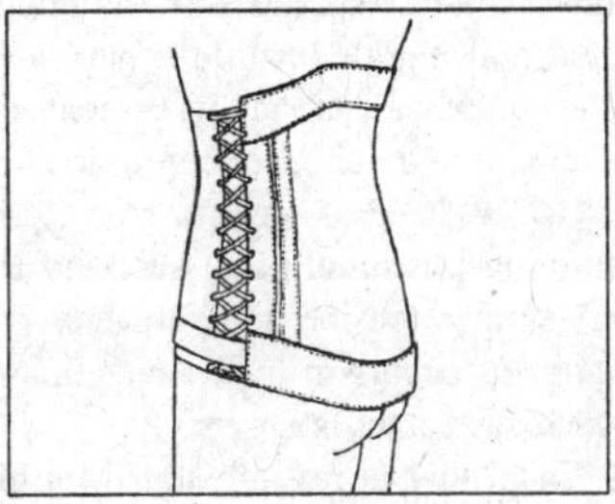

heavier and more rigid. Close fitting of the pelvic and thoracic band is crucial for stability and comfort. It is more durable and restricts lateral flexion.

Lumbosacral corset This is a fabric corset that has adjustable locings reinforced laterally. The belt is essentially a male corset. This corset should

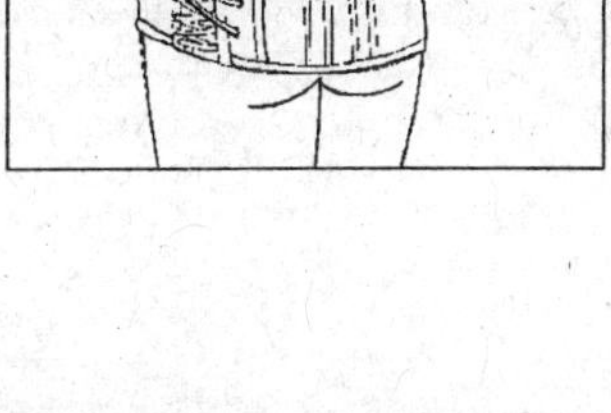

extend just above the lower ribs and anchor beneath the curve of the buttocks. Firm compression of all surfaces and abdominal compression are essential for proper fit. It is used in severe backache.

Lumbosacral plexus The nerve plexus that innervates the lower limbs; originates from spinal nerves L_1 to S_4.

Lumen The space within a tubular structure through which a substance passes.

Luminance contrast The amount of light reflected by an object relative to its surroundings.

Lumpectomy The surgical removal of a breast lump and also a margin of healthy breast tissue.

Lunar month A period of 4 weeks. Because a lunar month usually corresponds to the length of the menstrual cycle, it is often used for calculating fetal development.

Lung bud The endodermal origin of the bronchi and lungs in the fetus.

Lung function test It is a method to check working of lungs. Some tests measure the volume of air inhaled and exhaled while others analyse the contents of exhaled air and its contents comparing with arterial and venous composition.

Lung surfactant A mixture of lipoproteins (containing phospholipids) secreted by type II lowers surface tension and perevents collapse of the lungs as occurs in hyline membrane disease, in which surfactant is absent.

Lungs Each lung is invaginated from hilum into the closed sac of pleura. Pressure of 7 mm Hg is necessary to keep the lungs inflated. Right lung has 3 lobes and left two lobe. If the free flow of air into and out of lung is obstructed, the intrapulmonary pressure will be increased beyond normal range of (40 to+40 mm Hg).

Lunula A general anatomical term for a small crescentic or moonshaped area. The thin lamina fibrosa on either side of Arantius's nodules of the semilunar cusps of the aortic valve.

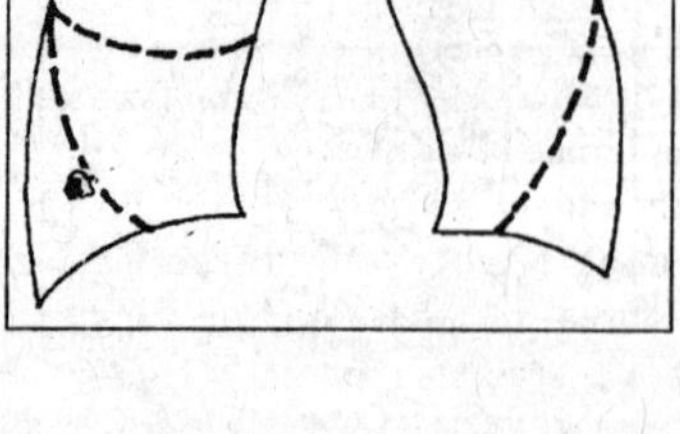

Lupus A nonspecific term originally used to designate various types of tubeculosis of the skin, later extended to mean any skin condition characterized by chronic destructive lesions with ulceration, hypertrophy, and degeneration. Alone, the term now may mean any specific form, such as lupus vulgaris, lupus tuberculosus, or disseminated lupus erythematosus.

Lupus erythematosus, chronic In the chronic form discrete white scaly macules and plaques occur on molar area and on the bridge of nose in a butterfly fashion. Oral lesions may precede or follow the skin lesions.

These include multiple white plaques with dark reddish purple margins looking like leucoplakia, ulceration of plaques may be seen. Microscopic picture shows hyperplasia and hyperkeratosis of epithelium with dense lymphocytic infiltration. Lesions of oral mucous membrane have similar microscopic features, hyperkeratosis or parakeratosis, basophilic degeneration of collagen.

Lupus vulgaris It is the most common form of cutaneous tuberculosis and runs a very prolonged course. It usually begins in childhood and causes extensive destruction of tissue. It starts as a reddish brown macule which changes slowly, over the months and years and finally presents with raised, flat, hyperpigmented irregular shaped patches. These indurated nodules are covered with very fine adherent scales.

The patches show healing with tissue paper like scarring. Nodules may ulcerate causing atrophic depigmented scars, lesions may produce hard, thick, depigmented usually crusted warty vegetative growth.

Luschka's body or glomus Coccygeal body.

Luster The characteristic of an opaque object reflecting light from its surface, causing it to look bright and shiny; a common appearance for polished metals.

Luteal phase The stage in menstrual cycle that is initiated following ovulation, at which time a corpus luteum is formed. It has a 14 days life span and secretes mainly progesterone and estradiol.

Luteinization The formation of a golden body corpus luteum in the ruptured follicle.

Luteinizing hormone (LH) A hormone secreted by the anterior pituitary that stimulates ovulation and preogresterone secretion by the corpus luteum, and readies the mammary glands for milk secretion in females; stimulates testosterone secretion by the testes in males.

Luteolysis The destruction of the corpus luteum through the dissolution of cellular structure. Thus luteolysis interferes with the function of the corpus luteum in progesterone secretion.

Luting The process of attaching one structure to another with use of an intermediate agent, such as a cement or wax; dental restorations are attached to teeth by this process.

Luxation A dislocation. For example, dislocation of the temporomandibular joint occurs when the head of the condyle moves anteriorly over the articular eminence and cannot be returned voluntarily.

Luxation of teeth It is defined as abnormal displacement of teeth. It can be intrusion and extrusion. Intrusion refers to the abnormal displacement of teeth into bone while extrusion refers to abnormal displacement of teeth out of bone. Crown of intruded tooth appears shorter while clinical crown of an extruded tooth appears longer than adjacent.

Lyases Enzymes that catalyze the removal of a group from a molecule to form a double bond, or the addition of a group to a double bond.

Lyme disease A complex disease that affects multiple systems of the body and results from exposure to the tick-borne pathogen borrelia burgdorferi. First stage is of expanding erythematous rash usually centred on the tickbite known as erythema chronicum migrans. Secondary eruptious may develop at other locations. Patient will develop malaise, fever, headache, muscleache and lymphadenopathy. Cardiac involvement develops in about 10 % cases. Oral doxycycline for 20 days will serve the purpose.

Lympatic vessel A large vessel that collects lymph from lymphatic capillaries and converges with other lymphatic capillaries and converges with other lymphatic vessels to form and thoracic and right lymphatic ducts.

Lympatic tissue A specialized form of reticular tissue that contains large numbers of lymphocytes.

Lymph Clear or yellowish fluid derived from interstitial fluid and found in lymph vessels. The composition of lymph can be regarded as a transudate of plasma,

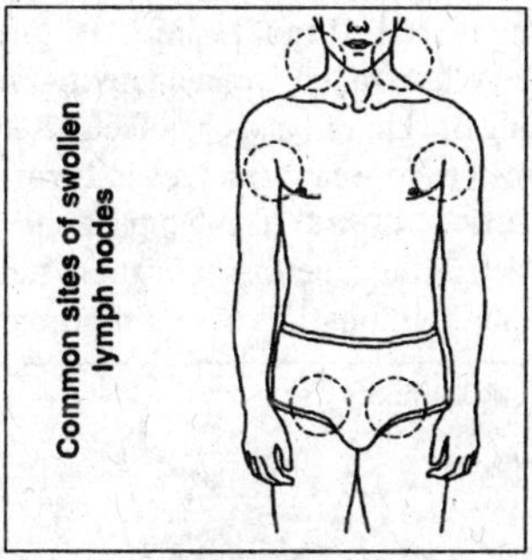

through a membrane which is partly permeable to protein. The electrolyte and crystalloid content is same as that of plasma, while protein content is approximately half of plasma. Lymph on standing clots. After fatty meal intestinal lymph becomes milky known as chyle.

Lymph glands Head & Neck Prominent lymph glands are sub mental, sub mandibular, cervical, parotid and retroauricular gland of clinical interest.

Lymph node Encapsulated mass of lymphatic tissue found along lymph vessels; functions to filter lymph and produce lymphocytes.

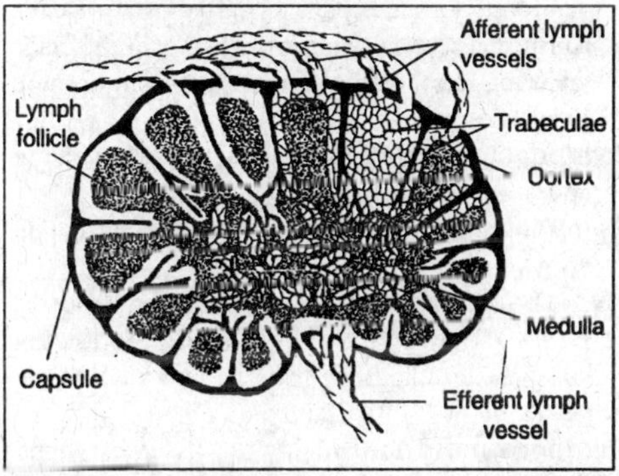

Lymph node metastasis It is rare in younger age group. It may be single or multiple, hard, nodular lymph nodes, initially mobile but gradually becoming fixed in one of cervical chains. Metastases from head and neck tumour most commonly involve deeper jugular chain at superior venous angle. Lymph gland metastases are generally bilateral.

Lymph node syndrome It generally occurs in patients under 5 years of age and is characterised by erythema of oral mucosa, dry and fissured lips, prominent red lingual papillae producing strawberry like tongue, conjunctivitis, fever and reddening of skin of hands and feets. Aetiology is not known and disease resolves in two weeks.

Lymph nodes, breast The lymphatic drainage of breast determines the dissemination and also its treatment. Lymphatic vessels drain mainly to

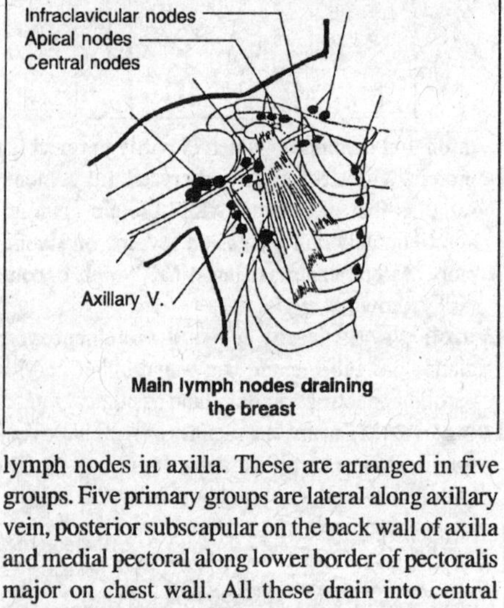

Main lymph nodes draining the breast

lymph nodes in axilla. These are arranged in five groups. Five primary groups are lateral along axillary vein, posterior subscapular on the back wall of axilla and medial pectoral along lower border of pectoralis major on chest wall. All these drain into central group lying in fat of axilla.

Lymphadenectomy Excision of a lymph node or nodes.

Lymphadenogram A roentgenogram of the lymph nodes.

Lymphadenography Roentgenographic visualization of the lymph nodes, following injection of radiopaque material into a lymphatic vessel.

Lymphadenoid Resembling the tissue of lymph nodes; lymphadenoid tissue..

Lymphadenopathy Disease process affecting a lymph node or lymph nodes.

Lymphadenosis Hypertrophy or proliferation of lymphoid tissue.

Lymphadenotomy Incision of a lymph node.

Lymphadenovarix Enlargement of the lymph nodes from the pressure of dilated lymph vessels.

Lymphangiography It is the lymphatic system by injection of contrast medium. The procedure serves to visualise lymph vessels in upper and lower extremities, the thoracic duct and regional lymph nodes in axillary, inguinal, paraaortic glands, etc. If lymph vessels are visualised, then water soluble contrast media is used and for lymph nodes oily contrast material is used. *Oily lymphangiography* is used in staging of malignant lymphomas and in chylothorax. *Water-soluble lymphangiography* is used in primary and secondary lymphoedema. Due to invention of CT and MRI now routine lymphangiography is not done.

Lymphangioma It is a tumour or tumour-like growth that may occur anywhere on the skin or mucous membrane of oral cavity. In mouth it is seen most frequently on tongue. When superficial they present as a cluster of colourless, thin walled, soft excrescences on the mucosa. When deep seated they produce a diffuse enlargement of tongue and surface may become smooth and devoid of papillae. Tongue may be enlarged. Microscopically, oral lymphangiomas consist of large thin-walled lymph containing spaces. These do not undergo malignant change and do not respond to radiation or sclerosing solutions. Surgical excision is the choice of treatment.

Lymphangioplasty Surgical restoration or correction of lymphatic vessels.

Lymphangiotomy Incision into a lymphatic vessel.

Lymphangitis Inflammation of lymphatic vessels. Acute lymphangitis is evidenced by painful subcutaneous red streaks along the course of lymphatics.

Lymphatic capillaries Tiny, blind-ended tubes distributed in the tissues spaces.

Lymphatic drainage A specific type of massage that enhances lymphatic flow.

Lymphatic duct Terminal vessel into which lymphatic vessels empty lymph; the duct then empties the lymph into the cirulatory system.

Lymphatic space A tissue or vessels filled with lymph.

Lymphatic system A system that plays a critical role in the functioning of the immune system, fluids and large molecules from tissues spaces and fat-related nutrients from the digestive system to the blood.

Lymphatic tissue Tissue that is responsible for manufacturing lymphocytes and monocytes; found mostly in the lymph nodes, thymus, and spleen.

Lymphatic vessels Vessels that carry lymph to its eventual return to the circulatory system.

Lymphedema Edema due to accumulation of excessive amounts of lymph, which is secondary to obstruction of the lymphatic system in conditions such as cancer, elephantiasis, or abnormalities of the lymphatic structures.

Lymphoblast A lymphocyte in its germinative stage; a developing lymphocyte.

Lymphoblastoma A neoplasm of the lymphoid tissue, made up of lymphoblasts. It is a malignant tumor that may arise in a single lymph node or in groups of nodes, sometimes leading to lymphatic leukemia.

Lymphocele These are collection of lymph fluid in nonepithelialised cavities. These develop after 12 months of surgery.

Typical collections are paraaortal, paracaval and parailiac region. Small lymphocele often shows spontaneous regression.

Lymphocyte Nongranulocytic leucocyte involved in the immune system; there are several types of lymphocytes with diverse functions, including antibody production, allergic reactions, graft rejections, tumour control, and regulation of the immune system. The primary white blood cells of immune system i.e. B-lymphocyte, B cells, T lymphocytes and T-cells.

Lymphocytic lymphoma Primary oral lesion may arise in hard palate, gingiva or tonsil. It usually develops in adults. Males are affected more. Clinically the lesion is a palatal or gingival hyperplasia or a tumour mass. Ulceration, necrosis and foul breath are common. Microscopic study shows that tumour mass consists of masses of round cells. Mitoses are variable. These are mistaken for inflammatory lesions. These are radiosensitive. Remissions are temporary.

Lymphoedema It is caused by accumulation of fluid in extracellular fluid compartment and in limbs it accumulates in subcutaneous tissue. There will be pitting on pressure over lower part of tibia in early lymphoedema. Later on this oedema becomes non-pitting oedema.

Lymphokine A class of chemicals produced by T-cells that activate macrophages and other immune cells; promote phagocytosis and inflammation. Cytokine produced by lymphocytes. Contribute to cell-mediated immunity.

Lymphoma A general term for malignant neoplasms of the lymphoid tissues.

Lymphopathia Any disease of the lymphatic system.

Lymphopathy Disease of the lymphatic system.

Lymphopenia Deficiency of lymphocytes in the circulating blood. It may be related to thymic hypoplasia and is associated with agammaglobulinemia.

Lymphotoxin Synonym for the tumor necrosis fact ß (TNFß).

Lyophillization The process of simultaneouly freezing and drying materials under a vaccum.

Lyse Disintegration of a cell.

Lysis Destruction of a cell's plasma membrane or of a bacterial cell wall, releasing the cellular contents and killing the cell.

Lysogen A bacterial or other cell carrying a viral prophage and having the potential of producing and releasing bacteriophage under proper conditions.

Lysogenic Relating to or having the property of lysogeny; capable of producing a full burst of progeny virus.

Lysogeny The heritable, stable potentiality of bacteria to produce and release bacteriophages due to the presence of a prophage within the bacterial cell.

Lysol It is most commonly used general purpose disinfectant.

Their chief use in laboratory is for sterilising surgical instruments, discarded cultures, floor and furniture. It is good for sterilisation of excreta or contaminated secretions from tuberculosis.

Lysosome Membranous organelles containing various enzymes that can dissolve most cellular compounds; hence called digestive bags or suicide bags of cells. Organelles containing degestive enzymes and responsible for intracellular digestion.

Lysozyme It is an antibacterial enzyme found in both parotid and submaxillary secretions. It is formed in basal cells of ducts. Lysozyme splits bacterial cell walls in the glycopeptide region containing muramic acid.

This a basic protein of low molecular weight formed in relatively high concentration in polymorphonuclear leucocytes as well as in most tissue fluids except CSF and sweat. Human tears contain large quantity of lysozyme and egg white is its commercial source. Lysozyme acts as a mucolytic enzyme splitting sugars. It plays a role in the intracellular destruction of some gram-negative bacteria.

Lytic Having to do with or involved in lysis.

Lytic phase A mode of virus interaction with cells in which the virus undergoes a complete replicative cycle with the production of many progeny virus particles and subsequent release of these virus upon the lysis of the cell.

M

Mac Donald's measurement Measurement of height of uterine fundus with a tape measure, the distance from symphysis pubis to fundus.

Maceration Skin that becomes abnormally soft and breaks down because of prolonged exposure to moisture. Softening of a solid by exposure to water or other fluid; usually pertains to the skin.

Mackenrodt's ligament Cardinal lateral cervical ligament of uterus.

Mackintosh It is double coated rubber sheet to be spread over bed in case of children and certain surgery cases to avoid spoiling of bed linen. As regards its washing it can be spread and washed with soap water on either surface. Then rinse it with plain water. It has to be dried in shade and not in bright sun. These are not to be folded many times for drying or hanged on hook. When dried dusting powder should be sprinkled before storing.

Macroanalysis Chemical analysis using 0.1 to 0.2 gm of the substance under study.

Macrobe A eukaryotic organism, either single-celled or multicellular, that is visible to the unaided eye.

Macrocheilitis Inflammation and swelling of the lips.

Macrodontism macrodontia

Macrogametocyte The cell that gives rise to a macrogamete.

Macrogynecomastia A dome-shaped breast enlargement greater than 5 cm in diameter that resembles the middle and late stages of normal female development.

Macrolactone A lactone ring that typically contains 14 or more atoms.

Macrolevel A level of analysis that focuses on the larger forms of social behavior; for example, social systems, social institutions, or the relationship between social institutions.

Macromolecule A large molecule, often containing thousands of atoms, a term that usually refers to protein, RNA, and DNA.

Macroorchidism A condition of larger than normal testis size.

Macrophage Literally, large eater; a large cell that ingests and destryos particles by an engulfing process known as phagocytosis; macrophages are an active component of the immune response.

Macrophagy The process of feeding on or ingesting relatively large amounts of material.

Macrophthalmia Abnormal enlargement of the eyeball.

Macroprosopia Excessive size of the face.

Macroshock Harmless distribution of low-amperance electricity over a large area of the body.

Macrosis Increase in size.

Macrosomia The condition of having greater than normal fetal size or weight; commonly definied as a weight of 4,500 g or more after 38 weeks of gestation.

Macrostomia An abnormally large mouth sometimes associated with lateral facial cleft.

Macrovascular Large blood vessels of the body.

Macula One of the sensory structures in the vestibule, consisting of hair cells and a gelatinous mass embedded with otoliths; responds to gravity.

Macula lutea It appears as a dark brown area at the posterior pole of the eye. it appears more brown than the surrounding retina. This is thin and the underlying pigment epithelium and choroid is seen through it. It lies 3.5 mm lateral to the edge of the disc. At macula there are numerous ganglion cells arranged in several layers and the outer molecular layer is thicker and there is progressive disappearance of rods which are replaced by cones.

Macular Pertaining to a small, discolored patch or spot on the skin that is neither elevated above nor depressed below the surface.

Macular rash A skin discoloration characterized by circular or oval spots which are not raised above the skin surface.

Maculate Spotted or blotched.

Macule A circumscribed spot not raised above the level of the skin, which is not palpable, such as a freckle.

Maduramycosis It is also known as mycetoma caused by variety of fungi. Organism enters the body through trauma. Lesion appears most commonly on the foot and is known as Madura foot. It gives rise to a painless papule at the site of inoculation. It later changes to deepened nodule, vesicle or abscess over months rupture and produce fistula, discharging viscid, oily exudate containing yellow or white and rarely black or red granules. Then entire area becomes woody, indurated and covered with open sinuses or atrophic scars.

Maffucci's syndrome The syndrome is manifested by unilateral nodules on the small bones of the hands and feet and on the long bones, fracture of the bones on trivial injuries, dilatation of the veins, and angiomatous tumours on the extremities and trunk.

Magendie, foramen Median aperture of fourth ventricle.

Magical thinking A conviction that thinking equates with doing. Occurs in dreams in children, in primitive people, and in patients under a variety of conditions. Characterised by lack of realistic relationship between cause and effect.

Magnesia core porcelain A type of porcelain composed of up to 50% magnesia crystals; used to make a core or body on which an enamel layer will be fired; the benefit to of this material is a much higher strength than conventional feldspathic porcelain.

Magnesium It is essential for the formation of bones and teeth. It is required for muscle contraction, for transmission of nerve impulses and for the activation of many enzymes. Body contains about 35 gm.

The recommended daily intake of magnesium varies from 350 to 400 mg in adult. Dietary sources are green, leafy vegetables, nuts, grains and sea food. Magnesium carbonates and magnesium oxides are ingredients of antacids. Symptoms of deficiency include anxiety, restlessness, tremors, palpitations and depression. Kidney stones may be formed. Too much magnesium may cause nausea, vomiting, diarrhoea, dizziness and muscle weakness. Very large amount may lead to heart damage.

Magnesium sulphate It is used as an anticonvulsant drug in pre eclampsia and eclampsia. It lowers BP causing vasodilatation.

Magnetic resonance imaging Technique for producing an image by using atoms subjected to a strong electromagnetic field.

Magnitude estimation A technique for measuring perceptual experience by having persons assign numbers to indicate the "magnitude" of an experience.

Magnocellular nucleus of the medulla A part of the brainstem that sends inhibitory impulses to the motor neurons of the spinal cord to produce the paralysis of REM (rapid eye movement) sleep.

Main bearing struts The struts of a subperiosteal implant designed to transfer functional load to basal bone.

Mainstream implant dentistry The use of any professionally accepted modality in uncomplicated, predictable treatment applicable to most implant candidates.

Mainstreaming Inclusion of mentally retarded children in normal classroom settings. Provisions are made for a slower rate of presentation and greater structure in the learning tasks, rather than special education per se.

Maintenance Continuing care after completion of treatment procedures.

Maintenance phase Series of appointments after initial therapy for periodic re-examination and additional therapy as needed to keep the teeth and periodontal tissues in health without recurrence of disease.

Maintenance therapy It is a careful monitoring of dosage during a course of treatment with drugs in order to maintain a patient's condition fit and chances of symptoms to reappear become low. Maintenance dose is lower than therapeutic dose.

Major amputation Any amputation through a long bone of the upper or lower extremity, a disarticulation of hip or shoulder.

Major depression A temporary or chronic mental disorder characterized by five of following feelings-sadness, inability to enjoy things, sleep disturbances, appetite disturbance, fatigue, difficulty in concentrating and suicidal acts.

Major depressive disorder Depressed mood or loos of interest in activities in combination with three or more additional symptoms such as loss of fatigue, feelings or worthlessness, thoughts about death or concentration problem.

Major histocompatibility (MHC) Antigens Surface proteins on white blood cells and other nucleated cells that are unique for each person (except for identical siblings) and are used to type tissues and help prevent rejection.

Major histocompatibility complex Specialised membrane proteins that are characteristic to each individual and present antigen to T cells.

Major minerals Essential nutrient minerals required daily in amounts of 100mg or higher.

Major renal injuries These have cortical laceration more than 1 centimeter. Deep laceration will go up to collecting system. It will create palpable mass, muscle tenderness, flank pain or colic. Such patients are in clinical shock and become surgical emergencies.

Major tranquilizer A type of drug that blocks the dopamine-2 (D_2) receptor and is used mainly for treating schizophrenia; also called a neuroleptic drug.

Mal Prefix for bad or ill.

Mal occlusion It is a position of maxillary and mandibular jaws to each other that is abnormal or out of proportion.

Mal prohibita An act or omission that is wrong only because it is prohibited or directed by the law.

Malabsorption It is the impaired absorption of nutrients, vitamins or minerals from the diet by the lining of small intestine. It may be due to lactose intolerance. In pancreatitis production of enzymes required for digestion and absorption of fats are decreased. Removal of portions of small intestine can cause malabsorption. Common symptoms are diarrhoea and weight loss in severe cases. Treatment depends on the cause.

Malacia The morbid softening of a part or tissue.

Malacic Marked by malacia or abnormal softness.

Maladie A disease.

Malaise A general feeling of discomfort or uneasiness.

Malar Pertaining to cheek or the zygotic bone.

Malar elevator To elevate or reposition of zygomatic bone.

Malaria It spreads by the bite of anopheles mosquitoes. Disease results in shaking chills and fever when red blood cells infected with parasites rupture to release more parasites into blood stream. It occurs in tropics. Incubation period is usually a week or two. Except for *Plasmodium falciparum* this fever has 3 stages—a cold stage of rigors, hot stage in which temperature may reach 105°F and finally a sweating stage that drenches the bedding and brings down the temperature. Severe headache, general malaise and vomiting may accompany the attack. At the end of attack patient is left weak and tired and sleeps. In many cases parasitised red blood cells rupture at the same time in each cycle and fever develops cyclically occurring every other or every third day. *P. falciparum* that affects all ages of RBCs whereas the others affect young or old RBCs. *Falciparum* affects more proportion of blood cells and is more severe. It may be fatal within a few hours of first symptoms. Fever is prolonged and more irregular. Kidneys become failed. Spleen enlarges and brain is affected. Destruction of RBC may lead to haemolytic anaemia. Chloroquine is drug of choice and in resistent cases, combination of pyrimethamine and sulphadoxine (Fancidar) may be given. In severe cases even exchange blood transfusion may be done.

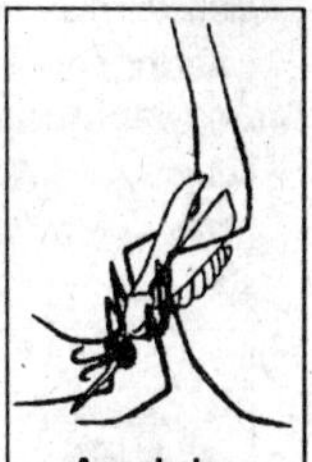

Anopheles

Malarial dysentery Malignant tertian malaria may manifest itself by severe diarrhoea. There may be occasional blood and mucus similar to bacillary dysentery. Sigmoidoscopy may show a diffuse or patchy hyperaemia. In severe cases scattered haemorrhagic areas are seen. Blood smear shows parasites.

Male catheterisation Catheter is longer one 20 to 22 cm having thinner lumen. Catheter is lubricated for 8 to 10 cm and penis is held at 60° angle. Position of patient is dorsal recumbent. By right hand the catheter tip is introduced gently for about 8 cm. If there is urethral obstruction the

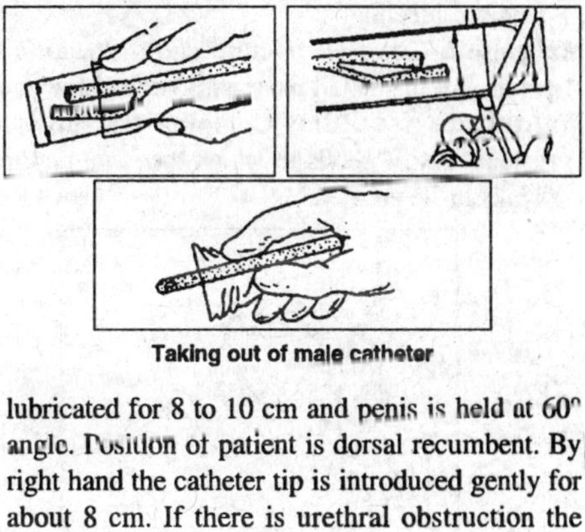

Taking out of male catheter

catheter may not go in, so never apply pressure. If catheter goes in urine flows.

Male resolution stage Suddenly loss of testicular congestion takes place. Scrotum becomes thin and penis decreases to 50% larger than unstimulated state.

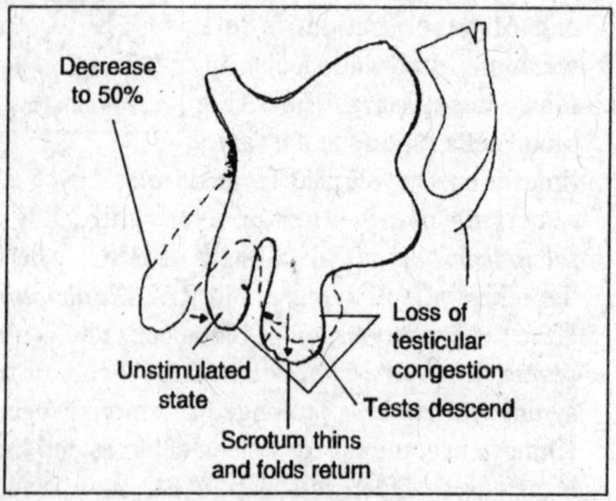

Male-male competition Competition among individuals of the chosen sex for access to individuals of the choosy sex.

Malformation Irregular or anomalous formation or structure of parts of an organism.

Malformations, arteriovenous These are arteriovenous fistulae consisting of mesh of abnormal thin vessels. These can occur in any part of cerebral cortex but mostly are found in posterior half of hemispheres forming a wedge-shaped lesion extending from cortex to ventricular lining. Patient may present with intracranial bleed, seizures, focal neurological deficits, headache and impaired higher functions. CT and MRI are better to diagnose bleeding.

Malgaigne Complex fracture and dislocation of pelvis. An unstable injury with vertical fractures.

Malgaigne fracture Complex fracture and dislocations of pelvis in which there are multiple breaks in ileum arch.

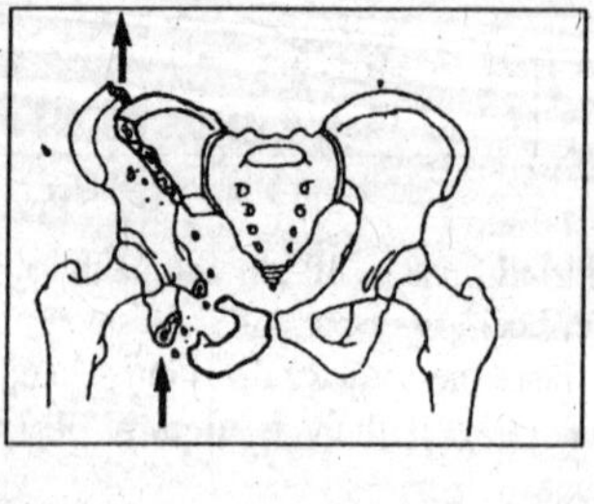

Malignant Tending to be progressively worse and to result in death. Having the properties of anaplasia, invasion, and metastasis; said of tumors.

Malignant angina There develops rapidly progressive swelling of peritonsillar tissue usually during or after a bout of tonsillitis spreading to soft tissue of lateral pharynx and deep fascial compartments of neck. Patient develops dysphagia with progressive dyspnoea. Mediastinal involvement may occur.

Malignant diphtheria It is characterised by extensive membrane with huge enlarged submandibular and cervical lymph nodes giving rise to bull neck. There is mouth breathing. The tongue protrudes out. Breath becomes foul. Voice becomes worse. Pharyngeal mucous membrane becomes red and oedematous, skin becomes pale and cold. Purpuric spots may be seen in neck and anterior chest.

Malignant hyperpyrexia In it heat production exceeds heat loss in body to cause a rise of temperature of at least 2° centigrade/hour. It is characterised by cyanosis, mottled rash, muscle rigidity, hypercapnia, hypervenilation, dysrhythmias and pyrexia. Exhaustion and cardiac failure result in death.

Malignant hyperthermia Due to inhalent anaesthetics and muscle relaxants. Temperature rises 1°C every five minutes. Death may result due to acidosis tachycardia and hypotension.

Malignant lymphoepithelial lesion In it epithelial component undergoes a malignant transformation. However, it is not associated with Sjögren's syndrome. It generally develops in females. Parotid gland is the most commonly affected organ. Under microscope it reveals undifferentiated carcinoma of poorly differentiated adenocarcinoma in a stroma of cells of the lymphoid series. It metastasises to cervical glands.

Malignant lymphoma Malignant lymphoma can arise in aggregation of lymphoid tissue, i.e. lymph nodes, diffuse lymphoid tissue of the body such as lingual and pharyngeal tonsils and lymphoid tissue of gastrointestinal tract. Certain tumours are more common in certain age groups. Hodgkin is more common between 20-40 years of age. Early symptoms include enlargement of external lymph nodes. Malignant lymphomas may be caused by virus. These may be classified into Non-Hodgkin's lymphoma, Hodgkin's disease and special types of lymphoma.

Malignant meningitis Multiple cranial nerve palsies can develop by direct extension of nasopharyngeal carcinomas, lymphomas or plasmocytomas or by local extension of a blood-borne metastasis from bronchus or breast. Malignant cells may be found in CSF. There will be low sugar in CSF. Anaplastic gliomas or medulloblastomas may seed down the meninges in a similar way.

Malignant neoplasm A tumor that grows in an uncontrolled manner, invading surrounding tissue; metastasizes and may cause death if untreated.

Malignant nephrosclerosis It is accompanied by cardiovascular changes. There is no history of acute or subacute nephritis. Headache specially on waking with vomiting is associated with precordial pain, breathlessness and nocturnal paroxysmal dyspnoea. There may be an epileptiform convulsion. BP is very high with 240/130 mm Hg or even more.

Left ventricle is hypertrophied. Radial and brachial arteries are contracted and hardened. In late stage, stress and failure of left ventricle are shown by attack of oedema of lungs. Failing vision is due to changes in fundus. Specific gravity of urine is fixed at 1012. Blood urea may be normal. Symptoms of incipient uraemia become more marked with loss of appetite and body weight.

Malignant oral tumour Malignant oral tumours such as carcinoma, lymphoepithelioma, osteogenic sarcoma, malignant salivary gland tumour, metastasise and kill the patient. Even some benign tumours of the maxilla such as chondroma can prove fatal by local extension to cranial base.

Malignant otitis externa There develops lancinating ear pain of increasing severity. Aural discharge usually emanates from a granulating area of floor of external auditory canal. Fistula forms at the junction of cartilaginous junction.

Malingerer Someone who pretends to be sick or in pain.

Malingering Person pretends to be ill to avoid work or undesirable situation. Soldiers in army malinger to be suffering by backache or so to be relieved from army which otherwise is very difficult. Person may malinger to avoid responsibility or a feared event.

Malleable A characteristic that allows a metal to be compressed and condensed on itself to change its shape without fracturing; similar to ductility, but specifically referring to a compressive force applications.

Mallet It is a metallic hammer used for striking on a gauze or a chisel to remove chips of bone during mastoidectomy to open up the mastoid antrum.

Mallet finger It is a fixed flexor deformity of the distal interphalangeal joint of finger. This results from either a rupture of extensor tendon at its insertion or an avulsion fracture of base of distal phalanx. When patient holds out his or her hand, with the fingers extended the peculiar deformity is obvious—the distal phalanx of affected finger remains 15° to 20° flexed. Distal phalanx can be extended passively and not actively.

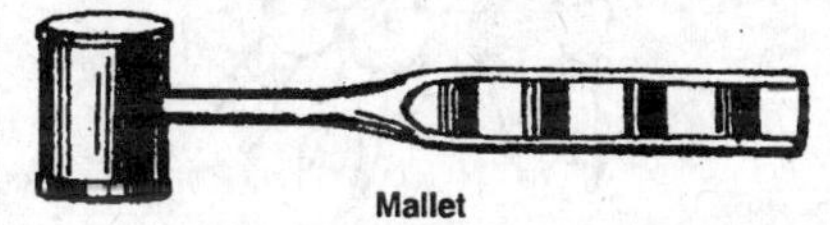
Mallet

Mallet finger and toe deformity Injury is usually a blow to the end of extended finger or a crush. There may be a complete rupture of tendon or an avulsion fracture at the base of distal phalanx involving area of insertion of extensor tendon. Splint is used continuously for 6 to 8 weeks.

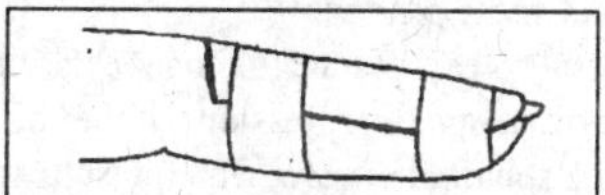
Splint

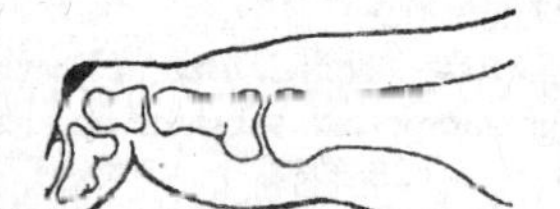
Mallet-toe

Malleus The most lateral of the middle ear bones, attached to the tympanic membrane, the hammer.

Mallory-Weise syndrome In this syndrome severe itching and vomiting produce gastrooesophageal mucosal tear with bleeding, haematemesis, perforation, and mediastinitis.

Malnutrition Condition resulting from a lack of proper nutrients in the diet.

Malocclusion It is an abnormal relationship between the upper and lower sets of teeth when they are closed. Ideally, upper incisors and canines slightly overlap the lower ones. The outer ridges of lower premolars and molars fit into hollows in the corresponding upper teeth except for the foremost incisors.

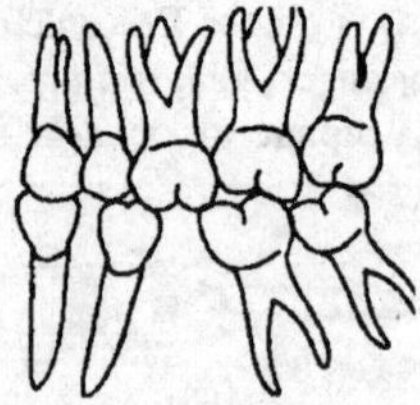

Malocclusion due to loss of mandibular first occlusion

This helps in food to be eaten and chewed efficiently. Malocclusion develops in childhood when jaws and teeth are growing. Some may develop it due to thumb sucking beyond a certain age. Malocclusion requires treatment to improve appearance.

Malpighian tubule An excretory organ of terrestrial insects and most acarines.

Malpractice Professional negligence resulting from improper discharge of professional duties or failure to meet the standard of care, which results in harm to a client or patient.

Malpraxis Malpractice.

Malt The major raw material, used in brewing that provides the appropriate substrate and enzymes needed.

Malunion Fracture which unites in a position of deformity is said malunion. There may be significant anglulation at the site of fracture. It may be caused by imperfect reduction or failure to stabilise a satisfactory reduction. Malunion is cosmetically annoying and may impair its function.

Mamelon Rounded end on one of the enamel-forming groups on the incisal edge of incisors. These are usually worn away with use.

Mammalian Relating to or designating a mammal.

Mammary Relating to or involving the mammary glands.

Mammary gland The gland of the female breast responsible for lactation and nourishment of the young.

Mammillary Refers to the mammillary bodies.

Mammogram An X-Ray of the breast that can identify abnormalities before they can be felt by a woman.

Mammography It is the radiographic examination of soft tissues of breast. Adequate contrast is difficult to obtain in the breast due to very low differences in attenuation between the soft tissues. There is only the small difference in atomic numbers between malignant tissue and normal breast. Detection of small attenuation difference is best achieved with low X-ray energies. Breast compression decreases scattered radiation.

Mammoplasty It is a surgical cosmetic operation to reduce the size of large, pendulous breasts or to enlarge small size breasts. Cosmetically, it may be repaired after surgery. Incisions are not visible. Nipple scar and scar below breast are generally not seen. Immediate results are usually excellent but internal scar tissue often eventually forms around the implant.

Managed care A systemj of administrative controls, the primary goal of which is to reduce the costs of medical care.

Managed care practices Cost-containment strategies used to plan and coordinate a patient's care to avoid delays, unnecessary services, or overuse of expensive resources.

Management The use of available resources to achieve a predetermined goal.

Mandamus A court order compelling public officers to do their legally mandated duties.

Mandate An authoritative command; a formal command from a superior court or official to an inferior one.

Mandible Lower jaw; a horseshoe-shaped bone, bilaterally consisting of a vertical component ramus, a horizontal component joined in a midline body and symphysis, and a condyle that articulates to the temporal bone of the skull (TMJ).

Mandibular arcs Circular or elliptics arcs created by closure of mandible.

Mandibular block This may be required for extraction of several teeth of lower jaw or for removal of second or third molars. A single well-placed injection makes one-half of the lower jaw and tongue analgesic except for central incisor which gets some nerve supply from other side. With the mouth open palpate the anterior border of ramus of mandible, the retromolar fossa and internal oblique ridge. Needle is inserted just medial to ridge for a distance of 1.5 cm. 2 ml or 3 ml solution is injected.

Mandibular foramen Opening on the medial aspect of the vertical ramus of the mandible, approximately midway between the mandibular and gonial notches; may be located posterior to the middle of the ramus. It contains interior alveolar vessels and the inferior alveolar nerve.

Mandibular nerve block It is done for facial and intraoral procedures.

Mandrel Part of the handpiece that holds a disk, stone, or cup. It is usually a shaft with a screw at the end to change the disk.

Maneuvering Procedure used by obstetrician in assisting delivery manually.

Mania One of the principal features is loss of self-control. It is accompanied by an exaggerated sense of wellbeing. Patient becomes talkative, restless and optimistic. In acute mania onset is usually rapid with tongue tremor. The stage of excitement is soon reached. Chronic mania is suspected when patient's restless excitement, incoherent conversation and disordered conduct continue. Delusions become more prominent and auditory hallucinations may be a feature.

Manic depressive psychosis in pregnancy This is a king of infantile excessive dependency on the patient's love object. When she loses this love object, she develops a sense of worthlessness exhibiting depression. The severe psychotic episode occurs more during puerperium. Infanticidal and suicidal tendencies are very strong amongst the manic depressive psychotics. A severe depressive psychosis after the first child in a young woman will not recur following second child.

Manic state A condition of extreme elation, sometimes so marked and inappropriate that it requires special treatment. The individual may have inappropriately optimistic expectations or new ideas that will "change the world". The state is one condition in the bipolar disorder, which also includes depression.

Manifest content The remembered content of a dream or fantasy, as contrasted with latent content, which is concealed and distorted.

Manifestation That which is made evident, especially to the sight and understanding.

Manikin Model of the human body or a part used for teaching purposes.

Manipulation A manual procedure that involves a directed thrust to move a joint past its physiologic range of motion without exceeding the boundaries of anatomic integrity. Audible joint cavitation noise is commonly produced by this procedure.

Mankin score A severity classification scale for disease course of osteoarthritis.

Mannitol It is an osmotic diuretic drug. It is used for short-term in glaucoma. It reduces fluid retention. It is given in brain tumour or in intracerebral haematoma. It is used to treat kidney failure in shock. Side-effects of mannitol are headache, nausea, dizziness and confusion.

Mannitol (eye surgery) Mannitol is given IV. Its dose is 2 gm per kg body weight, 30 minutes to achieve hypotonus. During infusion patient may complain of angina like pain in chest and headache. It is useful in cases of acute congestive closed angle glaucoma and that too to produce hypotony to produce surgery.

Mann-whitney U test A nonparametric significance test used to compare two groups of ordinal tata. It is analogous to the student's t-test for continuous data.

Manometer An instrument for measuring pressure or tension of liquids or gases.

Manslaughter Unlawful killing of another person.

Mantoux test It is an intradermal test in which 0.1 ml of 1:10,000 dilution of tuberculin is injected into skin over the forearm. If there is no reaction, larger dose is given 0.1 ml of 1:2000. It is characterised by delayed appearance and of long duration. It usually occurs after several hours of injection and maximum response may be seen in 1 or 2 days. The reaction is considered definitely positive if there is induration of at least 10 mm in diameter. Erythema is usually present. False-positive and false-negative tuberculin test do occur.

Manual expulsion of placenta The third stage of delivery is pushing out of placenta. Placenta was a lifeline of fetus throughout pregnancy. Cord is separated a few moments after the baby is born. It is painless because there are no nerves. Cord is clamped firmly on the baby's side so that there is no bleeding. Once the placenta has separated and

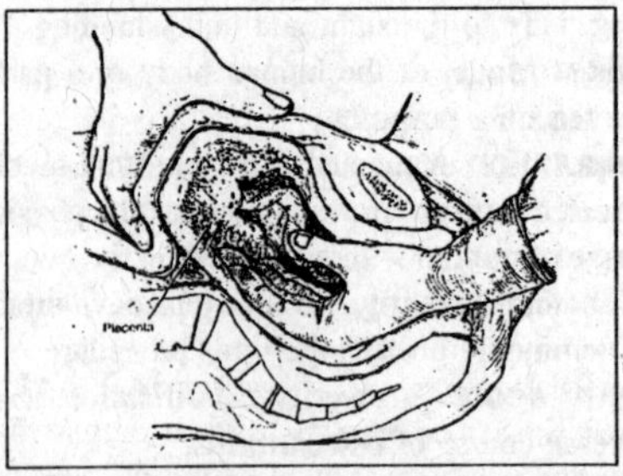

moved down through the open cervix into the vagina mother will feel another urge to push. Placenta is to be examined for its completeness. Retained placenta may be a source of infection and recurrent bleeding so it has to be taken out manually.

Manual hyperinflation A greater than normal inflannation induced with a manual resuscitator bag.

Manual rotation A manoeuvre used to turn the fetal head by hand from a transverse to an anteroposterior position to facilitate delivery.

Manual therapy Therapeutic application of manual force. Spinal manual therapy broadly defined includes all procedures in which the hands are used to mobilize, adjust, manipulate, apply traction, massage stimulate, or otherwise influence the spine and paraspinal tissues with the aim of influencing the patient's health.

Manual traction It is applied by the therapist usually for 15-60 sec. or as a suddent thrust.

Mapping Delineation or representation of anything, the locating of the relative position of genes on a chromosome.

Marasmus Patient is markedly emaciated. Body weight is less than 60% of expected weight for that age. Fat in the adipose tissues is severely depleted. Skin becomes wrinkled. Skin is dry and inelastic. Abdomen is distended due to wasting. Midarm circumference is reduced. Bony prominences become obvious. Child becomes irritable. It is a severe form of protein calorie malnutrition. It is widespread below the age of 3 years. Children become stunted and emaciated. They have loose folds of skin over buttocks and hands. There will be sparse, brittle hair, diarrhoea and dehydration. High-calorie protein diet is helpful.

Marathon therapy A method of group therapy based on the premise that it takes longer than 50 minutes for the patient to discard his or her defences. Marathon therapy may continue for several days.

March gangrene Anterior tibial compartment syndrome which results in muscle ischemia.

Marche a petit pas 'Walk with small steps' Hesitant gait. associated with frontal lobe disease.

Marchesani's syndrome An autosomal disorder with short stocky stature, spade-like hands with short stubby fingers, thick skin and hair, and ectopia lentis.

Marchiafava-Micheli syndrome The syndrome is characterised by abdominal and lumbar pain, normocytic normochromic anaemia, splenomegaly, haemoglobinuria, and haemoglobinaemia which is accentuated during sleep.

Marey's law Increased pressure in aortic arch causes bradycardia.

Marfan syndrome It is an autosomal dominant condition. Patient is tall, slender with elongated bones. Muscles will be weak with hypermobility. One can notice dislocation of lens, high-arched palate, myopia and glaucoma. Atrial septal defect (ASD) and mitral valve lesions are commonly noted.

Marginal leakage The movement of salivary components and bacteria toward the pulp along the interface or margin between a dental restoration and the cavity wall.

Marginal ridge Ridge or elevation of enamel that forms the boundary of the occlusal surface of a tooth.

Marginal sinus rupture A disorder of placental attachment, a mild type of abruptio placentae in which slight separation occurs at the edge of the placenta in the region of the marginal sinus of the mother.

Marginal zone The outer area of the splenic periarteriolar lymphoid sheath (PALS) which is rich in B cells, particularly those responding to thymus independnet antigens.

Margraine An emulsion of fat from variety of vegetable, animal or marine oils with 16% water, flavoured and coloured.

Maria santon disease Cliedocranial disease.

Marie sainton syndrome This is a benign hereditary disease inherited as autosomal dominant trait. Respiratory distress may occur in newborn. Mental retardation, epileptic attack, hemiplegia and spastic paraplegia may be there. Maxillary teeth are underdeveloped and crowding of teeth of upper jaw is seen. Thorax is narrow and ribs are short and 13 pairs are noted.

Marijuana It is the dried leaf and flowering top of Indian hemp plant *Cannabis sativa*. When marijuana is smoked, effects occur within minutes. Effect lasts for one and half hour. Physical effects include a dry mouth, mild reddening of eyes and increased appetite. Main subjective feelings are of wellbeing and calmness. Some on occasion may develop depression. User starts dreaming and relaxed. Imagination increases and sights and sounds become more vivid. Large doses may result in panicky stage. Regular user may become addict.

Marijuana toxicity Marijuana is one of the preparations of the leaves and flowers of the plant *Cannabis sativa*. Approximately 10 to 50 % of smoked THC is absorbed compared to 3 to 6 % by ingestion. Peak THC plasma levels after inhalation are achieved within a few minutes but peak clinical effects are delayed by 20 to 30 minutes. The features of intoxication appear soon after smoking *ganja* or *charas* and within half an hour after swallowing bhang. Anxiety lasts for 10 to 30 minutes.

There develops panic, fear of death and restlessness. This is followed by calm, euphoria and exhilarated behaviour. Person feels light. Patient laughs uncontrollably after 2 to 4 hours. Patient later becomes lethargic and drowsy. Other symptoms include increased appetite, tremors, hallucinations and altered vision. Features of toxicity disappear within hours hence it does not require much of treatment.

Marital functioning Term includes how spouse and couples think about, feel about, and behave in their marriage.

Marital rape Rape involving the legal or common law spouse or ex spouse of victim.

Marketing The advertising and other promotional activities required to sell a product or service.

Marking test The raised point at the apex of the head of an intramucosal insert that marks the gingiva to indicate the location of its planned gingival receptor site.

Marmalade Jam made from citrous fruits.

Marriage The legal union of two individuals.

Marrow The soft connective tissue found within the inner cavity of certain bones that produces red blood cells.

Martin syndrome This is an autosomal dominant disorder. Clinical features include mental retardation, large ears and hypertelorism. X-ray will show microcephaly, absent premaxilla, cleft lip and palate and spinal deformity.

Marvel test A maneuver used to assess the integrity of the transverse humeral ligament.

Masculine protest Term coined by Adler to describe a striving to escape identification with the feminine role. Applies primarily to women but may also be noted in men.

Masculinisation There is appearance of male characters, i.e. growth of hair on face and body, deepening of voice in females. It is due to hormonal disturbance. Treatment includes female sex hormones.

Masculinize To cause an individual to develop the secondary sexual characteristics of a mature male, as by the administration of androgens.

Masenteric patches Clusters of lymph nodes on the walls of the small intestine; also called peyer's patches.

Mask Oxygen can be given by means of a mask. Disposable polythene mask is light, handy and

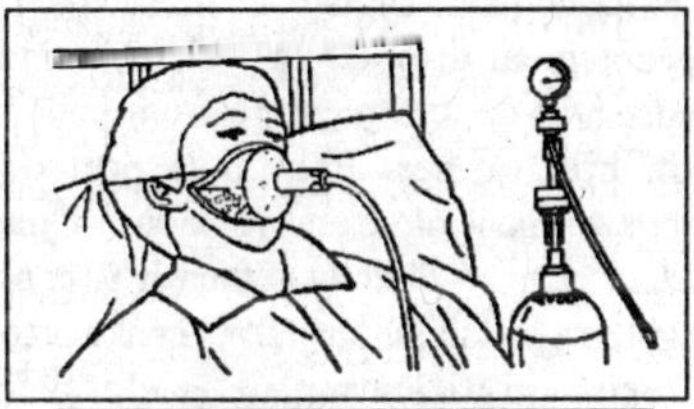

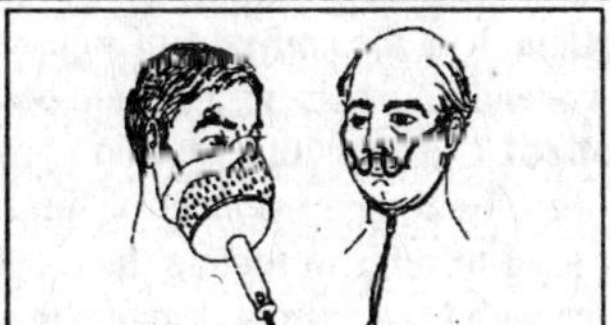

cheaper. It is disposed off after use so no sterilisation is required. When mask is connected to oxygen supply the flow of oxygen inflates a cuff around mask which fits closely. When oxygen supply is cut it deflates. Another is vent mask. It is designed to provide accurate control of oxygen concentration.

Mask ventilation It refers to assisted ventilation with a face mask. Technique is simple, quick and requires little invasive action. It is used in hypoventilation, hypoxemia and respiratory arrest. Face masks are made of rubber or plastic and are available in a variety of sizes.

Masked mastoiditis In case of otitis media after antibiotics pain and discharge is cured. The membrane fails however to return to normal stage and patient's hearing remains impaired. In severe cases following apparent response to antibiotics patient shows signs of general malaise, anorexia, listlessness and complaints of headache. There may be tenderness over mastoids. Persistence of pain or deafness or discharge indicates unextinguished infection. Persistent deafness is the most usual. Occasionally there is low fever. The patient is unwell, manifesting slight tenderness, anorexia, lethargy or headache. There may be tender mastoid.

Masochism It is the term derived after the name of author Sacher-Masoch a nineteenth century Austrian who wrote novels describing joys associated with torture and abuse of sex. It may involve verbal abuse.

There are certain females who achieve orgasm when they are insulted in worst possible matter. Sadomasochism, sadism or masochism. It is a psychological disorder in which the individual persistently derives pleasure from pain inflicted upon him or her. Pain is a prelude to or accompaniment of sexual relations or may itself produce orgasm directly. When it is consciously sought as a part of the sexual act or as a prerequisite to sexual gratification, it is classified as a paraphilia. It is the converse of sadism, although the two tend to coexist in the same person.

Mass effect The effect of a space-occypying lesion with the closed environement of the cranium, is often used to refer to tumors, but in the case of patients with head trauma. If refers to hematomas that result in further brain damage as a result of pressur and shifting of the brain.

Mass number The total number of protons and neutrons in an atom of a chemical element.

Mass reflex Sudden, abnormal and prolonged activation of somatic and visceral reflexes throughout the spinal cord, resulting from an extreme state of motor neuron facilitation.

Mass spectrometer Device used to analyse mixture of substances according to molecular weight.

Mass transfer The movement of a given amount of fluid or the material carried by the fluid. In bioreactors, it refers to the dispersal and solubilization of nutrients and gases in the fermentation medium.

Mass/charge ratio The mass/charge ratio is the mass of a fragment divided by the number of charges it carries. In most instances only one charge is involved, and the mass charge ratio is, therefore, generally equal with the mass of the fragment.

Massage The term used to designate certain manipulations of the soft tissues of the body's these manipulations are most effectively performed with the hands and are administered for the purpose of producing effects on the nervous, muscular and respiratory systems and the local and general circulation of the blood and lymph.

Massage belt Now a days different types of massage belts are available in market to massage particular part of body.

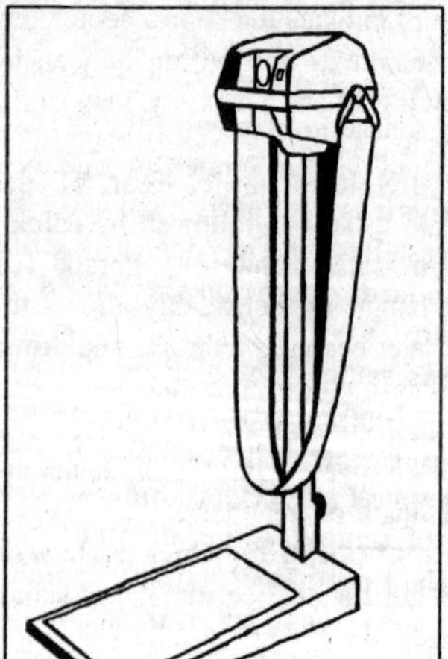

Massage chair A specially designed chair that allows the patient to sit comfortably during the massage.

Massage couch It is of different shapes and sizes. Folding types are also available.

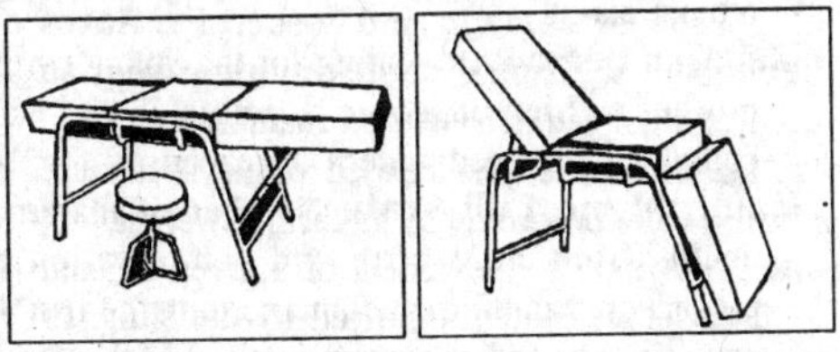

Massage environemnt An area or location where a massage is given.

Massage mat A cushioned surface that is placed on the floor.

Massage routine The step-by-step protocol and sequence used to give a massage.

Massage table A specially designed table that allows massage to be done with the client lying down.

Masseter Masticatory muscle which serves to close the jaws.

Massive blood transfusion Transfusion of 5 units of blood in one hour or transfusion of 10 units of blood in one hour or transfusion of 10 units of blood in 6 hours or replacement of blood volume with transfused blood within 24 hours.

Mast cell A type of connective tissue cell that produces and secretes histamine and heparin and promotes local inflammation. Loose connective tissue cell.

Mastalgia A general term for any recurring or persistent sensation of pain in the breast that is not associated with an immediate trauma.

Mastectomy It is a surgical removal of full or a part of breast. It is generally done in case of cancer. The standard operation is called radical mastectomy.

It involves removal of affected breast, chest muscles, and underarm lymph nodes. When certain chest muscles are left operation is known as modified radical mastectomy. Simple mastectomy consists of removing the affected breast and sometimes a portion of axillary lymph nodes. Surgeon may leave skin intact for further reconstruction and reconstructive surgery. Every operation is done under general anaesthesia. Healing is usually very good after lumpectomy and quadrantectomy.

Master cone Solid substance, usually guttapercha or silver, used to fill the space once occupied by the pulp in endodontic treatment.

Master genes A term for flagellar genes regulating the expression of all the other flagellar genes, sitting at the top of the hierarchy.

Mastery model In social learning theory, an individual who demonstrates complete competence in a given task. The mastery model succeeds to a high degree and therefore may be an inappropriate model for the beginning learner, except for the inculcation of positive attitudes toward the task.

Mastication A series of highly coordinated functions that involve the teeth, tongue, muscles of mastication, lips cheeks, and saliva, in the preparation of food swallowing and digestion.

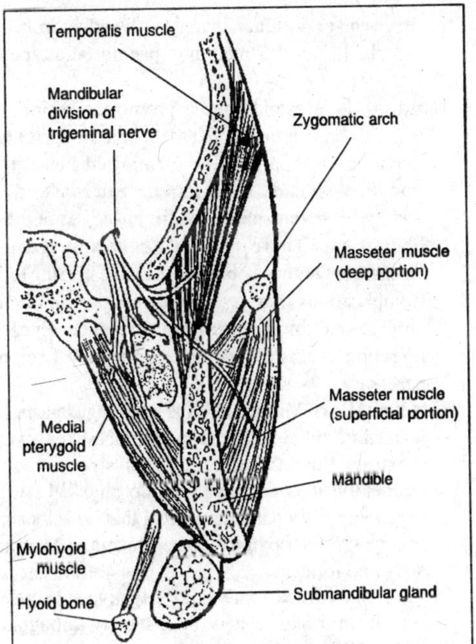

Muscles of mastication

Mastitis It is the inflammation of breast tissue. It generally occurs during breast feeding when bacteria enter the breast through nipple. Changes in levels of sex hormones can cause mastitis. Symptoms include pain, tenderness and swelling.

Breast becomes red and engorged. It may result in breast abscess. Acute mastitis clears in a few weeks with sensitive antibiotic. In chronic mastitis there may be diffuse lump. Symptoms are worst during second half of menstrual cycle. Breast tenderness caused by chronic mastitis generally requires no specific treatment.

Mastoid process Nipple like projection of the temporal bone behind ear.

Mastoid retractor It is used during mastoidectomy operation for retracting the skin, subcutaneous

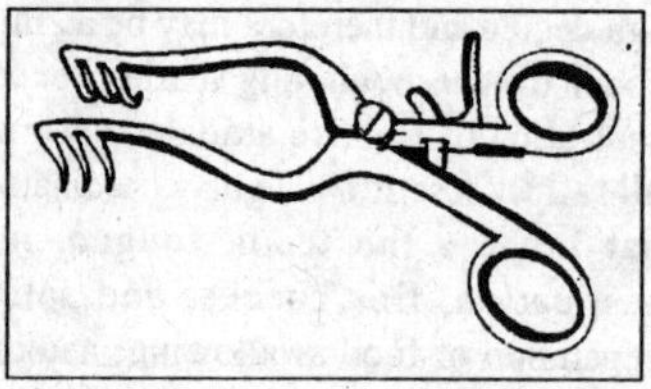

tissue and periosteum. It controls bleeding from cut vessels. It is a self-retaining, haemostatic type of retractor.

Mastoiditis Mastoid bone is prominent behind the ear. This bone is connected to the middle ear. Otitis media is an inflammation of mastoid bone. The infection spreads from middle ear Mastoiditis results in severe pain, swelling and tenderness behind ear. There may be fever and creamy discharge. There may be a progressive hearing loss. Complications may result in meningitis and brain abscess. Antibiotics are drug of choice. Even if infection persists mastoidectomy may become necessary.

Masturbation Masturbation is reaching orgasm by manual stimulation. It is seen as a release for sexual tensions that a teenager feels strongly and frequently. It is practically of no physical harm. Psychologically person may feel that he is loosing energy. On the contrary person learns to love his body and reflexes.

Matching events Acute major negative events that arise from or are related thematically to ongoing role conflicts.

Mate attraction The use of specialized acoustical, visual, or chemical signals (pheromones) to attract mates from a distance, sometimes over several hundred meters or more.

Material alba Soft white deposit on teeth with poor dental hygiene.

Materialism Phiolosophical position that holds that behavior can be explained as a function of the nervous system without explanatory recourse to the mind.

Maternal Relating to, involving, or derived from the female parent.

Maternal behaviour Caring for the young by the mother, which in some animals involves a complex, unlearned pattern of responses.

Maternal mortality rate Number of maternal deaths from child birth and complication of pregnancy, childbirth and puerperium, the first 42 days after the end of pregnancy per 100 thousands live birth.

Maternal surface placenta It is dull red with a rough and shaggy layer, It presents lobulated appearance consisting of number of cotyledons. There may be greyish areas due to deposit of calcium.

Maternity blues It is a state of mild depression, anxiety and slight intellectual clouding on third day after delivery. The weapiness, tension and sense of being slow for several days persist. This may well be an emotional effect of the drop in hormonal levels after parturition.

Maternity nurse practitioner A speciality nurse practitioner who provides prenatal care for uncomplicated pregnancies, postpartum care, contraception counselling, and management of minor problems. Also called Obs-Gyn nurse practitioner.

Mating system The typical pattern of reproductive behavior and parental care in a given species, or the social structure resulting from this.

Matrix The intracellular substance of a tissue; for example, the matrix of bone is calcified, whereas that of blood is liquid.

Matrotrophic Relating to or characterized by matrotrophy.

Matter Anything that occupies space.

Mattress overlays Layers of foam or other devices placed on top to the mattress.

Maturases Proteins sometimes encoded within self-splicing introns, that assist in the splicing reaction.

Maturation In biology, a process of cell division during which the number of chromosomes in the germ cells is reduced to one-half the number characteristic of the species.

Mature cataract When the entire cortex is opaque and swelling of lens subsides it is known as mature cataract. The nucleus shows only progressive sclerosis. It does not show an iris when light is being thrown from side. Visual acuity is reduced to hand movements or even to perception and projection of light. There is white reflex from pupil and there is no iris shadow. There is no red glow.

Mature follicle A relatively large, fluid-filled follicle containing a secondary oocyte and surrounding granulosa cells that secrete estrogens. Also called a Graffian follicle.

Mature milk Milk that is usually present after approximately ten days following birth. Volume and content of the mature milk adapts to the growth needs of the infant.

Maturity Being fully developed physically or emotionally.

Maturity of fetus Length of fetus will be 20 to 25 inches. Weight will be 2.5 to 3.5 kg. There will be thick hair on head. Nails will project beyond the fingertip. Eyebrows and eyelashes are separated. The membrana pupillaris has disappeared. Eyelids are not adherent and testes are within scrotal sac. Surest sign of maturity is presence of centre of ossification at the lower end of femur.

Maurer's dots Aggregate in the cytoplasm of erythrocytes infected with *Plasmodium flaciparum.*

Mauriceau Smellie-Veit A method of assisting with the delivery of the aftercoming head in a breech delivery. Two fingers of the left hand are placed firmly over the mandibles to flex the head. The right hand is placed over the back, with the fingers over the shoulders to guide the shoulders and head. The torso is elevated slowly with flexion of the head maintained by the maxillary pressure. Suprapubic pressure is applied by an assistant during these manoeuvres to aid the descent of the head into the pelvis and eventually with the suprapubic and maxillary pressure, the occiput is delivered.

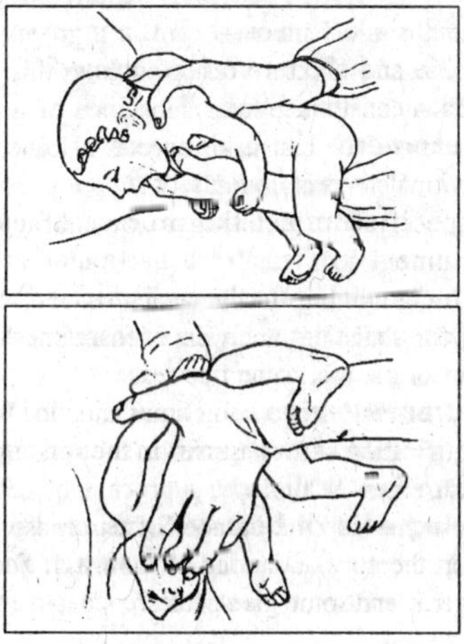

Mauriceau-Smellie-Veit manoeuvre This is also known as jaw flexion and shoulder traction method. It can be applied whether or not the hair at the nape of the neck is visible.

Maxilla Irregulary shaped bone forming half of the upper jaw made up of the two maxillae.

Maxillary Pertaining to the maxilla.

Maxillary tuberosity A rounded prominence of bone that extends posterior to the third molar region; appears radiopaque.

Maxillectomy Excision of the maxilla.

Maxillitis Inflammation of the maxilla.

Maxillodental Pertaining to or affecting the maxillae and the teeth.

Maxillofacial Pertaining to the maxillae and the face.

Maxillofacial prosthetics The art and science of anatomic, functional, and cosmetic reconstruction, utilising nonliving substitutes, of those regions in the maxilla, mandible, and face that are missing or defective.

Maxillopharyngeal Pertaining to the maxilla and the pharynx.

Maximal expiratory flow-volume curve The expiratory portion of the flow-volume curve generated during a forced expiratory maneuver.

Maximal oxygen uptake The maximum amount of oxygen that can be consumed by the body per unit time during heaving exercise.

Maximum The greatest value that can be obtained.

Maximum exposure limit Workplace exposure limit which must not be exceeded.

Maximum flexibility The strain associated with stress at the elastic limit is called maximum flexibility and is a measure of maximum elastic strain that can be produced.

Maximum heart rate Highest limit for heart rate during exercise

Maximum oxygen consumption (Vo_2max) The maximum amount of oxygen taken up by the lungs, transported to the tissues and used to do work.

Maximum permissible dose The maximum radiation an individual can recieve within a specified period without harm.

Maximum voluntary ventilation The volume of air breathed, when an individual breathes as fast and as deeply as possible for a given time (e.g., 12 or 15 seconds).

Mayo, vein Prepyloric vein.

McArdles disease There is a deficiency in myopenosphorylase. Patients develop generalised muscular cramps and stiffness after exercise. Blood lactate and pyruvate fail to increase as they should on exercise as the enzyme deficiency prevents breakdown of muscle glycogen, Vigorous exercise may be accompanied by myoglobinuria.

McDonald's measurement Measurement of the height of the uterine fundus with a tape; the distance from symphysis pubis to fundus.

McGill pain questionnair The MPQ is a commonly used test for the measurement of Pain. the questionnaie, basically, has three classes of ward descriptors to assess the subjective pain. It also, has an intensity score, a body diagram and an assessment of pain releative to activities and pain patterns. The three main measures are the pain rating index (PRI) the number of words chosen (NWC) and the present pain intensity (PPI).

McMurray Sign A test used in the evaluation of meniscal tear.

McMurry osteotomy Proximal femoral osteotomy described for treatment of osteoarthritis of the hip.

McNema chi-square test A modification of the chi-square test for use with paired data. The formula is (b - c - 1)2/(b+c).

MCT Medium-chain triglycerides; distinguished from other triglycerides by having 8 to 10 carbon atoms; are easily digested.

MD Doctor of Medicine.

Mead An ancient drink made of water and honey.

Meals on wheels Community program that delivers food to homebound people.

Mean The average value, calcuted as the sum of all of the observed values divided by the total number of observations.

Mean arterial blood pressure The average of the arterial blood pressure; it is slightly less than the average of the systolic and diastolic blood pressure, because diastole lasts longer than systole.

Mean arterial pressure Average arterial B.P. throughout the cardiac cycle.

Mean deviation The average of the absolute value of the deviations of all observations from the mean.

Mean square Another name for variance, which is defined as a sum of squares divided by the appropriate number of degress of freedom.

Measles It is a viral illness that causes a rash and fever. One attack usually confers lifelong immunity. The measles virus is highly infective. The disease spreads through droplets. Incubation period is 9 to 11 days. The illness starts with fever, sore eyes and cough. After 3 to 4 days a red rash appears on head, neck and chest. Lymph glands may be enlarged. After 3 days rash starts to fade. Complications include orchitis, mastoiditis and pancreatitis.

Measles vaccine Measles is the most common of the eruptive fevers. Generally it is given between

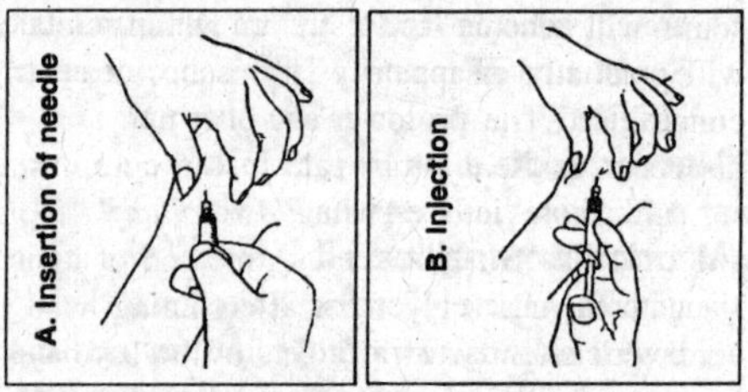

9 months and 12 months. It is a freeze-dried live vaccine and should be kept below 8°C. 0.5 ml subcutaneously is given.

Measurement The assignment of numbers to individuals, objects, events, or situations according to specified rules; the process of using an instrument to measure a particular attribute, assigning numbers to the attributes, and using the data for statistical analysis. Measurement can be a part of the assessment process.

Measurement bias Bias resulting in distorted quantification of exposures or subjectivity of the measurement scale.

Measurements of beauty Some say that beauty lies in the eyes and mind of a viewer. Some like long hair and some gives preference to a charming

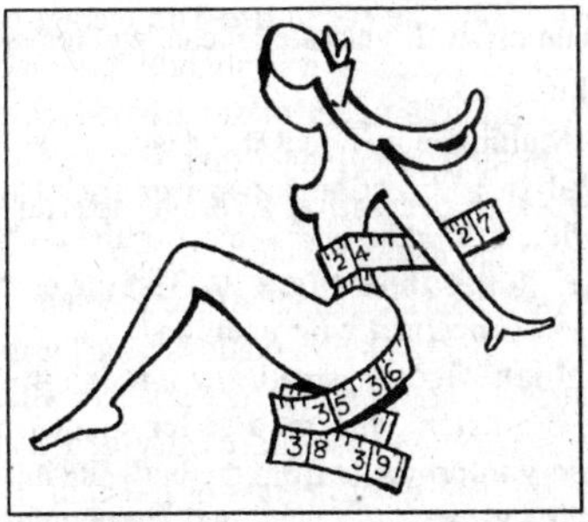

face. As regards measurement, three measurements are excepted : Loin 24 inches, hip and breasts 36 inches each.

Measuring of blood pressure To measure blood pressure apply the cuff around the arm just proximal to elbow. Inflate until pressure registers about 200 mm Hg. Blood flow is occluded and brachial artery may no longer be palpated in the cubital fossa. Place the stethoscope over brachial artery in the cubital fossa. Slowly deflate the cuff and listen for soft first beating sounds, i.e. systolic pressure. As pressure is reduced still further, the sound will become louder and more distinct but will gradually disappear as blood no longer is constricted. The pressure at which the sound disappears is the diastolic pressure.

Meat Any edible flesh, especially that of mammals.

Meat conditioning After an animal has been slaughtered, muscle glycogen breaks down to lactic acid which tends to improve the texture and keeping qualities of meat. Meat which has been left until these changes have occured is 'conditioned'.

Meat curing Pickling with aid of sodium chloride, sodium nitrate and some sodium nitrite which inhibits the growth of clostridium botulinum.

Meat extract The water soluble part of meat that is mainly responsible for flavour. It is rich in B vitamins.

Meat factor Factor used to determine the fat free meat content of sausages and similar meat products from a nitrogen estimation 100xN/3.4 applies to both pork and beef.

Meatus Opening through a body part.

Meatus, urethral External urethral ostium in male.

Mechanical axis The line that is perpendicular to the transverse axis of joint.

Mechanical axis of lower limb A line drawn from centre of femoral head to the centre of ankle joint normally passes through the center of knee joint. If

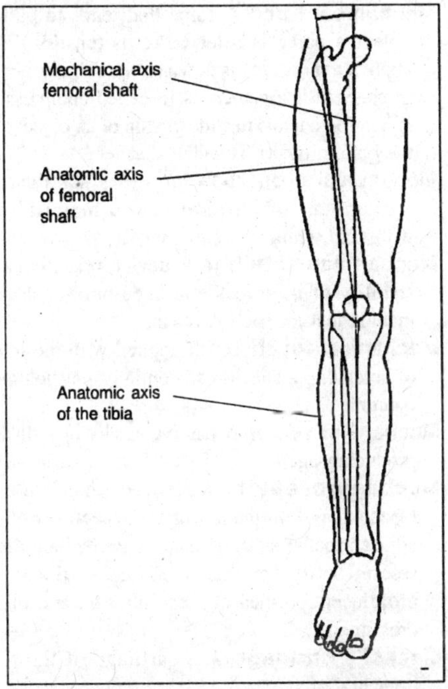

it does not then there is unequal loading of medial and lateral compartment of knee resulting in osteoarthritis.

Mechanical digestion The crushing and twisting effects of teeth and peristalsis that divides foods into smaller pieces.

Mechanical exercisers There are many aids to active exercise varying from a simple skipping rope to complex spring mechanism. There are ergometers that have been designed for resistive exercise where

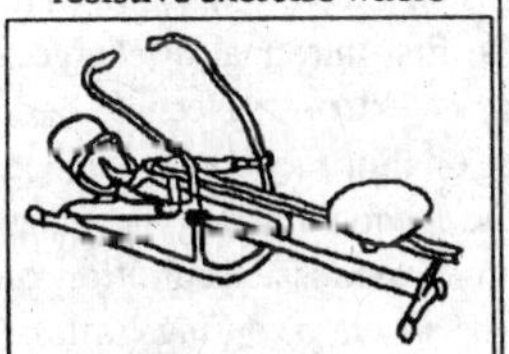

A rowing machine

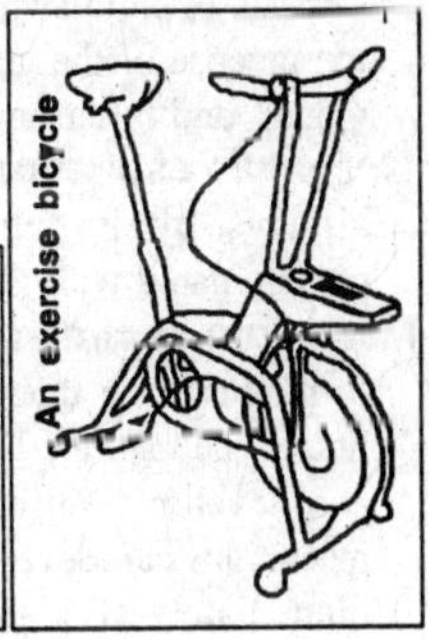

An exercise bicycle

resistance can be measured. Ergometer cycle and ergo rowing exercisers are most useful. Resistance is measured in kilograms or pounds.

Mechanical force A force that tends to pull an object a party is referred to as tensile. When application of force is down on the subject tending to squeeze it together is to called compressive. When force tends to slide the top of an object over the bottom then it is called shear.

Mechanical properties Properties that relate to the amount of stress a dental material can withstand within the oral cavity.

Mechanical stabilizer A device that increases stability of the prosthetic knee unit, such as a manual lock or friction brake.

Mechanical touch Touch applied with the intent of achieving a specific anatomic or physiological outcome.

Mechanical vector A passive carrier of a disase-producing agent.

Mechanoreceptor Receptor that detects mechanical deformation of the receptor itself or adjacent cells; stimuli so detected include those related to touch, pressure, vibration, proprioception, hearing, equilibrium, and blood pressure.

Meckel's cartilage The cartilage of the first branchial arch.

Meckel's diverticulum It is a common congenital anomaly of digestive tract. It is a small, hollow, wide mouthed sac protruding from ileum. There are usually no symptoms unless infection supervenes. There may be painless bleeding which may be sudden and severe. Treatment includes removal of the diverticulum.

Meconium Greenish anal discharge from the fetus; consists of fluid swallowed, epithelial cells from the mucosa of the gut, mucus from the intestinal glands, and bile from the liver.

Meconium aspiration The act of sucking into the airways, by the fetus in utero, amniotic fluid contaminated with the first intestinal discharges.

Meconium aspiration syndrome Neonate born to mother with thick or thin meconium stained liquor can aspirate the meconium into the lungs and develop respiratory distress. Aspiration of meconium can develop *in utero*, during birth or immediately after birth. It can cause chemical pneumonitis. If untreated it can lead to respiratory failure.

MED Multiple epiphyseal dysplasia.

Medial In a direction toward or forward of the midline or middle of an object or the body.

Medial geniculate nucleus The major thalamic region concerned with audition.

Medial lemniscus A pathway through the core of the brainstem, the medial lemniscus carries sensory information from the body, including fine touch and pressure, pain, and temperature.

Medial meniscus Knee Meniscus in medial compartment. It is a crescent shaped, fibrocartilaginous structure, triangular in vertical section. It is wider posterioly than anteriorly and having a complete peripheral capsular attachment.

Medial or internal rotation Turning the anterior surface of the extremity toward the midline of the body.

Medial or septal papillary muscles Muscles that are variable in their origin from the wall of the right ventricle.

Medial pontine reticular formation A brainstem nucleus that is responsible for initiating REM (rapid eye movement) sleep.

Medial shelf A medial patellar plica.

Medial surface The inner side.

Medial tibial stress syndrome The first area of tibial pain is located on its middle and lower one-third. It becomes tender. The second area is middle half of posteromedial border of tibia. There is microtraumatic elevation of the periosteum, due to jerk of attached muscle area may become thickened and palpable.

Medial umbilical ligaments The remains of the intra-abdominal umbilical arteries of the fetus.

Medialis A general anatomical term denoting a structure situated nearer to the median plane or the midline of a body or structure.

Median The middle observation when data have been arranged in order from the lowest to the highest value.

Median episiotomy It commences from the centre of the fourchette, the incision extends posteriorly for about 2.5 cms. During delivery incision may prolong causing third degree tear. In this bleeding is less, repair is easier and there is less discomfort to the patient.

Median nerve It is a branch of brachial plexus. It supplies the muscles of forearm and hand. It carries out bending movements of wrist, fingers and thumb rotating the forearm and palm inward. This carries sensations from 3½ fingers, thumb, index finger, middle finger and a part of ring finger. Nerve may be damaged in Colles' fracture. It results in numbness and muscle weakness.

Median palatal suture The immovable joint between the two palatine processes of the maxilla; appears radiolucent.

Median rhomboid glossitis It appears as smooth, flat, depressed or elevated nodular area just anterior to circumvallate papillae. It may be diamond shaped or irregular in outline. Area is devoid of papillae. It is believed to be a developmental anomaly caused by persistence of the tuberculum impar. When area is slightly depressed it may accumulate debris and become a source of inflammation. Microscopic sections reveal a covering of stratified squamous epithelium that is free of lingual papillae.

Mediastinum, posterior compartment of the inferior division That portion of the mediastinum bounded by the bodies of the fifth through the twelfth thoracic vertebrae posteriorly, the pericardium anteriorly, the diaphragm inferiorly, and the superior division cranially; contains the esophagus and thoracic aorta.

Mediastinal pleura The serous membrane overlying the mediastinum.

Mediastinum The space between the pleural cavities occupying the centre of thoracic cavity is the mediastinum. It contains, heart, great vessels, oesophagus, trachea, vagus nerve, lymph nodes and phrenic nerve.

Mediastinum, inferior division The part of the mediastinum that extends from a line passing from the fourth thoracic vertebra to the lower border of the manubrium downward to the diaphragm; subdivided into anterior, middle and posterior compartments.

Mediastinum, middle compartment of the inferior division That portion of the mediastinum bounded by the pericardium anteriorly and posteriorly, the superior division superiorly, and the diaphragm inferiorly; contains the heart and great vessels.

Mediator A variable that explains how, why or when to expect a relationship between a predictor and a criterion.

Mediator of inflammation Chemical released or activated by injured tissues and adjacent blood vessels; produces vasodilation, increases vascular permeability, and attracts blood cells; includes histamine, kinins, prostaglandins, and leucotrienes.

Mediatstinum, anterior compartment of the inferior division That portion of the mediastinum bounded by the sternum anteriorly, the pericardium posteriorly, the superior division cranially, and the diaphragm inferiorly; contains the ascending aorta.

Medicaid A program funded by general tax revenues of the federal and state governments. The benefits are considered to be social welfare, instead of social insurance.

Medical Related to medicine.

Medical asepsis Practices that confine or reduce the numbers of microorganisms.

Medical commons Shared medical resources. An attempt by one individual or group to maximize its own welfare by using more than its fair share of the medical commons would necessarily diminish the good that others can derive form it.

Medical consultation Consulting another medical man on the request of one to further evaluate and treat a patient.

Medical fomentation It may be simple when boiled water is used for fomentation and medicates when drug is added to boiled water for fomentation. It is applied to unbroken skin. Areas of application should be larger.

For joint stiffness or inflammation for whole of joint and some areas above and below joints are covered. For fomentation of breast nipples should be spared. Purpose of medical fomentation is to promote suppuration, to increase circulation, to relieve pain, to relieve swelling and to relieve congestion.

Medical history The relevant medical disease which might affect patient's present pregnancy such as cardiac ailment, T.B. and pyelonephritis. Rubella virus has a marked teratogenic effect in early gestation.

Medical impairement A alteration of health status.

Medical indemnity insurance It is a broad based cover for professional liabilities. It looks after and protect the professional interest of insured doctor. To arrange, conduct and pay for the defence of such doctors. It identifies the insured doctor in respect of any loss or expense directly arising from actions, claims, proceedings and demands against him on grounds of professional negligence, misconduct, etc.

Medical information system A hospital wide, automated data-gathering system.

Medical model The view that mental illness, like physical illness, has its origin in conditions of the body. One implication is that the alleviation of mental illness should be accomplished by medical practitioners.

Medical necessity Patient's conditions to be treated are recognized ones, and the examinations, tests, and treatments are based on scientific studies and principles that are generally accepted by the profession at large as being necessary and appropriate for proper diagnosis and treatment of patients with the particular conditions presented.

Medical nutritional therapy The use of specific nutrition services to treat an illness, injury, or condition.

Medical record department It is the section which provides systems and services for filling, maintenance and retrieval of primary or secondary record of patients. Index health and drugs card are prepared.

Medical records Written collection of information about a person's health problems, the care provided by health practitioners, and the progress of the patient.

Medical services Medical care performed by physician, nurses and other personals.

Medical waste A general term for material generated as a result of patient care, diagnosis, treatment, or immunization. It may or may not be hazardous.

Medically indigent persons People whose incomes are too high to be eligible for Medicaid, who do not receive medical insurance in their hobs, and who are not able to pay for individual medical care insurance policies.

Medicare A program that is asministered by the federal government. It pays for the health benefits of most individuals who are 65 years of age or older and of individuals who reveive social security benefits due to disability.

Medication Use of medicine or medicamants for treatment of a disease.

Medication administration record Agency form used to document drug administration.

Medication order Name and directions for giving a drug.

Medicinal paraffin A mineral oil of no nutritive value as it is not affected by digestive enzyme and passes through unchanged enzyme.

Medicolegal It relates with medical matters that come before the courts. Medical evidence is required about injuries, death and its cause, mental competence of person and a person's right to confidentiality concerning his illness, etc. It deals with tests in determining paternity and the mental status of giving dying declaration.

Medicolegal autopsy It is the postmortem examination of dead body for the purpose of identifying marks of scar. Shape of scar indicates nature of weapon causing injury. Age of wound if corresponds to the date of attack may have values as circumstantial evidence.

Medio lateral episiotomy The incision starts at the fourchette and is directed posterio-laterally either to the patients left or right about an inch away from the anus. The length of incision should not be more than 3 cm.

Meditation It is a disciplined concentration of thought. It includes breathing exercises. It is on the principle of holistic medicine. It makes body supple.

Mediterranean lymphoma This is a generalised lymphoma of small intestine first described in Medi-terranean region. The subepithelial region is diffusely and densely infiltrated with normal plasma cells with excessive lymphocytes. Villi are flattened out and the crypts widely separated. Epithelium is somewhat stretched. There is severe malabsorption. Overt steatorrhoea is commoner than watery diarrhoea. Vomiting and tetany are common. Clubbing is frequent. In a few cases oedema, fever, a palpable abdominal mass and ascites occur. Laparotomy is essential.

Medium A substance which provides nutrients for the growth and multiplication of micro organisms.

Medium chain triglycerides These are used in treating various aspects of malabsorption syndrome.

Medulla Latin for "marrow"; hence the inner portion of an organ in contrast to the outer portion or cortex.

Medulla oblongata Inferior portion of the brainstem that connects the spinal cord with the brain; contains nuclei of cranial nerves plus autonomic control centres for heart rate, respiration, etc.

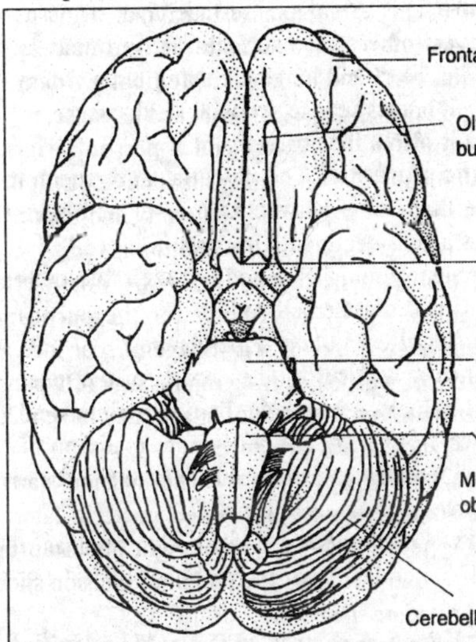

Medullary The hollow core of the diaphysis of a long bone in which marrow is found.

Medullary cavity Hollow area inside the diaphysis of the bone that contains yellow bone marrow.

Medullary Index The ratio of the diameter of the medulla of a hair to the whole diameter of the hair. The medullary index in human hair is almost always less than 1/3; in animal hair it is usually greater than 1/3.

Medullary rhythmicity area Portion of the respiratory center in the medulla oblongata that controls the basic rhythm of respiration.

Medulloblastoma It accounts 20 % of childhood tumour arising in vermis of cerebellum. These are believed to be of fetal external granular cell origin. Leptomeningeal seeding over convexities and down the spinal canal is common. Cytogenetic analysis often shows changes in chromosomes 1 and 17. Methotrexate is effective and an initial ventriculo-peritoneal shunt is often necessary.

Mefloquine It is similar in several respects to quinine although it does not intercalate with plasmodial DNA. It is used for malaria chemoprophylaxis, to treat uncomplicated *Plasmodium falciparum* and chloroquine resistant *plasmodium vivax* malaria. When used for prophylaxis dose is 250 mg and after 3 weeks 125 mg/week to reduce toxicity. It should not be given to a patient who is having liver and kidney impairment.

Megacolon It causes gross distension of colon. The most common cause of megacolon is behavioural due to chronic dyschezia, repeated failure to answer calls to stool, long standing inadequate bowel training and sometimes associated with chronic laxative abuse. Faecal incontinence and spurious diarrhoea due to impaction of inspissated stool may occur. Treatment is difficult.

Megadoses Amounts exceeding those considered adequate for health.

Megakaryocyte Large cell in red bone marrow that gives rise to platelets.

Megalocornea Cornea over 30 mm may be a congenital anomaly and is sometimes associated with embryontoxon. In contrast to buphthalmos the eye with a megalocornea has nomal intracorneal pressure, a flat cornea, normal limbus, astigmatism.

Megavoltage In ionizing radiation therapy, voltage greater than 2 megavolts.

Mehlis' gland A group of unicellular glands that empty into the ootype region of flatworms.

Mehta angle A radiographic measurement of rib vertebral angle. It gives a clue to develop scoliosis.

Meibomian glands Tarsal glands.

Meiosis The process by which the chromosome number is halved during the formation of gametes (sex cells). Consists of two cell divisions that result in four cells, each of which contains half the number of chromosomes as the parent cell; occurs in the testes and ovaries.

Meissner's corpuscles These are tactile end organs which are encapsulated. These are ovoid and measure about 100 mm in length. Each has a thin connective tissue capsule. These are exteroreceptors and subserve two-point discriminative touch. These are most numerous in dermal papillary ridges of the palmar surfaces of fingers, toes, hands and feet and are fewer in lips, eyelids and tip of tongue.

Melancholia A historical term that designates the presence of decreased appetite, weight loss, complete lack of pleasure, insomnia and depression more on early morning.

Melanin An endogenous, nonhemoglobin-derived, brown-black pigment synthesized from tyrosine in melanocytes. Tyrosinase catalyzes the oxidation of tyrosine to dihydroxyphenylalanine (dopa), and dopa is polymerized and then coupled with protein to produce melanin. The pigment is normally found in the basal malpighian layer of the epidermis and mucous membrane of the gingivae and remainder of the oral cavity. Melanin is also found in pigmented nevi (moles) and their malignant counterpart, melanocarcinoma.

Melano stimulating hormone Median lobe of pituitary gland produce one hormone, melanocyte-stimulatry hormone.

Melanocyte Cells found mainly in the stratum basale of skin that produce the brown or black pigment melanin.

Melanocyte-stimulating hormone (MSH) Peptide hormone secreted by the anterior pituitary; increases melanin production by melanocytes, making the skin darker in colour.

Melanoid Resembling melanin; of dark color.

Melanoma A tumor made up of melanin-pigmented cells. The term is commonly used to refer to malignant melanoma.

Melanosome Any of the granules with the melanocytes that contain the pigment melanin.

Melanphore A cell that transports melanin granules from melanocytes to peripheral cells, such as epidermal cells and phagocytes.

Melatonic A hormone, secreted by the pineal gland, that helps set the timing of the body's biological clock.

Melatonin A hormone secreted by the pineal gland that produce lightening of the skin in lower vertebrates and that may contribute to the regulation of gonadal function in mammals. Secretion follows a ciradian rhythm and peaks at night.

Melena Blood, which changes into a dark, tarry substance as it moves through the stomach or small intestine.

Melkersson-Rosenthal syndrome Main symptoms include triad of recurrent facial nerve paralysis, ipsilateral facial swelling. Often there is severe facial pain. Family history is common. The syndrome gives rise to recurrent facial paralysis, soft non-pitting oedema of the lips, oedema of upper face, buccal cavity and other parts of body.

Membrane It is a smooth surface layer of tissue that covers other tissue surfaces. It surrounds an organ, i.e. heart and lungs including brain. Many such membranes secrete synovial fluid and serum. Hymen is also a membrane.

Membrane potential The potential difference or voltage that exists between the inner and outer sides of a cell membrane. It exists in all cells but is capable of being changed by excitable cells (neurons and muscle cells).

Membranoid Resembling a membrane.

Membranous labyrinth The portion of the inner ear that is located inside the body labyrinths and separated from it by the perilymph; made up of the membranous semicircular canals, the saccule and utricle, and the cochlear duct.

Membrum Or Member, of the body; used as a general anatomical term to designate one of the limbs.

Memory It is to remember what has happened in the past. It has three stages—registration, long-term memory and recall. Stimulating the brain with electrodes can evoke different memories from the same site. Still disturbances of the temporal lobe and limbic lobe typically cause memory disorder. Mechanisms of storing memory are also unknown. It may be held within the chemical structure of some substance within brain cells possibly spare DNA which is not utilised to hold the genetic code. A good memory is usually a part of high IQ although some may have vertically photographic memory. Disturbances of memory can result from a problem at any of 3 stages. Most disturbances involve an inability to recall past events. Loss of memory is known as amnesia.

Memory cell Lymphocyte derived from a B-cell or T-cell that has been exposed to an antigen; when exposed to the same antigen a second time, the memory cell rapidly responds to provide immunity.

Memory response Immune response that occurs when the immune system is exposed to an antigen against which it has already had a primary response; results in the production of large amounts of antibodies and memory cells; also called a secondary response.

Memory span The maximum number of words, syllables, or digits recalled after a single presentation, whether presented in an auditory or visual manner.

Memory trace The neural modification inferred to underlie memory.

Membrane potential The voltage across a cell membrane.

Menadione It is a synthetic compound having greater vitamin K activity than the naturally occurring vitamin.

Menarche It is the first mensturation which marks the onset of puberty in the female. It usually occurs between the age of 11 and 16 years.

Meniere's disease It is characterised by recurrent episodes of vertigo which may be prostrating usually preceded by or associated with tinnitus or a sense of fullness in ear. The disorder is due to increased endolymphatic pressure. After each episode hearing loss is increased and eventually may be lost totally. Treatment is unsatisfactory. In severe cases labyrinth is destroyed. It is a disorder of inner ear resulting in recurrent vertigo, deafness and tinnitus. Mostly only one ear is affected. It is caused by increase in amount of fluid in the membranous labyrinth. Disease is uncommon in young age. Symptoms include sudden attack of vertigo of great severity which results in fall of a person on ground. There develops deafness, tinnitus and a feeling of pressure or pain. Audiometry helps in diagnosis. During attack person should rest in bed. Hearing tends to deteriorate progressively.

Meningeal carcinomatosis Diffuse infiltration of meninges occurs in patient with cancer including Hodgkin's lymphoma, leukaemia, melanoma and adenocarcinoma of lung, breast and GIT. Clinical features include seizures, headache and cranial nerve paralysis. CT shows diffuse enchancement of meninges at the base of brain and over hemispheres. CSF shows malignant cells and increased protein and reduced sugar.

Meninges There are three membranes that cover and protect the brain and spinal cord. Outermost layer is dura mater which is tough and fibrous. The middle layer is elastic and weblike and is known as arachnoid mater. Innermost layer is pia mater which is separated by subarachnoid space layer. Inflammation of meninges is known as meningitis.

Meningioencephalitis An inflammation of the brain and its membranes.

Meningioma It is a benign tumour developing from meninges. The tumour arises from arachnoid layer and usually becomes attached to dura mater. Symptoms include headache, vomiting and impaired mental function due to raised pressure. CT scanning and MRI are good tool to diagnose it.

Meningioma of optic nerve It is a primary mesodermal tumour of optic nerve sheath. These form cells of arachnoid around the optic nerve. It presents with early visual loss and proptosis follows later. There is painful ocular movement in upward direction. Fundus examination may show a swollen or atrophic disc. Surgical remedy is useful.

Meningitis It is the inflammation of meninges. Viral meningitis is relatively mild than bacterial. Symptoms include vomiting, headache and impaired mental function. In meningococcal meningitis the main symptom develops very quickly within hours. It is followed by drowsiness and loss of consciousness. While in tuberculous meningitis person may become sick for several weeks. It is diagnosed by CSF examination. Viral meningitis requires no treatment and is not serious.

Meningocele It is the protrusion of meninges of the spinal cord under the skin due to congenital defect in spine. Meningocele is less serious than myelocele which is the protrusion of spinal cord and meninges both.

Meningovascular syphilis It usually occurs within 5 to 10 years of primary infection. There becomes infiltration and thickened meninges with lymphocytes and plasma cells when it reaches a resonable size it is known as gumma. These contain fibroblasts, histiocytes and giant cells. Central lesion will be necrotic. There will be intimal proliferation in small arteries.

Combination of meningeal and vasculitic lesions leads to cranial nerve palsies. Meningovascular syphilis may also affect spinal cord. CSF findings are normal.

Menis corrhesis Repair of meniscus.

Meniscal radial tear A linear disruption of the meniscus that runs perpendicular to its margins.

Meniscectomy The surgical removal of meniscal cartilage.

Menisci Wedge-shaped fibrocartilages in certain synovial joints.

Menke's kinky hair syndrome It is characterised by sparse and brittle hair, bony changes, and retarded growth.

Menogingivitis Gingivitis occurring in conjunction with the menstrual cycle.

Menometerrhagia Uterine bleeding irregular infrequency and amount.

Menopausal symptoms It is the cessation of menstruation due to reduced production of oestrogen hormone by ovaries. In India, it occurs between the ages of 40 and 50 years. The follicles in ovaries stop producing ova. Hot flashes and night sweats occur in about 70 per cent of menopausal women.

These symptoms occur with varying frequency and severity. Vagina becomes dry. Vagina itself shrinks and loses elasticity and becomes prone to minor infections.

Sexual act becomes more painful. Body and scalp hair become dry and brittle and fall out more easily. Other symptoms are poor memory, poor concentration, anxiety and loss of interest in sex. Hormonal replacement therapy (HRT) is recommended in some cases.

Menopause During this period genitals undergo atrophy and regression. Ovaries become shrunken and their surfaces grooved and furrowed. Fallopian tubes atrophy and cilia disappear. Uterus becomes smaller. Vagina becomes smaller and conical. Vaginal epithelium becomes pale, thin and dry. Vulva atrophies and vaginal orifice becomes smaller.

Skin of labia minora and vestibule becomes pale and dry, pubic hair become scanty. There may be gradual diminution in amount of loss of blood with each regular period until they disappear or there may be gradual increase in spacing of periods. There will be hot flashes and sweating. Flashes are waves of vasodilatation for about 2 to 3 minutes and then severe sweating develops. Palpitation and mental depression are common features. Increased hirsutism is adrenal in origin. Slight degree of hypothyroidism is also noticed with lowered BMR, raised cholesterol, brittleness of hair, dryness of skin, lassitude and reduction of mental concentration.

Menorrhagia It is an excessive loss of blood during menstruation. Sixty ml blood is lost in one cycle. When loss is more than 300 ml it is known as menorrhagia.

It is caused by imbalance of progesterone and oestrogen. Fibroids may result it. D and C is performed to investigate cause of bleed.

Menses Loss of blood and tissue as the endometrium of the uterus sloughs away at the end of the menstrual cycle; occurring at about 28 day intervals in the nonpregnant female of reproductive age.

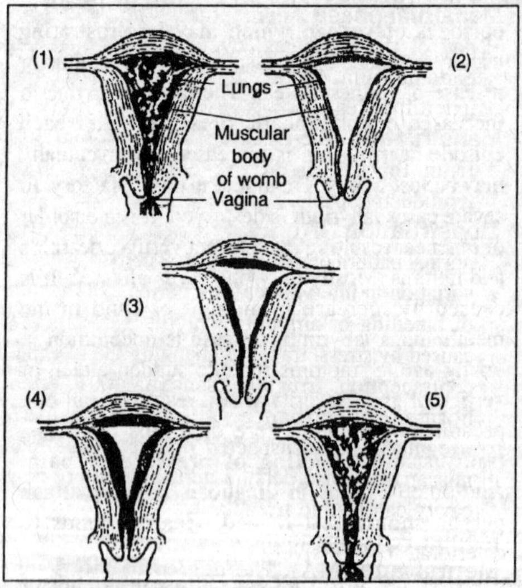

(1) *Menstruation* : showing disintegraton and shedding of the lining of the womb
(2) *After menstruation* : showing very thin and smooth lining to the womb
(3) *About the middle of the cycle* : showing the lining becoming thicker in its stage of growth
(4) *Just before menstruation* : Showing thick lining of the inside of the womb
(5) *Menstruation* : Same as stage (1)

Mensrea Having a guilty mind, the intent to harm that is required for most crimes.

Menstrual cycle Normal cycle varies from 3-5 days every 21-35 days. It may be grossly irregular. Normal pattern suggests a normal hypothalamic-pituitary ovarian function.

Menstrual extraction The aspiration of endometrium performed in a very early pregnancy without cervical dilatation usually a small canula and syringe or other low pressure suction.

Menstrual flow It is the loss of blood, mucus, and the discarded cells of endometrium. During fertile years normal women menstruate between 300 and 500 times. Each menstrual period lasts 3 to 7 days and the amount of vaginal discharge measures 6 to 8 ounces. The actual amount of blood loss per day is 15 ml or half an ounce.

Menstrual history Some women are careful of recording their menstrual period and some are not. The date of her last menstrual period, regularity of her period, the amount of loss in the last period and history of taking oral contraceptive may provide significant information.

Menstrual phase Approximately the 1st to the 5th day of the menstrual cycle, during which the endometrium, blood, glandular secretions and unfertilized eggs are expelled.

Menstruation The discharge of blood and tissue from the uterus at the end of the female reproductive cycle.

Menstruation, irregular It is a variation from normal pattern of menstruation. There may be wide variation in interval between periods, the duration of bleeding or amount of blood lost. It may be caused by stress, travel or changing the method of contraception. Irregular menstruation is often a hormone disturbance. A common cause of irregularity is unsuspected pregnancy and early miscarriage. Disorders of uterus, ovaries or pelvic cavity can lead to irregularity.

Mental Pertaining to the mind.

Mental age (MA) The degree of intelligence exhibited by an individual in relation to the age norms established for the particular test. A boy is said to have a mental age of 8, for example, if his performance on a standardised intelligence test equals that of the average child of 8 years, according to the norms. His chronological age (CA) might be greater or less than his mental age.

Mental control Control over ones own thoughts and feelings.

Mental defense Same as ego defense mechanisms, or defense mechanisms.

Mental disorder From a purely medical standpoint this term denotes a wide range of psychological and behavioral disorders. From a legal perspective, mental disorder is as defined in law; division, mental illness such as schizophrenia, mental impairment typically assessed in terms of intellectual capacity, psychopathy, and 'other disorders.

Mental foramen An opening or hole in bone located on the external surface of the mandible in the region of the mandibular premolars; appears radiolucent.

Mental fossa A scooped-out depressed area of bone located on the external surface of the anterior mandible; appears radiolucent.

Mental function Intellectual or cognitive abilities of an individual, including initiative, attention, concentration, memory, problem solving, and judgment.

Mental health A mental state marked by the absence of personal discomfort and socially disruptive behaviour. The emphasis is not upon an enduring set of traits but rather upon the capacity for adapting to environmental conditions, working productively with other or alone, and attempting to improve society as well as one's own personal condition.

Mental protuberance A more or less distinct the triangular prominence on the anterior inferior surface of the body of the mandible, on or near the median line.

Mental retardation It is the impaired intellectual function which results in an inability to cope with normal duties of life. Such persons have IQ below 70 up to the age of 18. The more severe grades of retardation should have specific cause like Down's syndrome. The mild retarded persons generally do not show any psychological symptoms except that he or she is overall 'slow', studies are impaired and emotions are expressed in child-like manner. But he or she is hyperactive and does repetitive movements. There is no specific means of eliminating the intellectual deficit but special training and behaviour enhances the skill. Family support is crucial.

Mental ridge A linear prominence of cortical bone located on the external surface of the anterior portion of the mandible; appears rdiopaque.

Mental status assessment Technique for determining the level of a patient's cognitive functioning.

Mental status evaluation Standard bedside clinical tests used to examine mental functions.

Mentalism Of the mind; an explanation of behavior as a function of the mind.

Mento vertical diameter It is 13.75 cms from the point of chin to the highest point on vertex.

Mentolabial Pertaining the the chin and lip.

Mentor An individual who counsels or teaches a younger or less experienced person.

Mentum The chin.

Meralgia paresthetica A painful paresthesia in the lateral femoral cutaneous nerve of thigh. It is manifested by burning, tingling and numbness in the distribution.

Mercury poisoning All forms of mercury are harmful except the amalgam in dental filling. Liquid metal is absorbed very slowly while mercury vapour is readily absorbed into body via lungs. Inhalation of mercury vapour results in shortness of breath. Mercury compounds may cause severe inflammation in skin. Swallowed mercury may result in diarrhoea, vomiting and abdominal pain. Once entered in body, mercury accumulates in brain and kidneys. Mercury deposited in brain may result in tiredness, incoordination, excitability, tremors, and severe vision impairment. Deposits of mercury in kidneys may lead to kidney failure. Treatment includes chelating agent like penicillamine to detoxifying mercury.

Mere exposure A Psychological phenomenon in which liking tends to increase as a person sees more of something or someone.

Meric technique A chiropractic system in which a clinical problem is considered in terms of which zone, or body segment innervated by a pair of spinal nerves, it occurs. All tissue of one type within a zone is considered a mere.

Merkel Type of cell in the epidermis of hairless skin that makes contact with a tactile (Merkel) disk, which functions in touch.

Merocrine Gland that secretes products with no loss of cellular material; an example is water-producing sweat glands.

Meromelia Congenital absence of any lower part.

Meromixis A condition in which stratification of the water mass in a lake is maintained during the whole year, often due to a solute concentration gradient.

Merozoite One or many cells resulting from schizogony.

Mescaline In Mexican deserts a cactus which rarely grows more than 3 inches, provides the most popular drug mescaline. Virgins will chew the bottoms and then soak them in water to prepare a powerful ceremonial drink which would be used in sexual initiation. Mescaline also has powerful hallucinogenic qualities and is an addictive drug.

Meschan angle A diagnostic method for measuring the degree of spondylotisthesis at L_5S_1.

Mesencephalic aqueduct The channel that connects the third and fourth ventricles of the brain; also called the aqueduct of Sylvius.

Mesencephalon The midbrain, which contains the corpora quadrigemina and the cerebral peduncles.

Mesenchyme An embryonic connective tissue that can migrate, and from which all connective tissues arise.

Mesentery Double layer of peritoneum extending from the abdominal wall to the abdominopelvic organs; conveys blood vessels and nerves to abdominopelvic organs; hold and supports abdominopelvic organs.

Mesentric artery occlusion Acute mesentric artery occlusion can be thrombotic or embolic. In thrombolic there may be gradual weight loss, abdominal pain and leukocytosis. Embolic occlusion results in sudden severe adbdominal pain with vomiting and diarrhoea.

Mesial Situated in the middle; median, toward the middle line of the body or toward the center line of the dental arch.

Mesicocclusion In which the mandibular first molar is anterior or mesical to the position of class I malocclusion.

Mesiobucco-occlusal Pertaining to or formed by the mesial, buccal, and occlusal surfaces of a tooth.

Mesiocervical Pertaining to the mesial surface of the neck of a tooth.

Mesiodens The most common supernumerary tooth, appearing singly or in pairs as a small tooth with a cone-shaped crown and a short root, between the maxillary central incisors; they may be erupted, impacted, or even inverted.

Mesiodistal Pertaining to the mesial and distal surface of a tooth.

Mesiogingival Pertaining to or formed by the mesial and gingival walls of a tooth cavity, called also mesiocervical.

Mesiognathic Malposition of one or both jaws ahead of the frontal plane or forehead.

Mesiolabial Pertaining to or formed by the mesial and labial surfaces of a tooth, or the mesial and labial walls of a cavity preparation of a tooth.

Mesiolingual Pertaining to or formed by the lingual an demsial surfaces of a tooth, or the lingual and mesial walls of a tooth cavity preparation.

Mesiolinguo-occlusal Pertaining to or formed by the mesial, lingual, and occlusal surfaces of a tooth, or the mesial and occlusal walls of a tooth cavity.

Mesionincisodistal Pertaining to the mesial, incisal, and distal surfaces of an anterior tooth.

Mesiopulpolabial Pertaining to or formed by the mesial, pulpal, and labial walls of a cavity preparation of a tooth.

Mesioversion Deviation of a tooth from the structures being joined together by internal hydrostatic pressure. In bacteria, invaginations of the membrane form internal organelles known as mesosomes.

Mesmerism It is a form of hypnosis. Anton Mesmer, an Austrian physician who called it 'animal magnetism' a natural power which can be developed by most setting themselves at that level.

Meso Prefix meaning middle.

Meso selectivity The ability of a catalyst or reagent to distinguish between two chemically identical but stereo-chemically different parts of a single molecule that contains chiral centers and a symmetry plane.

Mesoderm Middle germ layer of the embryo that produces connective tissue, blood, bone, cartilage, and muscle.

Mesolimbic fibers Dopaminergic fibers projecting to the limbic system formm the ventral tegmental nuclei.

Mesomelic Pertaining to or affecting the midportion of the limb.

Mesonephric duct Another name for the wolffian duct, an embryological duct draining the mesonephros.

Mesophile Literally, middle lover; an organism that grows optimally at temperatures considered to be in a moderate range; i.e., between 20 and 50°C.

Mesophilic Growing optimally at temperatures between 20 and 50°C.

Mesorrhine Having a nasal index between 48 and 53.

Mesosalpinx The external layer of mesothelium and loose connective tissue covering the oviduct.

Mesovarium Mesentery of the ovary; mesentery which attaches the ovary to the posterior surface of the broad ligament.

Messenger RNA A type of RNA that contains a base sequence complementary to a part of the DNA that specifies the synthesis of particular protein.

MET (metabolic equivalent) The rate of energy expenditure requiring an oxygen consumption of 3.5 ml of oxygen per kilogram of body weight per minute (3.5 ml/kg/min). This unit corresponds to the basal metabolic rate while sitting.

Meta analysis A statistical technique which summariges the results of several studies into a single estimate giving more weight to results from larger studies. Literally, an analysis which goes beyond the initial analysis; an analysis which attempts to incorporate other analyses within it. In psychological research, a meta-analysis may attempt to integrate results from many independent investigations, thus providing an overall analysis of the disparate findings. The aim is to provide a common basis for comparisons and an overall conclusion.

Metabolic Relating to, involved in, or affected by a process of metabolism.

Metabolic acidosis Acidosis refers to excess of acid or base deficit. It may result from diabetic ketosis, renal failure, infantile diarrhoea, after severe exercise, during cardiopulmonary byepass, shock and following cardiac arrest. Clinical signs include gasping, respiration and cold blue hands and feet. There may be clouding of consciousness and hyperkalaemic effect on ECG. There will be depression of all functions including vasomotor and respiratory. Cardiac and respiratory functions will be depressed along with hypoxia and dysrhythmias. Blood clotting is retarded. The body compensates by increased pulmonary respiration to remove CO_2 and by increased renal excretion of hydrogen ions. Treatment includes infusion of sodium bicarbonate IV. It may be given as 2.7% solution.

Metabolic alkalosis It may result due to ingestion of large amount of bicarbonate or citrate and in pyloric stenosis with loss of acid. Body compensates by under ventilation and increased renal biocarbonate excretion. Hypokalaemia occurs with excessive renal potassium and chloride loss. Potassium and chloride deficits are replaced with potassium chloride up to 150 mmol/day. More commonly ammonium chloride is given which is safe and effective and is given over 1 hour period. Dose (in mmol)=

$$\frac{\text{base excess x body weight (kg)}}{3}$$

Metabolic disease Any dysfunction caused by a defect in the hormonal or chemical reactions of body cells.

Metabolic disorder of bone It may be osteoporosis or osteomalacia and rickets. There may be hyperparathyroidism or renal osteodystrophy.

Metabolic energy equivalent Measure of energy and oxygen consumption during exercise.

Metabolic equivalent (MET) A rating of energy expenditure for a given activity based on oxygen consumption. One MET equals 3.5 ml of oxygen used per kilogram of body weight per minute.

Metabolic flux The rate at which material is converted via metabolic reactions and pathways.

Metabolic Genotype The complete set of metabolic genes identified in a genome. The utlization of the metabolic genotype under a given condition characterizes the metabolic phenotype.

Metabolic heat production The rate of transformation of chemical energy into heat in an organism.

Metabolic rate The total amount of energy produced and used by the body per unit of time.

Metabolic tolerance Reduced sensitivity to a substance that results from the increased ability of cells to metabolize the substance

Metabolic water Produced in the body by oxidation of food. 100 gm fat produces 107 gm of water while 100 gm of protein produces 41.3 gm of water.

Metabolism The sum total of the chemical changes occurring in the body, chemical process of transforming foods into complex tissue elements and of transforming complex body substances into simple ones, along with the production of heat and energy.

Metacarpal block A technique for digital anesthesia.

Metacarpal bones These are five long cylindrical bones within body of hand. On the palm these are covered by thick layer of fascia while on the back

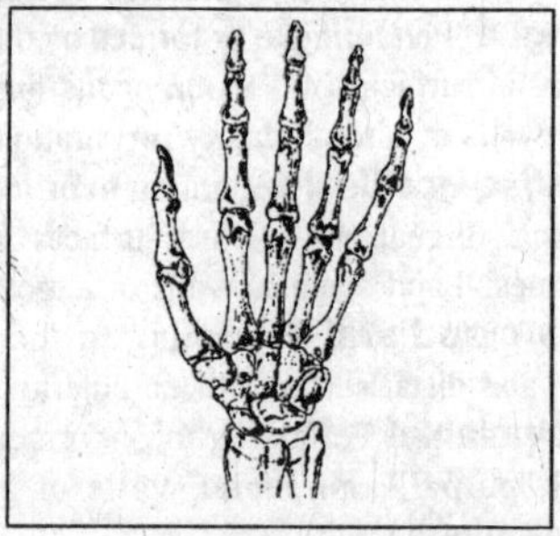

can be felt through skin. The heads of the metacarpal bones form the knuckles, standing out prominently when hand is clenched.

Metacarpal sign An accessory sign of gonadal dysgenesis.

Metacarpophalangeal Of relating to metacarpophalangeal joint.

Metacarpus The region of the hand between the wrist and the phalanges, including the five metacarpal bones that support the palm of the hand.

Metacyclic Describing a form of parasite infective to its vertebrate host, e.g., metacyclic trypomastigote.

Metacyclogenesis The developmental and biochemical transformation, occuring within the sand fly midgut, of the noninfectious procyclic promastigote into the highly infectious metacyclic promastigote.

Metal Metal has certain set of characteristic including high thermal and electrical conductivity, ductility, opacity and lusture. These can be casted into many different shapes. They can be used as crowns to replace the outer coronal structures of tooth. Inlay, onlay and bridges can be made out of it.

Metal base Metallic portion of a denture base forming a part or all of the basal surface of the denture. It serves as a base for the attachment of the acrylic resin part of the denture base and the teeth.

Metal fume Gaseus metal oxide that comes primarily from activities in occupational settings, such as welding without adequate ventilation.

Metal fume fever An acute syndrome that is usually characterized by flu-like symptoms occurring a few hours after exposure to metal fumes.

Metal resistance The ability of a microorganism to survive toxic effects of heavy metal exposure by means of a detoxification mechanism usually produced in response to the metal species concerned.

Metal tolerance The ability of a microorganism to survive toxic effects of heavy metal exposure because of intrinsic properties and/or environmental modification of toxicity.

Metallic Pertaining to, consisting of , or of the nature of metal, as in luster, resonance, hardness, or appearance; made of metal.

Metallic bond The primary chemical bonds holding a metallic material together, characterized by rigid positive cores with loosely held electrons than can carry energy in the form of electricity and heat.

Metallophilic Having an affinity for metal-containing stains.

Metallurgy The science, art, or technology dealing with the process involved in the separation of metals from their ores, the technique of making or compounding the alloys, the techniques of working or heat-treating of metals, and the mining of metals; the science dealing with the study of the physical properties and internal structure of metals and alloys.

Metamerism Division of the body into segments; as in insects.

Metamorphic Relating to or involved in a process of metamorphosis.

Metaphase Second state of mitosis, during which the nuclear envelope and nucleolus disappear.

Metaphyseal Relating to metaphysis.

Metaphyseal flaring An abnormal enlargement of metaphyseal ends of long bones seen in rickets.

Metaphysis Growing portion of a bone.

Metaplasia It is a reversible change in which one adult type cell is replaced by another. Common example is change from columnar to squamous epithelium. Metaplastic epithelium is benign.

Metapsychiatry The interface between psychiatry and such psychic phenomena as parapsychology, mysticism, altered states of consciousness, and nonmedical healing.

Metapsychology The branch of theoretical or speculative psychology that deals with the significance of mental processes; the nature of the mind-body relationship; the origin, purpose, and structure of the mind; and similar hypotheses that are beyond the realm of empirical verification.

Metarteriole A small blood vessel that emerges from an arteriole, passes through a capillary network, and empties into a venule.

Metastasis It is a way in which cancer spreads around the body. Cells detaching from malignant tumour travel through the blood stream in the lymphatic system. Replication of cell then results in formation of new cancer. Cancers of muscle and bone spreads by blood stream while lung and breast by lymphatics. The shifting of a disease or a neoplasm from one part of the body to another remote from the original location.

Metastasis to lungs More circumscribed and multiple nodules are secondary to cancer of breast and abdominal organs. Sarcoma of any part of body may give rise to deposits in lungs. There will be increasing cough, dyspnoea and cyanosis Much respiratory distress occurs when larger area of lung is involved. Haemoptysis is more with primary lung carcinoma. Pleural effusion may be seen. X-ray shows cannon ball appearance.

Metastasize Transfer of disease from site to other mostly malignant cell.

Metastatic calcification This results from hypercalcaemia caused by hyperparathyroidism, vitamin D intoxication. Addison's disease, bone tumours and hypercalcaemia affect the blood vessels, kidneys, lungs and stomach.

Metastatic neuroblastoma It is one of the common malignant tumour of infancy and childhood. It is a tumour of embryonic neuroblastic tissue and usually arises in the adrenal medulla. It commonly metastasise in both the orbits. X-ray shows osseous lesion. There are increased catecholamines in urine.

Metastatic tumors of placenta Malignant melanoma is the commonest. Hematogenous spread is common.

Metastatic tumours Metastatic tumours are far less than oral primary tumours. Roughly 72 per cent oral metastasis occur in mandible and 18 per cent in maxilla. About 20 per cent of jaw metastases are from a primary cancer in breast and 15 per cent from thyroid. Clinically metastatic lesion may produce swelling, pain, loosening of teeth and paraesthesia. On X-ray it may have ill-defined borders and moth-eaten appearance. Metastatic tumour patients with acute leukaemia and have leukaemic infiltrates in jaw.

Metastatic tumours of liver Majority of hepatic malignancy is metastatic in origin mostly from carcinoma of breast, lung and colon. There may be massive enlargement of liver. Metastases which outgrow their blood supply become centrally necrotic.

Metatarsal arch The arch that extends across the ball of the foot; also called the transverse arch.

Metatarsal bar Strip of firm material attached transversely to the outer sole immediately posterior to a point corresponding to the metatarso-phalangeal joints; intended to relieve weight bearing on those joints.

Metatarsal bone These are five long, cylindrical bones within foot. These are held in arch with the help of ligaments. March fracture results in fracture of head of second metatarsal. The metatarsophalangeal joint at the base of the big toe is commonly affected by gout.

Metatarsal formula It is a description of three metatarsal types according to their length. The index plus minus type in which the first metatarsal is equal in length to the second. The index minus type in which first metatarsal is shorter than second and index plus type in which first metatarsal is longer than second.

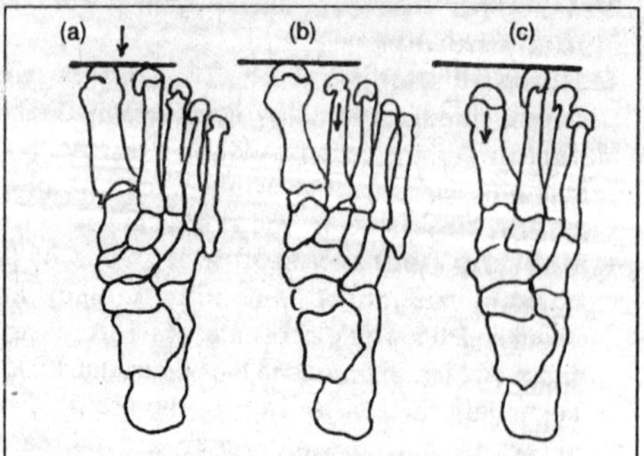

(a) Indus plus = minus (b) Indus plus (c) Indus minus

Metatarsalgia Pain in region of metatarso phalangeal articulation is a frequent complaint. It is common in women who wear heels that are too high to permit lateral deviation of foot.

Metatarsus The region of the foot between the ankle and the phalanges that includes the five metatarsal bones.

Metatarsus adductus This deformity involves the angulation of the meratarsal bones towards the midline (medially).

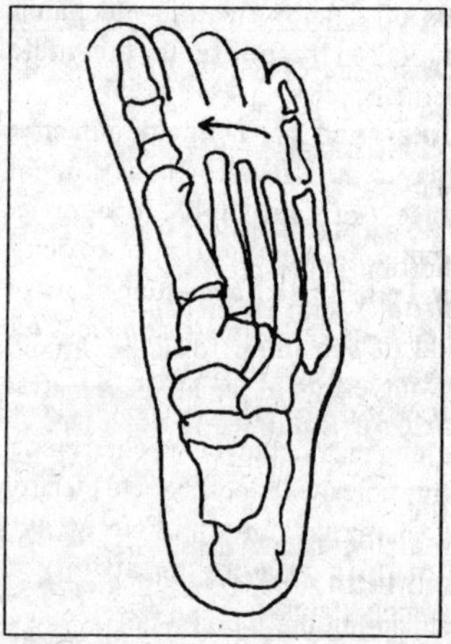

Metatarsus primus atavicus A congenital foot deformity in which there is abnormal shortening of first metatarsal.

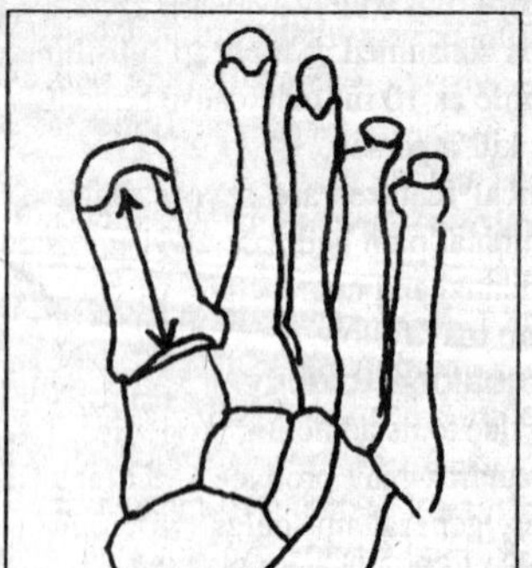

Metatarsus primus varus Congenital deformity in which first metatarsal deviates toward the midline. An angle greater than 10 degrees is abnormal and diagnostic.

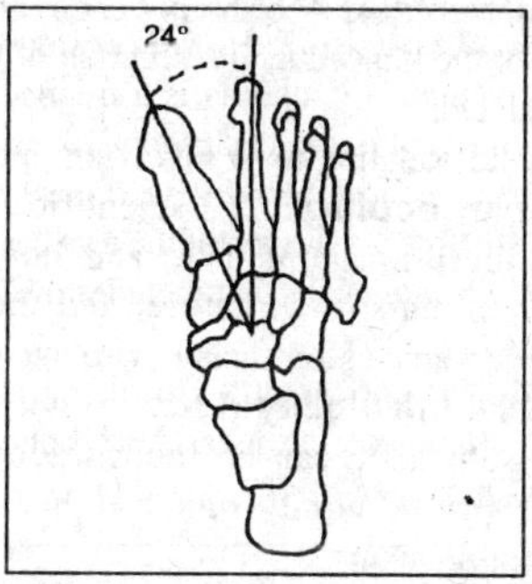

Meter A measure of length in the metric system; equal to about 39.5 inches.

Meter dose inhaler Puffs of metered medication or inhalations.

Metered-dose inhaler Canister that contains medication under pressure.

Metestrus A term classically used to designate the period of subsiding follicular function or rest following estrus in female mammals.

Methadone Synthetic compound with opiate properties used as oral substitute for heroin and morphine.

Methanal Formaldehyde.

Methanofuran A coenzyme that serves as a carbon carrier during the initial reduction of CO_2 in the methanogenic pathway.

Methanogenesis The process of methane formation by methanogens.

Methanol It is widely available as a solvent of paints and is consumed as a cheap substitute of ethanol. As little as 10 ml may cause blindness and 30 ml may kill a person.

Clinical features are severe malaise, vomiting, abdominal pain and loss of visual acquity. Pupils are dilated and nonreactive. Coma and circulatory failure may follow.

Methaqualone toxicity It is a commonly abused drug due to its addicting properties. Twenty tablets of mandrax may produce toxic effects. In normal doses, general muscular twitchings, myoclonic jerks and convulsions occur. Seizures may continue for 4 to 5 days after ingestion. Respiratory depression is less frequent than with barbiturates. However hypotension is more common and myocardial infarction may occur. ECG may show flat T-waves and prolong QT-interval.

Methods The steps, procedure, and strategies for gathering and analyzing data in a study.

Methotrexate It is an anticancer drug used in the treatment of lymphoma and certain form of leukaemia. It is also used to treat some cancers of uterus, breast, ovary and testis. In some resistant cases of rheumatoid arthritis it is tried. It may also cause anaemia, increased susceptibility to infection and abnormal bleeding.

Methotrexate intoxication It is an antimetabolite anticancer drug. It is also useful in rheumatoid arthritis. For adults maximum intrathecal dose is 12.5 mg. For cancer patient dose is 40 mg/sq. metre 2 to 3 times a week. Initial features include burning pain in legs followed by seizure, headache, neck rigidity and vomiting. A few patients may develop renal failure.

Methylation The biological mechanism by which inorganic forms of selenium are reduced to the Se (II) state and receive methyl groups from a carrier protein, resulting in the formation of volatiles such as dimethylselenide.

Methylene blue Blue dye that becomes colourless when reduced.

Methylotroph An organism that grows aerobically with one-carbon compounds as its carbon and energy source.

Methylotrophic Capable of utilizing a variety of simple methylated compounds as sole source of carbon and energy.

Methyltheobromine Caffeine.

Methylxanthines A class of drugs (e.g., aminophylline) that have diuretic, vasodilator, and cardiac stimulant properties.

Metoclopramide It is an antiemetic drug used to relieve nausea and vomiting caused by anticancer drugs, radiation therapy or anaesthetic drugs. It is often given with a premedication. It is used to treat heartburn also.

It reduces nerve activity in part of brain, stimulating vomiting. It increases the speed with which fluid is passed from stomach. Adverse effects may include rash, dryness of mouth and agitation. Large doses may cause sedation.

Metoprolol It is a cardioselective beta-blocker drug used in the treatment of angina pectoris and hypertension. It is also used in hyperparathyroidism. It may be given following myocardial infarction. It results in lethargy.

Metraterm The muscular, distal portion of the uterus of digenetic trematodes.

Metrazol shock treatment It is rarely used treatment in which a convulsive seizure is produced by intravenous injection of Metrazol. Introduced by von Meduna in 1934.

Metromenorrhagia Excessive bleeding, often prolonged, at abnormal and frequent intervals.

Metronidazole In aerobic microorganism it is converted into an active form by reduction of its nitro group.

It binds to DNA and prevents nucleic acid formation. It is bacteriostatic. It is well absorbed and is eliminated by urine. Half-life is 8 hours. It is widely effective against anaerobic organism. It is useful in trichomoniasis, amoebiasis, giardiasis and anaerobic vaginosis. Dose is 400 mg eight hourly.

Metropathia hemorrhagica Long period of amenorrhoea followed by heavy menstrual loss with bulky uterus. Pregnancy test is negative.

Metrorrhagia Variable amounts of bleeding at abnormal and frequent intervals.

Mettalic fatigue The repeated application of stress to an object causes tiny cracks to be generated into the metal with each stress the cracks grow until the material breaks.

Micelle A spherical aggregate of bile salts that dissolves fatty acids and monoglycerides so that they can be absorbed into intestinal epithelial cells. Tiny emulsion droplets of fatty acids, monoglycerides, cholesterol, and fatsuluble vitamins mixed with bile salts.

Miconazole It is an antifungal disease to treat tinea skin diseases such as ringworm, athlete's foot and vaginal candidiasis. Miconazole in the form of cream may cause burning sensation.

Micro surgery This surgery involves minute, delicate or not easily accessible tissues. These operations include transplanting lens and transplanting a new cornea. Restoring a severed limb by rejoining disconnected blood vessels and nerves and rejoining obstructed fallopian tubes.

Microabrasions Tiny cuts that provide an entrance for microorganisms.

Microaerophiles Micro organism that can grow in low concentration of oxygen.

Microatelectasis The absence of gas in a very small part of the lungs due to resorption of the gas from the alveoli.

Microbial Relating to or involving microbes.

Microbial ecology The scientific study of the distribution, abundance, and interactions of microorganisms in nature, and the impact of microorganisms on their environment.

Microbial infallibility A term for the premise that any substance can be biodegraded under the appropriate conditions by the appropriate microorganisms.

Microbiology This is the study of microorganisms. Microbiology began in 17th century. Louis Pasteur (1822–1895) and Robert Koch (1843–1910) were the pioneer workers. Microbiology continued to progress with the discovery of virus, the development of vaccines and antibiotics against many diseases. Microbiologists have played an important role in the study of genetics by pioneering techniques of genetic engineering. It is the branch of biological science which deals with the study of minute organisms which cannot be seen by naked eyes. Human eyes cannot see structures smaller than 1/1000 of an inch.

Microboides Cytoplasmic, membrane-bounded vesicles containing peroxide forming and peroxide-destroying enzymes; includes lysosomes, peroxisomes, and glyoxysomes.

Microcephaly It is an abnormal small head, usually associated with mental retardation. It may be the result of damage of brain before birth by rubella. It may also occur if the skull bones fuse too early. It is not treatable. The small head reflects failure of normal brain growth. These patients may have mental retardation and seizures. Secondary microcephaly may be of traumatic, vascular or infectious aetiology as in herpes simplex, rubella and toxoplasmosis.

Microchemistry Chemical reaction or phenomenal studies on very small amounts of material.

Microchips Microfabricated silicon devices that have traditionally been used for making relatively inexpensive but complex electronic circuits.

Micrococcus These are gram-positive, spherical cocci occurring in groups of 4. Each cell is 1 micrometre in diameter and is little larger than staphylococci and are often surrounded by capsule or pseudo-capsule.

They are strict aerobes. These are found in respiratory tract or on skin and can be extracted from cervical adenitis, dental abscess and pulmonary suppuration.

Microcomputer A smaller version of a computer, usually consisting of a microprocessing unit assembled on a printed circuit board with memory and auxiliary circuits.

Microcornea It is a congenital anomaly below 10 mm and occur in microphthalmos. An acquired microcornea may develop with atrophy of globe and is associated with a marked opacification. Severe corneal scar may also flatten the cornea.

Microcurie A unit of radioactivity, being one-millionth (10^{-6}) curie, or the quantity of radioactive material in which the number of nuclear disintegrations is 3.7 x -10^4 atoms per second.

Microcyst A very small cyst.

Microcyte An abnormally small erthrocyte, i.e., one 6 μ or less in diameter, such as seen in microcytic anemia.

Microdose A very small dose.

Microfilaria The juvenile, first-stage larva of filarial nematodes.

Microglia Small neuroglial cells that become phagocytic and mobile in response to inflammation; considered to be macrophages of the central nervous system.

Microgram One millionth of a gram.

Microlevel A level of analysis that focuses on the smaller forms of social behavior; for example, everyday interaction with the family.

Micron Unit of linear measurement; one-thousandth of a millimetre.

Micronemes Small, thin, anterior organelles that secrete their contents on a parasite's surface at the start of the invasion process.

Microorganism These are single celled living organisms too small to be seen by naked eye The main pathogenic micro organisms are bacteria which cause certain types of pneumonia, typhoid, diphtheria, etc.

Virus causes numerous infections including AIDS. Fungi causes ringworm and thrush.

Microphthalmos It is a condition in which there is small eye with many other defects. It is usually associated with coloboma. A pure microphthalamic eye is due to arrested development of globe in all directions after the embryonic fissure has been closed. Eyeball is small. There may be glaucoma and hypermetropia. Vision is subnormal with nystagmus and strabismus.

Micropore A tiny pore; e.g., a small, single invagination anterior to the nucleus with an apparent clathrin coat presumed but not yet demonstrated to be involved in phagocytosis.

Micropsia With paresis of accommodation especially unilateral ones patient will see objects smaller because the increased impulse for accommodation will elicit the impression of closeness of the objects. The same holds for palsy of covergence, which produces convergence micropsia.

Microscope It produces enlargement of small objects. Microscope may be one lens simple instrument to compound microscopes and high powered electron microscope. The single lens microscope may date as early as 15th century when it was capable of magnifying upto about 300 times. Greatest of the early microscopists was the Italian Marcello Malpighi (1628–1694) who is regarded as the founder of present day histology. At the end of 16th century two lens microscopes were introduced. For such instruments enlargement is 1500 times. Electron microscopes are light microscopes except that they use a beam of electrons instead of light and electromagnetic lenses instead of glass ones. Another instrument is fluorescence microscope to study chemical composition of cells. Operating microscopes are low powered compound microscopes with several modifications.

Microshock Low-voltage but high-amperage electricity.

Microsleep A brief period of sleep lasting a second or so.

Microslide The slide on which objects for microscopical examination are mounted.

Microsome A minute particle of a cell rich in nucleic acids, being a vesicular fragment of the endoplasmic reticulum. Small bodies derived from the protein synthesis apparatus of the cell when the cell is rather violently disrupted, for example by sonic shock waves or grinding with abrasives.

Microsphere The minute, round structural element used in the process of surface treatment of certain implant interfaces, often for the formation of porosities to increase surface area and retention.

Microstomia Abnormal smallness of the mouth.

Microsurgery This surgery involves minute, delicate or not easily accessible tissues. These operations include transplanting lens and transplanting a new cornea. Restoring a severed limb by rejoining disconnected blood vessels and nerves and rejoining obstructed fallopian tubes.

Microsyringe A syringe fitted with a screw-thread micrometer head for the accurate control of minute measurements.

Microthrix A specialized microvillus that projects from the outer, limiting membrane of the tapeworm tegument.

Microtome It is a device or machine which cuts material into very thin slices for examination under microscope. Objects are usually embedded in wax or synthetic resin.

Microtomy The cutting into thin sections.

Microtonometer A small tonometer for measuring the oxygen and carbon dioxide tension in the blood.

Microtubule Hollow tube composed of tubulin; microtubules help provide support to the cytoplasm of the cell and are components of certain cell organelles such as cilia and flagella.

Microvascular Small blood vessels of the body.

Microvasculature The portion of the vasculature of the body comprising the finer vessels, sometimes described as including all vessels with an internal diameter of 100 microns or less.

Microvilli The brushlike border made up of epithelial cells found on each villus in the small intestine; increases the surface area for absorption of nutrients.

Microvillus One of the minute projections of the cell membrane that greatly increases the surface area of the cell membrane.

Microwave An electromagnetic wave of very high frequency and of short wavelength, considered by some authorities as ranging between 1 millimeter and 1 meter, or between 1 centimeter and 1 meter.

Microzone A 'beam' of excitation of Purkinje cells by granule cells.

Micturition Urination.

Micturition reflex Contraction of the urinary bladder stimulated by stretching of the urinary bladder wall; results in emptying of the urinary bladder.

Mid foot Mid foot is made up of tarsal bones namely the navicular, medial intermediate and lateral cuneiform bones and the cuboid. Joint exist between them.

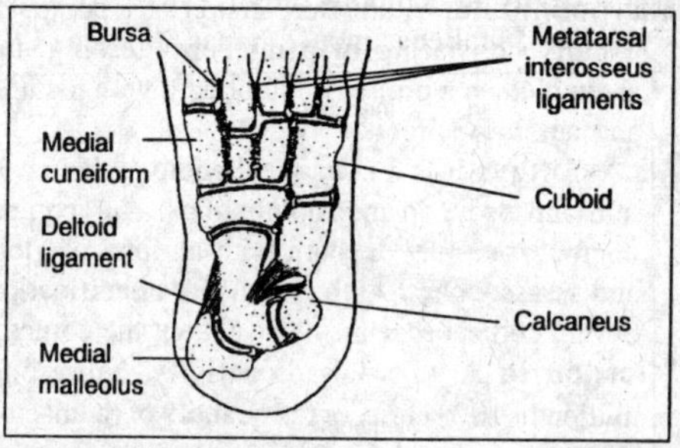

Mid forceps operation Forceps are applied on the fetal head which after engagement has descended with its leading part to or below the level of ischial spine. Axis traction forceps is convenient to apply.

Mid stance Begins at single limb support and progresses to when the body is over and in front of the stance limb.

Mid swing Extends from maximal knee flexion to when the tibia is vertical.

Mid tarsal joint The transverse tarsal joint.

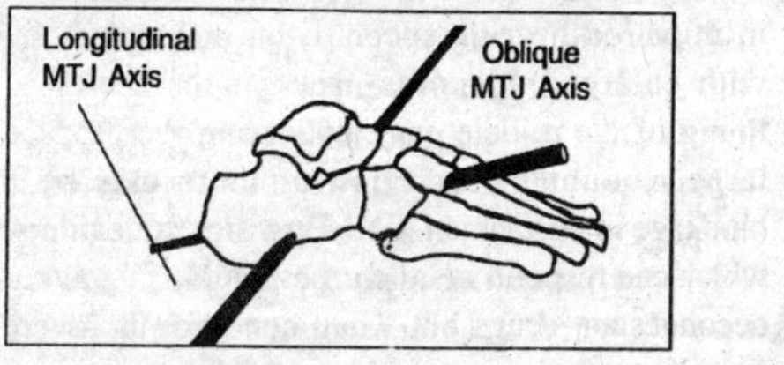

Midarm circumference Measurement used to assess skeletal muscle mass.

Midazolam It is a water soluble preparation which combines fast onset of sedation, rapid recovery, good amnesia, minimal irritation of veins and no risk of secondary sedation. Dose is 5 to 7 mg intravenously useful for night sedation before surgery.

Midbrain A short, narrow constricted portion of the brain stem, just below the thalamus, which connects the pon sand the cerebellum with the forebrain. Among its structures, it contains the center for visual reflexes, the nucleus of the mesencephalic root of the trigeminal nerve, the nucleus of the trochlear nerve, and the nucleus of the oculomotor nerve.

Middle cardiac vein A vein that receives blood from tributaries from both ventricles; runs in the posterior interventricular sulcus.

Middle ear Middle ear consists of ossicles located in a cavity of temporal bone. There are three ossicles : malleus, incus, stapes. Malleus is a

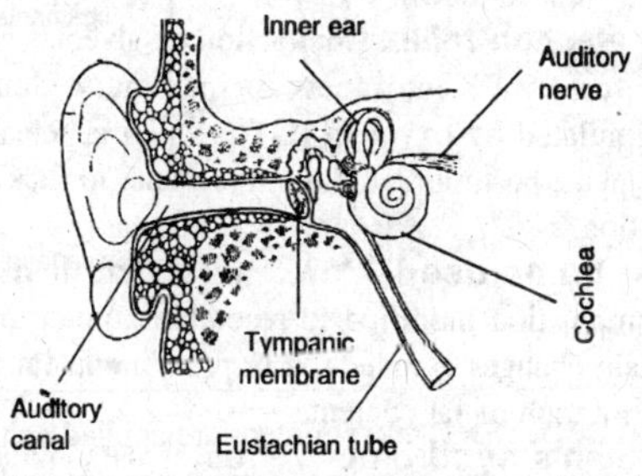

Structure of the ear

hammer-like bone attached to the tympanic membrane and the incus. The stapes is a stirrup-shaped bone that connects to oval window of internal ear. The eustachian tube is a canal that extends from inferior surface of middle ear to back wall of throat.

Middle ear, effusion Fluid accumulation can result in impaired hearing specially in children along with enlarged adenoids. The mucus secreting lining of the middle ear cavity may overproduce large amount of secretion or there may be a blockage in eustachian tube. First sign is deafness, which can respond in mild cases simply by putting decongestant drugs but when condition is severe myringotomy, i.e. opening in ear drum.

Middle lobe syndrome It includes chronic cough, wheezing, recurrent infection, haemoptysis, chest pain, and atelectasis.

Middle temporal gyrus (MT) The region of the occipital lobe in which motion perception is integrated.

Midsagittal A cut or plane that divides the body or any of its parts into two equal halves.

Midsagittal plane Invisible vertical line or plane that divides the body through the sagittal suture into equal right andleft portions.

Migraine It is a headache lasting for two hours to two days accompanied by disturbances of vision and vomiting. There may be multiple attacks at different intervals. It is more common in women. The exact mechanism is not known.

Stresses like anxiety, anger, shock, change of climate may precipitate it. In common migraine headache develops slowly mounting to a throbbing pain and is made worst by slightest movement or noise. Pain may be on one side of head. Vomiting gives relief. If it occurs more than once a month then dispirin with antiemetic may be helpful. Ergotamine may also be given. If migraine attacks occur more than once a month prophylactic drugs, i.e. beta-blockers and calcium channel blockers may be helpful.

Migratory glossitis Geographic tongue is characterised by one or more irregular areas of desquamation on the tongue. It may have an allergic basis. The filiform papillae in the bald spots are missing but fungiform papillae remain. These heal but new areas appear in another part of tongue thus the name wandering rash. The bald spots on the tongue may change size and shape within two hours. Lesions do not respond to treatment but disappears spontaneously.

Mikulicz's disease It is characterised by swelling of salivary and lacrimal glands. Lesions consist of unilateral, bilateral or multiple involvement of salivary glands. The parotid enlargement may be accompanied by enlargement of minor salivary gland. Mikulicz's disease is usually seen as asymptomatic swelling with duration of a few months to many years. It may appear as single or multiple nodule. Size of swelling varies from time to time. The disease may be diffuse and nodular. Spontaneous regressions occur.

Mild mental retardation A category of mental retardation in which the individuals have a subaverage intelligence quotient ranging from 55 to 69 and typically require intermittent support; generally allows individuals to master academic skills ranging from third to seventh grade slowly.

Milla White cysts 1.2 m.m. in size from distended sebaceons glands.

Miliaria Heat rash occurs due to failure of sweat to reach the surface. In hot and humid environment there may be increased production of sweat. When sweat is not able to come, out it produces the condition. It may be an occupational hazard to farmers working in field. Wearing undue heavy clothing can produce the condition. It presents with acute inflammatory eruptions on trunk, upper extremities and is accompanied by itching, burning and irritation. Repeated scratching may lead to excoriation and secondary infection.

Military time Time base on a 24 hour clock.

Milium It is a benign, very small-sized epidermal cyst of unknown origin. It occurs spontanously following various types of epithelial trauma. Pathologically there is downgrowth and cystic expansion of epidermis and cyst contains keratin and lipid containing debris.

The condition gives rise to multiple number of milia as tiny, white, slightly elevated cystic excrescence. Lesions occur on the eyelids, forehead and temples. Lesions are firm in consistency and when punctured or pressed hard between the fingers they express white material. No treatment is required for condition.

Milk 1. A white fluid secreted by the mammary gland, forming the natural food for young mammals. 2. the milk produced by cows, goats, sheep, and certain other domestic animals that is used for human consumption, either in the natural state or processed into dairy products, such as butter cheese, or yogurt.

Milk alkali syndrome There is hypercalcaemia accompanied by alkalosis. It may result by excessive long-term intake of calcium containing antacid drugs and milk in case of peptic ulcer. It is characterised by alkalosis hypercalcaemia and transient renal insufficiency. Person may have nausea, vomiting, headache, irritability, dizziness and confusion. It develops during milk alkali therapy for peptic ulcer. Eyes may show band-shaped keratopathy, conjunctivitis and calcification.

Milk drip Milk drip means introducing milk through stomach tube or Ryles tube either by passing through mouth or nose. It is done in severe case of peptic ulceration causing haematemesis or any corrossive poisoning in stomach. Introduce Ryles tube to stomach and fix it to the cheek of patient. Milk from bottle is allowed to flow down through the tube to make it air free. The drops of milk per minute is regulated. If cold milk is desired you can wrap the milk bottle by ice cold cloth. Remember milk drip is never given as an IV drip but milk infusion to stomach by drip-like method can be given.

Milk ejection The activation of a process by which contractions of the myoepithelial cells in a mother's breast propel milk along the duct into the lactiferous sinuses. Also called let-down reflex and milk let-down.

Milk ejection reflex Contraction of alveolar cells to force milk into ducts of mammary glands, stimulated by oxytocin (OT), which is released from the posterior pituitary in response to suckling action.

Milk humanised Cows milk that had its composition modified to resemble human milk. Main changes is reduction in protein content and restoration of fat content.

Milkman's syndrome A form of osteomalacia presenting with multiple pseudofracture of the bones lying in close contact with the arteries.

Milk-toned Dried skimmed milk added to a high fat milk such as bufffalo milk to reduce the fat content but maintain the solid fats.

Milli litre One-thousandth part of a litre, usually abbreviated ml. It is approximately equal to one cubic centimetre.

Milliampere (mA) Unit of electric current; 1/1000 of an ampere. In radiography, milliamperage determines the number of electrons available at the filament.

Milliard reaction Enzymatic oxidation of phenolic substances such as occurs in cut surface of apple.

Milligram One thousandth of a gram.

Milling The term milling refers to conversion of cereal grain into its derivative e.g. wheat into flour, brown rice to white rice.

Milney Mirrays' instrument It is 13.75 inches long. The cephalic curve should be large enough to grasp the fetal head without compression allowing a maximum separation of 3.3 inches in the center. The maximum separation between the points of blades is one inch. The shank measures 2.5 inches.

Mimicry Copying the behaviors of others.

Mind A nonmaterial entity that is proposed to be responsible for intelligence, attention, awareness, and consciousness.

Mind/body therapies Systemic psychological and self help experiences designed to impact upon psychological, emotional, behavioral and physical functioning.

Mind-body problem Problem of how to explain how a nonmaterial mind can command a material body.

Mineral A nonorganic homogeneous solid substance, usually a constituent of the earth's crust. m. jelly, petrolatum'.

Mineral salts Inorganic salts, including sodium, potassium, calcium, chloride, sulphate etc.

Mineralization The complete degradation of an organic compound to simple inorganic constituents, such as carbon dioxide, water, ammonia, chloride and sulfate.

Mineralocorticoid A steroid hormone released from the adrenal cortex; acts on the kidney to increase the rate of sodium reabsorption from the nephron and potassium and hydrogen ion secretion into the nephron of the kidney; an example is aldosterone.

Minerals These are chemical elements which must be present in the diet for the maintenance of health. At least 13 minerals are essential, i.e. potassium, sodium, calcium, magnesium, phosphorus, iron, zinc and copper, etc. Inorganic nutrient necessary for normal metabolic functions.

Minerva jacket Mernerva technique for fixation of the cranium to chest provide the greatest restriction of segmental cervical spine movement. Minerva jacket provides similar minimization of the parallelogram like broching effect. The Minerva's advantage is due to extent of chest fixation. It however does not allow substantial control of capital flexion and extension.

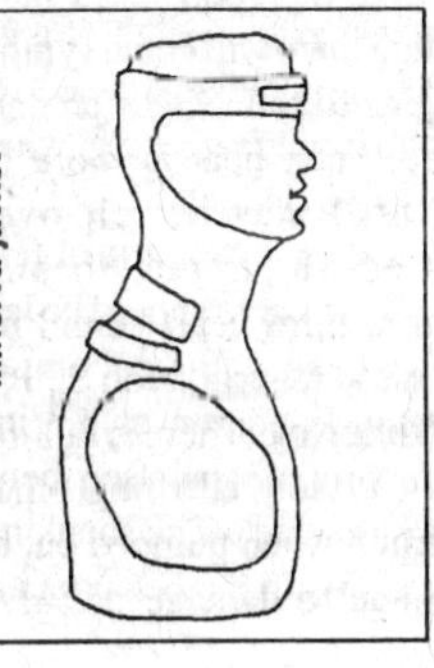
Minerva jacket

Minimal Blocking concentration Lowest concentration of local anesthetic agent that will block a nerve in vitro within 10 minutes.

Minimum The Lowest value which is obtained.

Minor depression Clinically relevant depressed mood not fulfilling the diagnostic criteria for major depressive disorder.

Minor renal injuries It may be contusion, perirenal hematoma or small laceration of renal parenchyma less than 1 cm in length that does not extend into collecting system.

Minor tranquilizer A sedative hypnotic drug promoted primarily for use in the treatment of anxiety.

Minority A part of population numerically less than 50%.

Minoxidil It is a vasodilator drug to treat severe hypertension. Prolonged treatment stimulates hair growth specially useful in male type of alopecia.

Minute ventilation The volume of air expired per minute. Total volume of air inhaled and exhaled per minute; about 6000 mL.

Miosis 'Constriction' of the pupil.

Mip Macrophage infectivity potentiatior, a legionella protein with activity as a cistrans peptidyle proly isomerase that is needed for full expression of bacterial virulence.

Miracidium The ciliated larva that emerges from the egg of digenetic trematodes.

Miracidium of schistosoma Eggs are usually released into the lumen of the hosts or an housing adult worm and pass to exterior through feces, sputum or urine. If the egg is deposited in water, it completes its development and a free swimming meracidium.

Mirror effect Reflection of all the ultrasound waves from tissues. It may produce a mirror image effect nearly duplicating the image.

Mirror neuron A neuron that fires when a monkey observes a specific action being made by another monkey.

Misalignment Not in proper alignment.

Miscarriage It is a loss of fetus before 22nd week of pregnancy or before viability to survive outside the uterus without artificial support. About 10 to

20 per cent pregnancies end in miscarriage. It may be as a result of chromosomal abnormalities or major developmental defects. Severe maternal illness or exposure to toxin may result it. Inadequate secretion of progesterone or autoimmune disorder may also be responsible. Symptoms of miscarriage are cramping and/or bleeding. Spotting and severe pain can be symptoms of threatened miscarriage. Ultrasound examination may be helpful. If medicines are not able to help then D&C is the solution.

Miscible Capable of being mixed.

Misdemeanor Minor criminal offense.

Missed abortion This is called when ovum dies and is retained in the uterus for eight weeks or more. When dead embryo is surrounded by blood clots covering the chorion, it is referred to as blood mole. Presenting clinical features include, brownish vaginal discharge, decreasing size of breasts and disappearing of morning sickness.

Missed incontinence It is a combination of stress and urge incontinence. It is thought that long standing stress incontinence may lead to urge incontinence and present as a mixed condition.

Missionary position It is the man on top sex position. The term originated in Polynesia where Christian missionaries approved the position. It is the most common position in the world.

Misting Blood which has been reduced to a fine spray, as a result of the energy or force applied to it.

Mistress She is a woman who provides sexual services and companionship to a man who may or may not be married, usually on a long-term basis. In return she gets financial support and a place to live.

Mistrust It results in acute emotional tension and behavioral signs of unmet needs.

Mitchell's osteotomy It is done for hallux valugus. A step cut is made in the first metatarsal neck and

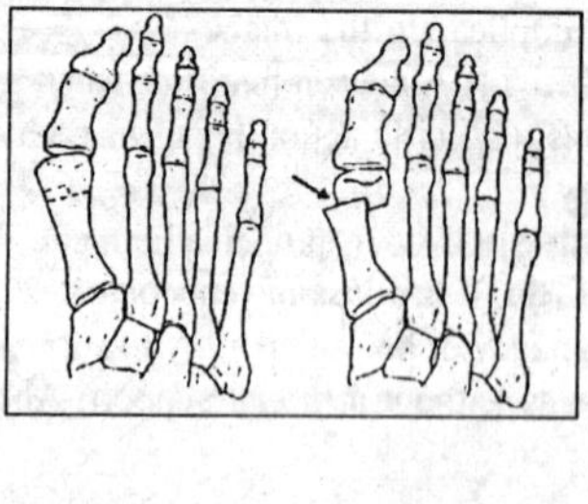

the metatarsal is transposed laterally. This reduces the effective inter metatarsal angle, reducing the degree of hallus valgus.

Mitered corner A triangular folded corner of a bedsheet, used to prevent the sheet from pulling out from the mattress.

Mitochondria It occurs in the form of granular rods or filaments in every type of cells and plays a role in production of enzymes present in cytoplasm of many cells. They are composed of phospholipin and glutathione combined with proteins. These provide requisite energy from oxidative processes in the cells.

Mitochondrial enzyme Enzyme involved in the exchange and transport of energy within the mitochondrion.

Mitochondrion An organelle within the cell that provides energy for cell process.

Mitogen Any factor that induces mitosis or cell replication; e.g., a protein derived from plants that is used in the laboratory to stimulate cells to divide.

Mitogenic Relating to or stimulating cell division.

Mitosis It is the way in which most of cells divide so that the chromosomes within the nucleus of original cells are exactly duplicated into two daughter cells. It can be seen in a cell culture under microscope. A minority of cells may not get the half of original cell of chromosomal material. This process is called meiosis and occurs in formation of egg and sperm cells.

Mitral incompetence Rheumatic fever accounts for most of cases of mitral insufficiency. Bacterial endocarditis results in destruction of valve. Due to incompetence of mitral valve blood leaks from left ventricles into left atrium during systole resulting in increased pressure. During diastole entire volume of blood leaks into left ventricle. For long time there will be no symptoms till cardiac output begins to fall. Slight precordial bulge may be present. Apex beat is more down than out. Systolic thrill may be felt over mitral area. Accentuated M_1 is due to posterior leaflet regurgitation. third heart sound may be audible. In severe mitral regurgitation S_3 is very explosive.

Mitral insufficiency There is failure of mitral valve of the heart closely allowing blood to leak back into left atrium when pumped out of left ventricle. It may be due to damage of valve in rheumatic fever. The symptoms are shortness of breath, fatigue may be along with palpitation. Later on there may be swelling on ankle. ECG and echo studies help in diagnosis. Diuretics and digitalis are helpful. If nothing helps, heart valve surgery may be useful.

Mitral stenosis Rheumatic fever is the cause. The resistance of narrow lumen of mitral orifice gives rise to high left atrial pressure. High pressure in left atrium gives rise to left atrial hypertrophy and dilatation.

Pulmonary arterial pressure also rises which puts great strain to right ventricle which hypertrophies and dilates. Dyspnoea is main symptom and may be of different grades. Palpitation is often distressing due to tachycardia. Haemoptysis is common. Patient may complain of cough and angina.

Mitral valve Also known as the bicuspid valve; located between the left atrium and ventricle.

Mitral valve prolapse An inherited disorder in which a portion of a mitral valve is pushed back too far (prolapsed) during ventricular contraction due to expansion of the cusps and elongation of the chordae tendineae.

Mitteleschmerz Low abdominal pain occurring at ovulation.

Mittelschmers Low abdominal pain occurring at the time of ovulation.

Mixed cochlear neural tinnitus Tinnitus may be unilateral or bilateral and can be marked at the auditory threshold or 10 to 12 dB above threshold. The masking level and frequency are variable and tinnitus may occur in all frequencies. Vestibular findings are nonspecific.

Mixed dentition Complement of teeth in the jaws after the eruption of some of the permanent teeth but before all the deciduous teeth are absent.

Mixed dysarthria When two or more types of dysarthria coexist, the term mixed dysarthria is used.

Mixed lucent, opaque A term used to describe a lesion that exhibits both a radiolucent and radiopaque component.

Mixed nerve A nerve that contain both motor and sensory nerve fibers.

Mixis The production of a new genotype by combination of genes from two sources.

Mixotrophy The fact of obtaining nutrients through a combination of organic and inorganic sources.

Mnemonic Having to do with memory.

Mnemonic devices Memory systems or techniques, designed to improve memory by the use of special rules, association, or other methods of organising the materials.

Mobile cabinetry Equipment that can be moved about the treatment area to provide close working surfaces and drawers for chairside assisting in four-handed dentistry.

Mobility Horizontal and, to a lesser degree, axial movement of a tooth in response to various forces, with return of the tooth to its original position, once the pressure is removed.

Mobility base A wheelchair support and movement system; consists of the tubular frame, the legrests and armrests, foot supports, and wheels.

Mobilization Process of making a fixed part movable. A form of manual therapy applied within the physiological passive range of joint motion, characterized by nonthrust increase in passive joint play.

Mobilometer An instrument for measuring the consistency of liquids.

Mobius syndrome It is a congenital bilateral palsy of motor cranial nerves mainly the sixth and seventh nerves. This may be associated with anomalies of external ear, mental retardation and paresis of masticatory muscles.

Modality Any of the specific sensory entities, such as vision, smell, taste, or touch.

Mode The most commonly ovserved value in a distribution (i.e., the value with the highest number of observations).

Mode of transmission Manner in which infectious microorganisms move to another location.

Model A theory that specifies relationships between variables but does not have a deductive component; used interchangeably with *conceptual framework.*

Model trimmer Grinding devices with an abrasive wheel used for trimming or shaping plaster or stone casts or models.

Modeling Behavior management technique that allows one person through observation to learn a desired response from another person.

Imitation or observational learning that involves copying the behavior of others.

Modified Stillman's technique Toothbrushing technique developed to simply massage the gingiva; the modified Stillman's method now includes cleaning the entire tooth. It is recommended for those patients with gingival recession and/or puffy gingival tissue.

Modified standing position Position in which the upper half of the body is leaning forward.

MODS Multiple Organ Dysfunction Syndrome.

Module A cell column in the cerebral cortex.

Moist heat It is more effective than dry heat. Moist heat sterilises at lower temperature in a given time and in shorter time at same temperature. Moist heat kills microorganisms by coagulating and denaturing their enzymes and structured proteins. Low temperature of 63°C for 30 minutes is used in pasteurisation of milk. It kills *Mycobacterium tuberculosis* at this temperature. For Streptococcus 60°C for one hour is required.

Molal Pertaining to the number of moles of solute per kilogram of solvent.

Molar One of the 12 teeth distal to second bicuspid three in each quadrant.

Molar solution One mole of solute dissolved in water to give a total volume of 1,000 mL.

Molasses Residue left after repeated crystallisation of sugar.

Molded splint Orthotic device made of rigid material.

Mole The number of grams of a chemical that is equal to its formula weight (atomic weight for an element or molecular weight for a compound).

Molecular Relating to or occurring at the level of the molecule.

Molecular mimicry The production of or covering by hostlike molecules, especially on the body surface of a parasite.

Molecule Two or more atoms of the same or different type joined by a chemical bond.

Molecule crowding A term to denote a dense population of molecules.

Moleskin Adhesivebacked tape used for some forms of skin traction. A soft material, often with an adhesive backing, used especially on the feet to protect against chafing.

Molluscum contagiosum It is an infectious type of warty growth over the skin produced by poxvirus. The condition presents with multiple but may also be single, small, smooth skin coloured or pearly white waxy almost translucent raised umbilical papules. The size of papules vary from pinhead to bean size. Papules are solid and firm and express cheesy material when squeezed hard. Condition is usually asymptomatic.

Molluscum fibrosum It occurs in connection with the terminal filament of cutaneous nerves. The lesion appears as multiple cutaneous nodules particularly over the chest, admomen or back. Nodules are multiple, small, discrete, firm, sessile or pedunculated. But there is no hypertrophy of skin. Pigmentation of skin is present.

Monandrous Describing species in which females generally mate only once during their lifetime.

Monangle Having only one angle, such as a chisel.

Moncement synergy Manner of operation of the primary motor cortex.

Monckeberg's medial sclerosis It is a diffuse form of arterial disease which occurs after 50 years of age. It is characterised by fibrosis, fatty degeneration and later calcification of muscle coats of larger arteries of limbs and their branches. It is a result of ageing and it causes lengthening, tortuosity and hardening of arteries but does not diminish their calibre.

Mondor's syndrome It is characterised by thrombophlebitis of the superficial veins of the breast and chest wall, knot-like cordons of the subcutaneous veins extending along the lateral thoracic wall.

Monestrous Having a single fertile cycle during a given mating season.

Monestrum The ovulatory pattern in which there is only one ovulation per breeding period.

Mongolian spots Round or oval, dark, bluish black spots over the back and buttocks which do not disappear on pressure. It occurs in congenital primary pigmentary disorder in young children which disappears later on spontaneously.

Mongolism Down's syndrome is recognisable at birth. Newborn is small with muscular hypotonia with laxity of joints. Head is rounded and relatively short. Face and nose are flattened. Iris may show white flecks.

Mouth is small and tongue protruding. Hands are short and wide with stumpy fingers. Muscular hypotonia and mental retardation are responsible for delayed mile stones. Speech is delayed and defective.

Monilial vaginitis It is the inflammation of vagina caused by candida albicans.

Moniliasis This is due to gram-positive fungus, *Candida albicans* which grows well in acid medium and in presence of carbohydrates, so it is more common in pregnancy and diabetes. There is profuse discharge and intense pruritus vulva becomes sore and oedematous. There may be white patches or plaques of cheesy material adherent to vagina which when removed leaves multiple petechia like haemorrhagic areas. Better personal hygiene and nystatin are helpful.

Monitor Screen attached to a computer to show data output.

Monitoring The overall surveillance of a patient by methods employing the senses of touch, sight, hearing, or smell or by means of devices that operate chemically, physically, or electronically to measure the adequacy of the various physiologic functions.

Monoclonal antibodies Identical antibodies derived from a clone of genetically identically plasma cells. Immunoglobulin of a single specificity produced by an expanded clone of plasma cells.

Monocular blindness Blindness in one eye.

Monocular crescent The C-shaped monocular visual field.

Monocyte A large white blood cell active in destroying bacteria or foreign matter that has entered the body.

Monogamous Having the behavior pattern of monogamy; matting with only one of the opposite sex.

Monogamy A matting pattern in which one male mates with one female for one or more reproductive cycles; in some species this behavior also involves cohabitation, the cooperative rearing of young, and the exclusion of strange males and females from the territory.

Monolayer A single layer of oriented lipid molecules.

Monomer A single molecular unit of longer, more complex molecule. Monomers are joined together to form dimers, trimers, and polymers; the hydrolysis of polymers eventually yields separate monomers.

Monomorphic adenoma It is a soft, mobile, painless, slow growing swelling. Tumour is rare. Sialography may show displacement of ductal system.

Mononeuritis multiplex There is multiple involvement of number of different nerves in different limbs at one point of time. Most common cause is leprosy. Patient presents with dermal lesion before classical neuropathy develops. In tuberculoid form granulomas form within peripheral nerves, resulting in local palsies. Some nerves may become thick and palpable. Nerve infiltrates may also occur with leukaemia and lymphoma. Local destruction by carcinoma often occurs.

Mononuclear phagocyte A cell of bone marrow origin,larger than lymphocyte which can phagocytose foreign material and present it to lymphocytes to bring about an immune response.

Mononuclear phagocyte system A system comprising blood monocytes and tissue macrophages.

Monophyodont Having only one set of teeth, all being permanent.

Monoplegia Paralysis of one limb resulting from upper motor neuron disease.

Monorchism The condition of having one testis.

Monosaccharide Simple sugar.

Monosaccharides A sugar composed of a single carbohydrate unit; glucose, fructose, and galactose are monosaccharides.

Monosynaptic reflex A reflex requiring one synapse between sensory input and movement.

Monotherapy Treatment with a single drug, contrasted with combination therapies using more that one drug at the same time.

Monounsaturated far A fatty acid that contains one double covalent bond between two of its carbon atoms; it is not completely saturated with hydrogen atoms. Plentiful in triglycerides of olive and peanut oils.

Monounsaturated fatty acid A fatty acid containing a carbon chain with one double bond.

Monozygotic Pertaining to or derived from a single zygote identical twins.

Monozygotic twins (A) There can be two implantations, two placentas and two sets of membranes. (B) One blastomere only with two inner cell masses, one fused placenta, one chorion and separate amnious (C) There can be separation of inner cell masses with fused placenta and single amnion and chorion.

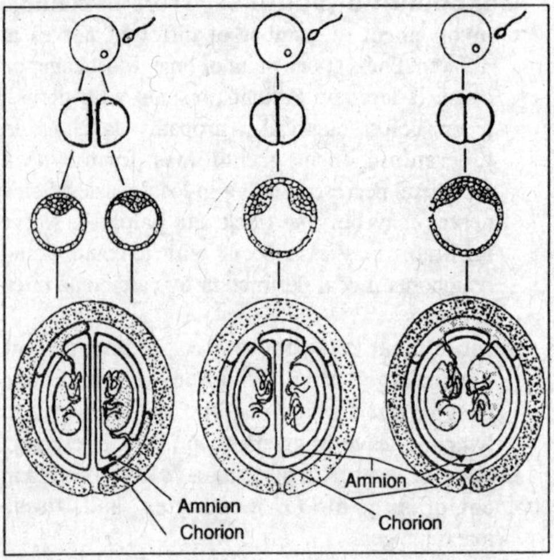

Monro, foramina Interventricular foramina of brain.

Mons pubis A fatty tissue pad covering the symphysis pubis and covered by pubic hair in the female. Prominence formed by a pad of fatty tissue over the symphysis pubis in the female.

Mons veneris A firm cushionlike formation of subcutaneous fatty tissue and loose connective tissue over the symphysis pubis.

Monster A fetus or infant with such pronounced developmental anomalies as to be grotesque and usually nonviable.

Montgomery straps Strips of tape with eyelets.

Mood A pervasive and sustained emotion that, in the extreme, markedly colours one's perception of the world. Common examples of mood include depression, elation, and anger. The subjective component of emotions in contrast to affect. The loss of capacity to experience pleasure, a core symptom of depression.

Mood disorder A mental disorder characterized by a disturbance in mood.

Mood episodes Mood syndromes that have no known cause other than the mood disorder.

Moore fracture A fracture of distal radius with dorsal subluxation of ulna.

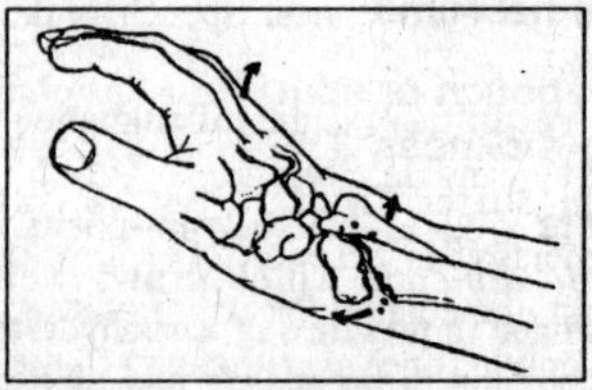

Mooren's ulcer It is a rare degenerative type of ulcer. It affects elderly person and progresses to involve whole of cornea. it commences as one or more grey infiltrates breaking to form ulcers, which further coalesce to form one big ulcer. The ulcer is characteristic as there is overhanging in advancing edge, undermining the epithelium and superficial lamellae. Usually both the eyes are involved, may not be at one point of time. Topical antibiotics and steroids are not effective.

Moral treatment A philosophy and technique of treating mental patients that prevailed in the first half of the nineteenth century and emphasised removal of restraints, humane and kindly care, attention to religion, and performance of useful tasks in the hospital.

Morals Rules or standards regarding what is right or wrong.

Morbid obesity Pathological state in which an individual weighs greater than 100 pounds over ideal weight.

Morbidity Incidence of a specific disease, disorder, or injury.

Morbidity rate The incidence of nonfatal cases of a given disease in the total population at risk during a specified period of time.

Morbus gallicus Literally, the French disese; the most common name given to a new disease that appeared in Europe in the late 15th century; many physicians and historians now identify morbus gallicus as syphilis.

Morgagni syndrome It is an autosomal dominant disorder usually seen in females. There develops trunkal obesity, fatigue, headache, lethargy and vertigo. Females develop hirsutism and menstrual disorder, visual loss and cataract. It is characterised by virilism, obesity, and hyperostosis frontalis interna in adult women.

Morgue A unit of a hospital with facilities for the storage and autopsy of the dead.

Morison, pouch or space of Hepatorenal recess.

Morning sickness The great majority of primi gravida suffer from it but in subsequent pregnencies it is absent. Some develop nausea, vomiting immediately on rising or after their first meal. Vomiting once over, there is no other problem. This lasts only for a few weeks. General health is not affected.

Morning stiffness This term describes theprolonged generalized stiffness that is associated with the inflammatory arthritis upon awakening. The stiffness is indicative of systemic involvement. The duration of the stiffness correlates with the intensity of the disease. This generalized stiffness is in contrast to the localized stiffness, seen in osteoarthritis, that results from inactivity.

Moro reflex Startle response of the newborn.

Morph The form or shape of an organism; e.g., the specific form of a given individual or the characteristic form of a species.

Morphine An opiate alkaloid produced by opium poppy that acts in the brain and peripherally to cause analgesia, euphoria and reduced alarm. They induce tolerance and dependence. It is derived from Greek word for juice and is used for last 2000 years. It is derived from poppy head. It depresses awareness, anxiety, pain sensation and respiration. It stimulates vomting centre and secretion of antidiuretic hormone. It depresses vascular tone and peristalsis. It stimulates bronchoconstriction, bowel sphincter, biliary spasm and fallopian spasm. Patient may develop both tolerance and dependence. In addicts withdrawal symptoms come on in about 8 hours after the last dose and are very distressing. 100 mg orally is effective and it raises the pain threshold, elevates mood and usually causes euphoria. It is more effective against dull, continuous than against sharp intermittent pain. It is more effective against visceral pain than bone and muscle pain. It constricts eye pupil by central and not peripheral action. Respiratory rate is decreased. It produces postoperative vomiting, constipation and respiratory depression.

Morphoea It is a localised form of scleroderma. It presents with one or more well-defined, deeply indurated, hard, thickened round or elongated white or yellow plaques, patches or spots surrounded by dusky red borders. Lesions develop on forehead. Affected skin appears rigid, inelastic, atrophic and shiny. Lesions may spread slowly or regress spontaneously on skin but will never regain normal appearance. When developed over joint, it restricts its movement.

Morphogen A substance existing in a concentration gradient along the body axis that specifies position along the axis.

Morphogene A gene that directly or indirectly controls the development of body form.

Morphogenesis The process through which an organism, or a body part, acquires its characteristic form or structure.

Morphological Relating to or based on body shape or form.

Morphological sex The sex of an individual as determined by the body shape and characteristic with appropriate secondary sexual characteristics. In the case of a true hermaphrodite, the individual has a mixture of the body and secondary sex characteristics of both sexes.

Morphology The science that deals with form and structure without regard to function.

Morsal Taking part in mastication; Also applied to the masticating surfaces of a bicuspid or molar.

Morsus A bite by a human being.

Mortality Incidence of deaths.

Mortality rate Death rate.

Mortar A bell-shaped or urn-shaped vessel of glass, orion, porcelain, or other material, in which drugs are beaten, crushed, or ground with a pestle.

Mortician Person who prepares the body for burial or cremation.

Mortise joint Anklo type joint.

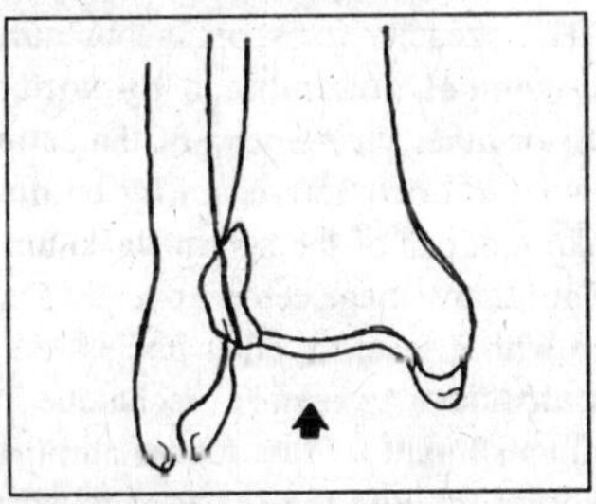

Morton's neuroma A neuroma of the plantar digital nerve caused by trauma to the nerve as it passes between the metatarsal heads.

Morton's syndrome It presents with shortened first metatarsal bone, tenderness at the base of the second metatarsal, and hypertrophy of the second metatarsal bone.

Mortuary It is a special section of hospital which deals with keeping of dead bodies temporarily. Here in some cases of doubtful death and accident postmortem may be done to establish the cause of death.

Morula The fertilized ovum at the 16 cell stage 3 days after conception. It is travelling from the Fallopian tube into the uterine cavity prior to implantation.

Morvan's syndrome The syndrome presents with sensory and trophic changes in the peripheral parts, muscular weakness, and difference in pain and temperature sensation.

MOS Markers of Occupational Stress.

Mosaicism The fact of having two or more cell lines of different genetic identity.

Mosquito It is a small flying insect found in tropics which bites to mammals and draw blood out of it. It is the female mosquito which carries infective organisms. Mosquitoes spread malaria, filaria, encephalitis and yellow fever.

Mother cell The compartment of the sporangium, which engulfs the forespore, syntehsizes spore coat proteins and lyses when the mature endospore is formed.

Mother-baby couple care An organisation of postpartum units that includes rooming-in or satellite nurseries with the same nurse caring for mother and baby.

Motile Capable of spontaneous or voluntary movement.

Motility The capacity for spontaneous movement; i.e., movement not induced by wind, water currents, or other phenomena of the surrounding environment. Locomotive ability conferred by whip-like motions of the sperm flagellum.

Motion The relative displacement over time of a body in space with respect to other bodies.

Motion palpation Assessment technique in which an examiner monitors the degree and quality of joint motion through the sense of touch while a joint is in active or passive motion.

This process is widely used technique in chiropractic analysis.

Motion range of lumbar vertebra Range of motion of lumbar vertebra and torso in as regards lateral inclination is 40 degree from S_1 though C_7. Limit. of rotation is 30 degrees, forward flexion is 90° degrees and backward extension upto 30 degrees.

Motion sickness It is a condition produced in some people by road, sea or air travel. In some persons it may be a feeling of uneasiness and headache. In severe cases there may be excessive sweating, salivation and vomiting.

Motion sickness is caused by effect of any constant pronounced movement of organ of balance in inner ear. To avoid it, one should not focus on nearby objects. Various antiemetic drugs can be taken to avoid motion sickness. Cyclizine or Avomin may be taken about an hour before start of journey to avoid it.

Motivation A need or desire that energies and directs behavior.

Motivational hierarchy A hierarchy of needs which human beings presumably fill successively in the order of lowest to highest. The five levels are : physiological needs, safety, love and belonging, self-esteem, and self-actualisation.

Motive An urge to attain some goal object, such as food when hungry, or some goal, such as becoming an engineer. Similar to drive except that drive has no clearly defined incentive.

Moton economy Elimination of unnecessary movement.

Motoneuron A specialized nerve cell in the spinal cord or brainstem that directly connects to muscle.

Motor apraxia A condition in which the person's ability to perform skilled, purposeful movement is impaired.

Motor area-4 In brain it occupies only the anterior lip of Rolandic fissure in man. Pyramidal tract takes origin from pyramidal cells including Betz cells of this area. It is responsible for individual movements.

Motor block Loss of voluntary movement caused by regional anesthesia .

Motor end plate Portion of the sarcolemma of a muscle fiber (cell) that receives neurotransmitter liberated by an axon terminal.

Motor learning Learning of a motor skill.

Motor memory The storage of motor programs or sub-programs for later retrieval and use.

Motor nerve A collection of nerve fibers that leave the spinal cord and brain and carry commands to muscles to make them contract.

Motor neuron Transmits nerve impulses from the brain and spinal cord to muscles and glandular epithelial tissues.

Motor neuron disease Disease of spinal cord/ brainstem motor neurons.

Motor paralysis Paralysis of the voluntary muscles.

Motor paretic gait Paralyis often influences gait in characteristic way. The paretic leg is exposed to weight bearing for shorter periods than healthy leg with central hemiparesis. There is circumduction, the leg is extended at the knee with slight plantar flexion of the foot.

Motor plan The combination of several motor programs into an action strategy.

Motor point The point of entry of a motor merve into muscle.

Motor point block Administration of a local anesthetic to a motor point within a muscle. Allows for more specificity than a nerve block.

Motor program A set of commands that, when initiated, results in the production of a coordinated movement sequence.

Motor projection areas Also called motor areas, this term has reference to the primary brain areas involved in the control of body movement. The cortical tissue at the rear or the frontal lobe is presumed to be most directly involved. The concept of projection refers to the relevance of specific areas for specific body movements.

Motor sequence A sequence of movements preprogrammed by the brain and produced as a unit.

Motor set Posture adopted prior to movement.

Motor unit The functional unit of neuromuscular system. It consist of anterior horncell, its axon, and all muscle fibres innervated by axon.

Mould 1. Form in which an object is cast or shaped. 2. The term used to specify the shape of an artificial tooth or teeth.

Moulding of fetal head It is the alteration in shape of the pliable vault of skull. This occurs due to over riding of skull bones at the surfaces. The engaging diameter is shortened by about 1.25 cm and compression in diameter is followed by expansion in another.

Moulding of head It occurs in normal delivery to allow some degree of adjustment to pressure.

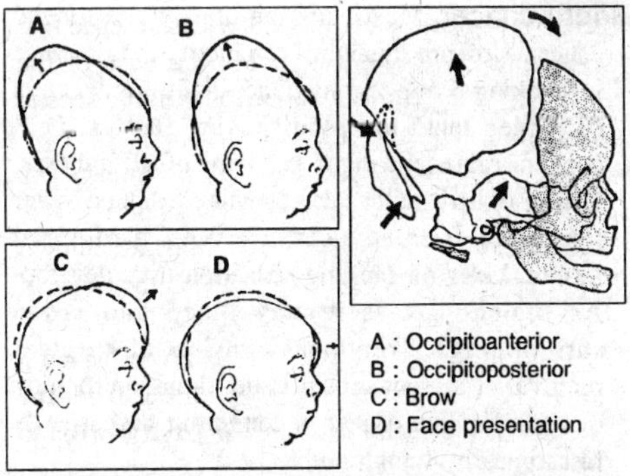

Mountain sickness It is an illness that can affect mountain climbers, hikers who attend the height of more than 8000 feet too rapidly. It is caused by reduced atmospheric pressure and reduced oxygen affecting nervous system. To avoid it one should climb gradually. Symptoms of disease are short-lived and are headache, dizziness and impaired mental process. In severe cases, fluid collects in lungs leading to severe breathlessness and froth.

Mounting The preparation of specimens and slides for study.

Mourning Reaction to a loss of a love object (important person, object, role, status, or anything considered part of one's life) consisting of a process of emotional detachment from that object which frees the subject to find other interests and enjoyment.

Mouth An opening or aperture; specifically, the anterior opening to the digestive tube.

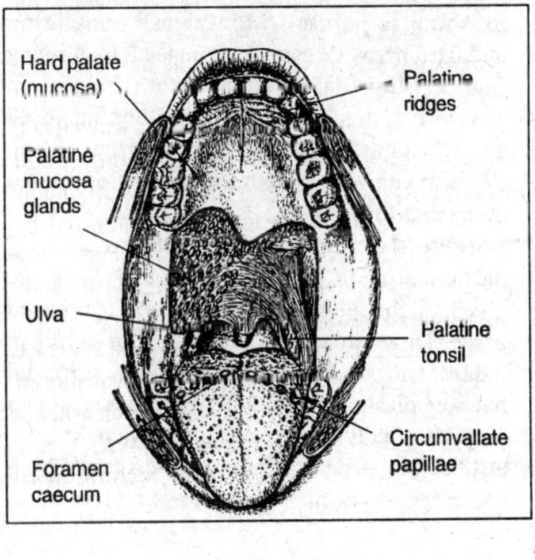

Mouth cancer Most common are lip and tongue cancer. Most are squamous carcinomas. Main cause is smoking. Poor oral hygiene, ill-fitting dentures or jagged teeth are predisposing factors. Oral cancers represent eight per cent of all cancers. Cancer of lip usually starts as white patch on lower lip. Lesion is small ulcer or a deep, hard edged fissure. Later on burning sensation may develop. As tumour grows it may bleed and erode surroundings. Treatment consists of surgical removal of all cancerous tissue, radiation therapy or both. Tongue cancer is dangerous and spreads fast to nearby lymph nodes.

Mouth dry It may be due to inadequate production of saliva. Dry mouth may be due to fear or salivary gland infection. Anticholinergic drugs may also lead to it. Radiation therapy also results in dry mouth. Dry mouth may result difficulty in speaking.

Mouth ulcers It is an open sore caused by a break in the mucous membrane lining the mouth. Ulcer may be round, oval, shallow, or yellow spots with an inflamed red border. Previously most common ulcer was of chancre followed by herpes simplex and cold sores. Mouth ulcer may be first stage of cancer. Any ulcer not healing in 6 to 8 weeks should be re-examined and investigated.

Mouth wash It is a solution to rinse the mouth. If used vigorously removes loose food debris from the tooth. Most antiseptic mouth washes intend to combat bad breath. But if used for long periods may irritate the mouth. In case of gingivitis even brushing is painful. Mouthwash containing hydrogen peroxide can clean the teeth by forming foams. Fluoride mouthwash are helpful in preventing dental caries strengthening tooth enamel and acting directly against plaque. Warm saline mouthwash helps in inflammation caused by tooth disorder.

Mouthguard Resilient intraoral device worn during participation in contact sports to reduce the potential for injury to the teeth and associated tissue. These protect the dentition from direct or indirect trauma. These are made from semirigid but soft plastics. Commonly used material is a polymer of polyvinylacetate and polyethylene.

Mouthstick A device held in the mouth by a handicapped person which allows the person to perform certain basic functions without the use of the hands. The devices include simple mouth-held sticks which permit only the most rudimentary activities, prostheses with grasping devices which are operated by use of the jaws.

Movement at elbow Movements which occur at elbow are flexion and extenion. The normal range is O° to 150°.

Movement of force Product of force and distance (moment arm) from any point to the action line of force.

Movement of Forearm When the palm is facing up the two bones are parallel. Palm up is called supination. When the palm is turned down the radius is crossed over the ulna. Palm down is called pronation.

Movement of vertebral column Lateral flexion of spine occurs in coronal plane and head and trunk bend towards one side. Rotation is movement in transverse plane. Extension of spine occurs in sagittal plane. Head and trunk bend backward.

Movement synergy Manner of operation of the primary motor cortex.

Movement therapies Aerobic exercise is related to decreased psychosexual stress.

Movement time The interval between initiation and completion of movement.

Movements It includes skeletal movements and movements of soft tissues and body organs. Skeletal movements consist of a change in position of two bones brought about by shortening of muscles attached to bones. Even in fairly simple movement several muscles are active, some contracting to initiate and others to maintain a movement. All voluntary skeletal movements are initiated in cerebrum called motor cortex. Signals are sent down the spinal cord along nerve fibres and from there along separate nerve fibres to appropriate muscles. Control depends on information supplied by sensory nerves. Skeletal movements can occur as a reflex action in response to certain sensory warning signals.

Movements of thumb Thumb is a very important part of hand in assisting its function. Movements include flexion, adduction, palmar abduction, opposition, ulnar adduction and radial abduction.

MRI Magnetic resonance imaging is a technique that provides high quality cross-sectional images of organs and structures within body without X-rays. During imaging patient lies inside a massive hollow, cylindrical magnet and is exposed to short bursts of powerful magnetic field. The protons of the body's hydrogen atoms normally point randomly in different directions but in magnetic field they line up in parallel to each other like rows of tiny magnets. If the hydrogen nuclei are then knocked out of alignment by strong pulse of radio waves they produce a detectable radio signals. Magnetic coils in the machine detect these signals and a computer changes them into an image based on strength of signal produced by different type of tissues. Tissues containing lot of hydrogen produces a bright image. No hydrogen produces black image. MRI also produces images in any planes. It is more useful in studying brain, spinal cord and knee joints.

M-RNA-Messenger Ribonucleic Acid It has the message to synthesize the protein encoded in the gene.

MS Mass Spectrometry

Mucigel Gelatinous material on a root surface, derived from plant sources mucilages, as well as microbial cells, soil colloids, and soil organic materials.

Mucilage Gelatinous organic materials released by a plant in the root cap region, derived from the Golgi apparatus, polysaccharide hydrolysis, and epidermal materials.

Mucin Secretion of the mucus or goblet cell; a polysaccharide protein which, combined with water, forms a lubricating solution called mucus, contained in saliva.

Mucobuccal fold Mucobuccal reflection; line of flexure of the oral mucous membrane as it passes from the mandible or maxillae to the cheek.

Mucocele The mucocele is a mucus containing cyst occurring in salivary gland. Cyst is initially seen as a small, circumscribed, elevated, translucent, bluish lesion of mucosa. If deep seated it can be palpated as a circumscribed, freely movable lesion. Lesion can occur anywhere except in anterior half of hard palate. Lip and tongue are the preferred sites. As soon as these appear to have healed they recur. Cycle of rupture, discharge and recurrence may go for months. Microscopically the fully developed lesions consist of cystic cavity filled with a basophilic homogeneous material—mucus. Round, swollen and degenerating cells are dispersed throughout this material.

Mucociliary transport The action of the cilia in mobilizing the mucus overlying the mucosa of the tracheobronchial tree.

Mucocutaneous Referring to an area of both exterior skin and mucus membranes, as at the borders of the mouth.

Mucocutaneous junction The transitional area where the skin and mucous membrane meet.

Mucogingival defect Improper shape of the gingiva or alveolar mucosa.

Mucokinetic An agent capable of enhancing the mobilization of mucus.

Mucolabial fold Line of flexure of the oral mucous membrane as it passes from the mandible or maxillae to the lip.

Mucolytic Destroying or dissolving mucus; an agent that destroys or dissolves mucus.

Mucomembranous Pertaining to or composed of mucous membrane.

Mucoperiosteal full-thickness flap All soft tissue in an area is incised and elevated.

Mucopurulent Characteristic of a combination of mucus and pus.

Mucopurulent conjunctivitis It often occurs in epidemic form and is called as pink eye or red eye by the patients. It is contagious and spreads directly by the conjunctival secretion and indirectly by fleas, fingers and use of common towels. Disease reaches its peak in 3 to 4 days. There is tendency for spontaneous recovery. There will be red eye with discharge. Discharge may be mucus, watery and mucopurulent discharge is seen in the fornix or at the margins of lids. Patient complains of a feeling of foreign body sensation. Person develops photophobia and matting of eylashes.

Mucor mycosis The fungus initially enters the paranasal sinuses. It extends cribriform plate to the CNS to involve the orbit and anterior fossa. Fungus invades blood vessels to cause haemorrhagic necrosis. CT shows haemorrhagic infarction or enhancing mass

Mucosa Mucous membrane consisting of the epithelium and connective tissue that line cavities opening to the outside of the body; many contain mucous glands, which secrete mucus.

Mucosa-associated lymphatic tissue (MALT) Lymphatic nodules scattered throughout the lamina propria (connective tissue) of mucous membranes lining the gastrointestinal tract, respiratory airways, urinary tract, and reproductive tract.

Mucosal Pertaining to the mucous membrane.

Mucosal lupus There develops clusters of round nodules in mucosa. The mucosal lesions are painless and progress very slowly with or without ulceration. There may be heavy scarring.

Mucosal split-thickness flap Epithelium and part of the underyling connective tissue are incised and separated from the remaining connective tissue and periosteum.

Mucositis Inflammation of mucus membrane.

Mucosocutaneous Pertaining to a mucous membrane and the skin.

Mucostatic An agent that arrests the section of mucus.

Mucosus otitis It is a mild otitis media with mild symptoms and a protracted course. There will be slight fullness and earache. Otoscopy shows a pale, thickened, doughy flaky tympanic membrane. There develops an infection with type III pneumococcus mucosus.

Mucous Pertaining to or resembling mucus.

Mucous membrane It is a surface layer of membrane upon other tissue which secretes and produces the lubricating and slippery fluid mucus. It is made up of epithelium containing multiple tiny glands. Many vessels and cavities like oral and vaginal are lined by mucous membrane.

Mucoviscidosis A disease of the exocrine glands, occurring chiefly in children but also in adults; so called because of the abnormally viscous mucoid secretions associated with the condition. It is transmitted as a recessive trait, and a characterized by obstruction of the pancreatic ducts, chronic pulmonary disorders, high levels of sodium chloride and potassium in the sweat, and susceptibility to infection.

Mucro The pointed end of a part or organ.

Mucus Viscid liquid which lubricates and protects mucous membranes from noxious elements, composed chiefly of mucin, a protein-carbohydrate complex, water inorganic salts, desquamated cells, and leukocytes. It is produced by gastric, intestinal, salivary, and other mucous glands.

Mucus membrane Tissue lining the oral cavity containing muscus glands.

Mucus-trap suction Suction using a catheter with a mucus trap; used to aspirate the newborn without the mucus being drawn into the nurse's mouth.

Muffuci's syndrome A rare congenital disorder of enchondromatosis with hemangiomatosis.

Muller's duct Paramesonephric duct

Mulling Final step of mixing dental amalgam.

Multiarticular Pertaining to or affecting several joints.

Multicellular Composed of many cells.

Multicentric Having many centers or points of origin.

Multicontaminated Contaminated by several different species or types of microorganisms.

Multicultural diversity Unique characteristics of ethnic groups.

Multienzyme system A group of related enzymes participating in a given metabolic pathway.

Multifactor studies Experimental investigation of the influence of several variables simultaneously. These variables may be additive, meaning that their total influence is equal to the sum of the separate influences, or interactive, in which case the influence of any one variable depends upon the presence, absence, or level of another variable. Multifactor studies are generally more complex than the traditional single-factor experimental design.

Multifactorial Pertaining to or due to many factors.

Multifidus There has been controversy regarding role of the smaller intersegmental muscles in stabilising lumbar spine. The multifidi span only

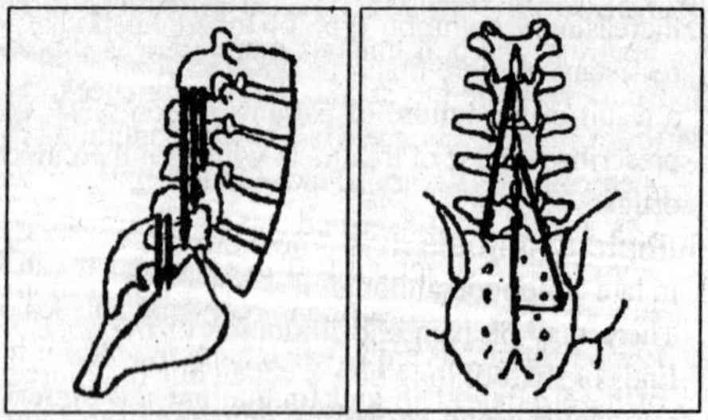

2 to 4 segments and lie very close to midline and centre of rotation of motion segment. The force vectors of multifidi indicate that they can generate posterior rotation in a sagittal plane.

Multifocal Arising from or pertaining to many foci.

Multifocal osteomyelitis The simultaneous occurence of acute or chronic bone injection at multiple bone sites.

Multiformat camera It is a camera used to transfer electronically acquired images into film. The camera contains an image projector which projects the image to be documented onto a predefined area of film which is exposed accordingly. Operator has several options for subdividing the film into different areas.

Multigated acquisition imaging (MUGA) It is a technique of nuclear cardiology. In it information from each of many cardiac cycles is combined to allow study of regional ventricular wall function. It helps in determining ejection fraction.

Multigravida A woman who has been pregnant more than once.

Multi-infarct dementia A cortical infarct due to occlusion of internal carotid may result in hemiplegia and focal deficits of aphasia. A lacunar infarctions may result in pure hemiplegia without cognitive impairment. Bilateral lacunate infarct may result in bilateral pyramidal lesions inducing shuffling short stepped gait. There may be some degree of dysarthria. There will be inappropriate weeping or laughter.

Multilobar Having numerous lobes.

Multiple Occurring in or affecting various parts of the body at once.

Multiple baseline design A single-system design in which several subjects are studied after baselines of varying lengths.

Multiple drug-resistant tuberculosis An increasingly common type of tuberculosis that is resistant of more htan one antimicrobial agent as a result of the failure of patients to completer the prescribed course of treatment with antituberculous drugs.

Multiple exostosis It is a hereditary disease seen in late childhood although it develops early in life. There may be pain and limitation of movements. Ends of shaft of long bones widen due to failure or remodelling and exostoses develop from there. Direction of growth is aways from epiphysis. Shortening of bone is frequently noted. Malignant degeneration is shown by fuzziness and irregularity of its outline.

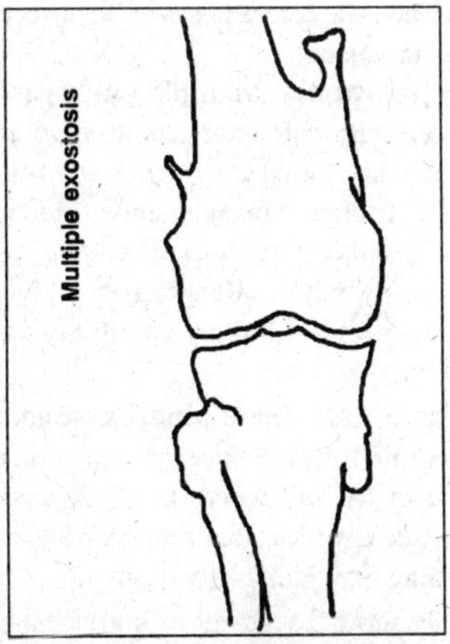

Multiple linear regression Method used in multivariable analysis if the dependent variable and all of the independent variables are continuous.

Multiple myeloma It is a malignant condition. It is characterised by the uncontrolled proliferation and disordered function of cells called plasma cells in bone marrow. As abnormal plasma cells expand within bone they cause pain and destruction of bone. It may cause numbness and paralysis when spines are affected. X-ray shows multiple punched-out areas and treatment includes anticancer drugs. 20 per cent patients with full care survive for five years.

Multiple organ failure Condition in which two or more organ systems gradually cease to function.

Multiple orgasm This is the ability to experience repeated orgasms without a refractory period between them. Only females have such capacity. Men require recovery period of several minutes or hours. Women are most likely to achieve multiple orgasm after they reach the age of 35 which is the peak of their sexual potency. Multiple orgasm may occur in second trimester of pregnancy when there is increased vasocongestion.

Multiple personality Memory disorder associated with history of abuse.

Multiple personality, disorder A rare mental disorder characterized by the development and existence or two or more relatively unique and independent personalities in the same individual.

Multiple placenta In a single pregnancy organ is divided into two lobes. One of the varieties of double lobed placenta is placenta bipartita and other is placenta duplex.

Multiple polyposis Multiple polyposis may be associated with osteomas, epidermoid cysts and soft tissue tumours and glioblastoma/ medulloblastoma. Management of adenomatous polyps involves search of whole colon by colonoscopy when adenomas are discovered anywhere in colon. Follow up all cases to watch for malignancy.

Multiple sclerosis Onset is rare before adolescence and after mid fifties. Plaques of demyelination can occur virtually any where in CNS. Person may develop sudden black out and blurring of vision. Every thing may look misty or grey.

MRI may show a segment of high signal in optic nerve in 85% of acute cases. The mean lesion length is about 10 mm. The hallmark of plaques in brainstem is impairment of balance and coordination of limb. Person may develop vertigo. Demyelination of afferent and efferent pathways in brainstem results.

A common site for a plaque is high in the posterior columns. Plaques are often symmetrical, tingling may occur in both upper limbs, hands and inner aspects of forearms.

There may be transient dysarthria or ataxia. This phenomenon may last only 20 to 30 minutes. In advanced multiple sclerosis euphoria may develop. Social disinhibition, impaired memory and frank dementia may afflict those with large zones.

Multiple sleep latency test Assessment of daytime sleepiness.

Multiplistic thinking A form of thinking in which all knowledge about the world is divided into certain categories, such as right, wrong, or unknown.

The individual understands that everything in the world has a significant element of uncertainty about almost everything. With this uncertainty in mind, the student may come to the pessimistic conclusion that nothing can be known or that all answers are equally uncertain.

Multipolar neuron A nerve cell with many processes originating from the cell body.

Multirooted having many roots; said of molar teeth.

Multisystem atrophy A neurological disorder frequently misdiagnosed as Parkinson's disease.

Multivariable models Statistical models that have one dependent (outcome) variable but include more than one independent variable.

Multivariate analysis A term that is frequently used incorrectly, it refers to methods for analyzing more than one dependent variable as well as more than one independent variable.

Mummification It is a desiccation of body and may occur in hot regions. Due to high temperature and moving air fluids of body evaporates rapidly and ordinary process of decomposition ceases. The tissues dry and shrivel. The skin hardens and becomes leathery in 12 to 24 hours.

Mumps It is an acute viral illness of childhood. There is inflammation and swelling of the parotid on one or both sides. Serious complications are uncommon. This spreads in airborne droplets. There is an incubation period of two to three weeks. Person can spread the virus to others for about a week before and up to two weeks after symptoms appear. Child first complains of pain in the region and has difficulty in chewing. Gland on one or both sides becomes painful and tender. Fever and headache may be there. Child may complicate with meningitis. A less common complication is pancreatitis causing abdominal pain and swelling. Male child may develop orchitis. Only one testis is affected and becomes tender. Subsequently the affected testis shrinks to smaller than normal size.

Munching An immature chewing motion that incorporates an up and down, vertical jaw movement.

Muramic acid A compound in bacterial cell walls, consisting of lactic acid and glucosamine joined by an ether linkage.

Murein Peptidoglycan, an outer layer of the bacterial cell wall; a biopolymer crosslinked by peptide bridges that are linked to the lactyl group of the muramic acid residues.

Murine Pertaining to mice.

Murmur An abnormal sound produced within the heart.

Murphy's sign The patient is asked to take deep breath and the examiner palpates the right upper quadrant. Murphy's sign is positive when a touch to the gall-bladder instantly elicits pain and an arrest in breathing. It is seen in the cases of inflammation of the gall bladder.

Muscarinic receptor A subtype of acetylcholinergic receptor; historically, activated by muscarine.

Muscle Elastic tissue that moves the joints by helping them fix, extend, or rotate, depending on how the joints are designed.

Muscle balance A state of equilibrium that exists when there is a balance of strength of opposing muscles acting on a joint, providing ideal alignment for movement and optimal stabilization.

Muscle contraction headache It is associated with occipital pain or pain radiating to frontal area. It may be caused by spasm, injury or inflammation.

Muscle dystrophy It is a muscle disorder of unknown cause in which there is slow degeneration of muscle fibres.

A blood test may be performed to look for high levels of certain enzymes released from the damaged muscle cells. EMG and muscle biopsy helps. There is no effective treatment.

Muscle endurance and strength Patient performing on bicycle increases cardiovascular and muscular endurance. A slow gradual build-up is

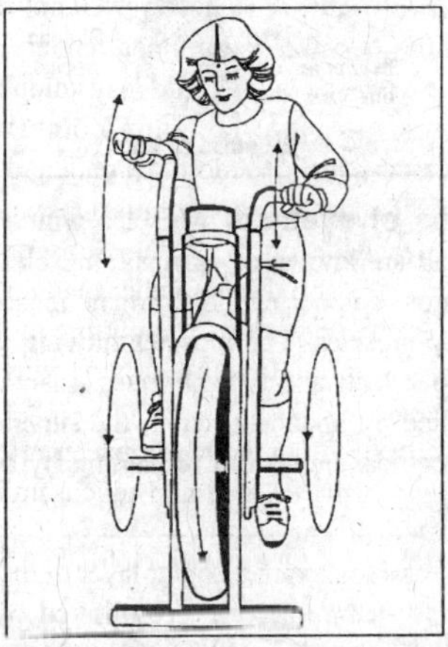

important to avoid overuse injury. Each programme should begin with a short session of 5 to 10 minutes and progress according to patient's tolerance.

Muscle fatigue It is usually defined as inability to maintain the required or expected force output. It may also be described as a loss of force generating capacity of muscle.

It is also described as an impairement in the force and power generating capacity of muscle with decline in maximal force and in the rate of force development as fatigue sets in. The marked slowing of muscular relaxation is another feature.

Muscle fiber The specialized contractile cells of muscle tissue that are grouped together and arranged in a highly organized way.

Muscle grades A relatively subjective means of assessing muscle strength.

Muscle hook It is used to engage the muscle during the squint surgery or surgery involving the extraocular muscle like detachment surgery.

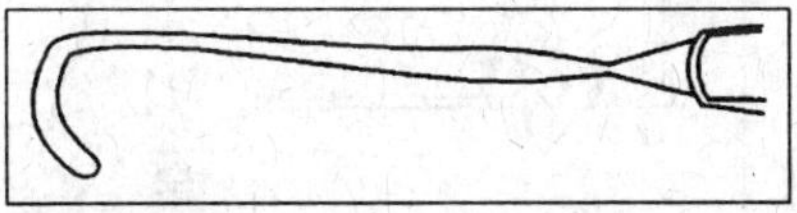

Muscle imbalance Inequality in strength of opposing muscles; a state of muscle imbalance exists when a muscle is weak and its antagonist is strong; leads to faults in alignment and inefficient movement.

Muscle load The actual resistance an exercised muscle overcomes.

Muscle relaxant These are the drugs which relaxes the muscles and are used for premedication before surgery. These are used for muscular spasm.

Muscle relaxant drugs It is a group of drugs to relieve muscle spasm and spasticity. These are generally used in combination with analgesics to relieve muscle spasm. These generally block nerve signals from the brain and spinal cord that stimulate different muscles to contract. These may result in drowsiness.

Muscle spasms Sudden, forceful, involuntary muscle contractions.

Muscle spindle This is a fusiform body 1.4 mm long and 0.1-0.2 in diameter, lying between the muscle bundles with its long axis. Large nerve fibres pass to the spindle, break up into branches and lose their medullary sheaths. The spindle also receives efferent fibres with usual motor end plates. These are known as stretch receptors. These are absent in muscles of face and tongue. Sensory organs within skeletal muscles composed of intrafusal fibers. They are sensitive to muscle stretch and provide a length detector within muscles.

Muscle strength It is evaluated by isometric contraction of muscle or group of muscle against resistence offered by examiner. Nearly every muscle or muscle group of head and neck region can be evaluated by this method. Muscle hypertrophy and atrophy can be noted and may indicate myofacial pain.

Muscle strength training To effect gains in strength the muscle must be progessively overloaded. Greater demand is put on the muscle

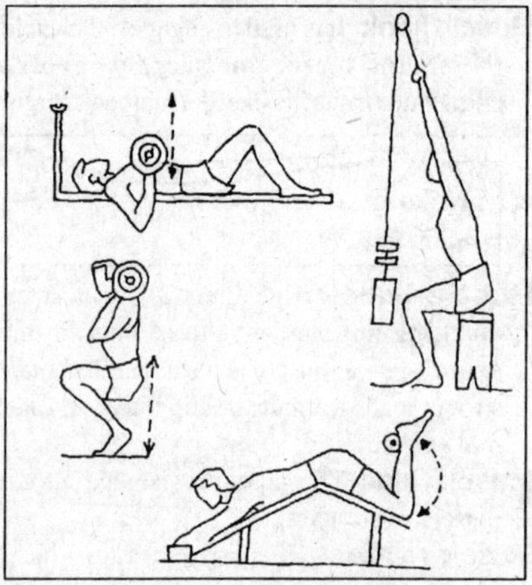

which is greater than normally required or used such as maximum voluntary contractions. Training stimulus should be varied, e.g. alternating high repetitions at low loads with sessions using heavier loads and fewer repetitions.

Muscle Testing of larynx The larynx during swallowing. Examiner lightly grasp the larynx with the thumb and the index finger on the anterior throat to determine the fact of elevation and its extent.

Muscle tissue One of the four major tissue types; consists of cells with the ability to contract; includes skeletal, cardiac, and smooth muscle.

Muscle tone This is the ongoing action of a muscle or group of muscles with purpose of controlling or preserving some position. Muscle stretch is perceived by muscle spindle receptors, relayed by sensory nerve fibres to the spinal cord, activating the anterior horn cells which in turn stimulates the muscle fibres. Catecholamines, hypocalcaemia and alkalosis increase muscle tone while hypoxia, hypotension and anaesthesia reduce muscle tone.

Muscle trimming Shapping of an impression material by the manipulation or action of the tissues adjacent to the borders of an impression.

Muscle twitch Contraction of an entire muscle in response to a stimulus that causes an action potential in one or more muscle fibres.

Muscles One of the contractile organs of body that affects movement of various body parts. Muscle can be skeletal, cardiac or smooth. Skeletal muscle is voluntary.

Muscles of back There are six pairs of large muscles in the back, i.e. trapezius major, trapezius minor, psoas, quadratus lumborum, sacrospinalis and latissimus dorsi.

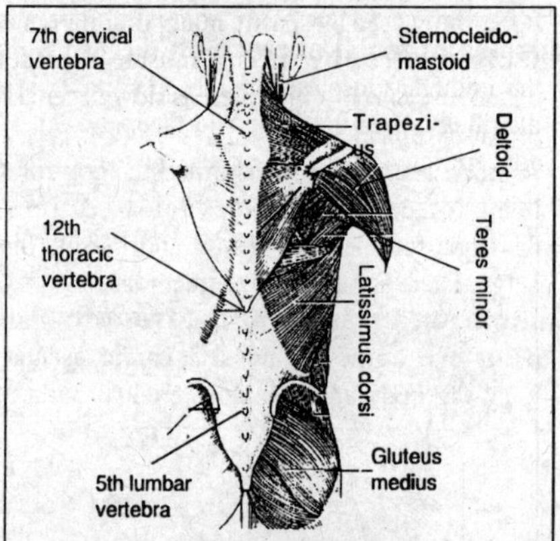

Muscles of back

Muscles of eyeballs Muscles which move the eyeball are known as extrinsic muscles including elevator of upper eyelid. Intrinsic muscles are the ciliary muscles. The muscles moving the eyeball are four recti and two obliques. Lateral rectus is supplied by abducent nerve, the superior oblique by trochlear nerve and remaining by oculomotor nerve.

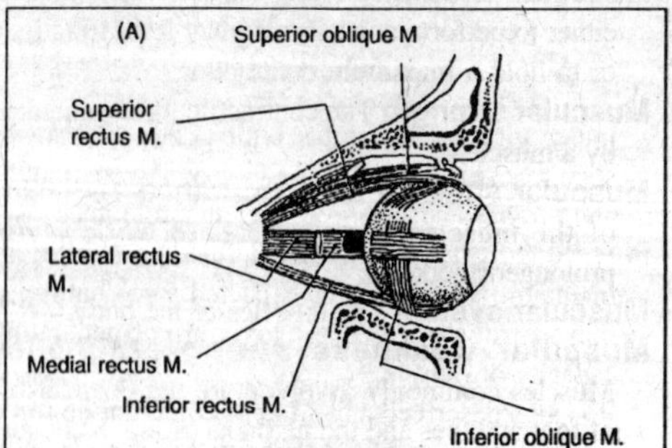

Muscles of eye

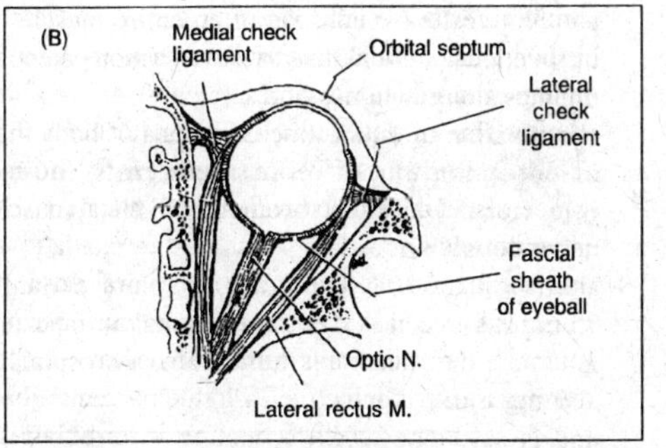

Muscles of facial expression Frequently called the mimetic muscles; variable in contour, widely distributed over the scalp and face, and espeically concerntrated about the orbits, outer ear, and lips.

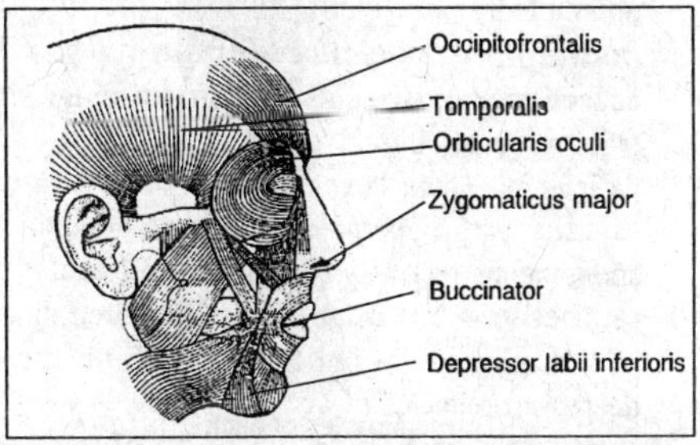

As a group they have only one bony origin in the facial skeleton. The muscles from a circular rim around the perimeter of the facial bones and extend anteriorly as a tube of tissue in which the lumen narrows and terminates in the orbicularis oris.

Muscles of mastication Powerful muscles that elevate and rotate the mandible so that the opposing teeth may occlude for mastication.

Muscular endurance The capacity of a muscle either to perform at a submaximal level to fatigue or to hold a maximum contraction.

Muscular strength The contractile force generated by a muscle.

Muscular strength and endurance The ability of the muscles to perform hard work and/or prolonged work.

Muscular system The muscles of the body.

Muscular weakness during pregnancy Muscles commonly involved are the dorsiflexors of foot and toes and the paroneal group. Knee jerk is often diminished on the affected side. In severe cases weakness and pain continues after labour. Full recovery takes about a year.

Muscularis Two layers of muscle surrounding the digestive tube that produce wave-like, rhythmic contractions, called peristalsis, which move food material.

Muscularis mucosa The inner, thin layer of smooth muscle found in most parts of the digestive tube outside the lamina propria.

Musculo A prefix meaning muscle.

Musculo skeletal Pertaining to muscle and bony skeleton.

Mushroom intoxication Toxic mushrooms account for 50 to 100 of about 5000 species. Short incubation period mushroom poisoning is rapid acting and affects autonomic nervous system. It produces sweating, lacrimation, blurred vision, miosis and watery diarrhoea. Treatment is supportive and atropine is limited to severe poisoning. Symptoms subside in 24 hours.

Music therapy It has been shown to produce physiologic relaxation effects. It is employed in operation theatres now a days.

Must in wine making, expressed grape juice or the mashed grape before and during fermentation.

Mustard foot bath Mustard is available in two forms : white mustard and black mustard. The volatile oil of white mustard is a powerful rubefacient and oil of black mustard is external irritant. If a poultice or mustard is left over the skin for long time it may cause intense pain and blister. It helps in to draw blood to the surface of body to combat effect of bad cold and infection.

Mutagen A chemical or physical agent that induces genetic mutations.

Mutagenesis The generation of mutations; any alteration or aberration in the native sequence of DNA that results in permanently inheritable changes in the organism.

Mutagens Chemical substances which damage the sturcture of DNA cell and can develop into a cancer cell.

Mutant An organism that carries a mutation; i.e., an altered or new genetic sequence that is inheritable.

Mutases Enzymes that catalyze the transposition of functional groups.

Mutation An abrupt, inheritable change in the nucleotide sequence of an organism. Mutations include base pair substitutions, deletions, duplications, transpositions/translocations, and inversions. Mutations can arise spontaneously and can also be induced by certain chemicals and by radiation. The rates of spontancous mutation in viruses and bacteria are controlled by DNA replication and repair enzymes.

Mutism Condition of being unable to speak.

Mutual Reciprocal.

Mutual orgasm It is the simultaneous orgasm at the same time. Many couples prefer it. However, preoccupation with this will hamper the sexual enjoyment. There may be some advantage to the woman achieving several separate orgasms, the first and the last of which may be made to coincide with man's ejaculation.

Mutual pair In a group, two members mutually attracted. They prefer one another's company and show no preference for other group members.

Mutualism A symbiotic relationship in which each partner is physiologically dependent on the other.

Myalgia It means pain in muscles. It is common in influenza and in rheumatic disorder, Systemic lupus erythematosus (SLE) and polymyalgia rheumatica. Myalgia is a main symptom of polyomyositis and causes of inflammation.

Myasthenia 'Muscle weakness'.

Myasthenia gravis It is an illness characterised by periocular, facial, bulbar and girdle weakness. It is associated with presence of antibodies to acetylcholine receptor protein. Antibodies are found in 85 per cent of patient. The titre of antibodies is lowest in patients with purely ocular myasthenia, intermediate in those thymic hyperplasia and highest in those with a thymoma. The external ocular muscles are first to be involved causing ptosis and diplopia. The shoulder girdle muscles are frequently involved. It becomes difficult to raise hand above head. Person may feel difficulty in chewing meat. Ophthalmoplegia is a common presenting symptom. Generalisation to other muscles usually begins within 2 years of onset. Fatiguability is a prominent feature. Chewing at the end of meal is more tiring. During the course of taking history progressive casuality of speech may be noted. Facial muscles may become flattened and jaw sags. Tongue may waste in a typical way developing furrows. Short-acting anticholinesterase edrophonium can be injected intravenously. Weakness will reverse in 1 to 5 minutes along with many of clinical features. One minute after an initial dose of 2 mg further 8 mg of edrophonium chloride is given by bolus injection. Patient should be warned of uncomfortable intestinal peristalsis, fasciculations and lacrimation. Neostigmine in an oral dose of 15 mg has an action that is no longer than 2 hours. Alternate day treatment with prednisolone up to 100 mg a day is effective in inducing remission, and is associated with a decline in circulating concentrations of antiacetylcholine receptor antibody. Immunosuppression can also be accomplished with azathioprine 2 to 5 mg/kg/day or with cyclosporin 6 mg/kg/day. Thymectomy is undoubtedly effective.

Myasthenia gravis pseudopara-lyticus It is caused by impairment of neuromuscular signal transmission based on acetylcholinesterase deficiency. There develops rapid decline in vocal capacity with hypernasal speech to aphonia with spontaneous recovery following brief rest.

Myasthenic syndrome It is an acquired disorder of neuromuscular junction in which there is decreased released of acetylcholine.

Mycelium The vegetative body of a fungus, composed of a cumulative mass of hyphae.

Mycetoma A chronic cutaneous and subcutaneous infection resulting from direct implantation of actinomycetes or true fungi. These are inflammatory masses within prior lung cavities usually from

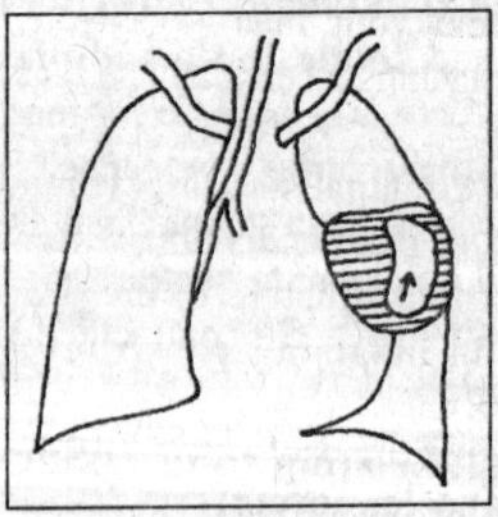

chronic. T.B. They are due to fungal injection especially aspergillosis. Patient develops hemoptysis.

Mycobacterium A bacterial genus containing at least 30 different species, including M. tuberculosis and M. leprae, the causative agens of tuberculosis and leprosy, respectively. Members of this genus are also opportunistic pathogens and are common causes of infection in AIDS patients. Although this group of bacteria is positive by gram stain, the bacteria are not true gram-positive organisms, but are classified as acid-fast bacilli, a staining characteristic that is attributed to the unique cell wall of mycobacteria.

Mycobacterium avium-intracellular An aerobic, nonmotile bacteria containing gram-positive, acid-fast, straight, or slightly curved rods.

Mycobacterium leprae It is mentioned in Vedas in 1500 BC as 'kusht rog'. The bacilli are straight or slightly curved 4-6 mm long and 0.3 to 0.5 mm in diameter. These are arranged in bundles or clusters like matchstick pack or pack of cigars. These are acid and alcohol fast. The organisms may be stained uniformly or may show beading. These are non-motile non-sporing and non capsulated. It causes leprosy.

Mycobacterium tuberculosis Occurrence of tuberculosis in bones of some Egyptian mummies suggest that tuberculosis is a disease of an ancient times. Tubercle bacilli are slightly curved rod-shaped organism measuring 2 to 4 micrometre. The ends are rounded, pointed and rarely expanded. These are acid-fast bacilli. Acid-fastness is partly due to presence of mycotic acid. Affected lymph glands show tubercle bacilli.

Mycology The scientific study of fungi.

Mycoplasmal Of pertaining to, or caused by mycoplasmas.

Mycoplasms Members of the class Mollicutes, a group of prokaryotic microorganisms resembling bacteria but lacking a cell wall and thus of variable morphology.

Mycorrhiza A mutualistic association coevolved between a host plant and a fungus localized in the root or root-like structure of the plant; this aids the plants in obtaining phosphorus and other elements.

Mycorrhizal Relating to or taking part in a relationship of mycorrhiza.

Mycosis A disease caused by the active invasion of living tissue by actively growing fungi Also mycotic infection.

Mycosis fungoides It is a T cell lymphoproliferative disorder that primarily invades the skin but may evolve into generalised lymphoma. It is caused by the proliferation of dermal reticuloendothelial cells. Histological changes are not specific. It gives rise to generalised persistent itching until the condition becomes fatal. In premycotic stage it gives rise to a variety of lesions, local and generalised such as papules, plaques, bullous eruptions. In infiltrative type there are well-defined areas of infiltration of skin. Lesions may ulcerate. Splenomegaly and enlargement of lymph nodes are common. In tumour stage there are nodules of various size. Nodules tend to breakdown in early stages and produce deep oval ulcers with necrotic greyish base.

Mycostasis A stopping inhibition of the growth of fungi; fungistasis.

Mycostat An agent that inhibits the growth of the fungi; fungal.

Mycotic hypopyon ulcer It may be the result of infection with fungus such as *Aspergillus fumigatus* or *Candida albicans*. In this corneal ulcer is dry and surrounded with satellites and yellow line of demarcation and mild hypopyon. There is marked circumciliary congestion. Vascularisation is absent usually medical therepy is not sufficient. Therapeutic keratoplasty is considered the treatment to save the eye.

Mydriatics Drugs which when applied locally dilate the pupil of the eye, Myotics constrict it.

Myelencephalon The posterior portion of the hindbrain that contains the medulla oblongata.

Myelin Lipoprotein derived from multiple layers of cell membrane encasing the axons of myelinated neurones.

Myelin sheath A lipoprotein envelope made by wrappings of the cell membrane of a Schwann cell or oligodendrocyte around an axon

Myelination The nerve fibres receive their myelin sheath at different ages and it is only after myelination that they begin to function . The peripheral nerves and nerve roots become myelinated in the first half of fifth month of fetal life. The sensory tracts of cord become myelinated first. Pyramidal tracts do not get myelinated. Myelination is not complete until about second year of life when child learns to walk.

Myelitis It is the inflammation of spinal cord. It may be the result of viral infection. Illness starts suddenly with headache, fever, neck stiffness and pain in back. Transverse myelitis is a type of myelitis in which there is inflammation of spinal cord. Common symptoms are back pain and gradual paralysis of legs.

Myelo Prefix pertaining the spinal cord.

Myeloblastemia The presence of myeloblasts in the circulating blood.

Myelocele A form of spina bifida associated with an open neural tube.

Myelofibrosis Fibrosis of bone marrow.

Myelogram A graphic representation of the differential count of cells found in a stained representation of bone marrow.

Myeloid Pertaining to bone marrow.

Myeloid epulis Pathologically it is an osteoclastoma arising from the mucoperiosteum of gum. Microscopically it consists of fibrocellular tissue scattered through which multinucleated giant cells are seen. It commonly occurs between the age of 10 and 25 years. It is common in lower jaw near the angle of mandible. It is rapidly growing painless tumour presenting under the gums. Swelling is soft and sessile, surface is smooth and lobulated. The overlying mucous membrane of gum becomes hyperaemic and oedematous. It looks dark red and plum coloured and may bleed and ulcerate. Extension of bone occurs both externally and internally. Draining lymph nodes are not enlarged.

Myelopathy Compression of spinal cord or cauda equina.

Myelophthisis An inflammation of spinal cord and roots of spinal nerve.

Myelosuppression Suppression of the production of the blood cells from the bone marrow.

Myenteric plexus A network of sympathetic and parasympathetic nerve fiber located in the muscularis tunic of the small intestine; also called the plexus of Auerbach.

Mylohyoid ridge A linear prominence of bone located on the internal surface of the mandible; appears radiopaque.

Myo Prefix indicating muscle.

Myoarthropathies It is caused by use of muscles of mastication unphysiologically. There will be faulty loading of temporomandibular joints (TMJs). Otalgia and tinnitus may occur in addition to headache and neck pain. Emotional disturbance may be there.

Myocardial contractility Force with which the myocardium contracts. On it stroke volume and cardiac output depends.

Myocardial degeneration It may cause reduced tonicity causing dilatation of heart. There may be failure of contractibility causing circulatory inadequacy and irregularities of rhythm. On exertion there is undue dyspnoea, marked lassitude, palpitation and angina of effort. Cardiac irregularities include premature beats often exaggerated by exercise. Auricular fibrillation and occasionally auricular flutter may be there. Dyspnoea may be present at night, cardiac impulse is feeble and heart sounds are poor and radial pulse week.

Myocardial infarction It develops when there is no blood supply to the segment of heart muscle due to occlusion of one of branches of coronary artery. Most commonly occluded are anterior descending branch, right coronary artery, left coronary artery and left circumflex artery. Infarction does not involve the right ventricle, usually coronary thrombosis is the most common cause. Typical retrosternal pain of angina pectoris is present but unlike angina pectoris it starts at rest, persists longer and is not relieved by coronary dilators. Breathlessness, cough, frothy and blood-stained sputum may be present. Due to cardiogenic

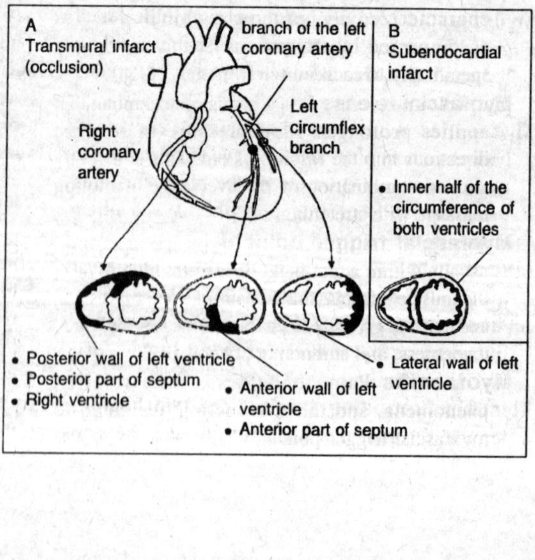

shock limbs may become cold, severe sweating, restlessness and confusion may be present. Fever may rise upto 39°C with leucocytosis and high ESR.

BP is low and continuously slows down. Pulse is high. Central cyanosis may be present. Abnormal Q wave is diagnostic of infarction.

Myocardial infarcts-Types Myocardial infarct is ischemic necrosis of myocardium. It may be either transmural or subendocardial.

Myocardial metabolism Myocardial O_2 consumption is normally about 30 mL/min.

Myocarditis It is the inflammation of heart muscle. It is a feature of rheumatic fever. Acute pericarditis accompanies myocarditis. Most of mild cases may clear up with corticosteroid. Exercise is to be avoided in case or myocarditis.

Myocardium The middle and thickest layer of the heart wall, composed of cardiac muscle.

Myoclonus Shocklike contraction of part of a muscle, an entire muscle, or a group of muscles.

Myodesis Method of muscle stabilization following amputation in which the cut muscle is sutured to periosteum or bone.

Myoepicardial mantle A thickening of the splanchnic mesenchyme around the outside of the endocardial heart tube.

Myofascial closure Mehtod of muscle stabilization following amputation in which muscle is sutured to fascia; often used in combination with myoplasty.

Myofascial pain syndrome Pain syndrome characterized by pain in regional muscles accompanied by trigger points that refer pain specifically to each muscle.

Myofascial release It is a hands on technique that applies prolonged light pressure in specific directions into the fascial system. This is a gently applied combination of passive range of motion massage with stretching.

Myofascial trigger point Hyperirritable spot, usually within a taut band of skeletal muscle or in the muscle's fascia, that is painful on compression and that can give rise to characteristic referred pain, tenderness, and autonomic phenomena.

Myofascitis Pain, tenderness, other referred phenomena, and the dysfunction attributed to myofascial trigger points.

Myofibril A fine longitudinal fibril of skeletal muscle consisting of sarcomeres, composed of thick (myosin) and thin (actin) myofilaments, placed end to end.

Myofibrillar Pertaining to the fine longitudinal fibrils occurring in skeletal or cardiac muscle fibers.

Myofibrosis Replacement of muscle tissue by fibrous tissue.

Myofilament An ultramicroscopic protein thread helping to form myofibrils in skeletal muscle; thin myofilaments are composed of actin, and thick myofilaments are composed of myosin.

Myogeloses These are local hardenings of muscles which are painful on pressure. These may be of two types : one is thread like another is round or

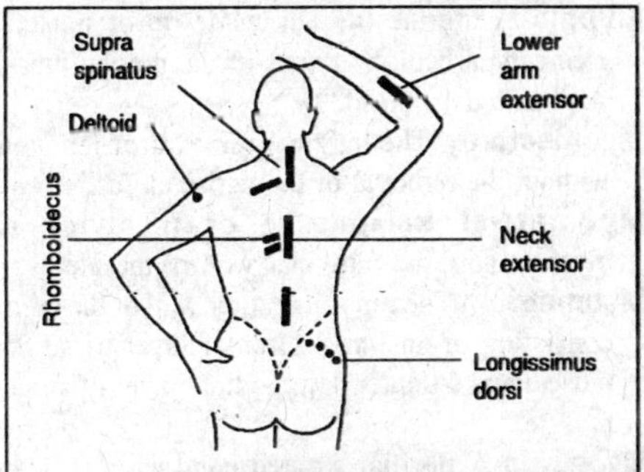

Myogelosus points

oval. Entire muscle may also be hardened because of surplus of metabolic wastes. Emotion and muscular tension may also result it.

Myogenic Originating within muscle cells; used to describe self-excitation by carfiac and smooth muscle cells.

Myogenic pain Pain stemming from dysfunctional muscular activity as part of motor behaviour in relation to stress, posture, movement and emotion.

Myogenic rhythm The intrinsic, spontaneous rhythm possessed by each cardiac myocyte.

Myoglobin Iron containing molecule with molecular weight 17000 similar to hemoglobin but binds only one molecule of 0_2 per molecule.

Myoglobinuria There is presence of myoglobin in the urine. It colours urine red and results from muscle breakdown.

Myognathus A developmental abnormality characterized by the presence of a supernumerary lower jaw attached to the normally placed mandible.

Myogram A recording of electrical activity within a muscle.

Myography Recording of muscular contraction.

Myokymias Waves of contraction that repeatedly affect new fibres and pass over muscles or muscle groups are called myokymias. There may be a symptom of continuous fibre activity. In the face appear as facial myokymia.

Myolipoma Myoma containing fatty or lipomatous elements.

Myology The study of muscles, and the body of knowledge relating thereto.

Myolysis Degeneration or disintergration of muscle tissue.

Myoma A uterine tumour made up of muscular elements; a benign tumour of the uterine muscle. Also called a fibroid.

Myomectomy The surgical removal of leimyoma without the removal of the entire uterus.

Myometrial Relating to or involving the myometrium, the muscular wall of the uterus.

Myometrium The muscular outer wall of the uterus, consisting of an inner, circular layer of smooth muscle and an outer, longitudinal layer of smooth muscle.

Myoneme A fibrillar striated contractile structure located in the cytoplasm of some protozoa ciliates, sporozoa, dinoflagellates. They are partially responsible for cell contraction.

Myoneural junction The junction between a motor neuron and a muscle fibre.

Myopic eye Myopic eyeball is too long thereby the retina is placed far backward than its normal position. In myopia the parallel rays coming from distant object have come to focus before reaching the retina, focus is formed in front of retina. So myopic cannot see the distant objects but can see clearly near objects.

Myoplasm The contractile part of muscle cell.

Myorhythmias These are rhythmic twitches occurring with a frequency of 1 to 3 per second, repeatedly affecting same muscle group with definitive but not pronounced movements. Myorhythmias of short duration are found as harmless in the region of orbicularis oculi. Around the mouth they can cause rhythmic protrusion of tongue. Hiccough is a myorhythmia of diaphragm.

Myosalpnix The muscle layer of the oviduct.

Myosin A thick myofilament protein that together with actin causes muscle contraction.

Myosin myofilament One of the two major kinds of protein fibres of a sarcomere; thick filament, resembles bundles of gold clubs.

Myositis Inflammatory disease of striated muscle.

Myositis ossificans circumscripta A localised area of myositis ossificans that occurs without a history of trauma.

Myotasis Stretching of muscle.

Myotatic reflex 'Muscle touching'. Tendon reflex.

Myotatic unit A group of agonist and antagonist muscles that function together as a unit because they share common spinal reflex responses.

Myotome Myotomes are only approximations of nerve root innervation. Positive signs of neurological involvement include diminished or loss of sensation, muscle weakness, muscle wasting and decreased or absent deep tendon reflex.

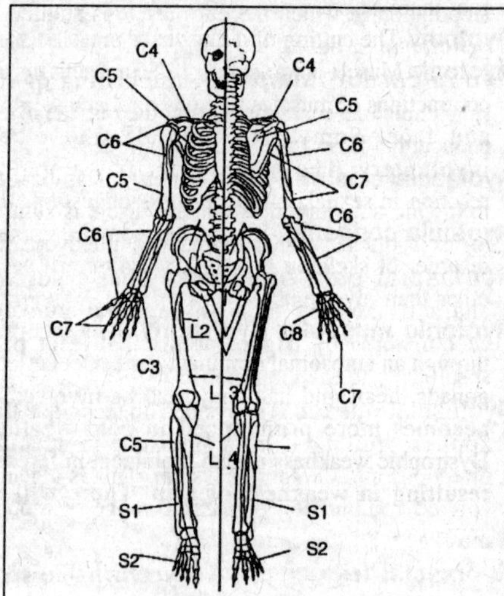

Dermatomes : anterior view.

Myotomes and dermatomes Positive signs of neurological involvement includes diminished or loss of sensations, muscle weakness, muscle wasting and decreased or increased deep tendon reflex in the distribution of affected nerve root. Dermatomes

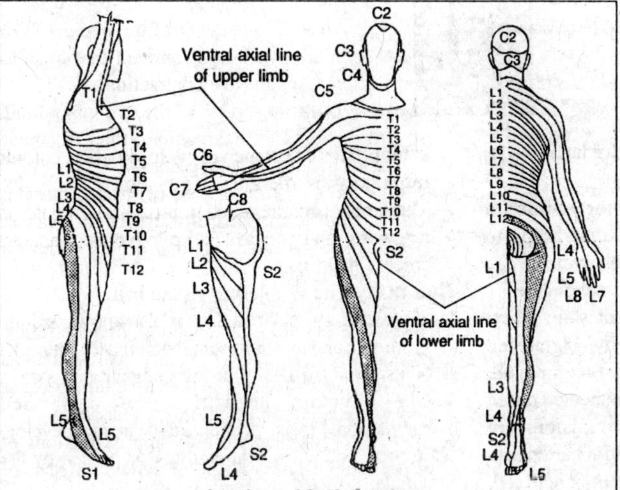

Anterior and Posterior view

and myotomes are only approxi-mation of nerve root innervation.

Myotomy The cutting of a muscle or muscle tissue.

Myotonia Muscle contractions; in sexual activity, the contractions of muscles in the genital areas, limbs, and face. Some are voluntary and others involuntary. The other major physiological reaction in sexual activity is vasocongestion.

Myotonia congenita It is an autosomal dominant disorder of skeleton muscle. No symptoms occur other than myotonia.

Myotonic muscular dystrophy It is inherited through an autosomal dominant gene. Ocular lens, gonads, heart and hair may also be involved. It becomes more pronounced in cold weather. Dystrophic weakness is also prominent in forearm resulting in weakness of grip. There will be premature baldness in a male distribution, premature cataracts, atrophy of testicles and cardiomyopathy, Mental retardation is common. Tendon reflexes are depressed or absent and nerve conduction shows slowing of velocity. Muscle biopsy shows nuclei lying in centre of muscle fibres and splitting of it. Type I fibres tend to be atrophied and type II hypertrophied. Severe disability results in 15 years.

Myplasty Method of muscle stabilization following amputation in which muscle is sutured to muscle; the cut flexor and extensor muscle are surgically attached; often used in combination with myofascial closure.

Myringotomy knife It is a slender, angulated instrument. It has short lancet-shaped blade at the tip. It is used for incising the tympanic membrane. Indications of myringotomy are excessive pain, imminent perforation and increasing hearing problem.

Myxedema Condition caused by deficiency of thyroid hormone in adults.

Myxobacteria Aerobic, free-living, rod-shaped gliding gram-negative bacteria that grow primarily in soil, on tree bark, on herbivore animal dung, and on decaying vegetation. Their distinguishing characteristic is the formation of multicellular structures called fruiting bodies.

Myxospore An asexual, dormant cell produced within the fruiting body.

N

Nacrcotic analgesic drug A drug that has sedavite and pain-relieving properties.

NAD Micotinamide adenine dinucleotide; a coenzyme derived from niacin that helps to transport electrons from the Krebs cycle to the electron-transport chain within mitochondria.

Naevi These are a primary lesions of skin. Naevi are occasionally seen in oral cavity. Pigmented naevi are of four types—junctional, compound, intramucosal and blue. These are pigmented raised Lesions of 0.1 to 0.5 cm in size. Lesions are asymptomatic and are mostly located at hard palate and lip. The essential component of junctional, compound and intra-mucosal types is the naevus cell and its location is based upon the distinction between these three types. The naevus cell is a small, round or polyhedral cell with distinctly outlined homogeneous or clear cytoplasm and a centrally located nucleus. Cells are usually found in clusters. Blue naevus is a rare type of pigmented lesion which occurs as a single, smooth, firm, round bluish area of less than 1 cm in size.

Nail These form dorsal surfaces of tips of fingers and toes. These help limit distortion of phalanges during mechanical stress. Body of nail covers the nail bed and nail production occurs at nail root. The deepest portion of nail root lies very close to periosteum of bone of fingertip. A portion of stratum corneum of the fold extends over the exposed nail nearest the root forming eponychium.

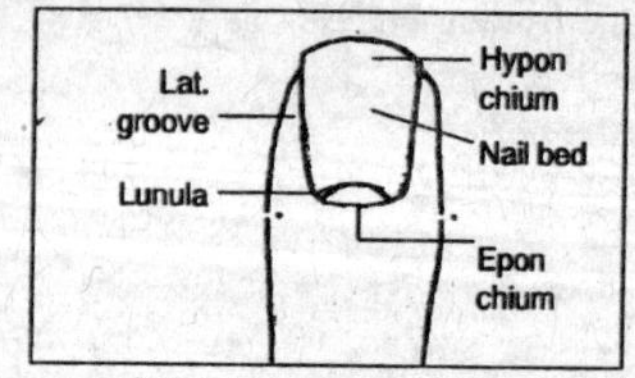

Underlying blood vessels give the nail its pink colour but near root these vessels may be obscure leaving a pale crescent known as lanula. The free edge of nail extends over a thickened stratum corneum, the hypochonium. Body of nail consists of dead, tightly compressed cells packed with keratin. These become yellow in jaundice, chronic respiratory disorders, thyroid dysfunction or AIDS. These may become pitted in psoriasis, irregular in ringworm and concave in koilonychia. Anaemia colours them pale.

Nail body The visible part of the nail.

Nail patella syndrome This is also known as little syndrome and is an autosomal dominant syndrome. Nails are dystrophied or are congenitally absent. One develops nephritis, proteinuria and haematuria. Ptosis, glaucoma and cataract develop.

Nail root The part of the nail that is hidden by the cuticle.

Nailing The operation of fixing or fastening of a fractured bone with a nail.

Nalidixic acid It is an antibiotic to treat and prevent urinary tract infection. It is very effective antibiotic. Adverse effect includes nausea, increased sensitivity to sunlight and blurred vision.

Nalorphine A drug that blocks opioid receptors.

Naloxone Half-life is 75 minute. It is a pure competitive anta-gonist at all opioid receptors. It induces an acute withdrawal syndrome in opioid dependent patient. Given IV it causes reversal of opioid induced respiratory depression in 1-2 minutes. It acts for about one hour after an IV of 100 to 200 micrograms. Naloxone is also used to counter excess opioid effects after surgical analgesia and child birth. It is derived from potent oxymorphone which is 10 times as strong as morphine. It was synthesised in 1972. It is more effective antagonist of narcotic-induced respiratory depression. Duration of effect is lesser. It has no intrinsic agonist activity. It also prevents the impairment of psychomotor performance of low doses of alcohol. It can be used in opiate-induced respiratory depression. It may cause acute pulmonaray oedema and even sudden death.

Nandrolone It is an anabolic steroid and is used in the treatment of short stature. It may be used to treat certain types of anaemia. Possible side-effects include swollen ankles and aggressive behaviour.

Nanogram One thousand millionth of a gram.

Nanometer A measure of length in the metric system; one billionth of a meter.

Napkin rash It develops due to wet or soiled napkins. Prolonged contact with ammoniated urine can produce the condition. Condition produces superficial inflammatory reaction over thigh, genitalia, perineum and lower abdomen. Lesion may be vesicular or ulcerative in severe form. In males tip of penis may become irritated and crushed. *Candida* and bacteria may cause secondary infection.

Narcissism (narcism) Self-love as opposed to object-love (love of another person). In psychoanalytic theory, cathexis (investment) of the psychic representation of the self with libido (sexual interest and energy). An excess interferes with relations with others. To be distinguished from egotism, which carries the connotation of self-centredness, selfishness, and conceit. Egotism is but one expression of narcissism.

Narcoanalysis Use of drugs such as sodium amytal and sodium pentothal to facilitate communication, remove certain inhibitions and bring about verbal release. However, this procedure is not a fact finding instrument and the hidden truth is not revealed under the influence of drugs.

Narcolepsy It is the intense desire to go to sleep. It happens during active conversation too. About 30 % persons have family history. There is apparent close relationship of gene for narcolepsy to HLA system.

There is no association with autoimmune disease. It has relationship with multiple sclerosis.

Narcoma Stupor or coma produced by narcotics.

Narcosynthesis Psychotherapeutic treatment under partial anaesthesia, such as induced by barbiturates. Originally used to treat acute mental disorders occurring in a military combat setting.

Narcotic Any drug which dulls senses and reduces pain, whose extended use may produce drug dependence, including heroin, morphine, meperidine, and methadone.

Nares The openings into the nasal cavity; also called the nostrils.

Naris Nostril, the opening into the nasal cavity.

Narrative The story, implicit, or explicit that contextualizes and gives meaning to human conduct.

Narrative charting Style of documentation generally used in source-oriented records.

Nasal Thin, vertical bony septum separating the right and left nasal cavities.

Nasal airway Flexible, curved piece of rubber or plastic with one wide or trumpetlike end and one narrow end that is inserted through the nose into the pharynx.

Nasal aperture Opening of the nasal cavity in the skull.

Nasal bones Bones that form the bridge of the nose.

Nasal cannula Hollow tube with prongs that are placed into the patient's nostrils for delivering oxygen.

Nasal catheter A flexible, smallbore tube inserted into the oropharyns by way of the nose.

Nasal cavity Cavity divided by the nasal septum, and extending from the external nares anteriorly to the nasopharynx posteriorly; bounded inferiorly by the hard palate.

Nasal cavity, Olfactory region The superior nasal concha, the intervening septum and roof of the nasal cavity.

Nasal cavity, respiratory region The inferoposterior portion of the nasal cavity bounded by the olfactory region superiorly, the vestibular region anteriorly, and the posterior nasal apertures posteriorly.

Nasal cavity, vestibular region The area extending from the nares backward and upward about two thirds of an inch to the limen nasi.

Nasal conchae Three scroll-like bones-the superior and middles bones, which rise from the ethmoid bone, and the inferior bone, which emanates from the facial bone.

Nasal congestion There may be partial blockage of nasal passage due to congestion or allergy. A simple effective method of alleviating procedure is to inhale the steam from a pot of hot water. This loosens mucus which can be blown out. Decongestant drugs in form of nasal drops and sprays are used but withdrawal reaction is also known.

Nasal packing forceps It is an angulated plain forceps. The tip of the forceps is blunt and non-toothed. It is used for anterior packing of nasal cavity in case of epistaxis with the help of it local anaesthesia by means of Xylocaine gauze packing. Packing should be removed daily.

Nasal polyposis Main symptoms include unilateral or bilateral nasal airway obstruction occasionally varying in intensity. Hyposmia or anosmia is common in severe cases. Rhinoscopy shows glazed, smooth walled reddish, localised excrescence of nasal mucosa. These are usually multiple and bilateral.

Nasal septal deviation Unilateral or bilateral constant and variable impediment of nasal respiration depending on the site and severity of septal deformity. Hyposmia is rarely present. Headache can present. Nare will be deviated, occasional proneness to epistaxis and snoring develops.

Nasal septum It is a partition inside the nose that divides it into two portions. It consists of cartilage at front and bone at the back. Both are covered by mucous membrane. Deviated septum may be present by birth or may be caused by blow. If deviation is severe, breathing is obstructed. The septum can be straightened by surgery. Hole may be eroded in septum by tuberculosis and cocaine.

Naso Prefix referring to nasal.

Nasoantral Pertaining to the nose and the maxillary antrum.

Nasoantritis Inflammation of the nose and the maxillary antrum.

Nasobronchial Pertaining to the nasal cavities and the bronchi.

Nasociliary Pertaining to the eyes, brow, and root of the nose, as the nasociliary nerve.

Nasociliary neuralgia These develop unilateral pain in the lateral nose and sometimes in the eye near the medial canthus, combined with swelling of ipsilateral nasal mucosa. Patient develops spontaneous ocular pain and tenderness.

Nasofrontal Pertaining to the nasal and frontal bones.

Nasogastric tube A type of tube that is placed through the nose into the stomach.

Nasointestinal tube Tube that is inserted through the nose for distal placement below the stomach.

Nasolabial groove Groove which connects the lip and nose.

Nasolacrimal Pertaining to the nose and lacrimal apparatus.

Nasolacrimal duct Duct that leads from the lacrimal sac to the nasal cavity.

Nasomanometer A manometer for measuring intranasal pressure.

Naso-oral Pertaining to the nose and mouth.

Nasopharyngeal air space An air space viewed on a panoramic film; appears as a diagonal radiolucency superior to the soft plate and uvula.

Nasopharyngeal angiofibroma This is a vascular tumour mainly occurring in males. A juvenile nasopharyngeal angiofibroma may extend from the nasopharynx to the oral cavity. It is noncapsulated and expansile. It produces nasal obstruction and may appear as a mass in palate. Microscopic features consist of numerous blood vessels surrounded by dense fibrous stroma of fibrous connective tissue. Surgical excision and radiation are methods of therapy.

Nasopharyngeal suction Purpose of suctioning is to maintain a patent airway by removing accumulated secretions. When air passages are obstructed by vomitus or secretions, it may prove

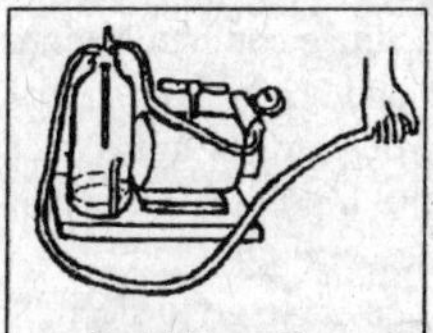
Portable suction

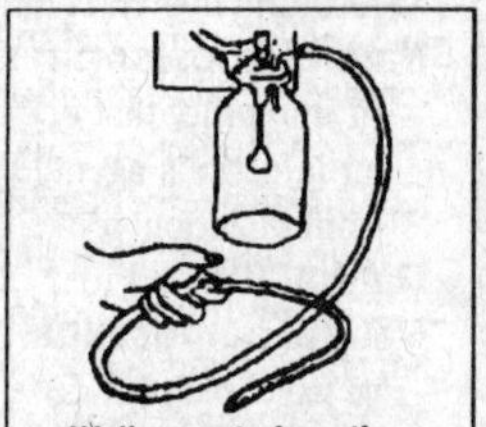
Wall-mounted suction

to be a life-saving device. Pharyngeal suctioning involves the upper air passage of nose, mouth and pharynx. Deep suctioning of lower respiratory passages stimulates the cough reflex and removes secretions from trachea and bronchi.

Nasopharyngeal suctioning Removal of secretions from the throat through a nasally inserted catheter.

Nasopharyngoscope A lighted, telescopic endoscope for use in examination of the nasopharynx and the pharyngeal end of the auditory tube.

Nasopharynx Part of the respiratory tract forms the upper section of pharynx. During swallowing the nasopharynx is sealed off by the action of the soft palate. The nasopharynx contains opening of eustachian tubes and adenoids. The adenoids can enlarge to such an extent that nasopharynx becomes completely blocked and child feels difficulty in breathing.

A malignant tumour of nasopharynx may result in recurrent nose bleeding, a persistently running nose and a change in voice. There may be bloody discharge from nose, double vision, facial pain and paralysis of one side of face.

Nasorostral Pertaining to the rostrum of the nose.

Nasotracheal suctioning Removal of secretions from the trachea through a nasally inserted catheter.

Natal Pertaining to birth.

Natrium Sodium.

Natriuresis The urinary excretion of sodium; commonly designates enhanced sodium excretion, which may occur in certain diseases or as a result of the administration of diuretic drugs.

Natriuretic A chemical compound that may be used as a means of retarding the tubular reabsorption of sodium ions from glomerular filtrate, thereby resulting in greater amounts of that ion in the urine.

Natural booster phenomenon An augmentation of immunity that occurs with periodic exposure to an infectious agent. This effect may be lost when immunization prevents exposure.

Natural fibers Fibes of animal or vegetable origin.

Natural homosexual period It is the term applied to psychosexual development preceding the onset of puberty. When boys tend to socialise with boys, girls frequently have crushes on girls of their own age or a little elder woman or teacher. The period ends with the awakening of their heterosexual interest in adolescence.

Natural killer cell Leucocytes that play a role in nonspecific immunity by specific lysis of cancer cells

Naturalistic One term for qualitative research; refers specifically to the philosphy that qualitative researchers should study subjects in their natural setting.

Naturopathy A drugless system of therapy, making use of physical forces such as air, light, water, heat, massage etc.

Naughton exercise test protocol A graded treadmill exercise test protocol consisting of stages of variable (tester choice) duration with incremental speed and grade change at each stage.

Nausea Feeling that usually precedes vomiting.

NBD (nucleotide binding domain) Part of the ABC protein transporter involved in energy coupling. This part is hydrophilic, highly conserved and is involved in ATP binding and hydrolysis.

Near death experience An altered state of consciousness usually occurring after traumatic injury and is often recalled.

Near response Passive thickening of the lens, miosis, and convergence, combined for close-up viewing.

Near-obligate parasite An organism that survives mainly as a parasite in its natural habitat.

Nearsightedness Myopia.

Nebuliser It is a device that converts drug solution into continuous fine aerosol which can be inhaled directly into lungs. It delivers high doses of inhaled medication. It uses normal tiding breathing. Wet

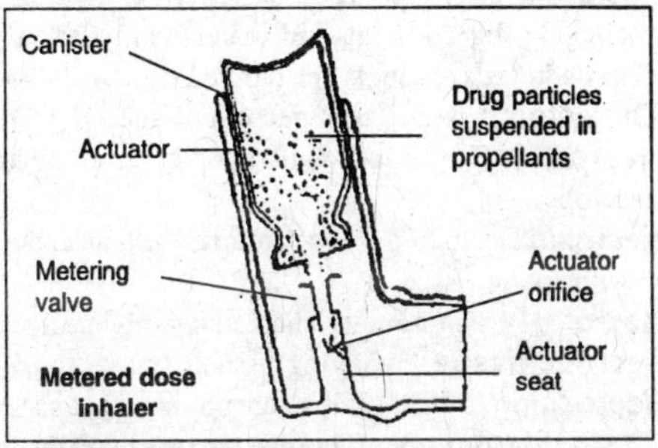

Metered dose inhaler

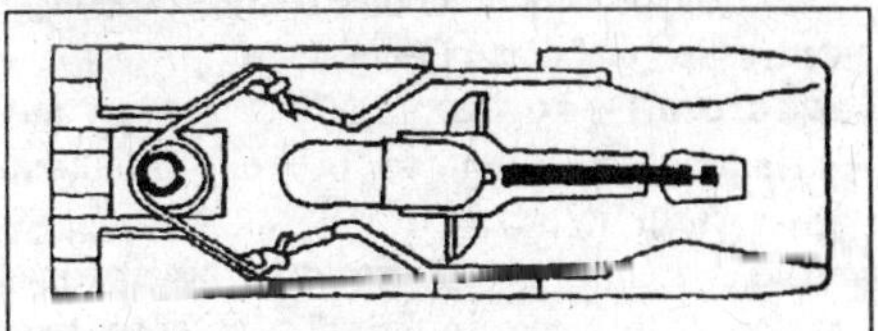
Dry powder inhaler

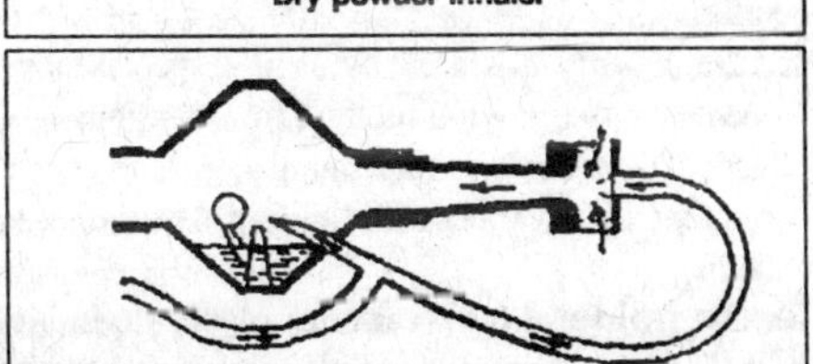
Jet Nobuller

aerosol is the choice of therapy. Patient Like to inhale the most which moistens their dry mucus membrane.

Nebulization Vaporization or dispersion of a liquid in fine spray.

Necessary cause Precedes a disease and has the following relationship with it: if the cause is absent, the disease cannot occur.If the cause is present, the disease may or may not occur.

Neck It supports head and is a passage between head, brain and body. Strangulation kills by compressive major blood vessels and by cutting off the air supply to lungs. Decapitation kills because it cuts through the spinal cord, it severs trachea, oesophagus and major blood vessels. Cervical vertebra is affected by cervical osteoarthritis. Cervical rib may result in pain, numbness and pin and needle sensation in hand. Neck pain of unknown origin is very common.

Neck of the rib The portion of the rib that extends from the head to the body of shaft of the rib.

Necking It is a milder form of petting, consisting of hugging, light kissing and manual stimulation of girl's breasts through her clothes.

Necrectomy Excision of necrotic tissue.

Necropsy Examination of a body after death; autopsy.

Necrosis Death of a cell or group of cells in contact with living tissue.

Necrotic Pertaining to or characterized by necrosis.

Necrotic tissue Nonliving tissue.

Necrotising fascitis It is an uncommon deep seated infection of subcutaneous tissue resulting in destruction of fat and fascia.

Nedocromil sodium Nonsteroidal anti-inflammatory agent to prevent immediate hypersensitivity reaction.

Needle A slender, sharp instrument, usually made to steel, with an eye for thread, used for sewing or suturing .

Needle biopsy It is done by using a special biopsy needle. This is a good method for doing biopsy of gland. Disadvantage is lacerating large blood vessel. Another disadvantage is yielding of small-sized sample.

Needle holder Many varieties of needle holders are available with or without catch, with straight or curved tips. These are used for passing sutures in the lid, superior rectus muscle, conjunctiva or corneosclera, or any surgery where suturing is required.

Needleless systems Intravenous tubing that eliminates the need for access needles.

Negative affectivity A stable personality associated with high level of negative mood.

Negative event Life events exerting a particular undesirable negative impact on a child.

Negative feedback A mechanism in the body for maintaining a stage of internal constancy, or homeostasis; effectors are activated by changes in the internal environment, and the actions of the effectors serve to counteract these changes and maintain a state of balance.

Negative pole In a battery, the pole with excess electrons.

Negative reinforcer A stimulus that induces a subject to respond in a manner that interrupts the response.

Negative staining A technique in which a particulate sample is surrounded by a solution of a heavy metal salt and allowed to dry; especially useful for small particles such as viruses.

Negativism Opposition or resistance, either covert or overt, to outside suggestions or advice. May be seen in schizophrenia.

Neglect Neglect of contralateral personal/ extrapersonal space associated with inferior parietal lobe disease.

Negligence Performance of an act that a reasonably careful person under similar circumstances would not do or, conversely, the failure to perform an act that a reasonably careful person would do under similar circumstances.

Negri bodies Rabies virus produces a specific cytoplasmic inclusions, the Negri bodies in infected nerve cells. Negri bodies are found most abundantly in pyramidal cell layer of cerebral cortex and Purkinje cell layer of cerebellum. Negri bodies may be round or oval in form when lying free in the cytoplasm. Negri body is stained by fluorescent antibody technique which also stains the small eosinophilic inclusion bodies. Negri bodies before rabies can be accepted as the cause of death.

Nelson's syndrome It presents with cranial nerve palsies and hyperpigmentation of skin following adrenalectomy.

Nematodes Nematodes are generally elongate, cylindrical and tapered at both ends. These are colourless and vary from 1 m.m. to 15 cms long. An elastic cuticles covers the body.

Neocortex A reference to the cerebral cortex, so named because neo means new and cortex means "bark." The neocortex is the cerebral cortex, markedly developed in human beings but less developed in lower animals. The subcortical regions are therefore regarded as older in evolutionary sense.

Neologism In psychiatry, a new word or condensed combination of several words coined by a person to express a highly complex idea not readily understood by others; seen in schizophrenia and organic mental disorders.

Neonatal Relating to or occurring in the period immediately following birth through the first 28 days of life.

Neonatal abstinence syndrome A cluster of physical signs exhibited by the new born exposed in utero to maternal use of substances such as heroin or cocaine.

Neonatal behavioral assessment scale A tool developed by Brazelton (1973) to evaluate newborn behaviour by measuring 27 specific behavioral items that fall into one of the six designated categories—habituation, orientation, motor maturity, variation, self-quieting abilities, and social behavior.

Neonatal cardio pulmonary resuscitation Prompt resuscitation is important to prevent permanent mental or physical handicap. Neonatal cardiac arrest is due to hypoxaemia.

Neonatal death Death of newborn within the first four weeks of life.

Neonatal hepatitis It is a term for a variety of hepatic disorders in the neonates involving prolonged conjugated hyperbilirubinaemia, hepatomegaly and variable degrees of hepatic dysfunction.

Neonatal mortality rate Number of death's among the born infants within four weeks of life per 1000 live births.

Neonatal myasthenia About 10 to 15 per cent of pregnant myasthenic mothers will give birth to infants.

These children suck poorly, cry poorly and are at risk from respiratory insufficiency. This phenomenon disappears after 10 to 20 days.

Neonatal nurse practioner She is skilled in looking after new born, both well and ill.

Neonatal period First month of life.

Neonatal sepsis The manifestations of neonatal septicaemia are often vague and nonspecific. There is an alteration in established feeding behaviour. Hypothermia is a common manifestation of sepsis while fever is infrequent. Episodes of apnoeic spells of gasping may occur. Cyanosis may occur. Cough is unusual.

Neonate Newborn, from birth to one month.

Neonatologist A physician who specializes in care of newborn upto 29th day of life.

Neonatology Study of diagnosis and treatment of disorders of newborn.

Neoplasm A new growth comprised an abnormal collection of cells, the growth of which exceeds and is uncoordinated with that of the normal tissues.

Neoplasm headache In malignancy headache may be an early prominent symptom. In meningioma (40%), pituitary adenoma (51%), glioblastoma (37%) and metastases (65%) may develop headache. Sudden onset of headache suggests haemorrhage into neoplasm. Headache may be intermittent with remissions.

Neoplasm of urinary tract Kidney tumours include wilm's tumor, renal cell carcinoma and transtitional cell carcinoma. Tumors of urinary

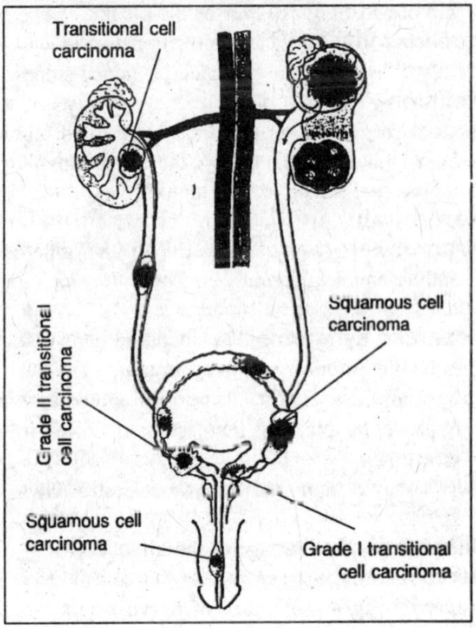

bladder includes transitional cell carcinoma, squamous cell carcinoma and adenocarcinoma.

Neoplastic Relating to or producing neoplasms.

Neoplastic enlargement of glands Clinically benign tumours are of long duration. They present as single nodule fixed to the overlying skin or mucous membrane. Recurrent lesions may be nodular. Benign tumours grow slowly and are asymptomatic. Malignant tumours are usually of shorter duration than benign tumours. These grow rapidly. Even if growth is slow sudden rapid activity may develop. These are fixed to the surrounding tissues. The overlying skin or mucus may be ulcerated. Malignant tumours of parotid gland may be associated with facial nerve paralysis. Regional lymph glands may be enlarged.

Neostigmine It is twice as powerful as physostigmine. It is also a depolariser and can cause on its own a depolarising type of block. When injected into a conscious patient it may cause muscular fasciculations. It is a direct stimulant of cholinergic effector cell. It has nicotinic effects and has a direct stimulant action on doses. It depresses autonomic ganglia. It also has muscarine properties. Dose is 2.5 mg and effect lasts for 2 hours. The muscarine effect especially bradycardia must be prevented by atropine. In anaesthesia 3 mg of neostigmine reverses the block.

Nephrectomy Surgical removal of the kidney.

Nephrolithiasis The presence of kidney stones.

Nephron A portion of the kidney; consists of the renal corpuscle, the proximal convoluted tubule, both limbs of Henle's loop, the distal convoluted tubule, and the collecting tubule.

Nephropathy Any disease of the kidney.

Nephrosclerosis It develops due to atherosclerosis and essential hypertension. There develops urea nitrogen retention in blood.

Nephrotic syndrome The condition gives rise to massive oedema, proteinuria, lipiduria, hypoalbuminaemia, hypercholesterolaemia, hyperlipidaemia, and increased susceptibility to infections.

Nephrotoxic Injury that is toxic or destructive to a kidney.

Nephrotoxicity Damage to the kidney cells.

Nerve A cordlike structure, visible to the naked eye, comprising a collection of nerve fibers which convey impulses between a part of the central nervous system and some other body region. It consists of a connective tissue shealth (epineurium) enclosing bundles (funiculi or fasciculi) of nerve fibers, each bundle being surrounded by its own sheath of connective tissue.

Nerve block It means to anaesthetise a region which may be small or large injecting either a peripheral nerve or a plexus. Nerve block provides its own muscular block. There are various specialised forms, brachial plexus, paravertebral pudendal block. Sympathetic nerve block may be used in vascular disease.

Nerve cell A cell capable of receiving a stimulus and propagating an action potential; a neuron.

Nerve conduction studies Nerve conduction studies provide quantitative information about neurological function in patients with a variety of neuromuscular disorders. Test can be performed

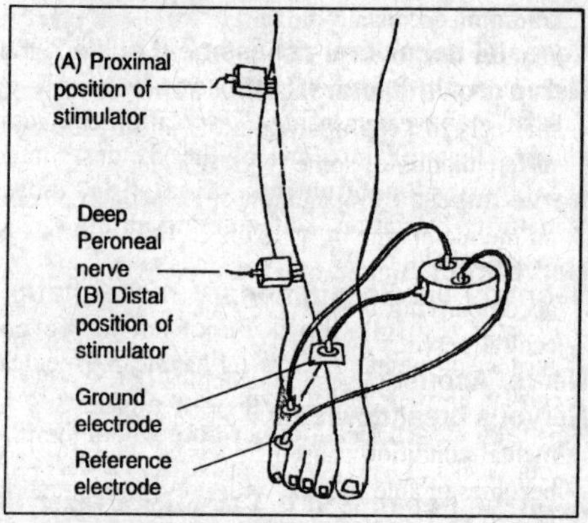

on motor and sensory nerves. In motor nerves, supramaximal stimuli are given at two sites and motor action potentials are recorded in the muscle supplied by nerve. Time between stimulus and onset of action potential is the motor latency. Motor nerve conduction is very helpful in the diagnosis of carpal tunnel syndrome and other compressive neuropathies. Nerve conduction studies are helpful in monitoring recovery or assessing success of surgical decompression.

Nerve conduction velocities It is determined by calculating the conduction velocity in meters per second in peripheral nerve. It is reduced in peripheral neuropathies.

Nerve fibre Nerve fibre consists of axon, thin membranous axolemma, myelin sheath and Schwann's sheath. Axon has a cytoplasm called axoplasm, within axoplasm are found neurofilament, mitochondria, endoplasmic reticulum. Protein synthesised in nerve cell body is transporated distally down the axon at a rate of 1 mm per day to even 300 mm per day.

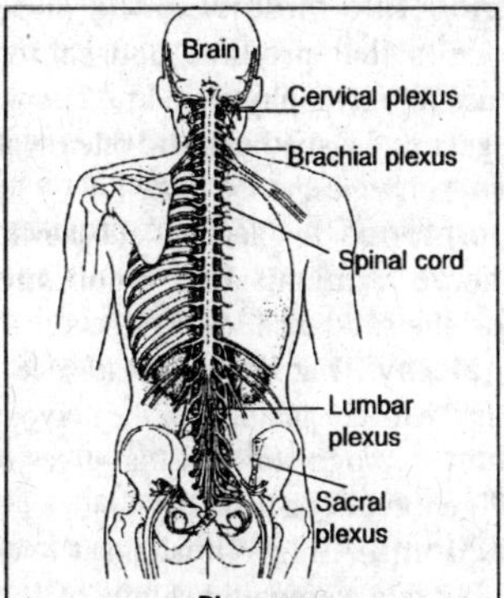

Plexuses

Nerve growth factor (NGF) A neurotrophic factor that acts to keep neurons alive and to stimulate differentiation of some types of neurons.

Nerve impulse Propagation of an action potential on the membrane of an axon.

Nerve tract Bundle of axons, their sheaths, and accompanying connective tissues located in the central nervous system.

Nerve, Acoustic Vestibulocochlear.

Nervous breakdown It is a lay man term used for mental condition caused by severe stress. Person becomes unable to cope with prevailing situation. It may be a part of mental illness.

Nervous diarrhoea Such diarrhoea may continue for years. There is usually no pain or tenesmus. Diarrhoea is recurring in the morning hours. Diet has little or no effect. Attacks are more during mental emotion or body fatigue.

Nervous dyspepsia The constant discomfort and distress of gastric disorder bring about neurasthenic and depressed state. Flatulence is common in anxiety neurosis. Anxiety and worry causes spasm. But it is wise to diagnose gastric neurosis until all clinical and special investigations have been done to exclude organic disease.

Nervous system The function of nervous system is to gather information about external environment as well as internal state, to analyse this information and to initiate appropriate responses.

The central processing unit for the system is central nervous system (CNS). Two of most important are the automatic nervous system (ANS) which is specially concerned with automatic regulation of internal body functioning, and somatic nervous system (SNS) which controls the skeletal muscles responsible for voluntary movement.

Nervous tissue One of the four major tissue types; consists of neurons, which have the ability to conduct action potentials, and neuroglia, which are support cells.

Nested design A design in which there are atleast two independent variables, but not all levels of the independent variables are crossed.

Netrins A class of tropic molecules.

Neural crest cell Cell derived during embryonic development from the crests of the neural fold; gives rise to facial structures, pigment cells, and peripheral nerve ganglia.

Neural dysgeusias There develops disturbance in taste. It results from damage to the peripheral nerves of the gustatory system. Afferent nerve damage can result from influenza and diphtheria. Section of chorda tympani may result it.

Neural plate Thickened region of the ectodermal layer that gives rise to the neural tube

Neural tinnitus The tinnitus is strictly unilateral and perceived deep within ear. It is constant and usually high pitched. Characteristic symptom is a masking level well above threshold of auditory level.

Neural tube A structure in the early stage of brain development from which brain and spinal cord develop.

Neural tube defect An abnormal opening in the brain or spine.

Neuralgia It is pain caused by irritation of or damage to a nerve. Pain develops in brief bouts but may be severe and can be felt along the nerve. In migraine neuralgia consists of attacks of intense radiating pain around the eye lasting for an hour. Postherpetic neuralgia has burning pain. Galossopharyngeal pain may respond to carbamazepine.

Neuralgia paraesthetica The lateral cutaneous nerve of thigh passes deep to or through the inguinal ligament. The nerve may be compressed by repeated exercise and constant pressure on sitting. Symptoms include unpleasant burning sensation and numbness in distribution of nerve. The border of impaired sensations are fairly sharply defined. There is no muscle wasting or weakness.

Neuralgia trigeminal There develops a severe unilateral cruciating pain in the area of face supplied by trigeminal nerve. Pain is transitory and stimulation of trigger zone may result it. There is no permanent treatment except glycerol injection into Gasserian ganglion.

Neuralgic amyotrophy First symptom is usually a deep, aching pain in shoulder and upper arm increasing in severity. The muscles most commonly affected are serratus anterior, deltoid and pericapsular muscles. Sensory loss is slight over axillary nerve . Recovery is often slow and incomplete. Cause of condition is unknown. It may recur.

Neurapraxia In nerve compression there may be a transient block of conduction due to invagination of myelin and subsequent demyelination of the axon over a short segment. In it there is no wasting accompanied.

Neurasthenia It is mainly characterised by fatigue and an element of anxiety. Tiredness of neurasthenic differs from ordinary exhaustion which is not relieved by rest. There is cortical inhibition. The patient becomes egocentric and introspective, the whole of his consciousness filled by abnormal physical sensation. Headache is typically a pressure type.

It is less bearable than pain. Sleeplessness adds misery to patient. All kinds of disturbances in the field of sex occur. Psychological factors are the primary cause.

Neurectomy Partial or total excision or resection of a nerve.

Neurilemma Nerve sheath.

Neurilemoma Lesions are asymptomatic. These appear as small sessile, smooth surfaced growths on oral mucosa. Microscopically it is an encapsulated tumour and fibroblastic proliferation. Number of Schwann cells lie together in groups forming what is called Verocay bodies.

Neurite Process of a neuron, whether axon or dendrite.

Neuritic plaques Deposits of amyloid protein and glial cells that collect in intercellular space.

Neuritis Inflammation of the nerves.

Neuro endocrine motorneurons Hypothalamic nerve cells that produce and secrete neuro hormones into hypophysial portal circulation and thus regulates the synthesis and release of anterior pituitary hormones.

Neuro hormones A chemical substance released from nerve terminals into blood stream that transport the substance to its targets.

Neuroanatomy That branch of science which is concerned with the anatomy of the nervous system.

Neuroblast A progenitor cell that gives rise to all the different types of neurons.

Neuroblastoma A highly malignant tumor of the nervous system, composed chiefly of neuroblasts, which may be located in the adrenal glands, in the sympathetic chain, as well as in the bladder and other visceral organs, and the lips nose and jaws. Typically, it is a lobular, soft lesion weighing between 80 to 150 gm, presenting as grayish mass with areas of hemorrhage and necorsis and, sometimes, foci of calcification.

Neurocanthocytosis There are abnormal red blood cells bearing spiky projections in peripheral blood. Syndrome includes seizures, tic-like vocalisations, biting of lips and tongue. There will be wasting of muscles due to peripheral neuropathy.

Neurocentral joints These are found in cervical spine C_3-C_7 and are best visualised in AP views. Osteophytes from these joints can project into the intervertebral foramina compromising nerve roots. They may also impinge on vertebral artery.

Neurochemistry Aspect of biological functioning related to chemicals which transmits signals from one nerve to another.

Neurochrome A blood borne signal of endocrine nature that is either derived directly from larger prohormones that consist of 3 to 100 or more amino acids released from nerve endings.

Neurocysticercosis This affects man in its larval form as the intermediate host of the pork tapeworm. Arachnoidal infestation causes meningitic syndrome and intracranial hypertension. Ventricular infestation causes obstructive hydrocephalus and parenchymal involvement causes mental disorientation and seizures.

Neurodystrophic Disease process within a nerve, resulting from trauma, circulation disorders, or metabolic diseases, e.g., a neurodystrophic factor (diabetes and pernicious anemia).

Neuroectoderm That part of the ectoderm that forms the neural tube and neural crest.

Neuroendocrine signature The concept that exposure to a stressor elicits a pattern of neuroendocrine response that is specific to that stressor.

Neuroendocrinology The scientific study of the interactions between the nervous system and endocrine system.

Neurofibril One of the delicate threads running in every direction through the cytoplasm of the body of a nerve cell and extending into the axon and the dendrites of the cell.

Neurofibril node A gap in the myelin sheath of a nerve fiber; also called a node of Ranvier.

Neurofibrillary tangles Tangles of neurofibrils, most numerous in Alzheimer's disease.

Neurofibrosarcoma Malignant schwannoma.

Neurogenesis The process of forming a new neuron. It involves the proliferation of neuronal progenitors.

Neurogenic Forming nervous tissue, or stimulating nervous energy.

Neurogenic claudication It is a disorder in which pain is brought on by walking and relieved by resting developed in one or both legs as a result of cauda equinal ischemia. There may be numbness, a burning sensation or a painful cramp. The affected limb is heavy and feels tired characteristic feature is that the distance walk can be increased by bending forward.

Neurogenic inflammation Triple response.

Neurogenic voice disorder It may be idiopathic. Symptoms include mild hoarseness to aphonia. Cord paralysis may be unilateral or bilateral, flaccid or rigid. Dyspnoea at rest is a feature of bilateral paralysis. Exertional dyspnoea may be ocular with unilateral paralysis.

Neuroglia Specialized supportive cells of the central nervous system.

Neuroglycopenia The direct effect of glucose deprivation on neurons in the CNS.

Neurohumoral reflex Reflex with neural afferent limb and hormonal efferent limb, e.g., the milk ejection reflex.

Neurohypophysial Relating to, occurring in, or involving the neurohypophysis.

Neurohypophysis Posterior pituitary gland.

Neurolemma Comprising chains of Schwann cells.

Neurolemmocyte A specialized neuroglia cell that surrounds an axon fiber of a peripheral nerve and forms the neurilemmal sheath; also called a Schawann cell.

Neuroleptic A medication having antipsychotic action affecting sensorimotor, congnitive, and psychologic function. It has a large number of actions. In acts in hypothalamus and brainstem reticular formation. It can control hyperactive and hypomanic states. It impairs consciousness and modifies abnormal behaviour in schizophrenic states. In large doses it causes dystonias. In moderate doses, it controls the muscle spasm of tetanus, large doses may make it worse. It reduces muscle spasticity due to other neurological lesions. It may precipitate epilepsy. Side-effects include drowsiness and lethargy.

Neuroleptic drug A type of drug that blocks dopamine-2; also called major tranquilizer.

Neuroleptic malignant syndrome A rare, idiosyncratic, and sometimes fatal reaction to high-potency neuroleptic drugs; most likely a result of dopamine blockade on the basal ganglia and hypothalamus. Symptoms include muscle rigidity and high fever. It is characterised by akinesia. There may be muscular rigidity, hyperthermia and labile BP. Controlling hyperpyrexia and maintaining circulation are necessary.

Neurologist A specialist in disease of the nervous system.

Neurology That branch of medical science which deals with the nervous system, both normal and in disease.

Neuroma When nerve is cut, both ends regenerate in an attempt to close the gap. Regeneration consists of a proliferation by Schwann cells and fibroblasts as well as the growth of axis cylinders. When axis cylinders contact the distal end of the nerve, repair is complete. If not, proliferation continues and a mass of fibroblasts is formed which constitutes a neuroma. The lesions usually appear initially as movable nodules in the oral mucosa. Treatment consists of excision.

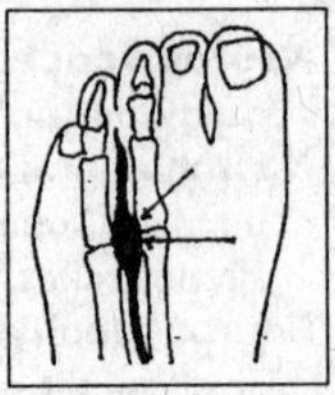

Neuromuscular Pertaining to muscles and nerves.

Neuromuscular functions Performance of motor behaviors.

Neuromuscular Junction (shun) and point of contact between the nerve endings and muscle, fibes.

Neuromuscular spindle These are spindle-shaped structures which are scattered among the large fibres of skeletal muscles. Each spindle consists of a thin connective tissue capsule which encloses 2 to 10 slender striated muscle fibre. The slender muscle fibres in the spindle are known as infrafusal fibres. These fibres are of 2 types : nuclear chain fibres and nuclear bag fibres.

Neuromyopathy A disease of nervous system and muscle.

Neuron Nerve cell, including its processes (axons and dendrites).

Neuron death The death of brain cells that can be due to disease or as part of normal development.

Neuron hypothesis The idea that the neuron is the basic unit of brain function.

Neuronal Relating to nerve cells.

Neuroparalytic keratitis It follows paralysis of trigeminal nerve. The common causes are trauma, surgery, tumour or injection with alcohol for trigeminal neuralgia. Cornea loses its sensitivity which is an important defence of cornea against degeneration, ulceration and infection. The corneal epithelium becomes dull and the epithelium is cast off, first at the centre and then over the whole cornea leaving a narrow rim at the periphery. The underlying substantia propria becomes cloudy, then yellow and finally breaks down to form a large ulcer accompanied with hypopyon. There is an intense circumciliary congestion. There is no pain as the fifth nerve is already paralysed. It heals early but breaks down rapidly, thus relapses are common.

Neuropathic joint Joint is damaged by a series of injuries which is not noticed because of neuropathy. It may develop in diabetes and untreated syphilis. When sensation to pain is lost, projective reflexes are not developed and joint may be damaged. Severe recurrent damage to a joint may lead to osteoarthritis. X-ray shows severe joint degeneration and deformity.

Neuropathic pain Pain with atypical characteristics.

Neuropathic ulcer These may occur on the sole or heel in foot. Ulcer is deep, penetrating ulcer-like arterial ulcer but it is painles and non-tender. It occurs at pressure areas. Surrounding tissues are healthy and have a normal circulation but are unable to appreciate pain. Peripheral pulse is present.

Neuropathogenic Disease within a tissue, resulting from abnormal nerve performance.

Neuropathy There is damage to peripheral nerves due to disease or damage. Symptoms caused by neuropathies include numbness, tingling, pain and muscle weakness depending on the nerves affected. Most neuropathies arise from damage or irritation to the axons or to their myelin sheath. There is no detectable cause.

Vitamin B deficiency, diabetes mellitus, alcohol consumption may result it. Damage to sensory nerve fibres may cause numbness and tingling often starting in the hands and feet and spreading towards centre.

Damage to nerves of autonomic nervous system may lead to blurred vision, impaired or absent sweating, episodes of faintness associated with fall of BP and sexual functioning. Treatment depends on underlying cause.

Neuropeptides A class of chemical neurotransmitters manufactured with instructions from a cell's DNA; thus a neuropeptide consists of a chain of amino acids that acts as a neurotransmitter.

Neurophysin The carrier protein for oxytocin and vasopressin that increases their half-life in blood.

Neurophysiology The study of the functioning of the nervous system.

Neuropsychiatry Referring to nervous and mental diseases.

Neuropsychology A general term used to refer to the study of the relation between brain function and behavior.

Neurosecretion A term applied to secretion of hormones by nerve cells.

Neurosis There is relatively mild psychiatric disorder in which sufferer remains in touch with reality. Neurotic symptoms are distressing to the affected person who is aware of a change from his usual psychological state. They tend to fluctuate in intensity often in response to social or personal stresses. No physical abnormality is seen.

Neurosis of pregnancy Disorder arising from mental conflict between sexual or aggressive drives and inhibiting social and cultural reality. Pregnancy itself may cause neurotic reactions. Hysterical symptoms appear in girls who had excessive 'babying' from their mothers.

Neurosurgery Procedures involving the cranium, brain meninges, cranial nerves, spinal cord and certebral column. It includes pain management too.

Neurosyphilis Invasion of nervous system by spirochaete occurs only in early course of syphilis. The majority of patients develop lymphocytic meningitis during second stage, i.e. six weeks of healing of primary chancre. During second stage person will have headache, neck stiffness, cranial nerve palsies, papilloedema and seizures. After secondary stage if untreated syphilitic infection will become asymptomatic. It usually causes subacute meningitis. CSF examination gives diagnosis. Syphilitic endarteritis involves the intracranial blood vessels to cause infarction. Clinically these patients present with acute stroke syndrome. CT findings are similar to cerebral infarction.

Neurothlipsis Direct or indirect pressure on a nerve, e.g., in the IVF through congestion of perineural tissues; in the carpal tunnel through direct ligamentous pressure.

Neurotic disorder A mental disorder in which the predominant disturbance is a distressing symptom or group of symptoms which one considers unacceptable and alien to one's personality. There is no marked loss of reality testing; behaviour does not actively violate gross social norms although it may be quite disabling. The disturbance is relatively enduring or recurrent without treatment and is not limited to a mild transitory reaction to stress. There is no demonstrable organic aetiology. In DSM-III-R. the neurotic disorders are included in affective, anxiety, somatoform, dissociative, and psychosexual disorders.

Neuroticism A personality characterised as emotional instability, physiological hyperreactivity and a lowered threshold for the experience of a variety of negative emotions such as anxiety, anger,irritation, depression and distress.

Neurotoxicity Refers to damage inflicted on target neurons by excess glutamate.

Neurotoxin It is a chemical that damages nervous tissue. Effects include numbness, weakness or paralysis of the part of body supplied by nerve. Neurotoxins are present in the venom of certain snakes. Some chemical poisons such as arsenic and lead are also neurotoxic.

Neurotransmitter A chemical liberated at a nerve terminal which activates postsynaptic and/or presynaptic receptors.

Neurotransmitter substance A chemical discharge into the synaptic space which influences the transmission of nerve impulses. It acts on the membrane of adjacent fibres, creating an excitatory or inhibitory condition by causing the adjacent membrane to become depolarised or more polarised. In the former case, a transmission occurs; in the latter, the nerve is more resistant to firing.

Neurotrophic factors A class of compounds that act to support growth and differentiation in developing neurons and may act to keep certain neurons alive in adulthood.

Neurotropic Something that has an affinity for the nervous system.

Neurovascular Pertaining to both nervous and vascular structures.

Neutral bath 34°C. Sedative effect-places no undue stress on cardiovascular or nervous system.

Neutral position Limb that is turned neither toward nor away from the body's midline.

Neutral position of the pelvis One in which anterior-superior spines are in the same transverse plane, and the anterior-superior spines and the symphysis pubis are in the same vertical plane.

Neutral solution Solution with equal numbers of hydrogen and hydroxide ions; has a pH of 7.0.

Neutral stimulus One which does not elicit the response in question. A puff of air to the eyeball, for example, is neutral stimulus for salivation. It does not evoke the salivary response automatically. Through repeated presentations with a stimulus such as meat, it could become a conditioned response for salivation.

A puff of air is not a neutral stimulus for the eyeblink, however it is an unconditioned stimulus in the case of the eyeblink.

Neutral thermal environment Environment in which body temperature is maintained without an increase in metabolic rate or oxygen use.

Neutrocclusion In which the mesical buccal cusp of the first maxillary molar lies adjacent to or in buccal groove of mandibular first molar.

Neutron A large neutrally charged particle found in the nucleus of an atom. Electrically neutral particles that exist together with positively charged protons in the nucleus of atoms.

Neutropenia Abnormally low levels of circulating white blood cells neutrophils that remove bacteria.

Neutropenic Having an abnormal decrease in the number of neutrophils, white blood cells, in the blood.

Neutrophil Leucocyte with granules that stain with neither basic nor acidic dyes; phagocytic white blood cell.

Neutrophile Middle lover; an organism that grows optimally in the neutral range of external pH, generally within pH 6-8.

Neutrophilic Growing optimally in the neutral range of external pH.

Nevus flammeus Permanent purple birth mark.

Nevus flammeus Permanent purple birth mark.

Nevus vasculosus Rough red collection of capillaries with a raised surface disappearing with time.

Newman-Keuls test A multiple-comparision procedure.

NEX measurement Distance from the nose to the earlobe to the xiphoid process.

Nexus A bond between members of a group; the type of bonds present in single-unit smooth muscles.

Neyman bias Same as Late look bias.

Niacin deficiency Niacin is important in intracellular oxidation and is found in meat, liver, yeast, milk and vegetables. Deficiency of it causes pellagra. Pellagra includes rough, scaly keratotic lesions on the exposed skin. Oral lesions consist of swelling, redness and ulceration of mucosa. Dementia, dermatitis and diarrhoea are the symptoms. Oral mucous membrane is inflamed and bleeds easily. Tongue is red and enlarged. Its papillae disappears giving it a bold appearance. Lateral margins show indentations by teeth. Microscopic sections reveal oedema, atrophy of papillae and infiltration by plasma cells and lymphocytes.

Niacin Therapy In gram quantity it may rise HDL and lower the LDL. As side effects it results in hot flashes and rashes. This therapy is contraindicated with gout, peptic ulcer and diabetes.

Niclosamide It is a drug for treatment of *Taenia*. The tablets are chewed well and taken with meals. The drug disintegrates the taenia in the gut. Mebendazole in double dose is more safe and useful.

Nicotinamide adenine dinucleo-tide (NADH) A base containing organic molecule capable of accepting hydrogen atoms and of transferring energy from glycolysis to the electron transport chain.

Nicotine It is a drug in tobacco acting as stimulant and is responsible for dependence. After inhalation it passes into blood stream. Nicotine in chewing is absorbed more slowly. Habitual smoking may slow heart rate to start then increases heart rate and narrows blood vessels resulting in high BP. It is the tar in tobacco smoke that damages lung tissue and causes lung cancer and peripheral vascular diseases.

Nicotine toxicity Nicotine is a water soluble alkaloid. The solution is intially clear but turns brown on contact to air. Tobacco leaves contain 1.5 to 5.4% in every leaf. A single cirgarette has 10 to 20 mg of nicotine. It is an extremely poisonous substance. Lethal dose of nicotine is 40 to 60 mg. Absorption of smoking one cigarette will be about 50 to 150 mg of nicotine. Nicotine acts by directly stimulating the central and peripheral acetylcholine receptors. Moderate intoxication presents with a burning in the mouth and throat.

The features include muscle fasciculations, miosis, salivation increased pulmonary secretions. In severe intoxications the patients develops hypotension and seizures leading to death due to respiratory failure.

Nicotinic receptor An acetylcholine receptor, historically activated by nicotine.

Nicotinic stomatitis It usually occurs on the palate. On palate it appears as a number of umblicated papules dispersed on a background of red mucosa but soon the mucosa becomes grey or white. The papules and the central depressions correspond to the orifices of salivary gland ducts. Under microscope it shows hyperkeratosis and parakeratosis but dyskeratosis is absent. The ducts of salivary glands show intraductal epithelial proliferation and plugging of lumina. Inflammatory exudates produce bumps and hyperkeratinisation produces the white appearance. Elimination of smoking treats the person.

NICU Neonatal intensive care unit.

Nidation Implantation of fertilized ovum in the uterine endometrium.

Nidus The point of origin or focus of a process.

Niemann-Pick syndrome In this syndrome there is loss of appetite and weight, retardation of growth, pigmentation of skin, occasional cutaneous xanthomas, hepatosplenomegaly, and perhaps lymphadenopathy.

Nifedipine It is dihydropyridine. Oral or sublingual dose is 10 to 20 mg 4 to 8 hourly. Action starts within 15 to 20 minutes. Main clinical use is as coronary and peripheral vasodilator. It antagonises intracellular calcium which is the necessary trigger for excitation-contraction coupling in vascular smooth muscle. It dilates coronary arteries in dosage which does not depress myocardial contractility.

Night fall Sex dreams involving sexual activities, attractive members of opposite sex, images of sexual features and sexual symbols accompanied by erection and or ejaculation in boys and men, and by vaginal lubrication and orgasm in women.

Night feeds It should neither be condemned nor forbidden. If babys' cry is not pacified by giving water then he needs feed being hungry. Feeding at night does not make a habit. If the baby is fed adequately during the day then he will not require feed at night.

Night guards These are special splints used for alleviation of bruxism and clenching. These are made of acrylic and completely cover the occlusal surfaces of teeth. These can be constructed for both jaws. Splints can be made thin to be comfortable while putting on. It stabilises mobile teeth.

Night mares It occurs in stage III or rapid eye movement (REM) sleep and presumbably reflect dreams with an unpleasant psychic content, certain drugs such as reserpine and L-dopa may result in it.

Night myopia In dusk, the refraction may change from –0.5 to –4.0 dioptres, usually around –20 dioptres. Night myopia is regularly found in young patients but only seen in older ones. Night myopia sometimes begins at an illumination that still allows clear vision. One of the causes is dilation of pupil in darkness which increases spherical aberration producing certain amount of myopia.

Night terror It has no significance but parents remain worried about the child. In stage III or IV of NREM sleep child cries out with a scream. During this period child becomes terrified with dilated pupils. It is a self-limiting disease.

Nightmare (dream anxiety attack) Anxiety-provoking dream occurring during rapid eye movement (REM) sleep.

Nihilistic delusion The delusion of nonexistence of the self, part of the self, or of some object in external reality.

Nippers A strong hinged pliers with cutting beaks.

Nipple It is the small protruberance at the tip of the breast. It contains tiny openings through which milk passes. Nipple and surrounding areola are darker.

Muscle in nipple allows it to become erect on excitation. An inverted nipple is usually an abnormality of development. Cracked nipples are common during last month of pregnancy and during breast feeding. Papilloma of the nipple is a benign tumour. Paget's disease of nipple appears initially as persistent eczema. Pus discharges from nipple in breast abscess.

Nipple discharge The spontaneous escape of fluid from the nipple.

Nipple secretion Fluid within the ducts of the breast collected by nipple aspiration or breast massage.

Nitremia Azotemia.

Nitric Pertaining to or containing nitrogen, applied especially to compounds containing nitrogen with a higher concentration than that contained in the nitrous compounds.

Nitric oxide Widely distributed in the body; plays role in the regulation of circulation; diffuses to the vascular smooth muscle cells; increases cGMP levels and induces smooth muscle relaxation.

Nitrification The biochemical oxidation of ammonium to nitrite and nitrate by microorganisms.

Nitrogen limitation The slower nitrogen assimilation that results from utilization of a single nitrogen source other than ammonia.

Nitrogen narcosis Compressed air at depth deeper than 20 meters exerts a narcosis characterized by euphoria, impaired cognitive functioning and neuromuscular coordination.

Nitrogen-balance studies Measurement of the amount of N entering the body compared to the amount excreted.

Nitrogenous A substance containg nitrogen.

Nitroglycerine It is used for treatment of angina. It has been used IV at a rate about 20 mg per minute. It can be used with halothene in anaesthesia. It produces relaxation of smooth muscle in vessel wall, especially in veins. In resonable dosage, it improves coronary perfusion. Intracranial pressure rises. Hypotensive effect comes gradually.

Nitrosamines Carcinogens which arise from reaction of amines with nitrites. They are produced in intestines and their production can be reduced by the presence of vitamin C.

Nitrous oxide It is a gas with a slightly sweetish smell. It is neither inflammable nor explosive. It produces light anaesthesia without depression. It reduces the requirement of more effective and toxic anaesthetic agent. Recovery time rarely exceeds four minutes even after prolonged use. But it is expensive and difficult to transport. For maintenance of anaesthesia it should be mixed with 30 per cent oxygen. It should not be given in case of any air-filled space which may move into it from blood. Such patients may be with pleural and pericardial effusion and intestinal obstruction. The side effect of nausea and vomiting increases with duration of anaesthesia. Cylinders are to be kept in below 25°C.

NMR Nuclear magnetic resonance.

Noble metal A metal made predominantly from metallic elements that do not corrode , such as gold, platinum, and palladium.

Nocebo effect Adverse side effect due to a negative psychological reaction of the patient to a pill or an injection.

Nociception Processes involved in percieving pain following stimulation of nociceptive nerve endings.

Nociceptive Responsive to noxious stimulation.

Nociceptors Nerve receptors that transmit pain impulses.

Nocioception The perception of pain and temperature.

Nocturia It is a disturbance of person's sleep at night by the need of passing urine. Drinking alcohol in the evening stimulates urine production and may result in nocturia. Enlargement of prostate may also cause it. Another common cause is heart failure and diabetes.

Nocturnal enuresis Bedwetting.

Nocturnal erection Normal physiological erection of penis occuring subconciously during rapid eye movement sleep cycle.

Nocturnal polysomnography Technique used to obtain physiological data during nighttime sleep.

Nod factors Symbiotic signal molecules synthesized in rhizobia by proteins encoded by nodulation genes; all share a similar lipochitin structure and have additional chemical substituents that allow the molecule to regulate root nodule formation, in particular host legumes at very low concentrations.

Nodal arrhythmias Arrhythmias arising from artrioventricular node. It is common during anesthesia.

Node A common ancestor, depicted as the intersection of two branches in a phylogenetic tree.

Node of Ranvier The area, every 0.1 to 1.0 mm, between adjacent oligodendrocytes, which forms myelin, of an axon in the central nervous system and between individual Schwann cells of the peripheral nervous system.

Nodular sclerosis In this fine or dense collagenous bands subside the lymphoid tissue into nodules. There are varying proportions of lacunar cells. Lymphocytes classic RS cells are rare. Prognosis is better.

Nodular vasculitis It is a chronic or recurrent nodular lesion of subcutaneous tissue. The nodules histopathologically show vasculitis with thickening and obliteration of blood vessels and fibrosis of subcutaneous tissue. It presents with slightly painful and tender erythematous nodules occurring chiefly on the calves of the legs. Nodules subside on bed rest and reappear on standing. Nodules may appear at varying intervals. There may be brown pigmentation along the superficial veins. Biopsy confirms the diagnosis.

Nodule A gall-like structure developed on the root or stem of legumes following infection by compatible rhizobia.

Nodules and tophi Rheumatoid subcutaneous nodule is firm, non-tender, well-demarcated and occurs over pressure points. While subcutaneous nodule of rheumatic fever by contrast is usually detected over the occipital region. Gouty tophi occurs particulary in relation to cartilage and seen arising from joints.

Nodulins Gene products expressed in host tissue during nodulation and N2 fixation.

Noise It is the sound that is disordered, unwanted which interferes with hearing. Any noise above the level of 20 decibels (dB) may cause damage. The louder the noise, the shorter the time required to damage. Exposure to a sudden very loud noise usually above 130 decibels can cause immediate and permanent damage. Occasionally loud noises can rupture the eardrum. Sound at 20 dB usually causes pain which is a warning that hearing may be damaged. Prolonged tinnitus after sudden cessation of noise is an indication that some damage has occurred.

High frequency sounds above 2000 Hz are found to be more damaging than low sounds. Hearing threshold is most marked around 4000 Hz. For continuous broad band and rapidly impulse noise, a 90 dBA sound pressure is typical of that which would be accepted as the minimum safe exposure 8 hours a day for 5 days a week. Steady state noise above 135 dBA is hazardous, no matter how short the duration is. A sound pressure level of 140 dB can be accepted as without risk for only 0.3 seconds a day.

Nominal dysphagia The area of brain in which language is organised extends over much of posterior, frontal, temporal and lower parietal regions of the dominant hemispheres. A lesion any where in this area will give rise to some difficulty in word finding, i.e. naming objects and is named as nominal dysphagia.

Nomothetic Relating to general or universal principles; opposite of *idiographic.*

Non ionic detergents A cleanser that acts by depressing the surface tension of water but does not ionize.

Non offending parent The non abusive parent who typiclly has the custody of the child.

Non shivering thermogenesis Process of heat production, without shivering by oxidation of brown fat.

Non thyroidal illness An illness not primarily affecting the thyroid gland assoiated with a decrease in plasma bioactive thyroid hormone.

Noncaseating A type of coagulation necrosis in which the necrotic material contains a mixture of protein and fat resembling cheese that is absorbed very slowly; typically occurs in tuberculosis.

Noncausal association The relationship between two variables is statistically significant, but no causal relationship exists, either because the temporal relationship is incorrect.

Nonconscious proprioception Sensory signals arising within the body that are not perceived, e.g., spinocerebellar tracts.

Non-consumation It is a failure to achieve satisfactory penetration during attempts of sexual intercourse. It causes great distress and may result from the muscular spasm of the woman, inability of the man to maintain erection, or psychological inhibition of the man in being overconsiderate in trying not to hurt the woman.

Noncoring needle Needle used to access implanted venous access device; it does not result in coring of the rubber diaphragm.

Non-corticated A term that refers to the periphery of a lesion; appears indistinct or ill-defined.

Nondifferential error Produces findings that are too high and too low in approxmately equal amounts, owing to random factors.

Nonelectrolytes Chemical compounds that remain bound together when dissolved in solution.

Nonessential amino acids (NEAAs) Amino acids manufatured by the human body.

Nonfeasance Failure to do an act that should have been bone.

Nonfluent aphasia A type of aphasia in which the flow of speech is slow and hesitant, vocabulary is limited and syntax is impaired. Articulation may be labored. Broca's aphasia is the most frequently occurring type of nonfluent aphasia.

Non-heme-iron Iron obtained from plant source.

Non-Hodgkin's lymphoma Non-Hodgkin's lymphoma (NHL) is of two types, nodular and diffuse. *Nodular lymphoma* is sometimes referred as giant follicular lymphoma characterised by proliferation of neoplastic cells in large nodules compressing remaining architecture of lymph nodes. It may change in diffuse form. Nodular lymphomas occur in oral cavity. *Diffuse lymphomas* are characterised by growth of neoplastic cells without a follicular pattern. These grow diffusely in lymph node and disrupt the normal pattern of node.

Nonhuman environment The physical surroundings of an individual..

Non-inflammatory oedema It appears whenever there is an increase in intravascular hydrostatic pressure and fall in colloid osmotic pressure. It may result due to impairment of flow of lymph.

Noninvasive techniques Methods that do not require entering the body of patient.

Nonmaleficence The moral principle of doing no harm.

Non-metallic restoration A restoration that does not have a metal component, e.g. composite or acrylic.

Nonnormative event Describes stressful events that occurs unexpectedly, leaving little or no time to prepare for them.

Nonnutritive sucking Sucking during which no milk flow is obtained.

Nonopioids Analgesics that do not contain opioids.

Nonparametric data Data for which descriptive parameters such as the mean and standard deviation cannot be obtained, because there is no measurement scale. No assumption is made about the underlying freuency distribution.

Nonpathogens Harmless and beneficial microorganisms.

Nonperiodic changes of FHR Accelerations or decelerations in the fetal heart rate that are not associated with uterine contractions.

Nonpolar Hydrophobic; describing molecules or groups that are poorly soluble in water.

Nonrandom Segregation Oriented distribution of chromosomes into progency cells; cosegregation of chromosomes and conserved cell structures.

Nonrebreather mask Oxygen delivery device in which all the exhaled air leaves the mask rather than partially entering the reservoir bag.

Nonregulatory behavior A behavior that is not required to meet the basic needs of an animal.

Nonsense mutation A single-base DNA mutation that changes the codon for an amino acid to a stop codon.

Nonshivering thermogenesis Process of heat production lasting no more than 10 seconds without change in colour or heart rate.

Non-specific lymphadenitis Bacterial and viral infection may result it. The secondary lymphadenopathies are clinically indistinguishable from one another. Main symptoms are tender, enlarged lymph glands at the mandibular angle.

Non-steroidal anti-inflammatory drugs (NSAIDs) These modify the responses caused by bradykinin. These inhibit synthesis of prostaglandin E and have direct analgesic effect on the higher centres. These reduce stickiness of blood platelets but may cause hypothrombinaemia in large doses, lowers blood sugar in low doses and may raise in higher doses. Indomethacin can be given per rectum for postoperative pain relief.

Nonstress test A test providing information about fetal well being, by using the external fetal monitor and evaluating the fetal heart rate for accelerations for the baseline rate.

Nonsuccedaneous Referring to permanent teeth that do not replace primary teeth.

Non-traumatic bursitis Diabetes and rheumatoid arthritis may lead to acute crystal bursitis. Appropriate aspiration and inspection of fluid for crystals will give diagnosis. Joint may become swollen with sympathetic effusion. Repeated bursitis needs surgical excision.

Nonverbal communication Exchange of information without using words.

Noradrenaline The main action of noradrenaline is to raise the blood pressure by constricting the arterioles and so raising the peripheral resistance. It is given by IV infusion to obtain a gradual sustained response because the effect of single IV injection will last only a minute or so.

Norepinephrine (NE) A chemical neurotransmitter in the brain, norepinephrine is found in one of the nonspecific ascending systems.

Norm Culturally expected behavior, appearance, or structure.

Normal Occurring naturally; not deviating from the standard.

Normal alignment knee Normal alignment of adult knee is slight physiological genu valgus. In an

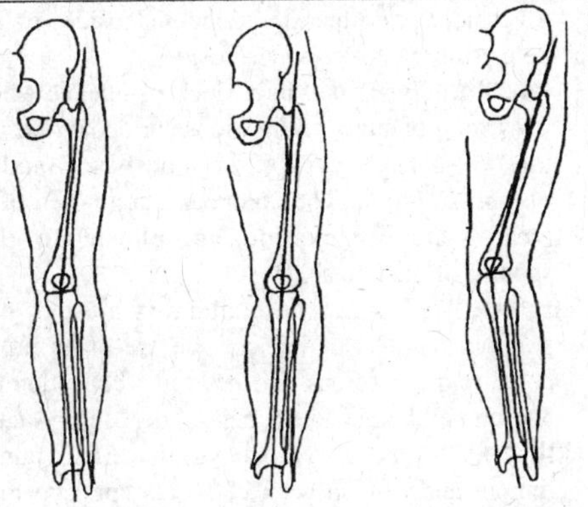

abnormal genu valgus alignment, the medial angle neasurement is more than 190° degrees. In genu varum the medial angle is less than 180 degrees.

Normal delivery It is a physiological process when foetus is expelled after 9 months. Head presents first.

Normal flexion of lumbar spine Straightening or flattening of the lumber spine.

Normal flora A term for the population of microbes that normally reside in a host and for the most part live in harmony.

Normal sinus rhythm The cardiac rhythm of depolarization that originatesin an proceeds from the sinoatrial node.

Normative event Term usually used to describe events that may be perceived as stressful but can be anticipated and planned for to reduce the effects of the stress. For example, the birth of a baby can be a stressful event for families, but they have several months to prepare for the new member's arrival.

Normocyte An erythrocyte that is normal in size, shape, hemoglobin content, such as seen in mormocytic anemia.

Normospermia A condition in which most ejaculated sperm are structurally normal.

Normotension Blood pressure below the criteria of normotension.

Normothermia 37° Centigrade.

Norplant It is contraceptive implant. Its six tubes filled with synthetic progestin are implanted in client's upper or lower arm. After insertion they are not visible.

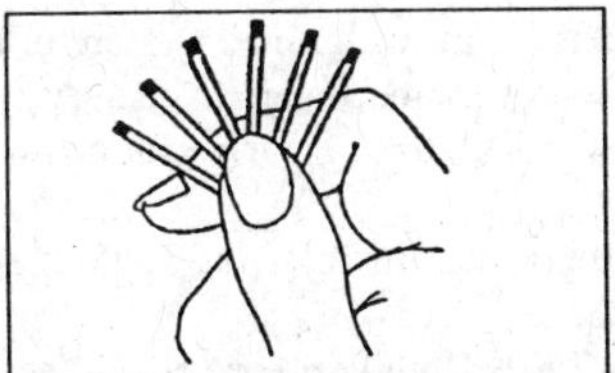

Contraceptive Implants

Nose bleed It is the loss of blood from mucous membrane that lines the nose specially in childhood. Most common cause is nose bleed, fragile blood vessels or dislodging crusts. Recurrent nose bleeds may be a sign of hypertension, a bleeding disorder or a tumour of nose and sinuses. Putting cold water

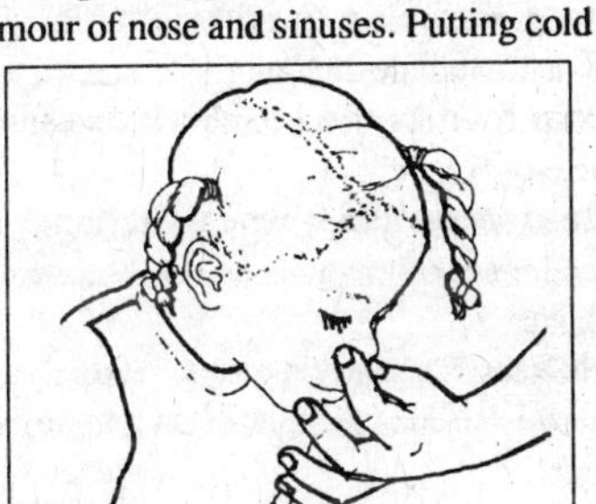

may help. To stop nose bleed apply direct pressure by firmly pinching both nostrils with a thumb and forefinger. The person should sit and lean slightly forward. If bleeding does not stop then it may be packed with gauge or may be cauterized the wound.

Nosocomial Denotes a disorder associated with being treated in a hospital, which is unrelated to the primary reason for being in the hospital.

Nosocomial infections Infections acquired while a person is being cared for in a hospital or other health care agency.

Nostril One of the external orifices of the nose.

Nostrum A quack, patent, or secret remedy.

Notary public Historically, a notary was a powerful public official who approved the filing of all official documents.

Notifiable disease A disease for which regular, frequent and timely information on individual cases is considered necessary for the prevention and control of disease.

Notochord A longitudinal flexible rod located between the gut and the spinal cord in all chordate embryos.

Noverbal communication Gesture or movement that indicates a reaction from another person, such as frowning, striking back with a fist, or folded arms.

Noxious Harmful, injurious, or detremental to health.

Nuchal cord Umbilical cord around neck.

Nuclear envelope Membrane that surrounds the cell nucleus.

Nuclear family A stereotypical structure of one mother, one father, and two children.

Nuclear lesion Lesion of a motor nucleus in the brainstem.

Nuclear medicine department Unit responsible for radionuclide imaging.

Nuclear membrane Membrane that surrounds the nucleus of a cell.

Nuclear pore Point where the inner and outer membranes of the nucleus comes together to form a hold.

Nuclease An enzyme that hydrolyzes in the internucleotide phosphodiester bonds in nucleic acids.

Nuclei Cluster of neurons.

Nucleic acid Molecule consisting of many nucleotides chemically bound together; deoxyribonucleic (DNA) acid and ribonucleic acid (RNA). Biologically occurring polynucleotides in which the nucleotide residues are linked in a specific sequence by phosphodiester bonds: DNA and RNA.

Nucleic acids The two nucleic acids are ribonucleic acid, found in the cytoplasm, and deoxyribonucleic acid.

Nucleocapsid It includes the capsid and the enclosed nucleic acid.

Nucleoid The bacterial chromosome when it is in a compact configuration, either inside a cell or as an isolated structure. In bacteria, the nuclear zone that contains the chromosome but has no surrounding membrane.

Nucleolus A dark-staining area with a cell nucleus; the site where ribosomal RNA is produced.

Nucleoplasm The protoplasmic contents of the nucleus of a cell.

Nucleoside A molecule composed of a heterocyclic nitrogenous base a nucleobase joined by an N-glycosidic bond to ribose ribonucleosides or 2'-deoxyribose deoxyribonucleosides.

Nucleotide Basic building block of nucleic acids consisting of sugar (either ribose or deoxyribose), one of several types of organic bases, and a phosphate group. The compound composed of a base, a monosaccharide, and phosphate; the subunit of nucleic acids.

Nucleus Cell organelle containing most of the genetic material of the cell; centre of an atom consisting of protons and neutrons; collection of neuron cell bodies in the central nervous system.

Null cell A type of lymphocyte that acts against tumour-and virus-infected cells; a lymphocyte that lacks the surface molecules of B-cells and T-cells.

Null hypothesis Testing the null hypothesis requires a computation to determine the limits within which two groups may differ in their results (e.g. an experimental and a control group—even though if the experiments were often repeated or the groups were larger no difference would be found. The probability of the obtained difference being found if no true difference existed is commonly expressed as a v-value, e.g. < 0.05 that the null hypothesis is true.

Nulligravida A woman who has never become pregnant.

Nullipara A woman who has never completed a pregnancy beyond 20 weeks of gestation.

Number A numeral that does not necessarily have quantitative meaning; it is a form of naming.

Number needed to treat The number of patients who would need to be treated, on average, for one of them to experince the beneficial effects of a particular type of treatment.

Numbness There is loss of sensation caused by interference to the passage of impulses along sensory nerves. It can occur naturally while sitting cross-legged. Multiple sclerosis can cause loss of sensation in any part of body. In a stroke, pressure on, or reduced blood supply to nerve pathways in brain causes loss of feeling on one side of the body.

Severe cold as in frostbite causes numbness by a direct action on the nerves. The distribution of the affected area may suggest the site and mechanism of nerve damage.

Numeral A symbol that does not necessarily have quantitative meaning; it is a form of naming.

Numerator data Data that define the events or conditins of concern.

Nummular eczema It is also known as discoid eczema. The condition may develop due to allergic manifestation. It is often found associated with dry skin in winter season. Condition generally begins with itchy, scaling or vesicular patches developed on dorsum of hands, extensor surface of arms, legs and thighs.

Later on they may form discrete, coin-shaped, erythematous, oedematous, vesicular and crusted patches. Plaques may enlarge leaving the centre clear space lesions appearing symmetrically. Patient complains of varying degree of pruritus but seldom leads to excoriation.

Nuptial plumage In many birds, especially males, an array of brilliant or showy feathers assumed at the onset of breeding, associated with increase in pituitary or gonadal hormones.

Nurse She is trained to look after those who need medical care either in hospital or at home. Some are superspecialists who have been trained in special branch, i.e heart, dental, operation theatre, etc. Senior ones concentrate on management and administration skill while others may be very good in special welfare.

Nurse egg A nondeveloping egg that is ingested by developing larvae.

Nurse midwife A registered nurse who is trained in the nurse midwifery.

Nurse practice act Statute that legally defines the unique role of the nurse and differentiates it from that of other health care practitioners, such as physicians.

Nurse practitioner A registered nurse with additional preparation in physical and psychosocial assessment, who provides primary care management for patients with common acute and chronic illnesses and developmental needs.

Nurse-client contract An agreement between the health professional and client to work together to attain goals that are determined by the client.

Nurse-managed care Pattern in which a nurse manager plans the nursing care of patients based on their illness or medical diagnosis.

Nurse-midwives These assist women with pregnancy and childbearing, either independent or with an obstetrician.

Nursing behavior Any of various maternal behaviors that facilitate suckling by young mammals.

Nursing care of dead body If patient dies on bed immediately cover the patient by a cloth from head to toe. Arrange to remove the body to a separate room.

This is done when doctor has already declared him dead. Record the exact time of death and close the eyes with tip of fingers. Pack the nostrils. While handing over the dead body to relatives give death certificate also.

Nursing care plan Written list of the patient's problems, goals, and nursing orders for patient care.

Nursing care planning It is the systemic assessment and identification of patient's problem, the setting of objectives and the establishing methods and strategies of accomplishing them. A care plan is written record of identified nursing problems and the nursing action to be adopted to meet the patient's needs. This also includes the method of evaluating the effectiveness of nursing actions.

Nursing diagnosis Health problem that can be prevented, reduced, or resolved through independent nursing measures.

Nursing implications Points the nurse needs to remember about a drug or to teach patients.

Nursing orders Directions for a patient's care.

Nursing process A goal-directed series of activities whereby the practice of nursing accomplishes its goal or alleviating, minimizing, or preventing real or potential health problems.

Nursing process-record Nursing process goes into details of patient's care and leaves no chance of negligence.

It ensures a complete record of patient's condition through out the stay of patient. It also mentions record of nursing care provided to the patient. It provides greater emphasis on social and psychological needs of the patients.

Nursing skills Activities unique to the practice of nursing.

Nursing team Personnel who care for patients directly.

Nursing theory Proposal on what is involved in the process of nursing.

Nutrient A biochemical substance used by the body that must be supplied in adequate amounts from foods consumed.

Nutrient canal A tiny tube-like passage way through bone that houses nerves and blood vessels; appears radiolucent.

Nutrient density The quality of protein, vitamin and minerals per 100 calories of food.

Nutrition Sum of processes by which an animal or plant absorbs or takes in and utilises food substances; ingestion, digestion, absorption (of products of digestion) of food materials through mucous membranes of the alimentary tract, transportation by blood and lymph to body cells where they are used or stored.

Nutritional category The classification of organisms based on their principal carbon and energy sources; microorganisms are classified into four nutritional categories; photoautotrophs, photoheterotrophs, chemoautotrophs, and chemoheterotrophs.

Nutritional stress A physiological, environmental or metabolic stress that is imposed on an organism to cause an neural, endocrine and metabolic response.

N-Way ANOVA See analysis of variance.

Nyctalopia Night blindness due to vitamin 'A' deficiency.

Nymphomania It is a compulsive insatiable need for sexual stimulation and gratification in women, frequently leading to promiscuity or to masturbation several times a day.

Nystagmus It is a rhythmical sequence of eye movements in opposite directions. The velocity of movement in each direction is often different. Nystagmus is usually not present when the eyes are in neutral straight ahead position. It is elicited by asking the patient to follow a moving target, i.e. examiner's finger. In Meniere's disease rapid movement is towards the side of lesion. Nystagmus induced by peripheral lesion is enhanced in dark. In destructive vestibular lesions closure of eyes usually abolishes nystagmus.

O

O. Felincus O Felineus and O.Viverrini are similar to that of C. Sinesis employing intermediate hosts of snail genus Bithynia as well as cyprimid fishes. Infection results from eating raw or improperly cooked fish.

OA Osteoarthritis.

Ober test Test used to evaluate contracture of hip band.

Obesity A person is considered obese when he or she is having 20 per cent more weight over the maximum desirable weight for his or her height and age. Obesity occurs when the net evergy intake is more than energy expenditure. Person's energy requirement is determined by his or her basal metabolic rate (BMR) and partly by his or her physical activity. Obese people may have a very low BMR or may need fewer calories because they are physically less active. Genetic factors play a part in the development of obesity. Hypertension and stroke are twice likely to occur in obese people than in lean person. Coronary heart disease is more common and adult onset diabetes mellitus is five times more common. Osteoarthritis may be precipitated or aggravated by obesity. Weight loss does not reverse the disease but does help to relieve stress and pain. Best way to reduce is to take less of food or increase physical activity.

Obesity hypoventilation syndrome A condition of acidemia and hypercarbia associated with reduced alveolar ventilation secondary to obesity; the chest wall is too heavy to move in the reclined position.

Object permanence In piagetian psychology, the capacity for memory. The child who has achieved object permanence understands that a given object may continue to exist even when it is not directly experienced. A memory, idea, or view of the object is carried around in the head. The development of object permanence is a necessary prelude to thinking, for thinking requires symbolic manipulation.

Object relations The emotional bonds between one person and another, as contrasted with interest in and love for the self; usually described in terms of capacity for loving and reacting appropriately to others.

Objective A microscope lens that magnifies the real image formed from an ocular lens and forms a virtual image in the focal plane of the microscope.

Objective data Facts that are observable and measurable.

Objective sign Signs which are perceptible to the external senses by feel, sight, hearing, smell and measurement.

Obligate Describing an organism that is restricted to a single type of environmental condition, behavioral mode, or the like.

Obligate intracellular parasite An organism that must live within the cells of its host to survive.

Obligate parasite An organism that has a parastitic phase as an essential part of its life cycle.

Obligate syntroph A microorganism that must interact mutualistically with one or more other microorganisms to metabolize a specific substrate.

Obligative anaerobe Microorganisms that can exist only in the complete absence of free oxygen because oxygen is toxic to it.

Oblique Slanting; inclined; between a horizontal and a perpendicular direction.

Oblique fissure The main or primary groove separating the upper and middle lobes from the lower lobe of the right lung and the upper and lower lobes of the left lung.

Oblique ridge Part of elevation of enamel on occlusal surface.

Oblique section A cut made at other than a right angle to the long axis of an organ.

Obscenity Language, gestures, pictures and films which are usually high sexually explicit that grossly violate the morals and standards of good taste in a particular society.

Observational learning Learning to behave by watching others.

Observe To see or notice; to watch attentively.

Obsession It means complete occupation of the mind by an idea inspite of the effort made by sufferer to drive it away. There are constant or frequent ideas due to some irresistible impulse in the mind of a person who is aware of absurdity of the same. It develops in persons of neurotic temperament. These are persistent distressing thoughts or impulses experienced as unwanted and senseless but irresistable.

Obsessive compulsive behaviour It is a neurosis in which person carries out repetitive, ritualised acts. The condition is partly inherited, but environmental factors also play a part. Certain forms of brain damage may also result it. Person suffers from both obsessions and compulsions, often accompanied by depression and anxiety. Obsessions are recurrent thoughts and feelings coming to mind involuntarily. Person is unable to ignore or resist them. Thoughts of violence, fears of being infected by germs or dirt and constant doubts develop. Compulsions are repetitive apparently purposeful acts that are carried out in a ritualised fashion. Person does not feel happy in doing activities. Seventy five per cent people respond to therapy very well.

Obsessive compulsive disorder Repetitive thoughts, images or impulses that are expressed as trusive or repetitive behaviour that are performed in response to an obsession or certain rules. It is a chronic illness dominated by obsessions and compulsions occuring in the absence of another psychiatric disorder.

Obsetric history Object is to find out the possibility of recurrence of previous complication arising in pregnancy or labour for which prevention may be useful.

Obstetric forceps Whatever may be the type of forceps, the action is essentially that of making traction. The blades compress the head but the amount of compression should be only so to have firm grip. More or prolonged force may cause intracranial damage. Presentation of fetus must be either a vertex or face with chin anterior. Head of fetus must be engaged and cervix must be fully dilated. Pelvic outlet has to be adequate too.

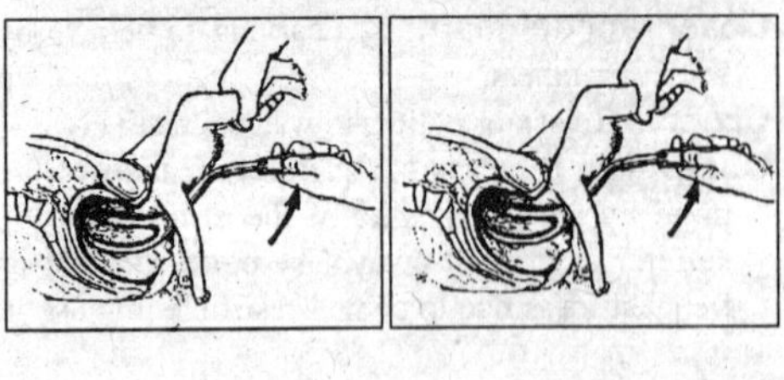

Application forceps should be considered when labour is complicated by maternal distress, fetal distress or prolongation of second stage. Obstetrical forceps vary greatly in design.

All types consist of two separate portions which are inserted into vagina sequentially. Each half consists of a blade proper which is applied to fetal head, a shank and a handle. The halves are joined by a lock. Before applying this membrane must be ruptured, cervix must be fully dilated and fetal head must be engaged.

Obstetric paralysis Birth injuries of brachial plexus that result in paralysis.

Obstetric shocks These are ruptured uterus, cervical tears extending to lower segment, vulval hematoma, PPH and inversion of uterus.

Obstetric yellow atrophy of liver It is a rare disease. Gross fatty changes are present in all liver cells except in narrow periportal zone. A light infiltration with small round cells is usually present. Patient develops severe vomiting, and epigastric pain. The vomiting becomes coffee ground in character, the jaundice deepens. Stupor progresses into coma. Prognosis is always grave.

Obstetrical outlet It is a segment between plane of least pelvic dimension and anatomical outlet.

Obstetrician A physician who specialises in the management of pregnancy, labour, and the period of confinement after delivery.

Obstetrics The branch of medicine that is concerned with the management of women during pregnancy, childbirth, and the puerperium.

Obstipation The absolute inability to pass stool.

Obstructed labour It refers to the cases in which spontaneous delivery through the natural passage is very difficult or impossible. Hydrocephalus, contracted pelvis, locked twins may be the cause.

Obstruction, prostate The most characteristic and usually first symptom of prostatic hypertrophy is slowness of urinary stream. Amount of residual urine increases resulting in urinary frequency. When infection occurs there is burning in urination and urgency. As obstruction increases urinary retention may take place. Blood in urine is uncommon. There may be fever and urine becomes cloudy. As urinary toxaemia develops patient's tongue becomes dry, red and swollen on occasions. Oedema may develop.

Obstruction, urine flow Most common causes are large calculus or tumour. Tumour of ureter,

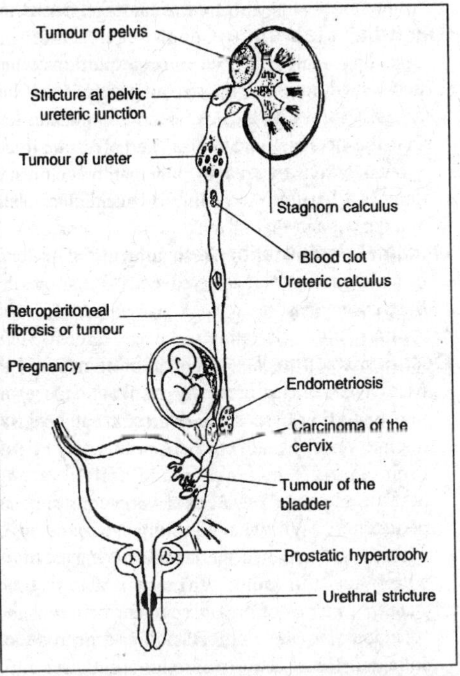

enlargement of prostate, urethral stricture, endometriosis and pressure of pregnancy over ureter may lead to obstruction of flow of urine.

Obstructive cardiomyopathy Here the ventricular system is massively hypertrophied. There is narrowing of inflow and outflow tracts of both ventricles. Clinically breathlessness, angina and syncope are present. Jerky pulse, prominent 'a' wave in jugular vein, biventricular hypertrophy, basal systolic thrill, late systolic murmur may be present. There may be double impulses at apex. ECG shows ventricular enlargement and conduction defect.

Obstructive jaundice The yellowish staining of the skin and sclerae by bile pigments that results from an obstruction to the flow of bile into the duodenum.

Obstructive sialadenitis It is associated with salivary stones or mucous plugs. In these cases the duct of gland is also inflamed. Sub maxillary and parotid glands are mostly involved. Involved gland is enlarged and painful specially just before, during and after meals. In chronic case gland becomes firm, painless and permanently enlarged. There may be stone in excretory duct. In a few cases of infection and scarring obstructive sialadenitis may develop. The interstitial tissue of gland lobules shows oedema and infiltration of plasma cells, neutrophils and lymphocytes. In long-standing disease a considerable amount of fibrosis and atrophy can lead to replacement of entire gland by connective tissue so that only the ducts of original glands can be seen.

Obstructive uropathy Obstruction increases susceptibility to infection and to stone formation. Untreated obstruction almost always leads to

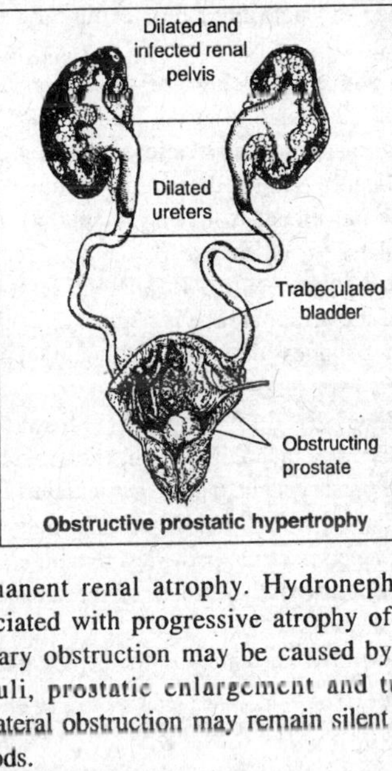

Obstructive prostatic hypertrophy

permanent renal atrophy. Hydronephrosis is associated with progressive atrophy of kidney. Urinary obstruction may be caused by urinary calculi, prostatic enlargement and tumours. Unilateral obstruction may remain silent for long periods.

Obsturator sign X-Ray sign of septic arthritis, a displacement of the obturator fat plane along the inner wall of pelvis.

Obtund To render dull or blunt; to render less acute.

Obtundent A chemical that has a sedative or numbing effect on a sensitive tooth; eugenol is a dental obtundent.

Obturation Act of closing or occluding.

Obturator Any occluding structure or a foramen so occluded, as with the obturator foramen of the hip.

Obturator foramen A large, oval shaped, opening in the pelvis between the pubis and ischium.

Obturator nerve block Performed to accompany sciatic nerve block or femoral nerve block or in the diagnosis of hip pain.

Occipit It extends from posterior fontanelle to the foramen magnum. Sub occipital region is region under occipital protuberance.

Occipital Pertaining to the occiput.

Occipital bone Bone in the posterior area of the skull that lies between the parietal and temporal bones. Forms the posterior base of the skull.

Occipital condyles The pair of bony prominence on the external surface of inferior aspect of occipit.

Occipital lobe Centre for vision is located on medial surface of occipital lobe surrounding calcarine sulcus. Area number is 17. There are association areas above and below the centre for vision, i.e. 18 and 19 related to visual perception. Following lesions in these areas objects are seen but their significance is not appreciated. A centre for control of eye movement is located in area no. 19 which modulates visual reflexes.

Occipital lobe, lesion In bilateral lesions of the tips of the occipital lobe is neglect or denial of the virtual blindness due to bilateral ocipital infarction caused by basilar artery occlusion. Neglect of blindness is due to preservation of some unconscious visual function, nicknamed 'blind sight' preserved in lateral geniculate bodies. In occipital blindness pupils react normally to light, as the anterior visual pathways remain unaffected.

Occipitalization Synostosis of the atlas with the ocipital bone.

Occipitoaxoid Pertaining to the occipital bone and the axis.

Occipitocervical Pertaining to the occiput and the neck.

Occipitocervical fusion Arthrodesis of the base of the occipit to C_1 vertebra.

Occipitofacial Pertaining to the occiput and the forehead.

Occipitomastoid Pertaining to the occipital bone and the mastoid process.

Occipitomental Pertaining to the occiput and the chin.

Occlude To close together. To bring the mandibular teeth into contact with maxillary teeth.

Occlusal Pertaining to the contacting surfaces of opposing units teeth or occlusion rims. Pertaining to the masticating surfaces of the posterior teeth.

Occlusal clearance Condition in which the oppsoing occlusal surfaces may glide over one another without any interfering projection.

Occlusal curvature Close observation indicates that the occlusal and incisal surfaces of all the crowns taken together in either arch would not contact a flat line. Curvature of mandibular teeth is concave and that of maxillary teeth convex.

Occlusal equilibration Reshaping of the occlusal or incisal surfaces of selected teeth to improve the bite; coronaplasty;

Occlusal load Bite force.

Occlusal trauma When the teeth are exposed to excessive occlusal forces, the resultant changes in the supporting tissues are referred to as occlusal trauma. The causes of occlusal trauma may be due to an absolute increase in occlusal force and because of some pathological conditions such as periodontitis. When a tooth is subjected to occlusal trauma, the forces that are most damaging are those which act in a lateral direction. Microscopic changes in areas of pressure are narrowing of the periodontal space, compression and necrosis of collagen fibres. Bone resorption continues until pressure is relieved and then a small amount of new bone is formed to reembed the fibres of periodontal ligament. In case of extreme tension, thrombosis of blood vessels can sometime be seen. The final result of these changes is that tooth moves out of the occlusal trauma. Occlusal trauma facilitates the spread of inflammation from the area of periodontal pocket into the underlying tissue.

Occlusion 1. Act of closure or state of being closed. 2. Any contact between the incising or masticating surfaces of the upper and lower teeth.

Occlusional harmony The nondistruptive relationship of an occlusion to all its factors.

Occlusive dressing Any bandage that covers a wound competely protecting it from exposure to air.

Occult Obscure or hidden from view, as, for example, occult blood in stools or urine.

Occult blood (faecal) It is the presence of faeces of blood that cannot be seen by the naked eye but can be detected by chemical test. It may be the result of oesophagitis, gastric inflammation/cancer or cancer of rectum. A thin film of faeces is smeared on a chemically coated paper and a drop or two of oxidising agent is placed on it. If blood is present in the faeces covered paper turns blue.

Occult fracture A fracture strongly suggestive by radiological signs but whose line is not visible until reperative bone changes have occured.

Occult sinusitis In paediatric age group main symptoms are dry cough, sniffing, lingering cold, anorexia and failure to thrive. Peak occurrence is from 7 to 12 years of age.

Occupation The active or "doing" process when one is engaged in goal-directed activity.

Occupational asthma A bronchospastic disease whose symptoms occur during periods of exposure to repiratory tract irritants in the workplace. The symptoms are usually less pronounced during peeriods away fromwork, such as weekends.

Occupational deafness Deafness brought on by noise in the workplace.

Occupational dermatitis It is an acute or chronic inflammatory process that is produced by direct contact on the surface of skin with chemicals, minerals, oils and animal origin. Condition produces intracellular oedema and intraepithelial vesicle formation. The onset is sudden with itching and erythema formation. Lesions are more where direct contact is there. There may also be hotness of area, exudation, crusting, excoriation and secondary bacterial infection. Treatment includes immediate withdrawal from offending agents. Topical application of corticosteroid is useful.

Occupational disease Any disorder caused by job related factors.

Occupational exposure standard Workplace exposure limit which will not damage the health of workers exposed to it by inhalation day after day.

Occupational marks Horny or rough hands are found in blacksmith and cultivators, rounded callosities in hollow of hands in shoe makers and horny callosities over shoulder in load carriers. Multiple needle pricks may be seen in tailors and varicose veins in traffic men.

Occupational medicine Branch of medicine which addresses the relationship of people to their work.

Occupational science A scientific discipline that studies the human as an occupational being.

Occupational therapist A person trained and licensed to provide instruction and supervision regarding median nerve paralysis.

Occupational therapy It may be a part of rehabilitation. Person learns a new skill for weakened part of the body. It helps in generating an attitude of creative independence to form medical care.

Occupational toxin A harmful chemical substance, present in the workplace, that acts on one or more types of cells within the testis to interfere with spermatogenesis of steroidogenesis or both.

Occupied bed While the patient remains in bed.

Ochronosis It is a rare autosomal recessive metabolic disease. Urine becomes black coloured on standing and person may have osteoarthritis, valvular heart disease, atherosclerosis and pigmentation of cartilage. Ocular symptoms include pigmentation of cornea, sclera and conjunctiva.

Ocona-z It is indicated for the treatment of moderate to severe dandruff and seborrhoeic dermatitis.

Ocular dominance columns Cell columns in the primary visual cortex activated by geniculostriate neurons.

Ocular dystrophy A rare form of muscular dystrophy that affects the extraocular and upper facial muscles.

Ocular nerve paralysis It produces a pattern of strabismus and diplopia. In 6th abducent nerve

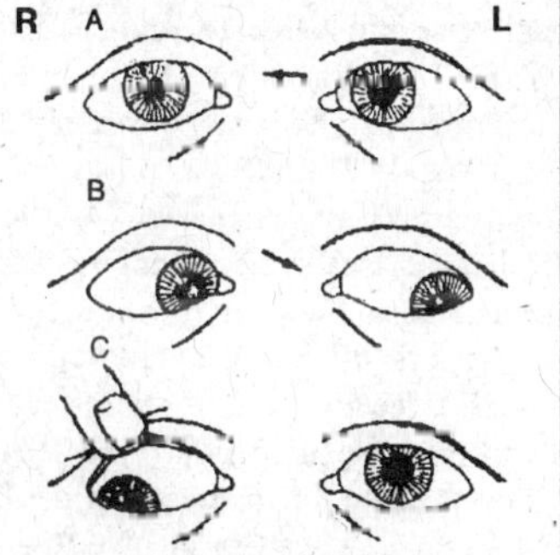

A Abducent nerve paralysis
B Trochlear nerve paralysis
C Oculomotor nerve paralysis

paralysis eye cannot look outward, with trochlear nerve paralysis eye cannot look downwards, with third nerve oculomotor lesion ptosis will develop.

Ocular pursuits The ability of the eyes to follow a moving object.

Oculocardiac reflex Bradycardia following traction on the extraocular muscles especially medical rectus.

Oculofacial Pertaining to the eyes and the face.

Oculomotor Refers to the oculomotor nerve.

Oculomotor hypokinesia Inadequate saccades associated with Parkinson's disease.

Oculomotor nerve It is the third cranial nerve. It stimulates only motor functions. It controls all the muscles which control eye movements except the two superior oblique muscles and the lateral rectus muscle. The nerve may be damaged during basal fracture or a disorder that distorts the brain, such as tumour. There may be drooping of eyelid, squint, dilatation of pupil, double vision and protrusion of eyeball.

Oculomotor skills Multiple coordinated eye movements produced by eye muslces; also known as ocular control or ocular motor skills.

Oddi, sphincer Sphincter of hepatopancreatic ampulla.

Odds ratio (OR) The odds of exposure in teh diseased group divided by teh odds of exposure in the nondiseased group.

Odontinoid Resembling a tooth; toothlike.

Odontoblasts Cell that forms the surface layer of the dental papilla that forms dentin of the tooth. Odontoblasts continue production for years after eruption.

Odontochirurgical A term formerly used to denote relationship to dental surgery.

Odontoclastoma Internal tooth resporption.

Odontodysplasia This affects both the ectodermal and mesodermal dental component. Any tooth may be affected but usually one or more quadrants are involved. There is defective dentin and enamel formation and discoloured, hypoplastic and hypocalcified teeth with short roofs. Tooth fails to erupt and radiolucent areas may be seen around their crowns. Pulp chambers are wide. Disorder may be bilateral as well as involve teeth in both jaws. Microscopically there is distortion of enamel matrix, absence of enamel rods and focal calcification in the connective tissue around the crown. The pulp contains calcifications.

Odontogenic An epithelial lined sac produced from tooth forming tissues.

Odontograph An instrument for recording the unevenness of the surface of tooth enamel.

Odontoid fracture These occur either through the isthmus or at the base of adontoid and are unstable.

Odontologist A dentist.

Odontoma These are composed of hard dental tissues. These are generally diagnosed in second decade of life and mostly occur in maxilla. Rarely these assume large sizes and produce deformity of normal jaw contours. These are slow growing and may persist without symptoms for decades. Two types of odontomas, compound and complex are having clearly outlined dense radiopacities often surrounded by a thin radiolucent zone. In the compound type crudely formed teeth of varying size and shape may be recognised in the radiopacity. In the complex type the radiopacity does not have a specific shape but appears as a disorganised irregular mass. Sometimes a cyst is associated with an odontoma. This cyst is lined by stratified squamous epithelium.

Odontophobia All kinds of phobic reactions related to dental treatment.

Odontoradiograph A roentgenograph of a tooth or of the teeth.

Odontoscopy The taking of dental impressions.

Odontosis The formation or eruption of the teeth.

Oedema It is an accumulation of serum like fluid in body tissues. Heart failure leads to blood congestion in the veins creating backward pressure in the capillaries. The backward pressure overcomes osmotic pressure in capillaries. This backward pressure causes more fluid to be pushed to tissues at various places. Nephrotic syndrome causes abnormal loss of proteins from blood which lowers osmotic pressure preventing enough fluid being drawn from tissues into the blood. Renal failure prevents salts being excreted allowing fluid to accumulate. When excessive fluid becomes more than 15 per cent it is evident as swelling. Treatment includes treating the causative pathology, restriction of salt and diuretic drugs.

Oedema glottidis Mucous membrane of the glottis is too adherent to allow much swelling. It covers below and above the cord. Onset is usually sudden attended by dyspnoea, dysphagia and inspiratory stridor. Diagnosis is on account of swelling at the back of tongue.

Oedipus complex A Freudian term representing the sexual attachment of a son for his mother, usually regarded as repressed and disguised in various ways. Also, it is assumed that the son will be jealous of the father because the father can have intimacies with the mother that the son is denied.

Oesophageal atresia A congenital defect in which the oesophagus ends in a blind pouch rather than a continuous tube to the stomach. It is characterised by excessive drooling, gagging, coughing, vomiting when fed, cyanosis, and dyspnoea. The condition is corrected by surgery.

Oesophageal carcinoma Alcohol and smoking are the cause of it. Most important symptom is dysphagia. At first solid foods are swallowed with difficulty and in course of time there may be difficulty with liquid too. Unless 75% of calibre of oesophagus is not involved dysphagia does not develop. Patient can locate the exact site of contraction and constriction. Later on food may be regurgitated. Metastatic lymph nodes are palpable in neck. There may develop hoarseness of voice.

Oesophageal contractility It is an indicator of anesthetic depth and brainstem integrity.

Oesophageal varices These are dilatation of normal submucosal oesophageal veins and are important collaterals of portal circulation. Bleeding from lower esophagus occurs.

Oesophagus The part of the digestive tract between the pharynx and stomach.

Oestradiol An oestrogen produced in ovarian follicles. It inhibits the release of follicle-stimulating hormone prior to ovulation.

Oestrogens These are responsible for the normal development of female genital tract, of breasts and female secondary sexual characters. These have less protein anabolic action than do androgens. Uterine bleeding may be stopped temporarily by giving large doses of oestrogens or may be started by sudden withdrawal. Oestrogens are necessary for the maintenance of normal pregnancy. Ethinyl oestradiol has a half-life of 13 hours and is the drug of choice since it is not rapidly degraded in liver and is effective orally. Oestradiol is weaker and is good for physiological replacement. For menopausal symptoms severe enough to demand treatment combined oestrogenprogesterone formulations are used for about a year.

Off flavours It is a term that describes the presence of an strange taste or aroma which is generally not associated with the food.

Office policy Written statement of the dentist's philosophy and policies defining the responsibilities of the patient and office staff.

Offset joint Knee joint in which the axis is located posterior to the midline of the leg; intended to increase knee stability.

Offsets Predictive mathematical conversions.

Oguchi's disease It is a type of congenital night blindness. After exposure to bright light the fundus assumes a white grey colour, especially around the optic nerve head and in macula. There is sometimes a more brownish discolouration. After remaining for about 2 to 3 hours in darkness ocular fundus becomes normal. Retinal vessels look darker.

OH 1. Oral hygiene; number describing the oral hygience condition of a tooth. 2. Abbreviation used in charting to indicate overhang in a restoration.

Oil A type of liquid lubricant.

Ointment It is a greasy, semisolid preparation that is applied to the skin. Most ointments contain petroleum or wax and have soothing, moisturising effect. These are thicker than creams. By occlusion they promote dermal dehydration and are also water miscible. Bases are composed largely of lipid by preventing water loss. Ointments contain fewer preservatives.

Olecranon Large process of proximal ulna that forms the posterior bony prominence of elbow.

Olecranon fossa A large depression on the posterior surface of the humerus.

Olecranon process The large bony process of the ulna; commonly referred to as the tip of the elbow.

Oleoinfusion A preparation made by infusing a drug in oil.

Olfaction The sense of smell

Olfactory tract The olfactory sensory tract of axons that conveys impulses from the olfactory bulb to the olfactory protion of the cerebral cortex.

Olfactory aura Epileptic aura accompanied by illusion of an odor.

Olfactory bulb The brain structure where most primary olfactory nerve fibers are first relayed.

Olfactory nerve It is the first cranial nerve which conveys smell sensations from nose to brain. Nerve endings are specialised in detecting stimuli. Nerve fibres pass from the receptors through tiny holes in the root of nasal cavity and comes together to form a bulb. Damage to olfactory nerve during head injury results in loss of impairment of sense of small.

Olfactory pit The olfactory pit that forms two recesses, one medial and one lateral. The lateral recess of the olfactory pit gives rise to the olfactory nerves, and the medial recess gives rise to the vomeronasal and terminal nerves.

Olfactory placode A thickening of the ectoderm on the lateral sides of the head of vertebrate embryos that gives rise to the nasal cavity.

Olfactory receptor Chemical receptors responsible for the sense of smell; located in the epithelial tissue in the upper part of the nasal cavity.

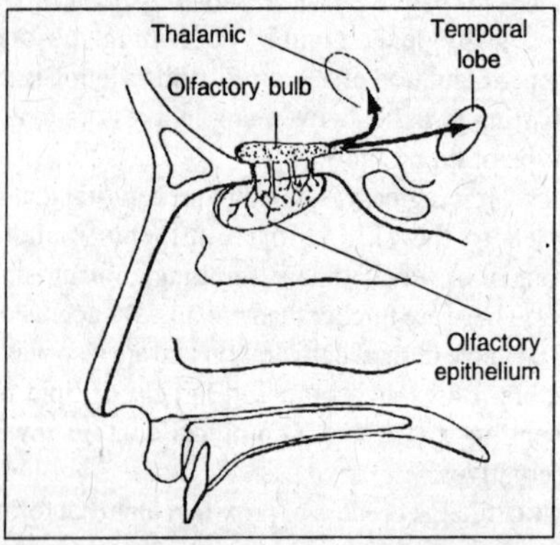

Olfactory receptors These are located in the lateral wall of nose and high up in nasal septum.

Olfactory system A collective term for the olfactory receptor cells in the olfactory epithelium of the nose, their axon that form the olfactory nerves, and the main olfactory bulb.

Olignonucleotide A short polymer of nucleotides, usually less than 50.

Oligo hydraminos When the liquor amni is deficient, a few ounces only so as to make fetus immobile or to restrict intrauterine movement. It may result due to placental insufficiency or due to renal agenesis. Uterus is found much smaller than expected. After the rupture of membranes liquor is thick, viscid and meconium stained. Intrauterine placental death may be due to placental insufficiency. Constriction of umbilical cord may occur.

Oligodendrocyte A neuroglial cell that supports neurons and produces a myelin sheath around axons of neurons of the central nervous system.

Oligodendroglial cell A glial cell in the central nervous system that provides myelin on axons.

Oligodendroglioma It is uncommon, slow growing primary brain tumour affecting adults. Symptoms of brain tumour are, i.e. headache and vomiting. Surgical removal of tumour in some cases can led to a complete cure. 30 per cent patients may survive up to five years.

Oligogalacturonate lyase One of a group of diverse, often cytoplasmic, enzymes that catalyze the eliminative removal of unsaturated terminal residues from D-galacturonate oligosaccharides.

Oligohydraminos In this liquor amnii is deficient in amount. There may be only 100 ml of fluid. Its cause is unknown. There is close relation between amnion nodosum, renal dysplasia and oligohydraminos. Amnion covering placenta may be studded with miliary, yellow grey nodules. Oligohydraminos may give rise to certain deformities, i.e. talipes spinal curvature, torticollis or ankylosis of joints. It is seen in potter's disease. It may result in mental deficiency by not providing nutrition sufficient to fetus. Fetal distress may develop during delivery.

Oligomenorrhea A condition in which menstrual cycles occur at infrequent or irregular intervals; specifically, intervals greater than 35 days apart. It is a scanty menstruation and is irregular in frequency. It generally develops during menarche and menopause. Hormonal treatment in other cases will be required.

Oligomer A short polymer, usually of amino acids , sugars, or nucleotides; the definition of "short" is somewhat arbitrary, but usually less than 50 subunits.

Oligomeric protein A multisubunit protein having two or more identical polypeptide chains.

Oligospermia There is deficiency in the number of sperms per unit volume of seminal fluid. There are normally more than 20 million sperm per ml.

Oligospermia is a major cause of infertility. It may be caused by orchitis, failure of testis to descend into the scrotum, varicocele, cigarette smoking and alcohol abuse. Gonadotropin hormone may be prescribed for shorter period.

Oligotroph Literally, small eater; an organism that is able to grow well in conditions of limited nutrients, thus, oligotrophic.

Oliguria There is production of a smaller than normal quantity of urine in comparison of fluids consumed. It may be simply due to excessive sweating in a hot climate. Renal failure may also result it.

Ollier's Layer The innermost layer of the periosteum.

Omental bursa The pocket-like sac inside the fold of the greater omentum.

Omentum It is a part of peritoneum. It comprises a large flap of membranous tissue hanging from stomach over the front of abdominal organs. It respresents second protective and insulating layer of the wall of abdomen.

Omeprazole Half-life is one hour. It produces a profound long lasting, irreversible enzyme inhibition of both basic and stimulated acid secretion.

A single 20 mg dose decreases acidity by 90 per cent over 24 hours. It is absorbed in small intestine. It is highly effective for ulcerative reflux oesophagitis and is a drug of choice for Zollinger-Ellison syndrome. Adverse effects include nausea, headache and diarrhoea.

Omnipaque The proprietary name of iohexol, a nonionic water soluble, contrast medium used in contrast study

Onanism Coitus interruptus. The term is sometimes used interchangeably with masturbation.

Oncocytoma It is a rare benign tumor affecting parotids in elderly. It consists of large eosinophilic cells with small compact nuclei.

Oncogene Gene that has the ability to transform a normal cell into a cancerous cell when it is activated.

Oncogenic Cancer causing.

Oncology A branch of medicine regarding the study of tumors.

Oncotic pressure Osmotic pressure exerted by plasma proteins. It is usually 25 m.m. Hg.

One-stage implant An implant equipped with its abutment/attachment component at the time of insertion, precluding the need for second-stage treatment to expose and/or attach the abutment/attachment component.

Onlay A dental restoration made from metal, ceramic or composite that is cemented within the tooth and extends to include a replacement of one or more cusps.

Onlay graft Augmentation by placing autogenous bone and/or appropriate substitutes on or over bone to increase depth, length, and/or width.

Onset of drug action Period of time after a drug is administered for it to produce a response.

Onset of labour The signs by which onset of labour is recognised are, painful uterine contractions, slight uterine haemorrhage, commencing dilatation of internal os and formation of bag of waters.

Ontogenetic Pertaining to the development of the individual.

Ontogeny The development of individual organism.

Ontological confrontation An experience that forces one to knowledge the reality and salience of death.

Onychectomy Excision of a nail and nail bed.

Onychitis Inflammation of nail matrix.

Onychocryptosis Ingrowing toe nail.

Onychomycosis It is a ringworm of nails specially of great toe nail. The lesion starts under the free margin or along the lateral portion of nail and causing discolouration, chalky deposit. There will be ridging and fissuring with black streaks. Nail plates become loose, brittle and separates from bed and breaks off. Finger nails also show similar changes.

Onychopathy Any disease of the nail.

Onychorrhexis A spontaneous splitting or breaking of nails.

Onychosis A disease or deformity of nail.

Oocyesis Ovarian pregnancy.

Oocyst A life stage in certain parasitic mircoorganisms when the parasite rapidly grows into a spherical cyst enclosed by an elastic membrane.

Oocyte Female gamete or sex cell; a secondary oocyte and a polar body result from the first meiotic division, which occurs prior to the time of ovulation; a zygote and a polar body result from the second meiotic division, which occurs following union of the sperm cell with the secondary oocyte.

Oogenesis The process of female gemete formation.

Oolemma The limiting plasma membrane of occytes.

Oophorectomy Surgical procedure to remove the ovaries.

Oophrectomy Surgical procedure to remove the ovaries.

Oospore The spore that results from fertilization of an oogonium, female sex cell. This spore form in phytophthora infestans is thick-walled and is the stage that is best able to survive adverse conditions.

Ootype A specialized region of the flatworm oviduct that is surrounded by Mehlis' gland.

Opacification The process of making opaque.

Opacity The state or quality of being impenetrable to rays or light.

Opalescent Showing a milky iridescence, like an opal.

Opalgia Facial neuralgia.

Opaque media Any contrast material introduced into a body cavity.

Open amputation An amputation with open wound edges.

Open anesthesia A form of general anesthesia in which no rebreathing of the expired gases occurs.

Open intermedullary nailing Procedure in which nail placement occurs after fracture site has been exposed.

Open skills Motor skills performed in a constantly changing, unpredictable environment.

Open system A system that exchanges, matter and energy with its surroundings.

Open wound Wound in which the surface of the skin or mucous membrane is no longer intact.

Open-end contract A contract that permits periodic revaluation of dental plan during the contract year.

Opening snap It is a high-pitched early diastolic sound best heard at left lower sternal border radiating to base of heart. It is produced by opening of diseased atrioventricular valve. An opening snap is the hallmark of mitral stenosis but disappears when valve leaflets are immobile due to dense fibrosis or calcification. An opening snap may occur when there is increased flow across arterioventricular valves as in left to right shunt and mitral or tricuspid regurgitation.

Opening wedge osteotomy A procedure used to correct an angular deformity.

Operant behaviour Any response which produces certain consequences —such as a food reward. It "operates" on the environment. The eliciting stimulus cannot be identified precisely, as it can in respondent behaviour. The operant response is said to be emitted rather than elicited.

Operant conditioning A type of conditioning which involves the modification of an operant response through reinforcements. A response which the organism emits is reinforced in certain ways, in accordance with certain schedules, and resulting changes in its rate of occurrence are studied. The rat's pressing a lever and the pigeon's pecking a disc are widely studied operants. The reinforcement is usually food, although a secondary reinforcer, such as a click previously associated with food, may be used.

Operating microscope It is used to perform surgery on small vessels, nerves, eye or ear

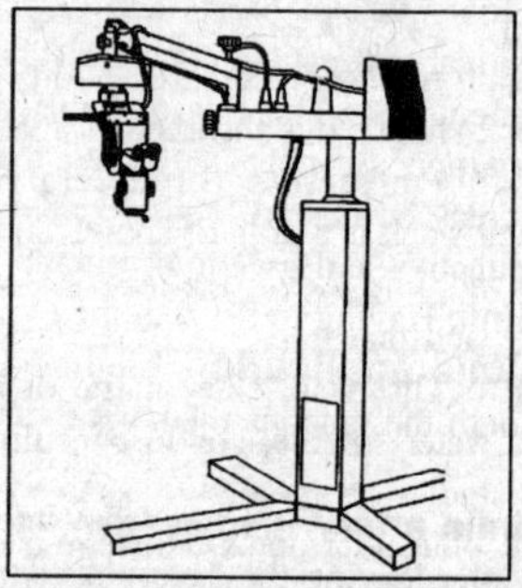

wherever a high magnification of the structures is needed. It is used by plastic surgeons, neurosurgeons, opthalmic surgeons.

Operating room A unit to be used for performance of surgery.

Operation Any surgical procedure.

Operational definition The meaning of a concept when it is translated into terms amenable to systematic observation and measurement, e.g. temperature defined by a thermometer reading under standard conditions.

Operations In the structure-of-intellect model of intelligence, this dimension concerns the processing of information. One operation for example is memory; another is convergent thinking: still another is divergent thinking.

Operative dentistry Operations to restore or reform the hard dental tissue.

Operative obstetrics Methods to expedite a complicated delivery and prevent harm to the newborn and mother, such a cesarean delivery or assisted delivery with forceps or a vacuum extractor.

Operculum Refers to any of the three opercula covering the insula.

Operon A unit of genetic expression consisting of one or more related genes and the operator and promoter sequences that regulate their transcription. A collection of contiguous genes that are transcribed together into a single mRNA molecule, together with any cis-acting regulatory sequences.

Ophthalmia neonatorum It is a preventable conjunctivitis. It occurs in newborn infant due to maternal infection of genital organs by gonococcus. Any discharge from infant's eye during first week should arouse suspicion as tears are not secreted in the first week of life. There becomes intense conjunctival congestion, watery discharge turning to purulent one. The lids become swollen and tender. Upper lid may hang over the lower lid. Lashes may be matted. There develops chemosis of conjunctiva and pseudomembrane formation.

Ophthalmic Having to do with the eyes.

Ophthalmic application Method of applying drugs onto the mucous membrane of one or both eyes.

Ophthalmic artery It arises from internal carotid artery after leaving the cavernous sinus. It enters the orbit along the optic nerve within dural sheath of the nerve. In the orbit it lies in the core of muscles with ciliary ganglion and lateral rectus to the outerside and optic nerve to the medial side. It passes forward giving branches and ends by dividing into nasal and frontal branches.

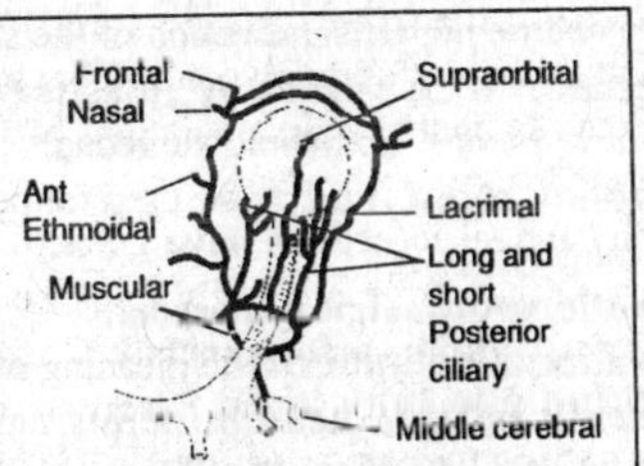

Ophthalmic artery and its branches

Ophthalmicus, herpes zoster It is caused by herpes zoster or varicella virus which affects the first division of trigeminal nerve. After infection virus remains dormant for months. The chief focus of infection is Gasserian ganglion from where the infection travels down.

There is severe neuralgic pain along the course of branches of ophthalmic division of fifth nerve. It is limited to one side. Neuralgic pain may be preceded by pain and fever. The area of skin supplied by ophthalmic division of fifth nerve appears red and oedematous. It is tender to touch. Vesicles are limited to the area of nerve supply. Intraocular pressure may or may not be raised. Neuralgic pain may persist for years.

Ophthalmologist Physician with specialised training and experience who specialises in the diagnosis and treatment of eye diseases, one versed in ophthalmology, the sum of knowledge concerning the eye and its diseases (obsolete term; oculist.)

Ophthalmology It is the study of eye and its diseases. It does not include only prescription of glasses but also the surgery of cataract, glaucoma and retinal detachment. Careful analysis of a person's field of vision can reveal defects indicating neurological damage.

Ophthalmoplegia It is a condition in which a group of muscles are paralysed. It occurs due to paralysis of third, fourth and sixth nerves. Diabetes, acute leukaemia, myasthenia gravis and acute cranial polyneuritis may cause it. There will be complete ptosis. There is no ocular movement in any direction. Pupil is dilated with no reaction to light, accommodation and convergence. The common causes for unilateral ophthalmoplegia are syndrome of apex or orbit of syndromes of sphenoidal fissure.

Ophthalmoplegic migraine Migraine is associated with impaired ocular motility and abnormal pupillary reactivity. It is more common in adolescence and in family history of migraine.

Patient develops unilateral pulsatile headache. Ocular headache disappears within a week.

Ophthalmoscope It is an instrument to examine the inside of eye. By means of a deflecting prism or a perforated angled mirror allows illumination

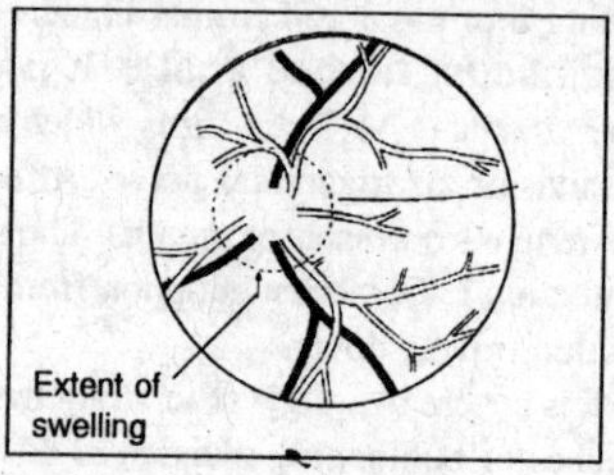

and viewing of entire area of retina, the head of optic nerve, retinal vessels and vitreous humour.

Ophthalmoscopy The ophthalmoscope provides a light source and an optical system to allow examination of fundus. The pupil appears pink. It

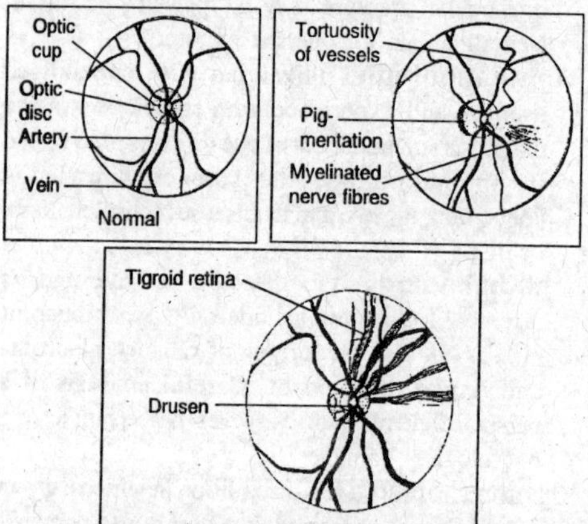

Normal variants

helps in diagnosing many eye pathologies and sequence of certain diseases such as hypertension, diabetes, etc. Doctors should be well versed with normal variations.

Opiate A generic term for drugs derived from exogenous sources producing effects like opium.

Opiate poisoning Opiates include the normal alkaloids of plant *Papaver somniferum* of poppy. Opium is derived from the milky fluid which exudes from cut surface of unripe seed capsules of poppy plant. The classic triad of opiate intoxication is pinpoint pupils, respiratory depression and coma. However in presence of hypoxia, hypothermia and pethidine poisoning pupils may be dilated. Cyanosis is late and is a serious sign. Hypotension may develop. Noncardiogenic pulmonary oedema is seen.

Opioid It is a dried juice of seed head of opium. The principal active ingredient in crude opium was isolated in 1806. Opium contains many alkaloids but important ones are morphine, codeine and papaverine.

Opisthogenia Defective development of the jaws following ankylosis of the jaw.

Opisthotonus Whole body arches backwards in a rigid spasm. Such state is seen in tetanus or in strychnine poisoning.

Opium It is a milky substance derived from the unripe seed pods of the poppy *Papaver somniferum*. Opium has an analgesic effect and may drowse a patient. It results in euphoria. Its important derivatives are codeine and morphine known as narcotic drugs.

Oppenheim sign Extensor reflexes of toes that suggest upper motor neurone or corticospinal motor paralysis.

Oppenheim's gait It is represented by a swinging motion of head, body and extremities on walking and is seen in disseminated sclerosis.

Opponenplasty Any surgical technique designed to restore the opposition function of thumb.

Opponens Any muscle of hand that brings opposing digits together.

Opponent-process theory An explanation of color vision that emphasizes the importance of the opposition of pairs of colors; red versus green and blue verus yellow.

Opportunistic Describing an organism that is not generally pathogenic but that can cause disease in a compromised host.

Opportunistic infection An infection with an agent that is not normally pathogenic but that can become so under certain conditions of a particular host.

Many fungal infections have been so described because they are more likely to cause disease in patients with impaired immunity.

Opportunistic infections Disorders caused by nonpathogens that occur in people with compromised health.

Opportunity costs In public health, the total value of the resources lost due to infectious diseases, valued in terms of foregone alternative uses. The use of opportunity costs is a core concept of economic analysis of disease burden.

Opposition Moving the thumb to touch the tips of the fingers; the movement used to hold a pencil to write.

Opsonin A substance coating an antigen either by antibody alone, or antibody plus complement components. This greatly increases phagocytosis by cells of the reticuloendothelial system.

Opsonization The action of some antibodies that renders bacteria and other foreing cells more susceptible to phagocytosis.

Opthalmia neonatorum Severe conjunctivitis in new born. May cause blindness even in rare cases.

Optic Pertaining to the eye.

Optic ataxia Deficit in the visual control of reaching and other movements.

Optic atrophy It is a common term used to describe the condition of optic disc when the optic nerve has degenerated. A damage to axons between the retinal ganglion cells and the lateral geniculate body results in optic atrophy. So in optic atrophy there is loss of axons. There is no regeneration of axon.

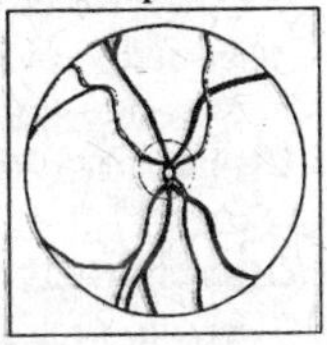

Optic chiasm The junction of the two optic nerves at which the axons from the nasal (inside) halves of the retinas cross to the opposite side of the brain. The structure in the brain which transmits visual information to both hemispheres; for each eye; it has connections with both the left and right hemispheres.

Optic disc The optic disc has only nerve fibre layer so it does not excite any visual impression known as blind spot. It appears as a nearly circular disc of 1.5 m.m. diameter. It appears pink. The depression in disc is called physiological cup. It varies in size and form. It increases in glaucoma.

Optic nerve It is the second cranial nerve, the nerve of vision. The optic nerve consists of a collection of about 1 million nerve fibres transmitting impulses from the retina to the brain. Two optic nerve converges at the optic junction behind the

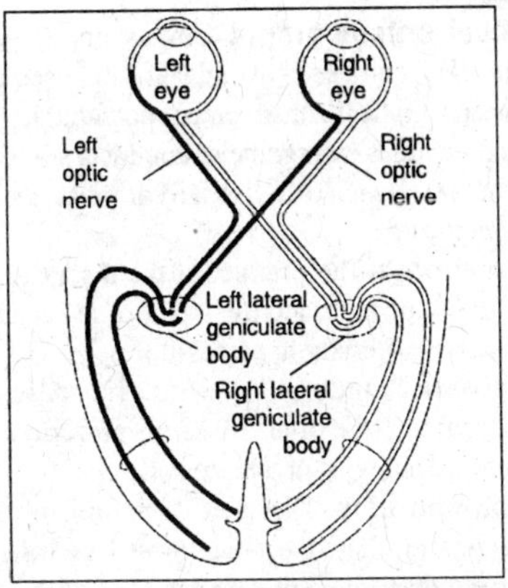

eyes where fibres from the inner halves of retina crossover. Disorder of optic nerves includes optic neuritis and optic disc oedema caused by external pressure from disease. The optic nerve covered with pia, arachnoid and dura traverses the optic foramen to enter the orbit and gets attached to sclera just above and 3 mm internal to the posterior pole of eye. The total length of nerve is 5 cm, the intracranial being 1 cm, the optic canal being 6 mm, intraorbital 3 cm, intraocular 0.7 mm In the canal the ophthalmic artery accompanies it to enter the orbit. In the orbit at optic foramen the origin of rectus muscles surrounds the optic nerve.

Optic neuritis There develops inflammation of optic nerve that often causes sudden loss of part of field of vision. It results in pain during eye movements and tenderness. Most common cause is demyelination of optic nerve and multiple sclerosis. It causes loss of vision, usually the central part of visual field, Vision improves in six weeks. Recurrent attacks usually causes loss of visual acuity.

Optic tract A bundle of axons that transmits nerves impulses from the retina of the eye between the optic chiasm and the thalamus. Inner half of each retina generates impulses that cross the opposite side chiasma. The result is that each half of brain both left and right, recieves visual impulses from nasal retina of opposite side from chiasma backwards to thalamus the pathways are inside the brain known as optic tracts.

Optical activity The capacity of a substance to rotate the plane of plane-polarized light.

Optical enhancement Covers improvements to imagery produced by optical as opposed to digital means. Optical enhancement potential is extensive and includes enlargement, contracts stretching and Fourier transform improvements by optical computing.

Optical path The product of the distance travelled by a ray of light and the index of refraction of the various materials it passes through.

Optician A technician who fits, adjusts, and dispenses corrective lenses on prescription of an ophthalmologist or optometrist.

Optimistic bias That part of optimism related to perception that one is at lower risk for negative events than average person.

Optimists People who generally expect to obtain favourable personal outcomes in the future.

Optimum pH The characteristic pH at which an enzyme has maximal catalytic activity.

Optokinetic drum It is a rotating drum covered with black and white vertical stripes parallel to the axis of rotation.

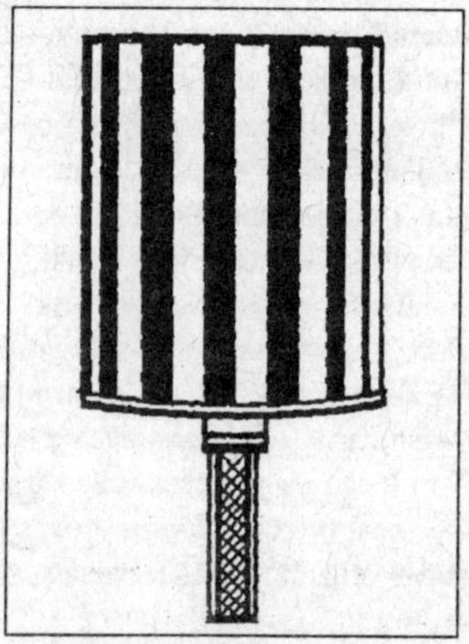

Optokinetic nystagmus It results when successive objects traverse the visual field. The eyes follow one towards the periphery in a slow motion until the successor object appears into the central field where on the eyes move back to primary position in a rapid movement. Clinically, it can be observed by asking the patient to gaze at a rotating drum marked with vertical stripes. There is response until the patient has enough vision to see the drum. It is abolished in complete blindness. So, it is a good test for monitoring.

Optometrist A person who practices optometry, tests the eyes for visual acuity, prescribes corrective lenses, and recommends eye exercises.

Optometry Measurement of the powers of vision and the adoption of prisms or lenses for the air thereof, utilizing any means other than drugs.

Ora serrata The jagged perpheral margin of the retina.

Oral Pertainng to mouth.

Oral airway Minimally flexible curved piece of plastic extending from the exterior of the lips over the tongue to the pharynx.

Oral bacteria The microorganism constant in oral flora of an individual.

Oral bioavailability The rate of, and extent to which, an active drug or metabolite enters the circulation by the way of the gastrointestinal tract.

Oral carcinoma 50 per cent intraoral carcinoma occur in tongue, 16 per cent in floor of mouth and remaining 34 per cent on alveolar mucosa. 60 per cent carcinoma lesions are seen as ulcers and 30 per cent as growth. Remaining 10 per cent are seen as white lesions. Lesions are indurated. Tumours of palate, gingiva and tongue are largest on size.

Oral cavity Mouth; the first portion of the digestive tract.

Oral character Behaviour traits pertaining to the mouth, such as excessive eating, smoking, and gossiping which presumably are related to early feeding experiences; a Freudian concept.

Oral contraceptives These are the drug of choice containing progesterone drug often combined with an oestrogen drug taken by women to prevent pregnancy. All types of oral contraceptives need to be taken on a monthly cycle for as long as woman wants. It is to be started on the first day of period or on the fifth day after bleeding starts. Some brands of pills contain seven additional pills which are of iron supplement so that the habbit of taking pill each day is not broken. Pill should be taken same time each day. A forgotten combined or phased pill should be taken as soon as remembered. Next day two pills to be taken. A different form of contraceptive should be used for seven days after missing the pill. If between 3 and 12 hours have elapsed from the time a minipill was due to be taken, pill should now be taken and for 48 hours additional contraceptive precaution should be used correctly. Oral contraceptive has a failure rate of one per cent. Oral pills are effective and do not interfere with spontaneity of sex. Oestrogen containing pills seem to protect against cancer of uterus and ovaries. These make periods regular, lighter and relatively free of pain. But oestrogen containing pills increase the risk of certain disorders so these should not be taken during hypertension, hyperlipidaemia and thrombosis. Possible side-effects are vomiting, nausea and weight gain.

Adverse effects usually disappear within a few months. If they persist it may be necessary to change a different brand.

Oral epithelium The epithelial covering of oral mucus membrane composed of strtified squamous epithelium of varying thickness and varying degress of keratinization.

Oral flora The microorganisms that inhabit the oral cavity of an individual, are usually saprophytic, and live together in a symbiotic relationship.

Oral frustration During the oral phase of early non verbal childhood development.

Oral histology Microscopic study of oral tissues.

Oral hygiene This is the method to keep the mouth and teeth clean and healthy. Good oral hygiene reduces the incidence of tooth decay. It prevents gingivitis and helps halitosis. *Personal care* includes important aspects of personal oral hygiene, i.e. daily removal of dental plaque by thorough toothbrushing and use of dental floss. Use of fluoride mouth rinse is a good oral irrigator. Dentures should always be kept clean. *Professional care* removes stubborn plaque and calculus by scaling and polishing.

Oral hygiene aids Assortment of materials, devices, and substances used intraorally to maintain good oral health.

Oral hygiene score Rating given to indicate the amount of plaque present in a patient's mouth. The oral hygiene score can be figured using the following formula; total number of disclosed tooth surfaces divided by the total number of tooth surfaces times 100% equals the oral hygience score. The lower the score, the more likely the oral hygiene habits are satisfactory.

Oral manifestation A symptom or sign of a disease in the oral cavity.

Oral melanotic nevi These are benign lesions of melanocytes which form circular brown to black patches about 5-6 m.m. across. They are asymptomatic but should be excised.

Oral motor control The ability to coordinate the movements of the tongue and mouth.

Oral pathology Branch of dentistry that deals with the study or oral diseases, especially the nature and function of the disease.

Oral route Drug administration by swallowing or instillation through an enteral tube.

Oral sex It is of two types. In felllatio a woman uses her mouth to stimulate man's organ while in cunnilingus a man uses his mouth to stimulate the woman's genitals. In both cases it includes, kissing, sucking and licking.

It is mostly disapproved on the ground that it is unnatural and unhygienic although woman can easily attain orgasm. If genitals are clean and healthy and if will is, there is absolutely no reason to discard the techinque.

Oral stage The first of Freud's psychosexual stages, in which personality development is significantly influenced by the conditions surrounding the intake of food. If this process is managed satisfactorily, the infant should develop an optimistic and trusting outlook. If not, feelings of uncertainty and pessimism are likely to arise. According to Freud, it is the earliest stage of psychosocial development lasting during first 18 months of life when the mouth is the principal erogenous zone and when the most important source of gratification is sucking during the feeding process.

Oral suctioning Removal of secretions from the mouth into the stomach.

Oral surgeon It is the doctor who treats deformity or injury of mouth, face and jaws. He specialises in operations on the teeth, jaws and other parts of mouth. Qualification needed is BDS plus specialised training. More complicated oral surgery includes orthognathic surgery to correct deformities of jaw, plastic surgery to correct cleft lip and palate and removal of certain types of tumours.

Oral surgery That part of dental practice which deals with the diagnosis and surgical and adjunctive treatment of the diseases, injuries, and defects of the human jaws and associated structures.

Oral temperature Temperature is generally recorded in mouth except in case of infants and unconsciousness, delirious or insane patient or in conditions where mouth cannot be kept closed. Ask patient to open mouth, put bulb of thermometer under the tongue and ask patient to close the lips only. Wait for a minute and note the temperature immediately.

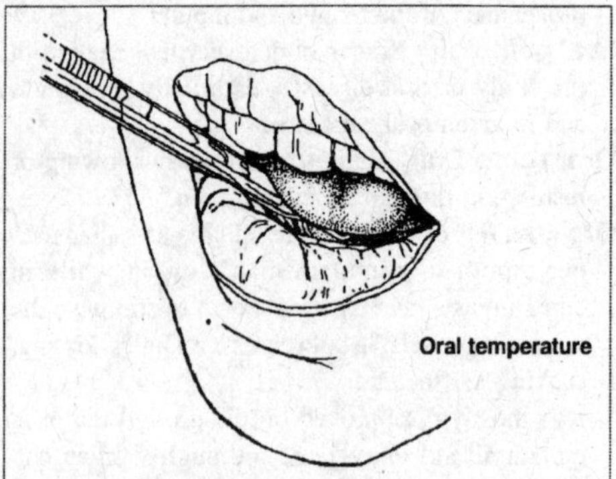

Oral temperature

Oral tuberculosis Main symptoms include flat, painful, mucosal ulceration with undermined borders. There will be greasy coating and swelling and redness of surrounding mucosa. It will result in difficulty in eating.

Oralogy Pertaining to the mouth.

Orbeli effect Increase in strength of contraction of fatigued muscle following sympathetic nerve stimulation.

Orbicularis oculi Facial muscle that causes a squint.

Orbicularis oris Muscular ring encircling the oral cavity which forms the lips. Facial muscle that puckers the lips.

Orbit It is the socket in the skull that contains eyeball along with protective pads of fat and muscles, vessels and nerves. Opening in back of orbit allows the optic nerve to pass from eyeball into the brain. Rarely bacteria may infect and cause cellulitis. The affected eye is protruded and is extremely painful, red and swelling. Orbital cellulitis is a severe disorder. Sports injury may fracture the orbit.

Orbital The region around the nucleus of an atom where each electron is most likely to be found.

Orbital cellulitis Orbital cellulitis is a purulent inflammation of the cellular tissue of the orbit. Most common cause is infection from neighbouring structures through venous stream from paranasal sinuses, nose, boils on face or lip, dental abscess or caries. There will be swelling of lids with chemosis of the conjunctiva. There develops proptosis of eyeball with severe pain in the orbit and on movement of eyeball. There will be fever with malaise. There is restriction of eyeball in all directions. Fundus may be normal or show features of optic neuritis.

Orbital dermoid cyst This is most common type of congenital orbital lesion, located in superior and lateral orbital region. These are slow growing benign lesions. These enlarge orbit. These contain fat and calcium causing hypodense and hyperdense lesions. These are sharply marginated and do not enhance on contrast.

Orbital haemangioma Clinical features include pulsatile proptosis and dilated vessels of eyelid and conjunctiva. There will be proptosis. Visual loss and ophthalmoparesis may develop. X-ray may show optic canal erosion or orbital calcification. CT shows retrobulbar sharply marginated mass.

Orbital septum A thin membrane containing collagenous and elastic fibres attached to orbital margin.

Orbital syndrome This involves pain and paraesthesias in the ophthalmic branch of the trigeminal nerve, ophthalmoparesis, proptosis and normal visual acuity. Skull X-ray shows erosion in orbital region.

Orbital thrombophlebitis There is thrombosis of orbital veins. Infection may come down from cavernous sinus. There is severe pain in orbit and surrounding areas accompanied with fever and malaise.

There is a swelling of lids, lips, dental caries or abscess. There is mild proptosis which may increase in short time. There is restriction of ocular movements in all directions. With proptosis the cornea is endangered with exposure keratitis. Optic atrophy follows optic neuritis. Patient may show signs of meningitis if infection has spread to cavernous sinus.

Orbital tubercle Small elevation on the orbital surface of the zygomatic bone.

Orbitonasal Pertaining to the orbit and the nose.

Orbitostat An instrument for measuring the axis of the orbit.

Orchitis It is the inflammation of testis. It may be caused by virus resulting in mumps. It is characterised by swelling and severe pain in the affected testis with a high fever. In epididymoorchitis tube carrying sperm is also inflamed. Antibiotics and analgesics help the person. Occasionally orchitis is followed by shrinking of testis.

Order-disorder transformation A change or rearrangement of the atoms produced in certain metals when they are heated above a specific temperature ;the transformation results in a more regular atomic arrangement and affects physical and mechanical properties.

Orderliness in nature An assumption that there are discoverable relations in our world; the world is not chaotic or ruled by chance.

The relationships among events are considered to be lawful, though the discovery of all the details of these relationships may be impossible. Without this assumption, scientific activity would appear to be useless.

Ordinal Scale A scale used to classify data into qualitative ordered categories; the values have a distinct order but are not separated by numeric distances.

Ordinal variables Medical data that can be characterized in terms of more than two values and have a clearly implied directin from better to worse but are not measured on a continuous measurement scale.

Organ Group of several tissue types that performs a special function.

Organ donation Most organs used as transplants are removed immediately after death but kidney is also taken from a living donor. Donation of kidney is confined to the relatives. The risk of donation is explained to donor and written well-documented consent is taken. The range of organs removed after death is eye, lungs, heart, liver, pancreas and kidneys. Most organs can be transplanted successfully only if removed carefully and immediately. People who want to donate some or all of their organs after death should make their intentions clear and sign a donor card.

Organ of Corti Specialised region of the cochlear duct consisting hair cells; produces action potentials in response to sound waves.

Organ of vision Eye is the organ of vision. Vision is made possible by the conversion of light rays

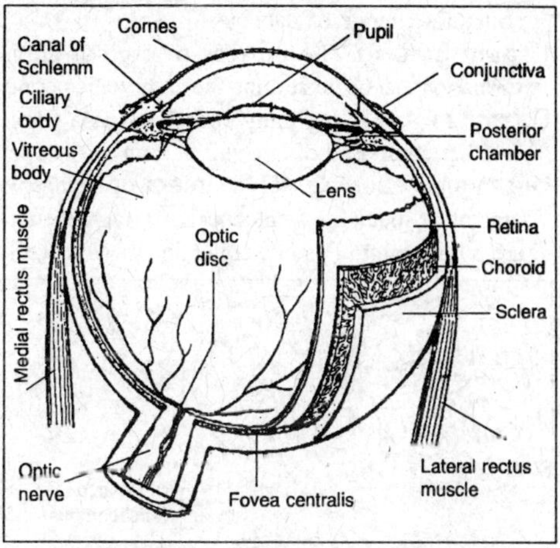

into nerve impulse. Light rays enter the eye through the cornea and pass through the pupil, crystalline lens and vitreous body to the retina. The light rays stimulate the sensory receptors in the retina to send impulses to the brain through the nerve to the occipital cortex where impulses are registered as visual sensations.

Organelle Specialised part of a cell performing one or more specific functions.

Organic Molecules that contain a carbon atom (carbon dioxide is an exception); originally defined as molecules extracted from living organisms; the original definition became obsolete when it became possible to manufacture these molecules in the laboratory.

Organic compound Compound that always contains carbon in which the atoms are held together by covalent bonds. Examples include carbohydrates, lipids, proteins, and nucleic acids (DNA and RNA).

Organic disease An illness caused or accompanied by structural changes in body organ.

Organic disorder A disorder related to an organ, such as the brain, or to the physical aspects of the whole organism. Sometimes having to do with the structure or function of a known anatomical unit.

For example, an organic psychosis is related to impairment in the structure of the brain, as in paresis.

Organic mental disorders Those conditions that are believed to be the result of physiological or structural change or damage.

Organification The process of orginal organ formation that occurs during the embryonic period.

Organism Any living thing considered as a whole whether composed of one cell or many.

Organisms causing pelvic infection Pyogenic organisms specially streptococci and staphylococci are pus forming. Pus is a collection of white cells

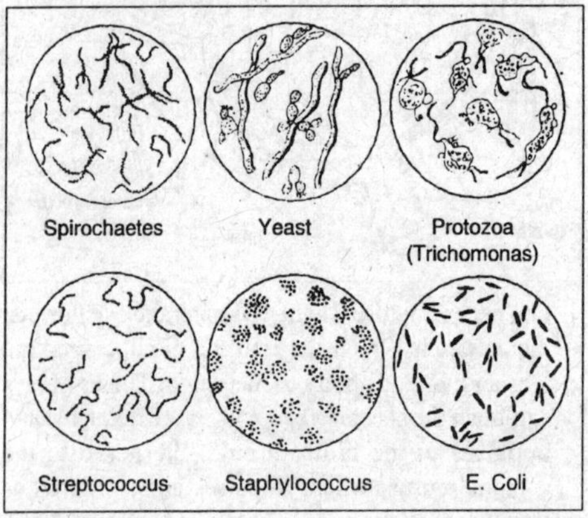

and dead bacteria. Cocci are minute dots under microscope. Some bacteria require oxygen for their growth and is called aerobic bacteria. Others grow in absence of oxygen and are known as anerobic bacteria.

Organogenesis The formation and development of the different organs, or of a particular organ.

Organophosphates Chemicals used as fertilizers.

Organotroph Literally, organic, eater an organism that derives its energy from organic sources; i.e., a heterotroph. Thus, organotrophic.

Organotrophy The fact of being an organotroph; deriving energy from organic compounds.

Orgasm Orgasm has been derived from Greek word *orgasmos* to swell or to be lustful. It is one of the most powerful and satisfying sensation that a human being can experience. It consists of an explosive discharge of accumulated neuromuscular tension. There is a drive towards release and person is not able to stop it. In male there is a seminal ejaculation while in females there is no emissio Male is quicker in reaching orgasm, its duratic is short and return to normal very quickly, whi in female orgasm lasts much longer, is slow come and slow to return to normal phase.

Orgasmic impotence It is the incapacity of th male to reach orgasm in spite of normal erectic and ejaculation which may be due to decline i sexual interest. It may be caused by immatu psychosexual development.

Orgasmic platform The thickened area c congested tissue that builds up and surrounds th lower third of the vagina during high levels c sexual arousal and just preceding orgasm.

Oriental sore A disease, also knwon as cutaneou leishmaniasis, caused by *Leishmania tropica.*

Orientation The ability to identify correctly persons places, current date, time and situation.

Orienting response Adjustments in attending; any response in relation to the reception of availabl stimulation, such as pupil dilation, increased hear rate, or a change in the electrical activity of th skin.

Orifice Entrance or outlet of any cavity in the body

Origin Less movable of the two points of attachmen of a muscle, usually the end attached to the more rigid part of the skeleton.

Origin of replication A chromosomal site that interacts with specific proteins to produce unwound DNA regions required to start polymerization of new DNA from existing template.

Oropharyngeal suctioning Removal of secretions from the throat through a catheter inserted through the mouth.

Oropharynx Portion of the pharynx that lies posterior to the mouth; it is continuous above with the nasopharynx and below with the laryngopharynx.

Orotracheal intubation It is the most common way of obtaining emergent airway control when ventilation by mask is not appropriate or possible. It gives an opportunity to apply positive pressure ventilation.

Orphan drugs Drugs that the pharmaceutical companies do not wish to develop either because they cannot be patented (e.g. lithium), because they are used only in rare conditions by very few people, or for a variety of legitimate economic reasons. In such cases, the federal government will work with the companies to make the drugs available to those who need them.

Orthdromic conduction A nerve impulse that moves in normal direction.

Orthodontic band Thin metal ring, usually stainless steel, that secures orthodontic attachments to a tooth.

Orthodontics That area of dentistry concerned with the supervision and guidance of the growing dentition and correction of the mature dentofacial structures, and includes those conditions that require movement of teeth and/or correction of malrelationships of jaws and teeth and malformations of their related structures.

Orthodontist A dentist who specialised in orthodontics.

Orthodromic Impulse conduction in a centrifugal direction, as distinct from antidromic conduction.

Orthognathic surgery Surgery to other relationships of dental arches and/or supporting bones, usually accomplished in conjunction with orthodontic therapy.

Orthograde transneuronal degeneration Neuronal degeneration in a proximodistal direction.

Orthograde transport Proximodistal axoplasmic transport.

Orthography Processing of letter shapes by the visual cortex.

Orthokeratology Method of fitting contact lenses altering the curvature of cornea specially in myopia.

Orthologous Describing genes that are related by descent from a common ancestor but that are divergent since organismal specification.

Orthomolecular treatment (mega-vitamin therapy) An approach based on the assumption that "for every twisted mind there is a twisted molecule" and that in some way psychiatric illness, and perhaps other illnesses, are due to biochemical abnormalities, resulting in increased needs for specific substances, such as vitamins. This treatment is of unknown and unproved efficacy.

Orthopaedics It is a surgical branch dealing with disorders of bone and joints, tendons and ligaments. They deal with fractures, dislocations, slipped discs, arthritis, etc. The branch of medicine that deals with the preservation and restoration of the skeletal system, articulations, and associated structures. Pertaining to the correction of deformities.

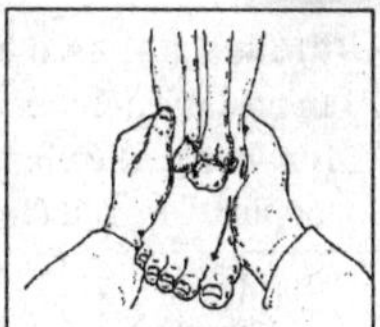

Fracture manipulation

Orthopedic appliance Any prosthetic, orthotic device or brace.

Orthopedic shoe A shoe designed with a variety of special features, a wide high toe box, a long counter, a large low heel.

Orthopedic surgeon A physician who practices orthopedic surgery.

Orthopedic table A table used for any orthopedic surgical procedure.

Orthophoria It is a condition of eyes in which there is a perfect balance of eyes with no duration even when fusion is disturbed. It is rare. Most of the cases show some kind of mild degree of heterophoria.

Orthopneic position Seated position with the arms supported on pillows or the arm rest of a chair.

Orthopnoea It is a dyspnoea at recumbent position which is partially relieved by sitting up. Patient puts extra pillows under head at night. It is due to increase in intrathoracic volume with rise in pulmonary, venous and capillary pressure which increase the pulmonary closing volume and reduce vital capacity.

Additional factor is elevation of diaphragm during recumbency resulting in lower end expiratory closing volume, resulting in significant alteration in alveolar gas exchange.

Orthopnoeic position This position is comfortable for patients with heart failure when the patient is breathless and finds difficulty in breathing. He or she is assisted to remain in position by help of a foot support in form of pillow. This helps to prevent bed sores caused by shearing force as the patient slips down the bed. A table is placed in front of patient. The patient comfortably leans.

Orthopsychiatry An approach that involves the collaborative effort of psychiatry, psychology, psychiatric social work, and other behavioural, medical, and social sciences in the study and treatment of human behaviour in the clinical setting. Emphasis is placed on preventive techniques to promote healthy emotional growth and development, particularly of children.

Orthoses It is used to redistribute a load to support an unstable joint or to provide a mechancial means for weak muscles. Simplest one is propylene moulded around the ankle and underneath the heel.

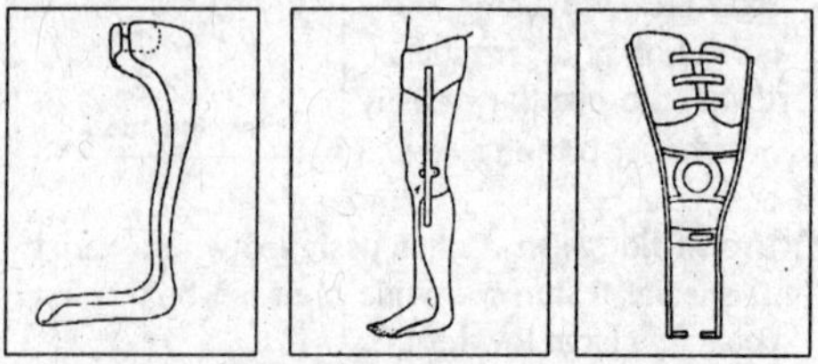

More complex orthoses supporting movement at the knee and ankle as well as foot may be used for those with cauda equina lesions.

Orthostatic hypotension A drop in blood pressure of 15 mm Hg or more when an individual reses from a sitting to a standing position.

Orthotic Pertaining to the use or application of an orthosis.

Orthotics Is the systematic methodology of straightening and improving function of the body or body parts by the application of an orthosis to the outside of body. Orthosis includes a number of devices such as braces, splints, calipers and corsets. An orthosis may be used for immobilizing a joint or body segment, restrict movement in a given direction, control mobility, assist with movement or reduce weight bearing forces. The primary principle behind the effects of an orthosis is the improvement of function.

Orthotopic heart transplantation Transplantation of the heart in which the native heart is removed and the donor heart is placed in its position.

OS Mouth

Os acetabula A round or oval accessory ossicle found on the superiolateral margin.

Os intermetatarseum An accessory bone of foot located between the proximal ends of the first and second metatarsals.

Os peroneum An accessory bone of the foot found in or adjacent to the peroneus longus tendon.

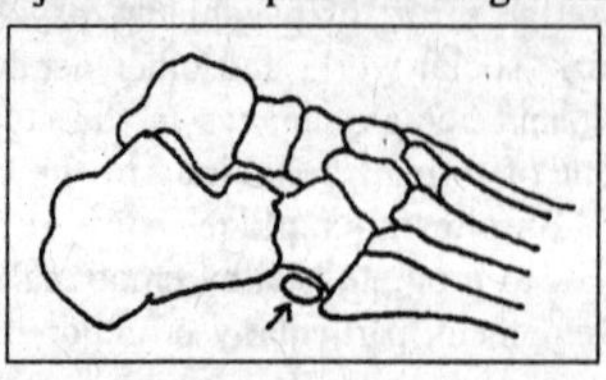

OS subfibulare It is located beneath the latera malleoli suggesting this was a seasamoid withi peroneus longus tendon.

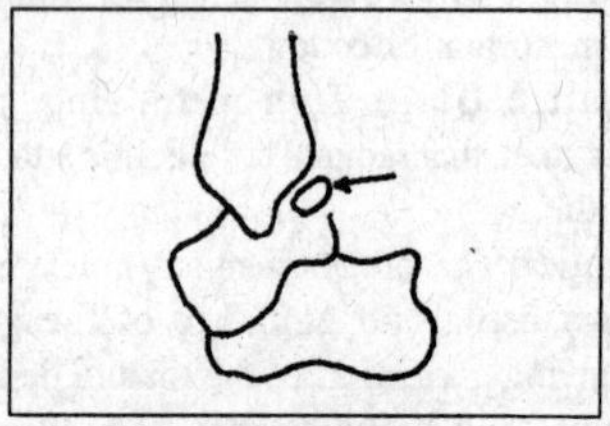

Os trigonum An accessory bone present variably and independently in the tarsus.

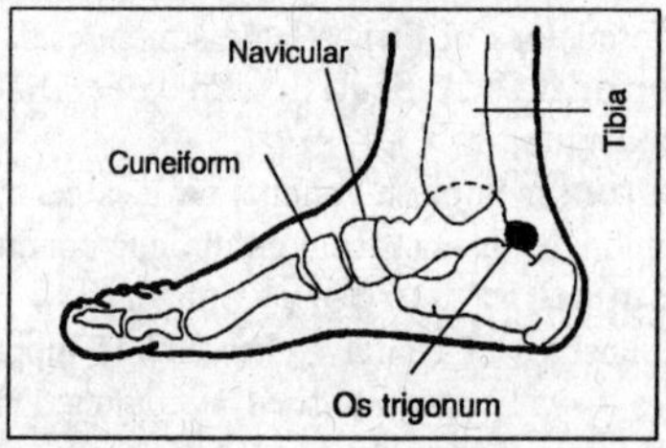

Os, external Uterine ostium.

Oscillopsia Vision in which objects appear to oscillate. It may be due to acquired nystagmus, neurosis and multiple sclerosis.

Oscilloscope A device that measures the flow of electrons to measure voltage.

Osgood-Schlatter disease It is the painful enlargement of tibial tuberosity bony prominence of tibia just below the knee. It is caused by excessive repetitive pulling of the quadriceps muscle on the patellar tendon. It clears up clearly without treatment.

OSHA Occupational Safety and Health Administration.

Oslander's sign It is the increased pulsation of lateral fornices of vagina. It may appear on eight week. It may be developed in other pelvic pathologies.

Osler's nodes These are semi-tender nodules 0.5 to 1.5 cm in diameter on the palmar and plantar aspects of finger and toe tips caused due to minute emboli of superficial terminal vessels or by arteritis of smaller vessels.

Osler's sign It is represented by small, tender, erythematous swelling in the skin and subcutaneous tissues of the hands and feet, and is seen in malignant endocarditis.

Osmolality Concentration of electrically charged particles per kilogram of solution.

Osmolarity The concentration of a solution in terms of osmoles of solutes per kilogram of solvent.

Osmophile Literally, lover of osmotic pressure; an organism that grow optimally in conditions of high osmotic pressure.

Osmophilic Growing optimally in conditions of high osmotic pressure.

osmoreceptor Receptor in the hypothalamus that is sensitive to changes in blood osmolarity and, in response to high osmolarity (low water concentration), causes synthesis and release of antidiuretic hormone (ADH). Sensory neurons that respond to changes in the osmotic pressure of the surrounding fluid.

Osmoregulatory Pertaining to water balance and related to hydromineral balance which also includes electrolytes.

Osmosis The passage of a solvent through a semipermeable membrane into a solution of higher molecular concentration, thus equalising the concentrations on either side of the membrane.

Osmotic diuresis Secretion of large amount of urine due to increased osmotic pressure resulting from hyperglycemia.

Osmotic pressure It is a pressure required to prevent migration of a solvent across semipermeable membrane into a solution of certain strength. If a mole of a compound which will not dissociate is dissolved in 22.4 litres of water it will exert an osmotic pressure of 1 atmosphere (760 mm Hg). An osmole represents the amount of substance which exerts an osmotic pressure of 22.4 atmosphere when dissolved in one litre of water. An osmole is the molecular weight of a substance in grams divided by the number of freely moving particles, each molecule liberates in solution.

Osmotic shock Cellular damage resulting from the rapid flow of extracellular fluid into the cell.

Osmotic thirst Thirst resulting from cellular dehydration that is produced by an increase in the osmotic pressure of the extracellular fluid relative to the intracellular fluid.

Osseointegration The process by which new bone forms at the surface of an endosseous implant, creating a strong adhesion to stabilize it within the tissue.

Osseous surgery Bone surgery. May be augmentive or resective.

Osseous tissue Bone tissue.

Ossicles The three small bones in the middle ear which amplify the vibrations of the eardrum and transmit them to the inner ear.

Ossification It is the process by which bone is formed, renewed and repaired. It begins in embryo and continues throughout life. There are three types of ossification : (*i*) bone growth during which a new bone is formed from epiphyseal cartilage, (*ii*) bone renewal which occurs as a part of normal regeneration process, and (*iii*) bone repair which fuses broken bones after fracture. It is something hardening into bone. It includes enclosing of special cells osteoblasts within matrix of connective tissue fibres and calcium salts in crystalline form. Each bone ossifies from different ossification centres.

Ossifluence Softening of bony tissue.

Ossiform Resembling bone.

Ossifying Changing or developing into bone.

Ossifying fibroma These have been given a wide variety of names. Clinically it may develop at any age but are most common in children. These are slow growing and painless but usually produces buccal or labial enlargement of jaw. There is facial deformity. Maxilla is more affected and migration of teeth takes place. Under microscope one finds presence of fibrous connective tissue of varying degrees of maturity. There may be a calcified material. Bone tissue forms foci of varying patterns.

Osteitis It is the inflammation of whole thickness of bone including marrow and cortex. Symptoms are pain, swelling and fever. Antibiotics help.

Osteitis condensi It is associated with bone formation rather than bone destruction. It occurs in middle age. Mandibulomolar area is the most commonly affected site. Usually there are no symptoms. It is associated with a tooth having pulp or periapical pathology in an old extraction site. Lesions appear as old localised opacities. Microscopic sections show dense bone trabeculae, narrow marrow spaces and mild infiltration of lymphocytes. Lesions require no treatment. If it is associated with a nonvital tooth, endodontic therapy of affected tooth may resolve the osteosclerotic area.

Osteitis fibrosa It is a rare disease of unknown origin. Medullary structures are replaced by fibrous dysplasia, brown pigmentation of areas of skin, from small freckle-like dots to large flat patches on thighs. There may be unilateral proptosis, papilloedema and optic atrophy.

Osteoarthritis It is a large joint disease of an old age. It is characterised by degeneration of the cartilage that lines joints or by osteophytes which lead to pain and stiffness. Lastly, joint may lose its function. Osteoarthritis causes pain, swelling, cracking and stiffness of one or more joints. Pain and stiffness may interfere with activities. Weakness of surrounding muscles may occur if pain prevents the joint movements. Affected joint becomes enlarged and distorted by osteophytes. There is pain on motion. X-ray shows cartilage loss and osteophyte formation. Non-steroidal anti-inflammatory drugs (NSAIDs) help the person.

Osteoarthrosis Non inflammatory bone disease

Osteoarticular Pertaining to or affecting bones and joints.

Osteoblast A cell that is associated with the mineralization of the bone matrix.

Osteoblastic Physiological activity that leads to the formation of specific bonce tissue, osteoblasts.

Osteoblastic activity The cells inbone responsible for new bone formation. Osteoblastic activity would thus indicate that the osteoblasts are active, and that new bone is being formed.

Osteoblastoma This is rare, solitary, painful lesion of long bone and vertebra may involve the jaw. Patients are between the age of 10 and 30 years. There will be solitary radiopacities of varying density. Under microscope one finds bone trabeculae with osteoid borders in a rich fibrous trauma. It is a local benign lesion. Excision is the treatment of choice.

Osteoblasts Cuboidal cells associated with the growth development of bone. In active growth osteoblasts form a continuous layer an old bone similar to a sheet of epithelial cells, when the bone growth is arrested, the cells assume an elongated appearance like fibroblasts.

Osteocalcin One of major noncollagenous proteins found only in bone.

Osteocartilaginous Pertaining to or composed of bone and cartilage.

Osteochondritis dissecans It is a degeneration of a bone just under a joint surface causing fragments of bone and cartilage to become separated from surrounding bone. It frequently affects the knee and usually starts between 15 to 20 years of age. Exact cause is unknown. It may be caused by damage of blood vessels due to injury. Separated fragment reattaches but usually forms a loose body within the joint. X-ray shows damage to joint and loose bodies if any. If a fragment has not completely separated the joint may be immobilised in a cast to allow reattachment. Loose bodies of knee are removed during arthroscopy.

Osteochondroma It is a benign tumour made up of a stalk of bone capped with cartilage. It grows from the side of the bone, usually at the end of a long bone. It develops in late childhood and early adolescence and stops growing when the skeleton has fully developed. If it is large, surgical removal may be necessary.

Osteoclasis The delibrate fracturing of a bone to correct deformity.

Osteoclasts Large multinucleated cells associated with the resorption of bone. Seen in irregular concavities within marginal areas of bone undergoing resorption.

Osteoconduction The process by which an inorganic material provides a bioinert scaffolding along which bone growth can occur.

Osteocyte A mature bone cell that maintains the daily activities of bone tissue.

Osteodynia Pain in bone.

Osteodystrophy Defective bone development associated with disturbances in calcium and phosphorus metabolism and renal insufficiency.

Osteoectomy, ostectomy Remo-valof tooth-supporting bone for correction of pockets and nonphysiologic bony contours.

Osteogenic Promoting the development and formation of bone, exclusively resulting from the action of osteoblasts.

Osteogenic sarcoma It is a malignant bone tumour developing during young adults. It spreads rapidly to the lungs. Long bones of legs and arms are commonly affected. Around knee is the commonest site. First symptom is painful visible swelling of the affected bone. As a complication of Paget's disease osteosarcoma develops in several bones. X-ray shows sunrays and periosteal elevation. Surgical removal followed by radiation therapy helps a patient. Anticancer drugs are also given.

Osteoinduction The induction of bone formation in the absence of a bony host site; for example, certain bone morphogenic proteins can cause pluripotential cells circulating in the blood supply to differentiate into osteoblasts to form bone in nonosseous tissues.

Osteointegration The mode of tissue integration around a healed functioning endosteal implant in which the prime load-bearing tissue at the interface is bone.

Osteology Study of bones, anatomy and their functions.

Osteolysis The dissolution of bone.

Osteoma It is a benign bone tumour. It is hard and small and may develop on any bone. It is harmless but surgical removal may be necessary. If it causes pressure symptoms, surgical removal becomes necessary.

Osteomalacia There is softening, weakening and demineralisation of bones in adults due to vitamin D deficiency. The development of bone needs adequate intake of calcium and phosphorus. But

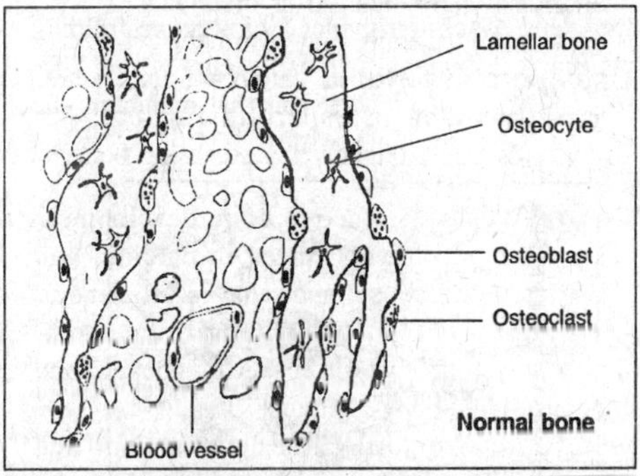

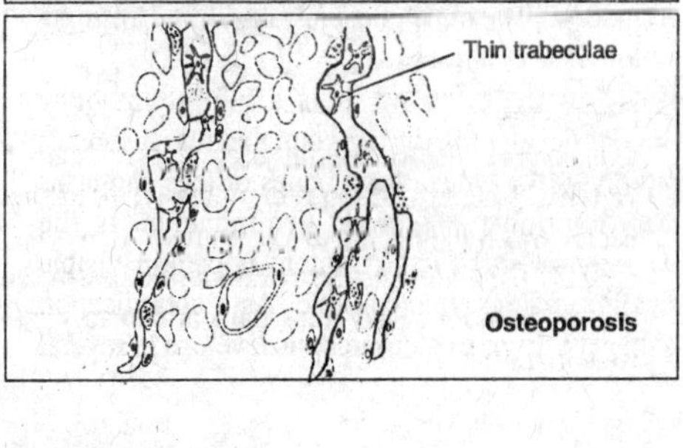

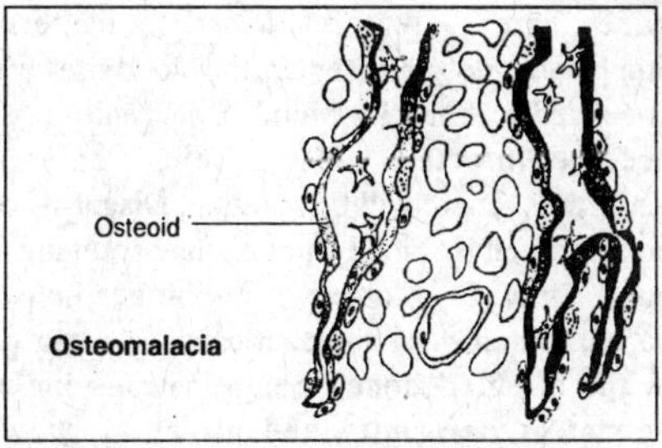

in deficiency of Vitamin D these will not be absorbed. Most commonly affected people are poor people who cannot afford balanced diet. If bones becomes thin may break easily. Densitometer can help knowing the bone density.

Osteomalacic pelvis It means softening bones due to deficiency of vitamin D, calcium and phosphorus. Due to progressive decalcification of bones there is replacement of the bony substance with soft osteoid tissue. Triradiate pelvis is the usual description given to such pelvis. Patient complains of dull to severe bone pain. There may be muscular wasting and waddling gait. Therapeutic response to vitamin D is dramatic.

Osteomyelitis It is the infection of bone by bacteria and may affect any bone. In children generally long

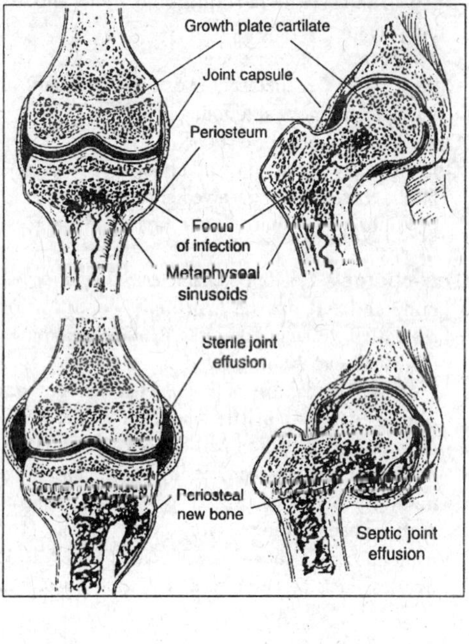

bones are affected. Mostly, bacterium *Staphylococcus aureus* enters the blood stream and is carried to bone by blood. Bone and marrow become infected causing fever, pain and tenderness. There will be swelling. Diagnosis may be confirmed by blood culture, bone scanning and bone X-ray. High doses of antibiotics help the patient. Chronic osteomyelitis causes constant pain in the affected bone. Complications include persistent deformity and arrest of growth. Suppuration may occurs. Antibiotics are also prescribed.

Osteon The basic unit of structure in adult compact bone, consisting of a central (haversian) canal with its concentrically arranged lamellae, lacunaem, osteocytes, and canaliculi. Also called a Haversian system.

Osteonecrosis The death of necrosis of a bone.

Osteopathology Patholy or disease of bone; also the field of study of diseases of bone.

Osteopathy It is a manipulative system of bone therapy specially in dislocation and fracture. It is helpful in pain and sprain too.

Osteopenia Reduced bone mass due to a decrease in the rate of osteoid synthesis to a level insufficient to compensate normal bone lysis.

Osteoperiosteal pertaining to bone and its periosteum.

Osteophage An osteoclast

Osteophyte Degenerative exostosis secondary to musculotendinous traction.

Osteoplaque A layer of bone.

Osteoplasty Reshaping of bone; alveoloplasty, plastic contouring of the alveolar process to achieve physiologic contours in the bone and gingival tissues.

Osteoporosis Condition characterized by a loss of bone cells. It can be a primary condition or associated with other diseases, therapies (steroids), or disuse can be improved or minimized with exercise. There is loss of protein matrix tissue from bone causing it brittle and easily fractured. Osteoporosis is natural part of ageing. By the age of 70 bone density decreases by 30 per cent. Bone naturally becomes thin as person ages. After menopause women are more prone for osteoporosis. Other causes include removal of ovaries, lack of calcium and certain hormonal

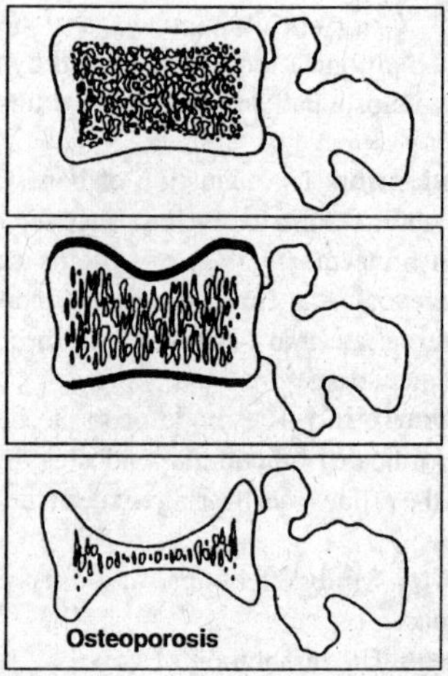

disorders. It is more common in smokers and alcoholics. In many cases it produces no symptoms. First sign may be a fracture just above wrist and femur neck. There may be spontaneous fracture of one or many vertebrae leading to a progressive loss of height.

Lost bone tissue cannot be replaced but calcium intake can be increased. Milk, milk products and green leafy vegetables are good source of calcium. Exercise also helps. After menopause hormone replacement therapy may also help.

Osteoporotic vertebra Vertebral fractures are the most common osteoporotic fracture. Many fractures go undiagnosed. Decreasing bone mass

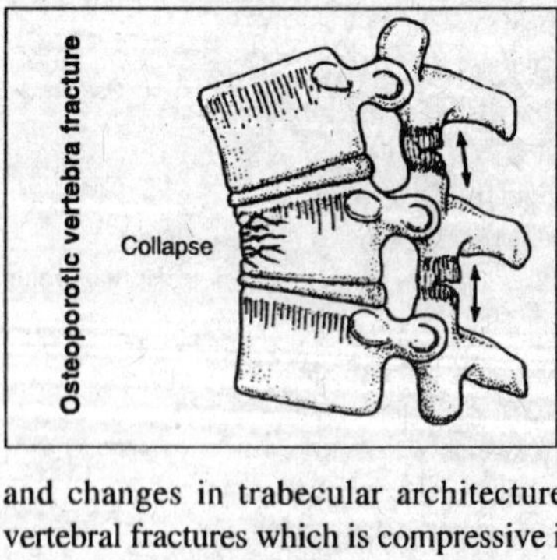

and changes in trabecular architecture lead to vertebral fractures which is compressive in nature. Biconcave fractures are also common. There may be acute pain with paravertebral muscle spasm and loss of function. Radicular pain is due to nerve root irritation.

Osteoradionecrosis Radiation of jaws during treatment of head and neck cancer can lead to long lasting damage to vascular, connective and bone tissues. Damage lowers the resistance of bone to infection and injury. The extraction of teeth or soft tissue infection after radiation can produce catastrophic bone destruction called osteoradionecrosis. Sequestration of bone, fistulae and ulceration of mucosa may be present. Teeth in area may show caries leading to pulp necrosis. Microscopic sections show sequestra.

Osteorathropathy Any disease of the joints and bones.

Osteorrhagia Brust hemorrhage from the bone tissue.

Osteosarcoma Osteogenic sarcoma.

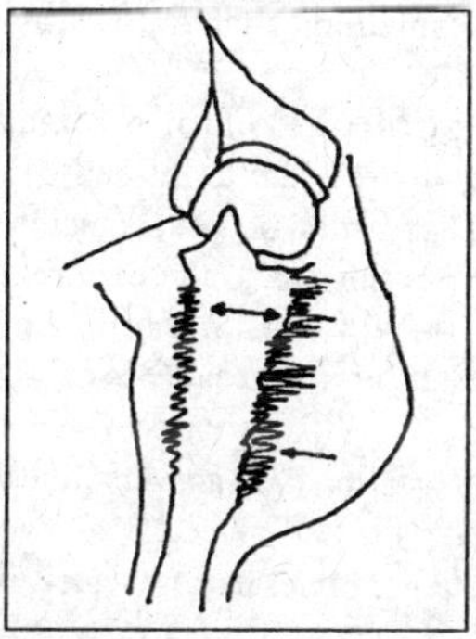

Osteosclerosis There is increased bone density becoming extreme white on X-ray. Local osteosclerosis may be a result of fracture or osteoarthritis. Chronic osteomyelitis may also result it. If it develops in all bones it is known as osteopetrosis.

Osteostimulatory Acting to stimulate, enhance, or accelerate the formation of bone in and around a host site, augmentation material, or endosteal implant.

Osteotome A chisel used to cut or expand bone.

Osteotomy In implant dentistry, a site prepared in bone for the placement of an endosteal implant.

Osteotrophy Nutrition of bone.

Osteotylus The callus enclosing the end of a broken bone.

Ostephytosis Formation of osteophytes.

Ostetitis pubis It is an inflammatory, overuse disorder of symphysis pubis. It is aggravated by kicking, runing or pivoting. Sit ups may also cause more pain. Local injection of corticosteroid is useful.

Ostomate Person with an ostomy.

Ostomy Surgically created opening.

Other oriented lies Lies told to benefit others.

Otic Having to do with the ear.

Otic application Drug instillation in the outer ear.

Otitic hydrocephalus Main symptoms include headache, possibly accompanied by ipsilateral facial paralysis or abducens paralysis occurring several weeks after resolution of an acute pain of otitis media. Nausea and vomiting are the systemic signs.

Otitic meningitis It is a major complication of otitis media. Two major features are headache and neck stiffness. Headache may be on the side of infection. Flexion of neck is resisted because of pain or discomfort arising from irritated nerve roots. Photophobia and cerebral vomiting may occur early as symptoms of cerebral irritation and raised pressure. Temperature is uniformly raised. Increased mental activity continues spilling over delirium. Final stage is of paralysis.

Otitis externa It is the infection of outer ear canal. It may be caused by bacteria or fungi which may produce persistent inflammation known as otomycosis. It causes redness and swelling of disease, discharge from ear and sometimes an area of eczema. If pus blocks the ear it may result in deafness. Thorough cleaning and drying is necessary. Antibiotics, antifungal and anti-inflammatory drugs will be helpful.

Otitis media It is an inflammation of middle ear cavity between ear drum and inner ear. Common cold is the disposing factor. Eustachian tube may be blocked due to inflammation or sometimes by enlarged adenoids. There may be infection of nose and throat. As a result fluid and pus remain in tube and are not drained. Children are generally affected. Acute otitis media is marked by sudden, severe earache, a feeling of fullness in ear and deafness. Sometimes there may be tinnitus. If ear drum bursts due to pressure, pus may be discharged. Healing takes time. Otoscopic study helps in diagnosis. Swab of discharge may be used for culture and sensitivity test. Antibiotics are helpful.

Otoantritis Otitis involving the attic of the tympanum and the mastoid antrum.

Otogenic brain abscess It is an intracerebral or intracerebellar accumulation of pus caused by pyogenic organisms derived from infection of middle ear cleft. It is a major complication of otitis media. It results in abscess formation resulting in fluctuating temperature and pulse, furred tongue, loss of appetite, general malaise and polymorphonuclear leucocytosis. There may be slow cerebral dysfunction, and loss of concentration, lethargy, drowsiness, capricious mood, irritability or apathy, vomiting and headache.

Otolaryngologist Medical specialist who treats the ears, throat, pharynx, larynx, nasopharynx, and tracheobronchial tree.

Otolith organs Bodies in the inner ear that provide vestibular information.

Otolithic membrane Thick, gelatinous, glycoprotein layer located directly over hair cells of the macula in the saccule and utricle of the inner ear.

Otoliths Small, hardened particles of calcium carbonate in the saccule and utricle of the inner ear, associated with the receptors of equilibrium; also called statoconia.

Otoplasty Pastic surgery of the ear.

Otopyorrhea A copious purulent discharge from the ear.

Otopyosis A suppurative disease of the ear.

Otorhinology That branch of medicine which treats disease of the nose and ear.

Otorrhoea It refers to discharge from external auditory canal of a material that is produced in auditory canal or middle ear. Discharge may be serous, mucous, purulent flaky, blood. The discharge may be odourless, otorrhoea may be continuous or intermittent.

Otosclerosis It is a disorder of the middle ear that causes progressive deafness. It is often inherited. It occurs when for unknown reasons an overgrowth of bone immobilises the stapes. It prevents sound vibrations passing to internal ear. It results in conductive deafness. In most cases both ears are affected. Sound is heard as muffled but is more distinguishable when there is background noise. Affected person wants to talk quietly. Hearing loss progresses slowly over a period of more than 10 years. Tinnitus is often present. A hearing aid is an excellent treatment for otosclerosis. The deafness can be cured by stapedectomy.

Otoscope It is the instrument for examining the outer ear. With the help of beam of light one can see the ear canal and ear drum for its infection and perforation.

Ototoxic Term referring to drugs causing sensorineural deafness.

Otto pelvis There are bilateral acetabular projections towards the pelvic cavity with narrowing of pelvis, suprapubic angle and bituberous diameter.

Outbreak Often used to denote a local epidemic (may be considered interchangeable with the term epidemic).

Outcome Something that follows as a result of consequence.

Outcome control Control of external events motivationally relevant to the self.

Outer ear That portion of the ear outside the cranium and extending inward to the ear drum.

Outlet of pelvis It is important to know the measurements of pelvic outlet to predict the nature of delivery. Three diameters are usually described : the anteroposterior, the transverse and the posterior sagittal.

Outliers Estreme values that are widely deviant from the mean.

Outline the line by which a figure or object is defined; a contour.

Outline form Shape of the area of tooth surface included within the cavosurface margins of a prepared cavity.

Outpatient A patient who comes to the hospital, clinic, or dispensary for diagnosis and/or treatment but does not occupy a bed. Pertaining to medical services rendered in a hospital without admitting the patient.

Outpatient surgery Operative procedures from which patients recover and return home on the same day.

Outpatients Persons who receive health care in a hospital department but return home in less than 24 hours.

Output Concerning computers, end result manipulation of information.

Outside density In social psychology, a measure of the number of people per unit of land space. The ratio concerns acreage and population, without concern for the availability or use of building.

Ova Female sex cells.

Oval Egg-shaped; having the outline of an egg.

Oval window A small, membrane-covered opening that separates the middle and inner ear.

Ovarian Relating to, involving or affecting the ovary.

Ovarian follicle It is one of niche within an ovary in which a single ovum develops. Each follicle secretes sex hormone oestrogen as long as ovum remains released. Only a few ova matures and are released from ovary rupturing their follicles. Ovarian follicles are also known as graafian follicles.

Ovarian hyperstimulation syndrome Condition caused by artificial stimulation of ovaries by gonadotrophin therapy to produce ovulation.

Ovarian ligament Fibro muscular cord which connects lower pole of ovary to the supero lateral angle of uterus.

Ovarian torsion and pregnancy Torsion of pedunculated tumor is the commonest complication. Usually it appears at 8 to 16 weeks when uterus is growing at a rapid rate. It causes sudden lower abdominal pain, vomiting and shock like features. almost simulating ruptured ectopic pregnancy.

Ovarian tumor and pregnancy Ovarian tumors with pregnancy are fairly common. It is difficult to diagnose ovarian tumors in the later half of pregnancy when tumor becomes abdominal.

Ovariectomy The surgical removal of the ovaries.

Ovary There is one pair of almond-shaped gland situated on either side of uterus below the opening of fallopian tube. Each ovary is about 30 mm long and 20 mm wide. It has narrow outer cortical layer and deeper medullary layer. Medulla contains spirally running arteries, lymphatics and nerves. It produces female sex hormones oestrogen and progesterone. Inflammation of it may be caused by mumps. Ovarian cyst may develop at any age and 95 per cent are benign. Polycystic ovary syndrome may produce male sex hormones leading to amenorrhoea, infertility and hirsutism.

Ovary cancer It is one of the major cause of death in women mostly who are not having any child. It may be primary or secondary growth extended from breast. Generally it does not cause any symptom until it is widespread.

First symptom is vague abdominal discomfort, digestive disturbances and abnormal vaginal bleeding. Ascites may develop. If growth is widespread only 20 per cent females will survive up to five years.

OVD Optical variable device.

Over feeding It occurs at the end of first week. Infant is fretful, passes frequent loose greenish stools containing undigested curds. Perianal region is excoriated. Baby may vomit after each feed.

Overall percent agreement The perventage of the total observations found in cells a and d of a 2 * 2 table.

Overbite Vertical overlapping of maxillary over mandibular teeth, usually measured perpendicular to the occlusal plane.

Overcompensation A conscious or unconscious process in which a real or imagined physical or psychological deficit generates exaggerated correction. Concept introduced by Adler.

Overdenture Complete or partial removable denture supported by retained roots to provide improved support, stability, and tactile and sensation and to reduce ridge resorption.

Overdenture abutment analogue A replica of an overdenture attachment/retention component for incorporation with a laboratory model for prosthesis fabrication.

Overdetermination The concept or multiple unconscious causes of an emotional reaction or symptom.

Overdeveloped film A dark film that results from excess development time—an inaccurate timer, not developer solution, an inaccurate thermometer or overactive developer.

Overdosage Administration of a drug or another agent in amounts that are greater than the standard or prescribed dosage.

Overexposed film A dark film that results from excessive exposure time, kilovoltage or milliamperage or a combination of these factors.

Overflow Incontinence Symptoms of overflow incontinence (urinary retention) include the involuntary continuous or intermiltent leakage of small amount of urine associated with over distension of bladder and may occur while the patient is awaked or asleep.

Overflow incontinence of urine Puerperal woman can hold an enormous amount of urine without complaint due to atony of bladder wall. Overflow occurs due to retention of urine. Early embulation helps to overcome atony of bladder.

Overgrafting The application of a second graft over a previously healed graft from which the epithelium has been removed, as a means of reinforcing split thickness grafts.

Overhydration Too large a fluid input that can put a burden on the heart.

Overjet Horizontal projection of maxillary teeth beyond the mandibular teeth, usually measured parallel to the occlusal plane. When not otherwise specified, the term is generally assumed to refer to central incisors and is measured from the labial surface of the lower central incisors to the labial surface of the upper central incisors at the level of the upper incisor edge. Unique conditions may sometimes require other measuring techniques.

Overlapped contacts Overlapped interproximal contacts appear superimposed over each other on a radiograph; results from using incorrect horizontal angulation.

Overloading circulation Sometimes in a haste or due to ignorance more blood or fluid may be introduced in short duration which may cause overloading of circulation. This causes cardiac distress and respiratory distress in presence of renal inefficiency.

Danger is more when large quantity of fluid is introduced rapidly. Pulses rise, respiration becomes rapid and shallow and one develops pain in chest and oedema.

Overriding The slipping of either part of a fractured bone past the other.

Oversew To close or join with sutures.

Oversight The application of appropriate laws, regulations, guidelines, or accepted standards of practice to control the use of a microorganism, based on the degree of risk or uncertainty associated with that organism.

Overstretch Stretch beyond the normal range or muscle length.

Overstretch weakness Weakness in a two-joint or multijoint muscle resulting from repetitive movements or habitual positions that elongate the muscle beyond normal range of muscle length.

Overt observation In the research method of naturalistic observation, any procedure in which the investigator's presence and intention is known to the research subjects. There is no effort to hide the research purpose or process.

Overthecounter drug(OTC) drug available to a consumer without a prescription.

Over-the-counter medication Nonprescription drug.

Overuption Supraclusion.

Overuse injury It is an injury that has been caused by repetitive movements of part of body. Epicondylitis is the common example of overuse injuries of fingers and wrist joints which may affect typist. Musicians are also affected by a variety of problems. Symptoms generally disappear with rests. It is possible to avoid pain and stiffness by altering technique.

Overuse syndrome It is a disorder characterised by pain, tenderness sometimes impaired function of muscle group and ligaments of repetitive action. It is common in typists and musicians playing instruments.

Oviductal transport The stage of oocyte or embryo transport that takes place in the oviduct.

Oviducts Uterine or fallopian tubes.

Oviparous Relating to or describing a mode of reproduction in which the female lays eggs that develop and hatch outside the body; e.g., birds.

Oviparous species Animals producing eggs that develop and hatch outside the body.

Ovomucoid A heat-stable mucoid in egg white, which represents about 10 percent of its protein content.

Ovotestis A gonad of certain invertabrates that supports the production of both eggs and sperm.

Ovovegetarian A vegetarian whose diet includes eggs.

Ovoviviparous species Animals producing eggs that develop within the maternal body to be born as live young.

Ovulation It is the development and release of ovum from follicle in the ovary. Ovulation occurs midway through the menstrual cycle and is regnlated by hormones. During first half of cycle follicle-stimulating hormone (FSH) causes several ova to mature in the ovary. At midcycle luteinising hormone (LH) causes one ripe ovum to be released. Follicle secretes progesterone during second half of menstrual cycle. After its release the ovum travels along the fallopian tube unless fertilisation occurs or is shed during menstruation. If a woman does not ovulate she cannot conceive. There is release of mature ovum by one of ovaries at the middle of regular menstrual cycles probably on 14th day. Ova travel down to a fallopian tube towards uterus. If in way it comes in contact with sperm, conception may take place.

Ovulation induction Any of various medical or surgical techniques used to cause ovulation.

Ovulatory Relating to or involved in ovulation; i.e., the release of a mature egg from the ovary.

Ovum It is a female sex cell and is produced by ovarian follicle. Each ovary contains thousands of immature ova, only one of which reaches maturation during early menstruation cycle. Mature released ovum travels down a nearby fallopian tube. Fertilisation generally takes place in fallopian tube forming a zygote. Very rarely 2 ova are released and may develop in twins. It is an eggshell of reproduction. Each cell measures about 1 mm in diameter. There are about one million immature ova present in each ovary at birth. Out of these only 200 per ovary mature to be released during woman's fertile years. If fertilisation occurs the ovum develops into an embryo.

Oxalate tubes It is used for blood chemistry and haematocrit estimation. *Potassium oxalate* 2 to 3 mg per ml of blood is required as anticoagulant. It may cause shrinkage of blood cells. *Double oxalate* is a combination of potassium oxalate and ammonium oxalate salts in the ratio of 2:3. It is used for erythrocyte sedimentation rate (ESR) and haematocrit. This is not to be used for NPN estimation. Trisodium citrate is used for ESR. For ESR 0.4 ml of liquid is taken to mix with 1.6 ml of blood to make total of 2 ml.

Oxalated blood Blood that has been prevented from clotting by addition of oxalate which combines with calcium.

Oxhemoglobin A compound formed from combination of hemoglobin with oxygen, used for transporting oxygen from the lungs to the tissue.

Oxidant Oxidizing substance.

Oxidase A hemoprotein that binds and reduces oxygen, generally to water.

Oxidation A term meaning combining of oxygen with another substance. Now defined as the process occurring when an element loses electrons or increased in valence number thereby losing negative charges and becoming more electropositive.

Oxidation-reduction reaction A reaction in which electrons are transferred from a donor to an acceptor molecule; also called a redox reaction.

Oxidative capacity The potential to combine elements or radicals with oxygen or to lose electrons.

Oxidative phosphorylation The formation of ATP using energy derived from electron transport to oxygen. It occurs in the mitochondria.

Oxidative stress The sum of the deleterious intracellular events associated with excess production or insufficient disposal of intracellular oxidants.

Oxidizing agent An atom that accepts electrons in an oxidation-reduction reaction.

Oximeter An instrument that determines the oxygen saturation of a blood sample photoelectrically.

Oximetery It is determination of arterial O_2 saturation of hemoglobin by measuring absorbance of light by blood.

Oximetry Procedure used to measure amount of oxygenated hemoglobin.

Oxmotic Relating to or involved in osmosis.

Oxycephaly Skull is elongated in a vertical direction with short transverse and anteroposterior measurements. It is due to premature ossification of all the sutures of skull. The anomaly is evident at birth and develops during first four years of life. Vertex is dome shaped, with a vertical forehead, absent superciliony arches, prominent nose, small upper jaw, heavy lower jaw and shallow orbits.

Oxygen It is a colourless, odourless gas that makes 20 per cent of earth's atmosphere. Oxygen is essential for all forms of life because it is necessary for the metabolic burning of foods to produce energy. Oxygen in the air is absorbed through lungs and into blood where it binds with haemoglobin in RBCs. Hence O_2 is distributed throughout the body. O_2 is used to treat hypoxia and anaemia. Generally oxygen is supplied in cylinders during

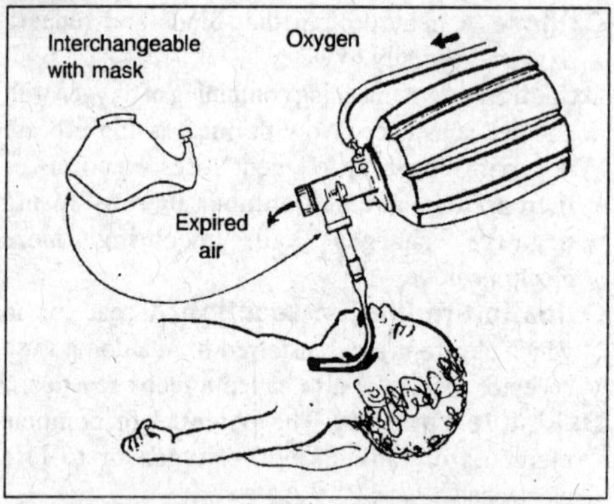

acute attack of hypoxia. John Mayow (1643-1679) of Oxford showed that a component of air was used up by a burning candle or by a live mouse. Modern use of oxygen was popularised in 1917 by JS Haldane. Medical oxygen is now manufactured by fractional distillation of liquid air. Oxygen is supplied in cylinders as the compressed gas at a pressure of 135. One volume of liquid oxygen is equivalent to 840 volume of gaze. Pipeline pressure of 410 kPa. Solubility in water at 37°C is 2 to 4% of volume. Critical temperature is 118.4°C with oil or grease it may cause an ignition. Oxygen content of air is 20.93%. In expired air content is 16.3%. While that of alveoar air is 14.2%. Partial pressure of oxygen in alveolar air is 104 mm Hg, in venous blood it is 40 mm Hg. Solubility of oxygen in plasma is 0.3 ml/HB. While of arterial blood it is 19.8 volume per cent. Oxygen saturation of arterial blood is 97% and oxygen tension in arterial blood is 100 mm of Hg.

Oxygen capacity of blood It is the power of normal haemoglobin content of blood to carry O_2 when fully saturated. Normally it is 19.8 cc per 100 cc of blood. It is estimated that one gram of haemoglobin when fully saturated will carry 1.34 cc of blood.

Oxygen concentrator A device used in health care that increases the proportion of oxygen gas in the air of the room in which it is placed—it is sometimes used in respiratory and other conditions that produce hypoxia (low oxygen concentration in the blood).

Oxygen consumption (VO_2) The volume of oxygen that is used by the tissues in one minute.

Oxygen consumption The amount of oxygen used by cells to meet metabolic needs.

Oxygen cylinder Oxygen cylinders are generally painted black. Small cylinder of 2 × 5" diameter

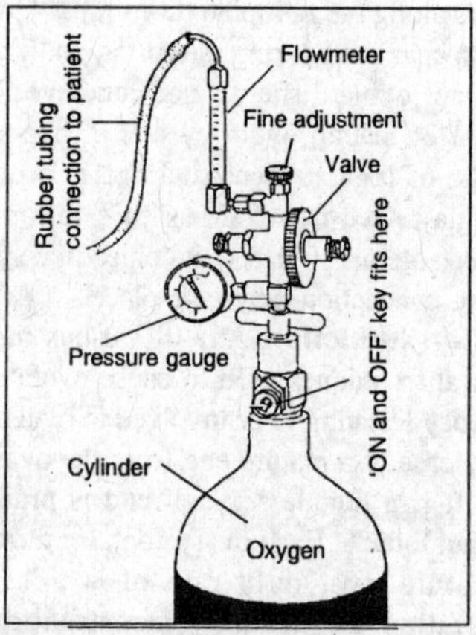

contains 24 cubic feet of oxygen while big cylinders 4" × 8" diameter contains 120 cubic feet of O_2. Gauge attached to the valve measures the amount of O_2 in cylinder. A flowmeter is attached to valve for easy adjustment and control of oxygen. When face mask is used 6 to 8 litres per minute O_2 is given.

Oxygen debt Continued increased metabolism that occurs in a cell to remove excess lactic acid that resulted from exercise.

Oxygen flux Amount of O_2 delivered to the tissues per unit time.

Oxygen mask A flexible mask that fits snugly and securely over the client's nose and mouth for delivery of oxygen.

Oxygen pulse The volume of oxygen extracted by the peripheral tissues or the volume of oxygen added to the pulmonary blood per heart beat.

Oxygen saturation Amount of hemoglobin that is fully saturated with oxygen expressed as percent of total available hemoglobin.

Oxygen tent It is a thin plastic tent-like structure which is suspended over patient and sides are tucked in firmly under bed clothings. Being airproof inside temperature may rise. It should not be allowed to rise above 70°F.

Concentration of oxygen is maintained at constant rate. A special humidifier is also incorporated into tent to maintain humidity of oxygen.

Oxygen therapy Giving oxygen is a major part of nursing procedure. It is given from oxygen cylinder in cases of obstruction in air passage, bronchial asthma, pneumonia and pulmonary oedema.

It is needed in peripheral circulatory failure, poisoning, drowning, chest injuries and during operation.

Oxygen toxicity Lung damage that develops when oxygen concentrations of more than 50% are administered for longer than 48 to 72 hours.

Oxygen transport Arterial blood carries about 20 mL of O_2 per 100 mL. 19.7 mL combined with hemoglobin 0.3 mL dissolved in plasma. In venous blood 15 Ml is carried per 100 Ml blood 14.9 mL combined with Hb. 0.1 mL dissolved.

Oxygen transport system The lungs, heart and blood vessels that conduct oxygen from the atmosphere to the mitochondria of cells.

Oxygenases Enzymes that catalyze reactions in which oxygen is introduced into an acceptor molecule.

Oxygenating agent Substance that liberates oxygen. Applied to tissues to kill anaerobic microorganisms.

Oxygopia Extreme sharpness of vision.

Oxyhaemoglobin It is combination of oxygen with haemoglobin and occurs in lungs as a normal part of breathing. It is in the form of oxyhaemoglobin that oxygen is carried by blood to the tissues of the body. With O_2 blood becomes brighter red.

Oxyhemoglobin saturation The ratio, expressed as a percentage of the amount of oxyhemoglobin in blood.

Oxymethylene Formaldehyde.

Oxyphilic Stainable with an acid dye.

Oxytocin Four drugs are currently available to increase the activity of uterus in labour : oxytocin, prostaglandin, sparteine sulphate and ergometrine. Oxytocin produces regular intermittent uterine contractions which are indistinguishable from normal labour contractions.

Half time of oxytocin in circulation is 10 minutes. Oxytocin helps in induction of labour, acceleration of labour, management of third stage of labour. Control of dose of oxytocin administered is of critical importance in induction and acceleration of labour, therefore 0.5 IU intravenous route is chosen in drip of 500 ml 5% dextrose. Overdose of oxytocin may result in fetal asphyxia.

P

P value The probability that the observed difference could have been obrained by chance alone, given random variation and a single test of the null hypotheses.

P wave Deflection of an ECG that occurs with depolarization of the atria.

P(PROM)H It is the measure of acidity or alkalinity of a solution. pH scale is from 0 to 14. pH 7 denotes neutrality. Below 7 is more acidic and higher the pH more strongly alkaline it is. Below 7.3 is called acidosis and above 7.5 alkalosis.

P.A Abbreviation for posteroanterior.

P-50 This is the oxygen tension needed to provide 50 % saturation of haemoglobin. Its value is an expression of shift of the dissociation curve to left or right. The dissociation curve may be altered by changes in pH. Carbon dioxide increase causes a flattening of curve to the right. An increase in temperature results in flattening of curve to the right. In hypothermia curve is shifted to the left.

Paalogism An unintentional or unnoticed fallacy.

PABA It prevents sun burn, prevents premature aging of skin. It provides protection in photosensitive disorders caused by UVB rays.

Pacemaker It is a device which supplies electrical impulses to heart to maintain heart beat. It consists of a small electronic device and power source connected to the heart via electrical wire. In a person's heart beat is maintained by sinoatrial node which sends out regular electrical impulses and trigger heart contractions. When sinoatrial node is not working properly pacemaker is applied. Pacemakers are of two types—fixed rate and demand. More advance pacemakers can increase heart rate when needed such as during exercise. Pacemaker is implanted using local anaesthetic. Vigorous exercise should be avoided for two weeks after operation.

Pachycheilia Thickness of the lips.

Pachydactyly Enlargement of digitis.

Pachyderma oris A benign white lesion of mucus membrane of buccal mucosa.

Pacinian corpuscle These are found in deeper layers of skin of hands, feet and penis and periosteum of bones specially in neighbourhood of tendons and joints. These consist of number of concentric fibrous coats externally arranged like the layers of an onion and encloses a soft cyclindrical core. Nerve fibre loses its medullary sheath. These are peripheral sensory receptors. These are elliptical about 1 mm long and 0.7 mm in width. These are encapsulated and capsule and are made up of 30 or so concentric lamellae of flattened cells. In the core of corpuscle is the termination of nerve fibre. The nerve fibre loses its myelin sheath as it enters the corpuscle.

Pack Treatment by wrapping a patient in blankets, sheets, or towels, wet or dry; also, the blankets, sheets, or towels used for this purpose.

Packing Gauze, sponge or other material used to pack a wound or cavity.

Paddles Wooden paddles attached to the limb are used to increase the surface area of a part to be moved against resistance.

Paediatrics It is the branch of medicine dealing with the health of children from birth to the age of 12 years. Care involves physically, mentally and socially.

Paedophilia It is a desire of an adult for sexual activity with a child. It is more common in males than females and treatment includes behaviour therapy or drugs to reduce sex desire.

Paget's disease It is a generalised bone disease of unknown cause and was described by Paget in 1876. Males after the age of 40 are more affected. Major development occurs in skull and the weight bearing parts of skeleton. Tibia is bent anteriorly and the femur outward. Person develops a waddling gait. Enlargement of head, headache, mental disturbances and loss of hearing and eyesight are the chief complaints. Alkaline phosphatase levels are increased. Oral involvement is common and jaw is frequently involved. Enlargement of alveolar ridge causes dentures to gradually lose their fit. Maxilla is affected more common than mandible. Teeth may migrate and occasionally loosen. In early stage an irregular radiolucency is seen. This turns to radiopacity and finally to dense, irregular highly radiopaque areas resembling cotton wool. The teeth show hypercementosis, pulp calcifications and loss of lamina dura. There is no treatment of Paget's disease. It is treated by calcitonin.

Paget's disease of spine It is characterised by massive osteoclastic proliferation with marked bone resorption. There is little osteoblastic activity. Osteoclastic proliferation is precipitated by RNA virus. Other features include enlargement of skull vault, bowing of tibia and shortening of stature. Monostatic forms are more common in vertebra. Surgical compression may be made.

Paget's of breast This is a malignant condition characterised by gradual destruction of nipple and development of carcinoma within breast usually close to nipple. At first nipple and areola become red. It is covered by scales and subsequently scales are detached and nipple destroyed leaving a flat bright red weeping surface.

PAH Para-aminohippuric acid; a substance used to measure total renal plasma flow because its clearance rate is equal to the total rate of plasma flow because its clearance rate is equal to the total rate of plasma flow to the kidneys. PAH is filtered and secreted but not reabsorbed by the renal nephrons.

Pain It is a localised sensation ranging from mild to severe and excruciating experience. The skin contains many nerve endings. Stimulation of these receptors leads to transmission of pain messages to brain. Nerve endings have different sensitivities, some respond only to severe stimulation such as cutting, piercing, others respond to warning stimuli. Blood vessels and tendons have these nociceptors. Most internal organs have a few if any nociceptors. Pain is usually associated with distress and anxiety while unexplained pain is often worse.

Experience of pain may be reduced by past experience. Cultural differences exist in expression of pain. Many adjunctives are used to describe different types of pain such as penetrating, throbbing, piercing, stabbing and cutting. If pain arises from an internal organ it is difficult for the sufferer to pinpoint its origin with any precision. Pain may be felt at a point some distance from the disorder. This is called a referred pain.

Pain and fatigue syndromes Multicausal and often chronic nonproductive patterns that interfere with well-being, activities of living and productivity.

Pain burning Causalgia refers to a burning pain in the area of previous injury or surgical procedure. It may follow after tooth extraction. A few days or weeks after socket becomes full of pain although the wound is completely healed. Pain is transitory and may be precipitated by emotional, visual and physical stimuli. Treatment is empirical.

Pain during 2nd stage at labour Uterine contractions are more painful, stronger, frequent and last longer. Uterine contractions last 1½ minutes and occur every two or three minutes. Bag of membranes usually ruptures. During the pains the length of the perineum from anus to vulva becomes lengthened and scalp appears at vulva.

Pain gate A hypothetical neural circuit in which activity in fine touch and pressure pathways diminishes the activity in pain and temperature pathways.

Pain intensity The degree or extent of pain perceived by an individual.

Pain management Techniques for preventing, reducing, or relieving pain.

Pain perception Conscious experience of discomfort.

Pain relief Method of treatment depends on severity, duration, location and causative factor. Acetaminophen and aspirin are widely used drugs to relieve headache and mild pain. Severe pain caused by injury, stones require treatment with narcotic analgesics.

Sports injuries are treated by non-steroidal anti-inflammatory drug (NSAID). Massage, ice-packs or poultice may be used for the relief of localised pain by muscle spasm, inflammation or injury. Surgical procedures to relieve pain may be adopted when everything fails.

Pain spot A point of the skin peculiarly sensitive to hurtful stimuli, which has a much lower limen for pain than adjacent regions.

Pain threshold Point at which sufficient pain-transmitting neurochemicals reach the brain to cause awareness of discomfort.

Pain tolerance Amount of pain a person endures once the pain threshold is surpassed.

Pain, myofacial This symptom complex is characterised primarily of pain and dysfunction around the temporomandibular joint and face. There are four groups of complaints, pain in temporo-mandibular joint area, muscle tenderness, limited opening and deviation on opening of jaw, and noise in TM joint. It produces occlusal disharmonies. Disease is produced by masticatory muscle's fatigue and spasm. Being of psychological origin, treatment is conservative with muscle relaxants and analgesics.

Painful arch syndrome Painful arch of foot.

Painful kidney Many serious diseases of kidney are not painful. A sense of dull aching in the loins may be present at the onset of acute nephritis and is frequent with pyelitis, pyelonephritis and oxaluria. Pain is severe when renal calculi is present. Perinephric abscesses are associated with lumbar pain and tenderness. In Dietle's crisis pain is on one side of kidney which is relieved on passing urine. A dull dragging pain in lumbar region relieved by rest in lying posture occurs with movable kidney. It is on affected side.

Painful micturition Pain may be present either during or immediately following the act of micturition. It is usually of vesical origin but may be of urethral too. Bladder spasm is felt in midhypogastrium so that as soon as patient has voided urine she again wants to pass it although bladder is empty. Gonococcal urethrtis causes scalding pain as the urine passes over inflamed mucous membrane. Painful micturition is a prominent symptom of cystitis where pain is felt at the end of micturition. Papilloma, carcinoma, stone and tuberculosis all may cause painful micturition and increased frequency of urine. It is when the patient passes small amounts of urine at short intervals and it may be accompanied with urgency of micturition. Symptoms always develop with cystitis which may be due to *E. coli* infection, stone or growth. Pressure on bladder due to pelvic tumours also causes it. Over distended bladder and neurosis may also cause if urine is sterile. Choice of treatment is of radical vulvectomy.

Painful sensation Perception of pain is usually tested clinically by pricking with a pin. This is mediated by free nerve endings of small myelinated fibres of 2 to 4 mm diameter conducting at 12 to 24 m/s. Impairment of pain perception can arise as part of peripheral neuropathy. Pain fibres may also be affected as they cross the spinal cord by tumour such as an ependymoma or astrocytoma within spinal cord.

Pain-induced aggression Aggressive behaviour following receipt of a painful stimulus. Various animals behave in this fashion, attacking any nearby object or event, regardless of its involvement in the painful stimulation.

Pain-spasm-pain cycle Steady contraction of muscles, which causes ischemia and stimulates pain, in turn, initiates more spasms.

Pair bonds Strong, lifelong attachments that occur between two. It includes "low" when speaking of humans.

Palaeocerebellum Having vestibular and spinal connections is concerned with the coordination of the reflexes of muscle tonus in its relation to maintenance of equilibrium.

Palantine Referring to palate.

Palatal bar A major connector that crosses the palate and unites two or more parts of a maxillary removable partial denture.

Palatal rugae The irregular ridges in the mucous membrane covering the anterior part of the hard palate.

Palate It is the roof of the mouth. It separates mouth from nasal cavity. It is covered with mucous membrane. At the rear is the soft palate, a flap of muscle and fibrous tissue that projects. During swallowing, the soft palate presses against the rear wall of the pharynx preventing food from being regurgitated into nose.

Palatine Pertaining to the palate.

Palatine bone Pair of bones in the skull that form the posterior part of the palate, a portion of the nasal cavity, and the floor of the eye.

Palatine raphe Line that delineates each half of the palate.

Palatine reflex Swallowing reflex paleencephalon (L. Edinger) Old brain; evolutionarily-ancient part of the brain in certain organisms including humans, such as the cerebellum and other areas not related to the cerebrum. Also known as metameric nervous system. Compare NEENCEPHALON.

Palatoglossal air space An air space on a panoramic film that appears as a horizontal radiolucency between the hard palate and the tongue.

Palatogram A graphic representation of the area of the palate contacted by the tongue.

Palatograph An instrument used in palatography.

Palatography The recording of the movements of the palate in speech.

Palatonasal Pertaining to the palate and the nose.

Paleontology A branch of biology which investigates organisms that existed in the past.

Paleopallium The olfactory cortex.

Paleopathology The technique of examining ancient skeletal remains to identify the disease suffered by historical populations.

Palilexia Abnormal frequent re-reading of words or phrases.

Palilogia An obsessive repetition of utterances or spoken phrases.

Palindrome A segment of duplex DNA in which the base sequences of the two strands exhibit twofold rotational symmetry about an axis.

Palinopasia Recurring visual hallucinations.

Palliate To reduce the severity of; to relieve.

Palliative Easing or reducing pain or discomfort without removing the cause.

Palliative care Care designed to relieve the symptoms of exacerbations but which results in no net improvement in the patient's stationary condition.

Pallidotomy Surgical lesion of globus pallidus, a treatment for Parkinson's disease.

Pallidum Refers to globus pallidus.

Pallium The cerebral cortex.

Pallor Paleness

Palm grasp Method of using the entire palm to hold a dental instrument; primarily used on bulky instruments such as rubber dam clamp forceps.

Palm oil Oil is expressed from pulp and kernel from a nut like fruit. It is an important source of migraine and contains large amount of fatty acids.

Palm-and-thumb grasp Grasp that is similar to the hold on a knife when one is whittling wood; the handle rests in the palm and is grasped by the four fingers while the thumb rests on an adjoining object.

Palmar Pertaining to the palm of the hand.

Palmar creases The typical creases in palm, flexure lines, best seen on flexing the digits are the radial longitudinal crease passing medial to thenar eminence. Palmists have tried to correlate these flexor lines with your life and fortune, etc. Persons

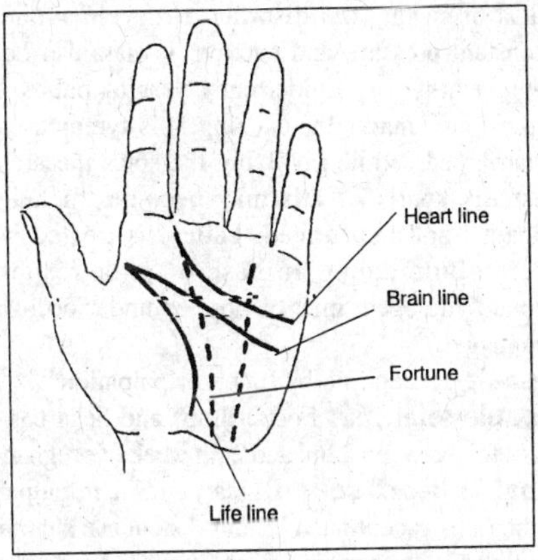

suffering from Down's syndrome have different pattern of lines.

Palmar grasp A means of holding an object in the palm of the hand; used by infants in ulnar orientation before radial orientation.

Palmar surface volar The palm of the hand.

Palmer Notation System Tooth-numbering system that codes the teeth with numbers and letters using brackets to indicate the arch.

Palmer/Zsigmondy system This system is based on the quadrant in which tooth is found. The teeth in each quadrant are numbered with 1 being central incisor and 8 being third molar. The primary dentitition is designated by using capillary letters in place of numbers with A being central incisor and 'E' the second molar.

Palmer's sign The regular and rhythmic contractions of uterus were noted and described by A C Palmer (1949) specially between 4 and 8 weeks. The patient is relaxed with legs draw up in Sim's position. Anteverted uterus should be defined and gently cupped between two fingers of right hand in vagina and left hand resting on lower abdomen. Consistency of uterus be estimated over a period of 2 to 3 minutes. Existence of an early pregnancy is suggested by regular, rhythmic contractions of uterus during which it becomes firm and clearly circumscribed contractions. After 10 weeks phases of relaxation become longer.

Palmoplantar keratoderma It is also known as keratosis plantaris. It may be congenital or acquired keratotic thickening of palms and soles. It is often familial disorder. It develops due to constant pressure and friction. It may also occur with ichthyosis. Epidermal layers of palms and soles show marked thickening. It is symmetrically distributed. While involving the soles the arch is usually spared. Nails may become thickened, opaque and malformed. Patient is treated with keratolytic agent. In case of poor response keratolytic agent may be applied under occlusive bandage.

Palpable Perceptible by touch or palpation.

Palpable fetal part Foetal limbs and head can be first felt between 22nd and 26th week of pregnancy.

Palpable heart sound Heart sound is palpable when it is accentuated in mitral stenosis; snapping giving rise to tapping apical impulse. Accentuated and palpable first heart sound is seen in left atrial myxoma. A_2 is palpable in aortic area in hypertension and P_2 is palpable in pulmonary hypertension.

Palpable voice sounds After percussion it is useful to palpate for voice sounds over the upper middle and lower zones of chest. It is tactile vocal fremitus and is best appreciated by placing ulnar border or flat of hand on the chest wall. This sensation is increased when there is consolidation which amplifies the transmission of voice sound. And in pleural effusion fremitus is absent and reduced where the lung is collapsed.

Palpate Feel.

Palpating fetal lie The fetal lie is the relationship of long axis of mother. Fetal axis can be detected by finding the two ends of fetus. Head is usually large, diffuse while bottom is soft. Back is firm and broad.

Palpation Lightly touching the body or applying pressure.

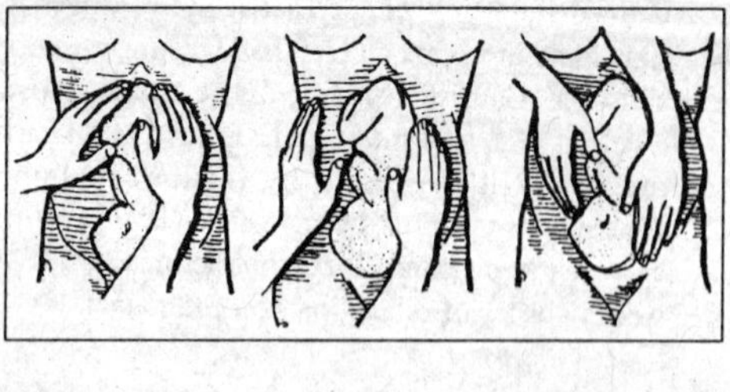

Palpation of carotid arteries The carotids lie anterolaterally in neck. One should palpate the

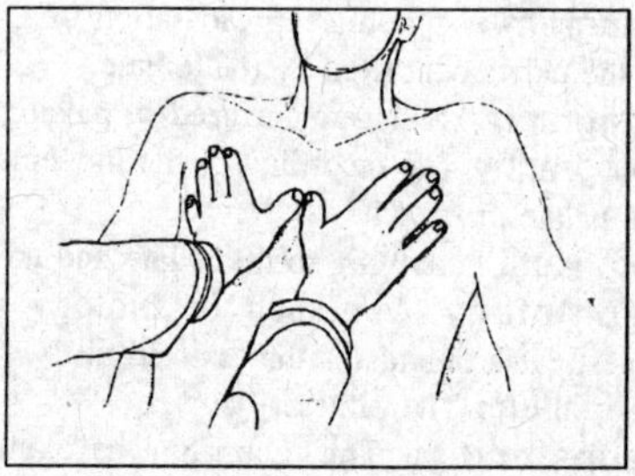

carotids one side at a time. Avoid palpating the carotid sinuses at the level of thyroid cartilage just below the angle of jaw since it may cause slowing

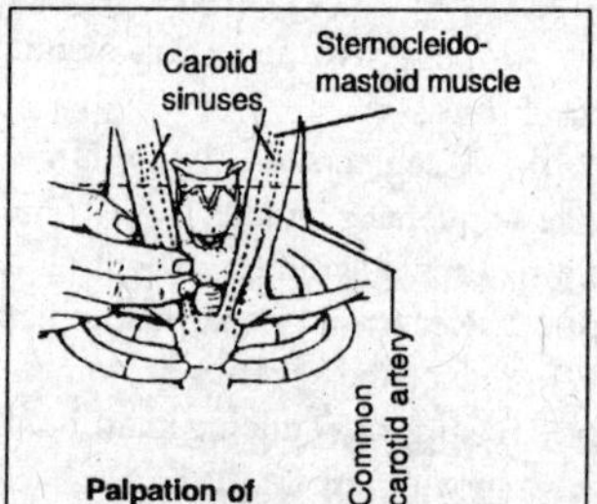

Palpation of carotid arteries

of heart rate. There should be symmetry of pulsation, strength and amplitute.

Palpation of thyroid If thyroid is palpable, it is normally smooth without nodules, masses or irregularities or bruits. Bruit is a gushing sound produced by blood moving through a narrow vessel.

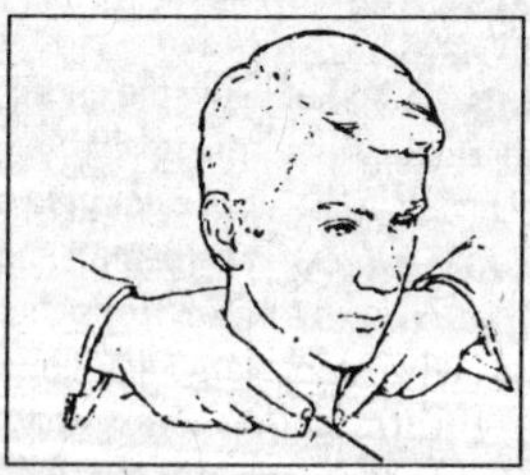

Palpation of uterus Place your abdominal hand on abdomen between umbilicus and symphysis pubis. While supporting the pelvic hand beneath the cervix, raise cervix and try to grasp cervix and try to grasp cervix upwards between two hands. Uterus is mobile in A-P plane.

Palpebra Portion of the conjunctiva that lines the inner surface of the eyelids; it is thick, opaque, and highly vascular.

Palpitation It is awareness of the heart beat. It is felt after strenuous exercise, in tense situation when heart beat is faster. When felt at rest it may be due to ectopic heart beat. It may be felt as a thumping in chest. Ectopic beats do not normally indicate heart disease. These are often caused by heavy smoking, alcohol or large consumption of caffeine. It may be a sign or arrhythmia, ectopic activity or forceful cardiac contraction as in aortic regurgitation and complete heart block.

Palsy, Bell's It is due to paralysis of muscles supplied by seventh nerve. Cause is unknown and may be associated with malignant tumour of parotid gland or may follow surgical procedures in parotid area. Some may be caused by herpes simplex type I virus. Paralysis is unilateral and on the affected side eyes cannot be closed, the mouth droops and saliva escapes from the corner of the mouth. Due to paralysis of fascial muscles patient is expressionless and has difficulty with speech and mastication.

Pan Prefix indicating all or the entirety.

Panacea A remedy for all diseases and difficulties. A cure-all.

Panachinar emphysema The diffuse, generalized destruction of alveolar structural components.

Pan-anxiety An all-pervading anxiety condition.

Panarthritis Any diffuse inflammatory disease of all the joints.

Panatrophy Diffuse atrophy; general atrophy.

Pancarditis Inflammation of all three layers of the heart, involving the endocardium, myocardium, and pericardium.

Pancoast syndrome It is due to involvement of brachial plexus due to apical carcinoma of lung. Clinically one develops pain in arm, shoulder and interscapular region. There will be wasting of small muscles in hand and arm. X-ray will show apical opacity on one side of chest.

Pancreas It lies retroperitoneally across posterior abdominal wall extending from second part of duodnuem to hilum of spleen. It consists of head, body and tail. Main pancreatic duct has many ductules and gradually tapers towards tail. Secretin and cholecystokinin are the principal regulators of pancreatic exocrine secretion. Enzymes

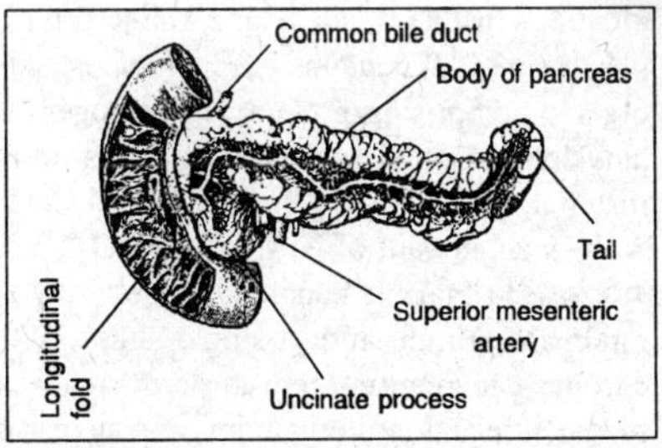

produced by pancreas are amylase, lipase, colipase, phospholipase and protease. Pancreatic secretion is rich in bicarbonate. The islets of Langerhans contain the hormone secreting cells. The beta-cells produce insulin, alpha-cells produce glucagon. D-cells produce somatostain and the PP cells produce pancreatic polypeptide. Ultrasound is an effective modality to examine pancreas.

Pancreas divisum It is a congenital anomaly and is failure of fusion of dorsal and ventral buds of the primitive pancreas. The main bulk of gland is drained by duct of Somtorini and accessory papilla. Such persons develop recurrent pancreatitis. If symptoms are severe, sphincterotomy of accessory papilla helps in reducing pain.

Pancreatic duct A single large tube that unites with common bile duct from the liver and gallbladder and drains pancreatic juice into the duodenum at the hepatopancreatic ampulla (ampulla of Vater). Also called the duct of Wirsung.

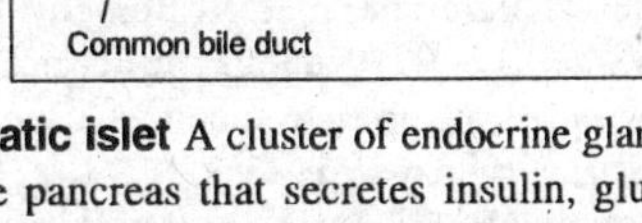

Pancreatic islet A cluster of endocrine gland cells in the pancreas that secretes insulin, glucagon, somatostatin, and ancreatic polypeptide. Also called an islet of Langerhans.

Pancreatic islets A cluster of cells within the pancreas that forms the endocrine protion and secretes insulin and glucagon; also called islets of Langerhans.

Pancreatic juice It is a clear alkaline fluid with a pH about 8.0. It contains 1.8% of solids and 0.6% organic comprising proteins, trypsinogen, lipase, amylase and other organic substances. Inorganic material, nearly 1.2 % is mainly Na, Cl and HCO_3 with small amount of K, Ca and HPO_4.

Pancreatitis In acute pancreatitis the gland usually returns to normal after a single attack. While in chronic pancreatitis there is permanent damage to structure and to the function of pancreas due to persistent inflammation which causes fibrosis. Most common cause is gall stones and alcohol abuse. It causes severe upper abdominal pain often accompanied by nausea and vomiting. Pain is radiated to back and is made worse by movement. Sitting may relieve pain. An attack lasts for about 48 hours. In chronic pancreatitis pain may last for days. There is no specific remedy for acute pancreatitis. Intravenous fluids are helpful. Nothing is to be given by mouth. In recurrent cases even surgery may be needed.

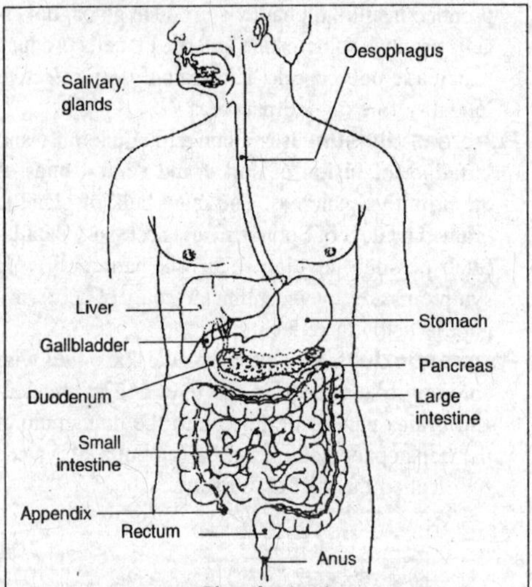

Digestive tract

Pancreazymin A hormone produced in the mucosa of duodenum which stimulates secretion of enzymes from pancreas.

Pancytopenia Reduction in all types of blood cells.

Pandemic An epidemic so widespread that it affects virtually the entire world.

Panel Group of tests.

Panerotic The potential for sexual arousal to arise from virtually any experience.

Panglossia A type of a normal garrulousness observed in psychotic patients, especially those in a manic state.

Panic attacks Expected attack of fears.

Panic disorder Recurring sudden episodes of intense apprehension, palpitations, shortness of breath and chest pain.

Pannus An inflammatory exudate overlying synovial cells on the inside of a joint capsule, which can damage the cartilage, usually occurring in rheumatoid arthritis or related articular rheumatism.

Panophthalmitis Whole eyeball is involved in panophthalmitis. It may occur due to endogenous metastasis or due to exogenous cause from infected wound usually due to perforating injury or an infected corneal ulcer. Infection may spread from anterior to posterior part of eyeball. Organisms are pneumococcus. There may be fever, headache and vomiting. Eyeball appears swollen and proptosed with lid swollen. Corneal wound appears yellow and necrotic with hypopyon with marked purulent discharge.

Panoramic Radiographic method in which a continuous image of both maxillary and mandibular dental arches and associated structures are obtained.

Panoramic film A radiograph that shows a large area of the mandible and maxilla on a single film.

Panoramic memory A form of hypermnesia characterized by vivid recollection of long stretches of life.

Panoramix An X-Ray system in which the source of radiation is placed inside mouth to expose a large film placed extraorally around the face.

Panoromic X-Ray External X-Ray which shows facial aspect of all teeth.

Panphobia Fear of everything.

Panpsychism A monistic doctrine that assumes reality is ultimately psychic in nature.

Pansystolic murmurs This begins with S_1 and ends after S_2. These are high pitched and regurgitant in nature. These are generated when there is flow between two chambers with widely different pressure throughout the systole. It happens between both ventricles in VSD or ventricles and atria in mitral and tricuspid regurgitation.

Pantagamy Group marriage.

Panus A lymph gland inflamed but not suppurating.

Pap test Screening test that detects abnormal cervical cells, the status of reproductive hormone activity, or the presence of normal or infectious microorganisms in the uterus or vagina.

Papanicolaon smears It is done with Ayre's spatula which should be applied to the carvix so that the spatula when rotated through 360° around the squamocolumner junction, scrapes off the superficial cells from the region. Smears obtained are classified as Negative - no malignant cells Doubtful - abnormal cells of doubtful significance Supicious - suspicion of malignancy Positive-cancer cells seen.

Papanicolaou test A cytological staining test for the detection and diagnosis of premalignant and malignant conditions of the female genital tract. Cells scraped from the epithelium of the cervix of the uterus are examined microscopically. Also called a Pap smear.

Papaver somniferum Botanical name of the opium poppy.

Paperless office A workplace in which information is entirely stored, manipulated and transferred electronically.

Papex circuit An 'emotional circuit of the limbic system first described by Papez.

Papilla A small, nipple-like process; projection of the dermis, containing blood vessels and nerves, into the epidermis; projections on the surface of the tongue.

Papillae Small buds concering taste in nodular form.

Papillary Having a small nipple-like or finger-like shape.

Papillary cystadenoma Warthin's tumour constitute 1 per cent of all salivary gland tumours. ninety percent patients are male. Tumour may arise in submaxillary gland or in neck. Gross specimens are encapsulated and cut surface shows cystic spaces with thick mucus. There are numerous cystic spaces whose walls are thrown into papillae and folds. These are lined by double layer of cells. Inner layer is columnar and outer is cuboidal and both are eosinophilic. Excision is the treatment of choice. If tumour is completely excised recurrence is rare. Malignancy is rare.

Papillary muscle Muscular projection from the ventricular walls of the heart to which the chordea tendineae are attached.

Papillate Marked by papilla-like or nipple-like projections.

Papillectomy Excision of a papilla.

Papilloedema It is a swelling of optic disc due to raised intracranial pressure. The most common cause is intracranial tumour near midbrain, haematoma, tuberculoma or an abscess. There may be headache becoming worse by coughing and

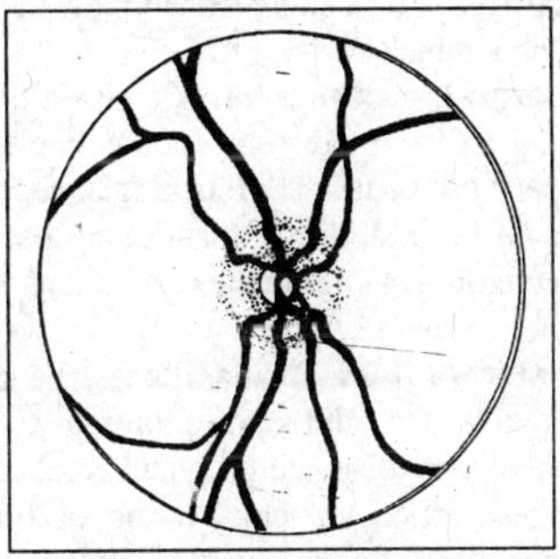

straining. Patient will be having vomiting without nausea. Consciousness may be affected and patient may complain of diplopia. Visual acuity remains normal and pupil reactions are normal until optic atrophy sets in. Ophthalmoscopy will show optic disc hyperaemic. There may be blurring of optic disc margin and filling of physiological cup filled. Optic disc will be swelled and numerous haemorrhages will be seen over disc and retina. Haemorrhages may be flame shaped and punctate. Posterior fundus may show numerous wool spots.

Papilloma Papilloma may be of central axis of connective tissue, blood vessels and lymphatics. Surface is roughened or composed of innumerable delicate villous processes. It may resemble malignant tumours as secondary growth arise by implantation.

Skin, colon, lip and tongue are common sites of lipoma.

Papillomatosis The development of multiple papillomas.

Papillomavirus One of a group of viruses causing common warts of various kinds. Certain types are also associated with various cancers; e.g., cervical carcimona.

Papoose board Means of restricting movements of an uncooperative child; consists of a flat board with soft fabric ties to deter the use of the limbs.

Papular rash A skin discoloration characterized by circular or oval spots that are raised above the surface of the skin.

Para Number of pregnancies that have progressed past 20 weeks at delivery. The term does not indicate whether the fetus was born alive or was still born.

Para axial Lying on the side of its long axis

Paracentesis Procedure for withdrawing fluid from the abdominal cavity.

Paracentral vision A form of vision that uses the retinal area immediately surrounding the fovea.

Paracervical block The blocking of neuropathways of pain by injecting a local anaesthetic into the parametrium at sites in the cervix. It abolishes pain in the uterus only.

Paracetamol It is a popular domestic analgesic and antipyretic for adults and children. It is a major metabolite of obsolete drug named phenacetin. Its analgesic efficacy is equal to that of aspirin but in therapeutic doses it has only weak anti-inflammatory effects. It inhibits prostaglandin synthesis in the brain but not at periphery. Half-life is two hours. It is very well tolerated by stomach and is inactivated in liver principally by conjugation as glucuronide and sulphate. Oral dose is 0.5 to 1 gm x 4 to 6 hour to a maximum of 4 gm in a day. A single dose of 10 gm may damage liver and kidney.

Parachromatopsia Partial color blindness.

Paracortex The part of an organ e.g. lymph node which lies between the cortex and the medulla.

Paracterine Chemical messengers that act locally in a general way in contrast to hormonal messengers that act via blood stream and to synaptic messengers that act as specialised interacellular junction.

Paradigm In biochemistry, an experimental model or example.

Paradigm shift A revolutionary alteration in the explanatory model that forms the basis of an entire discipline.

Paradox Evidence that appears to be inconsistent with or contradictory to the known facts of a particular phenomenon.

Paradoxia sexualis Sexual thoughts and behavior not consistent with the age of a person.

Paradoxical Other than that which normally occurs.

Paradoxical intention In logotherapy, a form of existential therapy, the patient is encouraged to assume the troublesome attitude or feeling. The confrontation, in a therapeutic setting, is presumed to assist the individual in gaining control over the aversive state.

Paradoxical pain It is a chronic pain which does not respond to opioid analgesic drugs in usual way.

Paradoxical sleep Sleep which occurs during the REM state, so-called because records of REM sleep are more similar to records of waking states than to records of other stages of sleep, but an individual in the REM state is difficult to awaken.

Paradoxical thinking Perverted or contrary cognitive precesses.

Paraesthesia It is a heightened sensitivity of sensation without evident cause. It produces advanced effect of heat and cold on the skin or pins and needles or tingling. Mostly it is caused by temporary pressure on the peripheral nerve. It may develop in neuritis.

Paraffin waxes These are obtained principally from high boiling point fraction of petroleum and are mixtures of saturated hydrocarbons containing from 26 to 30 carbon atoms. Ordinary commercial grades of paraffin melts in the range of 40 to 71°C. Melting temperature generally increases with increasing molecular weight. Paraffin waxes used in dentistry are refined waxes having oil less than 0.5 per cent.

During solidification there is volumetric contraction that varies from 11 to 15 per cent. Contraction is not uniform throughout the room temperature.

Parafollicular cell A cell type scattered in a network of loose connective tissue between the thyroid follicles of the thyroid gland which secretes calcitonin.

Paragasia An unintended action.

Parageusia A distorted sense of taste or a taste hallucination.

Paragonimiasis The larval stage of flukes may occasionally migrate to the brain rather than in lung and causes epilepsy, hemiparesis or hydrocephalus, Cysts are seen on CT. Treatment of choice is praziquantel.

Parahippocampal cortex Cortex located along the dorsal medial surface of temporal lobe.

Paralanguage Vocal sounds that are not actually words.

Paralexia A reading disorder characterized by the transposition of word order and the inclusion of additional words.

Paralinguistics The study of vocal qualifiers.

Paralipophobia Excessive fear of neglecting personal duty or obligations.

Paralle Extending in the same direction and at the same distance apart at every point so as never to meet, as in lines or planes.

Paralleling technique Intraoral radiographic technique in which the field is held parallel to the long axis of the tooth or teeth being radiographed while the x-ray beam is directed perpendicular at a right angle to the teeth and film.

Paralogous Describing genes that are related by descent from a common ancestor but that are divergent since an ancestral gene duplication. Their products generally serve similar functions in different organisms.

Paralysis It is the complete or partial loss of controlled movement caused by the inability to contract one or more muscles. Paralysis may be temporary or permanent. Paralysis of one-half of the body is called hemiplegia. Paralysis of all four limbs and trunk is called quadriplegia. Paraplegia is paralysis of both legs. Very common disorder causing paralysis is stroke in which damage to part of brain is caused by bleeding from or blood clotting in a vessel. Paralysis develops on the opposite side of brain damage. Hemiplegia can be caused by brain disorder in which part related to movement is damaged such as brain tumour, abscess encephalitis, etc. Paralysis can be caused by damage to the spinal cord from a fractured spine due to accidents. Disc prolapse may also result it. Muscular dystrophies cause progressive muscular weakness and may lead to paralysis. One has to treat the cause. For paralysed person confined to bed or a wheelchair nursing is useful.

Paralysis agitans Obsolete phrase for parkinsonism.

Paralytic squint Nonconcomitant strabismus is a condition in which there is dissociation of ocular movements. The deviation is irregular and varying in an incoordinate manner in different directions of gaze. In this condition the eyes do not remain in their normal relative position in all the movements of eyes. It is due to defect in the efferent pathway. The brain is able to command but the motor apparatus is unable to function due to lesion at the level of lower neuron. Most cases of paralytic squint are neurogenic. There is limitation of movement of eye in field of action of affected muscle during binocular movements. The change in postural attitude occurs to overcome the inconvenience caused by distressing diplopia. Vertigo may be felt by patient.

Paramedical workers These are pharmacists, nurses, lab assistants, physiotherapists and others who work in conjunction with doctors. In forces trained nursing staff and first aiders are in plenty.

Parameter A characteristic of a pupulation; estimated by sample statistics.

Parametric data Data for which descriptive parameters (typically the mean and standard deviation) are known and define the underlying frequency distribution of the data. The underlying distribution is often assumed to be normal, as provided in the central limit theorem.

Parametritis Pelvic cellulitis is usually related to an infected deep cervical tear due to lymphatic transmission of pathogenic organism. Infected injuries to the vagina and perineum may cause localised parametritis. Suppuration of parametritis may occur in 30% cases.

Parametrium The fibrous subserous coat of the supravaginal portion of the uterus, extending laterally between the layers of the broad ligaments.

Paramimia A form of apraxia characterized by inability to express feelings with appropriate gestures.

Paramolar A supernumerary molar, usually a small and rudimentary tooth, most commonly found in the maxilla, situated buccally or lingually to one of the molars or interproximally between the first or second and third molars.

Paranasal sinus Air-filled cavity within certain skull bones that connects to the nasal cavity; the four sets of paranasal sinuses are the frontal, maxillary, sphenoidal, and ethmoidal.

Paranoia Used to describe behavior characterized by delusions of persecution and/or delusions of grandeur.

Paranoia querulansi Obsolete phrase for litigious paranoia.

Paranoiac A person suffering from paranoia.

Paranoid litigiousness A delusional state that leads to continuous legal procedures against presumed enemies.

Paranoid type Pertaining to a type of mental illness in which the person has delusions, especially delusions of reference, such as imagining that people are doing things or saying things about him or her. A form of schizophrenia.

Paranomia A form of aphasia characterized by calling objects by incorrect names.

Paranormal experiences Those outside scientific explanation.

Paraparesis A partial paralysis affecting lower extremities.

Paraphimosis When the tight foreskin is retracted it may on occasion be difficult to return and a paraphimosis results. In this venous and lymphatic return from glans is obstructed and these structures swell alarmingly causing even more pressure within the obstructing ring of prepuce. Gentle manual compression may help, if it fails then circumcision helps.

Paraphrase Transform the client's words into the nurse's words, keeping the meaning intact.

Paraplegia Paralysis of the legs due to spinal cord injury.

Parapodium A standing frame designed to allow the patient the ability to sit when necessary. Ambulation is achieved by shifting weight and rocking the base across the floor. It is used for infants.

Parapraxia A condition characterized by loss of ability to perform purposive acts.

Parapraxis A faulty act, blunder, or lapse of memory such as a slip of the tongue or misplacement of an article. According to Freud, these acts are caused by unconscious motives.

Paraprosexia A fixed idea that does not change or advance.

Parapsis Perversion of the sense of touch.

Parapsoriasis It is a chronic condition of erythrodermic or scaly maculopapular dermatoses of unknown origin. Histopathological changes are non-specific. Changes show para-keratosis and acanthosis of epidermis. There develops erythematous, slightly elevated, sharply marginated and flat top papules or plaques. It develops mostly on trunk, thighs, arms and sides of neck. Face and scalp are never involved. Sometimes there may be generalised lymphadenopathy. Condition persists for years.

No effective treament is available. Ultraviolet radiation helps in acute phase.

Parapsychology The study of sensory and motor phenomena shown by some human beings (and some animals) that occur without the mediation of the known sensory and motor organs. The data of parapsychology are not accounted for by the tenets of conventional science.

Parasellar syndrome Unilateral frontal headache, ophthalmoparesis with no proptosis and normal visual acuity are seen. X-ray shows sella and petrous bone erosion. CT shows hyperdense enhancing parasellar and cavernous sinus mass.

Paraseptal emphysema The destruction of alveolar septa and the reduction in the number of alveoli involving the periphery of the pulmonary lobules.

Parasinodial Situated along the course of a sinus.

Parasite Any organism living in on any other living creature and deriving advantage from doing so. It causes disadvantage to host. The parasite derives nutritional requirement from host's blood or tissues or from host's diet which allows the parasite to reproduce and multiply. Some parasites cause certain symptoms or disease and may cause even death of host. Animal parasite includes parasites, flukes and lice. The scientific study is known as parasitology.

Parasitemia The presence of parasites in the blood.

Parasitic Pertaining to, of the nature of, or caused by a parasite.

Parasitism A symbiotic relationship in which only one of the organisms, the parasite, is physiologically depended upon the other, the host.

Parasitization Infection or infestation with parasites.

Parasitologist An expert in parasitology.

Parasitophobia Excessive fear of parasites.

Parasomnia A disorder of arousal, partial arousal or sleep stage transition. It may interfere with sleep and produce insomnia or day time sleepiness. Conditions associated with activities that cause arousal or partial arousal, usually during transitions in NREM periods of sleep.

Paraspasm A spasm of the corresponding muscles on both sides of the body.

Paraspastic Ataxic gait The characteristics of paraspastic gait are joined by clear ataxic elements such as stamping feet, sudden equilibrating movements of the trunk and slight retroversion of the knee. This is pathognomonic of multiple sclerosis.

Paraspastic gait Legs are usually extended. The feet drag audibly along the floor. Sometimes they move in scissors fashion with toes slightly inverted, i.e. pigeon toes.

Paraspecific Having curative properties in addition to the specific one.

Parasuicide An attempted but unsuccessful suicide, or suicidal gesture.

Parasympathetic nervous system It comprises autonomic nervous system distributed through out the body from the centres in cranial nerves of the brain. The system calms down the body after stress through anxiety or exertion. It slows down the rate of breathing and heart beat. It is also responsible for regulating the reduced level of neural activity during sleep.

Parasympatholytic A drug that inhibits cholinergic receptors of the autonomic nervous system.

Parasympathomimetic A chemical that produces effects similar to those of a parasympathetic nerve.

Parataxic distortion Sullivan's term for inaccuracies in judgement and perception, particularly in interpersonal relations, based on the observer's need to perceive subjects and relationships in accordance with a pattern set by earlier experience. Parataxic distortions develop as a defence against anxiety.

Parataxis In linguistics, joining phrases or sentences without conjunctions.

Paratenon The fatty areolar tissue between a tendon and its sheath. It carries vascular supply to the tendon.

Parathymia A distortion of mood, a schizophrenic disturbance characterized by reacting in a completely inappropriate manner, as in laughing when told that parents have died.

Parathyroid gland These are pair of glands, oval and pea sized adjacent to the two lobes of the thyroid gland in the neck. Gland produces parathyroid hormone which controls the level of calcium in blood. Even small variation can impair muscle and nerve function. If blood calcium level falls down the production of parathyroid hormone increases. If calcium level is too high the gland reduces their output. In rare cases, the gland may become overactive resulting in hyperpara-

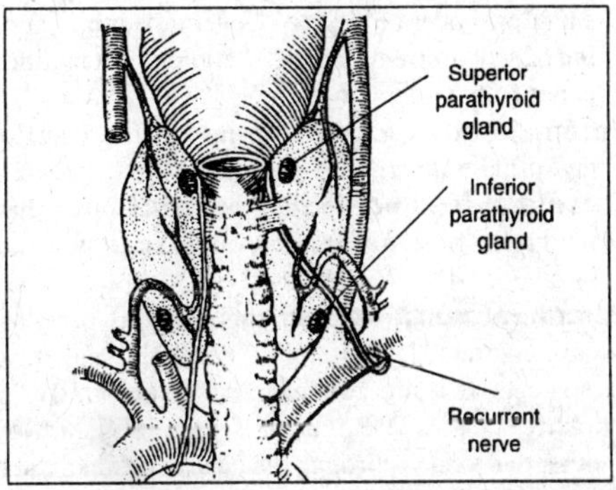

thyroidism resulting in osteoporosis and forming calculi in urinary tract. While in hypothyroidism it may cause spasm and seizures.

Parathyroid hormone Hormone released by the parathyroid gland that increases the concentration of calcium in the blood.

Paratomy A form of asexual reproduction in which complete individuals are produced prior to subdivision of the worm.

Paratrooper fracture A fracture of the distal tibial and fibular shaft.

Paratyphoid fever It is a form of typhoid fever caused by infection with *Salmonella paratyphi* A, B and C. It is caused by contaminated milk or drink.

Symptoms include rash, high fever, abdominal pain, etc. Chloramphenicol and ciprobid are drug of choice and for paratyphoid A B vaccine is also available for its prevention.

Paraventricular nucleus An important hypothalamic nucleus for the production of hypopsyiotropic factors.

Paravertebral Adjacent to vertebra.

Paravertebral ganglia There are 31 pairs of spinal nerves and only 22 to 23 ganglion in each sympathetic trunk. Because during development some of ganglion fuse to form a single ganglion. In neck there are 3 cervical ganglia. In thorax there are 10 to 12 ganglaon, in abdomen 4 and in pelvis 4 to 5.

Parenchyma The specific cells of a gland or organ contained in and supported by the connective tissue framework or stroma.

Parenchymatous goitre There is uniform, smooth and soft enlargement of thyroid gland, may be of small or moderate degree. General health is good but patient is often anaemic. Aetiology of condition is not fully understood.

Parental suit A legal action in which a court of law usually determines paternity.

Parenteral feeding Feeding by routes other than through the alimentary canal, such as intravenously.

Parenteral nutrition Nutrients, such as proteins, carbohydrate, fat, vitamins, minerals, and trace elements, that are administered intravenously.

Parenteral route Route of drug administration other than oral or through the gastrointestinal tract; administration by injection.

Parent-infant attachment A sense of belonging to or connection between a parent and infant.

Parerogis Psychotic manifestations such as delusions and hallucinations.

Paresis 'Weakness'. Incomplete paralysis.

Parietal Relating to the wall of any cavity; parietal serous membranes are in contact with the walls of cavities. The parietal bones forming part of the skull.

Parietal area It is situated between postcentral area in front and visual area behind and constitutes one of the large association areas of brain. Being surrounded by visual somaesthetic and auditory areas it is able to correlate items of information received from these sensory centres. It is responsible for the accurate knowledge of objects and their significance. It thus enables us to determine by the touch alone the size and shape of an object.

Parietal bone One of two bones that assist in forming the top and sides of skull.

Parietal layer The outer portion of the serous pericardium that is supported by the fibrous pericardium.

Parietal lesion, non-dominant An affected patient may feel that the limbs contralateral to a non-dominant parietal lesion are not his or her but belongs to some one else in the same bed.

Parietal lobe This lobe has numerous centres. The senses of heat, cold, touch, pain are located behind central sulcus. Sensory information of various parts of body is conducted to particular locations of these areas. Parietal cortex contributes to complex function. Disturbance of right side causes spatial agnosia, i.e. loss of orientation by individual in space and time. Agraphia is the loss of writing capability; and acalculia is the inability to make even simple arithmatic calculations. In apraxia, movements are not executed in right order. Loss of body image involves nonrecognition of side of the body contralateral to the damaged parietal lobe.

Parietal lobe lesion In it a single powerful visual stimulus such as finger movement may be readily perceived, but when it is accompanied by a similar synchronous stimulus in the opposite visual field, the stimulus in affected field is not attended but ignored. If there is a lesion of the left parietal lobe patient may be unable to recognise by touch alone, with his or her eyes closed, the nature of common object even a wristwatch or pen placed in his or her right hand, even though the sensory threshold tested with cotton wool is within normal limits.

Parietal pericardium Pericardium surrounding the heart like a loose-fitting sack to allow the heart enough room to beat.

Parietal peritoneum That portion of the serous membranes of the abdominal cavity lining the inner surface of the body wall.

Parietal pleura The serous membrane that covers the inner surface of the chest wall, the exposed part of the diaphragm and the mediastinum.
The pleural membrane that lines the thoracic cavity.

Parietal portion Serous membrane that lines the walls of a body cavity.

Parish nurse A nurse who works with a faith community and combines the activities of spiritual counselling with health promotion, disease prevention, and health maintenance for parishioners and families.

Parity The condition of a woman with respect to her having borne children.

Park's lines Growth lines in bones

Parkinson's disease It is a neurologic disease resulting in mask-like face, rigidity and slow movements. It is a brain disorder that causes muscle tremor, stiffness and weakness. Person develops a rigid posture. It is caused by degeneration of nerve cells within the basal ganglion. The disease starts as slight tremor of one hand, arm, or leg. In early stage tremor is worse when hand or limb is at rest. While in activity

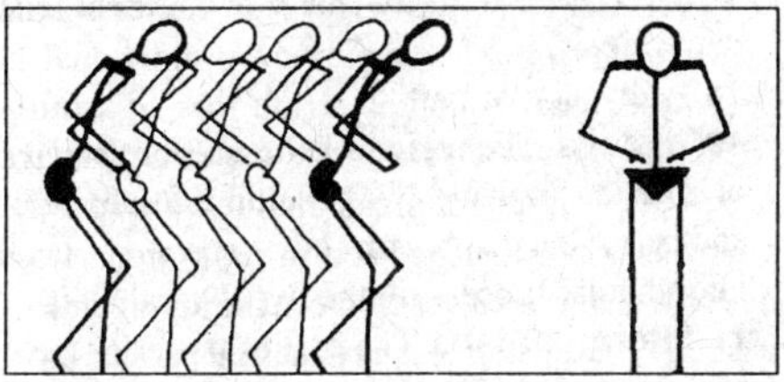

shaking virtually stops. Later both sides of body results in stiffness and weakness as well as trembling walk becomes imbalancing. Head shakes. Intellect is unaffected until late in disease. Speech may become slow and hesitant. Handwriting becomes small. Depression is common. There is no cure for Parkinson's disease. Levodopa sometimes help. The beneficial effects of this drug wear off very soon. Amantadine may also be added. Anticholinergic drugs may control tremors.

Parkinson's law "Work expands so as to fill the time available for its completion."

Parkinson's tremors This is a presenting feature in about 70 % cases. Tremor with a frequency of 4 to 5 C/S commonly begins in one hand with rhythmic movements of thumb across the index and middle fingers and *vice versa,* known as pill rolling tremors.

Later tremor spreads to foot on same side. Tremors persist when the limb is fully supported and disappears during voluntary movements. The tremor of Parkinson's may be brought out by asking patient to walk.

Parkinsonism A degenerative disease with primary involvement of the basal ganglia; characterized by tremors, rigidity, bradykinesia, and impairments of posture, balance, and gait. Onset is typically in the fifth or sixth decade of life.

Parmia A personality characteristic consisting of boldness, venturesomeness, and imperviousness to threats.

Parol evidence Oral evidence rather than written evidence. The parol evidence rule says that a written contract is presumed to be the final expression of agreement between the parties and other oral testimony cannot be used to vary the terms of the contract.

Parolfactory area A site of the cerebral cortex near the olfactory tract.

Paroneal Relating to fibular or lateral side of lower leg.

Paronia Disorder of judgement is the characteristic feature. The delusion is liable to lead the patient to assassination of some prominent person or even to attempt suicide. Megalomania is apt to develop as the disease progresses.

Paronychia It is an infection on distal phalanx that occurs along the edge of nail. The organism usually

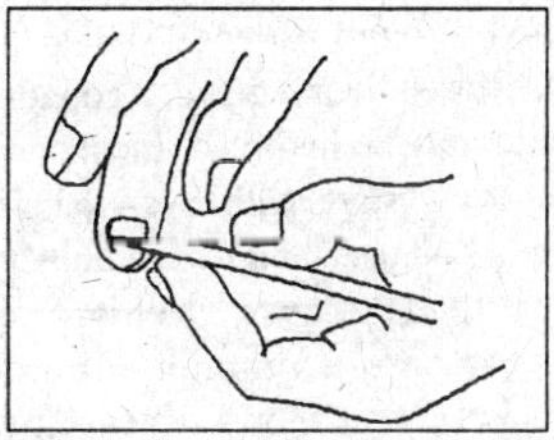

Staphylococcus is often introduced by biting the nail. Local signs of infection are invariably present such as redness, swelling and tenderness. Antibiotics if fails, surgical interference will be required.

Parotid fistula A salivary gland fistula may be internal or external. An internal fistula which opens inside the mouth does not give rise to symptoms, while external fistula is very rare and if develops gland is to be removed. It may be caused by rupture of parotid abscess. Sialogram with a watery solution of lipodol is done. Reconstruction of parotid duct is useful.

Parotid gland It is the largest of the three paired salivary glands situated in parotid mould. The gland is covered by inner true capsule and outer

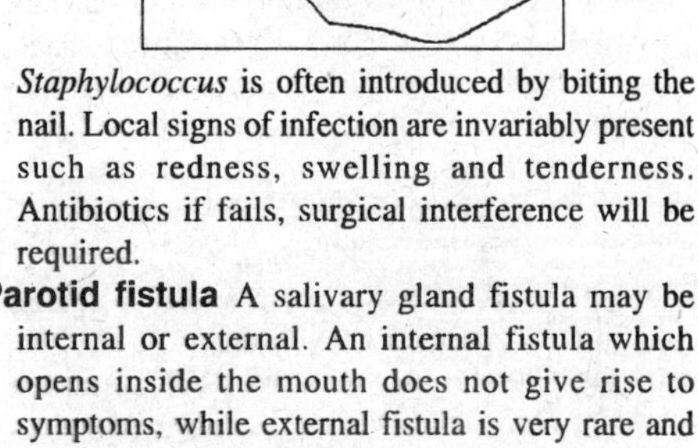

false capsule. True capsule is formed by condensation of fibrous stroma of the gland, while false capsule is known as parotid sheath and is formed by splitting of investing layer of deep cervical fascia. The superficial lamella of sheath is strong and is attached above to the zygomatic arch. The deep lamella is thin. It passes deep to the gland and is attached to the tympanic plate and styloid process. Parotid duct emerges from anterior border of gland and runs horizontally. Secretory nerve supply is via the auriculotemporal nerve carrying parasympathetic fibres from inferior salivary nucleus.

Parotitis Mumps is highly infectious and is transmitted through patient's saliva. It occurs in children. The salivary glands, gonads, pancreas and breasts may be involved. Incubation period is 2 to 3 weeks and starts with fever, malaise. Patients complain of bad taste and loss of appetite. Disease regresses in 10 days. Orchitis, otitis and pancreatitis are common complications. Microscopic section shows degenerative changes in epithelium of ducts, a few areas of acinar atrophy and presence of polymorphonuclear leucocytes. It does not require any treatment and healing is uneventful. It produces life long immunity.

Paroxymal attack A sudden onsent of symptoms.

Paroxysm Sudden attach or recurrence of symptoms of a disease, spasm or convulsions.

Paroxysmal atrial tachycardia (PAT) Recurrent episodes of rapid heart rate in excess of 100 beats per minute, with abrupt onset and cessation, originating from an ectopic focus in the atria.

Paroxysmal nocturnal dyspnoea Severe attacks of dyspnoea occurs at night which awaken the patient from sleep. Probably the absorption of oedema fluid from dependent position of body during recumbency produces pulmonary congestion. These patients have severe wheezing due to bronchospasm or may have actual pulmonary oedema with air hunger.

Paroxysmal tachycardia Here the ectopic pacemaker is located either in atrium, AV junction or in ventricle and rapidly discharges impulses varying from 150 to 250 per minute. According to location of pacemaker the condition is called paroxysmal atrial, AV junctional or ventricular tachycardia. In atrial and ventricular type the rate varies from 150 to 250 per minute, but in paroxysmal AV junctional tachycardia it is slightly less than 130 per minute. Symptoms include severe palpitation, fluttering sensation, syncope, precordial pain and breathlessness.

Parricide The killing of one's own parent, either patricide.

Pars A division or part.

Pars distalis The region of the adenohypophysis, or anterior pituitary, lying within the sella turcica and below the diaphragm sella, separated from the infundibular process by the hypohyseal cleft.

Pars interarticularis The part of posterior arch of a vertebra that lies between the superior and inferior articulars.

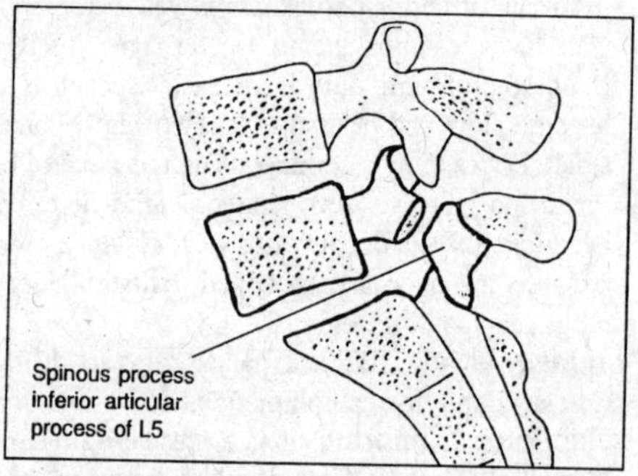

Pars intermedia The region of the adenohypohysis lying within the sella turcica, applied to the lower infundibular stem and the infundibular process and separated from the pars distalis by the infundibular cleft.

Pars planitis This is a chronic inflammation of the ciliary body. It occurs in young patients, is bilateral and produces fine precipitates. Synechiae do not develop. There is considerable infiltration at the inferior vitreous base leading to snow banking. Reduced acuity may be due to cystoid macular oedema.

Parsing The process used to assign words in a sentence to their syntactic categories.

Parthenogenesis Development of an unfertilized egg into a new individual.

Parthenophobia Excessive fear of girls or of virgins.

Partial agraphia Ability to write single letters but not words or phrases.

Partial airway obstruction Manual thrusts are indicated in the conscious patient with complete airway obstruction resulting in respiratory distress.

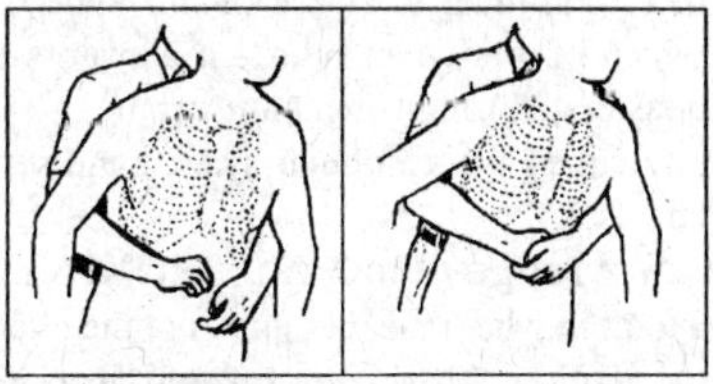

They increase intrathoracic pressure and blow the obstruction out of airway. Abdominal thrusts are given.

Partial anodontia Failure of teeth to form a part due to arrested tooth development.

Partial bath Washing only the areas of the body that are subject to the greatest soiling or that are sources of body odor.

Partial denture A dental prosthesis that restores one or more but not all of the natural teeth and/or associated parts and that is supported by the teeth and/or mucosa. It may be removable or fixed.

Partial expiratory flow volume A pulmonary function test that may be used to reveal low forced expiratory rates in children.

Partial pressure Pressure exerted by a single gas in a mixture of gases.

Partial rebreather mask Oxygen delivery device through which a patient inhales a mixture of atmospheric air, oxygen from its source, and oxygen contained in a reservoir bag.

Partial seizures A simple seizure of contraction of muscles in one part of body without loss of unconsciousness. Each muscular contraction is caused by discharge of neurons in the contralateral motor cortex. Muscular activity may remain localised or may spread to other parts. This is known as Jacksonian seizure.

Partial sight A seriously defective visual condition, often defined as acuity of less than 20/70.

Partial thickness burn Burn that damages only the epidermis (first-degree burn) or the epidermis and part of the dermis (second-degree burn).

Partial thromboplastin time The time is takes for a fibrin clot to form after calcium and a phospholipid have been added to a blood sample; a test of the intrinsic clotting system; activated partial prothrombin time.

Particulate matter Small solid particles disperesed in air. An example is the burnt matter that results from cigarette smoking or from fuel combustion, which often contains carcinogenic substances. Cigarette smoke contains 4000 chemicals.

Partilineage Familial descent considered through the male members.

Partis mollis Soft part anatomy, including skin, muscles, visceral organs.

Partition coefficient A constant that expresses the ratio in which a given solute will be partitioned or distributed between two given immiscible liquids at equilibrium.

Partner An alternative to the terms girlfriend, boyfriend, or spouse.

Part-object In psychoanalytic theory, refers to some anatomical part of a person which is viewed as a love object.

Parts of obstetric forceps It has two curved blades with fenestra, the shank, the lock and the handle.

Partunate period The hours following birth, when the neonate adapts to its existence as an independent being in a environment totally different from the uterine one.

Parturiphobia Excessive fear of the birthing process.

Parturition The act or process of giving birth, involving the expulsion of the products of conception, including the fetus and the placenta.

Party Any direct, named litigant in a legal proceeding.

Parulis A elevated nodule at the site of fistula draining a chronic periapical abscess.

Pascal's law It states that fluid pressure is exerted equally on all surfaces of an immersed body at a given depth.

Pass defect A lesion or fracture of pass interarticularis.

Passageway The birth canal through which the fetus travels.

Passionate love A state of intense longing for union with another.

Passivated The process by which an oxide film forms on a metallic structure to make it less active in terms of corrosion (i.e., enhances corrosion resistance); chromium -containing alloys are passivated by chromium oxide film formation.

Passive learning Incidental learning without making any active efforts.

Passive appraisal Ignoring a situation in hopes that it will go away.

Passive congestion liver It is a condition in which liver enlargement is due to the right sided heart failure. Liver is tender and sensation of weight and feeling of fullness is in hepatic region. Signs of general venous obstruction appear with ascites, oedema of legs, albuminuria, gastrointestinal symptoms and slight enlargement of spleen. Some degree of jaundice may be present.

Passive cutaneous anaphylaxis It is used for study of detection of antibodies. It is very sensitive test detecting as little as 0.1 mg antibody protein. Antibody is injected intradermally into normal animal and after a suitable period antigen mixed with dye is injected IV. Staining of skin occurs at the site of antigen-antibody reaction 4 to 24 hours afterwards. Dimension of it is a measure of intensity of reaction. It is used for IgG antibody.

Passive diffusion Physiologic process in which dissolved substances, such as electrolytes and gases, move from an area of higher concentration to one of lower concentration through a semipermeable membrane.

Passive Drop Bloodstain drop created or formed by the forced of gravity acting alone.

Passive exercise Therapeutic activity performed with assistance.

Passive forgetting A fading away of certain memories due to lack of interest or exercise.

Passive immunity Protection against an infectious disease provided by circulating antibodies made in another organism.

Passive insufficiency If you flex your knee while your hip is extended, you cannot complete the full range because the muscles dont have enough power. They have become actively insufficient.

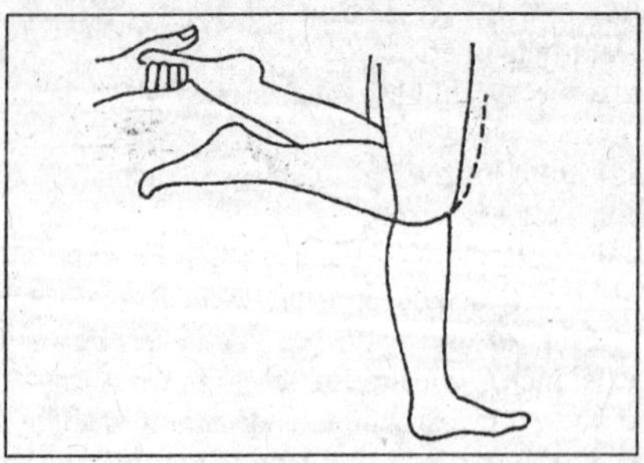

Passive joint movement Movement of a joint by the massage practitioner without the assistance of the client.

Passive motion In sensory psychology, the condition of travelling from place to place without any active movement on this part of the individual. The individual is aware of this type of motion, which occurs when riding in elevators and roller coasters, through mechanisms in the inner ear, particulary the vestibular system and semicircular canals.

Passive range of motion (PROM) Movement of a joint in which the therapist, not the client, effects the motion. Movement created at a joint by an external force.

Passive surveillance Reporting of disease by physicians, laboratories, and hospitals on a voluntary basis.

Passivism An attitude of submissiveness, especially in sexual relations, for example, male passivism.

Paste Vehicle that contains a drug in a viscous base.

Pasteurellosis Infection with microorganisms of the genus Pasteurella.

Pastoral stage That form of culture in which herds of sheep, cattle, etc., are maintained for livelihood.

Past-pointing Failure of pointing (a test for vestibular function).

Patau's syndrome It is chromosomal disorder like trisomy and is fatal in nature. Eye changes includes microophthalmia, cataract, coloboma, hare lip and cleft palate. There will be a single palmar transverse crease.

Patch A macule measuring over 1 cm of diameter.

Patchy dermatocele There is excessive overgrowth of endoneurium in the subcutaneous tissue. There is myxofibromatous degeneration of endometrium of the nerve and the affected nerve becomes enormously thickened. Clinically overlying skin may be thickened, oedematous, pigmented and adherent or it may be drawn out and folded. Sometimes the involved skin hangs down in pendulous fold. On palpation it resembles tortuous thrombosed veins due to the plexiform mass of thickened nerve fibres. It may undergo sarcomatous change.

Patella Small, shallow pan; the kneecap.

Patella alta A high riding or elevated position of patella.

Patellar reflex The reflexive tendency of the lower leg to extend when the knee joint is struck, usually by a rubber hammer.

Patellar tap A moderate effusion can be diagnosed by looking for patellar tap. The examiner's hands

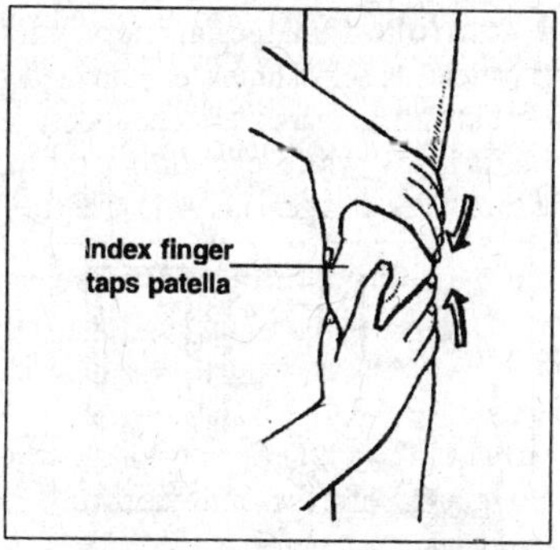

exert pressure downwards and towards the knee joint forcing any fluid behind the patella. The patella is then tapped with index finger.

Patellar tendon reflex The so called knee jerk.

Patellar tilt Refers to the angle of patella in the horizontal plane.

Patellar-tendon-bearing Refers to the modern total-contact below-knee socket that places moderate load on the patellar ligament.

Patency The condition of being wide open.

Patent ductus arteriosus Ductus arteriosus is normally present in the intrauterine life but closes soon after birth. When it does not close this condition arises. Here blood is shunted from aorta

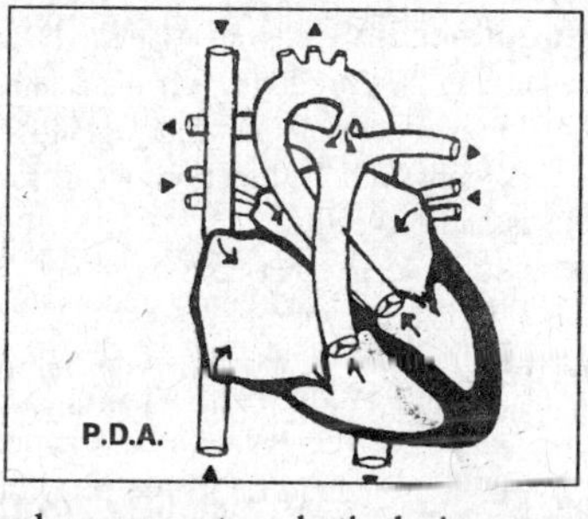

to pulmonary artery both during systole and diastole. Symptoms when present include dyspnoea, fatigue and cardiac failure. Left ventricular enlargement is seen. "Train in tunnel" murmur may be heard over left second intercostal space away from sternal border. Sometimes a middiastolic murmur or third heart sound may be heard over mitral area.

Paternity test It is to determine the controversial father of the child. In it genetic fingerprints from child and father are compared.

Pathic A person who assumes a passive role in any sexual act, especially when the act is considered a perversion.

Pathicism Male homosexual activity in which the passive partner simulates female behaviour and garb.

Pathocure The displacement of a neurosis by an organic disease. The opposite of pathoneurosis.

Pathogen A foreign agent that may result in clinical infection and disease if not eliminated by immune system.

Pathogen-derived resistance Resistance derived by expression of a gene or nucleic acid from the pathogen in a transgenic host, that interferes with the ability of the pathogen to complete its normal life cycle.

Pathogenesis The course of development of disease, including the sequence of processes or events from inception to the characteristic lesion or disease.

Pathogenic Anything that causes diseases or abnormality.

Pathogenic animals Large, multicellular organisms sometimes called *metazoa.* Most metazoa are worms that feed off human tissue or cause other disease processes.

Pathogenicity The ability of an organism to infect a host and cause disease.

Pathogenicity factor An agent of a virulent pathogen that in some ways mediates the extent of damage to the host.

Pathogenicity of an organism Calculated as the proportion of infected individuals who are clinically ill.

Pathogens Microorganisms that cause illness.

Pathognomonic A sign or symptom significantly unique to a disease as to distinguish the disease from other diseases.

Pathognomonic test A test whose results, if positive, are synonymous with having the disease.

Pathography The study of pathology.

Pathokinesis The dynamics, course, or development of an illness.

Pathologic barrier An adaptation of the physiologic barrier that allows the protective function to limit rather than support optimal functioning.

Pathologic grief Condition in which a person cannot accept someone's death.

Pathologic resorption Resorption of a tooth not associated with the normal shedding of deciduous teeth.

Pathological anatomy The study of structural changes caused by disease.

Pathological calcification Process of calcification in tissues.

Pathological vaginal discharge Infection with trichomonas vaginalis results in a thin yellowish discharge which has a few frothy bubbles. Monilial infection results in a white flacky discharge like thin cottage cheese. It creates intense itching. In secondary infection discharge may be yellowish.

Pathology It is the study of diseased organs while anatomy is the study of healthy organs and body. Pathology studies the effects of diseases and disorders on the body of humans. It helps in understanding the disease process and effects of treatment.

Pathomiosis Minimization by people of their diseases.

Pathopsychosis A psychotic condition that evolves from an organic disorder, such as general paresis or brain tumor.

Pathosis A pathological or morbid condition; a disease.

Pathotype A pathogen phenotype distinguished by differential reactions on hosts carrying different resistance genes.

Pathovar A subdivision of bacterial taxonomy within a named speices characterized by a pathogenic reaction of the bacteria in one or more hosts.

Pathways to goals Perceptions of alternative ways to achieve particular goals.

Patient A person who is ill or who is undergoing treatment. In dental practice, an individual who has established a professional and legally binding relationship with a dentist for the delivery of dental health care, after the dentist has accepted the person as the patient.

Patient controlled analgesia Technique where patient himself injects analgesic drugs according to severity of their pain.

Patient education Providing knowledge, i.e., dental information, to a patient to enhance dental health.

Patient-controlled analgesia Intervention that allows patients to self-administer pain medication.

Patient's screen In wards it is commonly used to provide privacy while examining the patient specially females. It is generally made of steel pipes

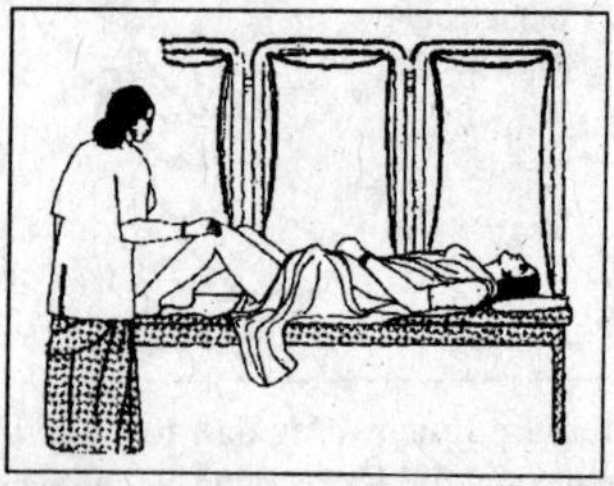

fitted with curtain cloth in three folds or more.

Patogen Any disease.

Patrick's sign A maneuver used in elvaluation of disorders of hip joint.

Pattern recognition The recognition of a specific pattern from a group of different patterns or displays.

Pattern waxes These waxes are to make inlays, crowns and pontics, bridges and partial denture attachments.

Pauwel's classification A classification of femoral neck fractures. Type I, II, III designate the angle of fracture.

Pavement epithelium Cells are flattened, larger and broader than they are high. It is distributed in alveoli of lungs, ducts of mammary glands and membranes of labyrinth. Its functions are diffusion and osmosis and protection.

Pavlik harness A device that hold an infants hips in flexion and external rotation.

Pavor diurnus A terror or fear reaction that may occur in a small child during his or her afternoon nap.

Pawl lock Knee lock consisting of a proximal segment having a pivoted bar that lodges in a notch on the distal segment.

PD Pocket depth distance from the gingival margin to the base a pocket.

PE Abbreviation for pulmonary embolism.

Peace keeping Acts undertaken by military personnel to maintain and ensure an established peace between two or more formerly warring parties.

Peak action Time it takes for a drug to reach its heghest dffective concentration.

Peak expiratory flow The maximum flow of gas at the beginning of a forced expiratory maneuver.

Peak level Highest effective concentration in the body of a drug.

Peak pressure In hallus after surgery peak pressure beneath the first metatarsal falls down. Procedures that destabilize the first metatarsophalangeal joint

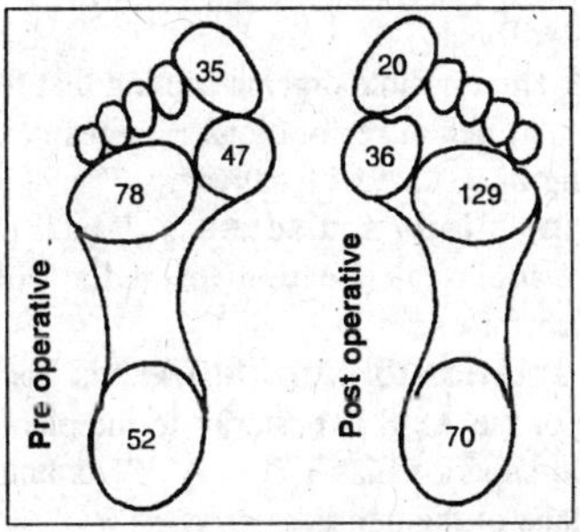

result in significant alteration of weight bearing pattern.

Pearson correlation coefficient A measure of strength of the linear relationship between two continuous variables.

Peaud'orange Dimpled skin condition that resembles an orange, associated with lymphatic oedema and often seen over the area of breast cancer.

Pectineal Pertaining pubic bone.

Pectoral Pertaining to the chest region.

Pectoral girdle Shoulder girdle; the scapula and clavicle.

Pectoralis major muscle An accessory inspiratory muscle arising from the medial third of the clavicle, from the lateral part of the anterior surface of the manubrium and body of the sternum, and from the costal cartilages of the first six ribs to insert into the lateral lip of the crest of the greater tubercle of the humerus.

Pectus carinatum A forward projection much like the keel of a boat of the sternum; pigeon breast.

Pectus excavatum A posterior displacement of the sternum; funnel chest.

Pedagogy Science of teaching children or those who have comparable congnitive ability.

Pedal Foot.

Pedal edema Swelling of the feet and ankles.

Pederasty Homosexual anal intercourse between men and boys with the latter as the passive partners. The term is used less precisely to denote male homosexual anal intercourse.

Pediatric dentistry Branch of dentistry that includes educating the child to accept dentistry; restoring and maintaining the primary mixed, and permanent dentitions; applying preventive measures for dental caries and periodontal disease; and preventing, intercepting, and correcting various problems of occlusion.

Pediatric intensive care unit (PICU) A unit that is speicifically designed for infants and children who require highly skilled medical care.

Pediatrician A physician who specializes in the care and treatment of children.

Pedicle Portion of a vertebra which extends from the body to the transverse process that connects and attaches the lamina to the body.

Pedicle erosion A thinning demineralization of pedicle seen on AP X-Ray of vertebra.

Pediculosis It is a parasitic infestation of skin produced by *Pediculus capites*, body louse or pubic lice. Head lices are transmitted through sharing combs. Pubic lice lives on pubic area, may be found in hairy areas of body. It gives itching which may be very intense. Prolonged infestation may lead to malaise and poor mental performance. Scratching may lead to excoriation over the affected areas. Gammabenzene hexachloride for 2 to 3 days is effective.

Pedigree Family tree; an ancestral line of descent.

Pedipalps Sensory and protective appendages associated with the mouthparts of chelicerates.

Pedodontics That branch of dentistry concerned with the aetiology, diagnosis, and treatment of oral diseases of children.

Pedophilia Adult sex with children.

Peduncle A stalk-like bundle of nerve fibers.

Peed group An assemblage of persons, all of whom are similar in terms of the purpose of the group.

Peer model In social learning theory, an individual who has mastered a given task, or nearly mastered it, yet has characteristics similar to the learner. For a child learning to do a certain arithmetic problem, another child of the same age and background, who has already mastered the task, may be more motivating and helpful than an expert mathematician, with whom the learner cannot readily identify.

Peer pressure It is a force that may contribute to teenage sexual experimentation or experimentation with drugs, smoke or alcohol. In male group it is important to demonstrate to one's peers that he is capable of attracting and/or seducing a girl.

Peer tutoring Students teaching other students.

Peer-group pressure Impact or influence of children's social groups on individual members, usually the power of the peer group of engender conformity.

Peizophilic Growing optimally at a pressure greater than atmospheric pressure and less that 50 MPa.

Pelagic Describing or referring to animals living in marine waters, especially those living within the ocean rather than on the surface or on the sea bottom.

Peliosis hepatitis It is characterised by presence of blood-filled lesions in liver. It may develop after use of anabolic steroids and oral contraceptives. Patients may remain asymptomatic or liver function test may be abnormal. Subcapsular lesions may develop.

Pelkan spur A radiographic sign of scurvy. It is a small bony spur protruding from lateral border of epiphyseal line at the junction with metaphysis.

Pellagra It develops in individuals eating maize due to deficiency of niacin. In addition imbalance of amino acids may play part in its causation. Prolonged treatment with isoniazid may also result

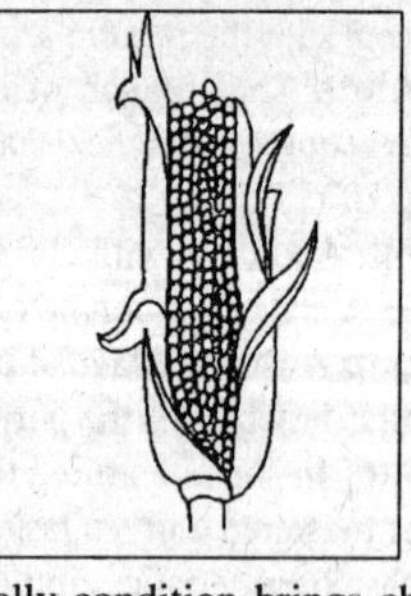

Maize

in it. Pathologically condition brings changes in mucous membrane and nervous system. In skin it produces marked keratosis in epidermis, increased vascularisation and chronic inflammation with oedema in dermis. Condition presents with dermatitis, dementia, and diarrhoea. There will be slightly swollen and sharply demarcated dull erythematous rash distributed symmetrically. Lesions may itch and give burning sensation. Affected skin appears depigmented. Later on lesions may become chronic atrophic with scales and skin may appear dry and shiny. Secondary infection may develop. Person feels weakness and fatigued. Nicotinamide 400 to 600 mg in divided doses will help.

Pellicle The invisible organic coating that forms on teeth and dental restorations as a result of their coming in contact with saliva .

Pelligrini stieda's disease X-Ray finding of heterotropic calcification in medial collateral ligament of knee.

Pelvic anterior torsion (tilt) Pelvis dorsal; the plane of the ASIS is posterior to the plane of the anterio-superior iliac spine (ASIS) is anterior to the plane of the public symphysis.

Pelvic belt A belt that encircles pelvis.

Pelvic cavity Space completely surrounded by the pelvic bones. Female pelvis is wider than male to accommodate fetus.

Pelvic colon It is continuous with descending colon. It begins from pelvic inlet.

Pelvic congestion syndrome All defined condition characterized by chronic pelvic pain not associated with menstruation generally associated with laparoscopy.

Pelvic contractures Disorders of pelvic muscles or fibrosis of supporting muscle tissue that cause an abnormal shortening of muscle tissue and make it difficult for the pelvic muscles to stretch.

Pelvic examination Physical inspection of the vagina and cervix, with palpation of the uterus and ovaries.

Pelvic exenteration Removal of the rectum, vagina, bladder, uterus, and cervix.

Pelvic Floor Muscle Strength Grading The test is performed with patient in hook lying position and relaxed. Gently insert the index and middle finger (with gloves on) into the vaginal canal. Instruct the patient to squeeze the pelvic floor muscles and hold the contraction as long and as hard as she can. To elicit maximal contrction of PEM instruct the patient like "Do not let me pull may fingers out". Or "Tighten your muscles as if you are trying to stop flow of urine". The muscle strength may be graded on the following scale:

0/5 No contraction.
1/5 Trace Contraction held less than 1S.
2/5 Weak Contraction held for 1-3S and/or fingers not elevated.
3/5 Moderate Contraction held for 4-6S and fingers elevated; repeat three times.
4/5 Strong Contraction held for 7-9S and fingers elevated; repeate three times.
5/5 Unmistkebly Rapid contraction with elevation for 7-9S; strong repeat four times.

Pelvic girdle The portion of the skeleton to which the lower extremities are attached.

Pelvic grip This is the best method of determining the presentation and attitude of head and engagement in case of cephalic presentation.

Pelvic Hematoma Hemorrhage in the retroperitoneal loose cellular tissue lying in the area between the pelvic brim and skin of the perineum is called pelvic hematoma. Infralevator hematoma is visible as vulval hematoma. Supralevator hematoma is rare and occurs in perivaginal tissue. It is marked by profound and sudden shock due to rapid retroperitoneal blood loss.

Pelvic inflammatory disease (PID) Collective term for any extensive bacterial infection of the pelvic organs, especially the uterus, uterine (fallopian) tubes, and ovaries.

Pelvic inlet It is bounded behind by sacral promontory, anterior border of ala of sacrum, iliopectineal lines of innominate bones and infront by crest of pubis and symphysis pubis.

Pelvic outlet The inferior opening of pelvis.

Pelvic posterior torsion (tilt) Angulation of the pelvis dorsal; the plane of the ASIS is posterior to the plane of the public symphysis.

Pelvic thrusts These are thrusting movements of both male and female partners during intercourse controlled by rhythmic contractions of the pelvic muscles and culminating into orgasm. The initial thrusts tend to be slow and shallow but as coitus progresses they become more rapid, deep and vigorous.

Pelvic traction A form of skin traction that provides traction through lumbar spine and reduces lumbar lordosis.

Pelvimeter It is used for measuring the external diameters of pelvis. It is done to rule out if any pelvic contraction is there. Different measurements are taken. Intraspinous is the distance between two anterior superior iliac spine. It measures 10 inches.

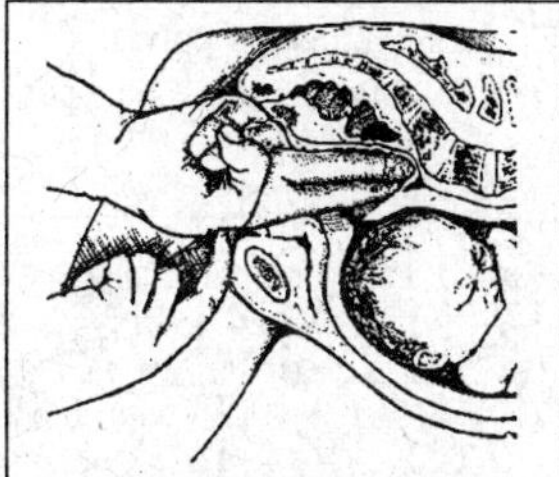

Diagonal conjugate measurement

External conjugate is the distance from depression below 5th lumbar vertebra to upper border of symphysis pubis which is normally 8 inches. Intertrochancteric diameter is the distance between outer surfaces of greater trochanter. It measures 12.5 inches. Distance between two outer most part of iliac crest is 11 inches.

Pelvis It is a funnel-shaped structure. It is one of the strongest joint comprising of 6 bones taking weight of spinal column. Women's pelvic cavity is broader because of child birth. It protects abdominal organs like bladder, uterus, etc. It contains two innominate bones which are joined

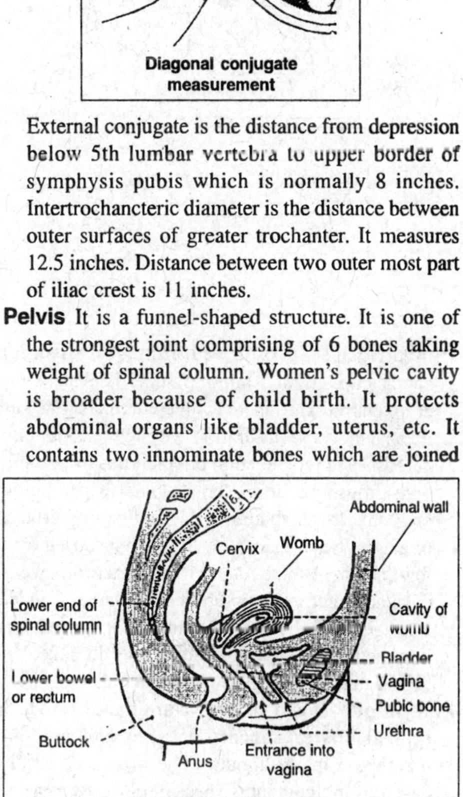

Female pelvic organs

by rigid sacroiliac joints to the sacrum. It is curved forward to join at pubic symphysis. Each innominate bone consists of three fused bones : ilium, ischium and pubis. Ischium bears most of the bodyweight. Pubis is the smallest bone. In women the pelvis is generally shallow and broad and pubic symphysis joint is less rigid than men. This helps in child birth. In men it is of larger built to bear a bodyweight. Fracture may be caused by road accident and considerable force is required to cause it. Osteitis pubis, i.e. inflammation is usually caused by repeated stress of pelvis.

Pelvis tilt Tilt of pelvis may be anterior, posterior or lateral.

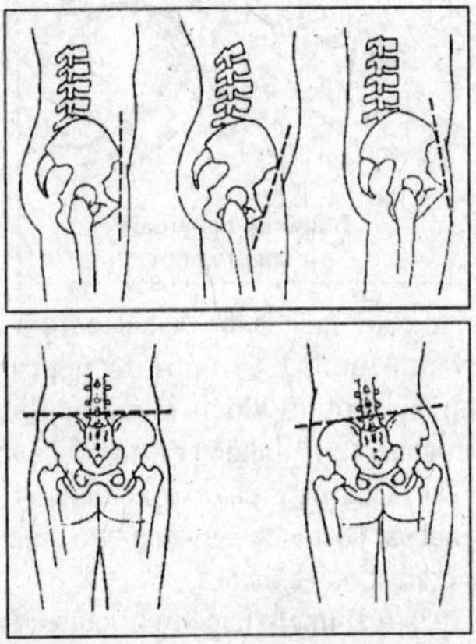

Pemphigoid It is an autoimmune disorder characterised by self-limiting, superficial blistering eruptions on skin. There is subepidermal bulla with no acantholysis, infiltration with few eosinophils, necrosis and regeneration of epidermis. It presents with diffusely scarred, large, dome-shaped bullae on groins, lower abdomen, thighs, flexural surfaces of extremities. Lesions may remain localised for a few months. Bullae may remian intact for several days and later may rupture leaving large denuded areas. Lesions heal spontaneously. Recurrence is very common. Topical steroids and dapsone 100 to 200 mg are helpful.

Pemphigus It is a serious skin disease in which typical blister appears on skin and mucous membrane in the mouth. The blister generally develops in the mouth. These often rupture easily, forming raw painful areas. Apparently unaffected skin may also blister on pressure. Skin biopsy gives the diagnosis. Usual treatment is with high doses of cortisone only over a long span of time. Antibiotics are helpful in secondary infection. In addition immunosuppressive drugs are given.

Pen grasp A grasp in which the instrument is held some what as a pen is held. Handle rests against a phalanx of index finger.

Penate Pertaining to a skeletal muscle fiber arrangement in which the fibers are attached to tendinous slips in a featherlike pattern.

Pendelluft Phenomenon believed to cause hypoxemia in flail chest.

Pendulum (Codman's) exercise Self-mobilization techniques that use the effects of gravity to distract the humerus from the glenoid fossa and gentle pendulum motions to move the joint surfaces.

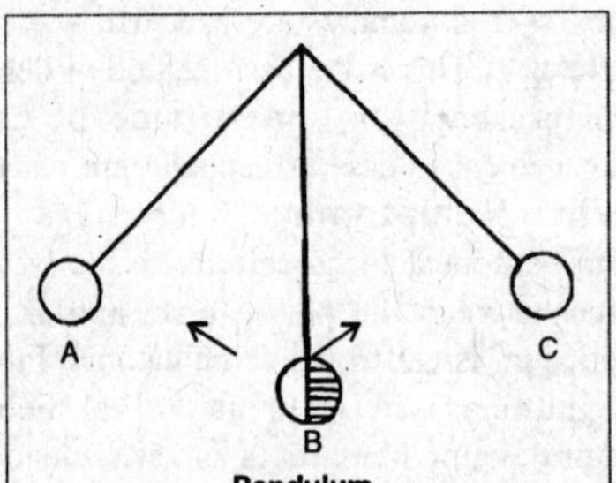

Pendulum

Pendulum test A test used to assess spasticity. A lim,b is extended and allowed to drop and swing like a pendulum; normal and hypotonic limbs swing freely, while spastic limbs are resistant to the motion.

Penetrability The ability of a beam of x-rays to penetrate matter, the degree of penetrability being determined by kilovaltage and filtration.

Penetrating wound Trauma that results in disruption of the continuity of the tissue at the surface of the body and extends into the underlying tissue or body cavity.

Penguin effect Similar to heat stroke syndrome caused by reduced ability to sweat in the center of tightly packed crowd.

Peniaphoia Morbid fear of poverty.

Penicillamine It reduces rheumatoid factor and also the concentration of immune complexes in plasma and synovial fluids. Half-life is three hours. It is incompletely but adequately absorbed following administration by mouth and undergoes metabolism by liver. Dose related impairment of taste is common. It may cause aplastic anaemia.

Allergic reaction tends to occur. If proteinuria is heavy drug may be discontinued.

Penicillin drug It is the first antibiotic group to be invented. Natural penicillin is derived from penicillium. All these chemical structures consist of thiazolidine ring and a side chain. These differ from each other mainly in side chain. Penicillins are bactericidal and act by interfering with bacterial cell wall synthesis. Penicillins are the drug of choice in pneumonia, lung and liver diseases. Most of the penicillins are ineffective against the microorganisms producing enzyme penicillinase. High doses are effective against rheumatic fever. Serious and occasionally fatal side effects are immediate hypersensitivity including anaphylactic shock and delayed reaction. Hence enquire about previous hypersensitivity reactions to penicillin and perform skin testing evaluation before giving penicillin injection. Penicillins are excreted in breast milk and may cause diarrhoea and allergic response in the nursing infant. Allergic reactions include wheezing, sneezing, urticaria, angioneurotic oedema, laryngospasm, vascular collapse and death.

Penile block Used to provide per and post operative analgesia for circumcision.

Penile cancer It is very rare and presence of phimosis increases the incidence. Smegma under the foreskin is considered carcinogenic. The most common site is glans penis. Most common histology is squamous cell carcinoma. It spreads through the lymphatic vessels. It manifests in early stages with painless induration, a nodule or indurated area.

Penile implant A rigid rod or inflatable device surgically implanted to permit men with erectile dysfunction to copulate.

Penile prosthesis Various devices, from a simple sheath to a self contained inflatable implant, to assist a male with erectile dysfunction to copulate.

Penis It is a male sex organ through which urine and semen passes. The penis consists of three cylindrical bodies of erectile tissue. Spongy tissue is full of blood vessels. Two of these cavernosa corpora lie on side and in the centre is corpora spongiosa. Through it urethra runs which carries urine and at times semen. Over the glans the skin forms a loose fold known as foreskin which in

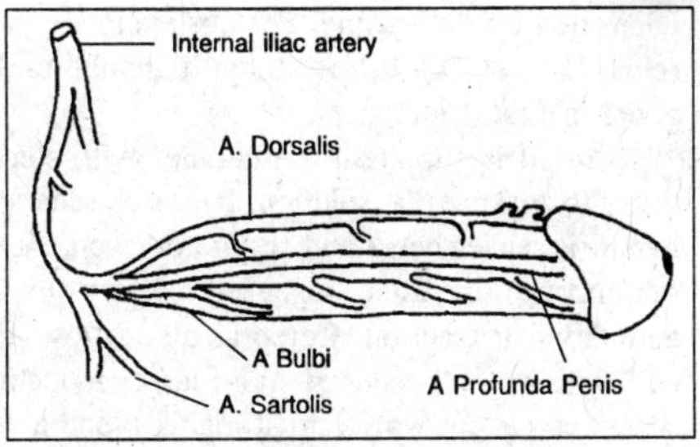

Muslims is removed just after birth. Inflammation of glans is known as balanitis. It may be affected by syphilis and gonorrhoea. In phimosis foreskin is too tight to move over glans.

Penis envy In psychoanalytic theory, envy by the female child of the male child's genitals.

Penis feminis The clitoris.

Penis pride A male feeling of superiority and power associated with the possession of a phallus.

Penis-vagnia fixation The reduction of all sexual activity to penile penetration of the vagina.

Pennate Pertaining to a skeletal muscle fiber arrangement in which the fibers are attached to tendinous slips in a featherlike pattern.

Penrose drain A thin walled cylinder of radiopaque latex used to drain purulent material.

Pentazocin toxicity Various features of toxicity includes seizure and coma, can occur within an hour of ingestion. Typical clinical triad of opiate toxicity, i.e. respiratory depression, CNS depression and miosis are not there. Mild to moderate CNS depression is seen in most of patients, coma is rare. Other CNS effects include unnecessary laughing dysphoria, anxiety, agitation and visual hallucinations.

Miosis is seen only in 20 to 25 % cases. Some patients have mydriasis. Hypertension is noted in 50 % cases.

Pentazocine It was first described by Archer in 1962. It is a narcotic analgesic derived from benzmorphinan. Analgesic potency of 30 mg is equal to equal doses of morphine and pethidine but does not result in vomiting. It raises blood pressure and does not influence pupil size.

It crosses placental barrier less easily than pethidine. It should not be given to narcotic addicts as it may produce withdrawal symptom. Hallucinations may follow its use but may be controlled by nalorphine. For postoperative pain relief 25 to 30 mg IM or orally. It should not be given in first trimester.

Pentothal It is supplied in ampoules with sterile water to make 2.5% solution. It causes sedation, hypnosis, anaesthesia and respiratory depression depending on dose injected. There is an anticonvulsant action. Cerebral blood flow and CSF pressure are reduced. With larger induction doses the patient wakes up at higher blood level. The greater the initial dose, the greater will be increments of drug required to maintain surgical anaesthesia. Acidosis reduces thiopentone concentration in plasma. About 70% of thiopentone in peripheral blood is bound to plasma proteins chiefly albumin and so is inactivated. The chief effect is repiratory depression depending on dose and rate of injection. Pupils first dilate then constrict. It is completely metabolised in body. Thiopentone anaesthesia except in shortest and most minor operation should always be accompanied by nitrous oxide and O_2. It produces smooth anaesthesia. Dose of thiopentone is O.1 to 1 gm. There is absence of delirium stage and relative freedom from vomiting and postoperative discomfort. Disadvantage is of laryngeal spasm and circulatory depression.

Peodeiktophilia Being sexually aroused by upsetting a stranger by exhibiting the penis.

Peplomer Surface projections of homo or hetero polymers of viral glycoprotein molecules on virus particles.

Pepsin Principal digestive enzyme produced by the stomach; digests proteins into smaller peptide chains.

Pepsinogen Component of gastric juice that is converted into pepsin by hydrochloric acid.

Peptic ulcer A peptic ulcer may develop in oesophagus, stomach or duodenum. It may be single or may develop in multiple. The lining of stomach and duodenum is constantly at risk of erosion due to gastric acid produced by stomach wall. Lower end of oesophagus is also at risk if acid reflux exists. Psychological stress and strain may play a part in causing ulcer. Many persons may not have symptom at all but many complain of a burning or growing pain which sometimes wakes them at 2 AM when stomach is empty. Pain of duodenal ulcer is often relieved by taking food but usually recurs a few hours later. There may be loss of appetite, belching, feeling of bloated nausea and vomiting. If not treated well bleeding may start. Chronic ulcer can cause extensive scarring of stomach. Barium meal examination and endoscopic examination help in reaching at diagnosis. Antacid drugs neutralise excess of acidity. Ranitidine/famotidine is ulcer healing drugs and is given for 6 to 8 weeks. Surgery when required is vagotomy. Substantial bleeding from an ulcer sometimes requires a blood transfusion.

Peptic ulcer and pregnancy Peptic ulcer rarely develop in pregnancy. Pregnancy has beneficial effect on course of peptic ulcer. Menstruation produces ill effects on ulcer symptoms but pregnancy exerts beneficial effect. Menopause brings about the severity of peptic ulcer. But acute abdomen due to perforation may be misunderstood as pain due to pregnancy.

Peptic ulcer, diet It should be frequently fed and should be soft, smooth and bland. It should be free from irritants. Raw, leafy, uncooked vegetables are to be avoided. Condiments, pickles, chutney, pepper and meat soups are to be avoided. Stimulating drinks like alcohol, tea, coca and coffee should not be consumed. Smoking is banned.

Peptic ulcer, perforation In first stage of peritonism there is irritation of peritoneum due to leakage of gastric juice in peritoneum. This stage lasts for 6 hours depending on the size of perforation.

There will be acute burning pain over epigastrium referred to tip of shoulder. In some cases pain gravitates down into right iliac fossa. There may be vomiting. Tenderness and muscle guard are constantly present. Second stage is stage of reaction, in reality a stage of delusion. As the irritant is diluted with peritoneal exudate the intensity declines.

Muscular rigidity will continue to be present and is obvious. X-ray will show air below diaphragm. Final stage is of definite peritonitis and there becomes little hope of recovery. Pulse rises in rate but falls in volume and tension. There will be persistent vomiting and board-like rigidity.

Peptide Any member of a class of compounds of low molecular weight that yield two or more amino acids on hydrolysis, and that from the constituent part of proteins.

Peptide bond A covalent chemical bond between adjacent amino acids in a polypeptide chain.

Peptide hydrolase Any of a group of enzymes that catalyze the hydrolysis of peptide bonds.

Peptide mapping The characteristic two-dimensional pattern formed by the separation of a mixture of peptides resulting from partial hydrolysis of a protein; also known as peptide finger printing.

Per rectal examination It is generally done to locate any growth. Anal canal is approximately 2.5 cm long and is bordered by external and

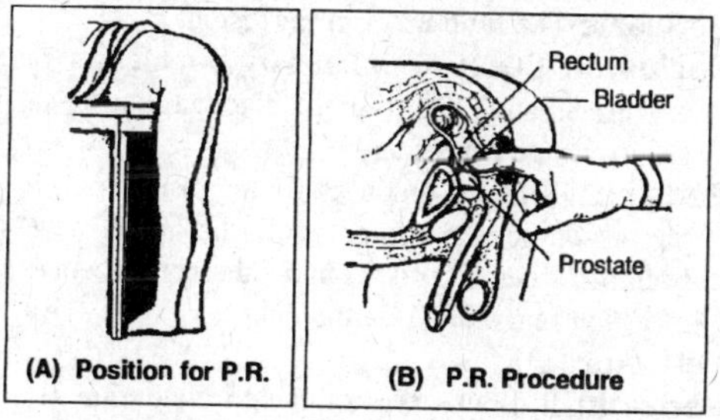

(A) Position for P.R. (B) P.R. Procedure

internal sphincters which are normally firm and smooth. It is done to know the anatomical situation of internal piles. Enlarged prostate can also be examined and felt per rectally.

Per vaginal examination It is a very common examination done by gynaecologist in married

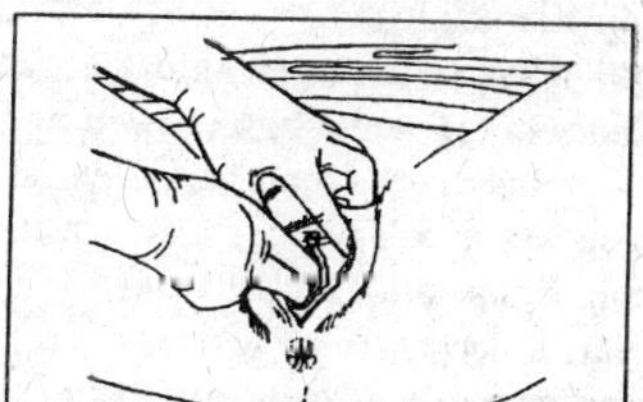

woman to know the cause of irregular bleeding, to know the fetal presentation, dilatation of cervix and many other gynaecological disorders.

Perceived intention The purpose which an audience attributes to the communicator's message. The issue concerns the motivation or aim behind the message.

Perceived stimulus The observer's experience, as a person looks at a particular visual configuration or listens to a series of sounds. The psychology of perception is concerned with the ways in which this experience corresponds to the distal stimulus, as opposed to the proximal stimulus.

Percent elongation The amount of permanent change in shape that an object may undergo before fracturing; a measure of ductility.

Percentile scale A simple scale based on 100% of the population of any group with which an individual is being compared.

Percept Mental image of an object in response to sensory stimuli.

Perception Being aware of something through the senses; seeing, hearing, feeling, tasting or smelling.

Perception deafness Inability to analyze or perceive sounds normally due to some impairment of the inner ear or auditory-nerve pathways leading to the brain.

Perceptual field All elements and aspects of the environment of which the individual is aware at any given point in time.

Perceptual masking Interference of one stimulus with another, preventing proper perception.

Perceptually handicapped Refers to a person who is learning-impaired because of deficits in the perception of sensory stimuli.

Percolation Process of filtration; seeping of a fluid through another substance.

Percussion (1) Striking or tapping a part of the body; (2) Type of chest physiotherapy performed by rhythmically striking the chest wall.

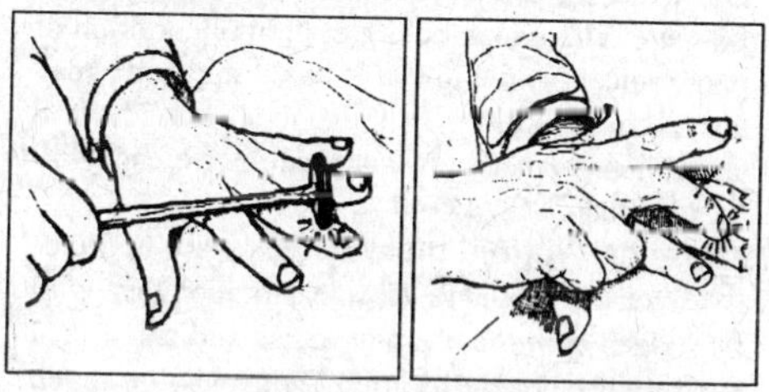

Percutaneous electrical nerve stimulation Pain management technique involving a combination of acupuncture needles and transcutaneous electrical nerve stimulation.

Percutaneous endoscopic gastrostomy (PEG) tube Transabdominal tube inserted into the stomach under endoscopic guidance.

Percutaneous endoscopic jejunostomy (PEJ) tube Tube that is passed through a PEG tube into the jejunum.

Percutaneous nephrolithotomy In it kidney is punctured under X-ray or ultrasound control with a needle. A tract is dilated into the kidney to gain access to the stone using graduated dilators up to a diameter of 1 cm and stone can be removed down

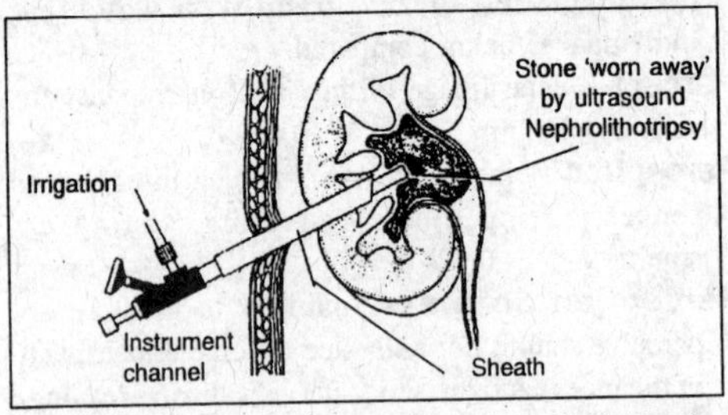

this tract. Stone removal is accomplished under direct vision within the kidney using special nephroscopes and a variety of grasping instruments. Stones up to 1 cm are taken out easily.

Percutaneous umbilical blood sampling (PUBS) A method of obtaining a sample of blood from the umbilical cord inside the placenta to study developments of various fetal biological parameters.

Perforating canal A minute duct through compact bone by which blood vessels and nerves penetrate to the central canal of an osteon; also called Volkamann's canal.

Perforation It is an irregular gap created suddenly due to weakness to part and increased internal pressure. There may be perforation of ear drum or peptic ulcer. Sometimes inflamed appendix may also perforate leaking its contents. It may result in shock hence emergency surgical interference will be required.

Perforation typhoid ulcer It takes place in 3rd or 4th week of typhoid fever. In perforation there will be sudden collapse, running pulse and subnormal temperature. In perforation there will be much local pain with dullness of right side of abdomen. Rigidity is a valuable sign of perforation of bowel.

Performance In social learning theory, an overt act. Performance is evidence of prior learning: it depends upon the availability or reinforcement. Learning, according to social learning theory, can occur solely through observation.

Performance components Sensorimotor, cognitive, psychosocial, or psychological elements.

Performance curve A graph representing the course of learning. Time or trials are plotted on the horizontal axis; the subject's performance is shown on the vertical axis. Also called a learning curve.

Performance test A type of test requiring noverbal or nonlanguage responses, typically using blocks and formboards.

Performance-based assessement Assessment of a particular skill based on observation of an actual attempt, as opposed to acceptance of a self-report of skill level.

Perfusate The fluid used for perfusion.

Perfusion Effect of pulmonary circulation in moving blood to and from the bloodgas barrier so gas exchange can occur.

Perhaps neurosis An obsessive neurosis in which the person is preoccupied with what might have been if the person had taken an alternative course of action regarding a past event.

Peri 'Around'.

Periactin It blocks serotonin and histamine H_1 receptors. It has the unusual effect of increasing appetite, probably via an action of serotonin in hypothalamus. It has been used in Cushing's syndrome and acromegaly.

Periapical Around the apex; in radiography, the type of film used to record images of the teeth and surrounding structures.

Periapical abscess A periapical abscess is associated with an acute onset, swelling, pain, reddening of overlying skin. There is elevation of tooth in socket which is extremely sensitive on percussion. Temperature rises. The involved tooth usually has a deep carious lesion, a fracture, a restoration or an inadequate root canal filling. Abscess may point intraorally or extraorally. Sometimes it may develop as gumboil. On X-ray there may be diffuse area of radiolucency not always restricted to single tooth. If there is already well-demarcated cyst, X-ray may show it as a sharp outline cyst. Periapical abscess is characterised by a necrotic pulp or a pulp densely filled by neutrophils. Periapical mass is solid. From the central area towards the periphery, there is gradual reduction in the intensity of polymorphonuclear infiltration. Bone trabeculae may show empty lacunae. Such is due to dead bone. Initial treatment of a periapical abscess consists of drainage. After acute symptoms subside root canal therapy is done. In some extraction tooth is to be extracted.

Periapical cyst A lesion characterised by an epitheliallined cavity or sac located around the apex of a nonvital tooth (also called a radicular cyst); appears radiolucent.

Periapical granuloma A lesion characterised by a localised mass of granulation tissue around the apex of a nonvital tooth; appears radiolucent.

Periapical radiograph Radiograph illustrating the tooth apices and surrounding structure in a specific intraoral area.

Periapical X-Ray Intraoral X-Ray showing 3-5 teeth.

Periarticular Situated around or about a joint.

Peribrachial area A nucleus in the brainstem that has a role in producing REM sleep.

Pericardectomy Excision of the pericardium.

Pericardial cavity Space between the visceral and parietal pericardium, filled with pericardial fluid; a cavity that surrounds the heart.

Pericardial effusion It is collection of fluid between pericardium. Symptoms include heaviness of precordium, dry cough, low-grade temperature, breathlessness and pain in right hypochondrium. Signs are detected when minimum amount of 500 cc of fluid accumulates in pericardial chamber. Normally it contains 5 to 20 cc of serous fluid. Patient may be dyspnoeic in propped-up position. Pulse is high of low volume.

Typical pulsus paradoxus may be present. Peripheral type of cyanosis may be present. Neck veins are engorged and non-pulsatile. During inspiration engorgement is aggravated. Oedema may be present. BP becomes low.

Pericardial fluid The serous fluid found within the pericardial cavity.

Pericardial friction rub A creaking sound caused by the rubbing together of the inflamed pericardial surfaces as the heart contracts and relaxes.

Pericardial membrane Serous membranes associated with the heart.

Pericardial sac The fibroserous membrane consisting of mesothelium and submesothelium connective tissue covering the heart and the beginning to the great vessels.

Pericardial tamponade A reduction of the venous return to the heart as the result of fluid in the pericardial space.

Pericardiocentesis The drainage of fluid from the pericardium by insertion of a hollow needle into the pericardial space.

Pericarditis It is the inflammation of pericardium. Pericardium is the membrane that encloses the heart. It may develop chest pain and fever. There may be effusion too in pericardial space. Fluid compresses the heart and restricts its movements. Long duration inflammation can result in constrictive pericarditis. Its cause may be bacterial, viral or tuberculous. Person will feel pain behind sternum sometimes radiating to shoulder. Constructive pericarditis may result in oedema. Anti- inflammatory drugs can relieve pain. Fluid may be drained out.

Pericardium It is a double layer membranous sac that surrounds the heart. Outer is fibrous one while inner one is softer. In between two layers there is fluid which reduces friction and acts as a cushion for heart.

Perichondritis Inflammation of the perichondrium.

Perichondrium A toughened connective sheet that covers some kinds of cartilage.

Pericoronitis Inflammation of the soft tissues surrounding the crown of an erupting tooth; frequently seen in association with erupting mandibular third molars and usually accompanied by infection.

Pericranial Pertaining to the pericranium.

Pericranitis Inflammation of the external periosteum of the skull.

Pericranium The external periosteum of the skull.

Peridinin A carotenoid pigment specific to most autotrophic dinoflagellates.

Peridontal file Miniature sized file used to remove small residual calculus.

Peridontal ligament The periosteum lining the alveoli (sockets) for the teeth in the alveolar processes of the mandible and maxillae.

Peridontal pocket Pathologically deepened gingival sulcus with peridontal disease.

Peridontal probe Instrument used for measurement of depth of gingival sulcus.

Peridontics Dentistry which deals with diagnosis and treatment of peridontium or gums.

Peridontitis Gingival disease involving bone.

Perietal lobe The cerebral cortex behind the central sulcus and beneath and parietal bone.

Perifascicular Surrounding or around a fasciculus of nerve or muscle fibers.

Periglandular Surrounding a gland or glands.

Perikaryon The cell body of a neuron.

Perikymata The numerous small transverse ridges on the surface of the enamel of permanent teeth, representing overlapping prism groups. With continued abrasion, the surface of the enamel becomes eroded and the perikymata become obliterated.

Perilaryngeal Situated around the larynx.

Perilymph A fluid of the inner ear that provides a liquid-conducting medium for the vibrations involved in hearing and the maintenance of equilibrium.

Perimeter stain A bloodstain that consists of only its outer periphery, the central area and having been removed by wiping or flaking after liquid blood has partially or completely dried.

Perimyositis Inflammation of connective tissue surrounding a muscle.

Perimysium The fibrous sheath enveloping each of the skeletal muscle fascicles.

Perinatal Pertaining to the period immediately preceding and following the birth of an infant.

Perinatal death Includes stillbirth and first week deaths.

Perinatal mortality It is defined as number of stillbirths and liveborn deaths within in the first week of life per 1000 total births, rises with rising parity. Toxemia of pregnancy and prematurity account for 60% perinatal deaths.

Perinatologist A physician who has specialised in the care of mother, fetus and infant during the perinatal period from 20th week of pregnancy to 4 weeks following child birth.

Perineal Area between the anus and genitals; the perineum.

Perineal care Techniques used for cleansing the perineum.

Perineal tears There are 3 degrees of perineal tear. First degree involves vaginal and perineal skin exposing perineal muscles. In second degree there is tearing of muscle of pelvic floor. Third degree tear involves the anal sphincter and lower part of rectum. Perineal tears should be repaired immediately after delivery to reduce blood loss and avoiding infection of the wound.

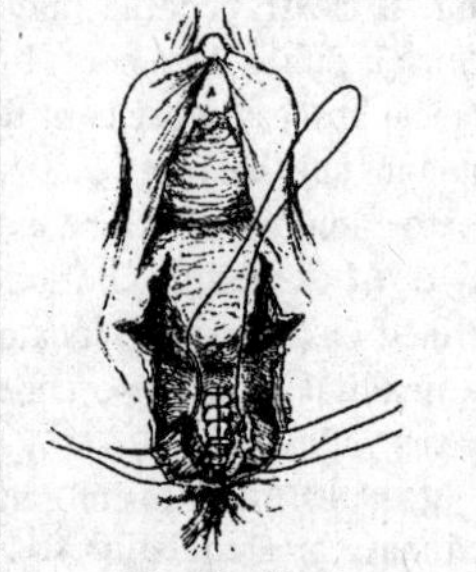

Repair of tears

Perineorrhaphy Suture of perineum, the operation for the repair of laceration of the perineum.

Perineum The pelvic flow; the space between the anus and the scrotum in the male and between and anus and the vulva in the female.

Period prevalence A measure that expresses the total number of cases of a disease known to have existed at some time during a specified period. It is the sum of point prevalence and incidence.

Periodic Recurring at regular intervals.

Periodic breathing Cessation of breathing lasting no more than 10 seconds without change in colour or heart rate.

Periodic paralysis These diseases are inherited as in autosome dominant trait showing episodic skeletal muscle weakness.

Periodicity Recurrence at regular intervals of time.

Periodontal Referring to structures surrounding the tooth, primarily in the alveolus.

Periodontal abscess A lesion that originates in a soft tissue pocket and is characterised by the accumulation of pus and destruction of bone; appears radiolucent.

Periodontal care For the patient with periodontal disease; consists of effective treatment for the elimination of disease and the creation of conditions conducive to the maintenance of periodontal health.

Periodontal disease Condition that results in destruction of the tooth-supporting structures and jawbone.

Periodontal dressing Periodontal pack; bandage for oral soft tissue.

Periodontal knife Interdental knife; surgical instrument with two beveled blades for incising marginal and interdental gingiva.

Periodontal ligament space A space that exists between the root of a tooth and the lamina dura; contains connective tissue fibres; blood vessels and lymphatics; appears radiolucent.

Periodontal probe Hand instrument with millimeter calibrations used for measuring pocket depth, attachment width, and size of soft tissue lesions.

Periodontalgia Pain arising in the periodontal ligament, usually as a result of infective or traumatic inflammation.

Periodontia 1. Plural of periodontium. 2. Periodontics.

Periodontics Art and science of examination, diagnosis, and treatment of disease affecting the periodontium; a study of the supporting structures, of the teeth, including not only the normal anatomy and physiology of these structures, but also the deviations from normal.

Periodontist Dentist with additional specialized education and training in diagnosis and treatment of the supporting structures of the teeth.

Periodontitis Inflammation of the tissues that support the teeth; result in the destruction of the periodontium.

Periodontium Tissues that invest and support the teeth, i.e., the gingivae, cementum of the tooth, periodontal ligament, and alveolar and supporting bone.

Periodontology The clinical science that deals with the periodontium in health and disease; that branch of dentistry concerned with the aetiology, diagnosis, and treatment of diseases of the surrounding and supporting structures of the teeth.

Perioperative care Care that patients receive before, during, and after surgery.

Periosteal elevator A surgical instrument used to strip soft tisue of bone.

Periosteal reaction Liner deposit of new bone by periosteum under elevted periosteum.

Periosteum It is the tissue that coats all the bones in the body. Periosteum contains small blood vessels that supply nutrients to bones and nerves. New bone formation is by periosteum. Inflammation of periosteum is known as periostitis. It results in swelling, pain and tenderness over the affected part.

Periostitis Inflammation of the bone in which the periosteum is predominantly involved.

Periovulatory Occurring around the time of ovulation.

Peripheral Situated away from a center or central structure.

Peripheral arterial disease An occlusive process involving the peripheral arteries.

Peripheral circulation Blood flow through all blood vessels that carry blood away from the heart (arteries), the capillaries, and all vessels that carry blood back to the heart (veins); consists of the pulmonary circulation and the systemic circulation; includes all blood flow except that through the heart tissue itself.

Peripheral field charting The patient is seated with his or her chin, resting over the chin rest, adjusted, to make him or her comfortable and the

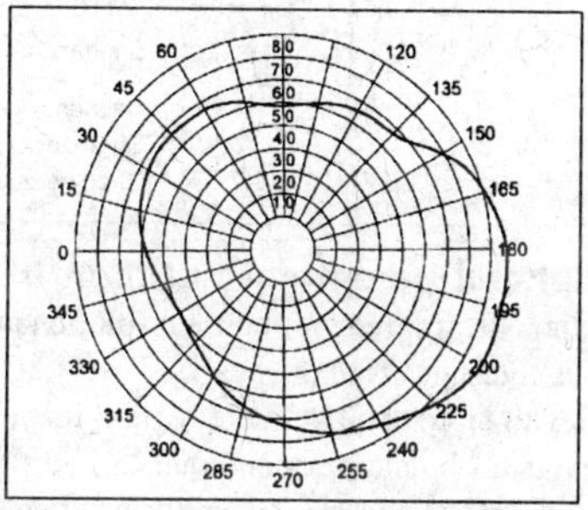

eye under examination in line with the fixation spot, situated at the centre of the arc, around which the arc revolves, the other eye occluded. A white test object 5 mm in size is brought in from the side at 15° intervals and the patient gives a signal by tapping the table, when he or she sees the test object. The readings are recorded by perforation with a sharp point, incorporated in all perimeters, on a chart at the back of the perimeter. Both eyes are tested.

Peripheral nerve One of a set of nerves that control sensory and motor functions of the body below the head; connects to the spinal cord.

Peripheral nervous system The spinal and cranial nerves, including the autonomic system. The nervous system which connects the brain and spinal cord with the receptors and effectors.

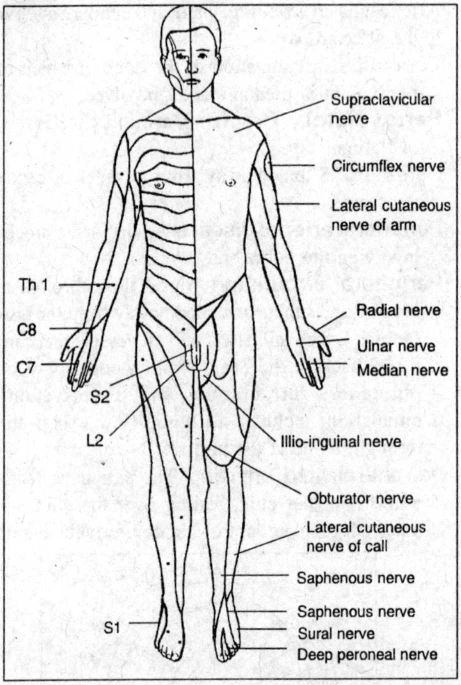

Peripheral parenteral nutrition Isotonic or hypotonic intravenous nutrient solution instilled in a vein distant from the heart.

Peripheral proteins Proteins that are loosely or reversibly bound to a membrane by hydrogen bonds or electrostatic forces; generally water-soluble once released from the membrane.

Peripheral receptors Physiological classification according to the form of energy to which they respond. *Mechanoreceptors*—respond to mechanical force, i.e. touch, pressure, stretch, position, sense; *Thermoreceptors*—which responds to heat and cold; *Photoreceptors*—respond to light; *Chemoreceptors*—respond to taste and smell.

Peripheral respiratory failure Respiratory rate more than 60 minute, intercostal or subcostal recession and expiratory grunt.

Peripheral vascular disease Restriction of blood flow takes place due to narrowing of blood vessels. In very severe case gangrene may develop and amputation may be needed. It may be caused by atherosclerosis. In it fatty plaques form on the inner walls of arteries. Hypertension and partially controlled diabetes may contribute in its formation. In atherosclerosis first symptom is usually tired feelings in leg muscles when walking and specially in calf muscles. Pain is relieved at rest. This procedure is known as intermittent claudication. Later on stage is reached when one feels pain even at rest and legs become numb and cold. Doppler study is the best tool to locate the disease, stopping of smoke, exercise and angioplasty may help. If gangrene has developed, amputation may become necessary.

Peripheral vestibular disorders It is characterised by attacks of paroxysmal vertigo associated with deafness and tinnitus. Attack occurs at any time without warning. A single episode of vertigo may be followed by a long period of freedom but often cluster of attack occurs over a period of weeks or months. Vertigo of each attack is violent and prostrating and is usually associated with nausea or vomiting. The sensation most often is of rotation but side to side swaying is also experienced. During attack person cannot stand and falls down. Deafness is fluctuating. Sensorineural loss is associated with distortion and intolerance for loud noise. After and between attacks, the hearing loss which is at first for a low tone, improves even to a normal level. Fluctuation of hearing level is very common. Music may be unbearably discordant. Tinnitus is low pitched.

Peripheral vision Visual experiences due to stimulation of the outlying portions of the retina.

Periphery Limit, boundary, or circumferential margin of a denture base.

Periphlebitis retinae It affects an apparently healthy young male adult. There is involvement of walls of blood vessels due to inflammation. Veins are affected more than arteries. Peripheral vessels are more involved. Retinal veins appear full and tortuous with sheathing. There is exudation under and around the vessel. Later on vessels becomes thin and attenuated appearing like thin cord with new vessel formation. New vessels may cause haemorrhages.

Periplasm The space between the cytoplasmic and outer membranes in gram-negative bacteria and between the cytoplasmic membrane and cell wall in gram-positive bacteria.

Periradicular Around or surrounding the root of a tooth.

Perirenal shaving Shaving the pubic hair in labour is commonly done to reduce wound infection and to improve wound approximation.

Perisinusitis Inflammation of the tissues around a sinus.

Peristalsis The wormlike movement by which the alimentary canal or other tubular organs with both longitudinal and circular muscle fibers propel their contents, consisting a wave of contraction passing along the tube.

Peristomal Referring to the area of skin surrounding a surgically created stoma.

Peristomal skin Skin around a stoma.

Peritoneal Relating to or involving the peritoneum.

Peritoneal dialysis This is the procedure for removal of end products of protein breakdown and other toxic material from blood of an anuric patient whose kidney is unable to excrete these substances through patient's own peritoneum as a dialysing membrane. The dialysing fluid is introduced into the peritoneal cavity and then removed by siphon method. It is indicated in acute and chronic renal failure, acute circulatory failure, poisoning and snake bite.

Peritoneal lavage Techniquè for diagnosing intra abdominal bleeding following blunt trauma.

Peritoneal membrane Serous membrane associated with the peritoneal cavity.

Peritoneal space Small, fluid filled space between the visceral and parietal layers that allows the layers to slide over each other freely in the abdominopelvic cavity.

Peritoneum It is a membrane which lines the interior abdominal wall and encloses and protects and supports the organs of abdomen leaving in between peritoneal cavity. Peritoneal glands secrete fluid lubricating the abdominal organs.

Peritonitis An acute or chronic inflammation of the visceral and parietal peritoneum occurs in a variety of conditions. Bacterial infection results from blood stream infection or by local spread from a neighbouring inflammatory focus such as appendicitis. In liver disease spontaneous bacterial infection of ascites occurs probably because of diminished ability of liver to remove *Escherichia coli*. Chemical peritonitis may result due to surgical power or gloves left inside. Chronic peritoneal infection may occur in patients on long-term chronic peritoneal dialysis. Symptoms may be of sudden onset following perforation of a duodenal ulcer or more gradual when there is peritonitis due to spread from local inflammatory focus. Pain is severe and constant. Vomiting is effortless and faeculent. Physical signs include fever, abdominal rigidity and absent or diminished bowel sounds.

Peritonsillar abscess It is rapidly increasing, typically unilateral throat pain, which become quite severe and radiates to ear. High fever, anorexia, eating difficulties, muffled speech and fetid breath develop. Head is tilted towards the affected side. Cervical glands become swollen. Respiratory impairment may develop.

Peritonsillar abscess drainage forceps It is a bayonet-shaped forceps used to drain peritonsillar

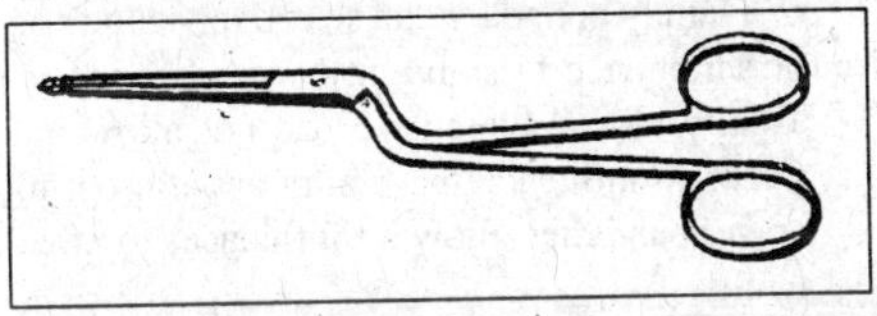

abscess. Incision is given at the junction of horizontal line passing through base of uvula and vertical tine along the anterior pillar.

Peritrichous Describing flagella that are uniformly distributed over the bacterial body.

Peritubular capillary The capillary network located in the cortex of kidney; associated with the distal and proximal convoluted tubules.

Peritubular tissue A layer of connective tissue and modified smooth muscle cells surrounding the seminiferous tubules.

Perjury The willful act of giving false testimony under oath.

Perkin's traction It is a type of skeletal traction used in the treatment of femoral shaft fractures that requires use of split bed.

Perky effect A tendency to falsely believe that an actual experience is due to imagination.

Perleche Single or multiple fissures and cracks at the corners of the mouth that may be caused by primary or superimposed infection with microorganisms, such as Candida albicans, staphylococci, and streptococci; poor hygience;

drooling; overclosure of the jaws in edentulous patients and in patients with ill-fitting dentures; riboflavin deficiency.

Permafrost Soil, subsoil, or other ground deposit that remains in a continually frozen condition, defined as a temperature below O°C for more than two years.

Permalcular vision A type of vision that uses the retinal area surrounding the macula.

Permanent dentition Thirty-two teeth of adulthood that either replace or are added to the complement of deciduous teeth.

Permanent set The amount of change in dimension that an impression material undergoes when it is removed from an undercut; a measure of accuracy.

Permastore The storage of material studies many years ago, such as foreign languages, that were never subsequently used.

Permeability of family boundaries The status of a family boundary that selectively allows access or admittance to some influences but not others. Totally closed boundaries do not allow outside forces to influence the family system, but totally open boundaries allow all influences to affect the family.

Permeable membrane A membrane that allows passage of substances.

Pernio It is also known as chilblains results from vascular disturbance when arterial spasms develop resulting in ischaemia. It causes damage to the capillaries and thrombosis. Exposure to cold weather gives rise to erythematous patches on fingers and toes but can also involve ear and face. There develops local oedema and blistering. There may be feeling of burring. Lesions are painful with itching. Affected part appears cold, clammy and cyanotic but colour disappears on pressure. Quick warming of affected part worsens the condition. Condition has no satisfactory treatment. The affected part may be massaged with rubefacient, peripheral vasodilator may play an important role in giving relief.

Peroneal muscles Plantar flexors and evertors of the foot; the peroneus longus forms a support arch for the foot.

Peroxisome Organelle similar in structure to a lysosome that contains enzymes that use molecular oxygen to oxidize various organic compounds. Such reactions produce hydrogen peroxide. Abundant in liver cells.

Perseveration Continued repetition of a meaningless word or movement.

Persistence A term for a mode of virus interaction with a population of cells in which a few cells are always in a lytic mode of infection, while the majority of cells care uninfected but potentially susceptible of lytic virus infection.

Persistent vegetative state Long-lasting state of decreased consciousness characterized by eye opening and return to sleep-wake cycles, but without any purposeful or meaningful behavior.

Personal accomplishments Feelings of competence and successful achievement in work.

Personal audit An oral or written interview or questionnaire designed to encourage respondents to asses their own personal strengths and liabilities.

Personal distance In interpersonal space, the second zone, ranging from 1 to 4 feet. Distances of this sort are common among people at small social gatherings, such as office parties and testimonial dinners.

Personal idiom Distinguishing behavior characteristics or mannerisms of an individual.

Personal protective equipment Garments that block the transfer of pathogens from one person, place, or object to oneself or others.

Personal space Distance of 6 inches to 4 feet.

Personal distance zone The physical distance comfortable for interactions with friends and acquaintances.

Personality The most characteristic integration of an individual's modes of behaviour, interest, attitudes, capacities, abilities, and aptitudes—the whole person as others know him or her. The characteristic way in which a person thinks, feels, and behaves; the ingrained pattern of behaviour that each person evolves, both consciously and unconsciously, as the style of life or way of being in adapting to the environment.

Personality breakdown Disintegration of the sense of self, leading to an inability to function normally.

Personality disorder The disturbance resulting from maladaptive personality traits causing functional impairment or substantial distress.

Personality formation The organization or structure of the components of an individuals character of personality.

Personality sphere The complete range of definable personality traits.

Personality trait A relatively stable and consistent behaviour pattern which is considered to be a characteristc component of an individual's personality.

Person-to-person contact Pathogens can often be carried in the air from one person to another.

Perspiration It is simple sweating. It is the part of controlling body temperature under the direction of autonomic nervous system, sweat glands deep in skin secrete salty water, lactic acid, urea and potassium. It cools the body. Cold sweats develop during tension and fear. In hyperthyroidism there should be an excess of sweating.

Perthes' test It is done to know whether the deep veins are patent or not. It should be done if patient complains of bursting pain in the lower leg on standing. A tourniquet is tied tightly around the upper part of the thigh while the patient stands, tightly enough to prevent any reflex down the vein. The patient is then asked to walk quickly for 5 to

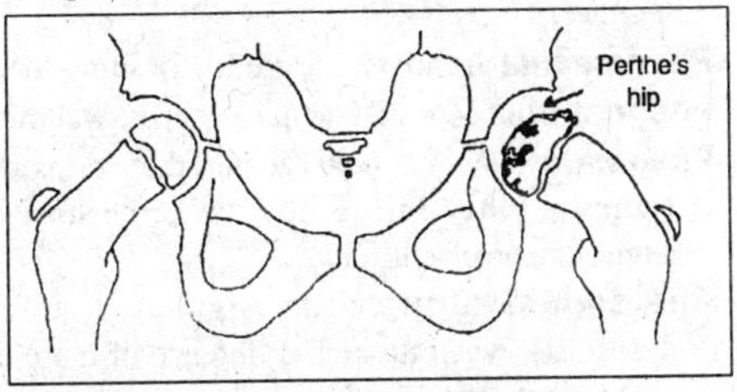

10 minutes. If the varicose veins shrink or disappear it indicates competence of the perforating veins and deep veins. If the varicose veins remain unchanged or become more distended, indicate that the perforating veins and deep veins are blocked.

Pertussis It is a type of infectious disease characterised by catarrh of entire respiratory tract producing paroxysmal cough and a typical stridor or 'whoop'. *Bordetella pertussis* is gram-negative anaerobic bacillus. It spreads by droplets. Incubation period is 6 to 18 days. Onset is insidious. In catarrhal stage it is like common cold. Signs of oral catarrh are present. Red eyes, fever and cough out of proportion is there. Leucocytosis is not present. In paroxysmal stage there are paroxysms of cough without any apparent inspiration ending in crowing inspiratory sound. Expulsion of large quantities of thick mucoid sputum and vomiting cough is more pronounced by night. Vomiting may occur at the end of bouts.

Perversion It is a deviation from normal. It is mostly used as an abnormal way of enjoying sexual activity. It includes bestiality, exhibitionism, fetishism and sadism. Psychotherapy helps the person.

PET Positron emission tomography.

PET Positron emission tomography.

Petals Strips of adhesive used to eliminate rough cast edges.

Petechiae Pinpoint, round, purplish-red spots that are not raised; caused by intradermal or submucous hemorrhage; a significant sign for various diseases.

Peter principle A satirical comment that in an organization, people often rise to their level of incompetence.

Pethidine Half-life is five hours. It has lower therapeutic efficacy. It does not suppress cough usefully. It does not cause constipation. It has little hypnotic effect and has a shorter duration of analgesia, i.e. 2 to 3 hours. It is extensively metabolised in liver and is excreted in urine. It results in vomiting. It has atropine like effects, including dry mouth and blurred vision. Its psychic effects are less constant and less marked than morphine. It is usually given orally 50 to 100 mg or IM 25 to 100 mg, its effects last 2 to 3 hours.

Petit mal Recurrent disorder of cerebral function resulting in some form of seizure. Petit mal seizure symptoms may range from no noticeable change in behavior to loss of consciousness and other functions.

Petit, triangle Lumbar triangle.

Petri plate A small, shallow dish of thin glass with a loosely fitting, overlapping cover, used for plate cultures in microbiology.

Petrissage Petrissage or pressure manipulations, cover several different massage strokes that are

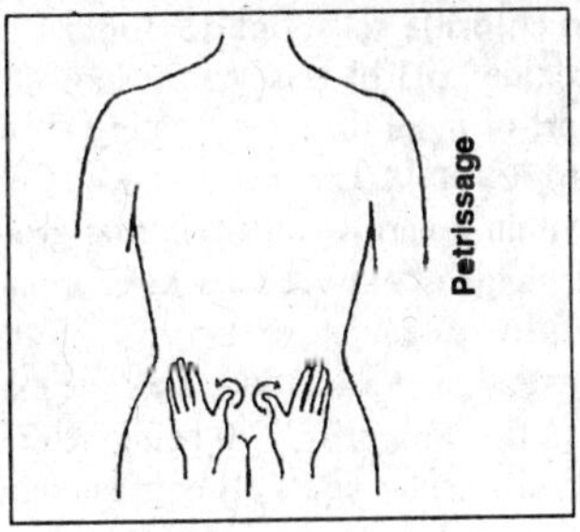

characterized by firm pressure applied to the tissues.

Petrositis It resembles air cells mastoiditis but differs in symptomatology because of its different anatomical relationship. It may be acute or chronic associated with acute and chronic otitis media. In masked petrositis the discharge will have ceased or diminished. The temperature will be normal or only slightly raised and he or she will be ambulant having headache and anorexia.

Peutz-Jeghers syndrome An autosomal dominant inheritance with generalised multiple intestinal polyposis, and melanin pigmentation in or about the body orifices, in the lips and fingers. Facial pigmentation fades after puberty.

Peyer's patches These are specialised sites for the reception of antigen and the priming of lymphocyte both T and B. Peyer's patches are present throughout small intestine. Peyer's patch consists of an aggression of lymphocytes covered by specialised thin membranous M cells which are flatter. Typhoid bacilli lodge in it.

Peyronie's disease It is the disease result of a focal fibrous proliferation of the tunica albuginea and the corpora cavernosa found mainly on the dorsum and at the root of the penis. Aetiology is unknown. Symptoms include pain during erection, penile deviation and difficulty during intercourse. If the blood circulation within corpora cavernosa is distended impotence may result.

PFM (porcelain-fused-to-metal) An esthetic dental restoration made by baking porcelain on to a metallic substrate used for support.

PFT Abbreviation for pulmonary function test.

pH The symbol of hydrogen ion (H^-)concentration, expressed in numbers corresponding to the acidity or alkalinity of an aqueous solution. The range extends from 14 ("pure" base) to O ("pure" acid), pH 7 being neutral; or from about 1 for 0.1 N hydrochloride to about 13 for 0.1 N Sodium hydroxide., pH of less than 7 indicating acidity and pH of more than 7 indicating alkalinity.

pH homeostasis The maintenance of intracellular pH within a narrow range, during growth over a wider range of extracellular pH.

pH scale A measure of the hydrogen ion concentration of a solution; the scale extends from 0 to 14.0 with a pH of 7.0 being neutral, a pH of less than 7 acidic, and a pH of greater than 7 basic.

Phage Short for bacteriophage a bacterial virus.

pHago A combining form denoting relationship to ingesting or engulfing.

Phagocyte This is a cell which has a capability surrounding, engulfing and digesting microorganism may be bacteria and virus. Phagocytes form part of body's immune system and are found in blood, spleen and lymph nodes. Granulocytes and monocytes are one of the phagocytes which go through the tissues and engulf organisms.

Phagocytic Relating to or having the property of phagocytosis; able to engulf and destroy foregin particles.

Phagocytosis It is the single most important component in the defence of body against invading organisms. Phagocytosis comprises ingestion and intracellular destruction of invading microorganisms.

Phagolysosome A host cell vacuole that forms after fusion of a phagosome with lysosomal vesicles.

Phagomania Insatiable desire to consume food.

Phagophobia Morbid fear of eating, or swallowing.

Phagosome A host cell vacuole that forms upon bacterial entry into a host cell; the host cell environment of ehrlichiae.

Phalangeal sign X-Ray sign of peripheral dysostosis, when there is difference of more than 2 m.m. between length of fourth metacarpal and combined length of ring fingers distal and proximal phalanges.

Phalanges The bones that make up the fingers and toes.

Phalangioma A term used to describe the appearance of a distal phalange of a patient's finger viewed on a radiograph as a result of improper placement technique; appears radiopaque.

Phalanx Any bone of a finger or toe.

Phallic mother In psychoanalytic theory, the fantasy among male children that the mother has a penis.

Phallic pride In psychoanalytic theory, the sense of superiority and even omnipotence experienced by boys when they discover that they have a penis and girls do not.

Phallic sadism Aggression associated with the child's phallic stage of psychosexual development.

Children interpret sexual intercourse as a violent, aggressive activity on the part of the male.

Phallic stage The period when the child becomes interested in his or her sexual organs. This stage, according to Freudian theory, is preceded by the oral and anal stages.

Phallus girl The fantasy of some transvestites of being a girl with a hidden penis.

Phantasmagoria The imagined process of raising or recalling the spirits of the dead.

Phantom A stimulus perceived that does not exist in reality.

Phantom limb It is a limb or part of it which even after being amputed feels that there is neural stimulation in the remaining portion of nerves. Such sensations usually fade after a few months.

Phantom pain Pain originating from the desensitized or amputated body part.

Phantosomia It is an olfactory halucination. Olfactory impression having an objective character but perceived in the absence of olfactory stimulus. Causes include schizophrenia, organic brain disorders and epilepsy.

Pharmacodynamics It concerns with drug action, what a drug does to body. The relationship between dose and response is frequently hyperbolic and lends itself to mathematical analysis.

Drug action may be due to chemical properties, e.g. chelating agents and antacids, enzyme inhibition, e.g. aspirin, neostigmine, penicillin and monoamine oxidase (MAD) inhibitors. In receptor action receptors are specific for certain drugs.

Pharmacokinetics The rate and efficiency of uptake, distribution, and disposition of a drug in the body.

Pharmacological effect A term for a condition in which a certain hormone responsible for stimulating the behavior under normal circumstances.

Pharmacologist One who makes a study of the action of drugs.

Pharmacology It is the science concerned with discovery and development of drugs. It deals with structure of drugs and ways in which they act and their doses and side effects. The practice of preparing drugs and books which lists drugs used in medicine is known as pharmacopoeia.

Pharmacometrics The comparative evaluation of drug activity, distinguished from bioassay in that substances with different chemical constitutions are compared.

Pharmacopeial Pertaining to or recognized by a pharmacopeia.

Pharmacopoeia It is an approved book of drugs, their compositions, doses, side effects and their constituents. It is very useful for pharmacists who work in hospital or in clinics.

Pharyngeal isthmus The space between the free edge of the soft palate and the posterior wall of the pharynx; the juncture of the nasopharynx and oropharynx.

Pharyngeal reflex test It is tasted by applying a stimulus with an applicator to the posterior pharyngeal wall or adjacent structures. Stimulus should be applied bilaterally. If positive, elevation and constriction of pharyngeal muscles will occur along with retraction of tongue.

Pharyngitis It is the acute inflammation of pharynx. It is mostly caused by viruses, bacteria mostly streptococci. Smoking and consumption of alcohol may result it. There may be discomfort when swallowing with fever, earache and tenderness. Lymph glands of neck may be swollen. Breathing may be difficult. Saline gargles are helpful. Pharyngitis clears up automatically still antibiotics and anti-allergics may help in certain cases.

Pharyngoplegia Paralysis of the pharynx.

Pharyngorrhagia Hemorrhage from the pharynx.

Pharyngoscope An instrument for examination of the pharynx.

Pharynx The part of the digestive and respiratory tubes superior to the larynx and oesophagus and inferior and posterior to the oral and nasal cavities.

Phase Part of a procedure or series of procedures that extend over time.

Phase difference A difference in phase sequence of two sounds waves, resulting in beats or alternating intensities.

Phase microscope A microscope that alters the phase relationship of light passing through and around object. Object can be seen without staining.

Phase variation Reversible switching on and off of the expression of a bacterial gene, resulting in different modifications of the cell surface; e.g., the phenomenon in several strains of E.coli in which the bacteria alternate between the fimbriated and nonfimbrated conditions.

Phases of Gait (RLA-Rancho Los Amigos, classification)

Phasic motor neurons a Motor neurons innervating squads of fast, glycolytic muscle fibers.

Phelebolith A calculus or concretion in a vein.

Phenazines Compounds based on the trycyclid phenzaine ring system; secreted by certain species of bacteria.

Phenobarbitone It was introduced in 1912 for having anticonvulsant activity. It is used to treat insomnia on occasion and for premedication too. With continued use it may result in behavioural abnormalities, lack of intelligence, impairment of surgery and loss of memory. It has slow absorption and excreted unchanged by kidney. In grand mal epilepsy 60 mg thrice daily is the accepted dose. It is not effective in petit mal epilepsy.

Phenol It is a corrosive aromatic hydrocarbon which is widely used as disinfectant. Pure carbolic acid consists of long, colourless, prismatic, needle like crystals. It has a typical odour. Minimal lethal dose is 1 gm or 20 ml of household phenol solution. Ingestion results in odour of carbolic acid in patient's mouth. There is intense burning sensation in mouth and throat. it is followed by abdominal pain and vomiting. Mucous membrane of lips and mouth becomes hard and white. Pupils become small, the temperature drops to subnormal. Respiration becomes slow and laboured. Cardiovascular depression results in pulmonary oedema and cyanosis. Cardiac arrhythmia is common in severe poisoning. Skin exposure may produce burning sensation followed by tingling and numbness. A white eschar is produced which falls of leaving a brown stain.

Phenomenal self The "self" as experience by an individual at a given time.

Phenomenologists Psychologists and philosophers who approach the study of human nature by seeking to understand consciousness.

Phenomenology The study of occurrences or happenings in their own right, rather than from the point of view of inferred causes; specifically, the theory that behaviour is determined, not by external reality s it can be described objectively in physical terms, but rather by the way in which the subject perceives that reality at any moment.

Phenomenon retention cyst This mucocele is a mucus containing cyst that occurs in salivary gland. Cyst is seen as a small circumscribed, elevated translucent bluish lesion of mucosa. If deep seated it can be palpated. Except in anterior half of hard palate the lesion can occur anywhere. Lip and tongue are the preferred sites. Superficial lesions frequently rupture, discharge a sticky mucoid material and collapse. As soon as they heal, they recur. Under microscope one can locate lesions consisting of cystic cavity filled with mucus. Round, swollen, degenerating cells are dispersed throughout the material. Treatment consist of removal of cyst as well as of associated gland.

Phenotype The sum of observable characteristics of an organism, based on its cellular or colonial morphology, biochemical structure, growth characteristics, and/or serological specificity, and resulting from the interaction of its genetic constitution with its environment.

Phenotypic Relating to the phenotype by one organism.

Phenylalanine-hydroxylase pathway An intrahepatic intermediary amino acid metabolic pathway.

Phenytoin Orally it is well absorbed. 90 per cent of it is bound to plasma albumin. It is hydrolysed in liver. At low doses half-life is 6-24 hours. Drugs that inhibit phenytoin metabolism include valproate, cotrimoxazole, isoniazid and chloramphenicol. Longer use results in impairment of learning situations, sedation to delirium, acute cerebellar disorders and convulsions. It may result in peripheral neuropathy and coarsening of facial features and hirsutism. Capsules for oral use should be taken with half a glass of water.

Phenytoin intoxication Phenytoin is used for the prevention of grand mal and psychomotor seizures and IV in the management of status epilepticus. Ingestion of 30 mg/kg is toxic but 100 to 150 mg/kg are not even toxic. The characteristic feature of phenytoin intoxication is the triad of nystagmus, ataxia and drowsiness. Symptoms start within one to two hours and are of brief duration. Psychological changes may be the first sign of toxicity. These include mood and behaviour changes. Nystagmus is very common. With the increasing toxicity of 30 mg/L ataxia occurs alongwith lacking of leg coordination and hyperflexion. Diplopia and slurred speech may be present At levels of more than 40 mg/L mental changes such as lethargy, confusion and disorientation develop. Decreased/cardiac toxicity with oral poisoning includes slow heart rate, reduced AV conduction resulting in AV block, ventricular fibrillation and direct myocardial depression.

Pheromonal Involving or describing a pheromone; i.e., a chemical used to transmit information between animals.

Pheromone A specific chemical produced by one organism to alter gene expression, or affect behavior, in a second organism of the same species.

Phialide A cell that develops one or more open ends from which conidia, phialospores are formed.

Philadelphia cervical brace It is of plastic, and comfortable to wear. It is good for stabilising the lower cervical vertebra. It has occipital, submental and upper thoracic contact points. It is uncomfortable during warm weather.

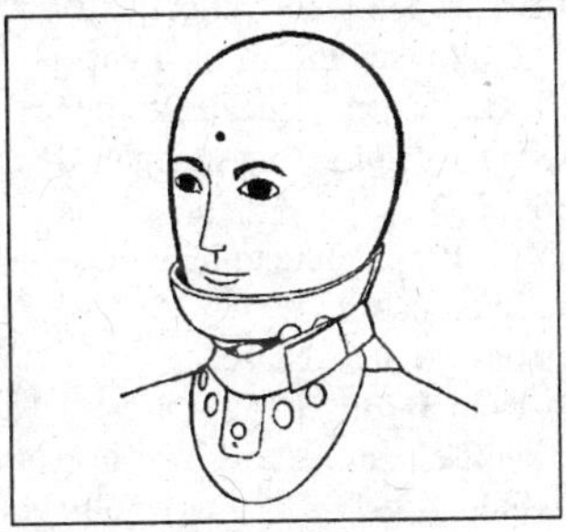

Philopatry Recurring use of the same reproductive sites during an individual's lifetime.

Philtrum Groove which connects the upper lip to the nose.

Phimosis A condition in which the opening of the foreskin is so small that it cannot be pulled back at all.

Phlebitis Inflammation of a vein or veins,

Phlebogram A radiograph obtained during phlebography.

Phlebotomy Incision of a vein; venesection.

Phlyctenular conjunctivitis It is an allergic condition caused by endogenous bacterial protein. Child is brought to the hospital for a nodule in eye. Discharge from eyes is usually watery. It increases with the involvement of cornea. Photophobia is prominent when cornea is involved. There are one or more nodules in eye located away from the limbus. Each nodule has congestion around it. There may be patches of eczema around lids, face, lips and near nostrils. Preauricular glands are enlarged.

Phlyctenular keratitis It is an allergic reaction to endogenous allergen, tuberculoprofien. First conjunctiva is affected then it involves corneal epithelium. Symptoms are minimal until the corneal epithelium is cast off. There may be one or more phlycten around the limbus. Some may be astriding the limbus other may be on cornea. Corneal phlycten is a grey nodule slightly raised from surface and looks yellow ulcer. Usually congestion is localised around phlycten. In some cases there may be associated conjunctivitis.

Phobic character Extremely inhibited, fearful persons. When faced with internal conflicts, such individuals resort to the defense mechanisms employed in phobic reactions.

Phobic reaction Neurosis characterized by persistent irrational fears of such an intense and dominating character that they interfere with everyday life.

Phobophobia Morbid fear of acquiring a phobia, or of being afraid.

Phon A unit of the subjective loudnes of sound.

Phonantograph A device that changes sounds into graphical waves.

Phonation First of the two basic mechnanical functions of the speech production. Phonation is the production of an acoustic signal.

Phoneme A minimal unit of sound that can signal a difference in meaning.

Phonemic paraphrsia In Wernicke's apshasia, the use of incorrect but similar sounding words.

Phonemics The study of sounds in any language.

Phonetic Related to speech sound.

Phoniatrics The study of speech habits, the science of speech.

Phonocardiography It is the technique employing contact microphones placed over chest for amplification and recording of heart sounds.

Phonogram A graphic or symbolic representation of speech sounds.

Phonological loop A memory store that can briefly retain speech-based information.

Phonology The study of the sound system of a language.

Phonophobia Exaggerated fear of sounds.

Phonopsia A condition in which certain sounds timuli elicit the subjective sensation of color.

Phonotaxis Locomotion oriented to a sound source.

Phootometer A light meter. An instrument designed to measure the intensity of light or to determine the light threshold.

Phoresis A nonobligatory form of commensalism in which one organism is mechanically carried by the other.

Phosphate Hypophosphataemia exists when serum phosphate is below 1 mmol/litre. Signs include confusion, disorientation, dysarthria, paraesthesia and coma. Oxygen dissociation curve shifts to left. There is poor O_2 transport with hypoxia, lactic acidosis and pulmonary oedema. There is poor leucocyte function. The maintenance requirement is at least 10 mmol per day in adult as sodium phosphate.

Phosphocreatinine A compound of creatinine with phosphoric acid; an intermediary energy source, that provides phosphate for the resynthesis of ATP from ADP.

Phosphodiesterase An enzyme that splits the phosphodiester bonds of some nucleotides.

Phospholipid Lipid with phosphorus resulting in a molecule with a polar and a nonpolar end; main component of cell membranes.

Phosphor A substance capable of emitting light when exposed to light and other radiations.

Phosphorelay A signal transduction pathway in which a phosphate group is passed along a series of proteins.

Phosphorescence Emission of radiation by a substance as a result of previous absorption of radiation of shorter wavelength; contrasts with fluorescence in that the emission may continue for a time after cessation of the ionising radiation.

Phosphorolysis Cleavage of a compound with phosphate as the attacking group; analogous to hydrolysis.

Phosphorylation The process of adding phosphorus to a dormant enzyme, thereby activating it. Occasionally perosphorylation deactivates an active enzyme.

Photoacoustic stimuli Flash light stimuli through closed eye and rhythmic noise stimuli through the ear at the same time.

Photoautotroph An organism that uses inorganic material as a source of carbon for growth, and light as an energy source.

Photochemical reaction center The part of photosynthetic complex where the energy of an absorbed photon causes charge separation, initiating electron transfer.

Photography and video recording Still photography although more accurate for measuring R.O.M. is time consuming and costly. Video recording through motion analysis systems are also available for measurement of joint motion. The application is more in research field.

Photoheterotroph An organism that uses organic material as a source of carbon for growth, and light as an energy source.

Photoma A visual hallucination in which sparks or light flashes are seen without external stimuli.

Photon The ultimate unit of light energy.

Photoperiod Number of daylight hours.

Photophobia Literally, fear of light; a movement away from light.

Photophobic Responding to light movement away from the light source.

Photophthalmia It is caused by ultraviolet rays specially from 311 to 290 m. It is caused by bright flash of short circuit, exposure to naked arc light during welding and reflection of ultraviolet rays from snow in snow blindness. There is latent period of 2 to 4 hours between exposure and occurrence of onset of symptoms and signs. On exposure oedema of corneal epithelium occurs. Then it is desquamated to form epithelial erosions. Person complains of severe pain, lacrimation and photophobia. There is swelling of conjunctiva and also lids in a severe case.

Photopic involving Substantial amounts of light; e.g., day-light.

Photopic luminosity The relative effectiveness of various wavelengths of light on visual acuity under light-adapted conditions.

Photopigment A pigment molecule that is sensitive to light types of photopigments including bacteriochlorophyll, carotenoid, flavin, retinal, or phycobilin.

Photopsia It is an important symptom of an acute posterior vitreous detachment. The patient complains of awareness of the flash of a light, a glow, a streak of light in form of an arc in his or her field of vision. This flash is for a fraction of second. This phenomenon of flash of light seen by patient is due to cerebral awareness of vitreous stimulating the retina. Vitreoretinal pathology has to be excluded.

Photopsin A protein in the cones of the retina. Along with retinence, a product of the breakdown of iodopsin upon exposure to light.

Photopsy The sensation of light flashes in the absence of actual light stimulation probably caused by mechanical stimulation of visual nerve tissue.

Photoreceptor A protein with an attached photopigment molecule that can absorb light energy.

Photoreduction The light-induced reduction of an electron acceptor in photosynthetic cells.

Photorespiration Oxygen consumption occuring in illuminated temperatezone plants, largely due to oxidation of phosphoglycolate.

Photoresponse A general term for the reaction of a cell to changes in the direction, quality, or intensity of light.

Photoretinitis Eclipse blindness is a burn of retina at the posterior pole, the macula. It follows looking at an eclipse of the sun with unprotected eye or exposure of the eye to the flash of short circuiting of strong electric current. The rays pass to retina where these are absorbed by pigment epithelium causing heating effect resulting in a burn of retina at macula.

Main symptom is an afterimage of strong light which may persist for long time. Patient sees a dark spot in the field of vision.

Ophthalmoscopy shows a pale spot at the macula with a brownish red ring around it. later there is pigmentation or small grey punctate spots or even both at macula.

Photosynthesis A series of processes in which light or other electromagnetic energy is covered to chemical energy to be used for the biosynthesis of organic cell malterials.

Phototaxis The oriented movement of a motile organism with respect to the direction of light. Phototaxis can either be toward (positive phototaxis) or away from (negative phototaxis) the light.

Phototherapy Technique for suppressing melatonin by stimulating light receptors in the eye.

Phototroph An organism that can use the energy of light to synthesize its own fuels from simple molecules such as carbon dioxide, oxygen, and water, as distinct from a chemotroph.

Phototrophy The fact or process of deriving energy from light.

Phototropism Growth or orientation in response to the location of light.

Phrenic nerve The nerve that stimulates the diaphragm to contract.

Phthisic type A body type described as thin and flat-chested, as were people suffering from tuberculosis.

Phthriasis Chronic blepharitis may be caused by pubic lice. On slit-lamp examination they can be recognised together with their eggs.

Phycobilin A photosynthetic pigment found in cyanobacteria.

Phyllocoenosis The association of a microorganism with the stem or leaves of a plant, which results in a benefit to one or both of the partners.

Phylloplane A collective term for the aboveground exposed surfaces of plants that are available for the colonization of microorganisms.

Phyllosphere A collective term for the leaves and stem of a plant that can be colonized by microorganisms.

Phylogenetic Relating to or involving phylogeny; describing an analysis that groups organisms according to evolutionary relationships.

Physeal bar A bridge of bone that forms the metaphysis to the epiphysis, crossing the physis. This results in a tethering of growth with possible angular deformity.

Physiatrics Physical therapy.

Physiatrist A physician who specializes in physical medicine and rehabilitation.

Physical Pertaining to the body, to material things, or to physics.

Physical abuse Physical violence directed toward an intimate partner including pushing, punching, kicking or chocking.

Physical addiction It is a drug produced condition characterised by tolerance and physical dependence.

Physical adjustment Harmonizing of the human organisms with its physical environment.

Physical assessment Systematic examination of body structures.

Physical dependence Physiological state produced by repeated administration of drug which necessitates the continued administration of drugs to prevent withdrawl symptom.

Physical education In rehabilitation, the use of physical condition, encourage, socialisation, and build morale.

Physical fitness A dynamic state of energy and vitality that enables one to carry out daily tasks to engaze in active leisure type pursuits and to meet unforeseen emergencies without undue fatigue.

Physical fitness The limits on the actions that the body is capable of making.

Physical function Sensory-motor skills necessary for the performance of usual daily activities.

Physical health The efficiency of body to function appropriately, to maintain immunity to disease and to meet daily energy requirement.

Physical restraint Any device, garment, meterial, or object that restricts a person's freedom of movement or access to one's body.

Physical signs Directly observable or measurable changes in an individual's organs or systems as a result of pathology or disease.

Physical sterilization The use of heat to disinfection.

Physical therapist Person skilled in technique of physical therapy.

Physical therapy Treatment of disorder or injuries with massage, heat, short wave diathermy, cold, light and water. Exercises are done with the help of physiotherapist. It is used to relieve physical stiffness of joints and to restore muscle strength. It reduces pain, muscle spasm and to bring strength after stroke or nerve injury.

Physical work capacity Physiologic maximal work performance defined as that level of performance beyond which the oxygen uptake fails to increase further with increasing work.

Physically correct In describing dolls, complete with external genitals.

Physician An authorized practitioner of medicine, as one graduated from a college of medicine or osteopathy and licensed by the appropriate board.

Physics The science that deals with natural laws and phenomena, but especially with matter and energy in terms of motion and force.

Physiologic contour Tissue shape that best promotes tissue health.

Physiologic race A group of isolates that share common pathogenic attributes. Isolates classified as a single race may or may not be genetically identical.

Physiologic resorption Resorption of teeth associated with the normal shedding of deciduous teeth.

Physiologic saline solution A 0.9% sodium chloride solution, which exerts an osmotic pressure equal to that exerted by the blood, and thus is compatible with blood.

Physiological Pertaining to physiology.

Physiological age A measurement of the level of development or deterioration of an individual in terms of functional norms for various systems.

Physiological anorexia Decreased appetite because of relatively decreased calorie need.

Physiological cycles Bodily activities that change regularly, usually in terms of inherent elements such as sleeping patterns.

Physiological jaundice This condition occurs in newborn infants and requires no treatment. It is due to relative deficiency of enzyme glucurongyl transferase, though red blood cell destruction and enteropathic circulation may be partially responsible. Jaundice does not appear before 24 hours and start disappearing after 7 days. It is maximum on the third day.

Physiological memory A memory for somatic experiences outside conscious awareness, for example, the memory of a conditioned-automatic-system response.

Physiological motion Normal changes in the position of articulating surfaces during the movement of a joint or region.

Physiological needs The most basic level of Abraham Maslow's hierarchy of needs; survival needs such as for food, air, water and sleep.

Physiology Science that deals with the functions of an organism or its parts.

Physiopathology The science of functions in disease, or as modified by disease; morbid or pathologic physiology.

Physiotherapy Treatment and prevention of disease using passive and active exercise, movements, vibrations and massage and application of hot/cold.

Physocele A tumor filled with gas.

Phytophthora A genus containing many important plant pathogens most of which are near-obligate parasites.

Phytoplankton The portion of the plankton community defined as plant life.

Pia mater This is separated from the arachnoid by subarachnoid space filled with CSF. Here local analgesic drugs are deposited in spinal analgesia. The pia closely invests the cord and sends delicate septa into substance. The pia mater ends as a prolongation, the filum terminale. Being filled with fluid and the spinal cord, it is also broken by nerve roots.

Pia-arachnoid The pia mater and arachnoid coverings of the cerebrum, considered as a single organ.

Pica An eating disorder characterized by the abnormal intake of specific substances such as clay dirt, cornstarch, or plaster. It may characterize the behavior of malnourished children or pregnant women.

Picking up In picking up, one or more muscles are grasped, lifted away from the underlying tissues, squeezed, and released. The grasping and releasing is performed in a circular motion, usually in the same direction as the muscle fibers.

Pickling A process used to clean oxides from the surface of a cast metal by warming in an acidic solution.

Pickling agents Substances used to impart, preserve or enhance the preservability.

Picornavirus A group of viruses with small RNA genomes, such as poliovirus.

Picture-interpretation test An examinatiо́n in which the participant must interpret a pictorial situation. Usually considered a test of intelligence.

PIE charting Method of recording the patient's progress under the headings of problem, intervention, and evaluation.

Piedmont fracture A fracture of radius at the junction of its distal and middle thirds.

Pierre Robin syndrome The syndrome presents with small mandible, cleft palate, and glossoptosis, often with congenital glaucoma and other eye defects.

Pigeon Toed In toeing position of feet.

Piggy back drip Medications to be given intravenously are often added to an existing intravenous line. Some primary administration sets have inlet port for adding medications or a second

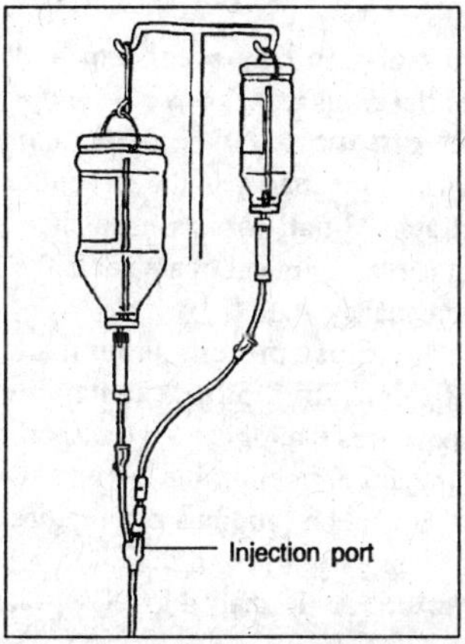

IV line. The advantage of this system for the busy nurse is that when solution in smaller bottle has been infused, the primary bottle begins to flow again without further adjustment. Do not clamp or alter the flow of primary bottle. It will not run until all fluid higher than this has been infused.

Piggyback infusion Method for administering intravenous medications intermittently; a piggyback IV set is a supplementary set tht connects with the primary IV tubing.

Pigment Any coloring matter in microbial, plant, or animal cells.

Pigment layer The layer of the epidermis that contains the melanocytes that produce melanin to give skin its color.

Pigmentation The colour of skin, hair, eye and iris depends on the contents of melanin. Melanin is produced be melanocytes. Africans have more content of melanin. Generalised deficiency of melanin produces albinism. In phenylketoneuria melanin level goes down making a person paler skinned and fairer haired. Eczema or psoriasis may result in lighter mingled with darker areas. Dark facial patches may be the result of certain perfumes. Darkening of skin in addition to sun exposure may be due to hormonal disorders like Addison's disease and Cushing's syndrome. Bile pigment bilirubin turns skin and urine yellow. Excessive iron turns skin bronze. Port-wine stain of skin may be due to haemangioma.

Pigmentation in pregnancy Hyperpigmentation occurs in 90% pregnancies. It may be generalised or loaclised only to areas of increased melanocyte density.
Darkening of skin may occur. Linea alba often becomes linea nigra. Chloasma develops.

Piles and pregnancy One of the commonest complaints in pregnancy is the discomfort due to hemorrhoids. Small loss is usual but massive bleeding is rare. Surgical treatment is the same as in non pregnancy state.

Pilin The invidiual protein subunit of a pilus organelle. Immature pilins, containing leader signal sequences that direct the transport of pilins across the inner membrane of gram-negative bacteria, are called propilins or prepilins.

Pillion A temporary artificial leg.

Pillion fracture A 'T' shaped fracture of lower end of femur.

Pilonidal sinus Pilonidal means a nest of hair. It is a subcutaneous track containing hair or their microscopic fragments. These are found most often in natal cleft overlying the coccyx or lower part of sacrum. It has been suggested that a developmental abnormality around the sacrococcygeal region leads to formation of an epithelial lined sinus which grows hair at puberty. Recently acquired theory has been approved that the sinus is nothing more than a foreign body granuloma, the foreign body being hair which penetrates the skin through abrasion.

Pilot drill The initial instrument used to establish angle of entry and depth of an implant osteotomy.

Pilot hole A relatively small hole that is drilled for either a self tapping screw or a tap.

Pilus A short, filamentous appendage extending from the surface of certain bacterial cells, composed, mainly of the protein pilin.

Pincer palpation Examination of a part by holding it in a pincer grasp between the tips of the digits, to detect taut bands of fibers, to identify tender points in the muscle, and to elicit local twitch responses.

Pinch graft A small, full thickness skin graft obtained by elevating the donar area with a needle and then taking off a small area with a knife.

Pinch roll test A fold of skin is pinched firmly between the thumb and index finger. Tension is applied to the skin fold as it is culled between the fingers in one direction and then in other. The pinch should never be released during manoeuvre. It is useful to find a true hypersensitivity in a small zone of involvement.

Pinched nerve A layman's term for radiculopathy produced by a herniated disc.

Pineal Pineal gland is part of the epithalamus.

Pineal body It is a rudimentary gland which is attached to the roof of third ventricle. It is a neuroendocrine organ which is concerned with photo sensitivity. It is a rich network of capillaries and connective tissue trabeculae. Special types of pinealocytes are found. True nerve cells are absent. Three types of biogenic amines are found in gland : serotonin, norepinephrine and melatonin. After the age of 16 granules of calcium and magnesium phosphates and carbonate deposit in the gland known as brain sand. These can be seen in X-ray of the skull and brain.

Pineal gland Endocrine gland located in the third ventricle of the brain; produces melatonin.

Pinguecula It appears as a yellowish triangular patches in the bulbar conjunctiva on either side of cornea in palpebral aperture. It appears first on nasal side and afterwards on temporal side. It develops on either side of limbus in a triangular form with the base towards the limbus.

Pinna The outer, fleshy portion of the external ear; also called the auricle.

Pinocytosis Cell drinking; invagination of the cell membrane forming narrow channels that pinch off into vacuoles. This allows for cellular intake of extracellular fluid and dissolved molecules.

Pins A general term for, pointed metallic implants.

Pinworm infestation It primarily affects children specially in temperate area. The female adult is one-third of an inch long. These lay eggs in skin around anus and movements of worm causes itching and tickling. Eggs are transferred from fingers to mouth. Swallowed eggs hatch in the intestine and worms reach maturity after 2 to 6 weeks. Antihelminthic drug is effective specially piperazine. Adverse effects include diarrhoea and nausea.

PIP joint Abbreviation for proximal interphalangeal joint.

Pipette A slender, graduated tube for measuring and transferring liquids from one vessel to another.

Piracy A behavior pattern in which an animal steals resources, such as food or nest material, from another.

Piries bone An accessory bone of the foot sometimes found anterior to the dorsal edge of talus.

Piriformis syndrome It is usually seen in females and occurs six times more than in males. The tight piriformis compresses the sciatic nerve producing pain in the buttock, back of thigh and calf.

Piriformis test The test is performed with patient in supine lying. The side under test is positioned with hip and knee flexed and the foot is across the opposite knee. The hip and knee is passively moved towards adduction while the examinee's other hand stabilizes the ipsilateral pelvis to prevent rotation. The test is positive if patient feels pain in the buttock or radicular symptoms if sciatic nerve is under compression.

Piroxicam Half-life is 45 hours and is completely absorbed from GIT and a proportion goes enterohepatic cycling which helps to maintain plasma concentration. Usual dose is 10 to 30 mg/day in divided doses and is used in rheumatoid disease and musculoskeletal disorder and gout.

Pisiform A small pea like carpal bone on the palmar side of hand that articulates with triquetrum.

Piskacek's sign It consists of asymmetric enlargement of the pregnant uterus due to enlargement of the cornual region over the implantation site

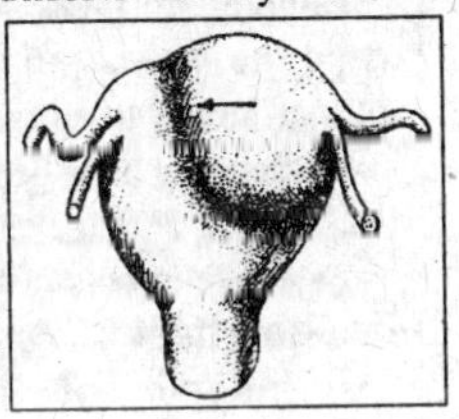

Pistol A small, short barreled firearm, that ejects the cartridge after firing.

Pit Small pinpoint depression in enamel.

Pit and fissure sealants Resinous material designed for application to the occlusal surfaces of posterior teeth to seal the surface irregularities and prevent ingress of oral fluids, food, and debris.

Pitch The highness or lowness of a sound as heard; related to frequency but also affected by loudness.

Pitting corrosion A specific type of corrosion process that occurs on passivated metals as a result of disruption of the oxide film, making the surface susceptible to localized and extensive electrochemical attack.

Pituitary crisis Acute systemic decompensation occurring in a patient with untreated panhypopituitarism that may be fatal if not rapidly diagnosed and treated.

Pituitary dwarf An individual of short stature, of relatively normal proportion, as the result of insufficient growth hormone secreted from the anterior pituitary.

Pituitary gland The pituitary gland regulates the activities of other endocrine glands and many body processes. It is a peasized gland hanging from the base of brain. It is attached by a short stalk. The pituitary consists of three parts : anterior lobe, intermediate lobe and posterior lobe.

Different lobes of pituitary secrete different hormones. Anterior lobe produces six hormones : growth hormone which stimulates growth, prolactin which stimulates production of milk, ACTH which stimulates hormone production by adrenal glands, TSH the thyroid stimulating hormone, and FSH and LH stimulating gonads. Posterior pituitary produces two hormones : antidiuretic homone (ADH) : which increases reabsorption of water in kidneys, and oxytocin which stimulates contractions of uterus during labour.

The intermediate lobe secretes one hormone : melanocyte which controls production of melanin.

Pituitary tumours These are not very common. Most are benign. But its enlargement is upward where it tends to press an optic nerve causing visual field defects. Tumour of anterior part may lead to excessive hormone production leading to acromegaly.

Excess of ACTH leads to too much of Cushing's syndrome. Increased prolactin leads to abnormal milk production. Tumour of posterior pituitary may disrupt production of ADH and lead to diabetes insipidus. MRI is noninvasive effective tool to diagnose the tumour. Treatment includes surgical resection followed by radiation therapy.

Pityriasis rosea It is a mild inflammatory but self-limiting disorder, condition begins with malaise, headache, mild fever and lymphadenopathy, Generally well-defined single red, patchy lesion covered with scaling develops.

Lesions show depression at the centre surrounded by more prominent pink borders. Condition is self-limiting and within a few days lesions begin to peel. Condition does not require any treatment except psychological appearance.

Pityriasis rubra pilaris It is a rare but chronic dermatological disorder is of unknown aetiology. There may be inherited metabolic disorder becoming worse in summer. Pathologically it presents with hyperkeratosis follicular plugs with occasional mast and plasma cells.

It presents with follicular, conical, pin head-sized, papules covered with scales or horny plugs and erythema. Much later generalised erythema and scaling develops. Skin looks glazed and atrophic. The lesion of palms and soles present with hyperkeratosis and fissuring. Nails become rough, thickened and striated which may crack or break. Lesions persist for years and then disappear automatically Patient is given large doses of vitamin A.

Pityriasis simplex It is also known as pityriasis alba. It is a benign skin disorder of unknown origin. Condition presents with hypopigmented macules of various sizes and shapes.

Patches are poorly demarcated and are covered with adherent scales. Sometimes margins of patches may show erythema. It does not produce any symptom and condition does not require any treatment.

Pityriasis versicolor It is a trivial, often unsightly, superficial mycosis caused by pityrosperum orbiculare. Severe perspiration and wearing too heaving clothes may favour the infection. Use of systemic corticosteroid may aggravate the condition.

Patient presents with brown, tan or white patches. In coloured skin hypopigmented macules and plaques may be seen. Lesions are delicately covered with fine scales specially on trunk. Lesions can develop anywhere but hands and feets are spared. Lesions may persist for some time or may resolve spontaneously.

Pivot joint A synovial joint in which the rounded head of one bone articulates with the depressed cup of another to permit a rotational type of movement.

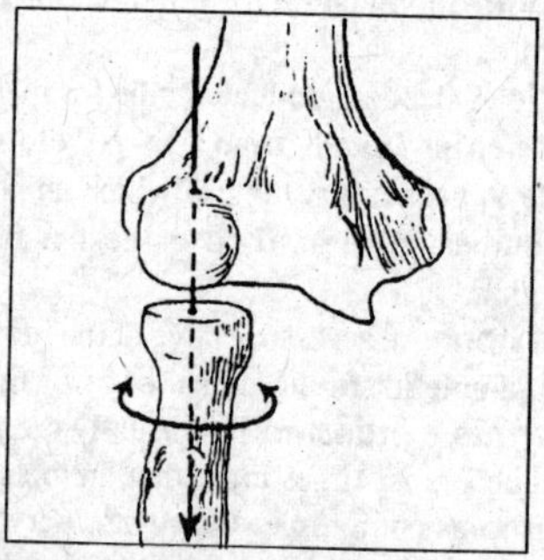

Pkexys Interwoven nerves or blood vessels.

Place code The system that codes information about sound frequencies in different locations on the basilar membrane.

Place theory The theory that the pitch of a sound is determined by the place on the cochlea that is maximally activated by a sound wave of a particular frequency; loudness depends on the number of activated fibres in each direction.

Placebo It is a chemically inert substance given in place of drug either to satisfy patient or as a control group in research studies. Person taking it believes that it will have positive effect. The placebo is made identical to drug in shape, size and tastes and person is kept in dark about placebo. Some patients respond to placebo. Literally, "to please". A pill of no medicinal value given to a male patient, for example, "to please him" or to make him think that he is taking medicine. Used in drug experiments to prevent subjects from knowing whether they have been given the drug or a control substance and thereby distributing equally the suggestive effects of taking the drug.

Placebo effect The production or enhancement of psychologic or physical effects using pharmacologically inactive substances administered under circumstances in which suggestion leads the subject to believe a particular effect will occur.

Placenta It is the organ which supplies mothers blood to the fetus in womb. It develops from chorion and is firmly attached to the lining of womb. By the end of pregnancy it is 8" wide and 1" thick. Shortly after the baby is born placenta is expelled out. Placenta acts as an organ of respiration and excretion of fetus. It carries oxygen from mothers circulation into fetus's circulation

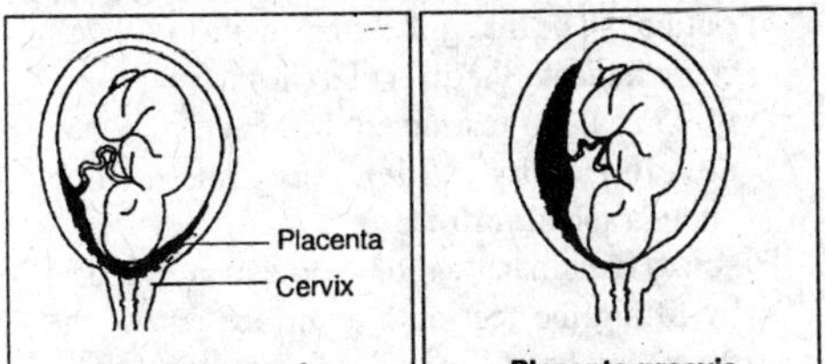

Placenta praevia (major grade) | Placenta praevia (minor grade)

and removes waste products. Placenta produces three hormones—oestrogen, progesterone and chorionic gonadotropin. Placenta praevia may result in painless bleeding.

Placenta acreta It is a morbid adherence of the placenta to the uterine wall since dividing line between the decidua compact and decidua spongiosa is absent. Hysterectomy may be needed.

Placenta annularis There is a wide ring of placenta surrounding the chorion.

Placenta at term It is a circular, flat, disc shaped spongy mass measuring 20 cms in diameter and 2.5 cm thick near the insertion of cord and abruptly becoming thinner at edges. It is made up of 15 to 20 polygonal shaped cotyledons each corresponding to a main villous system. It has a fetal and maternal surface.

Placenta biparita The placenta is incompletely divided into 2 lobes and the vessels extend from one lobe to other.

Placenta circumvallate Fetal surface of placenta presents a central depression surrounded by a ring of thick white tissue. The rigid ring of white tissue is made up of double fold of amnion and chorion with necrotic villi and traces of decidua.

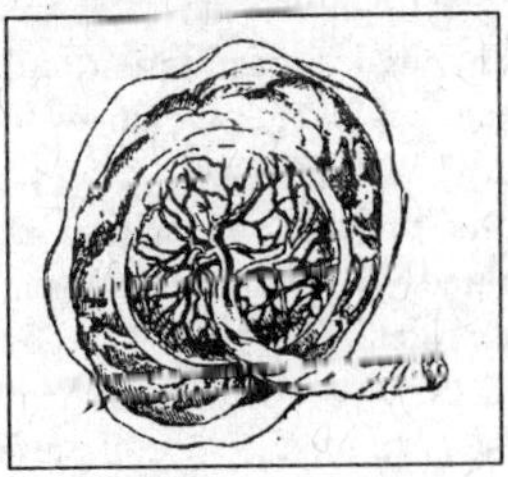

Placenta diffusa The placenta is thin, large and widely spread out. Signs of placenta previa occur in second and third trimesters. Bleeding may be severe in many cases. Abnormal placenta does not interfere with nutrition of ovum. Bleeding may be severe between 24-28 weeks.

Placenta duplex Two lobes are completely separated. Vessels remain intact in each lobe and unite just before entering the cord.

Placenta fenestra The placenta is oblong in size with a fold of varying size near the middle of placenta. It may be mistaken for a missing lobe.

Placenta praevia When placenta is partly or wholly over the lower segment it is known as placenta previa. In first degree lower edge of placenta does not encroches to the internal OS of undilated cervix. In second degree lower margin of placenta reaches to the internal OS in undilated cervix but with dilatation of the cervix the OS is partly covered by placenta and the membrane is exposed. In fourth degree placenta it completely covers the internal OS even with full dilatation of the cervix.

Placenta previa acreta In the lower segment of uterus placenta may be morbidly adherent to the uterine wall because of the poor development of decidua in lower segment. There is high incidence of placenta previa. Unsuspected free bleeding may be induced during lower segment casearean section.

Placenta succenturiata One or more accessory lobes are situated in the membrane at some distance from placenta. Between main lobe and accessory lobe there is a vascular connection which may be torn at delivery. It may lead to PPH.

Placenta velamentosa The umbilical cord is attached to the membranes some distance away from the placenta and fetal vessels traverse the membrane to reach the placenta. If there is doubt in prognosis vaginal blood smear stained with Kleihaur technique will show a high percentage of fetal blood cells.

Placental Relating to the placenta or to a placental mammal.

Placental analog An invertebrate counterpart to the mammalian placenta.

Placental blood flow About 500 to 700 ml of maternal blood enter the placental lake each minute spurting like an intermittent fountain to reach the chorionic plate diffusing back past fetal villi and finally out through maternal sinuses in the decidua. Any reduction in placental blood flow,

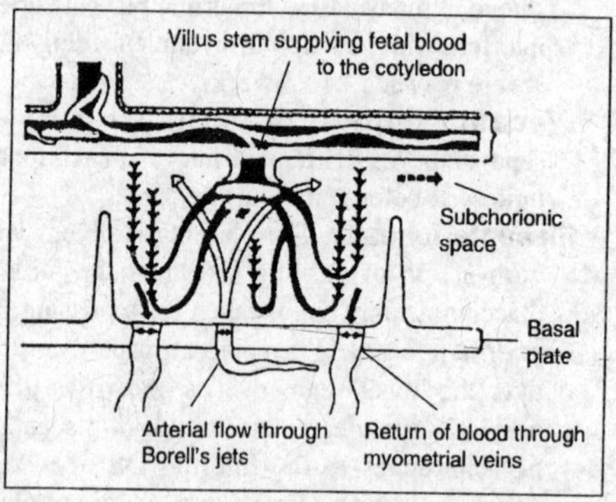

i.e. exercise, spasm of arteries or fibrin deposition may interfere with nutritional transfer mechanism of placenta. Fetus will have reduced levels of glucose and glycogen, amino acid and protein and fatty acids. Such infants are having less chances of survival.

Placental cyst It results as areas of degeneration and liquefaction in the placental sepate or in areas of intervillous fibrin. Contents may be clear & transparent. It is of academic interest instead of clinical importance.

Placental expulsion Uterine contractions expel the placenta into the vagina 5 to 20 minutes after delivery of an infant. It causes gush of blood from vagina and lengthening of cord as placenta descends into the upper vagina.

Placental immunity Refers to the placenta's ability to protect the unborn and the newborn child from many infectious and toxic agents in the mother. Syphilis is an example of an exception.

Placental infarct During last 2 months of pregnancy certain changes occur in fetal portion of placenta which result in formation of small solid areas known as infarcts. Multiple large areas of infarcts lead to placental insufficiency, fetal hypoxia and even death of fetus.

Placental separation Cardinal signs of placental separation are, globular shape of uterus, uterine bleeding, permanent lengthening or descent of umbilical cord and rise of fundus as placenta lies in the lower segment and lifts the uterus up.

Placido's disc The disc has black and white circles painted, alternately, with a central hole to observe. The surgeon looks through this central hole at the corneal images as reflected from a light behind the patient. The irregularities in the rings indicate the irregular surface of cornea. An instrument has been developed by which the image may be photographed for record.

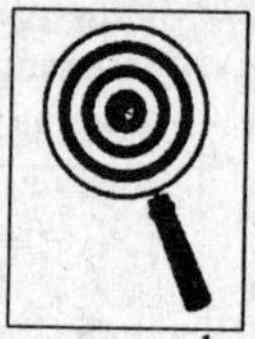

Placing In humans, a reflex movement characterized by lifting the feet onto a surface during the first three months of life.

Plafond fracture A fracture of distal end of tibia which extends into articular surface of tibiotalar joint.

Plain forceps These are used for tying the suture. These are also available with straight or curved tips, serrated or plain. The serrated inside of the ends gives a better and firm grip.

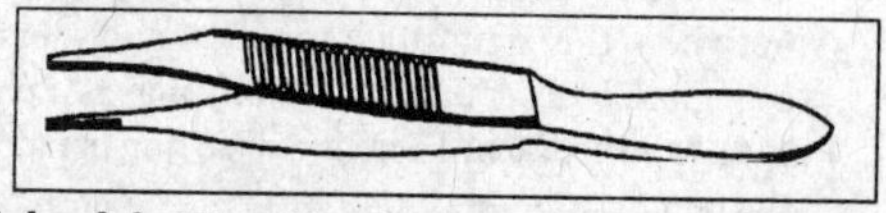

Plain vials When blood is required one anticoagulant is used. when only serum is required it is collected in plain vial. For one ml of serum 2.5 ml of blood is taken out.

Plain vial is used for blood chemistry like amylase, lipase, alcohol, bilirubin, calcium, cholesterol, creatinine, blood urea nitrogen (BUN), uric acid, serum glutamicoxaloacetic transaminase (SGOT) and serum glutamic pyruvic transaminase (SGPT). It is also used for VDRL, Australian antigen, cross-matching, Rh typing and *Coombs' test.*

Plaintiff The party to a civil suit who brings the suit seeking damages or other legal relief.

Planes Two-dimensional, flat surfaces, real or imaginary, at right angles to each other.

Planning It involves the selection or design of interventions in consultation and collaboration with the client, which facilitates the achievement of the desired objectives.

It is the process by which objectives are determined, interventions chosen, and the care plan is written.

Plant cell culture The production of plant cells in a bioreactor to produce useful products.

Planta flexion Flexion of the foot and toes towards the sole.

Plantar Pertaining to the sole of the foot.

Plantar aponeurosis It is a dense fibrous connective tissue that helps the longitudinal arch of foot.

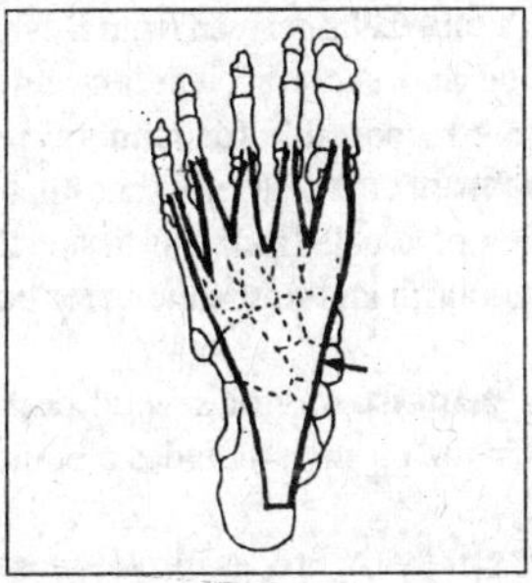

Plantar arch Plantar arch is necessary for proper weight bearing. One method to show overpronate is the wet foot test. Step in some water and then walk on dry pavement or cement. You will leave a

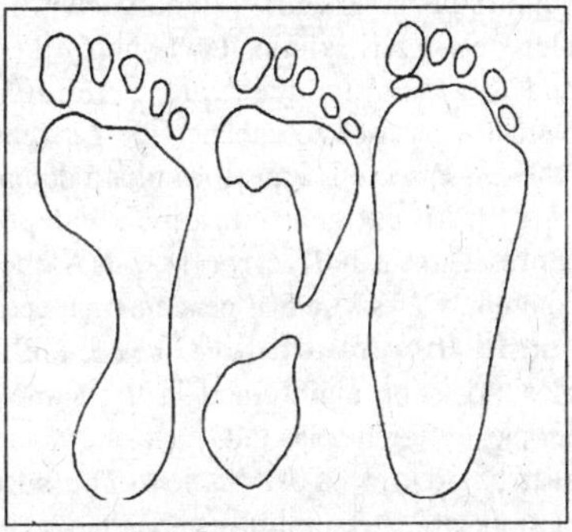

print of the weight bearing area of your foot. The ideal distribution shows the heel, the outer edge of the foot and forefoot. Your arch should not leave a print on the ground.

Plantar fascitis This usually follows prolonged strain caused by excessive standing or running on hard ground. There develops tenderness over the attachment of plantar fascia to the calcaneum. Raising the heal gives relief.

Plantar flexed first ray There is more causal position of first metatarsal head in relation to the plane of lesser metatarsal heads. It occurs in subtalar varus, forefoot varus or tibia vara. Fore foot remains unstable.

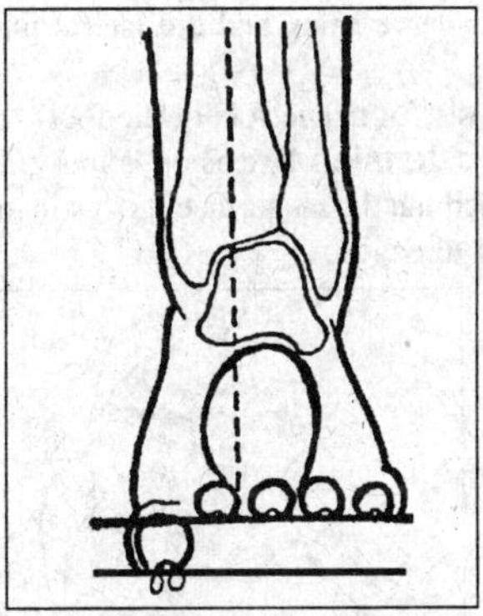

Plantar flexion The bottom of the foot is directed downward; this motion allows a person to stand on his or her tip-toes. Planter flexion is movement of

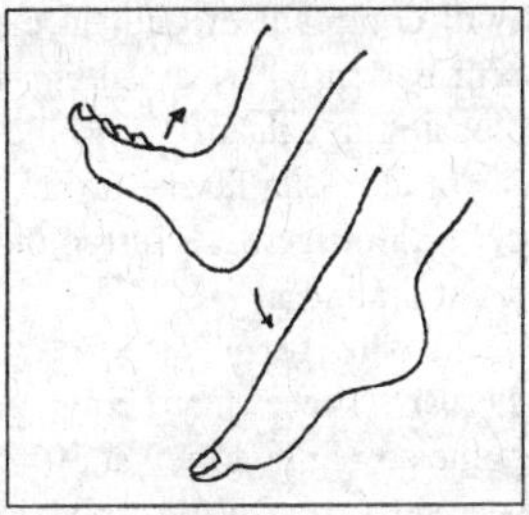

foot in which the planter surface moves in a caudal and posterior direction.

Plantar nerves The tibial nerve trunk crosses onto the sole of the foot. There it branches into the medial

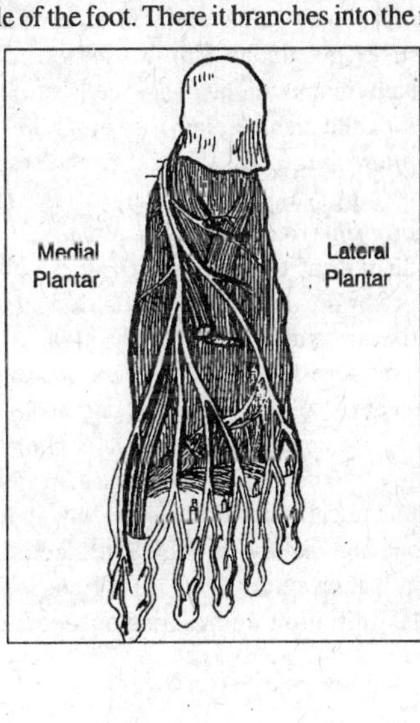

plantar nerve trunk and the lateral plantar nerve trunk.

Plantar surface The sole of the foot.

Planter extension Extension is movement of foot in which the dorsal surface moves in anterior and cranial direction.

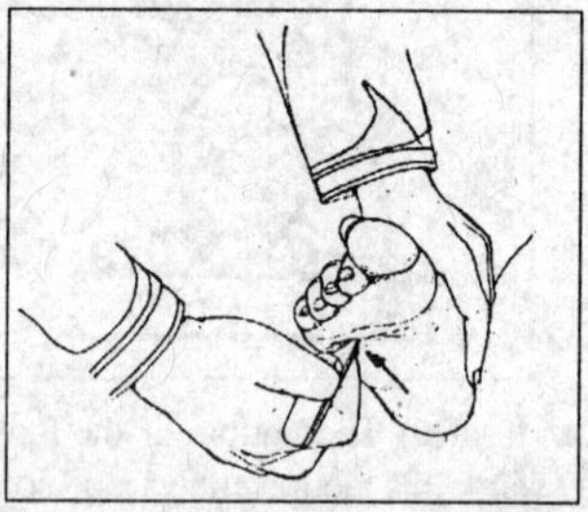

Planter fascitis After unaccostomed walking the patient will complain of pain in early morning. Fascia will be tensed by extending big toe. Pain may be located to calcaneum, to the head of first metatarsal or all along fascial layer.

Plantinic Pertaining to a compound containing quadrivalent platinum.

Plaque It is the term given to an area of atherosclerosis. These may be symptomless until they become so big that they start reducing blood flow in vessel or cause thrombosis. Plaques in coronary artery disease results in coronary heart disease.

Plaque, dental In the development of caries oral bacteria colonise the surfaces of teeth in the form of sticky gelatinous film that besides the bacteria contains mucus, desquamated cells and food debris. It is called dental plaque. *Streptococcus* is the primary bacteria. These proliferate in the supragingival dental plaque. *Lactobacillus acidophilus* bacteria also play a role in acid production of the plaque. Stickiness of plaque is caused by dextran which is produced by fermenting of dietary sucrose by *Streptococcus mutans*. Dextran forms about 10 per cent of weight and 33 per cent of volume of plaque and it traps all types of oral organisms. *Streptococcus mutans* acts on dietary fructose to produce lactic acid which causes enamel decalcification, at or below about 5.5 pH. Plaque and dietary carbohydrates are important in the initiation of enamel caries. Finally the rate of caries initiation and extension depends on the susceptibility of enamel. Some of plaque bacteria produce proteolytic enzyme which breaks down the organic portions of enamel and dentin.

Plasma Fluid portion of the blood (serum and fibrinogen) without formed elements; fluid portion of the lymph without its corpuscles or cells.

Plasma cells Cells derived from B lymphocytes that produce and secrete large amounts antibodies. They are responsible for humoral immunity.

Plasma membrane Membrane that separates the contents of a cell from the tissue fluid; encloses the cytoplasm and forms the outer boundary of the cell.

Plasma protein Any of several proteins normally found in the plasma; includes albumins, globulins, and fibrinogen.

Plasma spray A process involving deposition of metal powders that are totally or partially melted and then rapidly resolidify, forming a dense or porous coating.

Plasmapheresis It is the method of increasing the number of blood cells in blood count. From the blood plasma is skimmed out simply on standing and remaining concentrate is reinfused into patient. It is used to enhance the performance of athletes. Process is known as blood doping.

Plasmid An extrachromosomal, independently replicating, small circular DNA molecule; commonly employed in genetic engineering.

Plasmid incompatibility The inability of a plasmid to be maintained in the same host as another different plasmid.

Plasmocytoma, soft tissue The soft tissue plasmocytoma occurs in persons beyond the age of 40 years specially in males. Upper respiratory tract and oral cavity are sites usually affected. Lesion presents as a tumour mass or granulomatous lesion. Microscopically it consists of a dense aggregation of typical and atypical plasma cells. On electrophoretic studies on the serum show a sharp gamma peak. Some of these lesions are benign and surgical excision is the treatment.

Plasmodesmata Cytoplasmic connections between plant cells.

Plasmodium The genus to which the malaria parasites belong, notably P. falciparum and P. vivax. These organisms have two hosts; the vertebrate, in which two phases of a sexual reporduction occur, and a bloodsucking insect, in which fertilization between male and female forms of the parasite occurs, followed by a further phase of asexual reproduction.

Plasmolyzed Describing cells incubated in a hypertonic medium to retract the inner membrane and expand the periplasmic space.

Plaster A calcium sulfate hemihydrate mineral powder produced by heating gypsum to eliminate water; used as a model material in dentistry be mixing with water to reform gypsum.

Plaster boot Usually refers to a short leg cast.

Plaster of paris It is a quick drying calcium sulphate. It is used in dentistry to make impressions and used in applying plaster over broken bones to immobilise the part.

Plaster scissors Heavy scissors used to cut plaster bandages often serrated.

Plaster splints These are used generally in ankle fractures.

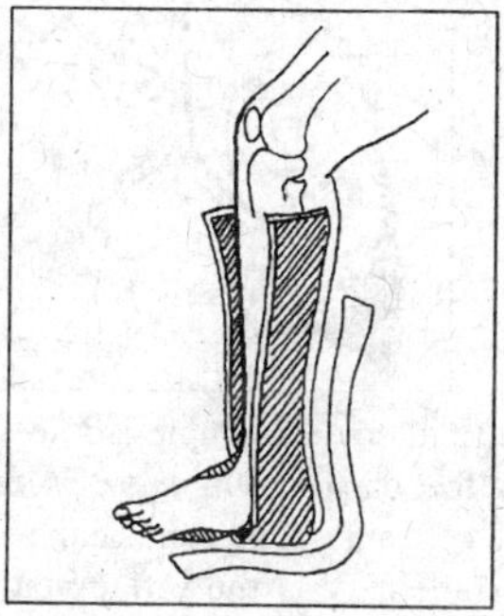

Plastic deformation A permanent strain or change in the shape of an object as a result of it being stressed beyond its elastic limit.

Plastic hallus valgus splint Pain over medical prominence of MTP joint may requre padding to relieve excessive pressure from shoe. Crescent shaped pad fabricated from a foam material is placed proximal to first MTP joint.

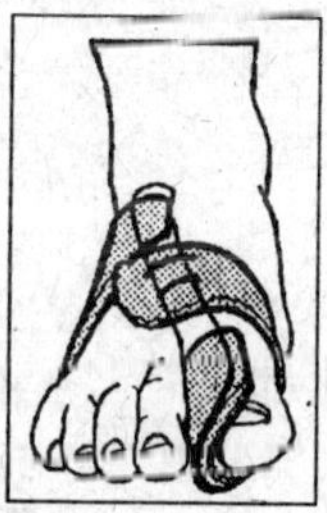

Plasticity Adaptation of an endogenous system so that the response of a system to a particular stimulus or set of stimuli changes.

Plasticizing Usually relating to polymeric materials becoming more plastic or deformable as a result of having or acquiring molecules that tend to keep polymer chains separated and thus less rigidly entangled.

Plastid In plants, a self-replicating or ganelle; may differentiate into a chloroplast.

Plateau Blood serum concentration reached and maintained after repeated, fixed doses of a drug.

Plateau sexual stage During this seminal fluid collects in prostatic urethra. There becomes a feeling of ejaculatory inevitability. Testes are fully elevated.

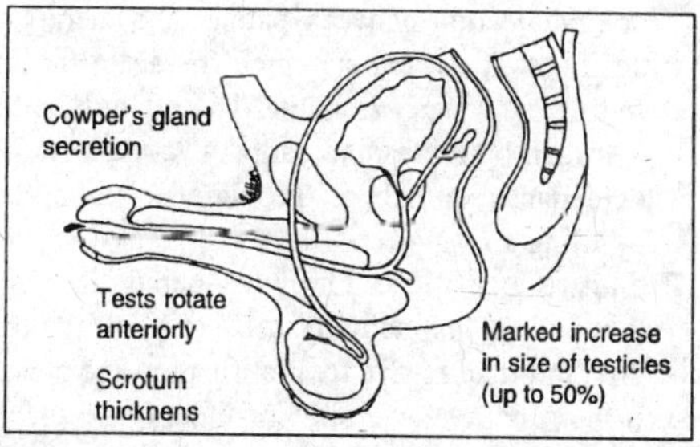

Platelet Minute fragments of cell derived from megakaryocytes; play an important role in haemostasis.

Platelet plug Accumulation of platelets that stick to connective tissue and to each other and prevent blood loss from damaged blood vessels.

Platform crutch It minimises stress on wrist and elbows because of distribution of body weight over the entire forearm. Stress on finger joint is minimised by thickened handles.

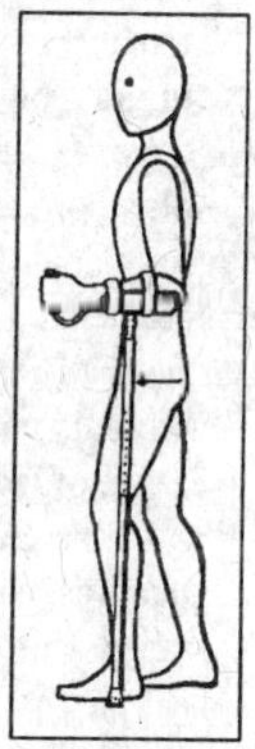

Platonic Pertaining to Plato; to resemble Plato in terms of thinking and feeling.

Platonic friendship A social relationship between two individuals of opposite or same sex, in which sexual relations or strong emotions are not evident.

Platonic love A type of love in which there is no overt sexual behavior or desire.

Platypelloid It is also known as flat pelvis. There is much larger transverse diameter than the AP diameter of the brim. Brim becomes kidney shaped. AP diameter of the brim is 9.2 cms and transverse diameter is 13 cms. Cavity of pelvis is roomy and side walls are divergent.

Platypelloid pelvis One of the four main types of female pelvis, having a flattened pelvic inlet.

Platypnoea Dyspnoea becomes worse when person stands than when lying flat is called platypnoea. It occurs with large pulmonary A-V malformation and in paralysis of intercostal muscles. Children with Fallot's tetralogy suffer from it.

Play therapy A treatment technique utilising the child's play as a medium for expression and communication between patient and therapist.

Pleadings A formal statement made to the court setting out a party's claims. The plaintiff initiates a lawsuit by a pleading called a "complaint." The defendant responds to the plaintiff's complaints by filing an "answer.

Pleasure principle The psychoanalytic concept that people instinctually seek to avoid pain and discomfort and strive for gratification and pleasure. In personality development theory, the pleasure principle antedates and subsequently comes in conflict with the reality principle.

Pleiotrophy The diverse effect of a single gene or gene pair on several organ systems and functions.

Pleniloquence A compulsion to talk incessantly.

Pleomorphic adenoma It is the most common tumour of parotid gland. It contains cartilaginous tissue besides epithelial tissue. It is a benign tumour but may change into malignancy at any time. It is adenoma of salivary gland with a pleomorphic stroma containing fibrous, lymphoid, myxomatous, pseudocartilaginous and epithelial elements.

It usually appears first in adult life of males. Patient presents with slowly growing painless swelling on a side of face for months or years without changing its size. Swelling is rounded with well-defined margins. Size varies from a pea-sized nodule to a large, almost pendulous mass.

Surface is generally smooth but may be lobulated too. Consistency is firm elastic to rubbery hard, not fluctuant and not translucent. It is not tender and not fixed to deeper structure. Cervical glands are not enlarged and there is no involvement of facial nerves.

Plerocercoid The larva from that develops the procercoid, as in Diphyllobothrium latum.

Plethysmographic tracings Recordings of variations in volume of body parts.

Pleura It is a thin membrane with two layers, one lining the outside of lungs and the other inside of the chest cavity. Fluid between two layers provide lubrication and helps in uniform expansion and contraction of lung during breathing.

Pleural Pertaining to the serous membranes associated with the lungs.

Pleural abrasion The excoriation of the mucous membrane of the pleura.

Pleural cavity Space between the visceral and parietal, filled with pleural fluid; a cavity that surrounds the lungs.

Pleural effusion It is an extra collection of fluid between two layers of pleura. It may be caused by pneumonia, heart failure, cancer and tuberculosis.

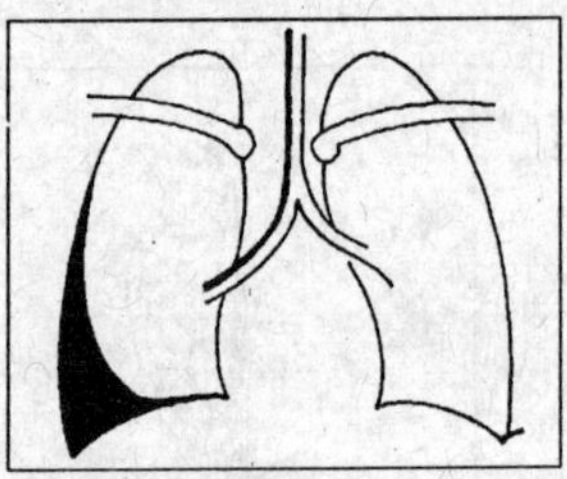

Extra fluid causes compression of lung tissue. It may affect one or both lungs. Excess fluid can be drained out and suitable medical treatment may be given. Pleurisy is the inflammation of pleural membrane. It is caused by lung infection. It causes a sharp chest pain. This pain may be referred to tip of shoulder. Treatment is of underlying cause.

Pleural fluid It is first detected in costophrenic angles. There may be actually 250 ml of fluid present before it is detected. Subpulmonic fluid collections are common in trauma.

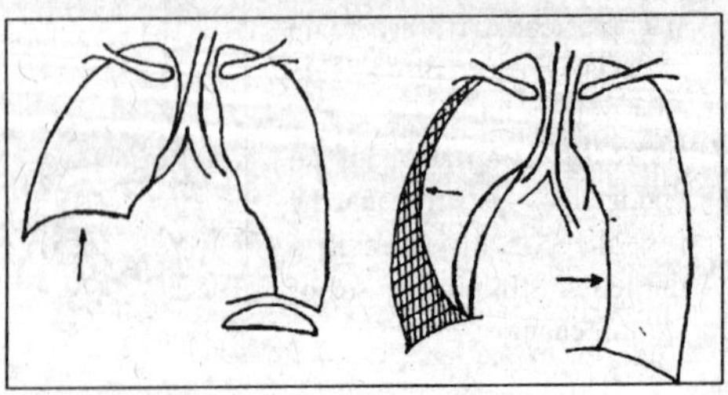

Pleural friction It is produced by two inflamed and roughened surface of pleura rubbing together. The sound has been likened to creaking of leather. It is generally heard both in inspiration and expiration. The sound is often intensified by pressure, and is not abolished by coughing.

Pleural membranes Serous membranes that surround the lungs and provide protection the compartmentalization.

Pleural pressure The pressure within the pleural space between the visceral and parietal pleurae.

Pleural space The space between the visceral and parietal pleuras filled with just enough fluid to allow them to glide effortlessly with each breath.

Pleurectomy The excision of the pleura, usually the parietal pleura.

Pleuritis Inflammation of the pleura that may be caused by infection, injury, or tumor.

Pleurodynia It is the pain in the muscles of chest wall but not related to lungs. An acute viral disease called epidemic pleurodynia is caused by Coxsackie B virus. It causes chest pain, headache, muscular tenderness and fever. Recovery is spontaneous and there is no effective treatment available.

Plexus An intertwining of nerves or blood vessels.

Plexus of auerbach Myenteric plexus.

Plexus, hypogastric Pelvic plexus.

Plica A ridge or fold of tissue.

Plica syndrome A clinical affection of knee joint in which plica becomes thickened and inflamed causing pain.

Plicae circularis Deep folds within the wall of the small intestine that increase the absorptive surface area.

Pliers Small tong-jawed princers for bending metals or holding small objects also used in dental work.

Plosive A category of speech sounds produced when the impounded air pressure in the portion of the vocal tract behind the constriction is released through the oral cavity.

Plugger An instrument used to compress the filling material in an apical direction.

Plumb line A line piece of cord to which is attached a plumb bob (a small lead weight). When suspended, it represents a vertical line.

When used for analyzing standing posture, it must be suspended in line with fixed points, namely, midway between heels in posterior view, and just anterior to the lateral malleolus in a lateral view.

Plume A term for dissolved contaminants emanating from a source region due to ground water transport proceses.

Plummer-Vinson syndrome It is a symptom complex that occurs most exclusively in middle age. It is associated with stomatitis, pharyngooesophageal ulcers, dysphagia and changes in nails. Oral lesions are similar to iron deficiency anaemia. There is leucoplakia with dyskeratosis, angular chelitis, atrophic glossitis and xerostomia. These persons are prone to develop cancer.

Plunger Part of a syringe inside the barrel that moves back and forth to withdraw and instill medication.

Pluralism A belief that multiple factors or principles must be considered to explain reality.

Pluralistic science A science composed of many different elements; it cannot be accounted for by a single system or approach, such as behaviourism, psychoanalysis, the humanistic approach, or cognitive psychology. A field of enquiry which is too diverse and amorphous to be approached by just one method or theoretical orientation.

Pluripotent stem cell Immature stem cell in red bone marrow that vies rise to precursors of all the different mature blood cells.

Plutomania An inordinate striving for money and possessions.

Plyometric exercise Plyometrics are quick, powerful movements that are used to increase the reactivity of the nervous system. Work performance can be improved by storing elastic energy in the muscle during the stretch phase and reusing it is mechanical work during the concentric phase. A quick transition from eccentric to concentric along with a high velocity stretch of high magnitude produces the greatest benefitcs. Plyometrics assist in developing power and speed and are used for sports persons at an advanced training stage.

Pnacreatic islets Endocrine portion of the pancreas; made up of alpha and beta cells among others.

Pneumatic compression device Machine that promotes circulation of venus blood and the movement of excess fluid into the lymphatic vessels.

Pneumatocele A thin-walled cavity within the lung; characteristic of staphylococcal pneumonia.

Pneumatosis cystoides It is seen with the appearance of large polyps on the contrast views. Sigmoidoscopic appearances are equally striking, bluish polyps bulging into the sigmoid colon. Cysts may appear in both small and large bowel at both submucosal and subserosal levels. They are lined by epithelium with low-grade inflammatory changes. Cause is not clear. Some cysts contain hydrogen and may be produced by gas forming anaerobes. Others contain oxygen and nitrogen. There may be gastric cancer, malabsorption syndromes, diverticulosis and scleroderma of small bowel associated with it.

Pneumococcal peritonitis It may occur by blood stream infection in patients with pneumococcal bacteraemia accompanying pneumonia. It can be a complication of nephrotic syndrome and in alcoholics.

Pneumococcus Gram-positive coccus, lancet-shaped, in pairs, encapsulated, non-motile and is non-sporing. It inhabitats in upper respiratory tract of man, causes infection primarily of respiratory tract, conjunctivitis, otitis media, peritonitis and meningitis. The growth on ordinary culture media is poor but it is greatly improved by addition of glucose, blood, serum or ascitic fluid.

Pneumoconiosis It is the lung disorder caused by inhalation of fine dust over a period of time. Asbestosis and silicosis are common. It is common in coal mine workers.

Pneumocystitis A protozoan infection, most likely to invade the body when the immune system has been compromised.

Pneumogram 1. The tracing or graphic record of respiratory movements.

Pneumomediastinum Air within the mediastinal tissues.

Pneumonectomy The surgical removal of a single lung.

Pneumonia There are mainly two types of pneumonia, broncho and lobar pneumonia. In bronchopneumonia inflammation starts in bronchi and bronchioles and then spreads to affect patches of tissue in one or both lungs. Most pneumonia are caused by virus or bacteria. Person develops fever, chill, shortness of breath and cough. Sputum is yellow-green. If pleurisy is also there pain increases while difficult breathing is potential complication of pleural effusion. One course of antibiotic and anti-inflammatory drug helps. Majority of patients improve within 2-3 weeks.

Pneumonitis Inflammation of the lung; may be caused by a virus, or may be a hypersensitivity reaction that occurs as a result of allergy to chemical or organic dusts.

Pneumophonia A voice disorder characterized by excessive breathiness.

Pneumotaxic area The region of the respiratory control center located in the pons of the brain.

Pneumotaxic center A mechanism in the central nervous system that controls breathing.

Pneumothorax In it air enters in pleural cavity from the lungs or from outside due to fracture of ribs or slab injury. Spontaneous pneumothorax occurs for no reason. It may cause chest pain or shortness of breath. Degree of breathlessness is

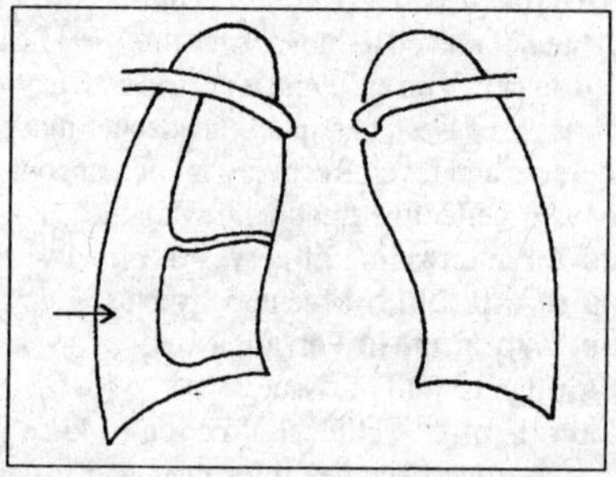

proportional to the size of pneumothorax. If there is continual leakage of air the pneumothorax may be bigger and is likey to produce tension pneumothorax which may be life threatening. X-ray shows pneumothorax and may show underlying cause. A small pneumothorax heals within a few days.

Pneumotiaxic area Portion of the respiratory center in the pons that continually sends inhibitory nerve impulses to the inspiratory area, limiting inspiration and facilitating expiration.

PO By mouth; orally.

Pocket A saclike space or cavity.

Pocket depth (PD) Distance in millimeters from the gingival margin to the base of a pocket.

Pocketing It is a characteristic feature of chronic periodontitis and is due to slower destruction of gingival soft tissues than of periodontal ligament and bone.

Pockets surrounds the teeth One wall is formed by cementum, the other by soft tissue replacing the destroyed bone and periodontal fibres.

Podagra Gouty pain in great toe.

Podiatrist A health care professional trained to diagnose and treat diseases and disorders of the feet.

Podiatry The diagnosis and treatment of foot disorders.

Podocyte Epithelial cell of Bowman's capsule attached to the outer surface of the glomerular capillary basement membrane; forms part of the filtration membrane.

Poggendroff's visual illusion Illusion in which two visible portions of a diagonal line overlayed by a rectangular dont appear to be continuous.

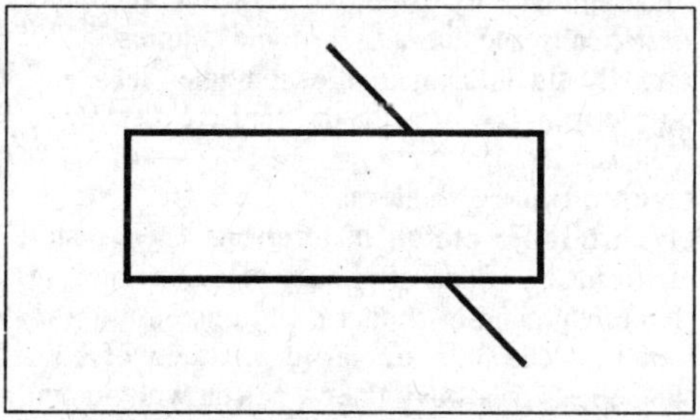

Poikilothermy The fact of having a body temperature conforming to the surrounding medium; being cold-blooded.

Point angle Angle formed by the junction of three walls at a common point; designated by combining the names of the walls forming the angle.

Point of entry The diagnosed access site. Point of entry usually refers to that point where an offender centered a building prior to committing an offense. However, it also sometimes refers to the entry piont of police, fire brigade and other persons after the incident.

Point of maximal impulse Point at which the heartbeat can nmost easily be palpated through the chest wall, usually along the leftmidclavicular line at the fourth or fifth intercostal space.

Point prevalence The frequency of the disease at a designed point in time.

Points of identification In fingerprint science, the minutiae or ridge characteristics that are used to compare two fingerprints.

Poison A substance that when it is ingested, inhaled, absorbed, applied, injected, or developed within the body may cause functional or structural disturbances.

Poisoning Number of metallic salts acts as a systemic poison. *Arsenic poisoning* results in gingivitis and stomatitis. There may be hyperkeratosis, hyperpigmentation and neurological disturbances. *Lead poisoning* leads to excessive salivation, metallic taste, swelling of salivary glands and a dark line along gingival margin. Microscopically, the lead line consists of granular pigment deposit in perivascular areas of submucosa and the basement membrane. Pigment is lead sulphide. *Bismuth poisoning* results in metallic taste, burning sensations of oral mucosa and a bismuth line and occurs with gingival margin in patients with poor oral hygiene. Microscopically, granular deposits of a black pigment is seen in submucosa. Metallic *mercury poisoning* leads to tremors and emotional instability. Oral manifestations lead to increased salivation, stomatitis, glossitis and swelling of salivary glands. In some cases, black line of gingiva is seen. *Silver contact* produces argyria. Skin and oral mucous membrane acquire an ashen grey hue. Microscopic sections show a deposit of fine black granular pigment in the subepithelial connective tissue. *Phosphorus poisoning* results in osteomyelitis of maxilla and mandible.

Poker spine Spinal deformity in which the vertebral column is relatively rigid and straight owing to the loss of normal lordosis.

Polar Hydrophilic, or "water-loving", describing molecules or groups that are soluble in water.

Polar body The smaller cell resulting from the unequal division of primary and secondary oocytes during meiosis. The polar body has no function and degenerates.

Polar brain damage Injury that results from contact between the surfaces of the brain and cranium. Most commonly affects the frontal and temporal lobes.

Polar covalent bond Chemical bond in which electrons are shared unequally between two atoms.

Polar molecule A molecule in which the shared electrons are not evenly distributed, so that one side of the molecule is negatively (or positively) charged in comparison with the other side. Polar molecules are soluble in polar solvents, such as water.

Polarity A aholistic health practice that encompasses some of the theory base of Oriental medicine and Ayurevada. Polarity is an eclectic, multifaceted system.

Polarized light The direction of an electric field, which is in a plane for plane-polarized light and rotates in a circle for circularly polarized light, as opposed to ordinary light whose waves vibrate in all directions.

Polarizing filters Filters which block out all transmitted light except that which is propagated in one direction.

Police power The power of the state to protect the health, safety, morals and general welfare of the people. The police power is the power to restrict the liberty of individuals to protect other individuals. Communicable disease laws are enacted under the police power.

Poliomyelitis Poliomyelitis is caused by a virus. This may lead to paralysis. Effective vaccine against it was prepared in 1950. Infected people pass large number of virus in faeces from where they may spread indirectly or directly via fingers to foods to infect others. Air-borne transmission also takes place. About 85 per cent of children having virus have no symptoms at all. After 3 to 5 days there is short illness with slight fever, sore throat, headache and vomiting. This lasts for a few days after which majority recover. In certain cases condition progresses often in the course of few hours to extensive paralysis of muscles. The trunk and lower legs are most frequently paralysed. If infection spreads to the brainstem the result may be difficulty in swallowing and breathing. There is no effective drug treatment for polio. Nonparalytic patients do not usually need treatment.

Poliomyelitis virus Poliomyelitis virus is like echo and coxsackie viruses, an enterovirus. These RNA viruses spread through faecal contamination of food and water. Some of them cause neurological disease. Poliomyelitis damages anterior horn cells. Polio virus may induce febrile illness without any neurological features. Some patients with an aseptic meningitis progress to paralytic illness often preceded by considerable muscle pain. Bulbar palsy, respiratory insufficiency and various patterns of lower motor neuron paralysis occur. There is no effective treatment in acute stage.

Polish A smooth and glossy surface produced by rubbing or friction or by the application of a substance, such as wax 3. A polishing agent.

Pollex The thumb

Pollution Impurity; the contamination of land, water, or atmosphere through the presence of noxious substances.

Polyacid-modified resin A chemically descriptive term for a compomer .

Polyadenopathy Any disease affecting several glands.

Polyandry Marriage of a woman to more than one husband at any time, a situation accepted historically and currently in some cultures.

Polyarthritis Inflammation of multiple joints.

Polyblennia The secretion of excessive quantity of mucus.

Polychromatic Exhibit many colors.

Polychromatic plates of Ishihara These plates are made up of dots of primary colours printed on the background of similar dots in a confusion of colours. The dots are set in a pattern of bold numericals or a wavy line. A person with normal colour vision can read the numbers or trace the wavy line correctly otherwise not . It is necessary that illumination should not be less than 50 foot candle for correct assessment.

Polyclonal antibodies A heterogenous pool of antibodies produced in an animal by a number of different B lymphocytes in response to an antigen. Different antibodies in the pool recognize different parts of the antigen.

Polycyesis A multiple pregnancy.

Polycystic ovarian syndrome A disease characterised by menstrual disturbances, obesity and polycystic ovaries.

Polycystic ovaries (PCO) Enlarged ovaries due to increased central stroma;.

Polycystic ovary syndrome Unexplained hyperandrogenic chronic anovulation.

Polycythaemia It is a condition of increased concentration of red blood cells in blood.

It may result due to loss of plasma or due to increase in RBCs. It may be due to disorder of bone marrow.

Polydipsia Excessive thirst that is fairly chronic.

Polydysplasia faulty development in several types to tissues or several organs or systems.

Polyembroy An asexual reproductive process whereby multiple individuals are produced from a single ovum.

Polyestrus Having two or more fertile cycles during a given mating season.

Polyether These are the stiffest of the elastomers when set. Liquid polymers are mixed with fillers to provide rigidity oils are added as plasticizers to enhance mixing.

Polygamous Relating to or characterized by polygamy; mating with several members of the opposite sex.

Polygamy A mating system in which a single member of one sex mates with a number of individuals of the opposite sex.

Polygene A group of nonallelic genes which individually have little effect but act cumulatively in exerting a phenotypic effect.

Polygenetic Having many sources, being controlled by many different genes.

Polyglot A person conversant in many languages.

Polygraph Apparatus for recording severe responses concurrently, such as a lie detector, in which changes in respiration, blood pressure, and the GSR are recorded simultaneously on a moving tape.

Polygraphy Polygraphy is one of the accepted terms used to refer to the use of a polygraph instrument in a specialized, systematic process to determine if a person is involved in, with holdding information about or 'laying' with respect to an event of interest.

Polygynous Relatng to or describing a species in which the male mates several times with two or more females during the same reproductive period

Polyhydria In it porphyrins are produced in excess. It combines with iron and protein globulin to produce red blood pigment haemoglobin. Urine is discoloured. Person develops skin blisters, neuritis and hypersensitivity to sunlight. Patient may develop abdominal pain too.

Polyketide A carbon chain containing multiple keta groups on alternate carbon atoms, derived from acetate, propionate, or butyrate units activated in the form of acetyle-CoA, methylmalonyl-CoA, and ethylmalonly-CoA, by the action of polyketide synthases.

Polykoria This is a rare condition in which two or more pupils are surrounded by a sphincter muscle. These pupil react.

Polylogia Continuous and usually incoherent speech.

Polymath A person of encylopedic learning.

Polymenorrhoea Bleeding at regular intervals less than 21 days.

Polymer A material that is made up of repeating units or mers. Most polymers are based up on a carbon backbone in polymer chain.

Polymerase An enzyme that synthesizes a nucleic acid polymer.

Polymeric formula Provides intact nutrients for example, whole proteins and long-chain triglycerides that require a normally funotioning gastrointestinal tract.

Polymerization shrinkage A contraction that accompanies the polymerization reaction often resulting in a loss of accuracy or a reduced fit.

Polymerize To chain together similar molecules to form a compound of high molecular weight.

Polymers Man made polymers were first introduced in early 1900s. Polymers are gigantic, long chain organic molecules. These are poor conductors of heat and electricity. They have tremendous strength in one direction.

Polymodal afferent Afferent neuron receptive to more than one sensory modality, e.g., touch and pain.

Polymodal association cortex Association cortex processing signals in more than one sensory modality.

Polymorphic Describing a protein for which amino acid sequence variants exist in a population of organisms, but the variations do not destroy the protein's function.

Polymorphism Ability to assume different forms, used by some animals for camouflage and mate attraction.

Polymorphonuclear leukocyte A granular leukocyte containing a nucleus with a number of lobes connected by thin, cytoplasmic stands. This type incudes nertrophils, eosinophils, and basophils.

Polymyalgia rheumatica This is a rare disorder of elderly. The cause is unknown arteritis in aorta and its branches is seen. There will be associated inflammmatory arthropathy.

Characteristic clinical features are pain and stiffness in shoulder girdle muscle that is most on first waking. Upper arm muscles are tender on squeezing.

Systemic features of loss of weight and depression are common. ESR is raised and person is anemic. Treatment is with corticosteroids.

Polymyopathy Any disease affecting several muscles simultaneously.

Polymyositis Inflammation of the muscles, involving multiple muscles.

Polymyxins The source of these antibiotics is *Bacillus polymyxa*. Only polymyxin B and polymyxin E are available. Clinically it is used against *Pseudomonas pyocyanea*.

Polyodontia The presence of supernumerary teeth.

Polyoncosis A condition characterized by the development of multiple tumors.

Polyorchid A male having one or more supernumerary tests.

Polyostotic Affecting several bones.

Polyp It is a growth of mucous membrane particularly in lower bowel, colon, nose and uterus. It may change in cancerous growth, surgery is indicated.

Polypeptide A long chain of amino acids linked by peptide bonds; the molecular weight is generally less than 10,000.

Polyphagia Excessive or voracious eating.

Polypharmacy The use of multiple medications, often inappropriately and excessively at the same time.

Polyphyodont Developing several sets of teeth successively through out life.

Polyploid An organism having more than two sets of chromosomes. Resembling a polyp.

Polyploidy The fact of having multiple sets of chromosomes.

Polyprotein A multicistronic protein translated from a single open reading frame. The polyprotein is subsequently cleaved into individual mature gene products.

Polyps Growths protruding from a mucous membrane.

Polysaccharide It is a form of carbohydrate that is a main source of energy. It contains many molecules of sugar used as storing energy in the form of glycogen. Starch is polysaccharide.

Polysensory units Neurons that respond to more than one type of stimulus.

Polysomnogram The continuous and simultaneous recording of physiological variables during sleep.

Polysomnography The all night recording of a variety of physiologic parameters (e.g. brain waves, eye movements, muscle tones, respiration, heart rate, penile tumescence) in order to diagnose sleep-related disorders.

Polyspermy The fertilization of the oocyte by more than one sperm.

Polysulfide It is an impression material supplied in two tubes.

One containing the base paste and the other containing the catalyst past. Both tubes contain the liquid polysulfide polymer.

Polytocous Producing more than one offspring at a time.

Polytropic Affecting many kinds of bacteria or many varieties of tissues.

Polyunsaturated fat A fatty acid that contains more than one double covalent bond between its carbon atoms; abundant in triglycerides of corn oil, sunflower oil, and cottonseed oil.

Polyunsaturated fatty acid (PUFA) A fatty acid containing one or more double bonds on the carbon chain.

Polyuria Production of an excessive amounts of urine.

Ponderal index The ratio of a person's height to the cube root of that person's weight.

Pons The part of the brainstem between the medulla oblongata and midbrain; contains relays between the cerebrum and cerebellum, as well as ascending and descending tracts.

Pontic An artificial tooth, usually made of metal, ceramic, or plastic, that is supported by a bridge to replace missing dentition.

Pontine sleep A phase of sleep during which dreaming takes place. Name is based on the pons' involvement in this phase of sleep. Also known as dream state.

Poor Posture Is a faulty relationship of the various part of the body which produces increased strain on supporting structures and in which there is less eficient balance of the body over its base of support.

'oor posture—wheelchair The poor postural foundation of wheel chair sling seat causes the

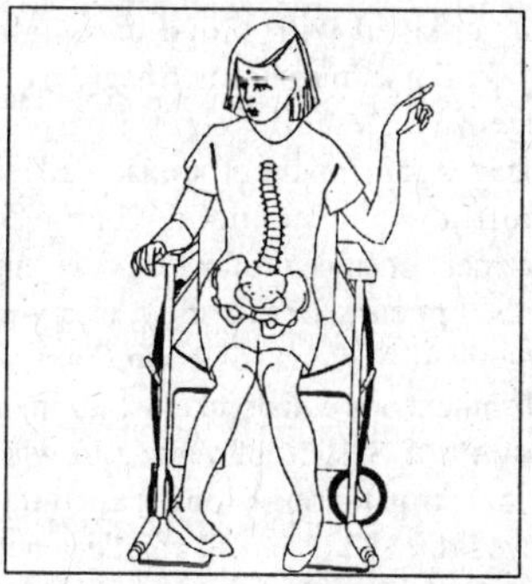

pelvis to lean to one side or the other, creating neck and trunk asymmetries. The legs are often internally rotated and fall into centre.

'OP Finger Splint For each finger, a piece of quick drying POP circular bandage 5 centimeters wide and 14-18 long is needed.

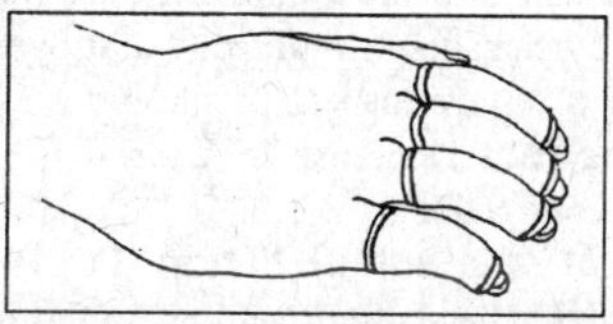

'op smear To obtain specimen for diagnostic testing.

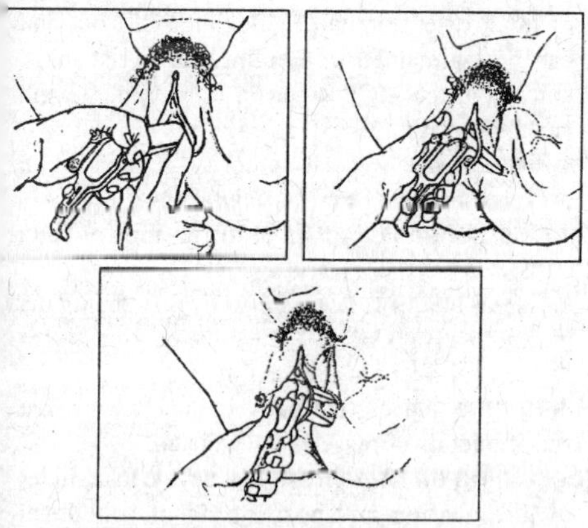

POP Thumb Splint Thumb splint should hold, the CMC joint in palmar abduction and opposition, MCP in palmar abduction and I.P. joint in extension POP must pass around the palm as well as around thumb.

Popcorn calcification Stippled calcification seen in chondrosarcoma.

Popliteal Behind the knee.

Popliteal line The fold or crease on posterior surface of knee joint.

Population A statistical concept that refers to all individuals or instances that theoretically could be available for study or measurement. Statistical inference involves generalising from the observation of some specified sample to the population. All the objects, events, or subjects in a particular class. For example, all the two-year-old babies in the United States comprise a population, and some babies from this group constitute a sample of the population.

Population attributable risk The risk in the total population minus the risk in the unexposed group.

Population genetics The discipline dealing with the biochemistry of inheritance.

Porcelain It is a specific type of ceremics. It may be crystalline or noncrystalline. It is very brittle, so they cannot be bent or deformed without cracking and breaking. They are used as insulators due to high melting points and low thermal and electrical conductivity.

Pore Pinpoint-size openings on the skin that are outlets of small ducts from the eccrine sweat glands.

Porencephalic cyst These represent fluid-filled cavities usually located in cerebral hemisphere. These develop in third trimester. It may be caused by intracranial haemorrhage, infarction, encephalitis and trauma. There may be mass effect and ventricular enlargement. There will be intracranial hypertension, head enlargement, seizures and neurological deficit. CT shows hypodense homogeneous sharply marginated non-enhancing lesion.

Pornolagnia An attraction to prostitutes as sexual objects.

Poroscopy The science of comparision and identification of friction Skin based on the placement, frequency and configuration of pores as they appear on the ridges. It is an extension of the process of identification based on minutiae.

Porosity An air bubble or void in a material.

Porous Characterised by pores and open spaces.

Porphin The parent compound of the porphyrins, a cyclic tetrapyrrole structure in which the pyrrole rings are connected by one-carbon methine groups.

Porphyria hepatica It is an inherited metabolic disorder in which there is an excess rather than a deficit of an enzyme hepatic ALA synthesis. Children are asymptomatic till they are exposed to the offending drugs or chemical agents. Colicky abdominal pain is the usual complaint. Patients may show evidence of polyneuritis and convulsions. Urine is colourless but later on darkens on standing. During acute attack urine is red.

Porphyrin Complex nitrogenous compound containing four substituted pyrroles covalently joined into a ring; often complexed with a central metal atom. A macrocyclic tetrapyrrole that has a conjugated double bond system conferring aromatic characteristics. In adults daily urine output is up to 0.1 mg and faeces up to 0.4 mg. In disease urine may contain 50-100 mg/daily. Actually in the synthesis of haemoglobin porphobilinogen forms porphyrins which with added iron produce haem; this links with globin to form haemoglobin. Less than 5 mg of porphyrin will not colour the urine. It is found in haemolytic and pernicious anaemia, so in liver disease. No symptoms arise from its presence.

Porphyrinogen A macrocyclic tetrapyrrole that is not aromatic because at least one of the links between adjacent pyrrole rings is saturated and the double bond conjugation system is interrupted.

Porridge A dish made of outer layer of wheat boiled in water or milk.

Port An aperture in a surface.

Port of entry Site where microorganisms find their way onto or into a host.

Portal hypertension There develops an increased blood pressure in the portal vein which carries blood from stomach, intestine and spleen to liver. The pressure in veins of upper stomach and lower oesophagus is raised causing oesophageal varices. The common cause of portal hypertension is the liver disease. Another cause is thrombosis in the vein. It may cause massive recurrent vomiting of blood and passing of black faeces. Ascites results in abdominal swelling and difficulty in breathing. Ultrasound is a reliable tool to diagnose.

Portal obstruction There will be flatulence dyspepsia, diarrhoea and constipation. Vomiting o mucus streaked with blood especially before breakfast. Sometimes haemorrhage may be due to enlarged anastomotic veins in lower end of oesophagus or in fundus of stomach. Bleeding from haemorrhoids is common. Congestion and enlargement of spleen follow. Ascites and oedema of legs appear. Urine may show albumin. Enlargement of veins of abdominal wall from establishment of a collateral circulation may occur.

Portal system System of vessels in which blood, after passing through one capillary bed, is conveyed through a second capillary network.

Portfolio test In consumer psychology, consumers are presented with a portfolio of advertisements, then tested for recall.

Portopulmonary shunting A potential complication of liver disease.

Portozoa One-celled organisms that are larger than bacteria and can infest human fluids and cause disease by parasitizing or directly destroying cells.

Portwine stain Permanent purple birth mark.

Poseiro effect Decrease in arterial BP during uterine contraction.

Position of safe immobiliation (POSI) is used immobilizing hand after fractures, strains or cruch injuries etc. It is important to use this position to prevent the common post traumatic contractures of MCP extension and IP flexion POSI of hand can be maintained in a splint with wrist in 30 extension, the MCP joints in maximum flexion and IP joints in full extension.

Position power Formal authority granted by an organization, as in high military rank.

Position sense Perception of the position of body parts.

Positional traction It is applied by positioning the patient in a way that will effect the relationship of the bony surfaces in the area treated.

Positioning Placing the body in such a way that specific joints of muscles are isolated.

Positioning stent A presurgical device that guides in the location and positioning of root form osteotomies.

Positive afterimage The brief continuation of a visual experience, especially the sensation of colour, after the stimulus has been removed.

Positive correlation A statistical concept indicating that increases in one variable are associated with increases in another variable; similarly decreases in the first variable are associated with decreases in the second. Among children of the same age, strength and exercise show a positive correlation. The more a child exercises the greater is the child's strength.

Positive effect Experiences high in the quality of joyfulness, happiness and cheerfulness.

Positive expiratory pressure mask A device used to increase the functional residual volume and enhance oxygenation in the treatment of some pulmonary disorders.

Positive feedback A feedback mechanism in which the response enhances the original stimulus.

Positive hit ratio An index of decision-making effectiveness; the number of successful applicants divided by the number of those selected by the procedure.

Positive induction Increased neural activity in a stimulated area due to preceding inhibition in neighboring areas.

Positive inotropic The property of being able to enhance the contractility of a muscle.

Positive predictive value The percentage of individuals identified by the test as positive who actually have the diagnosis.

Positive pressure Pressure, measured in mm Hg, that is greater than atmospheric pressure.

Positive pressure ventilation Mechanical ventilation that delivers compressed gas to the airways at greater than ambient pressure.

Positive reinforcement A procedure used to increase the frequency of a response by presenting a favorable consequence following the response.

Positive reinforcer A stimulus that increases the probability of a response.

Positive strand polarity An RNA molecule with a sequence able to be traslated by the cell's translational machinery, similar to a cellular mRNA.

Positivist criminology The study of the social causes of illegal behavior.

Positron emission tomography (PET) It permits examination of chemistry and metabolism in brain like stroke, dementia, epilepsy and mental disorder. One can know whether chemical or metabolic processes within brain might account for abnormal mental function and behaviour, including delusions, hallucination thoughts and behavioural disorders. It will be helpful in Alzheimer's disease and Parkinsonism. PET scanning of brain for oxygen and glucose metabolism can identify the site of epileptogenic focus which can be destroyed surgically. In patients with stroke PET can distinguish between reversible ischaemia and infarction. Quantitative imaging of hormone receptors by PET is equivalent to measurement of hormones in body fluids.

Possible diagnosis Problem that may be present, but more information is needed to rule out or confirm its existence.

Post and core Metal casting usually with a post in the canal or root, designed to retain an artificial crown.

Post dural puncture headache Headache occurring after dural puncture, spinal anaesthesia or lumbar puncture.

Post fix Meaning after.

Post hoc comparisons Tests that are used to make pair-wise comparisons of means after test has identified significant differences between more than two means.

Post mature baby A liveborn post mature infant is likely to show increased body length, hard skull bones, small fontanelles but child may be restless and alert.

Post operative After surgical procedure.

Post operative confusion It is very common while coming out of anesthesia. It may be due to hypotension and reduced cerebral blood flow, and metabolic disturbance.

Post operative dressing hallus valgus In it metarsal heads are firmly bound together with kling bandage and that great toe is rotated to keep sesamoids realigned beneath metatarsal head.

Post partum hemorrhage Primary symptom is abdominal discomfort or pain to which vaginal bleeding is secondary. Uterus is tender. Fetus can be palpated very well and may be alive or dead. Presenting part may be well down. Oliguria and albuminuria may develop.

Post streptococcal glomerulonephritis It is typically a sequlae of streptococcal throat developing 2-4 weeks after intial infection. Which recovers spontaneously. Clinical findings include oedema, proteinuria and oliguria.

Post term delivery Pregnancy prolonged more than 42 weeks of amenorrhoea. Post maturity is present when pregnancy is prolonged so far beyond term

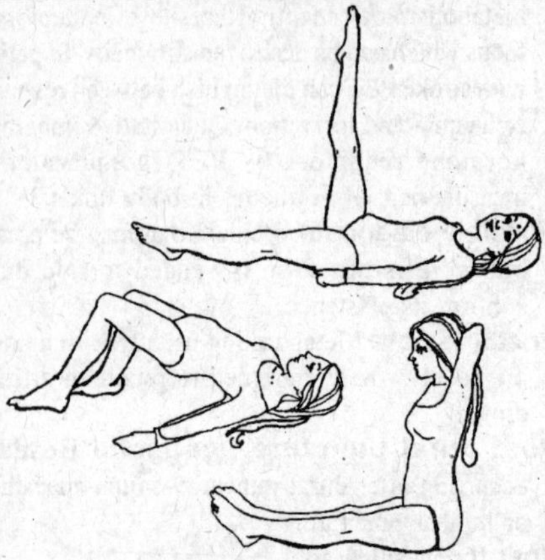

Post delivery exercise

that produces risk to fetus. It develops hypoglycemia and meconium is often present in liquor. At 42 weeks induction of labour is indicated.

Post term infant An infant born after 42 weeks of gestation.

Post traumatic distress disorder A psychological disorder that follows exposure to a traumatic event and is characterised by intrusive imagery sleep disturbances, poor memory and concentration.

Post traumatic stress disorder A psychological injury after violence, characterized by reexperiencing trauma, hyperarousal and withdrawl.

Postanesthesia care unit Area in the surgical department where patients are intensively monitored.

Post-burn contracture It is a contracture developing after burn. It occurs usually at junctional area, flexor aspects of the body involving nearby joint. It may be caused in case of deep burn involving the full thickness of skin where subcutaneous tissue is exposed. So healing does not take place by epithelialisation from the margins, but occurs by fibrous tissue which whe contracting leads to contracture. It may result i neglected cases of superficial burn which underg infections and ulcerations, the superficial burn i converted into a deep one and so heals by fibrosi Common sites of post burn contracture include neck, axilla, elbow, groin and knee. Early ski grafting prevents excessive scarring. It prevent infection.

Postanesthesia care unit Postsurgical recover area where clients are closely monitored an stabilized berfor discharge to a specific nursing uni or in the case of same day surgery to home.

Postcast cate Nursing interventions performed fo and with clients in casts or after cast removal.

Post-coital test A test of the cervical mucus withi 12 hours following intercourse. It permit evaluation of placement of spermatozoa, the qualit of cervical secretions, and their ability to suppor the life of spermatozoa.

Postcenetral gyrus Gyrus of cerebral corte located immediately posterior to the central sulcus contains the primary somatosensory area.

Posterioanterior view The image produced by the roentgen-ray beam as it passes through the patient from posterior to anterior.

Posterior That which follows; in humans, toward the back.

Posterior chamber The posterior chamber is a triangular space. The apex is formed by the edge of the iris which rests on lens. The base is formed by the ciliary processes and valleys in them. The posterior wall is formed by the anterior surface of the lens and anterior zonular fibres. The anterior wall is formed by the posterior surface of the iris.

Posterior circulation The vertebrobasal arterial system.

Posterior embryotoxon This is a congenital anomaly representing a grey white ring on the posterior surface of corneal periphery. Histologically, it is a hyaline protrusion at the border of Descemet's membrane and the trabecular meshwork.

Posterior fontanel A small, triangular fontanel between the occipital and parietal bones.

Posterior horn The posterior extension of spinal cord, grey matter; contains nerve cell bodies that receives input from primary sensory neurons and relay that input to the brain; also called the dorsal horn.

Posterior lumbotomy The patient is placed in lateral position, healthy side down and with 15 degree anterior rotation. Table breaks at the tip of 12th rib.

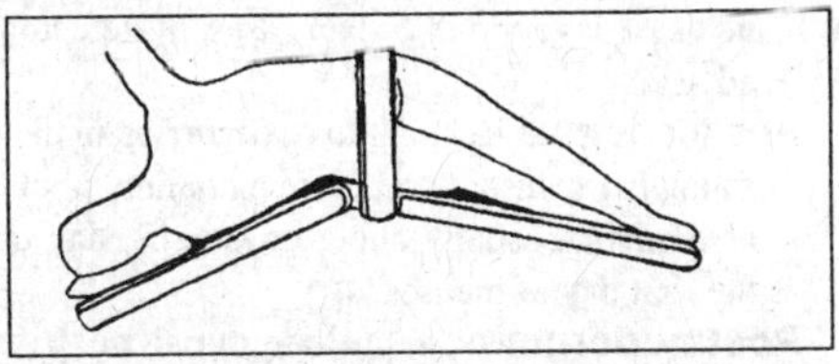

Posterior palatal seal Soft tissues along the junction of the hard and soft palates on which pressure within the physiologic limits of the tissues can be applied by a denture to aid in the retention of the denture.

Posterior pituitary The posterior portion of the pituitary gland, which consists of processes of nerve cells that have their cell bodies located in the hypothalamus; secretes oxytocin and antidiuretic hormone (ADH).

Posterior pituitary gland Known as neurohypophysis, site at which oxytocin and vasopressin are released in to general circulation.

Posterior probability Revised estimate of the probability of disease in a given patient following a diagnostic test or intervention.

Posterior pulmonary plexus A network of nerves formed by branches from the vagus nerves, the deep cardiac plexus and the second and fifth thoracic sympathetic ganglia, and the left recurrent laryngeal nerve supplying posterior branches of the bronchi and the pulmonary and bronchial vessels.

Posterior rhinoscopy mirror It consists of small circular plane mirror which is attached to the tip of a long, thin, angulated handle available in different sizes. Mirror is heated to avoid fogging. Patient is asked to open his mouth and tongue is depressed. The warmed mirror is passed behind uvula. Light is focussed on mirror and in reflected light structures can be visualised.

Posterior root An aggegation of sensory neurons fibers lying between a spinal nerve and the posterolateral aspect of the spinal cord; also called the dorsal root or sensory root.

Posterior root ganglion Ganglion located near the spinal cord; where the neuron cell body of the dendrites of the sensory neuron is located.

Posterior tibial pulse Pulse found between the malleolus and the Achilles tendon in the ankle.

Posterior tibial tendinitis The major job of posterior tibial muscle and tendon is to hold up the arch of foot. Tendon is attached to navicular bone. Athletes with flat foot put greater tension on the posterior tibial tendon and result in posterior

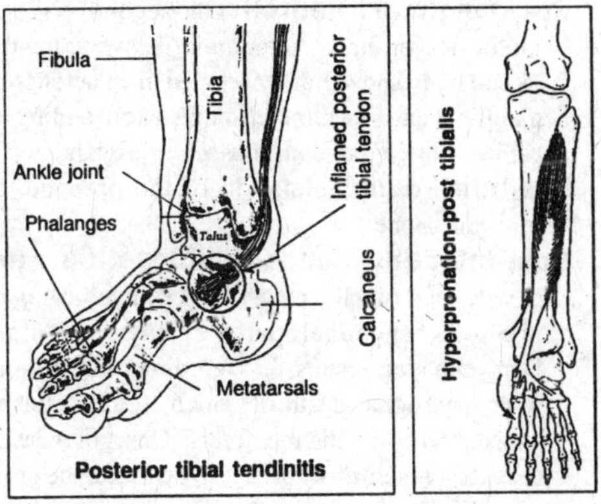

Posterior tibial tendinitis

tibial tendinitis. Posterior tibial tendinitis comes on gradually usually over 4 to 6 weeks. Pain is sharply localised at the tendon. It is tender. In such case one should stop exercise for 3 weeks. Posteromedial shin pain secondary to athletic overuse can indicate inflammatory microtrauma to the tendon of the posterior tibialis. Periosteal irritation and tibial stress reactions may also be suspected. Pain and swelling are present over the posteromedial crest of tibia along the origin of the postrior tibialis. Tenderness and crepitation may be found. Aetiology is excessive traction stress placed on posterior tibialis tendon with hyperpronation.

Posterm infant An infant born after 42 weeks of gestation.

Posterolateral herniation of disc Posterolateral herniation is the most frequent type of herniated disc often leading to compression or irritation of corresponding spinal root. It can compress the nerve root from either lateral or medial side. Bulging disc is due to merely an outward bulging of superficial fibres of the annulus fibrosus which are not broken. In herniated disc superficial fibres of annulus fibrosus are ruptured and nucleus pulposus is able to get exit and compromise the spinal nerve.

Postevent massage Massage provided after an athletic event.

Postganglionic Autonomic neurons whose cell bodies are located outside the central nervous system and receive synaptic stimulation from preganglionic autonomic neurons.

Postganglionic neuron The second visceral motor neuron in an autonomic pathway, having its cell body and dendrites located in an autonomic ganglion and its unmyelinated axon ending at cardiac muscle, smooth muscle, or a gland.

Posthitis An inflammation of the prepuce, or foreskin, alone.

Post-infectious encephalomyelitis After measles and rubella, a post viral demyelinating or allergic encephalopathy may develop. Demyelination results through direct infection of oligodendroglia, death of which would result in breakdown of myelin membrane. Onset of measles encephalomyelitis begins 2 to 7 days after the onset of rash. Alterations in conscious level, seizures, hemiparesis, ataxia and involuntary movements are frequent features. Neither hyper-immune 'g' globulin nor corticosteroid alter the course of post viral encephalitis. Mental retardation and late epilepsy are frequent residual features.

Postischemic Injury after decreased blood suply to a body organ or part.

Post-kala-azar dermal leishmaniasis It is a symptom or sequela of kala-azar caused by protozoa, *Leishmania Donovani*. Histopathologically subpapillary layer appears oedematous and vessels are enlarged, dilated and infiltrated with macrophages.

Condition gives rise to depigmented macules occurring on cheek, neck, legs. It may also produce erythematous patches on face. Skin lesions may show organisms or the LD bodies.

Postmaturity Overdevelopment, as of a postmature infant who was born after pregnancy has progressed beyond full term.

Post-menopausal bleeding Vaginal bleeding occurring anytime after six months of amenorrhoea in a women of menopause should be considered menopausal bleeding. Intermediate or prolonged use of unopposed oestrogen can cause post menopausal bleeding. Foreign body, cervical erosion, cervicitis senilis and tuberculous endometriosis, hypertension, malignancy of genital tract may give rise to postmenopausal bleeding. If no cause is found in certain cases, hysterectomy is advised.

Postmenstrual Relating to or occurring in the days following menses and before ovulation, in clinical assessments usually about days 6-12, day one is the first day of menses.

Postmodernism A philosophical position, it assumes that no definition, characteristic or attribute of something is fixed and invariant across either time or context.

Postmortem Occuring or performed after death; pertaining to the period after death.

Postmortem caloricity In it body temperature after death instead of coming down rises for an hour or two. It may happen in tetanus, cholera, rheumatic fever, liver abscess and injury to CNS. This rise of temperature is due to action of microorganism in living tissues and fluids of body and chemical changes after death.

When body instead of coming down to normal temperature after death shows a rise of temperature which persists for an hour or two. This may develop in cholera, tetanus, rheumatic fever or injury to CNS. Strychnine poisoning or CSF meningitis may develop it.

Postmortem care Care of the body after death.

Postmortem clots These are moist, smooth, rubbery, homogeneous, loosely or not at all attached to underlying wall.

These are of 2 types : (*i*) One, when blood clots rapidly a soft, lumpy, uniformly dark red slippery, moist red current jelly is formed, and (*ii*) when red cells sediment before blood coagulation starts a clot similar to first type at the bottom, and above this a pale or bright yellow layer of serum and fibrin is seen like chicken fat.

Postmortem interval The time interval between the date the individual was last seen, or death, and the date the remains of the body were recovered. This time interval is critical in many crime scenes when investigators are trying to establish the whereabouts of the accused at the time of the murder.

Postmortem stains Bright red stains in fair skin may mean poisoning by carbon monoxide or cyanide, dark chocolate ones are due to poisoning by one of methaemoglobin forming substances. Livid staining on face, neck and front of chest is usual in opium poisoning.

Postnatal After birth.

Postnatal period The period after birth and endings at death.

Postnecrotic cirrhosis Disease of any aetiology inexorably transforms a normal liver into patchwork of variably sized nodules alternating with broad septal scars. Most common cause is viral infection. Death is from usual complications of cirrhosis.

Postneonatal mortality rate Number of deaths between 28 days and one year of life per 1000 live birth.

Postoperative Occurring after operation; after surgery.

Postoperative care When the operation is over and patient returns from operation theatre, the post-operative care starts. Till the patient is unconscious never leave him unattended. Patient should be maintained in semiprone position. Tongue should not fall back.

Clean the throat. When the effect of anaesthesia passes off and he or she gains consciousness patient becomes restless and on occasion violent. He or she may try to remove bandage and drip, staff nurse has to take care. Never give any sedative or fluid and monitor vital signs.

Postoperative hypotension It may be due to reasons of cardiovascular, endocrine, respiratory and haemorrhage. The most common cause is hypovolaemia requiring infusion. Other causes may be injection of narcotic analgesic drug, vagal overactivity.

Postoperative jaundice This may be due to either a conjugated or an unconjugated hyperbilirubinaemia. Conjugated is more common and is possibly due to shock, septicaemia, type B hepatitis, phenothiazines, sulphonamides, erythromycin or halothane. Jaundice due to unconjugated fraction may result from haemolysis following transfusion.

This is asymptomatic and benign. It is associated with neither liver disease nor anaemia. Postoperative jaundice is likely to be due to bilirubin overload due to blood tranfusion.

Postoperative pain Pain relief is necessary for therapeutic reasons. Pain causes peripheral vasoconstriction and reduces sputum clearance. A severity of pain depends on site of operation, age, sex and premedication applied. Aspirin, phenylbutazone reduce skeletal pain and headache. These may not be given for longer time due to risk of papillary necrosis and interstitial nephritis and liver damage. Paracetamol is an active metabolite of phenacetin. It is analgesic and antipyretic and not anti-inflammatory. It inhibits prostaglandin synthesis within CNS. It does not cause gastric irritation and is relatively nontoxic in therapeutic doses. Five gram may be enough to cause hepatic necrosis.

Postoperative period Interval that begins after surgery is completed.

Postoperative shivering This can follow cyclopropane, ether, thiopentone, halothane or any combination of these, but is most common after halothane. It need not be due to heat loss and temperature remains near about normal. There is rise in metabolic rate with increased oxygen consumption upto 500% with increased cardiac work and fall in PaO_2. Intravenous pentazocine 30 mg and methylphenidate have been recommended. Diazepam 20 mg before operation is helpful.

Postoperative vomiting Vomiting may be central from causes acting on the brainstem and higher centres, peripheral from causes acting on gut and vestibule. It is mostly caused by chloroform, ether, cyclopropane, pethidine, trichloroethylene and halothane. Thipentone generally does not produce vomiting. Nitrous oxide and O_2 cause vomiting in 15% cases. Intradural and exradural blocks usually cause less vomiting. Hypoxia predisposes vomiting. Prolonged time and depth of anaesthesia are unfavourable factors. Vomiting is likely unless stomach is empty. Vomiting is most frequent after laparotomy and specially after operation on biliary tract.

Postoral Behind the mouth.

Postovulatory After ovulation; relating to or describing the events that follow expulsion of the oocyte from the follicle.

Post-papilloedematous optic atrophy Optic disc is greyish white or pale white in colour with markedly blurred margin and full physiological cup. Arteries become thin and retinal veins are full, tortuous and show a bend at the disc margin. There is degenerative change at macula. The vision is lost early and suddenly in a case of postneuritic optic atrophy while good vision is maintained for a long time in case of papilloedema.

Postpartum Term denoting first 6 weeks following child birth.

Postpartum blues Temporary, self limiting period of weepiness experienced by many new mothers within first few days after child birth.

Postpartum depression A term for a transient state of irritation, anxiety, restlessness, and tearfulness that occurs in the first few days after birth.

Postpartum estrus A condition in which a female ovulates and becomes sexually receptive immediately after parturition.

Postpartum psychosis Psychotic depression after childbirth, characterized by the loss of contact with reality, delusions, halluncinations, disorientation, sometimes anger, and possibly paranoia and strong aggressive feelings.

Postpartum thrombophlebitis It may manifest as pelvic thrombophlebitis. Puerperal infection of thrombosed veins at the placental site by pyogenic organism is primary origin of the condition. Then it spreads to uterine and ileofemoral veins. When veins of the uterine wall and broad ligament are involved the condition is called pelvic thrombophlebitis.

Postpartum traumatic neutritis Syndrome shows paralysis of some muscles of one or both legs with intense neuralgia and cramp like pains. If generally develops after labour.

Postperfusion syndrome The syndrome presents with fever, hepatitis, atypical lymphocytes in the peripheral blood, and occasional skin rash.

Post-phlebitis syndrome If deep vein thrombosis is not diagnosed in time and not treated properly, the surviving patient will have permanent damage of the vein with valvular destruction and incompetence. Permanent occlusion of femoral vein will lead to chronic swelling of leg, superficial varicose veins, eczema and gravitational ulcers.

Postpositivist The qualitative research tradition, resting on the assumption of multiple constructed realities.

Postprandial Describing the period after a meal.

Postraumatic amnesia Amnesia relating to events that occured after the trauma.

Postrotational nystagmus The nystagmus that occurs when rapid rotation of the body ceases.

Postsynaptic Situated distal to the synaptic cleft, as the postsynaptic neuron.

Postsynaptic inhibition The inhibition of a postsynaptic neurons by axon endings that release a neurotransmitter that incudes hyperpolarization (inhibitory postsynaptic potentials).

Postsynaptic neuron The nerve cell that is activated by the release of a neurotransmitter from another neuron and carries nerve impulses away from the synapse.

Postterm infant An infant born after the onset of 42nd week of pregnancy.

Posttranslational modification Covalent modification to a cellular component that occurs subsequent to its synthesis.

Posttraumatc amnesia State during the between injury and when the patient is able to memories on ongoing events.

Posttraumatic adjustment period The second reaction stage of adjustment to physical disablement or loss; this is usually the time during which psychologic effects of the traumatic experience are most felt by the patient.

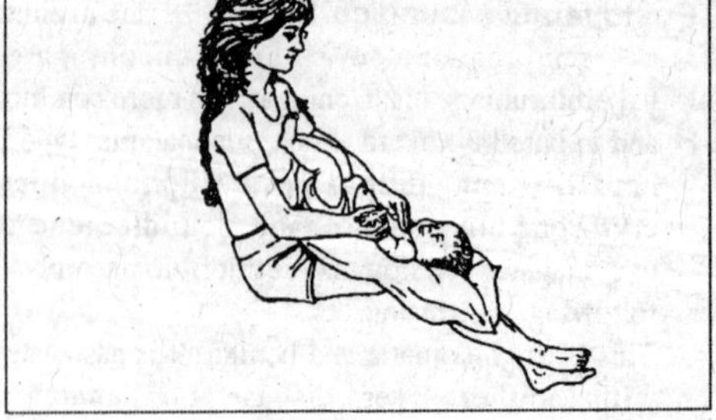

Posttraumatic epilepsy Seizure disorder following head trauma.

Posttraumatic stress disorder Psychopathologic reaction to a traumatic event; symptoms exhibited may include reexperiencing the traumatic event; numbing of responsiveness to, or reduced involvement with, the external world.

Postulate A fundamental assumption that does not require proof.

Postural Bowing is an apparent bowing that results from a combination of pronation of the feet, hyperextension of the knees, and medial rotation of the hips.

Postural (static) tremor Back-and-forth oscillatory movements of the body while patient maintains a standing posture.

Postural changes, old age With increasing years there are some common deviations from normal posture. In many elderly people there is an increase in thoracic kyphosis and associated flattening of

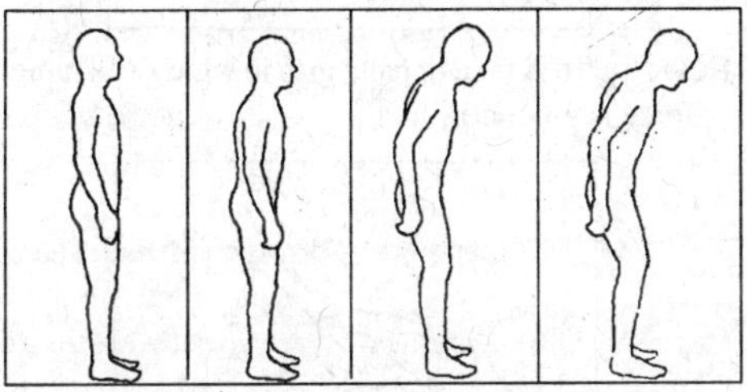

lumbar curve with posterior pelvic tilt or a compensatory increase in lumbar lordosis. The knee and hip joints become increasingly flexed and ankle joint is dorsiflexed.

Postural control The control, by skeletal muscles, of the relative positions of body parts with respect to gravity and to each other.

Postural drainage A means of clearing the airways of secretions by placing the patient in various positions so that gravity will assist in the flow of mucus.

Postural fixation Fixation of axial musculature prior to colunatry movement of a limb.

Postural hypotension Sudden but temporary drop in blood pressure when rising from a reclining position.

Postural muscles Muscles that support the body against gravity.

Postural reflex Any of a variety of tonic reactions or complex limb movements needed to support the body, shift weight, grasp objects, or maintain balance in a variety of situations, such as slipping on a floor.

Postural sway In standing there is continuous movement due to alternating action of antagonistic muscle groups resisting gravitational stresses,

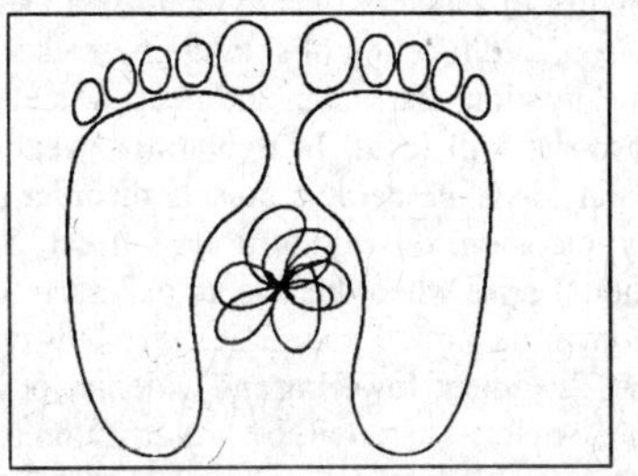

endeavouring to keep total centre of gravity of the body within body's base of support. This results in a slight anteroposterior swaying of the body approximately 4 cm. Postural sway would increase if the eyes are closed and the base of support is narrowed.

Posture Is a "position or attitude of the body, a relative arrangement of body parts for a specific activity or a characteristic manner of bearing the body". It may also be defined as a relative alignment of body segmetns in relation to each other and to the support suface.

Posture Position of the body, or the way in which it is held.

Postviral fatigue syndrome Chronic fatigue syndrome apparently triggered by a viral infection.

Postysnaptic inhibition Inhibition of a target neuron.

Potassium It is a mineral which with sodium and calcium maintains normal heart rhythm and regulates water balance. It is responsible for contraction of muscle and nerve impulses. Whole body contains about 140 gm of potassium. Whole grains, green leafy vegetables are good sources. Bananas and orange contain sufficient amount. Gastroenteritis results in hypokalaemia. Prolonged treatment with diuretic drugs and corticosteroids and excessive consumption of alcohol and coffee results in hypokalaemia. Symptoms of hypokalaemia include fatigue, drowsiness and muscle weakness. Excessive hyperkalaemia may result in numbness and tingling, muscle paralysis and heart failure.

Potassium depletion It results due to excessive loss from GIT, vomiting, diarrhoea and excessive loss in urine if diuresis is marked. Cirrhosis of liver, congestive cardiac failure, adrenal hyperactivity may result it. It results in clinical picture of lethargy, apathy, anorexia and nausea. Disordered function of smooth muscles may cause constipation, distension and ileus. Skeletal muscle disorder will result in hypotonia, weakness and paralysis while cardiac muscle disorder results in hypotension, dysrhythmia and arrest. Suspicion should arise when there is an excessive fluid loss from urinary or GI tract. ECG will show depression of ST segment, lowering and widening or inversion of T waves. There will be prolongation of PR and QT interval and appearance of U waves.

Potato It contains 70-80% water and gives about 300-380 kjoules or 70 to 90 calories per 100 gram. Protein content is 2 gm/100 gram but is of high biological value. Protein is tuberin. It is a good source of potassium. Vitamin C is 15-50 mg/100 gram.

Potency The ability of a male to obtain and maintain an erection and ejaculate.

Potential diagnosis Problem a patient is at risk for developing.

Potentiation Enchancement of one agent by another so that the combined effect is greater than the sum of the effects of each agent alone.

Potophobia Fear of drink.

Pott's fracture It is a serious fracture and dislocation of ankle. Tibia and fibula both may be fractured. Ankle ligament is teared. Treatment is to set broken bones and immobilisation.

Potter Buckey diaphragm A moving grid used to eliminate radiation scatter when X-Rays are taken.

Pouch An abdominal fold of skin around the mammary glands.

Pouches, perineal Perineal spaces.

Poultry All domestic birds used for human consumption such as chickens, ducks and pigeons.

Pounding Pounding is a movement is which the ulnar borders of the loosely clenched fists alternately and in rapid succession strike the part to be treated.

Poupart's ligament Inguinal ligament.

Pour resin It is poured into a processing mold made of agar hydrocolloid to form a denture base. Denture base made of these resins are processed quickly at room temperature.

Power Rate of performing work.

Power analysis Determination of the probability that a statistical test will result in the rejection of a null hypothesis that is false and should be rejected.

Power base chair Chair driven with the power of batteries.

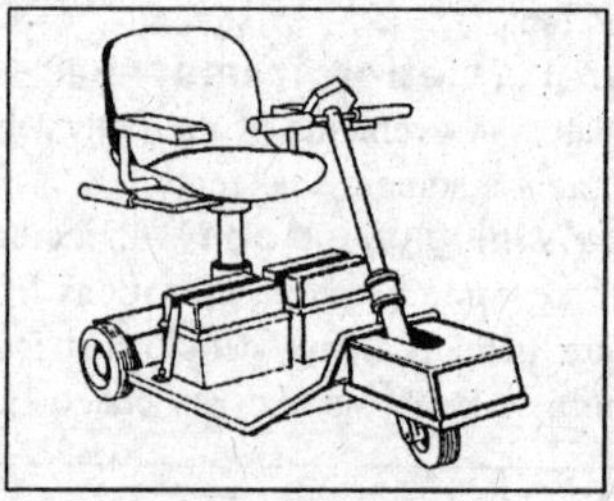

Power grip A type of hand grip in which a clamping force is produced.

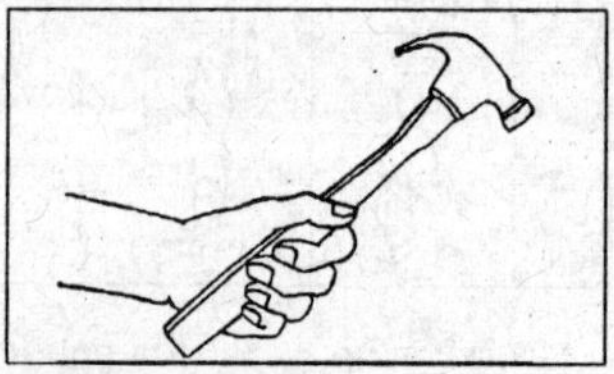

ppm- Parts per million.

Practical test A test that is relatively easy to perform and requires a minimum of equipment. One of the criteria for muscle length and strength tests.

Practice curve A graphic representation of progress in learning with trials plotted on the horizontal axis and successes or errors on the vertical axis.

Pragmatic language Those nonverval components of communication that influence the transmission of information.

Prana A term used in Ayurvedic medicine to represent life force energy.

Prandtl's Theorem When a fluid is flowing part of a body or surface, a layer of fluid can be seen adhacent to the surface and velocity of this fluid in relation to the surface is reduced so as to be non-existent. This region is called boundary layer.

Pratt's test It is a test for leg perforators. An elastic compression bandage is applied from toe to upper thigh which causes emptying of varicose veins. A tourniquet is then tied around the upper thigh above the bandage. Now tourniquet in position the bandage is unwinded in downward direction. Visible varix will develop over the site of constant leg perforator indicating incompetency of perforator.

Pravastatin An antihyperlipidemic agent; acts by inhibiting cholesterol synthesis.

Praxis The ability to conceive and plan a new motor act in response to an environmental demand.

Pre oxygenation Administration of 100% oxygen prior to induction of anesthesia. It increases the O_2 reserves in lungs and delays hypoaemia.

Prealbumin A plasma protein with a halflife of only 2 days used as a marker of nutritional status.

Precancerous It is condition which may lead to cancer. Ulcerative colitis in which there are no tumours but may lead to increased risk of malignant tumours. Secondly, there are benign tumours which tend to malignant themselves or are associated with development of malignant tumours elsewhere. Neurofibromatosis and tuberous sclerosis develop in brain. The third type comprises disorders like cancer cervix and leucoplakia of mouth and papillomas of bladder.

Precapillary sphincter A ring of smooth muscle fibers (cells) at the site of origin of true capillaries that regulate blood flow into true capillaries.

Precarious housing Substandard housing.

Precious metal A dental metal or alloy usually containing gold, platinum, or palladium or a combination of these noble and noncorroding metals.

Precipitate birth A birth that occurs without a trained attendant being present.

Precipitate delivery A delivery that occurs with undue rapidity (less than 3 hours) and usually without the benefit of asepsis.

Precipitate labour This may occur either spontaneously or due to oxytocic stimulation of uterus while inducing labour. It may be due to excessive force of uterine contractions and diminished resistance in the birth canal. Precipitate labour is unfavourable both to mother and fetus. Serious lacerations of cervix and perineum may occur and there is increased risk of shock, haemorrhage and sepsis. Fetus may develop brain injury. Oxytocin should be withdrawn immediately once the condition is recognised.

Precipitating factor Any factor which appears to cause a mental disorder, the most obviously disrupting event prior to emotional maladjustment. If an individual undergoes a divorce and shortly thereafter becomes seriously maladjusted, the divorce is said to be the precipitating factor. However, it is not necessarily, by itself, the reason for the disorder.

Precision The ability of an instrument to provide the same or a very similay result with repeted measurements.

Precision grip When an object needs to be manipulated in a finer type movement such as threading needle.

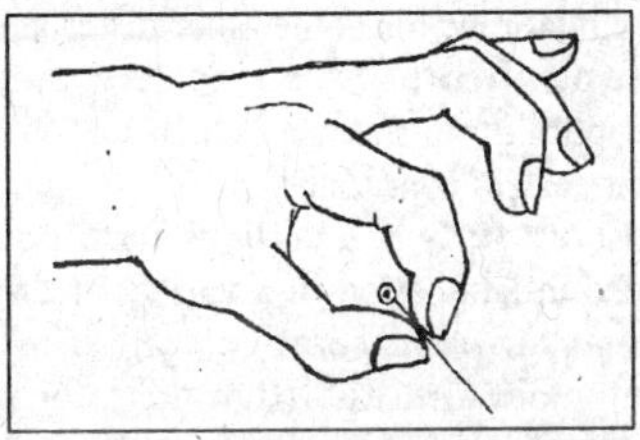

Precocial Relating to a relatively mature state at birth that requires minimal dependency on adult care, specifically, referring to a pattern of development in birds, in which the young can leave the nest shortly after hatching and are capable of feeding and thermoregulating largely independently.

Precocious Advanced in early sexual development.

Preconscious Thoughts that are not in immediate awareness but that can be recalled by conscious effort.

Precordial Of or pertaining to the precordium, which forms the region over the heart and the lower part of the thorax.

Precursor Chemical compounds which are converted in the body to useful chemicals.

Predental Preceding and preparing for the regular dental course of study, as predental education.

Predentin The soft fibrillar substance composing the primitive dentin and forming the narrow band of dentinal matrix immediately external to the layer of odontoblasts, in the inner layer of the circumpulpar dentin.

Predetermination Administrative procedure whereby a dentist submits a treatment plan to the carrier before treatment is initiated. Then the carrier returns the treatment plan, indicating the patient's eligibility, covered service amounts payable, application of appropriate deductibles, copayment factors, and maximum.

Prediction model A model, complete with coefficients, for use in predicting a particular outcome given the presence of a variety of independent variables.

Predictive theory A theory that is used to make predictions based on the relationships between variables.

Predisposing factors Circumstances conducive to maladjustment. If an individual has been phsycially ill and loses his job, the chances of emotional disturbances are increased. These conditions are called predisposing factors for they predispose the individual towards some other disturbance.

Predisposition A concealed but present susceptibility to disease, which may be activated under certain conditions.

Prednisolone It is a corticosteroid drug used to reduce inflammation in a variety of disorder like eczema, iritis, ulcerative colitis, asthma and rheumatoid arthritis. High doses or prolonged treatment may cause adverse effects like acne, hypertension, osteoporosis, diabetes and peptic ulcer. Corticosteroids are used to reduce inflammation.

Preeclampsia An abnormal condition of pregnancy characterized by high blood pressure, edema, and excessive protein in the urine; progression from this condition to eclampsia poses significant risk of fetal or maternal death.

Pre-eclamptic toxaemia It is a common hypertensive disorder of pregnancy. In hydatidiform moles, pre eclamptic features appear earlier. It is a disease of young primigravid women in later pregnancy. It covers those cases in which during pregnancy any 2 signs are present, hypertension, proteinuria and oedema. Hypertension and oedema are commonly found.

Preembryo The pluripotent dividing cells of the fertilized ovum prior to the beginning of cellular differentiation.

Prefilled cartridge Sealed glass cylinder of parenteral medication with a preattached needle.

Prefix A word element placed at the beginning of a root word to change the meaning of the word.

Preganglionic Autonomic neurons whose cell bodies are located in the central nervous system and that synapse with postganglionic neurons.

Preganglionic neuron The first visceral motor neuron in an autonomic pathway, with its cell body and dendrites in the brain or spinal cord and its myelinated axon ending at an autonomic ganglion, where it synapses with postganglionic neuron.

Pregenital In psychoanalysis, refers to the period of early childhood before the genitals have begun to exert the predominant influence in the organisation or patterning of sexual bahaviour. Oral and anal influences predominate during this period.

Pregnancy It is the period from conception to birth. Pregnancy begins with conception, fertilisation of ovum by a sperm and subsequent implantation of the egg. Smoking and alcohol should be avoided in pregnancy. During first trimester female develops vomiting, constipation, haemorrhoids and heart burn. During second trimester ankles swell and varicose veins may develop. Urinary tract infections are most common. Women may develop change in moods due to hormonal effects. Light exercise and sex can continue throughout pregnancy. Adopting different positions may make intercourse more comfortable.

Pregnancy tumour Hardly a few women during pregnancy develop gingivitis, tumour like growth on the gingiva which is identical to pyogenic granuloma. These are called pregnancy tumours developing in third month of pregnancy. These may regress automatically. Lesions are benign and excision after parturition is the treatment of choice.

Pregnancy, drugs Certain drugs taken during pregnancy may pass from the mother through the placenta to the developing baby. Drug treatment is to be weighed against the risk to the child. Smoking and alcohol both are harmful. Babies born to women who are IV drug abusers are at high risk of HIV. Certain drugs taken during late pregnancy may slow the rate at which baby grows. Tetracycline may affect developing teeth. Narcotic analgesics may cause breathing difficulty. Steroids can cause birth defects, specially cardiac malformations. Anti cancer drugs may result in abortion and metronidazole, diethylstilbesterol are suspicious of causing cancer.

Pregnancy-induced hypertension (PIH) A diagnostic label used to describe the syndrome of hypertension, edema, and proteinuria evident in certain pregnant women. Preeclampsia and eclampsia are two categories of PIH.

Prehallux A supernumerary bone of foot.

Prehension Prehensile related to the grasping and holding of an object.

Preiser's disease Osteonecrosis of navicular bone.

Prejudice A positive or negative attitude or opinion that is unsupported by evidence.

Preload Volume of blood that fills the heart and stretches the heart muscle fibers during its resting phase.

Premarital sex It has posed one of the thorniest social problem. Development of condom and other safe methods of contraception has brought more freedom to premarital sex. But adolescents may fail to take contraceptive measures or use them incorrectly. It may leave the young girl pregnant with the option of having an abortion, being rushed into marriage or becoming an unwanted unwed mother.

Premary intention Premary union of the edges of a wound, progressing to complete scar formation with granulation.

Premature atrial complex An extrasystole arising from an ectopic atrial focus that occurs before the usual or expected time of the normal depolarization wave.

Premature ejaculation It is not impotence but man ejaculates either before or immediately after interomission leaving his partner greatly unsatisfied. Erection takes place but ejaculation is almost instantaneously soon after the coitus begins. It is very irritating and unsatisfying to a woman specially.

Premature junctional complex An extrasystole arising from an ectopic atrioventricular nodal focus that occurs before the usual or expected time of the normal depolarization wave.

Premature labour This depends on the presence or absence of any cause that will interfere normal delivery. Baby weighing less than 2.5 kg, i.e. light for date is termed premature baby. Causes may be hydramnios, multiple pregnancies and cervical incompetence.

Premature ventricular complex An extrasystole arising from an ectopic ventricular focus that occurs before the usual or expected time of the normal depolarization wave.

Prematurity Early birth; usually clinically defined as a birth prior to 27 weeks of gestation.

Premaxilla The intermaxillary bone situated in front of the maxilla proper; carries the incisor teeth.

Premedication Its purpose is the administration of drugs to facilitate the induction and maintenance of and recovery from anaesthesia. Intramuscular sedative is given to reduce fear and anxiety before anaesthesia and operation. It reduces the amount of saliva and prevent undesirable reflexes, i.e. cardiac dysrhythmia due to drugs and afferent impulses. It helps in producing amnesia. The incidence of amnesia is low with opiate premedication. Opiate diazepam combination results in greater antegrade amnesia. But diazepamhyoscine combination is most effective though resulting in partial amnesia in only 25 % cases. With IV drugs amnesia is more prominent.

Premenstrual Referring to the days preceding the menstrual flow, usually about one week in clinical assessments, but symptomatic days may range from several days to two weeks.

Premenstrual magnification pattern (PMM) High severity symptoms of PMS, such as medical, psychiatric or other affective disorders, that occur during the postmenses phase and become worse during premenses.

Premenstrual syndrome This period begins after ovulation and takes place till periods start. It is a very common complaint. Imbalance between oestrogen and progesterone may be the cause. Similarly, deficiencies of vitamins E, B_6, magnesium or prostaglandin are suggested to be the cause. Symptoms of PMS include tension, irritability, depression and fatigue. There may be breast tenderness, fluid retention, backache and lower abdominal pain. Progesterone supplements are widely used.

Premorbid The functioning and condition of a patient prior to the present pathologic state; a reference point of the level of loss and deterioration.

Premunition A form of acquired immunity dependent upon retention of the infective agent.

Prenatal period The period after conception until birth.

Prenyltransferases A family of enzymes from different organisms involved in the synthesis of isoprenoid molecules by condensation of isoprene units.

Preoperational period The age from 18 months to approximately six or seven years; during this period, according to Piaget, the child's thinking tends to focus upon the most striking feature of an object or event, ignoring other aspects. The focus is upon states or conditions, rather than transformations or operations, hence the term preoperational thought.

Preoperative The period of time preceding induction of anesthesia and the beginning of a surgical procedure.

Preoperative assessment Generally anesthetist examines to exclude any chronic disease or disability which may be creating problem in performing surgery.

Preoperative checklist From that identifies the status of essential presurgical activities.

Preoperative medication Usually premedication having sedative effect is given 1 hour before operation. Combination of two drugs atropine and pethidine is used. Premedication helps the patient, the anaesthetist and the surgeon. After premedication patient should not go out of bed. He or she should lie comfortably.

Preoperative nursing care Nurse should tell relatives about nature of operation, approximate time taken, any postoperative requirement and requirement of blood if any. Psychological care includes morale boosting of patient to relieve his or her mental tension by feeding him certain information.

Patient should be assured. Nothing by mouth after midnight. Sedative if advised should be given at 9 PM. Nothing should be given by mouth. All jewelleries and false tooth should be got removed and recorded. Hearing aid should not be removed till the patient is anaesthetised and reinstated after becoming conscious.

Preparative period Time that starts when the patient is informed that surgery is necessary and ends when he or she is transported to the operating room.

Prepared childbirth The methods by which parents or partners actively participate in childbirth. Some approaches include the concepts and techniques of Dick-Read, Lamaze, and Bradley. Also called *natural childbirth*.

Prepartum Before parturition or birth.

Prepattelar bursitis An inflammation of bursa anterior to patella.

Prepolymerized resin fillers A reinforcing particle made from polymer and silica added to microfill composites to increase filler content.

Preprandial Before a meal.

Preprotein A term for a protein bearing a signal peptide prior to maturation by signal peptidase.

Prepubertal Before puberty.

Prepuberty Beginning sexual development.

Prepuce It is a foreskin consisting of skin tapering and covering the glans penis.

Glands on its inner surface secretes lubricating material. Removal of prepuce is known as circumcision.

Preputial ring The ring-like opening formed by the prepuce at the tip of the penis.

Preputial space The space between the glans penis and prepuce.

Presby (Gr. presbys old) A combining form meaning old or denoting relationship to old age.

Presbycusis It refers not only to the physiologic sensorineural hearing loss and the neural and central deterioration of old age but may be caused by cardiovascular and metabolic disorder. Marked initially by poor speech and later speech becomes disorted.

The acuity of hearing tends to show progressive impairment with advancing years. Person after the age of 65 develops some hearing loss of high tones. Typically the patient is either too intolerant of amplification or confused by multiple sounds or has difficulty in understanding speech.

This affects increased amplification in hearing aid. It is not correct that person will hear better if shouted at. More rewarding will be to speak in a normal articulated voice close to patient's ear.

Presbyopia It is a condition in which the near point of the emmetropic eye has receded so far away that it becomes uncomfortable to read or doing near working distance. It is an anomaly of accommodation and not the error of refraction.

Prescribe To designate or recommend a remedy for administration; to direct in writing the dosage, preparation and dispensing of a remedy or drug.

Prescription It is a written instruction from a doctor mentioning drug potency, dose and any special method of taking or applying it to pharmacist or medical drug dealer.

Presentation Term used to designate that part of the fetus nearest the internal os, or that part felt by the examiner's hand when doing the vaginal examination.

Presentation of fetus Normal presentation is occiput presentation and breech presentation is much less common. There will be face presentation

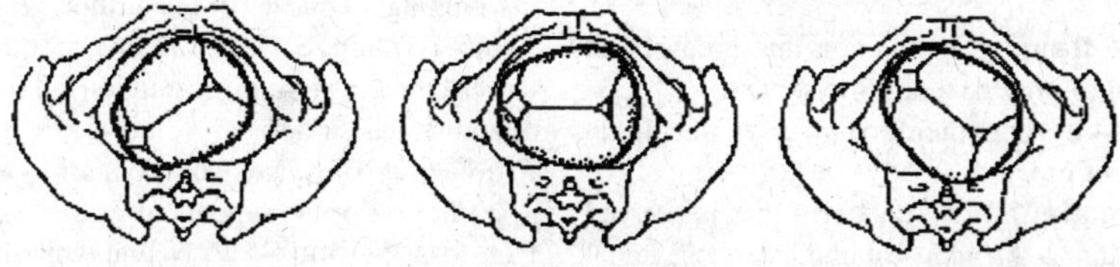

Left occipitoanterior — Left occipitotransverse — Left occipitoposterior

Left position in occiput presentations, with fetal head viewed from below.

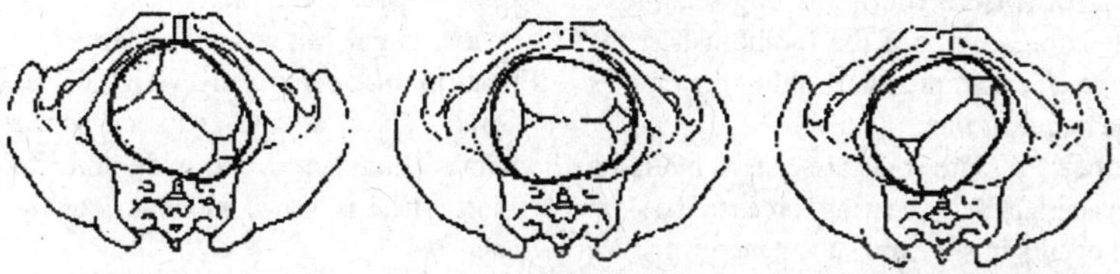

Right occipitoanterior — Right occipitotransverse — Right occipitoposterior

Right positions in occiput presentations

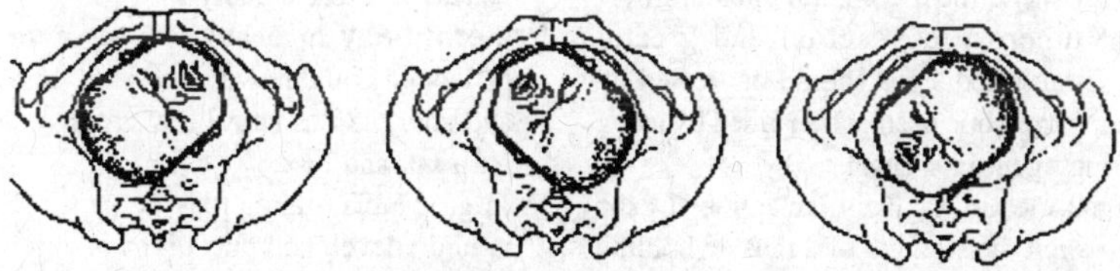

Left sacroanterior — Right sacroanterior — Right sacroposterior

Left and right positions in breech presentations

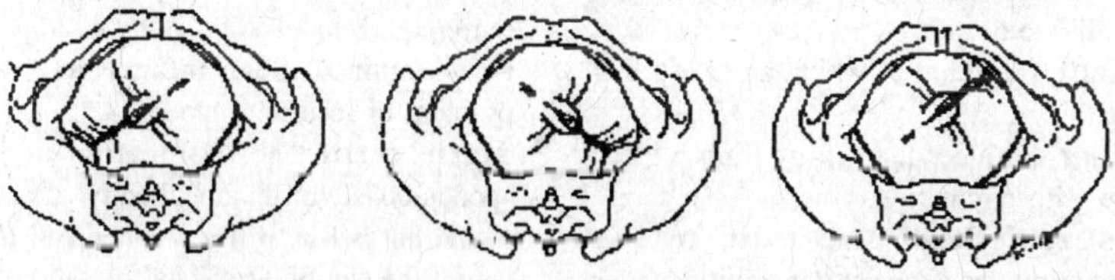

Left mentoanterior — Right mentoanterior — Right mentoposterior

Left and right positions in face presentations

too and each presentation is differently presented in different lie.

Presenting symptom Group of symptoms which patient complains to a physcian.

Preservative a chemical agent used to prevent microbial growth in finished products. It prevents their multiplication or kills them to prevent spoilage or contamination of the product with pathogens.

Preservice training Instruction that prepares an individual to provide a specific service.

Preset trays Armamentarium trays set up in sequence of use.

Press-fit implant 1. A root form that is pressed into position. 2. An endoseal implant whose initial recention is friction-dependent.

Pressor An agent that enhances vasomotor tone and increases blood pressure.

Press-roll technique Toothbrushing technique that involves placemnet of the toothbrush at the gingival line and with pressure rolling the bristles toward the occlusal line.

Pressue sores Pressure sores are caused by tissue hypoxia exacerbated by shearing forces to the skin. Ischaemia occurs in skin and subcutaneous tissues if the local pressure exceeds capillary perfusion. Frequent minor shifts in body position ensures that no area is hypoxic for a sufficient time to cause tissue necrosis. The most common sites are over the ischial tuberosities, sacrum and greater trochanter. Established sores should be treated by debridement of necrotic tissue often aided by using a desloughing agent like eusol.

Pressure In muscle testing, the force applied by the examiner to elicit the strength of a muscle holding in test position. Pertains to muscles grading fair +(6) or better.

Pressure coning Displacement of the cerebellar tonsils into the foramen magnum with compression of the medulla oblongata.

Pressure point The point at which an artery lies over a bone.

Pressure ulcer An ulcer that forms from a local interference with circulation.

Pressured speech Rapid, accelerated, frenzied speech. Sometimes it exceeds the ability of the vocal musculature to articulate, leading to jumbled and cluttered speech; at other times it exceeds the ability of the listener to comprehend as the speech expresses a flight of ideas (as in mania) or an unintelligible jargon.

Presthesis an artificial replacment for a missing part of the body.

Presumptive signs of pregnancy Signs that strongly suggest that a healthy woman is pregnant. These include menstrual suppression, nausea, vomiting, frequency of micturition, tenderness and other changes of breasts, "quickening," Chadwick's sign, pigmentation of the skin, and abdominal striae.

Pre-Swing The phase from heel off to when the toe pushes off of the support surface.

Presynaptic inhibition Neural inhibition in which axoaxonic synapses inhibit the release of neurotransmitter chemicals from the presynaptic axon terminal.

Presynaptic neuron A neuron that propagates nerve impulses toward a synapse.

Preterm babies Mostly weight is less than 2500 gram. The head and abdomen appear larger than limbs. Fontanelles are wide and skull bones are soft. There is loss of subcutaneous fat. Skin is thin and red.

Baby may appear jaundiced. Plantar creases are not visible before 34 weeks. Swallowing reflex is poor. Respiration is irregular and shallow. Baby is listless and reacts badly to feeding.

Preterm baby In many cases cause for early onset of labour is unknown. The skin of baby is tight and shiny. Soles show few creases and fine hair on trunk and face.

In girls labia minora may be gaped. Ear cartilage is underdeveloped and pinna is thin and floppy. There will be immaturity of nervous system. There is very little tone of muscles and child adopts a flexed posture.

Pupil reaction to light may be sluggish. This infant may require incubators. Baby's temperature is to be maintained. Such infants may develop the problem of recurrent apnoea.

Preterm birth The termination of pregnancy, spontaneously or therapeutically, after the fetus is viable but before it has attained full term, that is before the end of 37 weeks' gestation.

Preterm labour It is defined as one when a baby is born before 37 weeks of gestation calculated from the onset of last menstrual period. Most of the preterm babies weigh 2,500 grams or less.

Pretest Early use of a test solely for the purposes of evaluating that test, determining its strengths and weaknesses, and identifying the items which need to be eliminated or improved. Also, the use of a test to establish the initial performance of a group of subjects, before any programme or treatment has been introduced.

Pretragal Situated in front of the tragus.

Pretrial questioning Before a trial, asking the witness about the events in question, about a police line-up, or about the views of attorneys. It has been shown that pretrial questioning can prompt inaccurate recall on the part of witnesses.

Prevalence The number of persons in a defined population who have a specified disease or condition at a point in time, usually the time a survey is done.

Prevalence rate The proportio of persons with a defined disease or conidition at the time they are studied. This is not truly a rate, although it is conventionally referred to as one.

Prevention (1) Primary: focuses on preventing the occurrence of health problems; (2) secondary: designed to identify and treat health problems early: (3) tertiary; aimed at correcting health problems and preventing further deterioration.

Prevention (preventive psychiatry) In traditional medical usage, the prevention or prophylaxis of a disorder. In community psychiatry, the meaning of prevention encompasses the amelioration, control, and limitation of disease.

Preventive medicine A medical specialty emphasizing practives that help individuals and populations promote and preserve health and avoid in jury and illness.

Preventive mental health A movement aimed at providing assistance when individuals first experience maladjustment. The goal is to avoid emotional disorders or at least to treat them before they become serious.

Preventive resin restoration A restoration placed when there is a small occlusal lesion of a molar or premolar; caries is removed , and a small composite filling is placed and then sealed with a pit and fissure sealant by using the acidetch procedure.

Prevocational evaluation Testing of activities of daily living, learning abilities, and physical capacities needed to begin job training to earn a living.

Priapism It is an important circulatory disorder of penis characterised by persistent painful erection without sexual arousal. Disease is characterised by venous outflow obstruction involving both corpora cavernosa. This may lead impotency.

Prickly heat It is an irritating skin pinpoint rashes associated with profuse sweating. These are itchy spots on waist, upper trunk, armpits, etc. Mechanism of development of prickly heat is not fully understood. Sweat ducts may be blocked with debris. Frequent cool shower and sponging help. Irritating cheap soaps may not be used.

Prima Facie When all the necessary elements of a valid cause of action are alleged to exist. Once the plaintiff has established a prima facie case, the defendant will lose unless he or she can rebut one or more elements of the case.

Primal scene In psychoanalytic theory, the real or fancied observation by the infant of parental or other heterosexual intercourse.

Primaquine Half-life is 6 hours. It acts at several stages in the development of plasmodial parasite by interfering with its mitochondrial function. Its effect is to eliminate the hepatic forms of *Plasmodium vivax* and *P. ovale*. It is well absorbed from GIT. Adverse effects include nausea, abdominal cramps and haemolytic anaemia.

Primary Initial or first.

Primary acid-base disorder A disturbance of the normal acid-base balance to which other complications are attributable.

Primary acquired cholesteatoma If cholesteatoma is to be formed there must be a matrix of squamous epithelium from which to derive the squamous debris. The gradual accumulation of squamous debris in the invaginated pockets of pars flaccida is associated with gradual expansion of cholesteatoma. As it expands it causes erosion of bony walls. Principal symptom is chronic purulent otorrhoea. Some conductive deafness is inevitable.

Primary amyloidosis In it deposits of amyloid occur without any apparent cause. Usual affected sites include tongue, gingiva, heart and skin.

Tongue is involved in 50 per cent of cases. Tongue becomes enlarged and smooth. It may appear browny and indurated. Lateral borders of tongue are scalloped and focal amyloid deposits look yellow nodules. Infiltration of mucosa and gingiva becomes nodular. Treatment is conservative but may recur.

Primary antibody The antibody used to measure the concentration of ligand in biological samples.

Primary appraisal Where the person estimates the degree to which a particular event is a threat to their personal goal.

Primary bone callus First stage of fracture healing is formation of fibrous or temporary callus, i.e. inflammation, organisation of clot and removal of cellular debris. In the next stage immature bone trabeculae are formed in the connective tissue of callus. Stage is known as primary bone callus. Primary callus is composed of immature bone and is radiolucent. Primary callus not only bind the broken ends but extend beyond the fracture line in all directions.

Primary bronchi The main bronchi arising from the bifurcation of the trachea; right and left.

Primary care The first health care worker or agency to assess a person with a health need.

Primary carier The plan covering the patient as the employee.

Primary consistency State to which a dental material is mixed to allow the material to achieve flow and act as a leuting agent.

Primary dentition Teeth that erupt first and are usually replaced by the permanent teeth.

Primary dressing A dressing that comes in direct contact with the wound bed.

Primary emotions The emotions which are universal and innate such as fear, anger, sadness, joy and disgust. See secondary emotions.

Primary erectile dysfunction Some persons may have never been able to obtain erection and maintain it with a sex partner although they may be able to do so during masturbation at other occasions.

This is referred as primary erectile dysfunction while the secondary form includes those whose erectile capacity with a partner was at one time adequate but became impaired at some later stage due to some disease or psychologically.

Primary follicles The follicles present at puberty; covered with granulosa cells.

Primary gain The relief from emotional conflict and the freedom from anxiety achieved by a defence mechanism.

Primary germ layer One of three layers of embryonic tissue, called ectoderm mesoderm, and endoderm, that gives rise to all tissues and organs of the body.

Primary habitual aborters Women who aborted three times and aborted again in fourth pregnancy are called primary habitual aborters.

Primary host In parasitism, the host organism on which the sexual part of the life-cycle occurs.

Primary hypertension A heterogeneous syndrome; multiple factors contibute to the elevated blood pressure, including cardiac output, systemic vascular resistance, and sodium balance.

Primary hypotonic uterine activity The uterine contractions are weak and frequent and intrauterine pressure will be below 50 mg Hg. Causes include over distension of uterus due to multiple pregnancies.

Primary illness One that develops independently of any other disease.

Primary infertility An existing condition of infertility with no prior history of conception.

Primary IV infusion set It consists of a bottle of solution, a regular tubing set, a needle and an IV stand to hold the bottle. It consists of the spike end which is inserted into bottle, the drip chamber,

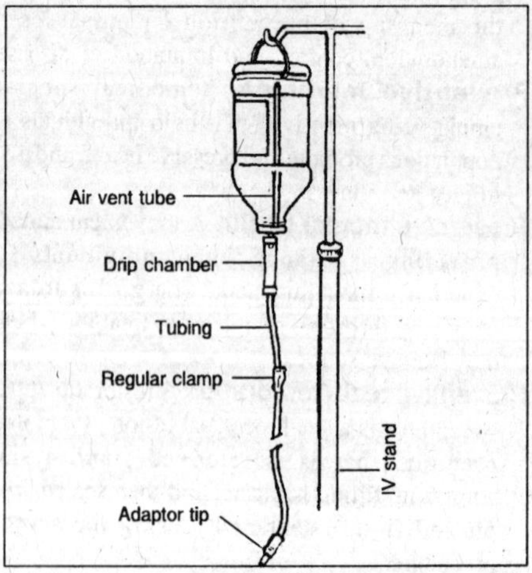

the tubing and a flow regulator or clamp. The spike and the needle adoptor at the end of tubing are covered with plastic protectors to keep them sterile. For blood transfusion it is generally not used because it requires a special set with a filter in drip chamber.

Primary mesothelioma These are most common in lungs but may affect peritoneum also. Asbestos may be an aetiological agent. Incubation period is very long.

Largely elderly males are involved. The symptoms are vague and non-specific. Major symptoms include abdominal pain and distension, anorexia and weight loss. Ultrasound may show peritoneal thickening and presence of free fluid. Prognosis is poor and person does not survive more than a year.

Primary metabolite Simple molecules and precursor compounds such as amino acids and organic acids that are involved in the pathways essential for life processes and the reproduction of cells.

Primary motives Any form of motivation which stem from the biological needs of the organism, such as the need for food, drink, and sleep.

Primary motor area A region of the cerebral cortex, in the precentral gyrus of the frontal lobe of the cerebrum, that controls specific muscles or groups of muscles.

Primary nursing Pattern in which the admitting nurse assumes responsibility for planning patient care and evaluating the progress of the patient.

Primary prevention Activities to avert the initial development of disease or poor health.

Programs that intervene with a population or setting to reduce the incidence and number of new cases.

Primary process In psychoanalytic theory, the generally unorganised mental activity characteristic of the unconsciousness. It is marked by the free discharge of energy and excitation without regard to the demands of environment, reality or logic.

Primary response Immune response that occurs as a result of the first exposure to an antigen; results in the production of antibodies and memory cells.

Primary sex characteristics The physiological features of the sex organs. A term for those characteristics that are essential for reproduction; i.e., the gonads and gametes.

Primary somatonsensory area A region of the cerebral cortex, posterior to the central sulcus in the postcentral gyrus of the parietal lobe of the cerebrum, that localizes exactly the points of the body where somatic sensations originate.

Primary spermatocyte Specialized cell that undergoes meiosis to ultimately form sperm.

Primary teeth These are known as milk teeth and appear at the age of six months and are gradually replaced by permanent teeth from about the age of 6 years. There are 20 primary teeth.

Primary tumor Tumor from which metastasis develops.

Primary virus pneumonia It occurs in epidemics. Onset is with dry paroxysmal cough, headache, muscle pains and a temperature of 101 to 103°F with a slow pulse and respiration rate. There may be pleuritic chest pain and some blood-streaked sputum. Temprature settles in 7 to 12 days but in more severe cases persist for 3 weeks.

Primary visual cortex The striate cortex (area 17;VI); it receives input from the lateral geniculate nucleus.

Primase An enzyme that catalyzes the formation of RNA oligonucleotides used as primers by DNA polymerases.

Primate space Diastema or gap in tooth row occasionally observed in primary dentition. Characteristic of almost all species of primate except man. Maxillary primate spaces accommodate mandibular canines and mandibular primate spaces accommodate maxillary canines when teeth are in occlusion. Reduced length of canines accompanied man's evolution, so canines no longer protruded beyond occlusal level and diastema was no longer functional.

Primates Vertebrates mammals with prehensile hands.

Prime mover The muscle directly responsible for producing a desired motion. Also called an agonist.

Primer effect A relatively long-lasting physiological response to a pheromone.

Primigravida A woman who is pregnant for the first time.

Priming A widely used measure of nondeclarative memory.

Primipara A woman who has given birth after a pregnancy of at least 20 weeks of gestation.

Primitive pulmonary vein The small venous conduit between the nonfunctioning lungs and the left atrium.

Primitive streak A shallow groove in the ectodermal surface of the embryonic disc; cell migrating through the streak becomes mesoderm.

Primordial cyst An epithelium lined sac containng fluid and appearing as a radiolucency in jaws.

Primordial dwarf Arrest of fetal growth during early embryonic life causes reduction in growth potential in the postnatal life. Children are slender with sharp features. Craniofacial disproportion is present. Bone age is normal or moderately delayed. There will be retardation of learning abilities in school.

Principal diagnosis The condition established after study to be chiefly responsible for the admission of the patient to the hospital or for outpatient treatment.

Principle cell Cell found in the parathyroid glands that secretes parathyroid hormone (PTH); cell type in the distal convoluted tubule and collecting duct of nephrons that is stimulated by aldosterone and antidiuretic hormone.

Principles Fundamental truths; rules; foundations.

PRIND Partially reversible ischemic neurologic deficits.

Prinzmetal's angina A form of angina that is not precipitated by cardiac exertion; generally is of longer duration, more severe, and associated with unusual ECG manifestations e.g., ST-segment elevation when compared with typical angina pectoris.

Prion The infectious agent that causes transmissible spongiform encephalopathies (TSEs). Prions do not contain informational nucleic acids. In 1996 Stanley B. Prusiner was awarded the Nobel Prize for Medicine for the hypothesis that prions consist of a modified form of the normal cellular protein called PrPc. Although the human forms of prion disease are rare, the recent epidemic of bovine spongiform encephalopathy dramatically raised the issue of transmissibility of these disease from affected animals to humans.

Prion disease Prion protein is the normal product of gene found in many organisms. It is bound to membranes. An abnormal form of prion protein is found is human brains with a variety of diseases. There may be neuronal loss, vacuolation of th cytoplasm, marked astrocytosis.

Prior art In patent law, the previous development in the field of an invention against which the novelty and non-obviousness of the invention are assessed, including prior developments that have been described, published, or otherwise disclosed publicly.

Prior probability The probability of dixease in a given patient that is esti9mated prior to the performance of laboratory or other tests and is based on the extimated prevalence of a particular disease among patients with similar sighs and symptoms.

Priority A first right established on emergency, need or choice.

Private practice Provision of occupational therapy services by an independent practitioner or group of practitioners.

Privilege A special legal status that prevents the privileged actor from being held legally liable for actions that would otherwise trigger liability.

Privileged communication A medical man in some cases disclose some professional secrets. It is done for the benefit of majority of people. Facts are written out and disclosed in an envelop on the top of which is written 'privileged communication'. Envelop is sent to proper authority.

Probate The judicial proceeding that determines the existence and validity of a will in the Probate Court.

Problem focussed coping Attempts to manage one's emotions during stressful periods.

Problem-oriented records Records organized according to the patient's health problems.

Procaine hydrochloride It is a local anesthetic agent introduced in 1904. It is less lipid solution than lingocaine with slow onset of mild anesthesia and shorter duration of action.

Procedural memory Memory for certain ways of doing things or for certain movements; this memory system is thought to be independent from declarative memory.

Procerus muscle A small slip of muscle originating as a continuation of the occipitofrontalis and attaching to the fascia covering the lower part of the nasal cartilage; muscle that wrinkles the skin of nose.

Process In anatomy, a marked prominence or projection of a bone. In dentistry, a series of operations that convert a wax pattern, such as that of a denture base, into a solid denture base of another material.

Process, odontoid Dens of axis.

Processing waxes These are used in bordering an impression tray. These have low melting point. These are generally coloured red. Boxing and utility waxes are hard and must be heated with a flame to be melted.

Proctology The branch of medicine that deals with the rectum and its disorders.

Proctolysis It is a fluid therapy by rectal route. Fluid is introduced drop by drop for a longer period. If the patient has lost more fluid it may retain 80 drops per minute. To start one cleansing enema is given to clean the rectal mucosa and for better absorption of fluid 5% glucose or hypotonic solution may be used.

Proctoscopy Different types of proctoscopes are available. The instrument after proper lubrication is carefully inserted using a gentle rotation into anus. The mucous membrane is inspected. It should be pink and glistening with thin rectal valves. Any ulceration, inflammation, polyp or tumour mass is noted and a biopsy taken. Haemorrhoids are recognised by asking the patient to strain and noting the presence of blue distended veins in 3,7, and 11 O' clock position. Anal fissure may be visualised but frequently it is not possible to undertake endoscopic examination unless patient is anaesthetised.

Proctotomy An incision into the wall of the rectum.

Prodromal Indicating the onset of a disease or morbid state.

Prodromal period Early or very beginning stage of an illness.

Prodrome A warning symptom indicating the onset of a disease.

Prodrug A drug that is given in an inactive form and thus has to be metabolized in the body to attain its active form.

Productive cough A cough that produces sputum or mucus.

Products In the structure-of-intellect model, a dimension which concerns the outcomes of intellectual activity. One outcome is classification, in which events are grouped, as in concept formation. Another involves systems, in which events are organised according to their function or operation. Overall, the products dimension concerns the result of the individual's intellectual efforts.

Proenzyme The inactive precursor of an enzyme; an enzyme that must be processed in order to exhibit catalytic activity.

Profession An occupation that requires training and specialized study.

Professional boundaries Limits seperating professional from personal relationship.

Professional misconduct It includes issuing certificates which are untrue, misleading or improper. One should not employ an unqualified assistant. Advertising or canvassing directly or indirectly to promote practice, accepting of professional bribe, involving in moral turpitude are all covered under misconduct.

Professional negligence It is a gross mistake made by a doctor while treating the patient. Doctors found guilty of professional negligence may be struck off the register of practitioners by medical council of country.

Professional secret Medical man is bound if asked by court to disclose secrets which have been confided to him professionally in connection with venereal disease, TB, etc. If medical man refuses he or she can be liable to be charged for contempt of court. Out of court doctor is not supposed to discuss and publicise patient's disease.

Professional touch Skilled touch delivered to achieve a specific outcome; the recipient in some way reimburses the professional for services rendered.

Professionalism The adherence to professional status, methods, standards and character.

Professorial position A standing posture in which the trunk is forward leaning, with the upper body supported on extended arms.

Progenitor cell A cell that is derived from a stem cell and acts as a precursor cell that migrates and produces a neuron or glial cell.

Progestagen A progesterone-like compound used to regulate reproductive activity.

Progesterone response element (PRE) A specific DNA sequence that is recognized and bound by the progesterone receptor.

Progestogen A progesterone derivative produced by the testis in vertebrates.

Progestomedin A factor that mediates the effects of progesterone.

Prognosis A forecasting of the probable course and termination of a disease and the response to treatment; the prospect of recovery from a disease as indicated by the nature and symptoms of the case.

Prognostic stratification Same as stratified allocation.

Program planning The process of designing an appropriate treatment program for a client.

Programmed approach A carefully prepared sequence of study materials. Common features include introducing new information on a step-by-step basis, requiring active participation by the learner, provision for immediate knowledge of results for the learner, and many opportunities for review.

Progress note Written or electronically recorded documentation of an individual's change in status or advancement toward goals.

Progressive bulbar palsy Rapidly lethal medullary variant of progressive muscular atrophy.

Progressive care units Units for patients who were once in critical condition but have recovered sufficiently to require less intensive nursing care.

Progressive multifocal leucoencephalopathy These are patients who are immunologically incompetent for any reason. It is caused by infection with a papova virus, a group of DNA virus. Multinucleated enlarged astrocytes are found in areas of focal demyelination. Initial signs are of foci of myelin destruction.

Personality change, cognitive impairment, hemiparesis, dysarthria and ataxia are found. Severe dementia follows. Headache and seizures are unusual. CT shows focal zones of decreased attenuation. They do not enhance after IV contrast. Disease is progressive and death may follow within 2 to 4 months.

Progressive relaxation Therapeutic exercise in which a person actively contracts and then relaxes muscle groups.

Progyny A form of sex differentiation in which all developing animals are at first female.

Prohormone A precursor of a hormone.

Projected blood pattern A bloodstain pattern that is produced by blood released under pressure as opposed to an impact, such an arterial spurting.

Projectile vomiting Vomiting that occurs with great force.

Projection A defence mechanism, operating unconsciously, in which what is emotionally unacceptable in the self is unconsciously rejected and attributed (projected) to others.

Projection areas Areas of the brain concerned with specific sensory and motor functions. Impulses from the sense organs are projected into the sensory areas of the brain; messages to the muscles are projected from the motor areas.

Projective tests Psychologic diagnostic tests in which the test material is unstructured so that any response will reflect a projection of some aspect of the subject's underlying personality and psychopathology.

Prokaryote A bacterium; a unicellular organism with a single chromosome, no nuclear envelope, and no membrane-bounded organelles.

Prokaryotic Generally, describing a cell whose DNA is not enclosed in a nuclear membrane, or an organism having this cellular feature.

Prolactin A hormone secreted by the pituitary that promotes lactation in the female and may stimulate testosterone secretion in the male. Prolactin secretion is in part controlled by inhibiting and releasing factors in the brain. Because dopamine is involved in the brain's inhibition of prolactin secretion, the measurement of serum prolactin has been proposed as a way of judging the efficacy of specific antipsychotic drugs that have been thought to act primarily by blocking dopamine's effects.

Prolactinoma These are micro-adenomas, diagnosed initially by serum prolactin above 2000 U/L. There will be delayed puberty or menstrual irregularities, galactorrhoea and infertility in women. It happens due to inhibition of secretion of luteinising hormone and blockade of the effects of gonadotrophins.

Prolapse Prolapse of small bowel through introitus is known as enterocele, of rectum is rectocele and of bladder cystocele.

Prolapse of cord When a loop of the cord slips the presenting part before the membranes rupture it is called presentation of cord, if descends after the rupture of membrane it is called prolapse of the cord. There is a serious threat to fetal life with prolapse.

Prolapse of disc during pregnancy It is caused by exaggerated lithotomy position used for forceps delivery. Disc prolapse is a flexon injury caused by exaggerated lithtotomy position. It may occur even in primigravida without any history of previous backache. Pain is felt in back of thigh.

Prolapse of gravid uterus Multiparity is an important cause. Under stretching of pelvic floor is an important contributing factor. Sudden prolapse of uterus can occur during pregnancy. Plastic ring pessary may be useful.

Prolapse of umbilical cord This is one of the emergency which calls for immediate delivery of child. In it loop of cord protrudes below the head of baby and appears in vagina, either inside the

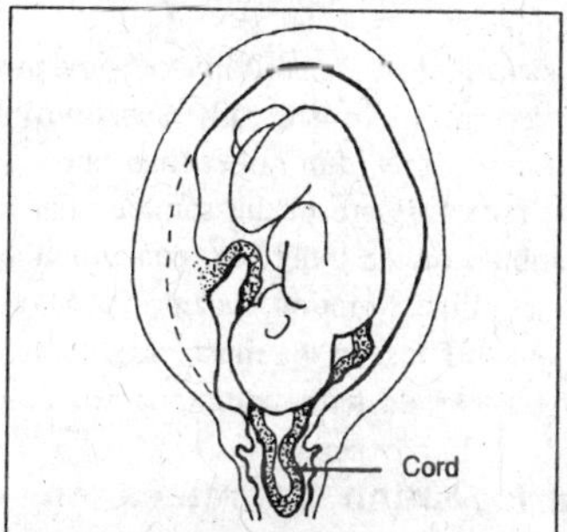

Cord prolapse

intact bag of membranes or if membranes have ruptured may be seen outside. If a loop of cord is below the head it will be compressed by the head and when head passes through pelvis during delivery it could cause sudden death by cutting off the supply of oxygen.

Proliferation Reproduction or multiplication of similar forms.

Proliferative retinopathy It develops due to 2 factors : vitreous haemorrhage and neovascularisation. Fibrous tissue proliferates into the vitreous. Neovascularisation is common in diabetes and Eales' disease. These new vessels have a tendency to bleed repeatedly causing vitreous haemorrhage. The neovascularisation arises from optic nerve head and along large retinal blood vessels. If not treated well it may lead to retinal detachment.

Prolonged latent phase of labour It is abnormal to exceed 20 hours in a primigravida or 14 hours in multigravida. Causes include unripe cervix, malposition, cephalopelvic disproportion and premature sedation.

Promastigate It occurs only in the insect vector and differs having elongated and long flagellum free anteriorly. Lone flagellum helps in locomotion.

Promethazine It is an antihistaminic drug used to relieve itching, urticaria and even in eczema. It may also be used in motion sickness and Meniere's disease. It has a sedative effect and may be used as a premedication and also during child birth.

Promiscuity A breeding pattern of multiple males mating with the same female.

Promontory Projecting process or eminence.

Promoter A sequence of DNA whose function is to be recognized by RNA polymerase in order to initiate the transcription of a particular gene. A typical E. Coli promoter, contains two conserved elements.

Pronate To turn the palm downward.

Pronation Rotation of the forearm, starting in the anatomical position, so that the anterior surface faces posteriorly.

Pronation and supination These movements occur at superior and inferior radioulnar joints. Pronation and supination are best assessed with the elbow flexed at 90°.

Pronator A muscle that pronates, that is, turns the hand palm posterior, starting in the anatomical position.

Prone Used to describe the body lying in a horizontal position facing downward.

Prone on elbows A position in which the individual lies on the stomach while propped on the elbows.

Prone on extended arms A position in which the individual lies on the stomach with the elbows straight and the weight on open hands.

Prone position The patient lies flat on bed with face downwards and hands kept folded over pillow.

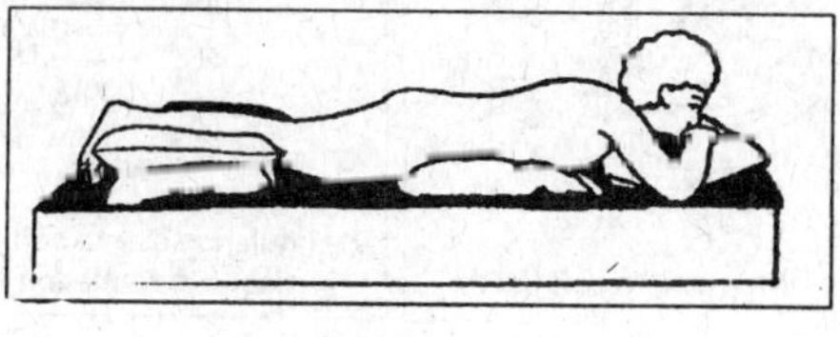

One pillow is given at head end for resting of chin and hands, one pillow under abdomen and one under legs. More or less no part of body rests on direct mattress. This position is useful in postoperative cases, operation over spine and tonsillitis. It prevents bed sores.

Pronucleus The haploid nucleus of a male spermatozoon or a female (egg) germ cell present in the fertilized egg before the male and female pronuclei fuse.

Pro-oxidant A substance which promotes oxidation.

Propagation The stage of an addition (free radical) polymerization reaction in which the polymer chain actually is formed , or propagated from the monomers.

Prophage A bacteriophage in an inactive state in which the genome is either integrated into the chromosome of the host cell or replicated autonomously. First stage of mitosis during which chromosomes become visible.

Prophetic religion A religioin which maintains that truth is revealed by prophecy.

Prophylacitic paste A paste containing polishing agents that is applied to teeth with a rubber cup and handpiece for cleaning purposes .

Prophylactic brace Brace used to prevent or reduce the severity of a joint injury.

Prophylactic knee braces These attempt to prevent or reduce severity of knee injuries, typically for a normal knee. These are of two basic designs. First is lateral bar with various hinge designs strapped to soft tissues and second is medial and lateral bars with plastic cuffs or straps. Many professional team uses these.

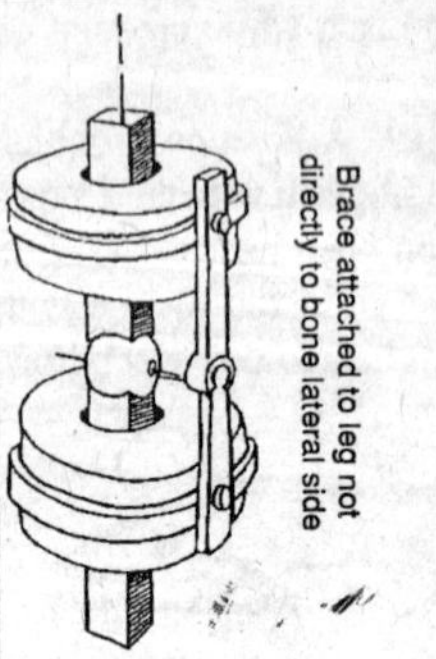

Strapped to soft tissue

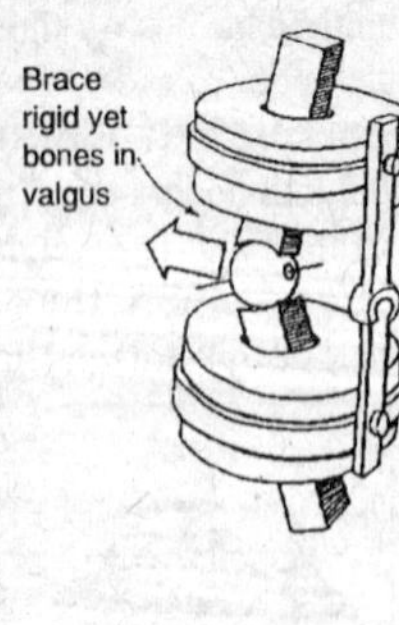

Angulation due to soft tissue deformation

Prophylactic odontomy Removal of precarious pits and fissures in posterior primary and permanent molars and their restoration with amalgam.

Prophylaxis The fact or process of preventing disease; efforts to prevent the spread of disease.

Proportion A fraction in which the numerator is a subset of the denominator; the formula is $a/a + b$.

Proportional hazards model A modification of multiple logistic regression to permit multivariable modeling of the data in a life table analysis.

Proportional hazards method A method used to testfor differences between Kaplan-Meier survival curves while controlling for other variables the method is also used to determine which cariables are associated with better survival.

Proposition A statement of the relationship between concepts. Sometimes used interchangeably with hypothesis.

Proprioception Sensitivity to body position and movement, more generally, sensitivity to stimuli coming from within rather than outside the body. The receptors are in the semicircular canals and vestibule of the inner ear, concerned with rotary and rectilinear motion, balance, and body position in space. Those in the muscles, tendons and joints are concerned with voluntary movement of the body and body parts.

Proprioception Exercises Are aimed at improving/restoring the sense of position and movement of the body, in particualr the limbs so that balance and co-ordination is optimized. The proprioceptive awareness can be enchanced by the use of rocker or balance activities, balls thrown and caught while balancing, jumping and landing from onto gradually more unstable surfaces, P.N.F. Patterns can also be used. Exercises with vision occluded place further demands on proprioceptive receptors and a better response can be achieved.

Proprioceptor A receptor located in muscles, tendons, or joints that provides information about body position and movements.

These are nerve endings which changes senses of events within the body. These transmit information to brain specially about coordinated voluntary movements.

Proptosis It is a passive protrusion of eyeball. Any space occupying lesion of orbit or oedema of orbital tissue pushes forward the eyeball resulting in proptosis. In pseudoproptosis there is no displacement of eyeball but eyeball itself is larger than normal eye giving an appearance of proptosis. It is seen in high axial myopia, buphthalmos. Orbital emphysema or orbital haemorrhage may result in acute proptosis.

Prosody The melody of speech; determined primarily by modifications of pitch, quality, strength, and duration, which are perceived primarily as stress and intonational patterns.

Prosopagnosia An inability to recognize faces or other visually ambiguous stimuli as being familiar and distinct from one another.

Prospective sohort study The investigator assembles the study groups in the present time on the basis of exposure, collects baseline data on them, and follows subjects over time for the outcomes of interest.

Prospective study Assessing predictor and outcome variables at some appropriate baseline and then reassessing outcome variables later in time.

Prostacyclin Prostaglandin PG 12 occurs in artery walls and inhibits the aggregation of blood platelets and formation of blood clots.

Prostaglandin It is a group of fatty acids made naturally in the body and acts in similar way as hormones. These were first discovered in semen but now have been isolated from uterus, brain and kidneys. These cause pain and inflammation in damaged tissue. These protects the lining of stomach and duodenum. Nonsteroidal anti-inflammatory drugs, such as aspirin relieve pain and inflammation by reducing prostaglandin production in tissues. Dimoprostone is E_2 prostaglandin used to stimulate contractions of the uterus for induction of labour.

Prostaglandins in termination of pregnancy Prostaglandins are a specialised group of hydroxyl fatty acids found in all mammalian tissues. Human semen is very rich in prostaglandins. E prostaglanduis is more potent than F prostaglandins. Prostaglandins have been shown to sensitize the uterus to oxytocin.

Prostate gland It is a solid, chestnut-shaped organ. It surrounds the first part of the urethra in male. It is situated under the bladder and in front of rectum. It produces secretions that form part of seminal

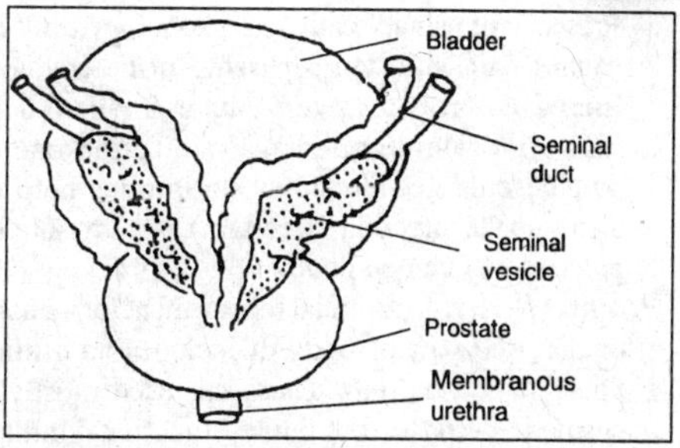

fluid during ejaculation. It weighs only a few grams at birth. Enlargement starts at puberty and at the age of 20 it is about 20 gm. In old age it further starts enlarging.

Prostatectomy Surgical removal of part or all of the prostate gland.

Prostatic abscess It is rare and results from inadequately treated bacterial prostatitis in elderly patient. Rectal examination reveals fluctuations and pain on palpation. It can spread to peristaltic tissue.

Prostatic carcinoma Incidence of it increases with age. In 95% of cases it develops in androgen-dependent peripheral glandular part of prostate. The prostatic capsule is a mechanical barrier. Beyond it, it may invade periprostatic and perirectal fat tissues, seminal vesicles, bladder floor and pelvic floor muscles. Lymphatic spread occurs through the periprostatic lymph plexus to the regional and juxtaregional lymph nodes. Haematogenous spread affects the skeleton. Lungs are mostly affected and liver rarely. Retroperitoneal lymph node metastases may cause urinary obstruction by encasing ureters.

Prostatic urethra The portion of the urethra that penetrates the prostate.

Prostatitis It is the inflammation of prostate gland mainly due to bacterial spread from urethra.

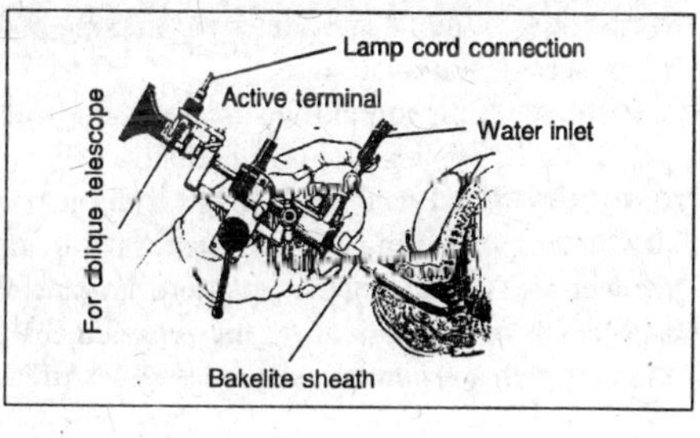

Presence of urinary catheterisation may result it. It causes pain and while passing urine frequency increases. It may even cause fever and pus discharge. Through rectal examination one can palpate enlarged prostate. Antibiotics help and clears up the infection. In certain cases transurethral prostectomy can be done.

Prosthesis It is an artificial replacement for a missing or diseased part of body. It includes an artificial upper or lower limb. These are used mostly for cosmetic purposes but limited functional utility is also there. Nowadays women use breast prosthesis after getting one breast removed due to cancer.

Prosthetic group A metal ion or an organic compound that is covalently bound to a protein and is essential to its activity.

Prosthetic sockets Sockets prescription should be specified by shape and material. Shape affects prosthetic suspension. Flexible sockets are made of soft, very pliable, thermoplastic material and are supported by a rigid carbon fibre enforced frame.

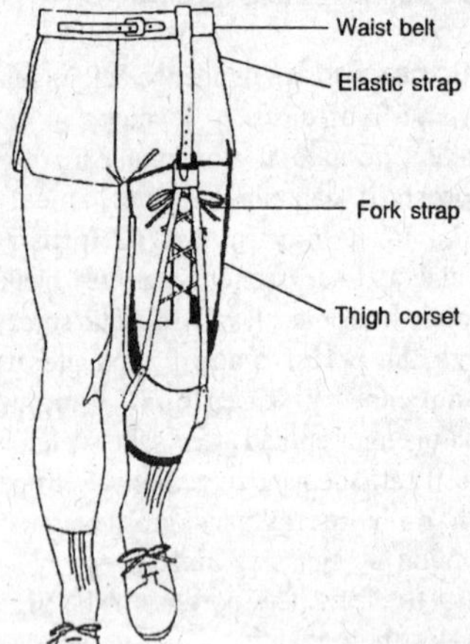

Prosthetic sockets

Prosthetics Artificial substitutes for missing body parts, such as artificial limbs.

Prosthetist A person skilled in prosthetics and practicing its application; prosthodontist.

Prosthodontics Prosthetic dentistry; the part of dentistry pertaining to the restoration and maintenance of oral function, comfort, appearance, and health of the patient by the replacement of missing teeth and contiguous tissues with artificial substitutes. Prosthodontics has three main branches; removable prosthodontics, fixed prosthodontics, and maxillofacial prosthetics.

Prosthodontics alloys These are comparable with gold alloys.

Prostitution Prostitution is the exchange of sex for money. The majority of prostitutes are women who sell their services to men. There are some men also who sale their body. This is an oldest profession of mankind.

Protease Protein-digesting enzyme.

Proteases Protein enzymes.

Protective muscle spasm A reflex muscle spasm by which nature "splints" or immobilizes a part to avoid movement that would cause further irritation of the injured structure.

Protective Sport Equipment This is a specifically designed equipment for a particular sport and specially indicated for protective function and used for prevention of sports injuries. The main features of such protective equipments are:

- To absorb and reduce the rate of transfer of energy as, in the high density foam rubber products that used in shoes, knee pads (volley ball) and thigh pads (foot ball) leg pads (circket) etc.
- The dispersion of impact injury, as in shin guards for soccer and hockey arm guards for cricket.
- The deflection of blows, as in helmets.
- The transmission of energy to other body parts, as in shin pads or in a baseball catcher's face mask.
- The protection of the face and eyes from penetrating equipment, as in fencing face masks and eye protectors in squash.
- The ability to limit excessive motions by mechanical or proprioceptive mechanisms, as in the use of sports tape, orthoses and braces.

Protective substance In freeze-drying procedures, smaller or larger molecular weight compounds that are dispersed into a suspension to protect biological materials from injury arising from freezing or drying.

Protein Nutrient composed of amino acids, chemical compounds made up to nitrogen, carbon, hydrogen, and oxygen. Upon burning one gram of protein in bomb calorimeter, 4 kcal energy in produced. Children have higher protein requirement as compared to adults. Growing children require 2 gm/kg proteins per day. While adults require half of that value

Protein complementation Combining plant sources of protein.

Protein efficiency ratio (PER) It is related to ratio between the gain in weight of weaning rats and the amount of protein consumed under the standardised condition provided that the concentration of protein in the diet is less than that required for maximal growth rate of animal. weight gain (gm) protein consumed (gm).

Protein enginerring The design, development, and production of new protein products having properties of commercial value.

Protein export The transport of proteins to extracytoplasmic compartments, including the exterior of the cell or to other cells.

Protein folding The process that newly synthesized polypeptides or denatured proteins produce functional conformation.

Protein hormone First messenger, provides communication between endocrine glands and target organs; triggers second messengers to affect the cell's activity.

Protein kinase C An intracellular serinetheonine kinase that catalyzes phosphorylation of intracellular proteins and alters their activities.

Protein losing enteropathy It refers to excessive, unselective loss of plasma proteins into the lumen of gastrointestinal tract. Despite compensatory increase in synthesis this is insufficient to keep pace.

The fall in plasma levels is greatest for proteins with a slow turnover rate. Serum levels are low particulary for albumin and 1gG. Albumin is responsible for most of colloid osmotic pressure of plasma and hence oedema and sometimes serous effusions occur. It can occur in almost in any inflammatory or ulcerative disease of GIT and in addition in various hypersecretory states.

Protein targeting The process by which newly synthesized proteins are sorted and transported to their proper locations in the cell.

Proteins These help to form supporting and protective structures such as bone, cartilage, skin, nails and hair. These are needed for growth of body and consists of amino acids. Proteins are of two types : class I proteins which are derived from animals containing all amino acids, and class II proteins of vegetable source. But proper consumption of mixed vegetable proteins make it near about class I proteins. Daily requirement of protein for human adult is 1 gm per kg of body weight. Growing children, pregnant ladies and active sportsmen need 1.5 gm/kg of body weight. Lack of protein in children results in kwashiorkor while excess of proteins are utilised as a source of energy only.

Proteinuria The presence of urinary protein in concentrations greater than 0.3 g in 24 hour urine collection or in concentrations greater than 1g/L in a random urine collection on two or more occasions.

Proteinuria in toxemia 5 gram or 10 gram per litre in 24 hours is indicative of heavy protein loss. Generally albumin is present but when larger molecules of protein are present, it indicates greater damage to kidneys.

Proteobacteria A kingdom of bacteria divided into five groups based on their 16S ribosomal RNA sequences; a group of bacteria diverse in their morphology, physiology, and life patterns.

Proteoglycan Macromolecule consisting of numerous polysaccharides attached to a common protein core, attract and retain large amounts of water.

Proteoliposomes Membrane vesicals made in vitro by incorporating detergent-solubilized membrane proteins into artificial bilayer lipid vesicles liposomes.

Proteolytic An enzyme capable of digesting proteins or polypeptides.

Proteome A collective term for the entire protein content contained in an organism.

Proteomics The study of the protein complement, or proteome, of an organism.

Proteotoxic Condition resulting in the misfolding or damage of cellular proteins.

Prothoracic gland An endocrine gland in the prothorax of insects that produces ecdysteroids.

Prothrombic Clot forming.

Prothrombin It is a proenzyme of thrombin produced in liver.

Prothrombin activator A protein formed by clotting facts from damaged tissue cells and platelets; it converts prothrombin into thrombin, a step essential to forming a blood clot.

Protocols Standard procedures.

Proton A large positively charged particle found in the nucleus of an atom.

Proton donor The donor of a proton in an acid-base reaction; that is, an acid.

Proto-oncogene Gene responsible for some aspect of normal growth and development; it may transform into an oncogene, a gene capable of causing cancer.

Protopathic system Refers to nerve fibers that allow perception of crude, nondiscriminative, poorly localized sensations such as pain and temperature.

Protoplasm A general term for the colloidal complex of protein that constitutes the living material of a cell. It includes cytoplasm and nucleoplasm.

Protoscolex The immature scolex found in coenurus and hydatid larvae.

Prototype An original form or model on which later refinements are based.

Protozoa One celled animal.

Protozoan One of the protozoa, free-living, unicellular, eukaryotic organisms that posses motility.

Protracted descent Delayed descent of the fetal head in the active phase of labour.

Protraction The movement of a body part, such as the mandible, forward on a plane parallel with the ground the opposite of retraction.

Protrusive occlusion An occlusion of teeth existing when mandible is protruded forward from centric position.

Provirus The double-standard DNA replicative intermediate of a retroviral genome found integrated into the host chromosome.

Provitamin A precursor of a vitamin; a substance from which the animal organism can form vitamin.

Proxemics Relation of space to communication.

Proximal Used to describe the relative position of something that is nearer the attachment of a limb to the trunk or nearer to the point of origin or attachment.

Proximal convoluted tube The first segment of a renal tubule.

Proximal convoluted tubule Convoluted portion of the nephron that extends from Bowman's capsule to the descending limb of Henle's loop.

Proximal renal tubular acidosis In this capacity of the proximal tubules to reabsorb bicarbonate is decreased so that large amounts of bicarbonate are delivered to distal tubules. There becomes growth retardation. Some calcium is liberated from bone. Rickets and osteomalacia may occur.

Proximodistal Progression from center outward or from midline to periphery.

Prssure palsy Paralysis resulting from prolonged external pressure.

Prudent Sensible and careful.

Prudent daily intake Daily amount of micronutrient which result in desirable plasma levels.

Prune belly syndrome An absence of abdominal muscles that results in a flabby distended and creased abdomen. May occur in the infant exposed to cocaine in utero.

Pruritus It is a subjective manifestation. Generalised pruritus also occurs due to several drugs and diseases. It gives rise to itching, resulting from scratching and rubbing. Surface may show excoriated papules, fissures and elongated crusts along the scratch. Pruritus ani and pruritus vulvae give rise to a localised pruritus.

PSE Psychological stress evaluator.

Pseudarthrosis Persistent abnormal movement at a fracture site interfers with function of a limb. Fibrous tissue in an untreated fracture is usually painful when stressed. Occasionally, a very firm fibrous scar forms so that it becomes indistinguishable from bony union. Scar may even be containing a cavity like joint, hence it is known as pseudarthrosis.

Pseudo Prefix meaning false.

Pseudobulbar palsy It may be due to bilateral pyramidal degeneration of motor neuron disease or demyelination of axons in multiple sclerosis. It is also caused by bilateral lacunar infarctions in internal capsule. There will be brisk tendon reflexes and extensor plantar responses, Gait becomes hesitant and shuffle with short steps.

Pseudo-cyesis It is an embrassing psychosomatic manifestation. Pregnancy fantasies may be intense in infertile women while pregnancy phobia in young girls is common. A frequent relationship between false pregnancy and depression has been postulated.

Pseudodementia A syndrome in which dementia is mimicked or caricatured by functional psychiatric illness. Symptoms and responses to mental status examination questions are similar to those found in verified cases of dementia. In pseudodementia, the chief diagnosis to be considered in the differential is depression in an older person vs cognitive deterioration on the basis of organic brain disease.

Pseudogout Similar to gout clinically, but in this condition the synovitis is due to deposits of pyrophosphate crystals.

Pseudohermaphrodite An individual with some of the physical characteristics of both sexes, but who lacks functioning gonads of both sexes; a true hermaphrodite has both testes and ovaries.

Pseudohypertorophy The increase in the size of an organ due to an increase of some tissue other than itself.

Pseudomaturation Ooctye maturation during atresia.

Pseudomembranous colitis There is inflammation of large bowel characterized by diarrhoea, abdominal pain, fever, blood + mucus in stool. On occasion it may be life threatening. It is caused by toxins produced by C. difficile while on treatment with clindamycin.

Pseudomenstruation Vaginal bleeding in newborn due to withdrawal of placental hormones.

Pseudopods Footlike extensions of the cytoplasm that enable some cells (with amoeboid motion) to move across a substrate. Pseudopods are also used to surround food particles in the process of phagocytosis.

Pseudo-spondylolisthesis It is without spondylolisthesis It is without spondylolysis i.e. without a defect in pars interarticularis. It occurs more frequently between L_4 and L_5 while spondylolisthesis occurs between L_5 and S_1.

Pseudotumour cerebri Increased intracranial pressure due to cerebral oedema may mimic brain tumour. Disorder is generally idiopathic. It may be associated with withdrawal of corticosteroid therapy.

Symptoms are of increased intracranial pressure. Ventricles appear small due to surrounding cerebral oedema. Corticosteroid therapy reduces oedema.

Psilocybin A psychedelic drug obtained from the mushroom Psilocybe mexicana.

Psoas abscess Extraperitoneal abscess that follows the course of iliopsoas.

Psoas muscle This is a bigger muscle which bends the hip upwards towards chest. It is composed of psoas major and psoas minor. The lower end of psoas minor is attached to the margin of pelvis while lower end of psoas major is joined to the prominence just below the neck of femur. Sometimes abscess may be formed in this muscle. Spasm of psoas muscle may result in pain.

Psoas spasm The patient lies face down. The examiner presses the pelvis to the table with one hand and grabs the ankle with other and the leg is moved vertically with thigh partially flexed. If it instantly gives rise to muscular spasm and resistance it indicates disease of psoas muscle, surrounding soft tissue or of lumbar vertebrae.

Psoriasis It is a skin disease of unknown cause. It develops white scaly patches on the skin, elbow, knees, scalp and other areas. Disease is chronic and presents remissions and exacerbations. It may be accompanied by arthritis. Microscopically it shows hyperkeratsis, and parakeratosis. Immunologic studies reveal lgG in the keratinised layer.

Psoriatic arthritis Characteristic feature is destruction of interphalangeal joint. Resorption of tuft of terminal phalangeal is seen. Osteolysis may progress to destruction of most of distal phalanyx. Periostitis is common. Phallanyx becomes dense. Erosion of bone is often seen as irregular bony paint brush excrescences.

Psyche A term often used interchangeably with mind; signifies the total organ that controls behavior.

Psychedelic drug A drug that can alter sensory perception.

Psychiatry It is a branch of medicine which deals with study, prevention and treatment of mental diseases and behavioural and emotional problems while psychology deals with normal behaviour and normal mental process only. Psychiatrist approaches the understanding and treatment of mental illness and emotional problem considering social and physical state. It has now many branches as child and adolescent psychiatry, social and community psychiatry. A treatment for mental illness is based on psychoanalytic therapy. Psychoanalysis can help neurosis and personality disorder. The treatment includes interviews between trained analyst and patient lasting for hours. Patient is encouraged to talk as freely as possible.

Psychic masturbation It is a type of sexual gratification through erotic images and fantasies without physical manipulation, even without touching the erogenous zones.

Psychic vaginismus It is a painful vaginal spasm, severe enough to prevent sexual intercourse. It may result from inhibitions instilled by the parents, fear as being hurt or association of STDs and AIDS.

Psychoactive drug A drug that produces behavioral or congnitive changes as a result of its action on the brain.

Psychoanalysis A theory of the psychology of human development and behaviour, a method of research, and a system of psychotherapy, originally developed by Freud. Through analysis of free associations and interpretation of dreams, emotions and behaviour are traced to the influence of repressed instinctual drives and defences against them in the unconscious. Psychoanalytic treatment seeks to eliminate or diminish the undesirable effects of unconscious conflicts by making the analysand aware of their existence, origin, and inappropriate expression in current emotions and behaviour.

Psychoanalytic practice Application of psychotherapeutic method characterised by emphasis on free association, transference and interpretation.

Psychoative drugs Drugs that enter the brain, producing changes in mood and feelings. All abused drugs are considered to by psychoactive, typically resulting in mood states that are subjectively reported as pleasant or euphoric.

Psychobiology The study of the interactions between biological and psychological processes.

Psychodrama A form of group therapy to explore a patient's personality, make up, interpersonal relationship, conflicts and emotional problem.

Psychodynamics The systematised knowledge and theory of human behaviour and its motivation, the study of which depends largely upon the functional significance of emotion. Psychodynamics recognises the role of unconscious motivation in human behaviour. The science of psychodynamics assumes that one's behaviour is determined by past experience, genetic endowment, and current reality.

Psychoendocrinology The study of the psychological effects of neuroendocrinologic activity. For example, it is known that the release and inhibition of pituitary hormones are mediated in part by brain monoamines, disorders of which have have been implicated in the pathogenesis of various psychiatric illness.

Psychogenic abdominal pain Disturbed parent-child relationship, too rigid discipline and authoritarian attitude of parents, over protection, rejection and sibling rivalry may cause emotional and behavioural disturbance. These children may use abdominal pain as attention seeking device. Pain is not associated with distress, fever, vomiting or diarrhoea. Pain is localised vaguely.

Psychogenic disorder An illness that is attributable primarily to a psychological conflict or to emotional stress.

Psychogenic impotence If a person has morning erection but does not have erection during intercourse then be sure that such patient has impotence of psychogenic disorder. Impotence continues till coital anxiety and fear of failure is not removed. Such sexual dysfunction arises from a sexually noncongenital environment created by either or both of partners.

Psychogenic otalgia Ear pain like disturbances of hearing and balance may have a psychogenic cause. Symptoms do not correlate with any organic disease or to specific nerve distribution.

Psychogenic sexual stimuli Stimuli processed through the higher brain centres that cause sexual arousal. These include sensory stimuli such as sight, sound, taste, smell, and touch, and cognitive events such as thoughts, fantasies, memories, and images.

Psychological abuse Damage in primarily emotional including physical and social isolation, extreme jealously, deprivation, degradation and humiliation.

Psychological addiction Refers to a behavioral pattern of compulsive drug use, the securing of its supply and high tendency to relapse after withdrawl.

Psychological function Ability to use mental and affective resources effectively in response to the requirements of a particular situation.

Psychological stress An emotional state of anxiety and hyper excitation that may have various origins and varies in its intensity.

Psychologist Usually, an individual who has completed a programme of graduate study in psychology and is engaged in research, clinical treatment, teaching, or other applications of psychology.

In most states, persons in private practice who call themselves psychologists must be certified or licensed by law.

Psychology The study of human behaviour.

Psychometrics The theory or technique of psychological measurement; the measurement of psychological differences among people and the statistical analysis of those differences.

Psychometry The science of testing and measuring mental and psychologic ability, efficiency potentials, and functioning, including psychopathologic components.

Psychomotor activation Increased behavioral and cognitive activity.

Psychomotor domain Learning by doing.

Psychomotor seizure Epileptic seizure that affects the temporal lobe and results in reduced motor activity.

Psychoparmacology The study of the mechanism of or therapeutic use of drugs that affect the functions of CNS related to behaviour and complex brain function.

Psychopathic personallty Symptoms appear in early life. Patient displays excessive emotions, temper tantrums, pathological lying and antisocial element. The intellectual levels are within normal limits. Aetiological factors are hereditary and environmental. Antisocial actions become more acute and more frequent.

Psychophysics The study of the relationship between physical units of a stimulus, such as amplitude, and its sensory, experienced qualities, such as loudness.

Psychophysiology The study of the relation between mind and body, behavior and physiology.

Psychosexual development A series of stages from infancy to adulthood, relatively fixed in time, determined by the interaction between a person's biologic drives and the environment. With resolution of this interaction, a balanced, reality-oriented development takes place; with disturbance, fixation and conflict ensue. This disturbance may remain latent or give rise to characterologic or behavioural disorders.

The stages of development are : *Oral* The earliest of the stages of infantile psychosexual development, lasting from birth to 12 months or longer. Usually subdivided into two stages—the oral erotic, relating to the pleasurable experience of sucking, and the oral sadistic, associated with aggressive biting. Both oral eroticism and sadism continue into adult life in disguised and sublimated forms, such as the character traits of demandingness or pessimism. Oral conflict, as general and pervasive influence, might underlie the psychologic determinants of addictive disorders, depression, and some functional psychotic disorders. *Anal* The period of pregenital psychosexual development, usually from one to three years, in which the child has particular interest and concern with the process of defaecation and the sensations connected with the anus.

The pleasurable part of the experience is termed anal eroticism. *Phallic* The period from about 2½ to 6 years, during which sexual interest, curiosity, and pleasurable experience centre about the penis in boys, and in girls, to a lesser extent, the clitoris. *Oedipal* Overlapping some with the phallic stage, this phase (ages four to six) represents a time of inevitable conflict between the child and parents. The child must desexualise the relationship to both parents in order to retain affectionate kinship with both of them. The process is accomplished by the internalisation of the images of both parents, thereby giving more definite shape to the child's superego.

With the internalisation largely completed, the regulation of self-esteem and moral behaviour comes from within.

Psychosis A major mental disorder of organic or emotional origin in which a person's ability to think, respond emotionally, remember, communicate, interpret reality, and behave appropriately is sufficiently impaired so as to interfere grossly with the capacity to meet the ordinary demands of life.

Often characterised by regressive behaviour, inappropriate mood, diminished impulse control, and such abnormal mental content as delusions and hallucinations. The term is applicable to conditions having a wide range of severity and duration.

Psychosocial stages Stages in the life cycle postulated by Erik Erikson.

Each of the eight stages poses a particular crisis or problem, usually pertaining to relationships with other people. The solution at each stage has repercussions for solutions at later stages.

Psychosocial theories Theories related to socialization and life satisfaction.

Psychosomatic These cause physical symptoms although exact cause is mental stress. Some allergies, high BP or peptic ulcers are made worse by mental stress.

Psychosurgery A neurosurgical intervention to destroy brain areas or sever connection between brain areas with the intent of modifying disturbances of behavior.

Psychosymbolic function Conscious and unconscious psychological function of an organ.

Psychotherapy A general category of treatment techniques for mental disorders; most psychotherapy uses talking as a tool and centers on the client-psychotherapist relationship to develop awareness and provide support.

Psychotocism A scale of Eysenck personality questionnaire. High score on this dimension have tendencies toward being criminal, hostile aggressive etc.

Low scores tend toward the confirmist, conventional and and altruistic.

Psychotropic drugs Drugs that directly affect psychic functions, behavior, or experience i.e., tranquilizers, mood-altering drugs, etc.

Psychrophile Literally, cold lover; an organism able to grow over the temperature range of below 20ºC down to below 0ºC, with an optimum range of 10-15ºC.

Psychrophilic Describing an organism having a growth temperature range of below 0ºC to 20ºC, and optimally at 10-15ºC.

PTCA Percutaneous transluminal coronary angioplasty.

Pterygium It is a triangular encroachment of the bulbar conjunctiva onto the cornea. Aetiological factors include dust, wind, chemical irritants, decrease of lacrimal secretion and solar radiation. Early change is the appearance of grey opacities in the cornea near the limbus with shrinkage of conjunctiva. Pterygium appears as a triangular fold of conjunctiva with overhanging upper and lower border and base merging into bulbar conjunctiva. Progressive pterygium is fleshy, thick and vascular. It may result in dim vision when it reaches the pupil. It can cause astigmatism.

Pterygoid Wing-shaped structure; two of the muscles of mastication, attached to wing-shaped bony projections.

Pterygoid muscles There are two pterygoids, lateral and medial one. Each one arises by two heads. Nerve supply is from mandibular nerve.

Ptosis There is drooping of upper eyelid which may cover pupil. It may be congenital or due to myasthenia gravis or injury. Levator muscle becomes weak. Acquired ptosis without cause may be a neurological sign.

Ptyalin A form of amylase in the saliva of human beings and some animals that catalyzes the hydrolysis of starch into maltose and dextrin.

Puberche Pubic hair appear a little after the onset of breast development. It develops in different stages :

(*i*) long, slightly pigmented straight or slightly curved downy hair along labia majora,

(*ii*) dark, coarse curly hair over symphysis pubis,

(*iii*) adult type of hair only around the labia and over pubes, and

(*iv*) area of pubic hair extends further to form an inverted triangle. Development is regulated by adrenal androgen.

Pubertal Relating to or occuring at puberty.

Puberty It is the period when secondary sexual characteristics develop and the sexual organs mature allowing reproduction possible. It underlies the emotional changes of adolescence between the ages of 12-15 years.

In females ovaries increase the secretion of ovarian hormones. Puberty is acompained by significant growth spurt and weight gain. First sign of puberty in girls is breast budding which occurs around 11 years of age. Pelvis starts becoming wider and fat start depositing giving roundness to female figure. Puberty completes when menses become regular at predictable periods. In boys puberty is headed by a sudden increase in rate of growth of testes and scrotum followed by pubic and facial hair. Boys increase secretion of testosterone, stimulates sperm production and causes prostate to mature. Typical male distribution of hair starts growing on chest and abdomen.

Puberty acceleration The acceleration of puberty in females of many mammalian species through direct contact with the adult male, or by exposure to a male urinary pheromone.

Puberty inhibition The delay of puberty among female mammals housed in groups due to direct physical interactions or to a female urinary pheromone.

Pubic symphysis The juncture between the two pubic bones in the pelvis which in some mammals is necessarily modified in order to facilitate delivery of relatively large fetuses.

Pubis The os pubis or pubic bone forming the front of the pelvis.

Public distance The study of personal interaction at distances beyond 25 feet. This distance is the fourth and last zone identified in studies of the use of interpersonal space. It is so-named because it commonly occurs in public gatherings, as when someone stops to observe another individual performing acrobatics in a public park.

Public health The science and the art of preventing disease prolonging life, and promoting physical health and efficiency through organized community efforts.

Public health nursing The practice of promoting and protecting the health of populations using knowledge from the nursing, social, and public health sciences.

Public space distance of 12 or more feet.

Pudendal cleft Cleft between the labia majora.

Pudendal nerve block It is used bilaterally to provide analgesia in obstetric cases.

Puedendal block It is usually only helpful for the final stage of labour and spontaneous delivery because it provides anesthesia only to lower portion of the vagina and introitus.

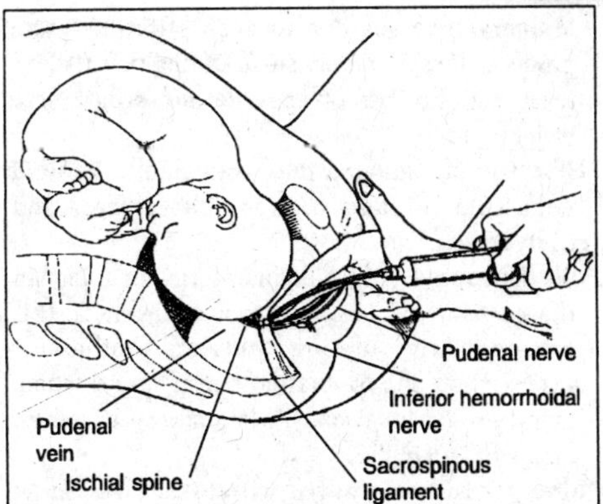

Puedendal block

Pueropera A woman who has just given birth.

Puerperal Relating to or occurring in the time immediately or shortly after birth; puerperium.

Puerperal arterial embolus It may occur with mitral stenosis. Clinical symptoms depend upon seat of blockage. Blockage of bifurcation of aorta causes sudden numbness of legs and loss of pulsation of femoral, popliteal and dorsalis pedis artery.

Puerperal cystitis It is an important cause of puerperal pyrexia. The bladder base and neck are exposed to stretching and brusing when labour is prolonged. Cystoscopic examination may reveal trauma, oedema and blood in trigone.

Puerperal fever Infection, accompanied by fever, which develops in a wound to the birth canal during delivery.

Puerperal infection It is the invasion of the genital tract by certain pathogenic organism within 14 days of postpartum. Fever may be due to pyelitis, mastitis, thrombophlebitis. T.B. pneumonia etc.

Puerperal pyelonephritis Hormonal changes in pregnancy and mechanical pressure of gravid uterus results in gradual dilatation of renal calyces and pelvis, sluggish peristalsis of ureter and stasis of urine. Bacterial invasion of parenchyma results due to ascending infection E. coli. It results in fever with chill and rigor.

Puerperium It is the period succeeding labour during which certain processes take place to restore genital organs approximately to the condition they were before pregnancy. During first 24 hours temperature rises due to absorption of waste products. Pulse becomes slow. During first 10 days there may be loss of appetite and progressive weight loss.

PUFA Poly unsaturated fatty acid tend to be liqid vegetable oil and reduces cholesterol and triglycerides.

Pulled muscle It is a layman term for a tear in fibrous tissue of muscle, tendon or ligament. It is caused while running, playing football or overexertion due to unusual stress. Fomentation, massage and local anti-inflammatory analgesic tube will be helpful.

Pulley Consist of grooved wheel that turns on an axle with a rope or cable ridding in the groove.

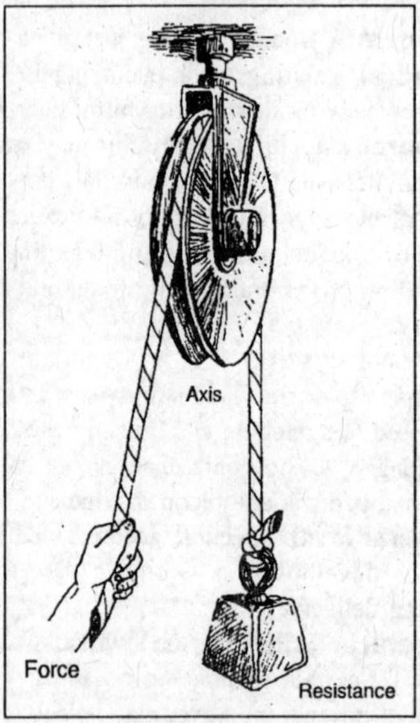

Pulley assisted stretching The healthy arm pulls down the one end of the pulley system and assists the affected arm in stretching. Changing the patients position under the pulley system permits assisted stretching in the various planes of motion.

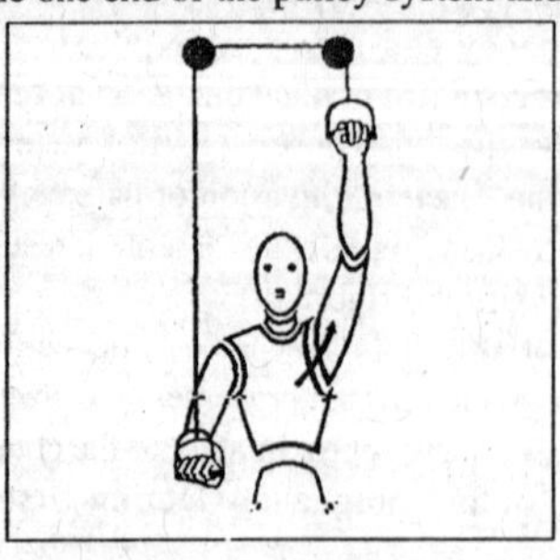

Pulleys Discrete anatomic thickening in the flexor tendon sheath.

Pulling osteochondritis Pull of a strong tendon on the growing area of a bone leads to detachment. Pain is felt on physical activity.

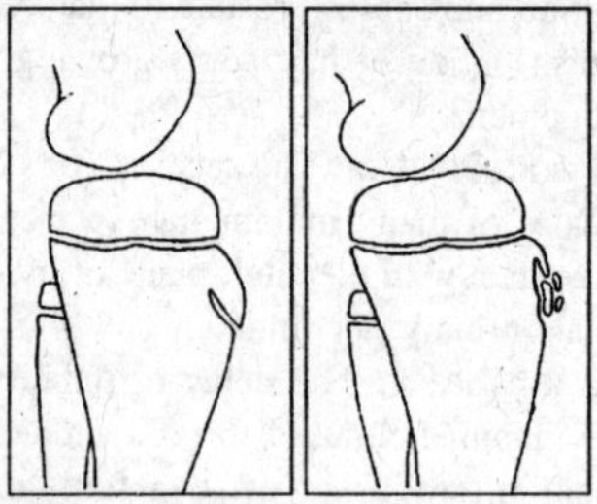

Pulmonary Pertaining to the lungs.

Pulmonary alveoli The final saclike dilatations of the terminal sacs in the lung.

Pulmonary arterial hypertension A condition of abnormally high pulmonary arterial blood pressure.

Pulmonary arteries These carry blood from right side of heart of lungs for oxygenation

Pulmonary arterioles The smallest subdivision of the pulmonary arterial tree before the pulmonary capillary bed.

Pulmonary artery Artery that carries deoxygenated blood from the right ventricle to the lungs.

Pulmonary artery catheter A thin, flexible, flow-directed, balloon-tipped catheter introduced into the pulmonary artery used to monitor cardiovascular pressures.

Pulmonary capacity The sum of two or more pulmonary volumes.

Pulmonary capillaries An intermeshed network of blood vessels, whose walls consist of a single layer of cells, in the septa and walls of the alveolar ducts and alveoli; the bridge between pulmonary arterioles and venules.

Pulmonary circulation Blood flow through the system of blood vessels that carry blood from the right ventricle of the heart to the lungs and back from the lungs to the left atrium. Its function is gas exchange. Flow of blood through the lungs is equal to that of systemic circulation. Pulmonary arterial pressure is about 1/6th of systemic value. Pulmonary blood volume is of the order of 500 ml about 20% of which constitutes a large capillary volume. It is affected by gravity. Exercise results in increased pulmonary blood flow and moderate rise in pressure in supine position. Pulmonary shunt reduces the rate of gas uptake with an insoluble agent. Pulmonary dead space reduces the rate of gas uptake with more soluble agent.

Pulmonary dysmaturity An insidious disease of premature infants beginning with mild respiratory symptoms after the first week of life. The cause is thought to be collapse of the bronchial tree, with partial airway obstruction following aspiration of small amounts of milk as a result of a poorly developed gag reflex. Also known as Wilson-Mikity disease.

Pulmonary embolism In medical ward it is due to heart disease and carcinoma. Prolonged bed rest in patients of hip fracture increases the risk. Condition is usually associated with venous thrombosis in leg and pelvis. Onset may coincide with getting up or straining at stool. Tachycardia is rise in central venous pressure. There will be distended neck veins, hypotension, cyanosis and sometimes gallop rhythm, X-ray may show right-sided cardiac enlargement, elevation of dome of diaphragm, clouding of costophrenic angle due to pleural effusion. Symptoms include faintness, dyspnoea, substernal discomfort, pleural pain, and haemoptysis. Pain is less severe than myocardial infarction. If the embolus is massive there is profound shock, sweating, pallor, air hunger, raised venous pressure and anxiety. Death may follow quickly.

Pulmonary fibrosis Focal fibrosis is due to irritation by dust as in pneumoconiosis. Lung parenchyma is replaced by fibrous tissue. In interstitial fibrosis the fibrosis is limited to the alveolar walls. Clinical features include progressive breathlessness leading to complete incapacitation. Central cyanosis may be present. X-ray will show evidnece of fibrosis. Breath sounds may be diminished and adventitious sounds may be present.

Pulmonary infarction It develops due to an embolus loading in one of the branches of pulmonary but can occur with primary thrombosis of pulmonary vessel. It may cause small area of peripheral infarction usually at base of lung. Emboli of small size cause sudden dyspnoea, pleural pain and collapsed with rapid thin pulse, sweating, a fall of BP and acute cor pulmonale. Patient become cyanosed. Haemoptysis may or may not be.

Pulmonary insufficiency Failure of the pulmonic valve to close completely, allowing regurgitation of blood.

Pulmonary interstitial edema The presence of an abnormal amount of fluid in the interstitial spaces of the lungs; pulmonary congestion.

Pulmonary semilunar valve The semilunar valve found at the base of the pulmonary trunk where it exits from the right ventricle.

Pulmonary thromboembolism It is a dangerous and insidious complication of venous thrombosis. It is the leading cause of death. The size of embolus determines the outcome.

Patients having prolonged convalescence, dehydration, pronounced blood loss, subacute bacterial endocarditis and heart block are prone to develop it. Chest pain after first week of puerperium is strong indication of it. Fatal case presents with dramatic suddenness of air hunger, cyanosis and pain resembling cardiac infraction. Death may ensue within a short time.

Pulmonary trunk Large elastic artery that carries blood from the right ventricle of the heart to the right and left pulmonary arteries.

Pulmonary vascular resistance Pressure resistance in the pulmonary vascular system.

Pulmonary veins The four veins returning oxygenated blood from the lungs to the left atrium.

Pulmonary ventilation The inflow (inspiration) and outflow (expiration) of air between the atmosphere and the lungs.

Pulmonary volume Lung volume, measured by spirometry; deviations from a normal value can be used to diagnose certain lung diseases; the pulmonary volumes are the tidal volume, inspiratory reserve volume, expiratory reserve volume, and residual volume.

Pulmonologist A physician specializing in pulmonary medicine.

Pulp Organ made up of blood vessles, nerves, and cellular elements, including odontoblasts, that forms dentin. It normally occupies the central portion of teeth.

Pulp canal Space in the radicular portion of the tooth occupied by the pulp.

Pulp cap The process of placing a medicament such as calcium hydroxide, over an exposure of the dental pulp.

Pulp cavity A cavity within a tooth that includes both the pulp chamber and pulp canals; contains blood vessels, nerves and lymphatics; appears radiolucent.

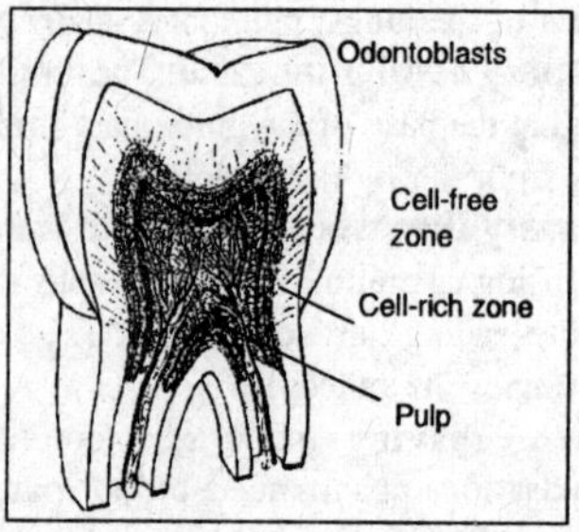

Pulp chamber Pulp cavity; space occupied by the pulp.

Pulp chambers of deciduous teeth Pulp chambers are large in relation to tooth size and pulp horns are well developed. The furcation of roots is also very much closer to the cervical area of crown.

Pulp extirpation The complete removal of pulp from the pulp chamber and root canal.

Pulp horn A small projection of vital pulp directly under cusp or developmental lobe.

Pulp stone A dystrophic calcification within the pulp cavity of a tooth, appears radiolucent.

Pulpal Pertaining to the pulp.

Pulpal floor Flat bottom or enclosing base of the prepared cavity nearest the pulp.

Pulpal obliteration Total calcification of the pulp cavity within a tooth, appears radiolucent.

Pulpitis Inflammation of the pulpal tissue of a tooth.

Pulpless Without pulp.

Pulpoma Tooth resorption. Internal.

Pulpotomy Surgical amputation of the dental pulp coronal to the dentinocemental junction.

Pulsating proptosis In pulsating proptosis the patient complains of a continuous rumbling sound like that of a sound from a waterfall. It can be heard and is due to arteriovenous aneurysm, the communication between internal carotid artery and cavernous sinus. Proptosis is reducible and patient complains of pain and due to stretching of branches of fifth nerve.

Pulse Wave-like sensation that can be palpated in a peripheral artery.

Pulse deficit Difference between the apical and radial pulse rates.

Pulse generator The cellular and molecular mechanisms that produce and sustain pulsatile neurosecretion; these mechanisms are currently unknown.

Pulse oximetry Noninvasive, transcutaneous technique for periodically or continuously monitoring the oxygen saturation of blood.

Pulse pressure The difference between the maximum (systolic) and minimum (diastolic) pressures; normally about 40 mm Hg.

Pulse rate Number of peripheral arterial pulsations palpated in a minute.

Pulse rhythm Pattern of the pulsations and pauses between them.

Pulse volume Quality of the pulsations that are felt.

Pulse volume recordings Changes in volume of blood flowing through a limb as measured by plethysmographic tracings to assess for blockage.

Pulseless disease It is a nonspecific arteritis involving aortic arch and peripheral vessels of young females. Exact aetiology is not known. Clinically it presents with consistutitonal symptoms like weakness, fever, arthralgia and

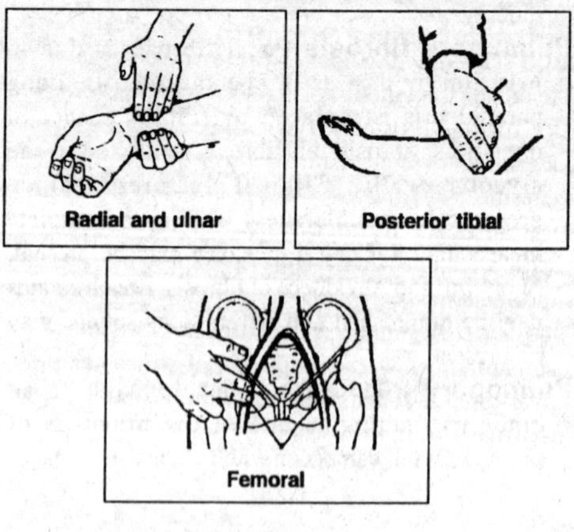

night sweats. When aortic arch is involved there may be blurred vision, syncope, pain along carotid artery with murmur and poor pulsation. When aortic arch is involved along with renal artery, patient will have hypertension with absence of pulse in upper limb called reversd coarctation syndrome. Funduscopy may show a wreath-like anastomosis around optic disc.

Pulsus alternans In this the arterial pulse alternatingly vary between stronger and weaker beats, detectable only with the sphygmomanometer, even though the rhythm of the pulse remains normal. It is found in left ventricular failure and also in arterial hypertension.

Pulsus bisferiens In pulsus bisferiens the arterial pulse shows two palpable beats, the former being weaker than the later. It is found in aortic regurgitation.

Pulsus paradoxus Marked decrease in arterial pulse volume during inspiration or a fall in systolic BP more than 10 mm of Hg is known as pulse paradoxus. It is noted in constrictive pericarditis, right ventricle infarction, severe asthma and superior vena cava obstruction. In some cases of obesity and pregnancy it can be noted.

Pulvianar A region of the posterior thalamus taking part in visual processing.

Punctum dilator It is used to dilate the punctum for syringing of the lacrimal sac.

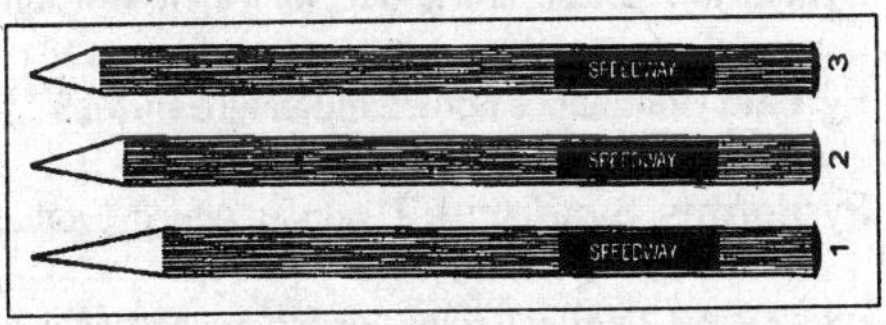

Pupil The opening in the center of the iris that regulates the amount of light entering the eye.

Pure motor syndrome Syndrome associated with a lacuna in the posterior limb of the internal capsule.

Pure sensory syndrome Syndrome associated with a lesion of the ventral posterior nucleus of the thalamus.

Pure tone A sound produced by a vibration of a single frequency, the amplitude of which changes over time as a sinusoidal function; a sine wave.

Purging Eliminating food through self-induced vomiting; seen in eating disorders.

Purine A nitrogenous heterocyclic base found in nucleotides and nucleic acids; containing fused pyrimid in and imidazole rings.

Purkinje cell A distinctive neuron found in the cerebellum.

Purkinje fibre A specialised cardiac muscle fibre that conducts action potentials through cardiac muscle; forms part of the conduction system of the heart. These form a network under the endocardium of ventricles and are clear quadrangular cells. The peripheral parts of cells only show cross-striations. The fibres run uninterruptedly from auricle to ventricle after piercing the auriculoventricular septum.

Puromycin An antibiotic that inhibits polypeptide synthesis by being incorporated into a growing polypeptide chain, causing its premature termination.

Purposeful activities Tasks that have meaning or anticipating outcomes.

Purposive sampling A sampling technique, commonly used in qualitative research, involving selection of individuals for diversity of views rather than for representativeness.

Pursed-lip breathing Form of controlled ventilation in which the expiration phase of breathing is consciously prolonged.

Purulent Containing pus.

Purulent drainage White-or green-tinged fluid.

Pus A fluid product of inflammation, which consists of a liquid containing leucocytes and the debris of dead cells and tissue elements liquefied by the proteolytic and histolytic enzymes. It is a thickened yellowish-green discharge from wound or so. It is a mixture of dead and live leucocytes. Presence of pus in blood causes septicaemia. There will be high fever with jaundice.

Putamen Outer part of lentiform nucleus.

Putanam's sign Apparent lengthening of limb.

Putrefaction This process begins when rigor mortis ceases. End of putrefaction is destruction of dead animal or vegetable matter. There is breaking up of complex organic compounds composing the tissues into simpler compounds largely gaseous by the action of bacteria. The chief gases formed are H_2, CO_2, H_2S, PH_3 and NH_4. Eventually all organic matter disappears and only a small quantity of inorganic matter remains. Soft parts are first to disappear. Skeletonisation will be complete in about a year. In 24 hours green patch appears on abdominal wall in right iliac region and spreads rapidly. Colouration spreads to face and later to limbs. Colour changes are also seen in viscera. The tissues specially those of the more vascular organs begin to soften and liquefy and gas in large quantities begin to form.

Putrifaction The decomposition of proteins by microorganisms under anaerobic condition.

Putty-wash An impression technique in which a putty -like materials is first used to make an initial impression, it then serves as a tray to carry a more fluid "wash" material, which reproduces the tissues more accurately.

P-Wave Deflection on an ECG that occurs with depolarization of the atria.

Pyelonephritis Inflammation of kidney as a result of bacterial infection.

Pyknodysostosis Autosomal recessive condition best known for osteosclerosis, frequent fractures, delayed closure of cranial sutures and short stature.

Pyknosis A shrunken nucleus with condensed darkened chromatin, usually characteristic of apoptosis.

Pylon A temporary prosthetic replacement.

Pyloric sphincter A modification of the musculais tunic between the stomach and the duodenum that functions to regulate the food material leaving the stomach.

Pyloric stenosis It is a constriction of terminal part of stomach upto pyloric sphincter. Such constriction may be caused by muscular spasm, ulceration of mucosal lining, tumour or any genetic disorder. It results in vomiting. Barium meal study helps.

Pylorus The small narrow section of the stomach that joins the first part of the small intestine

Pyogenesis Formation of pus.

Pyogenic Pus forming.

Pyopericarditis In case of TB and empyema and in some other conditions the fluid in pericardium becomes purulent or seropurulent in character. It will produce shivering attacks, profuse perspiration and a temperature with wide variation in a course of few hours. Frequency of sound is usually transient. It is often fatal. Clinical features include fever, anaemia and leucocytosis.

Pyorrhea Periodontitis.

Pyramidal tract Another name for corticospinal tract. Descending pathway of upper motor neuron concerned with voluntary movement.

Pyramid A pointed or cone-shaped structure, one of two roughly triangular structures on the ventral side of the medulla oblongata composed of the largest motor tracts that run from the cerebral cortex to the spinal cord; a triangular structure in the renal medulla.

Pyramidal cell A distinctive neurons found in the cerebral cortex.

Pyramids Triangular-shaped divisions of the medulla of the kidney.

Pyranose A simple sugar containing the six-membered pyran ring.

Pyrazinamide It is an antituberculous drug used in combination with other drugs. Its effectivity lasts for 2-3 months. It penetrates CSF, hence can be used in meningitis. Dose is 1.5- 2.0 gm. daily for 3 months.

Pyrazines These are about 50 which are highly aromatic.

Pyrexia Continuous body temperature above 37.5°C upto 39°C.

Pyriformis Syndrome Disorder which produces sciatica like syndrome.

Pyrogen Chemical released by microorganisms, neutrophils, monocytes, and other cells that stimulates fever production by acting on the hypothalamus.

Pyuria Pus in the urine.

Q

'Q' angle It is a clinical measure that is calculated by connecting the central point on the patella with the anterior superior iliac spine above and tibial tubercle below. The normal 'Q' angle with the knee in full extension is 15 degrees. Values greater than 20° are associated with pain.

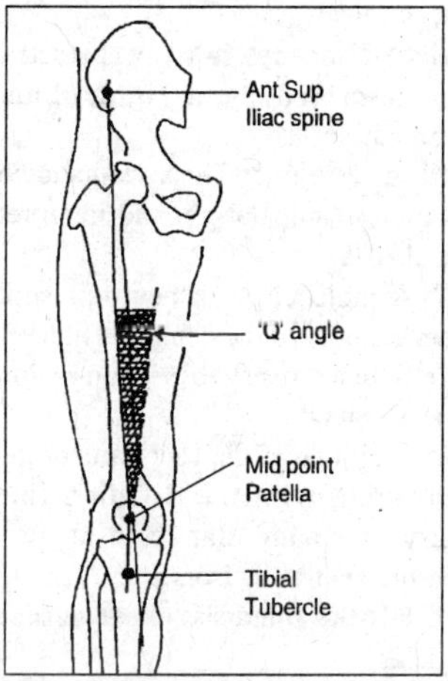

Q-fever It is caused by *Coxiella burnetii* a type of riketsia harboured by farm animals. It occurs in urine, faeces and milk.

It can be contracted by inhaling dust. Incubation period is 20 days. The illness begins suddenly with high fever, severe headache, muscle and chest pain and cough. In some cases pneumenia may develop and 30 per cent may develop hepatitis.

QRS complex Deflection on an ECG that occurs as a result of depolarization of the ventricles.

Q-sort A method of personality assessment in which the subject sorts a large deck of statements about human behaviour into categories, according to the extent to which they apply to him or her.

Quack One who is not a qualified doctor and misrepresent his ability and experience in diagnosis and treatment of disease or results to be achieved by his treatment

Quad coughing Assisted coughing with the therapist's support. In supine lying position the therapist's hands are placed below the patients sub-costal angle. The hands are pushed inwards and upwards as the patients attempt to cough. The therapist's force of hands assists in rapid exhalation of air and secretions may be expectorated.

Quadran One-quarter of a circle, the abdomen is divided into right upper and lower and left upper and lower quadrants by a horizontal and a vertical line intersecting at the umbilicus.

Quadrant One fourth of a circle. In dentistry, one fourth of the total dentition, consisting of all the teeth in half of one jaw, extending from the midling circumferentially around the arch and including the last molar. The four quadrants are the maxillary right, maxillary left, mandibular left, and mandibular right.

Quadrantanopsia Visual filled loss in a quarter of visual field of eye. Defect is usually bilateral.

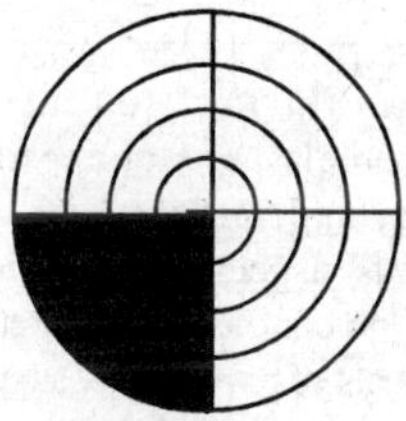

Quadrantic hemianopia Blindness in one quadrant of the visual field.

Quadratus lumborum It is often injured as a violent side bending movement. Person will complaint of pain in the region of injured muscle which is made worse on active side bending.

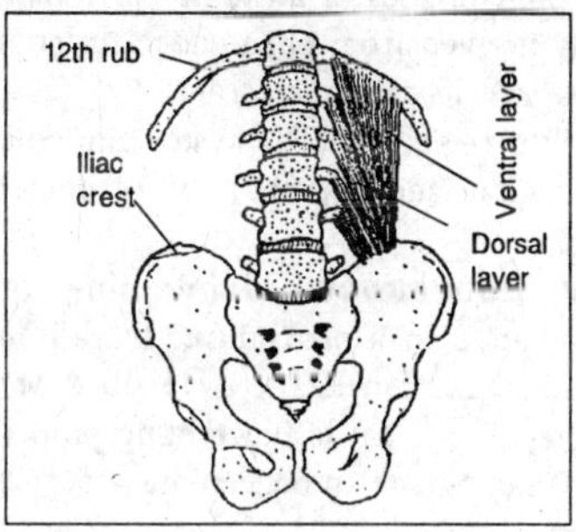

Quadriceps femoris Extensor of the lower leg.

Quadriceps muscles It straightens the knee. Common disorder is haematoma caused by direct blow. Sudden stretching of leg may tear muscle especially in older age causing pain and swelling.

Quadriplegia Paralysis of all four limbs e.g., tetraplegia.

Quadriplets These can be formed from one to four ova.

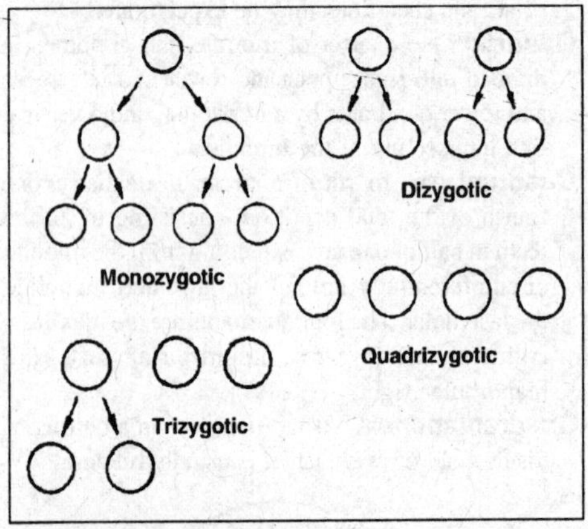

Qualitative Having to do with certain distinguishable aspects of experience— such as sour, blue, and middle C. These are called "qualitative" aspects of experience or merely "qualities", in contrast to the intensive or "quantitative" aspects of experience, such as the sourness of what is sour, the brightness of blue and the loudness of middle C.

Qualified Criteria that indicated when the goal is achieved.

Qualitative data Derived from family assessment and describes family's characteristics or qualities. The characteristics or attributes of a family are usually derived from open-ended questions and summarized in narrative form.

Qualitative research The systematic collection, organization, and interpretation of nonumerical data.

Quality assurance Maintaining optimal performance in a procedure. In radiology it describes certain tests to ensure that the radiographic system is functioning properly and that the radiographs produced are acceptable.

Quality of life The presence of personal and social positive well being.

Quality-adjusted life years A health status index that incroporates both life expectancy and the perceived impact of illness and disability on the quality of life.

Quantification The process of measuring intensity or degree. Psychophysics, for example, is quantitative in the sense that it deals with measuring stimulation and observable responses, often in terms of intensity. The assigning of numerical values.

Quantitative characteristic A characteristic that can be described by a rigid, dimensional measurement scale.

Quantitative research The systematic collection, organization, manipulation, and interpretation of numerical data.

Quantum A molecule of a neurotransmitter or a sufficient quantity of the neurotransmitter that will produce a just observable change in a cell's membrane voltage.

Quardrant Any one of the four parts or quarters of the denitition, with the dividing line of the maxillary or mandibular teeth at the midline between the central incisors.

Quardrantanopia Blindness of one quadrant of the visual field.

Quasi-experiment An experiment that does not allow subjects to be assigned randomly to treatment conditions.

Quatrantic hemianopia Blindness in one quadrant of the visual field.

Queckenstedt-Stookey test According to the test, in the thecal block, the pressure of cerebrospinal fluid is not increased on compression of the jugular vein. The test is positive in spinal cord compression.

Queen In a colony of social insects (e.g., bees, ants), a mature, fertile female that lays eggs.

Queer Queer has been reclaimed as a term to describe sexual orientation, to reflect the continuum of sexual practices and tastes.

Quenching -the process of plunging a hot metal part (or dental casting) in to cold water to cause a rapid cooling to room temperatures.

Questionnaire A series of items or questions presented to one or more individuals for the purpose of gathering information. The results are usually treated statistically.

Quickening It means coming to life, i.e. mother has come to know that something is moving in her womb which is alive. Many women do not experience it. It develops during 18 to 20th week. Fetal movements continue until the end of pregnancy.

Quincke's pulse In this the capillary pulse becomes visible as alternating reddening and blanching of the nailbed when pressure is applied to the tip of the nail. It is seen in aortic regurgitation.

Quinine It is the oldest treatment for malaria. There is high risk of adverse effects, including headache, nausea, hearing loss and blurred vision.

Quinine intoxication Quinine is an extract of the cinchona tree and is used in treatment of malaria particularly falciparum malaria. It is also used for the prevention of nocturnal cramps. The lethal dose of quinine is 8 gm for adults and 20 mg/kg for children. Early features of mild intoxication include nausea, vomiting, tinnitus, dizziness and vertigo. In severe cases patient develops hypotension and convulsions leading to death. Hearing is impaired and pupils become dilated. Visual blurring may occur in 2 to 24 hours. Optic disc may become pallor. ECG changes may occur as late as 22 to 34 hours and include prolonged PR and QT intervals. There is widening of QRS complex, transient bundle branch block and non-specific ST changes. Due to its oxytoxic action it may lead to abortion in case of pregnancy.

Quinke oedema It is an allergic, angioneurotic oedema based on anaphylactic type of allergic response or pseudoallergic process. It is paroxysmal, firm, nontender oedematous facial swelling particularly affecting the lids and lips appearing suddenly and regressing within 1 to 3 days. It recurs.

Quinolones Nalidixic acid is useful against urinary tract infection. Quinolones are well absorbed from gut and widely distributed in body tissue. Adverse effects are GIT disturbance and allergic reaction. These are bactericidal and active against gram-negative organisms, *E. coli, Salmonella sp., Shigella sp.*

Quinone A lipid-soluble hydrogen i.e., proton plus electron carrier that mediates electron transfer between respiratory chain components.

Quinsy It is an abscess around tonsil usually as a complication of tonsillitis. It causes painful throat, high temperature, headache, impaired speech and drooling. Lymph glands become swollen and tender. Uvula is displaced to the affected side. Antibiotics clear infection within a week. It usually occurs after tonsillitis, an abscess forms just outside the capsule of tonsil. Severe pain is felt in throat and swallowing may be almost impossible. The pain radiates to ear and down the neck. Fever may be high. The anterior pillar of fauces and the affected side are very red and oedematous and buldges forward. The cervical glands of same side enlarge and become tender.

Quota sample A sample which includes subgroups of people or items in the same proportion as they are represented in the population. If the population is one half red, one-fourth blue, and one-fourth green, the sample is composed of subgroups in these same ratios. Within each subgroup, the members of the sample are chosen on a random basis.

R

R

RA Abbreviation of rheumatoid factor.

Rabies It is also known as hydrophobia. It primarily affects animals and can be transmitted from rabid animal, specially dog to a man. The virus present in saliva, travels from the wound along nerve pathways to the brain where it causes inflammation resulting in delirium, painful muscle spasm in throat. Incubation period extends from a day to many months. Often person attempts to drink which induces violent, painful spasms in throat. Eyes and facial muscles become paralysed. Coma and death follow in three days to three weeks. Once symptoms have developed only symptomatic treatment is done by sedatives and analgesics.

Rabies encephalitis Rabies virus spreads along peripheral nerves to reach CNS. The initial neurologic symptoms are severe anxiety, speech and psychomotor overactivity followed by dysphagia, spasm of throat muscles while drinking. Coma gradually follows and death is sure in 4 to 7 days. Negri bodies are found mainly in hippocampus.

Rabies virus It belongs to genus Lyssa virus. It is rod-shaped virus to that vary in length from 60-150 nm and in width from 60 to 85 nm. It is bullet shaped in appearance. Particles are surrounded by membranous envelop with protruding spikes 10 nm long. It survives at 4°C for weeks and survives subzero degree for longer period. Thermal inactivation occurs at 37°C in 4 to 5 hours and 2 minutes at 100°C. Virus is inactivated by 1% formalin. Nitric acid is used in animal bite at places because it destroys virus rapidly.

Race Apparently straightforward, the concept of race has a complicated history. Sociologists now define race as a group of people with shared physical characteristics.

Rachialgia Pain in spine.

Rachiometer Apparatus for measuring spinal curvature.

Rachitic Pertaining to rickets.

Rad Acronym for radiation absorbed dose.

Radial angle Angle between distal radial articular surface to shaft or radius.

Radial bursae A common name for synovial shealth of flexor pollicis longus.

Radial flexion A range of motion exercise during which there is a bending of the wrist medially toward the thumb, maintains wrist mobility.

Radial glial cells Cells that form miniature "highways" that provide pathways for migrating neurons to follow to their appropriate destinations.

Radial neck The constricted area of proximal radius first distal to radial head.

Radial nerve It is a branch of brachial plexus. It straights the wrist so that the back of hand is in line with the forearm. It also conveys sensations

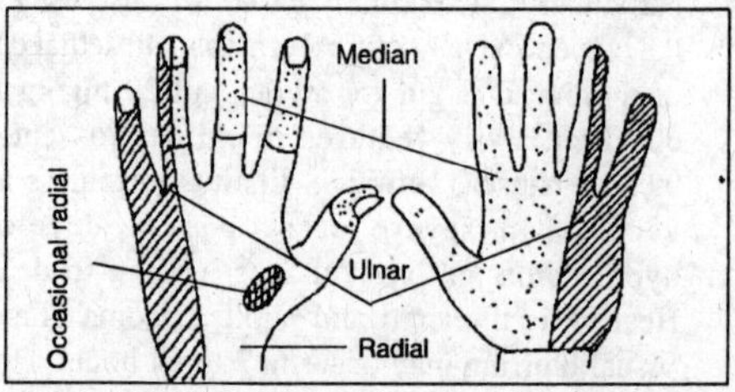

from back of forearm, back of thumb, second and third fingers and from the area at the base of thumb. Fracture of humerus and persistent pressure on the armpit due to crutch may result in wrist drop and numbness in the areas of skin supplied by radial nerve.

Radial pulse Pulse found in the forearm.

Radial surgery It is an extensive surgery aimed at eliminating a major disease by removing all affected tissue and any surrounding tissue that is diseased or may be diseased. Previously it was done to cure cancer. Radial mastectomy for breast cancer involved removing the entire affected breast along with chest muscles, under arm, lymph nodes and other tissues. In case of gangrene amputation is also a radical surgery.

Radial symmetry Symmetry in which the body parts are arranged radially around a central oral-aboral axis.

Radial Tunnel syndrome A compression neuropathy of radial nerve in the proximal fore arm.

Radial/ulnar nerve Radial nerve is considered a preparatory nerve because it controls wrist extension for positioning and stabilising the hand. The digital extensor open the thumb and finger in preparation for grasping or manipulating object.

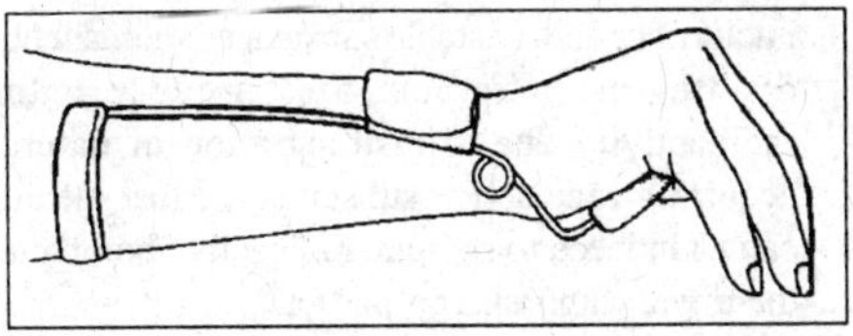

Ulnar nerve is known as power nerve. It becomes superficial at wrist and the hand through Guyou's canal. At that point it divides into a sensory and motor branch. Sensory branch is superficial and supplies sensation to the small finger and distal aspect of ring finger. Motor branch innervates hypothenar muscles.

Radiant heat exchange The net rate or heat exchange by radiation between an organism and its environment.

Radiation There are two main types of radiation : ionising and nonionising. Ionising radiation is capable of forcibly ejecting one or more electrons of orbit nucleus of an atom thereby emitting an ion which has an electrical charge and is capable of chemical combination with other ions. In body it can lead to biological damage. Nonionising radiation has a different effect on molecules. It shakes but does not impart enough energy to the atoms to displace electrons and form ions. There are three types of ionising radiation X-rays, g rays and particle radiation. X-rays are electromagnetic waves and are produced by special electrical machines. X-rays have no mass and no electrical charge but penetrating power which depends on their energy. While g rays are produced by spontaneous decay of radioactive material than machines. They have shorter wavelength and higher frequencies. On the other hand, particle radiation has mass and may also have electrical charge. It represents electrons, protons and neutrons.

Radiation cystitis It can result from any radiation treatment delivered to the pelvic area. Early symptoms are reversible but delayed sequelae may appear even years after therapy is finished.

Radiation enteropathy Because of its high rate of cell turnover the small intestine is the part of gastrointestinal tract (GIT) which is most vulnerable to radiation. When small intestine is damaged the colon is however damaged too. Damage to small intestine is worse if there is concomitant chemotherapy. Within hours there is epithelial necrosis, the villi are swollen and flattened and crypts shortened and there may be gross ulceration and inflammation. The serosa becomes damaged and thickened and adhesions form between adjacent loops.

In early stage, nausea and vomiting, colicky pain, diarrhoea containing blood and mucus may occur. Then follows a quiescent phase, usually of at least a year or more. Then it is followed by symptoms of subacute obstruction with colicky pain, nausea, vomiting and distension. Radiology shows hypermotility above lesions.

Radiation fog Darkening due to radiation from sources other than intentional exposure to the primary beam; for example, scatter radiation, or film storage not protected from radiation.

Radiation hazard It may develop from external source of radiation as well as internal source too. The effects of radiation depend on dose received and the duration of exposure.

Some forms of radiation damage always occur when the total radiation dose exceeds a certain threshold. Above this level one may develop radiation sickness, dermatitis, cataract or failure of certain organs. With increasing dose one may even develop cancer.

Radiation ionising Any electromagnetic or particulate radiation capable of producing ions, directly or indirectly, in its passage through matter.

Radiation proctosigmoiditis Injury to rectum particulary the rectum and sigmoid is said to occur in up to 25 % of patients. Risk of injury is largely dose dependent and is uncommon with a total dose of less than 4000 rads.

The individual lesion is inflammatory mucosal injury, but this is followed by a vascular injury with endarteritis, ischaemia and subsequent fibrosis and stricture formation. Early symptoms include diarrhoea, mucus discharge and bleeding with lower abdominal pain and tenesmus. Mucosa of rectum and sigmoid may be friable and ulcerated. Telangiectasis are common and characteristic features on sigmoidoscopy.

Radiation safety Methods used to protect persons from accidental injury from exposure in dental and medical setting.

Radiation sickness The effect of exposure to radiation depends critically on dose and time of exposure. Above acute exposure of 30 to 100 Gy there is rapid onset of nausea, vomiting, anxiety and disorientation and within a few hours the victim usually loses consciousness and dies as a consequence of direct damage to nervous system and oedema of brain. At doses of 1 to 10 Gy transient nausea and vomiting may occur but disappears early followed by relative wellbeing. After four weeks effects of radiation to the bone marrow and immune system begin to appear with repeated infection and pinpoint spots of bleeding under skin. Radiation up to 1 Gy in fractionated doses may not be fatal.

Radiation therapy The radiation as it passes through the diseased tissue, destroys or slows down the development of abnormal cells. Side by side some normal cells may also be damaged. Radiation therapy is often used after surgical excision of a malignant tumour as in breast to destroy any left over cancer cells. It is also used to reduce the size of tumour to relieve the symptoms of cancer which are not curable. If the benefits of destroying diseased tissue far outweigh the risk of damage to healthy tissue radiation therapy may be used over active thyroid gland. Some malignant tumours are treated not by radiation from an external source but by inserting radioactive material directly into the growth. Radiation used to treat thyrotoxicosis is given as a liquid form of radioactive iodine.

Radiator hypothesis The idea that the development of a new blood flow in early hominids improved brain cooling to such an extent that the brain was able to grow larger.

Radical An atom or group of atoms possessing an unpaired electron; also called a free radical.

Radical prostectomy Surgical removal of the prostate; the most used definitive treatment for prostate cancer.

Radiculopathy Compression of a single nerve root.

Radio neuritis Inflammation of a nerve that is due to exposure to radiant injury.

Radioactive nuclide perfusion imaging Radioactive labeled agents used with perfusion imaging to improve the assessment of coronary artery perfusion.

Radioactivity The emission of alpha particles or beta particles and or gamma rays that occurs when nuclei of certain unstable substances spontaneously disintegrate. Uranium ores produce natural radioactivity due to disintegration of naturally occurring radioactive substances. Most elements can be induced to become radioactive bombarding them with high energy particles.

Radiode An instrument for the therapeutic application of a radioactive source.

Radiograph It is an image produced on photosensitive film by exposing the film to X-rays. It is the actual film exposed while an X-ray refers to beam of energy. So, radiograph should be referred as an X-ray film.

Radiographic measurment of Joint Motion Radiographic techniques are used to study the range and type of motion taking place at various joints and also to check the validity of goniometry. The radiographic technique of measuring joint range has health risks of repeated exposure and are of high cost.

Radiography Diagnostic procedures that use x-rays.

Radioimmunoassay A measuement process by which a radiolabled analog of the drug being measured competes with unlabeled drug analyte and an antibody specifically recognizing that particular drug, or a family of chemically closely related substances.

Radioimmunoassay test A test of blood serum for pregnancy. It is very accurate from the eighth day after fertilisation.

Radiologic hidden tetrad Cervical spine injury may also be entirely soft tissue in nature and these injuries can be missed on initial examination. Complete and careful evaluation is necessary.

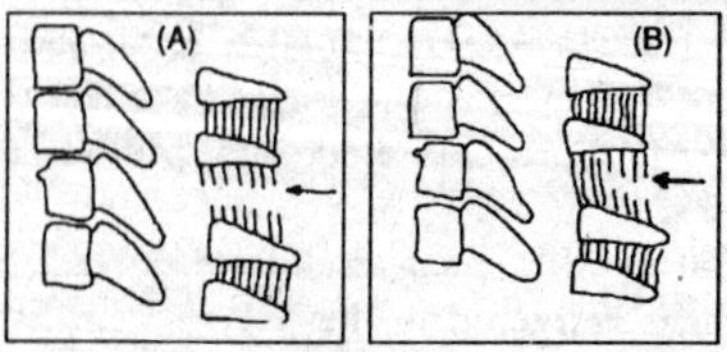

A Complete tear of posterior cervical complex
B Incomplete tear of posterior cervical complete

Radiologist A physician who specializes in radiology.

Radiology Branch of medical science that deals with the use of radiant energy in the diagnosis and treatment of disease.

Radiolucent Producing dark images on film because a large amount of radiation interacts with the film. Also refers to structures that are easily penetrated by x-rays.

Radionecrosis Tissue destruction that is due to exposure to radiation.

Radionuclide scanning It is a diagnostic technique based on the detection of radiation emitted by radioactive substances introduced into the body. Different radioactive substances known as radionuclide are taken up in greater concentrations by different types of tissue, so that specific organs can be studied. Such as thyroid takes up more of radioactive iodine. Radionuclide scanning can detect certain disorders better than other imaging technique. Technique is also able to provide information on functions such as blood flow, movement of heart walls, urine flow through kidneys and bile flow through liver. It is safe because it requires only minute doses of radiation.

Radionuclides Elements whose molecular structures are altered to produce radiation.

Radiopaque It appears white or light on X-ray. These are dense structures and absorb X-ray beam. A metallic restoration appears radiopaque because it is very dense and absorbs the radiation. As a result very less radiation reaches the surface of film resulting in white radiopaque area on film. Radiopaque structures are enamel, dentin and bone.

Radiopharmaceutical A radioactive pharmaceutical substance used for diagnostic or therapeutic purposes.

Radioresistant Relatively resistant to injury by ionising radiation.

Radiosensitive Relatively susceptible to injury by ionising radiation.

Radioulnar synostosis Synostosis between adjacent bones may occur anywhere in limb between carpal bones but in radius and ulna it is very common. It may cause difficulty in radius and ulna. If there is minimal functional disability no specific treatment is required.

Radium It has four naturally occurring isotopes : radium 226, radium 228, radium 224 and radium 223. Artificial radioisotopes have been produced too. Most important isotope is radium 226 which is produced by the decay of naturally radioactive elements of uranium series. Its half-life is 1,600 years and decays to form gas radon. During its decay radiation is emitted in alpha, beta and gamma rays.

Radius It is laterally placed and shorter of two bones of forearm. Shaft of radius articulates with lower end of ulna and with the upper bones of wrist. Head of radius articulates with lower end of humerus. Radius takes more of strain when weight is placed on the wrist and is a common site of fracture.

Radon It is a odourless, colourless, tasteless, radioactive gaseous element produced by radioactive decay of radium. It has three isotopes—radon 219, radon 220 and radon 222. Parent source of radon occurs in many materials such as soil, rocks and building material. So environment makes a largest source of radiation to human body.

Raffinose It is trisaccharide of glucose, galactose and fructose found in molasses.

Rage A state of intense emotional behaviour associated with uncontrolled destructive behaviour.

Raimiste's phenomenon An associated reaction in which abduction or adduction of the normal limb produces a similar response in the affected limb.

Rales These are continuous moist sounds due to presence of mucus or other fluid in the bronchial tubes. unlike ronchi they are heard during inspiration. Rales are of third types according to the size of tubes involved and the amount of fluid present : coarse, medium and fine rales. *Coarse* rales are produced in mediumsized bronchi where there is much sticky mucus as in resolving pneumonia or bronchiectasis. *Medium* rales are due to mucus in smaller bronchi. *Fine* rales are known as crepitus and occur when there is excess of moisture in terminal bronchioles.

Ramping In implant dentistry, the removal of bone at the alveolar ridge crest, to increase width to enable insertion of an endosteal implant.

Ramus The portions of the mandible that extend upward and backward from the horseshoeshoe body and terminate in two process; the articular condyloid process and the coronoid process.

Ramus Frame implant A mandibular endosteal implant consisting of a symphyseal plate/blade-like structure with a contiguous bar providing bilateral extension into the rami to support the prosthesis.

Rancid Food with a high content of fat giving disagreeable aroma or off flavour.

Rancidity Process of becoming rancid.

Random error Produces findings that are too high and too low in approximately equal amounts, owing to random factors.

Random groups Groups of subjects, usually large in number, formed on a random basis, generally for purposes of research.

Random sample The selection of subjects or items for research, on the basis of chance. The cases are chosen from the population in such a way that all of them presumably have the same chance of being selected.

Random sampling Entails selecting a small group for study from a much larger group of potential study subjects.

Randomization Entails allocating the available subjects to one or another study group and is generally used in clinical studies.

Randomized controlled clinical trials Studies designed to test a therapeutic measure. Subjects are randomly assigned to one of the lowing groups: (1) the intervention group, which will receive the experimental treatment, or (2) the control group, which will receive the nonexperimental treatment, consisting of either a placebo or a standard method of treatment.

Range The difference between the highest and lowest scores in a series.

Range of motion (ROM) The amount of movement available at a specified joint; measured by occupational therapy practitioners with a goniometer.

Range of motion, cervical vertebra Every joint has its limitations. Range of motion of cervical vertebra is extension and flexion 45 degrees, lateral inclination to 45 degrees and rotation to 80 degrees.

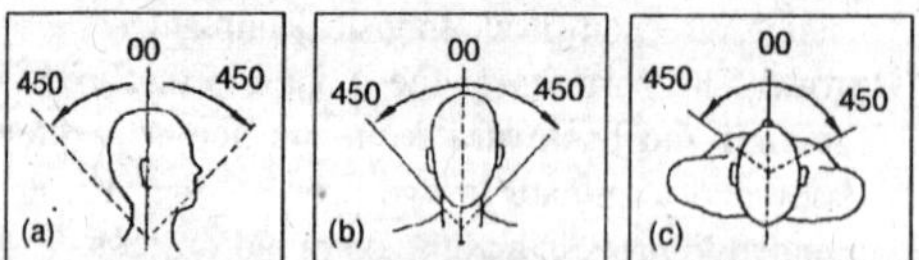

Range-of-motion exercises Therapeutic activity in which joints are moved.

Ranitidine It is an ulcer healing drug belonging to histamine 2 receptor antagonist group of drugs. It is useful in treating peptic ulcer and peptic oesophagitis. Side effects include headache, skin rash, constipation and lethargy.

Ranula It is a soft and bluish swelling stimulating frog's belly. The term ranula is derived from Latin word *rana* which means little frog. It is a mucous retention cyst arising from the mucous glands situated on the floor of the mouth and undersurface of tongue. Swelling is mostly unilateral. Spherical cyst varies from 1 to 5 cm in diameter but only the top half is visible. Colour is pale blue with semitransparent appearance due to presence of deep lingual vein. Surface is smooth and mucous membrane is mobile over the swelling. Edge of swelling is difficult to feel. Swelling is not tender. Fluctuation is present and transillumination test is positive. Cervical glands are generally not enlarged.

Ranvier, nodes Constrictions of the myelin of nerve fibers.

Raphe A ventral ridge on the penis denoting the edge of fusion of the two urethral folds.

Rapid Eye movement sleep The stage of sleep with highest brain activity. There is enhanced brain metabolism and vivid dreaming.

Rapid sand filtration A technique for puriying water by adding a flocculent called alum to the water before filtration, The flocculent coagulates and traps suspended materials, therby preventing them from passing through the sand with the filtered water. The flocculent is removed periodically by back flushing, and new flocculent is added to the nest batch of water.

Rapid-filling phase The phase that occurs once the mitral valve opens and the ventricular volume begins rising as the ventricle passively fills.

Rapidly adapting receptor A body sensory receptor that responds briefly to the onset of a stimulus on the body.

Rapport The feeling of harmonious accord and mutual, responsiveness that contributes to the patient's confidence in the therapist and willingness to work cooperatively. To be distinguished from transference, which is unconscious.

Rarefaction The thinning of bony tissue that can cause a decreased density to X-Rays.

RAS Return activated sludge; activated sludge solids returned from the final sedimentation tanks to the aeration tanks on a continuous basis.

Rash It is an area of red, inflamed skin or a group of spots. It may cause fever and itching. It may be localised or generalised. It may be in form of blister, macular, nodular, pustular according to type present.

It is a main sign of childhood infections like measles and chickenpox. Drug reaction due to barbiturates and antibiotics may also cause rashes. Purple red rash is particular of purpura.

Rashes of urticaria and dermatitis are due to allergic reaction. Soothing lotion and antihistamine drugs are useful.

Rate A proportion expressed over a particular unit of time, often multiplied by a constant to obtain whole number values.

Rate difference Similar to risk difference but applied to rates.

Rate pressure product An index of myocardial oxygen consumption determined by the product of heart rate and mean systolic blood pressure.

Rate-limiting factor Any enzyme that is in limited supply and so limits the are at which a chemical can be produced.

Rating of perceived exertion A subjective numerical scale of exercise intensity.

Ratio Expresses the relationship between two numbers by dividing the numerator by the denominator; the simple formula is a/b.

Ratio bias Bias resulting from differential recall of exposure to causal factors among those who have a disease as compared with those who do not have it.

Ratio scale Exhibits all three components of a real-number system: order, distance, and origin. All the arithmetic functions of addition, subtraction, multiplication, and division can be applied to ratio scales.

Ratio schedule A reinforcement schedule in which reinforcer delivery is contingent upon the performance of a specified number of responses.

Ratio variables The variables derived from a continuous scale that has a true 0 point.

Rational emotive behaviour therapy A brief psychotherapeutic treatment that realise on persuation and reason.

Rationalisation A defence mechanism, operating unconsciously, in which an individual attempts to justify or make consciously tolerable by plausible means, feelings, behaviour, or motives that otherwise would be intolerable. Not to be confused with conscious evasion or dissimulation.

Raw scores Scores obtained directly from the measuring instrument—the results of research or of a test administration which have not yet been treated by any statistical methods.

Ray amputation An amputation procedure in which the entire metacarpal or metacarpal with corresponding phalanges are ablated.

Raynaud phenomenon Painful blanching of the fingers in cold weather.

Raynaud's disease In it small capillaries of fingers and toes become contracted. Fingers are affected more than toes. Young women are affected more. On exposure to cold the digits turn white because of shortage of blood. At the time of attack there is feeling of tingling, numbness and burning in the affected part. In severe cases, walls of arteries becomes thick parmanently reducing blood flow and leading to painful ulceration or even gangrene. Parts should be kept warm. Vasodilator drugs may be given.

RDS Respiratory distress syndrome.

Reabsorption Process of absorbing again that occurs in the kidneys.

Reactant A substance that enters into ad is sltered during a chemical reaction.

Reaction An involuntary movement response to a stimulus; it appears in infancy and remains throughout life.

Reaction formation A defence mechanism, operating unconsciously, in which a person adopts effects, ideas, attitudes, and behaviours that are the opposites of impulses he or she harbours either consciously or unconsciously (e.g. excessive moral zeal may be a reaction to strong but repressed social impulse).

Reaction intermediate Any chemical species in a reaction pathway that has a finite chemical lifetime.

Reaction of degeneration When the motor nerve to muscle is cut it undergoes degeneration and after sometime it ceases to function. The muscle chronaxie rapidly increases and faradic current becomes ineffective to excite the muscle while the longer acting galvanic current produces a slow worn like contraction known as reaction of degeneration.

Reactive arthropathy A painful joint inflammation that can follow infection with a number of foodborne pathogens.

Reactive oxygen species One of the several oxygen derived molecules that have the potential to damage cellular proteins, nucleic acid and lipids.

Reactive schizophrenia A schizophrenic condition, the onset of which involves an acute and sudden reaction to severe environmental pressure.

Reactivity Physiological responsivity to an external stimulus.

Reactogenicity The undesired symptoms produced by a vaccine strain.

Reader's syndrome It is of two types migrainous and symptomatic. In migrane type patients are afflicted by episodes of unilateral pulsatile, supraorbital pain and paraesthesia. There may be ptosis or miosis. Some patients develop supraorbital pain suddenly and pain progressively worsens. There is trigeminal nerve involvement manifested by facial paraesthesia, decreased corneal reflex and tic-like bursts of pain and weakness of jaw muscles.

Readiness The time, resulting largely from maturational factors, when the organism is first capable of responding correctly to a task.

Reagent A chemical that is used in a chemical reaction or is used to make up a particular mixture.

Realistic conflict theory A theory from social psychology that suggests that direct competition for scarce or valued resources can lead to prejudice.

Reality principle In psychoanalytic theory, the concept that the pleasure principle, which represents the claims of instinctual wishes, is normally modified by the demands and requirements of the external world. In fact, the reality principle may still work on behalf of the pleasure principle, but it reflects compromises and allows for the postponement of gratification to a more appropriate time. The reality principle usually becomes more prominent in the course of development but may be weak in certain psychiatric illness and undergo strengthening during treatment.

Reality testing The ability to evaluate the external world objectively and to differentiate adequately between it and the internal world. Falsification of reality, as with massive denial or projection, indicates a severe disturbance of ego functioning and/or the perceptual and memory processes upon which it is partly based.

Reamer Instrument with a tapered metal shaft, more loosely spiraled than a file; used to enlarge and clean root canals. These are made by twisting tapering lengths of wire which have a triangular or square cross section to form an instruments with sharp cutting edge along the spiral.

Reappearance hypothesis The view that prior experiences are never completely forgotten; they are somehow stored in the brain as permanent records. According to this view, the full memory of a given event will appear whenever the individual is properly stimulated.

Rebase Process of refitting a denture by replacing the denture base material without changing the occlusal relations of the teeth.

Rebound phenomenon Absence of a check reflex; when resistance to an isometric contraction is suddenly removed, the body segment moves forcibly in the direction in which effort was focused.

Rebuttal Answering the allegations of an adverse party in a legal proceeding. If a charge is not rebutted, the court must accept is as true.

Recall The process of bringing a memory into consciousness. Recall is often used to refer to the recollection of facts, events, and feelings that occurred in the immediate past.

Receiving chambers Atria of the heart; receive blood from the superior and inferior vena cava.

Receiving room Presurgical holding area.

Receptive field Region of the visual world that stimulates a receptor cell or neuron.

Receptor A molecule that is located in the membrane or cytoplasm of cells of a target tissue to which a hormone binds; each receptor binds to a specific type of hormone, neurotransmitter, or other substance.

Receptor blocker A drug that can occupy a membrane receptor without activating it. It is devoid of any intrinsic activity.

Receptor cell A functionally specialized lymphocyte that produces a specific antibody.

Receptor desentization The process by which repeated stimulation of a receptor with an antagonist elicits a smaller response and or requires larger doses to acheive a similar spouse.

Receptor Evidence Evidene whose origin is unknown.

Receptor-G protein Guanine nucleotide-binding regulatory proteins (G proteins) are the links between the many different receptors on a cell's surface and their catalytic units or other effectors within the cell.

Receptor-mediated endocytosis A highly selective process whereby cells take up specific ligands, which usually are large molecules or particles, by enveloping them within a sac of plasma membrane. Ligands are eventually broken down by enzymes in lysosomes.

Recession Gradual drawing away of a tissue or part from its normal position, as the progressive exposure of the root surface by an apical shift of the gingiva.

Recessive In genetics, a gene that may not be expressed phenotypically because of the expression of a contrasting dominant gene.

Recessive allele Pain felt on the surface of the body but actually due to pain in one of the internal organs of the body.

Recessive inheritance The acquisition of a characteristic from both parents that is the result of an allele that must be carried by both members of a pair of homologous chromosomes.

Recipient tissue Tissue bed; area to which tissue gingiva, mucosa, or bone is added in a grafting procedure.

Reciprocal inhibition In behaviour therapy, the hypothesis that if anxiety-provoking stimuli occur simultaneously with the inhibition of anxiety (e.g. relaxation), the bond between those stimuli and the anxiety will be weakened. Inhibition of antagonistic muscles when the agonist is stimulated.

Reciprocal Innvervation Inter connections of neurons arranged so that pathways exciting one group of muscles inhibit the antagonistic neuron.

Reciprocity Licensure based on evidence of having met licensing criteria in another state.

Recognition Perceiving something as having been experienced before, as being familiar; a method of measuring memory.

Recombinant Relating to or resulting from recombination.

Recombinant DNA Synthetic DNA, formed by joining a fragmental of DNA from one source ot a portion of DNA from another.

Recombinant protein A product engineered for large-scale production by manipulating genes.

Reconstitution Process of adding liquid to a powered substance.

Reconstruction hypothesis The view that memories are not full and fixed images but rather reconstructions of prior events or experiences. The memory trace is not complete; it is a remnant of the past and must be used in reconstructing prior experience. The memory is assembled, rather than evoked *in toto*.

Reconstructive phase Portion of periodontal treatmen in which the teeth arches are brought to physiologic from. As they are indicated, reconstruction includes procedures for removal of decay; restoration of teeth with filling, inlays and onlays; endodontics; orthodontics; oral and maxillofacial surgery; implant therapy; and fixed and removable prosthodontics.

Recorded families Families where the parents have divorced, remarried and taken on stepfamilies.

Recording Process of writing information.

Recording electrode Needle or surface electrode used to record electrical activity from nerve and muscle.

Recovery from anesthesia It is the period from the end of surgery to when patient becomes alert and physiologically stable but still he may remain drowsy.

Recovery index Guide for determining a person's fitness level.

Recovery massage Massage structured primarily for the uninjured athlete who want to recover from a strenuous workout or competition.

Recovery oxygen consumption Elevated oxygen use following exercise, due to metabolic changes that start during exercise and continue after exercise. Previously called oxygen debt.

Recovery position Side-lying position that helps to maintain an open airway and prevent aspiration of liquids.

Recovery resistance The ability of plant tissues to grow away from an infection to produce a healthy shoot.

Recruitment The process of increasing the number of active motor units. Also called motor units summation.

Rectal administration of anesthesia It is an effective absorption of drugs due to richer blood supply. Drugs used include 0.4-0.5 mg/kg for cheking convulsions in children.

Rectal bleeding It is a bleeding from rectal canal. Colour of blood may range from bright red to dark brown or black. Haemorrhoids are the most common cause of rectal bleeding on the surface of faeces or on hand while cleaning rectal opening. Some disorders of the colon such as diverticular disease may cause dark red faeces. Cancer of intestine or polyps can cause bleeding. Ulcerative colitis, amoebiasis may cause bloody diarrhoea.

Rectal probe ejaculator It is a choice of therapy in case of person suffering from interruption of sympathetic inervation. It helps in erection and emission in certain cases. This procedure is popular in case of animal. Pulsatile ejaculation generally occurs.

Rectal suppository It is rectal medication for local effects and is solid at room temperature. When introduced it melts at body temperature and produces local effect.

Rectal temperature Temperature may be taken in the rectum by a rectal thermometer with a short blunt bulb. Turn the patient on one side. Lubricate

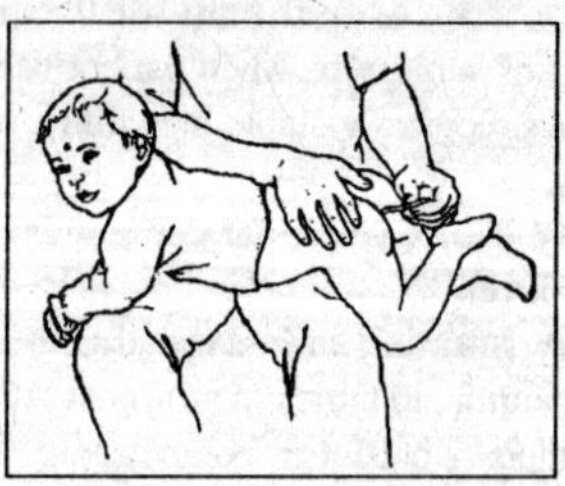

the thermometer bulb evenly for about 2 inches with Vaseline. Insert it in the rectum and let it be there for 3 minutes. Hold in place, then take it out and note the temperature.

Rectal tube Flexible tube inserted into the rectum to assist in relief of flatus.

Rectification Conversion of alternating current to direct current.

Rectilinear motion Motion in a straight line.

Rectovaginal examination It should be a part of rectovaginal examination. Lubricate fingers with

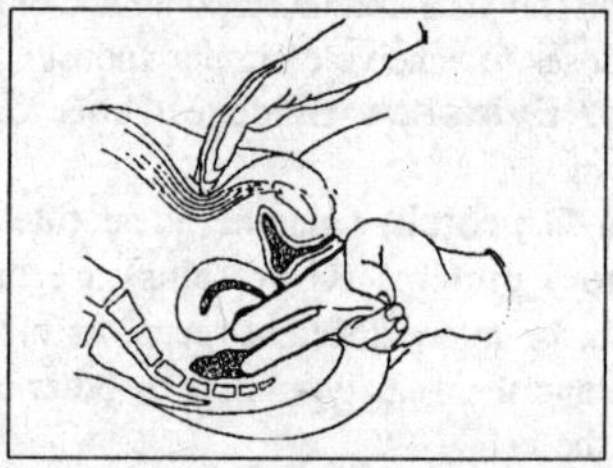

water soluble lubricant. As patient to relax anal sphincter to allow easy entry of examination finger. Check for any nodule or mass or bleeding.

Rectum It is a short, musclular tube that forms the lowest part of large intestine and connects it to anus. Faeces collects in rectum before it is expelled out. The urge to defaecate occurs when faeces distend the rectum. Pressure on rectal wall causes nerve impulses to pass to brain which in turn sends the messages to the muscles in anus to relax allowing defaecation. Inflammation of it is known as proctitis. Rectum can become obstructed due to narrowing caused by radiation therapy or pelvic infection. Rectal prolapse occurs when lining of rectum protrudes outside the anus. During rectal carcinoma bleeding develops during defaecation. There may also be a change in bowel habits, diarrhoea or constipation and sensation of incomplete emptying. Later on pain may develop. Sugery followed by radiotherapy is the only solution of it.

Rectus Straight.

Rectus abdominis Muscle that runs down the middle of the abdomen; protects the abdominal viscera and flexes the spinal column.

Rectus femoris site Injection area in the anterior thigh.

Recumbent measures Measurements taken while the subject is lying down or reclining.

Recumbent position In this position patient lies flat on bed with one pillow at the head end and legs extended. In case of low blood pressure this

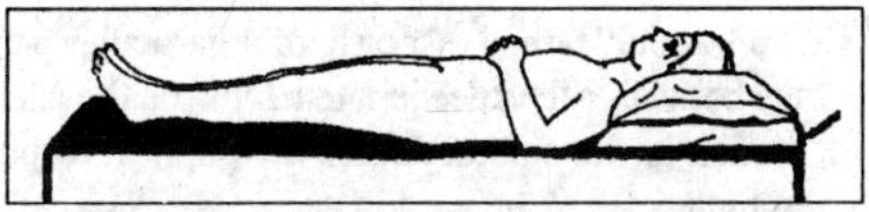

position can be used with two pillows at leg end. By raising the leg there becomes comfortable venous flow from lower extremity.

Recurrent Returning after intermissions.

Recurrent abortion Three or more consecutive first-trimester spontaneous losses of fetus.

Recurrent aphthous ulceration It is a chronic inflammatory disease characterised by repeated episodes of oval or round superficial ulcerations on the mucous membrane of inside lip, cheek, tongue and floor of mouth. Occasionally gingiva may be involved. Lesions are 2-20 mm in diameter and are painful. The lesions are self-limiting and heal spontaneously within 1-2 weeks. However, recurrences are common and more frequent. Treatment is symptomatic.

Recurrent laryngeal nerve It is the nerve that controls the muscles of vocal cord. Its fibres are being branched away from vagus nerve in the neck. It is called recurrent because it loops back to the larynx.

Recurrent mastoiditis It is a tender, erythematous swelling developing in the area of retroauricular scar left by a previous mastoidectomy. There is rapid fluctuation developing in lower half of scar.

Recurvatum A backward bending or curvature of a joint.

Recyling The reuse of waste materials as valuable raw materials for the production of new industrial products.

Red blood cells It is yellowish red, non-nucleated and perfectly elastic, biconcave disc. Its envelop consists of proteins and lipids and is responsible for its characteristic permeability. Average diameter of RBCs is 7.5 microns.

Red blood corpuscles These are 5000,000 per cu mm of blood. The total surface of corpuscles in blood is very large about 600 square metres per litre. Larger area helps in oxygen exchange. The characteristic biconcave shape of RBC is due to stroma of protein. The red cell is flexible and pass through small capillaries. Average life is 120 days.

Red eye The oral mucosa shows extensive white folded or smooth lesions that occur in the form of plaques. Lesions are asymptomatic. There are gelatinous plaques in the eye and red conjunctiva. Lesions undergo excerbation in spring and improve in late summer. If cornea is involved blindness may follow. Disease requires no treatment.

Red marrow It is highly vascular connective tissue which fills the interstices of cancelled bones. It contains large number of marrow cells which gives rise to erythrocytes of blood. Red marrow is found in medullary cavity of long bones and consist of reticular framework supporting numerous blood vessels.

Red nucleus An aggregation of gray matter of a reddish color, located in the upper portion of the midbrain. It sends fibers to certain brain tracts.

Redox The balance between oxidation and reduction states of cellular molecules.

Because some molecules must be oxidized when another is reduced and the overall redox balance is invioable.

Redox pair An electron donor and its corresponding oxidized form; for example, NADH and NAD.

Redubig bugs Characteristically a short three jointed probloseis protrudes from tip of the head. The insects feed primarily on body fluids of other animals.

Reducing agent An electron donor in a coupled oxidation-reduction reaction.

Reducing sugar A sugar in which the carboxyl carbon is not involved in a glycosidic bond and can therefore undergo oxidation.

Reduction The opposite of oxidation. Gain of an electron by an atom resulting in a decrease in positive valence or increase in negative valence.

Reductive stress Where a cell becomes relatively more reduced than normal. It is converse of oxidative stress.

Redundancy Jobless resulting from slack demand of labour.

REEDA Acronym for redness, ecchymosis, oedema, discharge and approximation. Useful for assessing wound healing or the presence of inflammation or infection.

Reef knot For tying a knot 'reef knot' must always be used. Take the ends of the bandage one in each hand, cross the end in the right hand under and then over the end in the left hand thus making a turn. Then cross the end now in the right hand

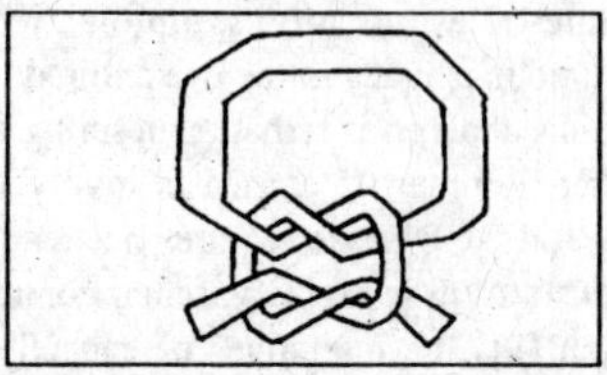

over and then under the end in the left hand thus making a second turn.

Reefing A surgical technique for the repair of slack or redunant soft tissues.

Reenactment Reliving an event as though it were happening at the moment.

Reevaluation Retest' a means of determining whether therapy intervention is effective and should continue, or not.

Reference electrode In motor nerve conduction velocity test, the electrode placed over the tendon of the test muscle. In monopolar recording of EMG, the inactive electrode placed over a neutral area.

Reference sample A sample that allows an absolute scientific or technical identification to be made of a test sample or a control sample. To serve as a reference sample, the material must be accompanied by scientific and/or technical evidence of its identity, composition or properties.

Referral Sending patient to a health care professional for specific diagnosis and treatment of a disease.

Referred autonomic phenomena Vasoconstriction/blanching/coldness, sweating, pilomotor response , ptosis, and/or hypersecretion that is caused by activity of a trigger point in a region separate from the trigger point. The Phenomena usually appear in the area to which the trigger point refers pain.

Referred pain Discomfort perceived in an area of the body away from the site of origin.

Referred trigger point Pain that arises in a trigger point but is felt at a distance, often entirely remote from its source of origin. The distribution of referred trigger point pain rarely coincides with the entire distribution of a peripheral nerve or dermatomal segment.

Reflect To push back tissues from an area.

Reflection (2) An interaction between some type of radiation and a surface that causes the radiation to be "bounced back" or off of the surface rather than penetrating it.

Reflex An unlearned response of a particular part of the body, like the knee jerk to a blow on the patellar tendon or the contraction of the pupil in response to light.

Reflex arc The most basic conduction pathway through the nervous system, connecting a receptor and an effector and consisting of a receptor, a sensory neuron, an intergrating center in the central nervous system, a motor neuron, and an effector.

Reflex reversal Term used to signify the 'change of sign'

Reflex sympathetic dystrophy (RSD) Burning pain, usually felt in a traumatized extremity, and often accompanied by symptoms and signs consistent with sympathetic hypertonia such as increased sweat gland activity, reduced temperature, muscle weakness, edema, and degeneration of skin and bone in the affected body part.

Reflex therapy Treatment that is aimed at stimulating afferent neuromuscular receptors.

Reflexive impotence Impotence caused by damage to reflex arcs.

Reflexive methods Massage techniques that stimulate the nervous system, the endocrine system, and the chemicals of the body.

Reflexology It was developed by Eunice Ingham in America during 1930's. Her theory was that the body is divided into 10 energy zones running the length and if there are blockages within these pathways, there is dysfunction within the body. She devised the foot charts showing the precise position of body's anatomy.

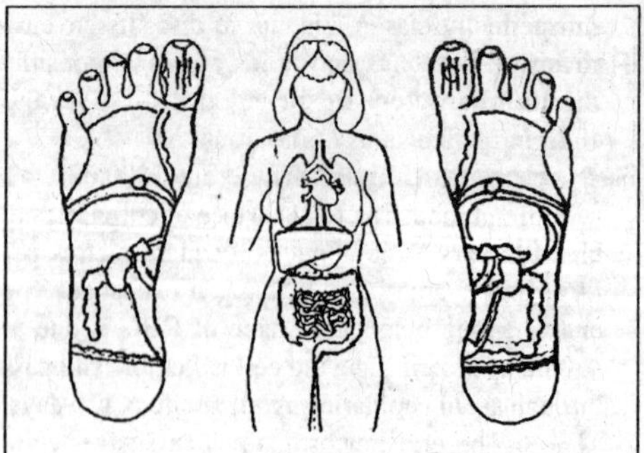

Different reflexology centers

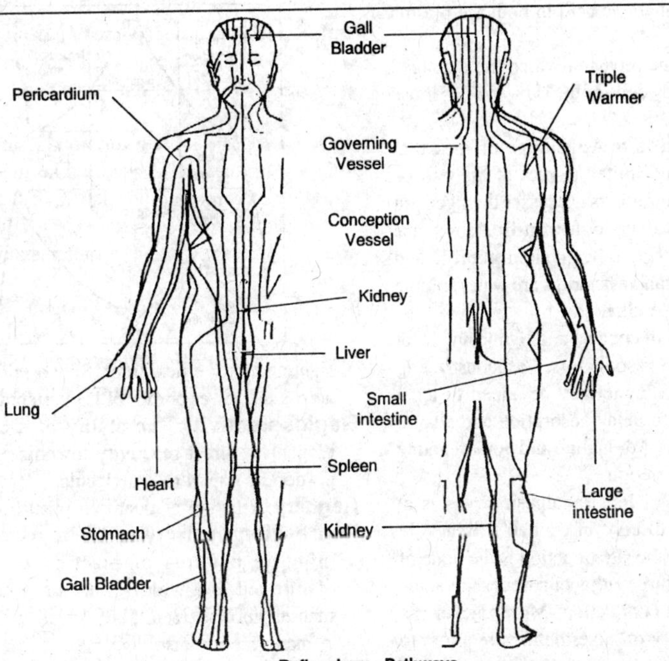

Reflexology - Pathways

Reflux Backflow, as in flow of stomach contents back into esophagus.

Refraction It is the bending of light rays as they pass from one substances to another. In reference to eye, refraction provides the mechanism by which an image is focused on the retina permitting vision. The term is also used to describe the testing of an eye sight. The change in direction of propagation of a wave when it passes from one material to another in which the index of refractions is different.

Refractive index The effect of a material object on the incident wave defined as the ratio of the velocity of light in a vacuum to that in the object.

Refractometer Device used to measure urinary specific gravity by measuring the amount of light that can pass through a drop of urine.

Refractory period Going back to an earlier, usually less adequate, mode of response. In hypnosis, behaving as one did at an earlier stage of life. The brief interval following response of a neuron or muscle fiber during which it is incapable of second response.

Reframing Redefining an event or situation so that it is manageable and controllable.

Refrigeration analgesia It is the application of cold to a localised part of body to block local nerve conduction of painful impulses. It is not to be confused with induced hypothermia, which is the application of cold in order to reduce the oxygen needs of tissues.

During temporary interruption of circulation. some use chilling and not refrigeration. Chilling interferes with conduction of nerve impulse analgesia, reduction of metabolic rate and oxygen requirement. It inhibits bacterial growth and infection.

Refrigeration anesthesia Use of cold to reduce pain sensation.

Refsum disease It is due to disturbance in phytanic acid metabolism. Clinical features include ataxia, atypical retinitis pigmentosa. There may be blindness, deafness, ichthiosis and conduction defects in heart. Protein levels in CSF are high.

Refsum's syndrome A rare autosomal recessive familial disorder characterised by marked accumulation of phytanic acid in both the plasma and tissue.

Regeneration Tissue repair in which the damaged cells are replaced by cells of the same type as those damaged.

Regional anaesthesia Advantage of it is that effects of drugs are limited to part of body to be operated upon. Aftereffects are lesser than general anaesthesia. Relative contraindications are children under 10. Not to be given in stuprose and psychotics. Local analgesic drugs are water soluble salts of lipid soluble alkaloids.

With the exception of cocaine and lignocaine local analgesic drugs are vasodilators, Vasoconstricting agents such as adrenaline may be added to local analgesic solution to delay absorption and also to prolong their action. Adrenaline and noradrenaline do not prolong the action.

The site of action of local analgesic drugs is at surface membrane of cells of excitable tissues. In a myelinated nerve the site of action is the node of Ranvier. Two or three adjacent nodes must be affected to prevent conduction. More thicker the nerve, more quantity of anaesthetic is required to block its conduction. Local analgesia may be of different types such as field block, nerve block, infiltration analgesia, intravenous local analgesia and central neural blockade.

Regional anatomy The division of anatomy concerned with structural arrangement in specific areas of the body, such as the head, neck, thorax, or abdomen.

Regional anesthesia The blockading of nerves that provides pain relief or prevents pain in particular area of the body while maintaining consciousness.

Regions of abdomen For the purpose of description of position of viscera, abdomen is divided into nine regions by means of a pair of vertical and a pair of horizontal planes. The transpyloric plane lies midway between the suprasternal notch and upper margin of pubic symphysis.

Transtubercular plane passes through the tubercle of iliac crest on either side of body through the upper border of L_5 vertebra. Vertical lines one on either side of the midline connecting the midclavicular and mid inguinal points are called

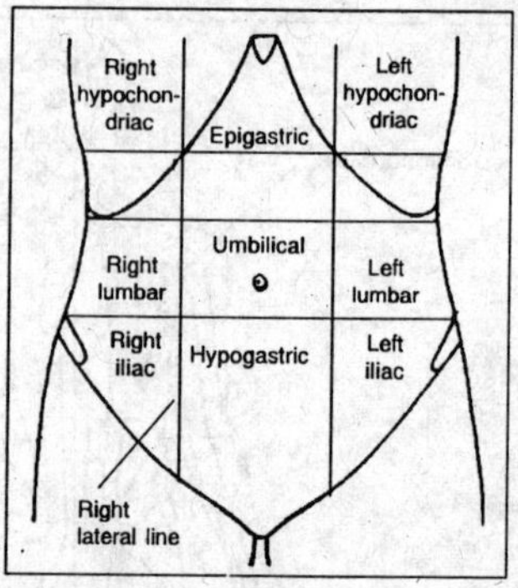

right and left vertical lines. Subcostal line passes across the lower border of L_3 vertebra.

Regioselectivity The ability of a catalyst or reagent to direct reactivity towards a particular portion or region of a molecule.

Registry A listing of qualified practitioners.

Regression Partial or symbolic return to more infantile patterns of reacting or thinking. Manifested in a wide variety of circumstances such as normal sleep, play, physical illness, and in many mental disorders.

Regulation A standard published by a governmental administrative agency under legal authority delegated to it by the legislature. Regulations have the force of law in both civil and criminal proceedings. Much of medical practice is governed by regulations rather than by statues.

Regulatory enzyme An enzyme having a regulatory functions through its capacity to undergo a change in catalytic activity by allosteric mechanisms or by covalent modification.

Regulatory gene A gene that gives rise to a product involved in the regulation of the expression of another gene; for example, a gene coding for a repressor protein.

Regulon A group of genes or operons that are coordinately regulated even through some, or all, may be spatially distant within the chromosome or genome.

Regurgitation Being passive act it is silent. Predisposing factors include, head down position if the cardia is inefficient, a stomach full of fluid, indwelling stomach or oesophageal tubes. Drugs favouring reflux include atropine, tricyclic antidepressants, phenothiazines and ganglion blocking agents. Tone of lower oesophageal sphincter is increased by ranitidine and metaclorpramide. Actually it is bringing up of food or liquid from the stomach as far as throat or mouth. Cause is indigestion but nausea is not felt. In heart failure backward flow of blood is noted.

Rehabilitation It is the treatment aimed at enabling a person to live an independent life following injury, illness or drug or alcohol dependence. Rehabilitation is done generally in residential places. Drug and alcohol rehabilitation centres help people through the period of withdrawal and providing psychological support. Restoration to former state of health, efficiency, and independent action; regeneration.

Rehabilitative brace Brace that allows protected motion of an injured joint that has been treated surgically.

Rehydration therapy It is the treatment of dehydration by giving fluids IV or orally with salt and glucose. The amount depends on the degree of dehydration. Oral rehydration solution (ORS) is available easily to be diluted in fixed amount of water and to be given. At home also oral rehydration solution may be prepared by adding one-half teaspoonful of salt, 2 TSF of sugar and half litre of water.

Reiger's syndrome It is an autosomal dominant hereditary disorder. It shows oligodontia and microdontia associated with iridial hypoplasia and anterior synechiae. Glaucoma may develop as a complication. Missing teeth also develop.

Reil, island Insula of cerebral hemisphere.

Reimbursement To pay back or compensate someone.

Reimplantation Replacement of tissue or a structure into the site from which it was previously lost or removed.

Reinforced composites These have been developed of produce onlays, crowns and three unit bridges. These can be reinforced with glass or polyethylene fibres.

Reinforced Kneading The basic kneading technique is performed with one hand on top of the other, to reinforce the stroke. It is useful for treating very large patients, when extra effort is required for effective treatment.

Reinforcement Generally, a reduction or satisfaction of drive; a reward. In classical conditioning, any instance in which a conditioned stimulus is followed by an unconditioned stimulus. In operant conditioning, any instance in which response is followed by favourable consequences; any event which increases the probability of a response.

Reinforcer In operant conditioning, any event that strengthens the behavior it follows.

Reiter's syndrome It is characterised by non-specific urethritis, conjunctivitis or less commonly uveitis and polyarthritis.

Relapsing (recurrent) fever Periods of pyrexia that alternate with normal temperatures; periods may last for a day or more.

Relapsing fever It is caused by bacterial disorder by lice or ticks. There develops recurrent episode of fever lasting for 8 to 10 days and again developing after a few days. Fever with shivering, headache, joints pain and skin rash may develop. There may be jaundice. Fever may even cause delirium.

Relatedness The proportion of genes shared among individuals that are identical by descent rather than simply identical in state.

Relationship Association between two people.

Relationship focussed copying Attempts to manage one's social relationship during stressful period.

Relative density Relative density of an object is the ratio of the weight of the object to the weight of an equal volume of water.

Relative humidity Ratio between the amount of moisture in the air and the greatest amount of water vapor the air can hold at a given temperature.

Relative movement In perception a visual cue to distance gained from the speed and direction of movement of objects in the environment. When they are moving, nearby objects seem to move more rapidly than distant objects; when the observer is moving, objects nearby move in the opposite direction, and those in the distance move in the same direction as the viewer.

Relative risk (RR) The ratio of the risk in the exposed group to the risk in the unexposed group.

Relativistic thinking A form of thinking which recognises that all knowledge must be understood and evaluated in a particular context. The complexity of knowledge is recognised, with the understanding that no single viewpoint can account for all explanations. The value of particular facts or theories depends upon the purpose for which they are used. The implication is that there are few absolutes; some evaluation or judgement must be made.

Relaxation Relaxation of mind and body helps in conserving energy. After relaxation one feels energetic. It prolongs life.

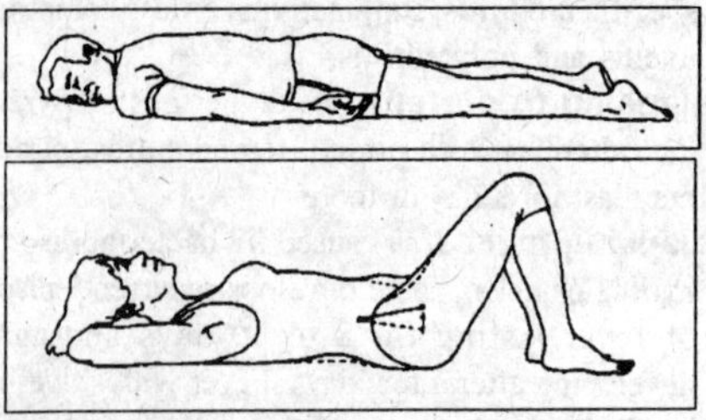

Relaxed (slouched) posture A posture characterized by a shifting of the pelvic segment anteriorly resulting in hip extension, and shifting of the thoracic segment posteriorly resulting in flexion of the thorax on the upper lumbar spine. An increased lordosis in the lower lumbar region, an increased kyphosis in the thoracic region, and a forward head are usually observed with a relaxed posture.

Relaxin A female hormone produced by the ovaries that increases flexibility of the public symphysis and helps dilate the uterine cervix to ease delivery of a baby.

Relearning Regaining a skill that has been partially or wholly lost. The saving involved in relearning, as compared with original learning, gives an index of the degree of retention.

Release Setting free of tissues.

Release factor A protein factor that promotes the termination of protein biosynthesis and release of the mRNA and newly synthesized polypeptide from the ribosome.

Releaser effect A rapid behavioral response to a pheromone.

Releasing factor A hormone that is produced by the pituitary gland and stimulates endocrine glands to release hormones into the circulatory system. Hypothalamic hormones that stimulate release of other hormones by the pituitary gland.

Releasing hormone A peptide that is released by the hypothalamus and acts to increase or decrease the release of hormones from the anterior pituitary.

Relevance Evidence is relevant when, if it were accepted, it could rationally affect, directly or indirectly, the assessment of the probability of the existence of a fact in issue.

Relevant question Polygraph test questions which refer directly to the crime under investigation.

Reliability Consistency of measurement; dependability as a measuring instrument. Reliability may be indicated by high correlation between test and retest scores for the same individuals.

Reliability coefficient A numerical value, or coefficient, indicating the stability of test scores, often obtained by administering the test twice to the same subjects and comparing the scores. The value can range from 0.0 to 1.0.

Reliable test A test that produces the same results on successive trials. One of the criteria for muscle length and strength tests.

Religion A system of beliefs centered around the concept of a supernatural being or force.

Religiosity A continuum with intrinsic religious motivation on one end and extrinsic religious motivation on the other end.

Religiousness Adherence to the beliefs and practices of an organized church or religious institution.

Reline To resurface the tissue side of a denture with new base material to make it fit more accurately.

REM Rapid eye movement.

Remaining dentin thickness The depth of dentin remaining between the pulpal floor of a cavity preparation and the pulp chamber .

Remedial Intended to correct something.

Remedial massage Massage used for minor to moderate injuries.

Remediation A remedy; correction of a fault or problem.

Remedies The means by which a court will enforce a party's rights or redress a wrong. These include payment of damages, injunctions, and ordering the parties to carry out specific actions.

Remineralization The restoration of mineral elements to a structure.

Reminiscence A normal, universal process of life review in the elderly prompted in part by the realisation of approaching death. The person reviews past life and conflicts and possibilities for their resolution. Depression, anxiety, regret, and despair may be persent.

Remission A decrease or arrest of the symptoms of a disease, also the period during which such decrease occurs. It is the period in which symptoms are distinctly absent. Person looks normal but after sometimes it may reappear again.

Remittent fever Fluctuations in temperature above normal without returning to normal between fluctuations.

Remodeling A continuous process of breakdown and renewal in bone; the final common pathway for adult bone loss or gain.

Removable appliance Orthodontic appliance designed to be removed and replaced by the patient.

Removable partial denture A denture that replaces several teeth (not an entire arch) and is not permanently attached to the remaining dentition, thus facilitating cleaning.

Removable Teeth Branch of prosthodontics that is concerned with the replacement and restoration of teeth and tissues with a prosthesis that can be readily removed.

Renal artery thrombosis White thrombus occurs in arteries. It is formed by platelet adhesions and aggregation with fibrin deposition in layers and

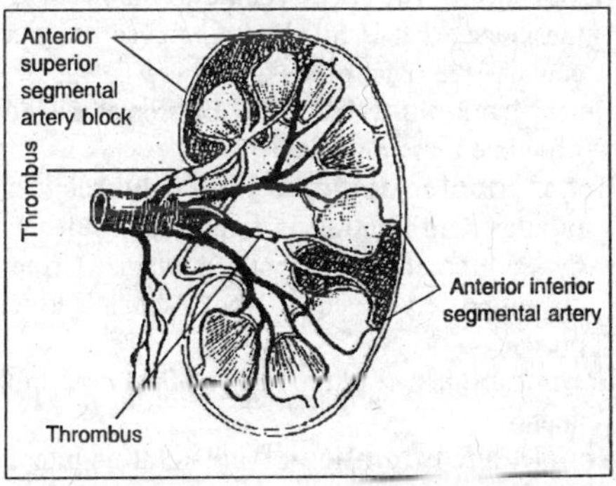

may in time occlude the artery. In kidney it may result in infarct in area supplied by respective artery.

Renal calculi Kidney stone results in intermittent spasm of severe pain on one side referred to back. If it is in ureter pain may be radiating towards its course. Each spasm usually lasts for several minutes. Antispasmodics helps the patient.

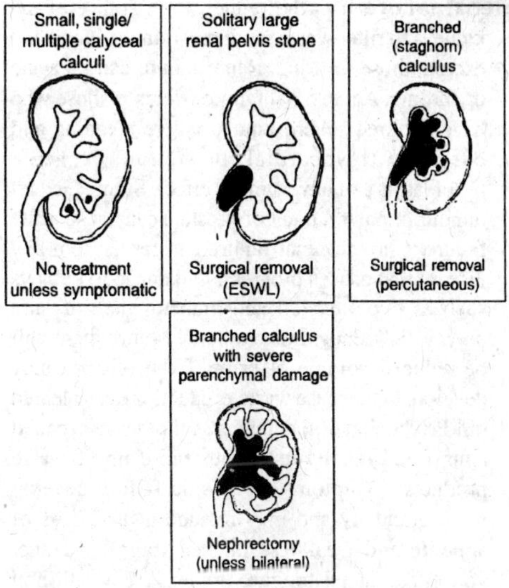

Renal capsule The connective tissue capsule that surrounds each kidney.

Renal colic Patient is seized with sudden pain starting in the loin radiating down to testis, groin and inner side of thigh. Testis of the affected side may be drawn up due to the same region. Tenderness can be elicited over the renal angle. Frequency of micturition may be present. Previous history of similar colic may be there.

Renal corpuscle The part of the nephron located in the cortex of the kidney.

Renal cortex It is pale, dense and homogeneous on macroscopic study. It contains 1 million renal capsules. and convoluted portions of renal tubules.

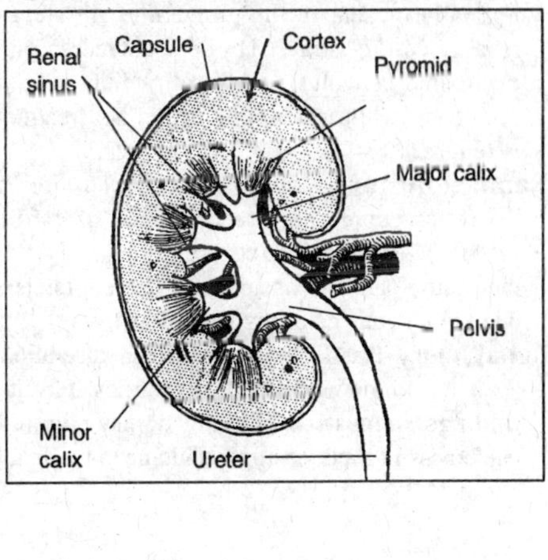

Renal failure It is the reduction in ability of the kidneys to filter waste products from the blood and excrete those in urine. Renal failure can be acute or chronic. Acute renal failure occurs in those who have suffered severe injury, severe bleeding and burns. A myocardial infarction or acute pancreatitis can have similar effect. Stone, bladder tumour or enlargement of prostate can cause acute failure. Chronic renal failure can result from any disease that causes progressive damage to kidneys such as hypertension and diabetes mellitus and polycystic kidney. In acute renal failure there will be reduced volume of urine. Even oliguria may develop. In that case waste products are not cleared off. Production of less than 50 ml of urine is called anuria and results in serious build up of waste products. Symptoms of chronic failure develop more gradually and may include nausea, loss of appetite and weakness. In last stage headache, vomiting, furred tongue, unpleasant breath and coma may develop. Kidney function tests help in diagnosis.

Renal fat pad The layer of adipose tissue that surrounds each kidney.

Renal glycosuria It is characterised by presence of glucose in urine at normal blood glucose level. Glucose metabolism and glucose tolerance test curve is normal. Glucose reabsorptive capacity of some of nephrons is reduced resulting in lowered glucose threshold while the maximum glucose reabsorption may be normal. The disorder is hereditary, asymptomatic and benign. When a small quantity of sugar is excreted in urine but blood sugar is not above normal. Glucose is normally present in the glomerular filtrate and renal glycosuria is caused by deficient reabsorption in proximal convoluted tubules. Condition is found accidently while examining urine. No treatment is required.

Renal infarcts Kidneys are favoured sites of infarctions since they receive 25% of cardiac output. Most renal infarcts are asymptomatic but they cause pain and haematuria. Large infarcts of one kidney may cause hypertension.

Renal injury This includes contusions, lacerations, shattered kidneys and pedicle injuries. Physical findings suggestive of renal damage include tenderness in flank or upper abdomen or palpable abdominal mass. Flank distension or ecchymosis may indicate a retroperitoneal collection of blood.

Renal insufficiency In this diseased or damaged kidney cannot cope with normal flow of blood. Waste products may collect along with oedema. Hypertension may develop it.

Renal medulla The inner portion of the kidney, including the renal pyramids and renal columns.

Renal oedema It occurs in legs and eyelids at the same time although oedema around eyes on rising in the morning first attract the attention. Urine examines feature of renal disease. Presence of many casts is strong evidence of renal origin. Patient looks pale or waxy.

Renal pelvis The inner cavity of the kidney that is formed by the expanded ureter and into which the major calyces open.

Renal plasma clearance rate The milliliters of plasma cleared of a particular solute per minute by the exertion of that solute in the urine. If there is no reabsorption of secretion of that solute by the nephron tubules, the plasma clearance rate is equal to the glomerular filtration rate.

Renal pyramid Coneshaped structure that extends from the renal sinus, where the apex is located, into the cortex of the kidney, where the base is located.

Renal sinus The cavity central to the medulla of the kidney that is filled with adipose tissue and contains the renal pelvis.

Renal transplantation The transfer of a kidney from one person to another.

Renal tubular acidosis In this disorder renal tubular acidification is impaired resulting in hyperchloraemic metabolic acidosis. Urine is inappropriately alkaline. Hypokalaemia is usually present.

Renal tubule One of the two principal parts of the nephron.

Renal vein thrombosis Unilateral or bilateral renal vein thrombosis is mainly seen in the neonatal period.

Dehydration, sepsis and shocks are the predisposing factors. Infants of diabetic mothers are also more susceptible. Gross haematuria usually follows. In bilateral cases oliguria and renal failure occur. Kidneys become large and palpable. Treatment is conservative.

Rendu-Osler-Weber syndrome The syndrome is characterised by small, thin dilated vessels in the skin and mucous membrane that blanch on pressure and tend to bleed spontaneously.

Reniform Shaped like a kidney.

Renin It is an enzyme involved in the regulation of blood pressure. When BP falls kidney releases renin which converts an inactive substance called angiotensinogen to protein angiotensin. It stimulates the release of hormone aldosterone which also increases BP. Blood pressure can be lowered by drugs that affect the reninangiotensin system such as beta-blockers which inhibit the production of renin and ACE inhibitors which interfere its action.

Renin-angiotensin-aldosterone pathway A mechanism for the control of aldosterone secretion by angiotensin II, initiated by the secretion of renin by the kidney in response to low blood pressure.

Renography It is a type of radio-nuclide scanning used for scanning the kidney. Radionuclide hippuran or peptic acid is injected into blood stream and passes in urine through kidney. Radiation count is done continuously during the procedure. The information is recorded graphically as a renogram. Both kidneys are examined for comparison purpose. It is done where obstruction of urine is suspected. Normally radiation count increases rapidly for 30 seconds after injection, rises more slowly for five minutes and then decreases as radionuclide passes into bladder.

Repair of laceration of birth canal Spontaneous lacerations of birth canal may be reparied either before or after delivery of placenta. Abrasions of lacerations which dont bleed dont usually require suturing.

Reparative dentin Dentin of an irregular nature formed below a carious lesion as a means of preserving pulpal intergrity.

Repellent Any chemical that causes a negative chemotaxis response.

Reperfusion Resumption of blood supply.

Reperfusion injury Damage to the cells caused by oxygen free radicals. During reperfusion free radicals react with the cells and form lipid peroxides leading to cell damage.

Repertoire The range of skills, aptitudes, or abilities that an individual posesses.

Repetition compulsion In psychoanalytic theory, the impulse to re-enact earlier emotional experiences, Considered by Freud more fundamental than the pleasure principle. According to Jones, "The blind impulse to repeat earlier experiences and situations quite irrespective of any advantage that doing so might bring from a pleasure-pain point of view."

Repetitive strain injuries Disorder that results from cumulative trauma to musculoskeletal structures.

Replacement Tissue repair in which the damaged cells are replaced by cells of a type different from those damaged.

Replacement culture The resuspension of a microorganism in a medium other than its growth medium.

Replant To replace a tooth or teeth that have been removed from the alveolus either intentionally or unintentionally, as in an accident.

Replantation Replacement of a traumatically or otherwise removed tooth back into its own alveolar socket.

Replantation of tooth It is the replacement of traumatically or exfoliated tooth in its own socket. The tooth is cleaned, its root canal is filled and it is inserted back into its socket and splinted. The root surface usually undergoes resorption. Repair follows by bone formation. Later tooth is ankylosed to the surrounding bone. These may be ueful for years.

Replication 1. The synthesis of a copy of a DNA molecule, using the original as a template. 2. the synthesis of multiple copies of virus genome transcribed from a complementary strand of RNA or DNA.

Replication cycle The series of steps that a virus or cell goes through to multiply itself.

Replicon A region of DNA that contains the origin for initiation of replication.

Repolarization The reestablishment of the resting membrane potential after depolarization has occurred.

Reposition The return of an abnormally placed part

Representative sample A sample or subgroup which accurately reflects the characteristics of the larger population. A representative sample of voters includes males and females, the elderly and the young.

Repressible enzyme In bacteria, an enzyme whose synthesis is inhibited when its reaction product is readily available to the cell.

Repression A defence mechanism, operating unconsciously, that banishes unacceptable ideas, fantasies, effects, or impulses from consciousness or that keeps out of consciousness what has never been conscious. Although not subject to voluntary recall, the repressed material may emerge in disguised form. Often confused with the conscious mechanism of suppression.

Repressor The protein that binds to the regulatory sequence or operator for a gene, blocking its transcription.

Reproduction The ability of a species to produce offspring, or the fact or activity of producing offspring.

Reproductive axis The intergrated system of reproductive organs and control systems.

Reproductive cell division Type of cell division in which gametes (sperm and egg cells) are produced; consists of meiosis and cytokinesis.

Reproductive competition The various behavior patterns such as aggression that males use to compete for access to females and for the opportunity to mate and to prevent other males from mating.

Reproductive cycle A recurring, predictable series of changes in physiological activity that characterize the process of reproduction in a given species; can be short-term or over the lifetime of the organism.

Reproductive function Any bodily or behavioral function dedicated to the production of offspring.

Reproductive success The number of an animal's offspring that survive to maturity, relative to the number produced by others in the same population.

Reproductive system, female These are the organs which makes a woman to produce ova, to have sexual intercourse. These organs lie in pelvic cavity. Ova is released by ovaries. Adjacent to each ovary is fallopain tube which carries ova to uterus. If on journey along the fallopian tube an ovum unites with a sperm fertilisation takes place. Later on it develops in uterus. Fertility begins at puberty and ceases at menopause.

Reproductive system, male The organs that enable man to have sexual intercourse and to fertilise ova with sperm. Sperms are produced in testes lying in scrotum. From each testis sperms pass into epididymis where these mature slowly and are stored. During orgasm semen is ejaculated from the urethra through erect penis.

Reproductive wastage Loss of the products of conception.

Rescue breathing Process of ventilating a nonbreathing victim's lungs.

Research Scholarly or scientific investigation or inquiry.

Research design The overall plan for collecting and analyzing data.

Research report A description of a scientific investigation, which includes a detailed statement of the purpose, method, results, and conclusions of the research.

Resect To surgically remove.

Resection Operation in which part of a tissue or an organ is removed.

Reservoir A host species or inanimate source that supports the long-term growth of a pathogen in nature, but that is not necessarily susceptible to disease caused by the pathogen.

Resident A client in a longterm or extended care facility.

Resident microorganism Generally, nonpathogens that are constantly present on the skin.

Residual urine The volume of urine in the bladder after a ormal voiding.

Residual volume The volume of air still contained in the lungs after a maximal expiration; about 1200 mL.

Residue A single unit within a polymer; for example, an amino acid within a polypeptide chain. The term reflects the fact that sugars, nucleotides, and amino acids lose a few atoms generally the elements of water when incorporated in their respective polymers.

Resilience Property of returning to the former shape or size after distortion.

Resin-modified glass ionomer A glass ionomer material modified by the addition of a resin monomer component to enhance its properties.

Resins Certain trees and plants produce exudates of natural resins. These are insoluble in water but vary in solubility. Shellac is produced by insects.

Numerous natural resins are blended with waxes to develop waxes for dental applications. The mixture produces harder products. Synthetic resins such as polyethylene and vinyl resins of various types are added to paraffin waxes to improve their toughness for dental applications. Natural resins such as dammar and kauri may be mixed with waxes. These may be used in organic solvents to produce film forming materials used as a cavity liner.

Resistance A force tending to hinder motion; in muscle testing, refers to resistance by the examiner or by gravity during test movements.

Resistance reflex Resistance to passive movement notably at the knee joint, produced by passive stretching of neuromuscular spindles. Compare with Assistance reflex.

Resistance to flow The force acting in opposition to the movement of a fluid or gas.

Resisted inhalation A technique of resisting movement of the diaphragm during inhalation for the purpose of increasing the strength of the diaphragm, either by manually resisting or with weights.

Resistence form Shape given to a prepared cavity to enable the restoration and remaining tooth structure to withstand masticatory stress.

Resitency It occurs when an individual is exposed to noxious circumstnaces but succeeds.

Resolution In microscopy, the ability to distinguish objects that are close together, defined as the minimum distance between points or parts of the object that appear as distinct points in the image.

Resonance The sound produced by percussing on a part that can vibrate freely.

Resorption Removal of bone or tooth structure by pressure; gradual destruction of dentin and cementum of the root, as the primary teeth prior to shedding, in orthodontic tooth movement, bone formation on one side compensates for resorption of bone on the other side.

Resource A general term for any environmental factor that enhances reproductive success and that is in short supply, relative to the number of potential users.

Resourceful compensation Adjustments made by the body to manage a permanent or chronic dysfunction.

Respect Communication of esteem, honor, or consideration of another.

Respiration It is the physiological process for carrying oxygen throughout the body by means of RBCs and collecting carbon dioxide and excreting it outside. It has two stages, inspiration and

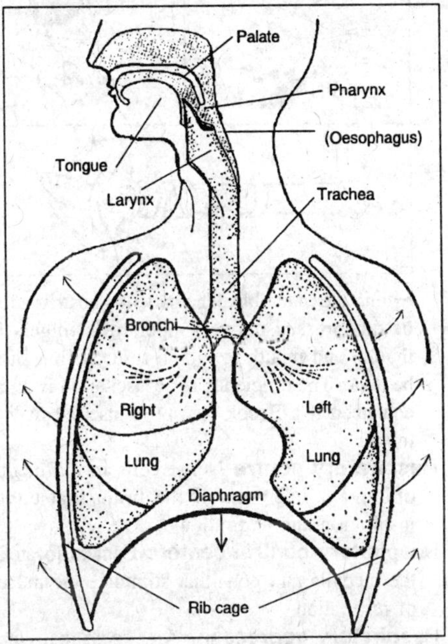

expiration and pause in between. To count the respiration, count the rise and fall of chest of upper abdomen for full one minute. The normal rate of respiration per minute is as follows, in newborn 40, at 1 year 30, between 2 to 5 years 24 to 28, adults 16 to 18, a little quicker in women than men. The ratio of respiration to pulse is usually 1:4.

Respiratory acidosis Acidosis due to increased arterial PC02 caused by alveolar hypoventilation.

Respiratory alkalosis This is caused by hyperventilation which causes hypocapnia and rise of blood pH. It results in reduction of cerebral blood flow and shrinkage of brain and reduction in cerebral oxygen tension. There will be noted fall of blood pressure, cardiac output and vasoconstriction. It results in increase in circulating RBCs. There will be loss of plasma from circulation and fall of plasma sodium and shift to the left of O_2 dissociation curve.

Respiratory arrest In respiratory arrest skeletal muscles become flaccid and pupils are widely dilated. The patient should be laid flat on the floor and his or her airway should be cleared, then

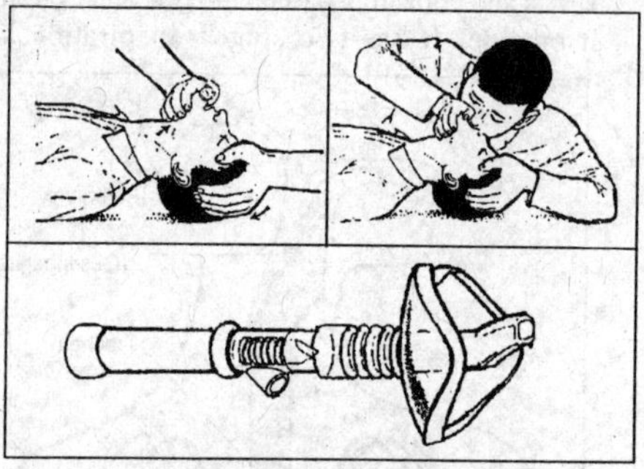

extend the mandible. The patient's nostrils should be compressed between operator's fingers and thumb, and mouth to mouth resuscitation should be done. The efficiency of resuscitation is greatly enhanced if a Brook airway is inserted over the tongue.

Respiratory centre Nerve cells in the medulla oblongata and pons of the brain that control inspiration and expiration.

Respiratory control centers Centers located in the medulla and pons that stimulate the muscles of respiration.

Respiratory depressant Any agent that acts to reduce the activity of the respiratory center or otherwise retard pulmonary ventilation.

Respiratory distress syndrome It is seen in preterm small babies at birth but may also be observed in babies of diabetic mother delivered by caesarian section. Infant develop it in first four fours after birth. There is poor peripheral circulation and extremities become pale and oedematous.

Respiratory distress syndrome (RDS) of the newborn A disease of newborn infants, especially premature ones, in which insufficient amounts of surfactant are produced and breathing is labored.

Respiratory droplet A droplet produced by high velocity airflow over the wet respiratory mucosa, generated by coughs, sneezes, and other forced expiratory maneuvers.

Respiratory failure The inability of the respiratory system to ventilate the alveoli.

Respiratory membrane Structure in the lungs consisting of the alveolar wall and basement membrane and a capillary endothelium and basement membrane, through which the diffusion of respiratory gases occurs. Also called the alveolar capillary membrane.

Respiratory mucosa Mucus-covered membrane that lines the tubes of the respiratory tree.

Respiratory muscle fatigue It is the inability of the respiratory muscles to sustain tension with repeated activity.

Respiratory muscles Muscles that are responsible for the changing shape of the thoracic cavity that allows air to move in and out of the lungs.

Respiratory quotient (RQ) Ratio of CO2 exhaled to O2 inhaled; depending on the net metabolic needs of the body, the ratio ranges from 0.7 to 1.0, and averages around 0.8; carbohydrate metabolism produces an RQ = 1; protein metabolism RQ = 0.8; and fat metabolism RQ = 0.7.

Respiratory rate Number of ventilations per minute.

Respiratory stimulant Any agent that enhances the activity of the respiratory center.

Respiratory system Respiratory organs are responsible for carrying oxygen from the air to the blood stream and for expelling waste products, i.e. CO_2. Air passes from nose to mouth via various respiratory passage to millions of alveoli in lungs. Oxygen passes through thin walls of alveoli into the blood stream and CO_2 passes from blood into alveoli to be breathed out. Diseases of muscles and diaphragm make it difficult to inflate lungs.

Respiratory therapist Health professional who helps patients increase respiratory function and/or overcome or cope with the effects of respiratory conditions.

Respiratory tract The two division of the respiratory system are the upper and lower respiratory tracts.

Respirofermentation Yeast fermentative metabolism in the presence of oxygen.

Respirometer A closed vessel in which oxygen consumption due to biological activity can be measured.

Respite care Provision of shortterm relief or time off for people providing home care to an ill, diabled, or frail older adult.

Respondent The party who argues against a petition or appeal.

Respondent condition A form of unconscious learning in which an organism learns an association between stimuli; also known as Pavlovian conditioning and classical conditioning.

Respondent conditioning (Pavlovian conditioning) Elicitation of a response by a stimulus that normally does not elicit that response. The response is one that is mediated primarily by the autonomic nervous system (such as salivation or a change in heart rate). A previously neutral stimulus is repeatedly presented just before an unconditioned stimulus that normally elicits that response.

When the response subsequently occurs in the presence of the previously neutral stimulus, it is called a conditioned response, and the previously neutral stimulus, a conditioned stimulus.

Respondent cuperior Principle that holds an employer liable for the negligent acts of an employee when carrying out the employer's order or serving the employer's interest.

Response An action, such as doing or saying something; involving the actions of a muscle or a gland.

Response bias A subject's tendency to give a certain response regardless of the stimulation. For example, a subject may have a tendency to answer "no" to questions, even when the negative answers are contradictory.

Another subject may be inclined to agree, regardless of the nature of the question.

Response regulator A protein containing a receiver domain, which brings about the final step in a signal transduction pathway resulting in regulation of the target of the system. Many response regulators are transcription factors that activate or repress gene expression upon phosphorylation of their receiver domain.

Rest Waking state characterized by reduced activity and reduced mental stimulation.

Restatement of content In the person-centred approach to counselling, a method of responding to feelings by rephrasing the person's statements, often in somewhat different words. the counsellor makes no effort at interpretation of feelings but rather, by restatement of content, shows that he or she understands and appreciates the individual's reaction.

Resting cell A quiescent, nongrowing cell.

Resting energy expenditure The energy expanded in a normal life situation while at rest, and energy used following meals and exercise.

Resting membrane potential The voltage difference between the inside and outside of a cell membrane when the cell is not responding to a stimulus; in many neurons and muscle fibers, it is –70 to –90 m/v, with the inside of the cell negative relative to the outside.

Resting metabolic rate The energy expenditure measurement as done for BMR but without a requiremnet of 12 hour fast.

Resting position The first stroke of the massage; the simple laying on of hands.

Resting potential The voltage across the cell membrane produced by a greater negative charge on the intracellular side relative to the extracellular side in the absence of stimulation.

Resting tremor Present when involved body segment is at rest; typically disappears or decreases with purposeful movement.

Restitution As the head is no longer flexed inside the birth canal, it rotates through 45° to return to the position that it held prior to internal rotation. Head is at right angles to shoulder.

Restless leg It is a syndrome resulting in burning, pricking or aching sensations in the muscles of leg. Symptoms become worse at night in bed and gets relief during movements. It tends to run in families specially in pregnancy, smokers and one who consume lot of caffeine. It may develop in persons having rheumatoid arthritis. Exact cause is not known, may be due to circulatory problem.

Restless legs syndrome Movement typically in the legs, but occasionally in the arms or other body parts, to relieve disturbing skin sensations.

Restoration A device or component used to replace tooth structure.

Restrained eating The chronic tendency to try to exert control over food intake.

Restraint Device used to immobilize a client or an extermity

Restratin alternatives Protective or adaptive devices that promote patient safety and postureal support, but which the patient can release independently.

Restrictive cardiomyopathy A disease of the myocardium characterized by marked endocardial scarring of the ventricles with resulting impaired diastolic filling.

Restrictive lung dysfunction An abnormal reduction in pulmonary ventilation.

Resuscitation Any procedure that restores that ability of an organism to grow and develop after sublethal injury.

Resynthesis The polymerization of nucleotides into excised region of damaged nucleic acids.

Retained placenta A condition in which the natural expulsion of the placenta is delayed for 48 hours or longer after birth.

Retained suppository In case of bronchial asthma aminophylline suppository is given. As anaesthetic suppository thiopentone is used to cause anaesthetic effect in children. As alternate route to IV steroid suppository hydrocortisone is used as suppository to produce desired effect in case of proctitis and ulcerative colitis.

Retarded ejaculation It is a persistent delay or failure in occurrence of orgasm and ejaculation despite the adequate erection. It can cause distress to both the partners. The man may feel inadequate and humiliated and may face climax to deceive his partner. On some occasion wife may welcome husband's delayed ejaculation to have sufficient time to reach the orgasm.

Retarded fetal growth Babies who weigh less than the mean minus two standard deviations for their gestational age are said to suffer from retarded intrauterine growth. Stationary weight growth or abdominal girth is suggestive of retarded growth. The volume of liquour amnii also decreases with impairement of placental function.

Retching Act of vomiting without producing vomitus.

Rete testis A network of ducts in the center of the testis associated with the production of spermatozoa.

Retention catheter Urinary tube that is left in place for a period of time.

Retention enema Solution held in the large intestine.

Retention form Provision made in a cavity preparation to prevent displacement of the restoration.

Retention of urine It is common after surgical symptoms on vagina and perineum. Postoperative oedema may cause obstruction of flow of urine.Retroverted gravid uterus between 12th and 14th weeks of pregnancy may cause it. Ectopic gestation, cervical myoma and spinal cord lesions may result it.

Retentive properties Ability of a dental material to resist movement or displacement under axial stress.

Reticular Reticular formation.

Reticular activating system (RAS) A portion of the reticular formation that has many ascending connections with the cerebral cortex; when this area of the area of the brain stem is active, nerve impulses pass to the thalamus and widespread areas of the cerebral cortex, resulting in generalized alterness or arousal from sleep.

Reticular cartilage Elastic cartilage.

Reticular formation In it bundles of fibres are not organised into well-defined tracts but are arranged in a sort of crisscross network, hence the term reticular. It is deeply placed in brainstem. Stimulation of reticular neurons of one side of brainstem produces bilateral somatic and visceral responses. Reticular formation is concerned with state of alertness and it influences the somatic and visceral motor activities.

Reticulation A cracking of the film emulsion that results from a drastic temperature difference between the developer solution and the rinse water.

Reticulocyte Immature red blood cells. Normal value for children is 1%.

Reticulocytosis An increase in the number of immature forms of red blood cell reticulocytes in the bloodstream.

Reticuloendothelial system Collection of cells that are capable of phagocytosis.

Reticulogranular pattern A network of granulelike shadows in a radiograph of an infant with infant respiratory distress syndrome.

Reticulonodular pattern A network of nodulelike shadows throughout both lungs the typical radiographic presentation of idiopathic pulmonary fibrosis.

Reticulum In ruminant mammals, a small pouch of that extends from anterior of the rumen. It collects either large feed particles for rumination or small particles for passage to the lower gut.

Retina It is the light sensitive membrane that lines inside the back of eye on which images are cast by the cornea and lens. Retina contains rods and cones which convert light energy into nerve impulses. Then it conveys these impulses back along optic nerve to brain. Rods are very sensitive to dim light.

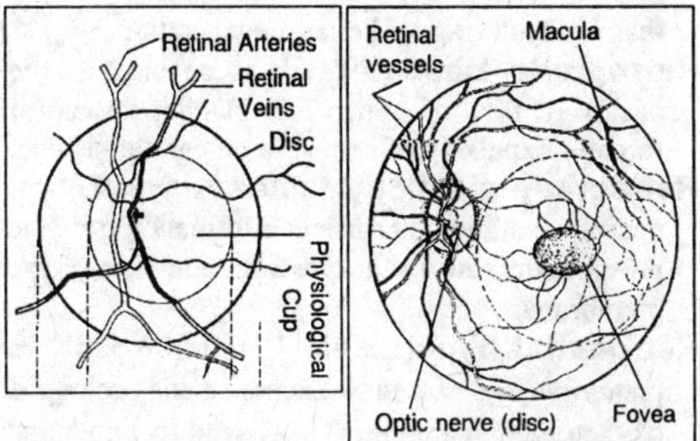

Posterior structures of the eye : the macula, optic nerve, and retinal blood vessels

Cones are less sensitive but are responsible for colour vision. Near the centre of retina is fovea where retinal vessels are absent. Retinal artery occlusion is caused by thrombus and if occlusion persists for long may result in blindness.

Retinaculum Dense, regular connective tissue sheath holding down the tendons at the wrist, ankle, or other sites.

Retinal detachment It is the separation of light sensitive inner surface of back of eye from outer layers. First retinal tear takes place which may be due to old age degeneration or by pulling on retina by contracting strands in the vitreous gel. Vitreous fluid collects between the delicate nerve membrane and underlying pigment layer. It may occur after major injury to eye. It is more common in highly myopics. Retinal detachment is painless and symptoms are exclusively visual. First indication is bright flashes seen with floaters at the edge of the field. Floaters are seen by release of blood pigment into vitreous gel. Sometimes affected person may be unaware unless black drop obscures vision. Retinal detachment is an emergency. Once detachment has occurred normal central vision may not be obtained again. Treatment is an emergency surgery.

Retinal detachment perimetery Size and location of a defect caused by retinal detachment relates to size and location of separated retina.

Retinal disparity The slight difference between the retinal images perceived by the two yes when a nearby object is viewed. The difference is caused by different locations of the two eyes. An important cue in some types of stereoscopic or depth vision.

Retinal ganglion cells Cells of the retina that give rise to the optic nerve.

Retinitis pigmentosa It is an inherited disease characterised by night blindness and constricted visual field. It is diffuse, bilateral, symmetrical dystrophy of retina. There is a predominant damage to rods which are responsible for night vision and peripheral vision. It is an inherited autosomal recessive, autosomal dominant X-linked recessive trait. Patient complains of difficulty in dim illumination.

Later on it becomes impossible to walk even in dim light or after sunset. Patient is not able to see from his or her lateral side. Everything is clear in the line of vision only with passage of time. There is loss of central vision also.

Retinoblastoma It is a malignant tumour of retina that affects babies and infants. It is seen as visible whiteness in pupil. Affected eye may be blind and later on strabismus may develop. It may spread from eye to orbit and along the optic nerve to brain. Treatment is removal by surgery and followed by radiation therapy.

Retinohypothalamic tract A direct projection from the retina that terminates in the suprachiasmatic nucleus of the hypothalamus.

Retinopathy A noninflammatory degenerative disease of the retina.

Retractile testis Testis that moves in and out of the scrotum.

Retraction The movement of body part, such as the mandible, backward on a plane parallel with the ground; the opposite of protraction.

Retraction ring It occurs in obstructed labour after membranes have ruptured. Upper segment becomes thickened and lower segment progressively thinner. When it rises abnormally high it is known as Bandl's ring.

Retrieval The process of locating information stored in memory and bringing it into awareness.

Retrieval failure Forgetting due to the inability to stimulate the memory, rather than the disappearance of the trace. The trace is presumed to be intact; but there is no appropriate cue for evoking it.

Retrobulbar block It allows surgery on the globe of the eye.

Retrobulbar neuritis Patient notices sudden onset of blurring of vision. Patient may complain of loss of intensity of colours. Visual acuity may go very low but complete loss of vision may not develop. Examination of central visual field will show central scotoma. Optic disc may become pink and swollen. There is a sudden total or partial loss of central field of vision usually in one eye. This is caused by inflammation of optic nerve. It may be caused by demyelination process in the nerve fibres similar to multiple sclerosis. Visual loss lasts for about 6 weeks. Repeated attacks may result in permanent loss. Corticosteroids are useful.

Retrocalcaneal bursitis Retrocalcaneal bursa is located between posterior angle of os calcis, and Achilles tendon may become inflamed and hypertrophied with repeated trauma. Symptoms consist of pain and tendernes in retrocalcaneal region. These symptoms develop either during running or just after it. It is the inflammation of

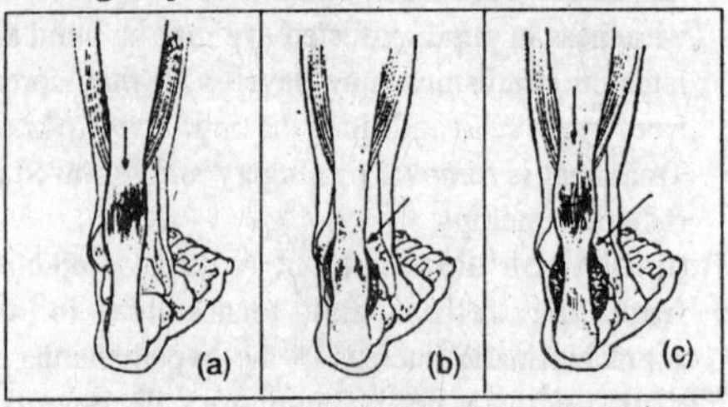

(a) Tendinitis (b) Retrocalcaneal bursitis (c) Combined

bursal. On occasion along, with it there may be Achilles tendinitis. Tendon becomes inflamed and thickened and adhere to the tendon. There may be fluid around tendon. Pain is a dominant symptom 2 to 6 cm above heel.

Retroflexion The bending backward of an organ on its axis, specifically the tipping backward of a uterus upon itself.

Retrograde amnesia The inability to recall earlier experiences, especially those preceding a traumatic event. After a brain operation or traumatic injury, the individual cannot recall preceding events, including those from childhood, but memories of events subsequent to the trauma are readily available.

Retrograde blood flow A flow of blood in the opposite direction from that expected ; e.g., the flow of blood in the spermatic vein toward the testis rather than away from it.

Retrograde degeneration Changes that occur in the proximal portion of a damaged axon only as far as the first node of Ranvier; similar to changes that occur during wallerian degeneration.

Retrograde ejaculation It is defined as the backward flow of semen into bladder instead of forceful expulsion of semen in antegrade fashion.

Retrograde plasticity factor A hypothetical neurotransmitter that carriers information from the presynaptic side to the postsynaptic side of the membrane.

Retrolental hyperplasia It is retinopathy in preterm babies caused by excessive and prolonged oxygen administration. It may lead to blindness. To prevent this oxygen content of inspired air should be kept below 40% and PO_2 should not be allowed to rise above 60-80 m.m. Hg.

Retrolingual Behind the tongue.

Retrolisthesis The posterior displacement of a vertebra in relation to one below it.

Retromandibular Behind the mandible.

Retromastoid Behind the mastoid process.

Retromolar pad Mass of tissue located at the distal termination of the mandibular residual ridge.

Retroparotid Behind the parotid gland.

Retroperitoneal Located behind the parietal peritoneum; includes the kidneys, adrenal glands, pancreas, portions of the intestines, and urinary bladder.

Retroperitoneal fibrosis This is a rare disease of uncertain cause chracterised by dense fibrosis behind the peritoneum in the area of 3rd and 4th lumbar vertebrae. It may compress ureter. The cause is unknown but 10 % have a malignant tumour of which carcinoid is the most common. Symptoms are vague such as renal colic, oliguric, renal failure and hypertension due to ureteric compression and oedema of legs. There will be backache and pain in legs due to lumbar nerve root involvement, weight loss, lethargy and fever. Mass may be palpable. There will be normochromic anaemia and ESR is raised in 50% cases. CT scan is useful.

Retropharyngeal Situated or occurring behind the pharynx.

Retrospective cohort study Cohorts are identified on the basis of past exposure and followed forward to the present for the occurrence of the outcome of interest.

Retrospective study A study in which the results of a number of similar cases already performed are reviewed. The cases can be related in terms of diagnosis, treatment plan, case presentation, longevity, or other criteria.

Retroversion The tipping backward of an entire organ; in the case the retroversion of the uterus, the turning back of the entire uterus in relation to the pelvic axis.

Retroverted Tilted or turned backward without being bent or flexed.

Retrovirus These viruses differ from DNA viruses in that they are occasionally associated with tumour production in their natural hosts. All oncogenic RNA viruses belong to the family of Retroviridae. Retroviruses are widespread in nature and cause leucosis or sarcoma in their hosts. The viruses are usually transmitted vertically from parent to progeny.

Retrovitreous haemorrhage It is also known as preretinal haemorrhage. It is located between retina and detached posterior hyaloid membrane. The blood remains fluid and changes its shape with change of position of the head of the patient. In standing position the subhyaloid blood takes up the position of boat. It impairs the visual acuity if the haemorrhage is located at or near the macula. There is rapid resolution of subhyaloid haemorrhage.

Reverse Trendelenburg's position Position in which the lower extremities are low and the body and head are elevated on an inclined plane.

Reverse genetics A term for techniques that allow the introduction of specific mutations into a gene.

Reverse isolation Protective isolation.

Reverse spiral bandage This technique can be used on an arm or leg. After applying bandage end tail is cut down and 2 ends are tied properly.

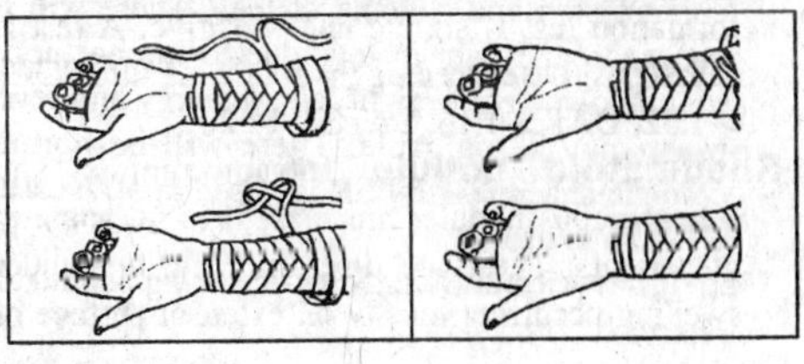

Reverse transcription A process in which RNA is converted to DNA by the reverse transcriptase enzyme.

Reverse transfer Act of transferring instruments or handpieces in an opposite direction; specifically transferring an earlier used handpiece with the pickup portion of the hand and receiving the used handpiece with the delivery portion of the hand.

Reversible reaction Chemical reaction in which the reaction can proceed from reactants to products, or from products to reactants; the amount of reactants relative to products is constant at equilibrium.

Review A critical review of data.

Reye's syndrome There is sudden development of profuse vomiting, anencephalopathy with stupor and acute fatty degeneration of liver. The cause of Reye's syndrome is unknown but is multifactorial. Aspirin seems to play important part in adult cases. CSF is usually normal. Cerebral oedema rather than hepatic failure is principal cause of death.

Rhabdomylosis An acute fulminating disease that destroys skeletal muscle.

Rhabdomyoma It is a rare soft tissue tumour of muscle. It occurs primarily in adults in floor of mouth. Histologic sections show circumscribed very vascular lesions that are composed of ovoid or elongated cells with granular eosinophilic cytoplasm in which cross-striations can be identified. Local excision is the treatment of choice.

Rhabdomyosarcoma It may develop in mouth with tongue the favoured site. Mass grows very fast and is associated with induration and haemorrhage.

Cervical lymphadenopathy develops. Microscopic features include the presence of highly bizarre cells. The cytoplasm of some cells shows cross-striations. The tumour is highly malignant. Its prognosis is poor.

Rhabdosarcoma It is the most common sarcoma in the paediatric age group and pelvis is the most common place after head and neck region. Large cauliflower like tumours with locally invasive growth pattern and early haematogenous and lymphatic metastases are typical findings.

Rheology The science of the deformation and flow of matter, such as the flow of blood through the heart and blood vessels.

Rheostat An appliance for regulating the resistance and thus controlling the amount of current entering an electric circuit; the dental unit control usually is located in a device operated by the foot.

Rhesus constitution The symbols CDE, cde have been used to express the six chief RH antigens. An individual carries the six main rhesus genes on two chromosomes three of which are dominant CDE genes and 3 are their alleles the cde which are recessive genes. A group of three genes are located in each chromosome.

Rhesus incompatibility Mainly fetus is affected but mother may also be affected. Fetus may show hemolytic anemia, grave jaundice and hydrops fetalis.

Rheumatic fever It generally follows throat infection with certain strains of streptococci. Children between 5-15 are most commonly affected. Throat infections should be treated well with suitable antibiotics. There develops fever with pain, inflammation and swelling of one or more larger joints. Several joints may be affected at one point of time. It may result in thickening and scarring of heart valves leading to narrowing and leaking of valves specially mitral valve. It may lead to mitral stenosis. Diagnosis is suspected when disease moves joints to joint. High doses of penicillin are needed. Sometimes corticosteroids and sedatives help the patient. Penicillin has to be used for years.

Rheumatic nodules Subcutaneous nodules appear on bony prominence like elbows, shin, occiput and spine. Pin head sized nodules are non-tender. These develop after 6 weeks of rheumatic fever. Patient may have carditis.

Rheumatic palsy Complete or incomplete, unilateral peripheral facial nerve paralysis developing within hours. Paralysis that is incomplete initially may become complete within a few days. 30% cases show taste disturbance or some degree of fine hearing impairment. There is no fever.

Rheumatoid arthritis It is an autoimmune disorder. Disorder usually starts in early adulthood or middle age. It is more common in women. Commonly involved joints are fingers, wrists and toes. These become painful. There is gradual onset with mild fever and generalised aches and pains preceding joint symptoms. Joint becomes swollen, red, warm, painful and stiff. Structures around joint becomes inflamed. When fingers are involved grip becomes weaker and becomes white on exposure to cold. In some cases soft nodules develop beneath

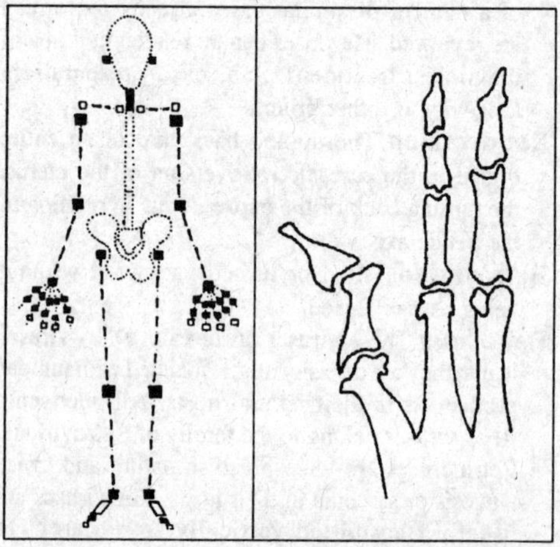

the skin. When knee is involved Baker's cyst, i.e. fluid-filled swelling may develop. Early morning stiffness of fingers is common. X-ray and blood tests are helpful in diagnosis. Non-steroidal anti-inflammatory drugs (NSAIDs) are given. Antirheumatic drugs such as gold or penicillamine may be given.

Rheumatoid arthritis fever Fever associated with juvenile rheumatoid arthritis is often low or absent in early part of the day and rises to high levels in afternoon and evening.

Rheumatoid carditis Inflammation of the heart as a result of a rheumatic disorder.

Rheumatoid factor It is positive in 80% cases of rheumatoid arthritis, systemic lupus erythematosus (SLE), chronic active hepatitis, sarcoidosis, fibrosing alveolitis and leprosy. While ehzyme-linked immuno-absorbent assay (ELISA) is the most sensitive test for rheumatoid factor, Latex formation test is simple and sensitive. A test is called positive exceeding the following titre SCAT > 1:32, DAT > 1:16, LATEX 1 : 20

Rheumatoid nodule Intracutaneous and subcutaneous nodules are present in one-quarter of patients. These are discrete, firm, nontender swelling occurring mostly on extensor surface of forearm. Intrapulmonary nodules may breakdown and can be mistaken for tumour or abscess.

Rheumatoid varient The seronegative sypondylo arthropathies.

Rhinitis It is the inflammation of membrane of nasal cavities. There will be watery discharge. It may develop due to allergy, cold or due to flu.

Rhinitis of pregnancy Increasing bilateral nasal airway obstruction, specially in second half of pregnancy caused by marked swelling of turbinate, mucosal and nasal discharge. Symptoms subside during the postpartum period.

Rhinology The study of the nose and its disorders.

Rhinophyma There develops coarsening of anterior nasal contour with firm, lobular, bluish red to reddish brown outgrowths like potato. It is of slow growth with no pain.

Rhinorrhea A discharge from the nasal mucosal lining.

Rhinovirus A genus of acid-labile viruses of which there are more than 100 antigenic types associated with the common cold in humans and foot-and-mouth disease in cattle.

Rhizo Nerve root.

Rhizobacteria A group of root-colonizing bacteria.

Rhizocoenosis The association of a microorganism with the root system of a plant, which results in a benefit to one or both of the partners.

Rhizoplane A root surface that can be colonized by microorganisms.

Rhizotomy Surgical sectioning of a nerve root close to the spinal cord.

Rh-negative Red blood cells that do not contain the antigen called Rh factor.

Rhodopsin A chemical substance which plays a significant role in visual adaptation, making the retina more sensitive to visual stimulation. When the lights are turned off and the room is suddenly darkened, at first the scene appears to be completely black, but gradually, through the influence of rhodopsin and pupil dilation, the individual's vision improves.

RhoGAM An injection of a special protein given to an Rh-negative women who is pregnant to prevent her body from forming anti-Rh antibodies, which may harm an Rh-positive baby.

Rhomboid glossitis This condition appears as a smooth, flat, depressed or elevated nodular area. It may be rhomboid, diamond-shaped or irregular in outline. It is supposed to be a developmental anomaly. When area is slightly depressed it may accumulate debris becoming a source of inflammation. Microscopic sections reveal a covering of stratified epithelium free of lingual papillae. If the lesion is elevated and interferes with function or it is depressed it should be excised.

Rhoptries Club-shaped, apical organelles of certain parasitic protozoa that release their contents into the nascent parasitophorous vacuole.

Rhythm method A birth control method relying upon abstinence from sexual intercourse before, during, and after the period of time the ovum is capable of being fertilised.

Rhythmicity The pattern of recurrence of a phenomenon.

Rhythmicity area A portion of the respiratory control center located in the medulla oblongata that controls inspitatory and expiratory phases.

Rib A curved slightly twisted strip of bone that forms part of skeleton of thorax.

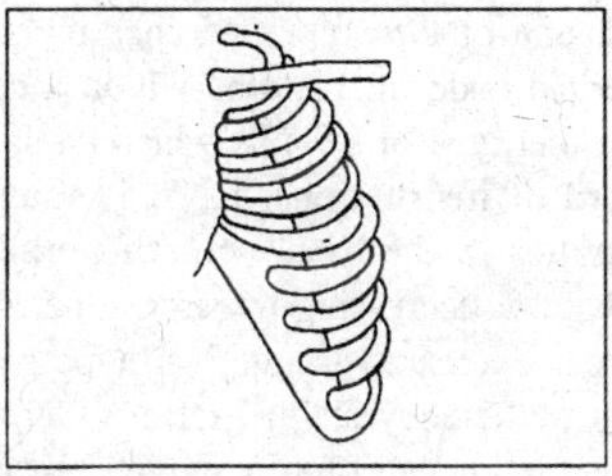

Rib belt An elastic support worn around the thoracic region.

Rib hump The prominence of ribs on the convexity of a spinal curvature.

Ribavirin An antiviral agent used to treat respiratory syncytial virus

Riboflavin Deficient intake or impaired absorption of B_{12} may lead to this condition. In general it causes atrophy of skin and mucous membrane. It may cause dermatitis and glossitis. The condition presents with dry scaling, cracking and fissuring of lips. It gives rise to erythematous, greasy seborrhoeic scales at nasolabial folds covering eyelids and ears. There may be malaise, weight loss, interstitial keratitis, dysphagia and magenta coloured tongue. Patient is adequately treated with riboflavin 10 to 30 mg daily orally.

Riboflavin deficiency Vitamin B_2 is found in eggs and green leaves. Its deficiency produces vascularisation of cornea, keratitis and later on corneal ulceration, cheilosis, and greasy dermatitis. Oral manifestations are seen in tongue and lips. Tongue becomes red and inflamed. Lips show fissures. Microscopic lesions show ulceration, oedema, infiltration by plasma cells and lymphocytes.

Ribonuclease A nuclease that catalyzes the hydrolysis of certain internucleotide linkages of RNA.

Ribonucleic acid (RNA) Type of nucleic acid containing the sugar ribose; involved in protein synthesis. There are 2 kinds of nucleic acids. Ribonucleic acid is so called because its sugar moiety is the pentose ribose. In RNA the purine bases may be adenine or guanine and pyrimidine bases, cytosine and uracil. Three types of RNA can be distinguished on the basis of structure : messanger RNA (m RNA), ribosomal RNA (r RNA) and transfer RNA (t RNA). Ribonucleic acid, one of two types of chemicals that carry inherited code instructions within a cell activity. The other type of is DNA which holds permanent record of instructions. RNA is found in large quantities in the basal cells of normal gingival epithelium decreasing towards superficial layers. RNA is decreased in gingival hyperplasia and in areas of leucocytic infiltration. DNA normally present in nucleus of all gingival cells is increased in gingival hyperplasia. The DNA and RNA activity of the epithelium at gingival margin is greater than in remaining oral mucosa.

Ribosomal RNA A form of RNA that makes up most of the structures (subunits) of the ribosome organelle of the cell.

Ribosome A cytoplasmic organelle composed of protein and RNA in which protein synthesis occurs.

Ribotype A specific profile obtained after hybridization of digested bacterial DNA with a ribosomal RNA or DNA proble.

Ribozyme An RNA molecule that can catalyze a chemical reaction.

Ribs These are flat curved protective cage around lungs. There are 12 pairs of ribs, each joined at the back of rib to a vertebra. Between the ribs thin sheets of muscles are attached to help to expand and relax chest during breathing. Spaces between the ribs contain nerves and blood vessels. Ribs can easily be fractured by fall and blow. Fracture causes pain increasing on breathing. Diagnosis is confirmed on X-ray. Healing is straight forward and strapping serves the purpose.

Rice bodies Loose bodies in joints.

Rickets Vitamin D helps in absorption of calcium and phosphorus. Deficiency of vitamin D produces rickets in the growing child and osteomalacia in adult. There is retardation of eruption of tooth, malpositioning of teeth, retardation of growth of mandible and class II malocclusion.

Rider's bone Occupational strain of adductor muscle causes development of so called, riders

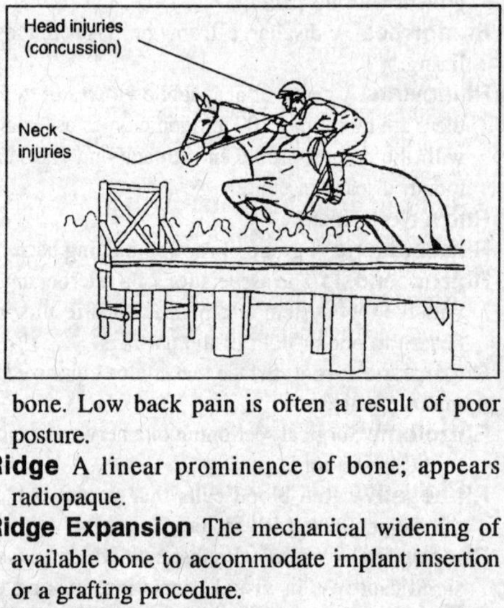

bone. Low back pain is often a result of poor posture.

Ridge A linear prominence of bone; appears radiopaque.

Ridge Expansion The mechanical widening of available bone to accommodate implant insertion or a grafting procedure.

Rifampicin Half-life is four hours and has bactericidal activity against the tubercle bacilli. It is also used in leprosy. It acts by inhibiting RNA synthesis. It is effective against mycobacteria which lie semidormant within cells. It has wide range of antimicrobial activity. It is well absorbed by GIT. It penetrates well into most tissues. It rarely causes serious side-effects. It raises plasma bilirubin. In a few cases it induces fatal hepatitis. It is antibacterial and is successfully used in tuberculosis. It is also used to treat leprosy and endocarditis. Some strains of bacteria quickly develop resistence when it is given alone. It results in harmless, orange coloured urine and saliva. Side effects include muscle pain, nausea, vomiting, diarrhoea, jaundice and itching.

Rifle A gun with a rifled barrel. It is attached to a stock and is normally fired from the shoulder.

Right Superior pulmonary vein the vein that returns blood from the upper and middle lobes of the right lung of the left atrium.

Right atrial catheter An indwelling intravenous catheter inserted centrally or peripherally and threaded into the superior vena cava or right atrium.

Right atrial pressure The blood pressure in the right atrium.

Right bronchus It is shorter and more in line with the trachea than the left bronchus. It enters the right lung at 5th thoracic vertebrae. It is wider than left and catheter passes more easily into it.

The main upper lobe bronchus given off within 2 cm of the commencement arises above right pulmonary artery. The opening is on a level with carina. The right bronchus leaves the trachea at an angle of 25°.

Right interior pulmonary vein The vein that returns blood from the lower lobe of the right lung to the left atrium.

Right lymphatic duct Lymphatic duct that empties into the right subclavian vein; drains the right side of the head and neck, the right upper thorax, and the right upper limb.

Right marginal artery A branch of the right coronary artery.

Right occipito anterior (ROA) The occiput is towards the right ileo pectineal eminence and the sagittal suture is in the left oblique diameter of the pelvic brim.

Right occipito posterior (ROP) The occiput points towards the right sacroiliac joint in the right posterior quadrant of the pelvis.

Sagittal suture is in the right oblique diameter of the pelvic brim.

Right occiptio lateral (ROL) The occipit points to the right side of pelvic brim midway between the right ileopectineal eminence and right sacroiliac joint. The sagittal suture is in the transverse diameter.

Right of refusal The entitlement of both of patient and the professional to stop the session.

Right pulmonary artery The right branch of the pulmonary artery distributed to the right lung; runs behind the ascending aorta, superior vena cava, and upper pulmonary vein but in front of the esophagus and right primary bronchus to the root of the lungs.

Right surface The right side of the heart that is in contact with the right lung.

Right ventricular failure There is inability of right ventricle to propel blood forwards resulting in enlargement of right atrium, enlargement of liver and oedema. Mitral stenosis is the most common cause. There may be palpitation or heaviness of precordium. There may be insomnia, blurring of vision, lack of concentration, lack of personality and drowsiness. There will be pain in right hypochondrium after meals, tightness of upper abdomen due to stretching of hepatic capsule. Urinary symptoms include of oliguria and nocturia. Venous pressure is high and arms to lung circulation time is increased.

Righting reaction An involuntary movement response to a stimulus; it serves to maintain the normal alignment of the head and body in space.

Right-left discrimination The ability to differentiate one side of the body from the other.

Right-left discrimination disorder The inability to identify the right and left sides of one's own body or of that of the examiner.

Right-to-left shunt When blood passes from the right to the left side of the heart without participating in gas exchange; intrapulmonary shunt.

Rigid dressing A mildly compressive total contact plaster wrap applied immediately following surgery to control oedema and pain specially in amputation stumps.

Rigidity It is the increased tone in one or more muscles causing them to feel tight. Part becomes inflexible. It may be caused by injury to muscle, arthritis and neurological disorder such as Parkinson's disease or stroke.

Rigor mortis It is the stiffening of muscles which result after death. It starts after 3-4 hours of death and is complete after 12 hours. Then it gradually disappears between 2 5 days. Sooner rigor mortis begins then sooner it passes off too. It helps in medicolegal cases to access the time of death.

Stiffness in rigor mortis is closely related to the coagulation of muscle plasma and formation of lactic acid which accumulates in the muscles. Reaction of muscle becomes acidic. It starts after the first stage of primary relaxation with a gap of 2 hours. Once body becomes stiff it remains so for 20 hours. It first appears in involuntary muscles than in voluntary group of muscles.

Rim sign X-Ray sign that strongly suggests the presence of posterior shoulder dislocation.

Rima glottidis The fissure between the vocal folds commonly called glottis.

Rima vestibuli The fissure between the vestibular folds.

RIND Reversible ischemic neurological deficits.

Rinderpest A morbillivirus that causes severe gastroenteritis in cattle, with inflammation and necrosis.

Ring apophysis The secondary centres of ossification. It develops in cartilaginous end plates of vertebral bodies.

Ring injuries An avulsion injury of soft tissues of ring finger.

Ringworm It is a fungal infection developing in groin, armpit, nails and trunk where humidity is there. There is ring-shaped reddened, scaly or blistery patches. Antifungal tube's application 3 to 4 times a day and keeping part dry help the patients.

Rinne's test Assessment technique for comparing air versus bone conduction of sound. Vibrating tuning fork is held near the pinna and then on the mastoid process. In cases of nerve deafness one hears the sounds through the bone louder than that is conducted through the air.

Riparian Relating to or occuring in the terrestrial area along river stream banks.

Risk Calculated as the proportion of persons who are unaffected at the beginning of a study period but who undergo the risk event during the study period.

Risk difference The risk in teh exposed troup minus the risk in the unexposed group.

Risk event Death, disease, or injury.

Risk factor An attribute associate with an increased likelihood for developing a specific disease among those individuals with the attribute compared to those individuals without attribute.

Risk ratio Method of calculating relative risk by creating a ratio of the incidence rate for one subgroup and the incidence rate for another subgroup; contrast with odds ratio.

Risser Ferguson method A technique for measuring the angle of scoliotic curve.

Risser localiser cast A type of body cast used for preoperative correction of scoliotic curve.

Risser sign Iliac apophysis is used as indicator of the degree of skeletal maturity.

Ritgen method Delivery of the infant's head by lifting the head upward and forward through the vulva, between contractions, by pressing with the tips of the fingers upon the perineum behind the anus.

Ritual A repetitive activity, usually a distorted or stereotyped elaboration of some routine of daily life, employed to relieve anxiety. Most commonly seen in obsessive compulsive neurosis.

Ritualism The need to maintain sameness and reliability.

Ritz stick A device used in determining the numerical size of shoes.

Rivinus, ducts Lesser sublingual ducts.

RNA Ribonucleic acid; a nucleic acid consisting of the nitrogenous bases adenine, guanine cytosine, and uracil; the sugar ribose; and phosphate groups. There are three types of RNA found in cytoplasm; messenger RNA (mRNA), Transfer RNA (tRNA) and ribosomal RNA (rRNA).

RNA splicing Removal of introns and joining of exons in a primary transcript.

Robert's pelvis There is congenital absence of both lateral masses of sacrum with synostosis of sacro-iliac joints. Pelvis is transversely contracted from brim to outlet. Caesarian section is indicated.

Robotics The science of mechanical devices that work automatically or by remote control.

Rocker bar A convex strip affixed to the sole proximal to the metatarsal heads.

Rocking Rhythmic movement of the body.

Rod A photoreceptor in the retina of the eye that is specialized for colorless, dim-light vision.

Rod vision It depends on presence of visual purple requiring a derivative of vitamin A. It is responsible to see in dim light.

Rodent ulcer It is the cancer of skin located on lip, face, nose, etc. To start spherical nodule will develop which will ulcerate and becomes deeper to damage structures.

Rods These are photoreceptors as they receive the light impulses and found in the sensory epithelium or retina. These have outer and inner limbs. Outer is made up of fine superimposed discs. It is here that rhodopsin is found. Each rod has got a fine rod fibre which is varicose at places. In the middle of the fibre is the red granule which is really the rod nucleus. Rod fibre terminates by absorbing in the molecular layer. They are responsible for vision in dim light.

Roentgen rays X-Rays.

Roentgenogram A film produced by roentgenography.

Roentgenography General term for procedures that use x-rays.

Roentgenology The branch of radiology which deals with the diagnostic and therapeutic use of x-rays.

Rogoff's sign In this sign palpation on the costovertebral angle produces pain and tenderness in acute adrenal insufficiency.

Rolandic fissure Central sulcus of cerebral hemisphere.

Rolando fracture Intra-articular fracture of base of first metacarpal.

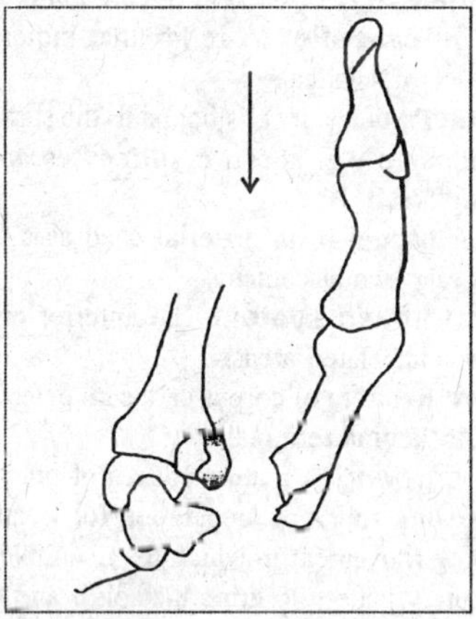

Role The behavioral expectations attached to a position.

Role conflict When efforts to fulfill demands associated with one role interfere with efforts to fulfill demands associated with other roles.

Role delineation The identification of the behavioral expectations associated with a role.

Role enactment Behavior demonstrated by a person in the performance of a role.

Role strain Difficulty in the delineation and enactment of a role.

Role transition Changing form one pattern of behaviour to another.

Role-performance family health model This view of family health is based on the view that family health is the ability of family members to perform their routine roles and achieve developmental tasks.

Roller board A device used in rehabilitation therapy that permits abduction and adduction of hip.

Rollover test A simple test for preeclampsia in which the diastolic blood pressure is recorded with the patient in a lateral recumbent position, then on her back. A positive result is indicated if diastolic blood pressure increases by 20 mm Hg or more.

Romano's sign Early symptoms of Chagas' disease, consisting of unilateral, periorbital edema and conjuctivitis.

Romberg's sign Inability to maintain standing balance when vision is occluded. It is positive when a patient cannot stand steadily with his eyes closed as it is seen in tabes dorsalis.

Ronchi These are continuous sounds produced when the lumen of bronchial tube is narrowed by swelling of mucosa by adherent sticky mucus and by spasm of bronchial muscle in asthma. These occur during inspiration, during expiration or both. Expiratory ronchi are characteristic of asthma. When low pitched these are known as sonorus and when high pitched are known as whistling.

Rongeur forcep A sharp, biting type of forcep designed to cut bone.

Root The interradicular bone resorpton in multirooted teeth due to periodontal disease.

Root canal treatment It is a dental procedure to save a tooth in which pulp has died or become untreatably diseased due to extensive caries. X-rays are taken to know the length of pulp cavity. Local anaesthetic may be given. A hole is drilled in the crown of teeth, the pulp is removed and crown is sealed with temporary filling. About one weak after dentist removes the filling to ensure that cavity is free of infection. If there is no infection permanent filling is done. If pulp cavity is not filled completely bacteria may enter leading to apical periodontitis.

Root compression Root irritation may be caused by facet joint inflammation/degeneration. Disc protrusion may also result it.

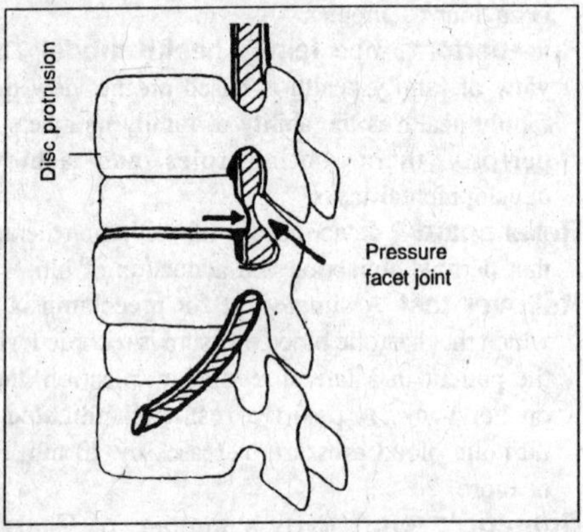

Root end cavity obturation To clean and obturate the root canal before root end resection is done generally with surgery cleaning and shaping of root canal is filled up with gatta parcha and then filled up.

Root end resection It refers to the removal of apical portion of root. Root, end can be resected and bevelled in many ways. Root may be shaved from beginning from the apex cutting down. In second technique resection is predetermined.

Root form An endosteal implant, generally cylindrical in shape, parallel-sided or tapered, threaded or unthreaded, that functions in the osteointegration mode of tissue integration.

Root pick Hand instrument which is used to locate and dislodge root fragments.

Root planing Use of instruments, primarily curets, to smooth the root surface until it feels like glass.

Root resection Removal of one root of a multirooted tooth.

Root word Part of a word that provides the fundamental meaning.

Rooting reflex A normal response in newborns when the cheek is touched or stroked along the side of the mouth to turn the head toward the stimulated side and begin to suck.

Rope's test A test used in joint fluid analysis.

Ropiness Tissue texture abnormality characterized by a cord-like feeling.

Rosacea It is a chronic inflammatory disorder of skin due to hormonal effects on sebaceous glands. It develops due to hyperplasia and overactivity of sebaceous glands of face. It is more common in menopausal females. Histological changes show vascular dilatation, low-grade inflammation, hypertrophy of sebaceous glands and formation of fibrous tissue.

It involves nose, cheeks and forehead. Trunk and back are not affected. Condition gives rise to recurrent episodes of bright red erythema and hot flushes. The lesion over tip of nose produces soreness, itching, burning and stinging. Condition also produces several ocular manifestations such as nonspecific keratitis.

Rose spots These are sparse, small maculopapular skin lesions which blanch on pressure, and are usually seen on the upper abdomen or anterior chest. These are seen in some cases of typhoid fever usually 2 to 3 weeks after the infection and last for a short period.

Rose's position An anatomic position, patient in supine with head over table edge in full extension.

Rosenmuller, fossa Pharyngeal recess.

Rosenthal, vein Basal vein of cerebrum.

Roses luteal reflex A reflex that indicates the presence of sciatica.

Rosettee Particles or cells bound to the surface of a lymphocyte e.g. sheep erythrocytes around a human T cell.

Rosin A natural resin material used as a filler in temporary dental cements.

Rostaral limbic system The anterior cingulate cortex and related areas.

Rostrum Rostrum of corpus callosum extends from genu to lamina terminalis.

Rotary chewing A mature pattern of masticatiion or chewing solids in preparation for swallowing; chewing movement in which the mandible moves in a rotary pattern to grind the solids and mix the bolus with saliva.

Rotary motion In sensory psychology, sensitivity to circular movement. Passive rotary motion occurs whenever an individual is automatically transported from one place to another, as in a swing or motorboat ride; sensitivity to this type of motion is mediated largely by the semicircular canals.

Rotating kinetic therapeutic table The patient is positioned and balanced on the table. The motor mechanism allows the patient to be rotated side to side thereby displacing weight and assisting to relieve pressure areas. Cervical traction may be applied by tension system at he head of bed.

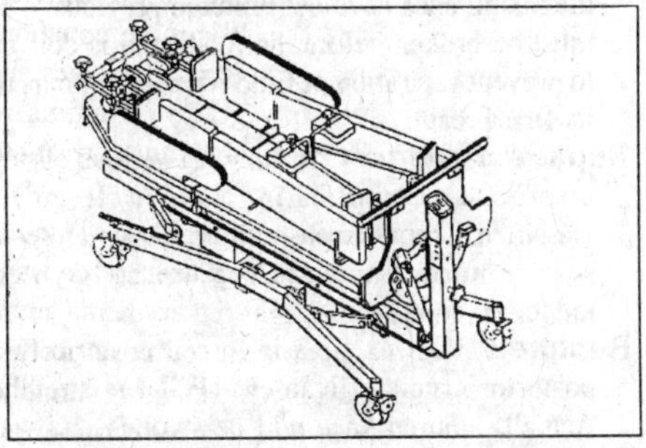

Rotation Movement around a longitudinal axis; for example, shaking your head "no".

Rotational speed The rate at which a bur or drill turns, expressed as the number of revolutions per unit of time.

Rotator cuff It is a structure around shoulder joint composed of four muscle tendons which merge with the fibrous capsule enclosing the joint. It may be torn due to fall or sudden forcible jerk. It may result in painful arc syndrome. A complete tear seriously limits the ability to raise arm and may even require surgical repair.

Rotatory instability A term used in classification of knee ligament.

Rotavirus It has been incriminated as a cause of diarrhoea in 25 to 50 % cases. Children have antibodies against rotavirus by the age of 5 years. Rotavirus affects the absorptive villous epitholial cells. Diarrhoea is attributed to loss of absorptive surface.

Rotoh's sign In this sign there is dullness in the 5th right intercostal space on percussion, and is present in pericardial effusion.

Rothmund syndrome An autosomal recessive disorder characterised by atrophic dermatosis, wasting of muscles, saddle nose, congenital bone defects, juvenile cataract, hypogonadism, and premature greying and loss of hair.

Rotoscoliosis Rotational curvture of the spine.

Round ligament pain Some will notice sharp growing pain caused by spasm of round ligaments associated with movements. It is more felt on right side. Local heat helps. Patient may be awaken with pain at night.

Round window A round, membrane covered opening between the middle and inner ear, directly below the oval window; also called the cochlear window.

Rounds Visit to patients on an individual basis or as a group.

Roux sign A diagnostic marker indicative that hip joint is riding relatively high.

Rubber dam It is a thin sheet of rubber which is placed over a tooth to isolate it from rest of mouth. Rubber dam punch is used to punch a small hole in rubber. The rubber dam is kept in place by a rubber dam clamp which is fixed on the tooth with rubber clamp forceps. Finally a rubber dam frame is used to support the sheet of rubber.

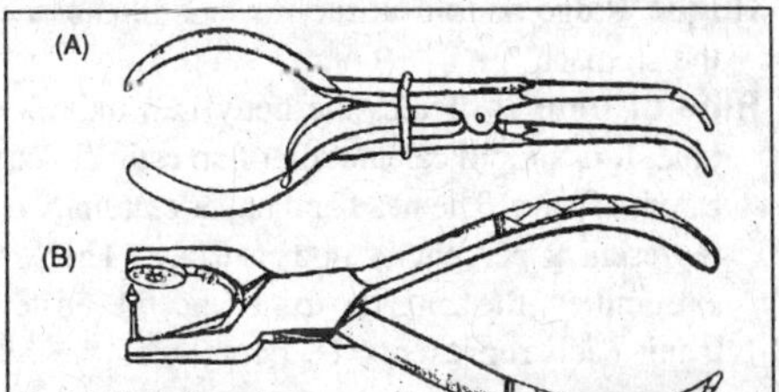

A. Rubber dam clamp
B. Rub punch

Rubefacient An irritant which acts locally on the skin and mucous membranes to induce by peremia. Most rubefacients may also exert vesicant effects when applied in high concentrations.

Rubella It is a viral disease of skin and oral manifestation occurs within 2 to 4 days. The oral lesions are called Koplik's spots which do not consist of vesicles. Oral lesions are a few but may occur as red macules. In German measles there may be erythema of mucosa or a few macules in posterior part of mouth.

Rubella embryopathy The risk of fetal infection is 50 % or higher when the mother acquires infection during the first four weeks of gestation. The risk declines with each successive month of first trimester. Growth retardation, deafness, microcephaly and mental retardation may occur in infants infected during the fourth month of gestation.

Rubescent Becoming red.

Rubin maneuver Fetal shoulders are rotated so that they may traverse the pelvis in an oblique fashion. It is accompanied with direct rotation dependent on which scapula pressure is applied to. This maneuver generally allows relief of mild to moderate dystocia.

Rubin's Test When semen test is within normal limits Rubin's test is performed to ascertain tubal patency. A controlled amount of carbon dioxide is administered under pressure. After an initial rise between 60 to 150 m.m Hg pressure falls as the gas flows through the fallopian tubes.

Rubro Projections from red nucleus.

Ruga Rigid folds which cover the hard palate.

Rugae Ridge or fold in the mucous membrane of the stomach

Rule of nine It divides the body into multiple of nine. It is a rapid calculation of an estimate of the extent of burn. The head and upper extremity each represent 9 percent of body surface. The lower extremities, the anterior trunk and the posterior trunk each represents 18 percent of the bdoy

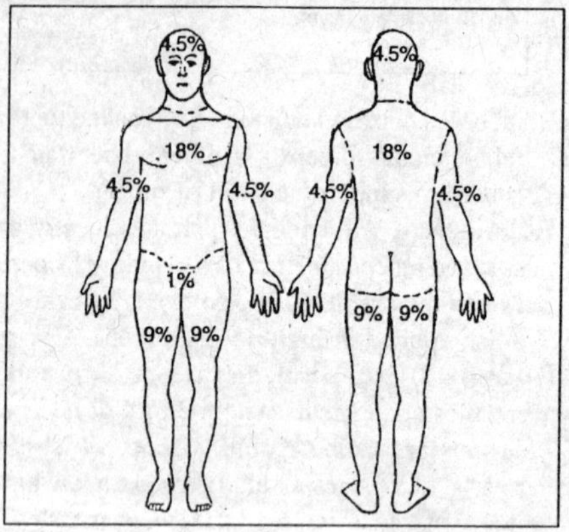

surface. These areas represent for 99 percent of body surface and perineum accounts for remaining 1 percent.

Rumination In psychiatry, obsessive preoccupation with ideas and recollections; also rare eating disorder of early childhood consisting of a return of food from the stomach without nausea or retching. It leads to loss of weight, failure to thrive, interference with growth and development, and, in about 25% of cases, death.

Rupture of the membranes The breaking of the amniotic sac, which may occur spontaneously and be the first indication of approaching labour. If the membranes have not ruptured previously, they must be broken before the fetal head is delivered to prevent aspiration of fluid when the infants take its first breath.

Rupture of uterus It is the most serious obstetric emergency complicating labour. It may be classified asspontaneous rupture, caesarian section scar rupture, traumatic rupture and syntocin induction rupture.

Ruptured PCL As tibia is forced posteriorly the posterior cruciate ligament (PCL) is stretched. Actually injured knee will be swollen and warm

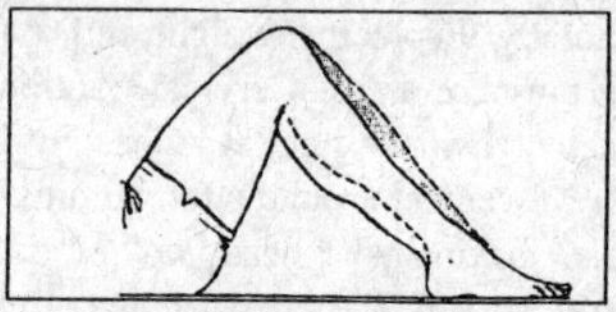

with a patient supine and both knees flexed to 90 degree, the injured knee will appear to sag posteriorly with a dip in infrapatella region.

Russel viper bite Russel vipers hiss loudly and continuously. Head is triangular. It is brown with deep, elliptical patches running in 3 rows. One bite is not sufficient to kill a person. Within minutes there develops severe local pain followed by swelling. Within 15-30 minutes often there is blood-stained discharge from the wound. Swelling and oozing occur within 24 to 36 hours. Victim starts bleeding from gums, kidney, nose and other sites.

Rust The disease that results from the interaction of a pathogenic rust fungus with a host plant. Although not strictly valid, the term is sometimes used to refer to the fungus itself.

Rutin An antioxidant vitamin like substance from the bioflavonoid group.

Rx—Thou take An order to take medicine as prescribed.

Ryle's tube This is commonly used for gastric aspiration or feeding purpose in hospitals. It has thin bore and 3 markings at various places to indicate the tip of tube in stomach, next to indicate body of stomach and third one to indicate tip of pylorus.

S

S.I. Joint It consist of two parts, a true joint and ligamentous attachment between two adjacent bones. The anterior inferior one half to two third of S.I. Joint is a true synovial joint. The iliac side is covered by hyaline cartilage 1 m.m. in thickness and the sacral side is covered by fibrous cartilage 3.5 m.m. in thickness.

S.I. units The international system of units.

S1 heart sound Normal "lub" (of "lub-dub") caused by closure of the mitral and tricuspid valves.

S1 root syndrome Pain radiates on the dorsal aspect of thigh and leg towards the heel and over lateral aspect of foot to 4th and 5th toes. Muscle weakness may be found in gluteus muscles. In severe case patient may not walk on toes of affected side. Achilles tendon reflex is weakened or abandoned. There is hypoaesthesia at the dorsal aspect of thigh and leg and lateral aspect of foot, and 4th and 5th toe.

S2 heart sound Normal "dub" (of "lub-dub") caused by closure of the pulmonic and aortic valves.

S3 heart sound Abnormal heart sound heat sound heard after "lub-dub" ("dub"), indicating ventricular noncompliance except in an athlete.

S4 heart sound Abnormal heart sound heard just before "lub" (of "lub-dub"), often indicating atrial noncompliance.

SA block It is due to excessive vagal tone from different neurohumoral factors. As no impulse is generated in SA node, heart as a whole will miss a beat. ECG will show complete absence of all complexes. In many cases it may not require any treatment.

Saber out Surgical approach to shoulder.

Sabin oral polio vaccine (OPV) A vaccine that provides herd immunity to poliomyelitis and has resulted in the apparent eradication of wild virus from the western hemisphere. The oral vaccine is made from live virus and has produced clinical illness under certain circumstances.

Sac Any pouch or bag like part.

Saccade Scanning movement of the eyes.

Saccadic eye movements Very rapid eye movements that occurs constantly and that change the focus on the retina from one point to another.

Saccharification A process in which a substrates is converted into low molecular weight saccharides by enzymes.

Saccharin White crystalline powder having a taste about 500 times sweeter than cane sugar, used as a calorie-free sweetener.

Saccular bronchiectasis A type of chronic dilation of the bronchi or bronchioles that appear to have a pouchlike shape.

Saccule The inferior and smaller of the two chamber in the membranous labyrinth inside the vestibule of the internal ear, containing a receptor organ for static equilibrium.

Saccule of the larynx A small pouch extending upward from the anterior aspect of the sinus of the larynx.

SACH foot Solid ankle cushion heel prosthetic foot.

Sacra cotyloid diameter It is a distance from mid point of sacral promontary to the iliopectineal eminence. It is 9.3 cms to the iliopectineal eminence. It is 9.3 cms.

Sacral agenesis A rare congenital abnormality in which all parts of sacrum are absent.

Sacral canal It is a cavity 10-15 cm. long and triangular in section. It runs the length of sacrum, itself is formed from five fused sacral vertebral.

Sacral inclination In spondylolisthesis a measure of degree of vertical orientation of the sacrum.

Sacral line A line drawn perpendicular to the level of iliac crest and through the center of sacrum on X-Ray

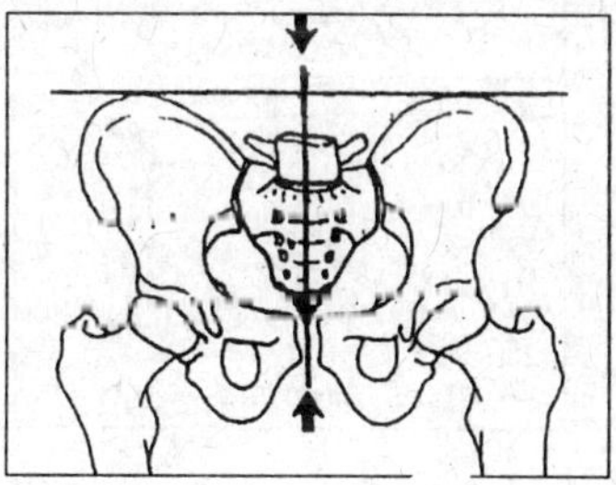

Sacral nerves The five pairs of spinal nerves that emerge from spinal column in sacrum.

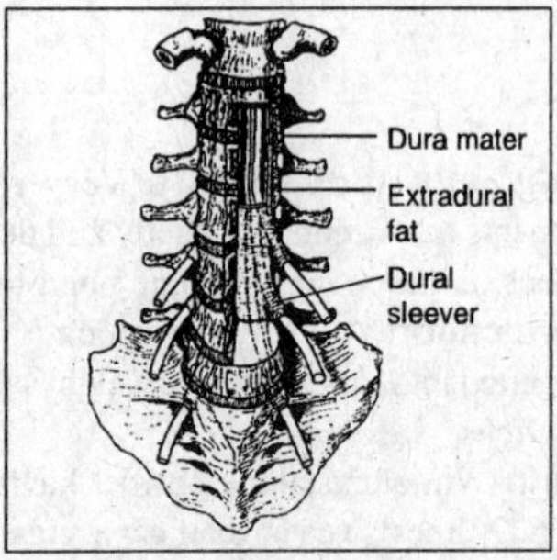

Sacral plexus A network of nerve fibers that arises from spinal nerves L4 through S3. Nerves arising from the lumbar plexus to form the lumbosacral plexus and supply the lower extremity.

Sacral promontory The superior surface of the body of the first sacral vertebra that projects anteriorly into the pelvic cavity; a line from the sacral promontory to the superior border of the pubic symphysis divides the abdominal land pelvic cavities.

Sacralisation It is the fusion of lowest lumbar vertebrae with upper part of sacrum. It may be a birth anomaly. It generally produces no symptoms and is found accidentally when X-ray is being done. Sometimes it may be performed in severe case of prolapse disc.

Sacroiliac joint It is a pair of rigid bones between each side of sacrum. Bony joint is lined by cartilage and have a small amount of synovial fluid.

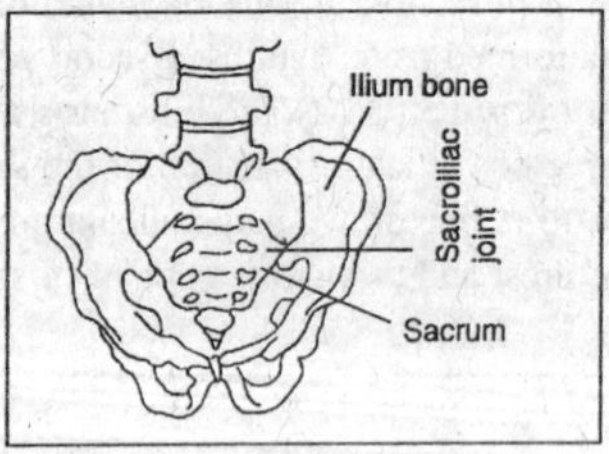

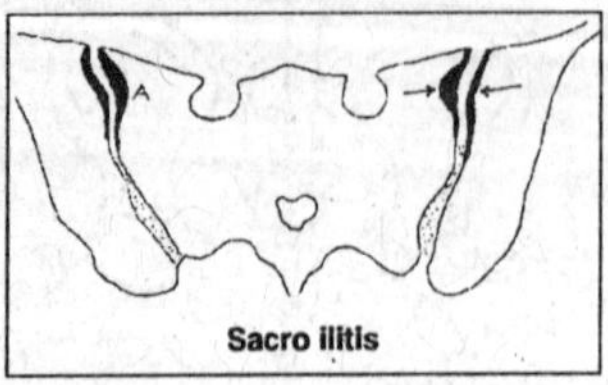

Sacro iliitis

Inflamed condition of it is known as sacroilitis. Sacroilitis may be caused by spondylitis or rheumatoid arthritis. It causes pain in lower back, buttock, groin and back of thighs. There may be fever and malaise. X-ray helps in diagnosis.

Sacrolema The cell membrane of muscle fibre.

Sacroplasm The cytoplasm within a muscle fiber.

Sacrum A triangular wedge shaped bone consisting of 5 vertebra fused together. It forms a back part of pelvis.

Saddle Part of a complete or partial denture that rests on the oral mucosa and to which the teeth are attached.

Saddle block The blocking of neuropathways of pain by injecting a local anaesthetic into the subarachnoid space in the spine. A true saddle block blocks pain in the perineum. A modified saddle block abolishes both uterine and perineal discomfort.

Saddle joint A synovial joint in which the articular surface of one bone is saddle shaped and the

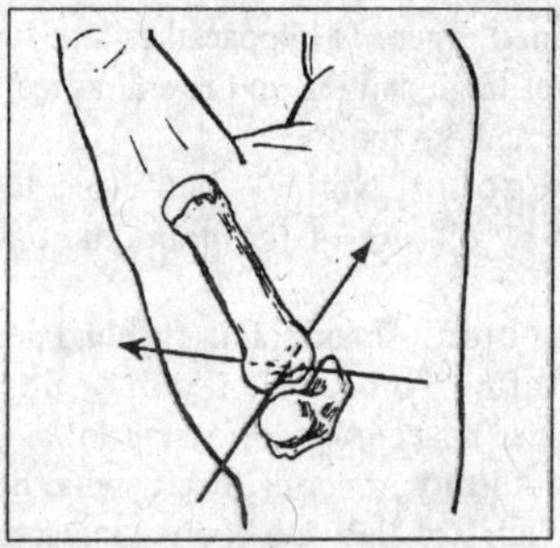

articular surface of the other bone is shaped like the legs of the rider sitting in the saddle, as in the joint between the trapezium and the metacarpal of the thumb.

Sadism Pleasure derived from inflicting physical or psychologic pain or abuse on others. The sexual significance of sadistic wishes or behaviour may be conscious or unconscious. When necessary for sexual gratification, classifiable as a paraphilia.

Sadomasochistic relationship Enjoyment of suffering by one person of an interacting couple with a complementary enjoyment in inflicting pain to the other.

Safe period It is the period of menstrual cycle when conception is least likely to result from intercourse without use of a contraceptive device.

Safe sex It is the procedure to take proper care to reduce the chances of getting sexually transmitting diseases. Nowadays due to prevalence of AIDS safe sex has become very important.

Only sexual intercourse is completely safe when it is between husband and wife. Known methods of transmitting sex are vaginal, anal or oral intercourse. To reduce the risk good quality condom should be used.

Safe touch Secure, respectful, considerate, sensitive, responsive, sympathetic, understanding, supportive, and empathetic contact.

Safety Measures that prevent accidents or unintentional injuries.

Sag sign A sign of posterior cruciate ligament instability.

Sage nail A solid reamed rod designed for the intramedullary fixation of bone of forearm.

Sagittal A vertical plane, extending from front to back. The midsaggital or median plane divides the body into right and left halves.

Sagittal axis A horizontal line extending from front to back, about which movements of abduction and adduction take place.

Sagittal plane A plane that divides the body or organs into left and right portions. Such a plane may be midsagittal (median), in which the divisions are equal, or parasagittal, in which the divisions are unequal.

Sagittal sutures It unites the two parietal bones.

Saha's classification A functional classification of the muscles of shoulder.

Said Specific adaptation to imposed demands (SAID) is the body's response to exercise, in that the more specific the demands made the more specific are the adaptations that occur. It has been shown by research that Iso-tonic, Iso-metric and Iso-kinetic strength gains are specific to the type of conraction used during training. However, a combination of all types of contractons in an exercise regime is more useful in increasing strength than any one alone.

Salbutamol It is a selective beta stimulator with little cardiac stimulant action.It is administered by metered aerosol inhaler, 100 microgram per time or IV. Maximal bronchodilatation occurs within 5 minutes and duration of effect is 4 hours. It can be given orally 2 to 4 mg, 6 to 8 hourly. It is used to treat asthma, bronchospasm and premature labour.

Salenius graph A graph of normal tibiofemoral angles in growing children.

Salicylate poisoning Mild salicylate toxicity occurs at a dose of 140 mg/kg. An acute ingestion of 360 mg/kg is considered potentially fatal. In acute salicylate overdose peak levels occur in 6 to 8 hours and plasma level may continue to rise for 24 hours. Person develops nausea, vomiting and epigastric distress. Later on tinnitus, headache, confusion, lethargy and fever occurs. Dehydration occurs due to vomiting. Respiratory alkalosis occurs due to hyperventilation. Due to renal compression, potassium is lost resulting in severe hypocalcaemia. In severe cases the patient develops hyperglycaemia and increased lactic acid level. In severe cases delirium, hallucinations, convulsions, cardiovascular collapse and coma.

Salicylic acid It is a keratolytic drug used in the treatment of skin disorder including dermatitis, eczema, psoriasis and is sometimes used in treatment of fungal infection. It may cause inflammation if used for long.

Salient Important to the issue at hand.

Saline agglutinin Agglutinates RH positive red cells suspended in saline. The agglutinin is the first antibody to appear in maternal circulation. These dont cross placenta being of larger molecule.

Saline solution 0.9% sodium chloride solution.

Saliva It is watery, slightly alkaline fluid secreted into the mouth by salivary gland and the mucous membrane of mouth. It contains amylase which is a digestive enzyme to breakdown carbohydrate. It keeps mouth moist and lubricates food to aid swallowing. In addition to amylase saliva contains chemicals such as sodium, potassium, calcium, chloride, proteins and mucins. It is a mixture of three pairs of glands. The submaxillary secretes most of protein mucin while parotid secretions contain none. The amount of secretion from each gland varies with stimulus and nature of food. Total quantity secreted daily is 1000 to 1500 cc. pH varies from 5.8 to 7.6. Total solids vary from 0.3% upto 1.4%. Chief organic constituent is mucin over 0.3%. The function of saliva is to provide amylase, moistening dry food and assisting deglutition by lubricating quality of mucin. On standing saliva loses CO_2 and deposits calcium phosphate and carbonate which are responsible for deposition of tartar. Saliva acts as backward tide to remove food, cellular and bacterial debris. It maintains integrity of tooth by providing minerals for posteruptive maturation. It forms a film of glycoproteins on teeth which reduces wear due to abrasion and attrition. IgA of saliva is effective against many bacteria and viruses. Lysozyme breaks up cell walls of susceptible bacteria. Several antibacilli system has been studied in saliva. Glycoproteins and mucoids produced by major and minor salivary glands form a protective coating for the mucous membrane. Primarily because of its bicarbonate content and secondarily of phosphate saliva works as a buffer against acidogenic micro-organism.

Saliva ejector Tubular plastic or metal-tipped suction tube attached to either a water or air pressure vacuum system; evacuates fluids from the oral cavity during a dental procedure.

Saliva-amount Total salivary fluid produced during a 24-hour period is 1000-1500 ml. About 90 per cent of it is derived from parotid and submaxillary gland, about 5 per cent from sublingual and 5 per cent from minor salivary glands. Flow of it is 0.05 ml/min/gland at rest and 0.5 ml/min/gland when stimulated. 80 to 90 per cent of daily production of saliva is the result of stimulation while eating.

Saliva-calculus formation Mineral contents of supragingival calculus are derived from salivary fluids. Calculus deposition is rapid and heaviest opposite the orifice of salivary glands. When calcium and phosphorus in saliva is high person becomes prone to form calculi. Persons who are heavy calculus formers have higher levels of saliva glycoproteins.

Saliva-composition Glucose is present in very low concentration. It is elevated in diabetes. Lipids and amino acids are also present in low concentrations. Saliva is slightly acidic prior to secretion. It becomes slightly alkaline on excretion from gland due to loss of CO_2. pH is elevated at high flow rates. The major component of saliva is amylase. There is virtually no amylase in sublingual or minor salivary gland secretions. Enzyme lactoperoxidase is antibacterial. Saliva contains epithelial cells from oral mucosa as well as leucocytes from gingival sulcus. The enzyme lactic acid dehydrogenase has been found in parotid saliva but not in submaxillary saliva. In saliva IgG to IgA ratio is 1 : 10 reverse of blood.

Salivary amylase Digestive enzyme found in the saliva that begins the chemical digestion of carbohydrates.

Salivary fistula An opening between a salivary duct and or gland and the cutaneous surface or into oral cavity.

Salivary gland-adenoma It is rare and develops in minor gland than major ones. It is seen as a small, freely movable, circumscribed nodule and develops after the age of 30. These are smallest and least aggressive of the epithelial salivary gland tumours. Microscopic sections show an encapsulated lesion composed of a monotonus succession of ducts. Treatment consists of excision and the lesion rarely recurs.

Salivary gland-mucocele It is a mucus containing cyst and is seen as a small, circumscribed, usually elevated, translucent bluish lesion of mucosa. When it is deep seated it can be felt as a circumscribed freely movable lesion. It can occur anywhere in oral cavity. Lips and tongue are preferred sites. The cycle of rupture, discharge and recurrence may go on months. These are formed because of traumatic rupture of excretory duct of a salivary gland. Treatment consists of removal of cyst as well as associated gland.

Salivary glands These are three pairs of glands that secrete saliva via ducts into mouth. Largest salivary gland parotid lies over the angle of jaw just below and in front of ears. Ducts open inside the cheek. The sublingual glands are situated in the floor of mouth. They form a ridge on each side

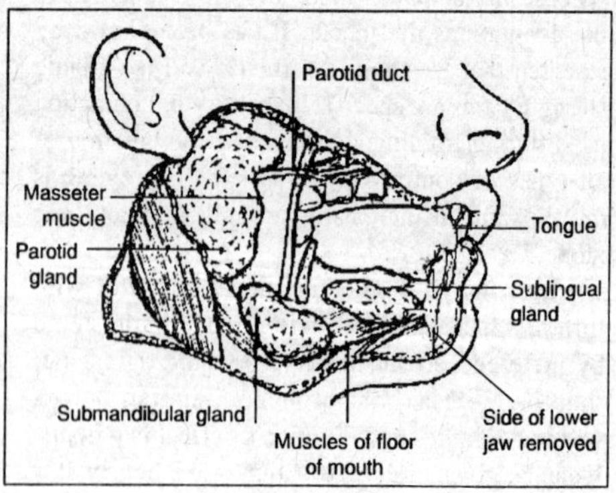

of frenulum. This ridge has a row of small openings through which saliva is secreted. The submandibular glands lie toward the back of mouth close to the sides of jaw. Their ducts run forward to open under the tongue in two small openings one on either side. Sometimes calculi are formed in these ducts which has to be removed surgically. Parotid glands may be affected by mumps. Insufficient secretion of saliva causes dry mouth.

Saliva-secretion Saliva secretion is controlled by salivary centre at medulla. There are superior and inferior salivary nuclei. Flow is generated mainly by unconditional reflex stimulation, primarily by tastebuds but masticatory, olfactory stimuli, oral pain and irritation can stimulate. Emotional and psychic factors also stimulate.

Salk polio vaccine An injectable vaccine that provides individual immunity to poliomyelitis by is less effective at interrupting transmission than is the live attenuated vaccine.

Salmonella These are gram-negative, non-spore forming, non- capsulated. Most strains are motile and grow very easily on ordinary culture media. These ferment glucose and mannitol with acid or gas. These do not ferment lactose or sucrose. Organisms are aerobic. Some strains of typhoid bacillus require trytophan. These cause typhoid fever.

Salmonella carriers About one-third of individuals having typhoid fever discharge bacilli for a period of 3 weeks after onset of illness and about 10 % for 8 to 10 weeks. They are convalescent carriers. A certain proportion continues to excrete typhoid bacilli for 6 months or more and many cases for years together.

Salpingitis It is the inflammation of fallopian tubes that run from ovary to the tip of uterus. Gonococcal infection also infects it. It results in severe abdominal pain, fever and frequent passing of urine. Abdomen becomes very tender. Patients keep her legs withdrawn and folded. Ectopic pregnancy and appendicitis may cause similar symptoms. Laparoscopic examination may help. As a complication pus may collect resulting in pyosalpinx. Pus collection within abdomen may result in pelvic abscess. Suitable antibiotics help, if not then surgery is the remedy.

Salt A substance that, when dissolved in water, ionizes into cations and anions, neither of which are hydrogen ions (H^+) or hydroxide ions (OH^-).

Salt appetite The behavior of selective ingestion of osmotically active solute.

Saltatory conduction The propagation of an action potential (nerve impulse) along the exposed portions of a myelinated nerve fiber. The action potential appears at successive nodes of Ranvier and therefore seems to jump or leap from node to node.

Salt-free diet It is a diet without salt. This diet is prescribed in case of high blood pressure, severe ascites, severe pitting oedema of legs due to any cause, preeclampsia, nephritic syndrome and nephritis.

SAM splint Structural aluminium malleable splint.

Sample A portion of a given population of organisms, objects, or events. In an incidental sample convenience is the chief criterion in selecting the portion of the total population, and therefore it is usually not representative of that population.

Sampling error The extent to which population parameters deviate from a sample statistic.

Sampling plan Process of selecting a portion of the population to represent the entire population.

Sampson's Nail An intramedullary nail for the treatment of fractures of the femoral shaft.

Sanatorium It is a specialised place for convalescent patients. These are admitted not only for treatment but for rehabilitation too. TB sanatoriums are common located at hill stations.

Sandblaster Device used in conjunction with air and small sand particles to reduce the smoothness on a surface.

Sandwich generation Having dependent children at home and dependent elders needing care.

Sanguineous Bloody.

Sanichair It a lavatory chair on wheels. Seat is shaped like a lavatory seat. Bedpan can be placed under the seat.

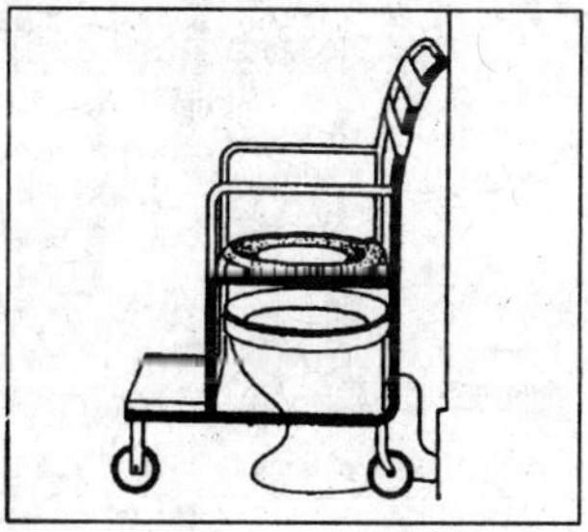

Sanitary pads These absorb moisture. Most women and grown-up girls wear them during menstruation to protect their clothing. The discharge contains some waste blood and these are used like bandage.

Sanitation The formulation and application of measures to promote and establish conditions favorable to health, specifically public health.

Sanitization Act of making something sanitary, or clean and free of dirt.

Sappey's veins Small veins in the falciform ligament.

Sarcoidosis A systemic granulomatous disease that predominantly affects the lungs with resulting fibrosis.

Sarcoidosis of nervous system It is a multisystem granulomatous disorder of unknown origin. There are epithelioid cell granulomas without caseation. Nervous system is involved in 5% cases. Most common neurological manifestation is cranial neuropathy may be accompanied by lymphocytic meningitis. Granulomas may affect the parenchyma of brain. Hypothalamus is the common site. Granuloma may invade the optic chiasma and result in visual defects. Some may cause seizures. Vasculitis may develop. Muscle biopsy shows granulomas in 50 % cases. Corticosteroids prove helpful in most of cases.

Sarcolemma The cell membrane of a muscle fiber (cell), especially of a skeletal muscle fiber.

Sarcoma Malignant neoplasm of connective tissue elements.

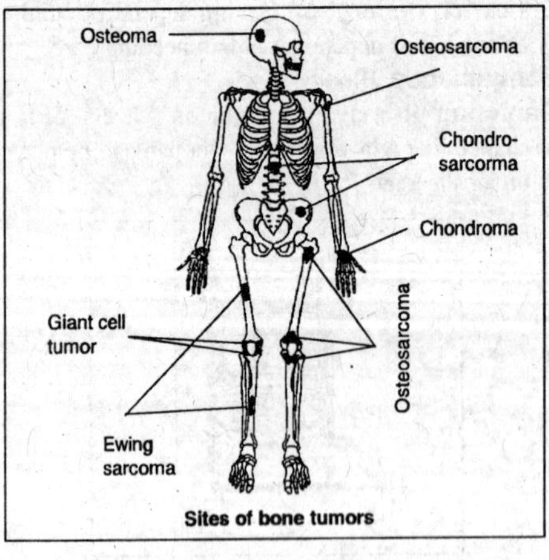

Sites of bone tumors

Sarcoma of Kaposi It is a rare tumour of blood vessels. Lesions are much more generalised and disseminated and 50 per cent AIDS patients show oral lesions.

Oral lesions are flat or raised, nontender, pigmented and reddish purple growth. Common sites are palate and oropharynx. Microscopic features are of spindle cells of which some show mitosis and atypical vascular channels.

Sarcomere The portion of a striated muscle fiber between the two adhacent Z lines that is considered the functional unit of a myofibril.

Sarcoplasm The cytoplasm of a muscle fiber.

Sarcoplasmic reticulum The endoplasmic reticulum of a muscle fibre.

Satellite Satellite cells in spinal ganglia.

Satellite spatter Small droplets of blood that are distributed around a drop or pool of blood as a result of the blood impacting the target surface.

Satiation The condition of being fully satisfied; without need or desire; gratified to an excess. In behaviour therapy, a mild form of punishment in which a stronger-than-normal desire is gratified in excess, thereby in some cases lessening the desire. For example, a child who is constantly pestering to stay up late at night may be allowed or even encouraged to do so on several successive occasions; subsequently, the tired child might lose the desire to stay up late and develop the habit of an earlier bedtime.

Satiety center A collection of neurons located in the ventromedial nuclei of the hypothalamus that, when stimulated, bring about the cessation of eating.

Satiety factor A factor that acts on the appetite regulating regions of the brain to indicate satiety or to reduce food intake.

Saturated fats Lipids that contain as much hydrogen as their molecular structure can hold.

Saturation The degree to which colour of a given hue is present, i.e. the degree to which it differs from grey of the same brightness. A highly saturated red, for example, is very red and a minimally saturated red is only barely distinguishable from grey.

Satyriasis Pathologic or exaggerated sexual drive or excitement in the man. May be of psychologic or organic aetiology.

Saucerization An operative procedure in which tissue is excavated from a wound to form a saucer like depression for the drainage of infected bone.

Sauna bath Sauna bath is available in two types : pannel sauna, and log sauna. *Pannel saunas* are made of outer and inner pannels of pine with an air space between. Air space is filled with an

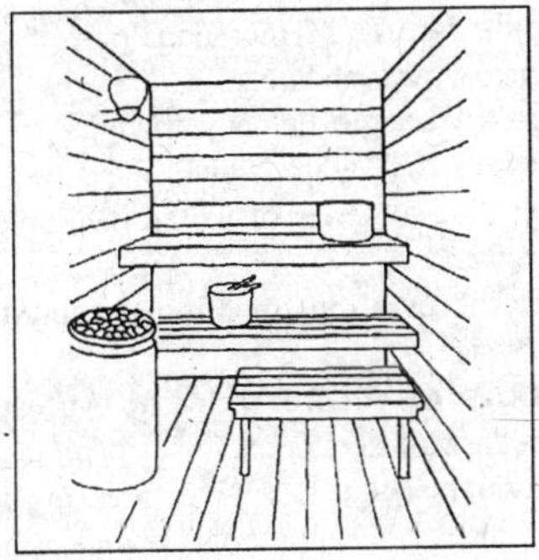

insulating material which insulates the bath saving electricity and preventing heat. *Log sauna* is made of solid wood. Heating is usually achieved electrically with stoves which have a space on top for a quantity of special stones. Heaters are controlled by thermostat switches. It is possible to preset to the required temperature.

SC joint Sternoclavicular joint

Scab A hard crust of dried blood, serum or pus that develops over a sore.

Scabies It is a parasitic infection produced by mite, *Sarcoptes scabie*, which lives upon the skin and is visible through naked eye. The infection can also occur through use of clothes and beddings of infected person when fertilised female mite burrows into stratum corneum and deposits eggs along with her irritating excreta into burrows and after hatching young larvae leave the burrows. The condition presents with papular or papulovesicular lesions on the skin but spare the head and neck. There are burrows which are greyish, linear, scaly lesions usually of about 5 mm long but also can be seen on flexors of wrists and elbows, axillary folds, nipples and lower abdomen. Itching is usual complaint which is more intense in night. Scratching may cause secondary and pyoderma. Scabicides kill the mite that invades epidermis.

Scala media Cochlear duct.

Scala tympani The interior spiral-shaped channel of the bony cochlea, filled with perilymph.

Scala vestibuli The superior spiral-shaped channel of the bony cochlea, filled with perilymph.

Scalar quantity Quantity having magnitude only, not direction.

Scalded skin syndrome The syndrome is characterised by extensive loosening of skin with or without bullae, peeling off large sheet of skin with slight trauma leaving denuded area, and extreme toxicity.

Scalene muscles A group of three muscles anterior, medial, and posterior scalenes acting as accessory inspiratory muscles to elevate the first and second ribs.

Scaler Hand instrument used to remove local irritants.

Scales A collection of horny material on the skin of different sizes.

Scaling Use of instruments with cutting blades to remove calculus from the tooth surface.

Scalp It is the region of skin and underlying tissue layers of head that is normally covered with hair. Scalp skin is tougher and is attached to an

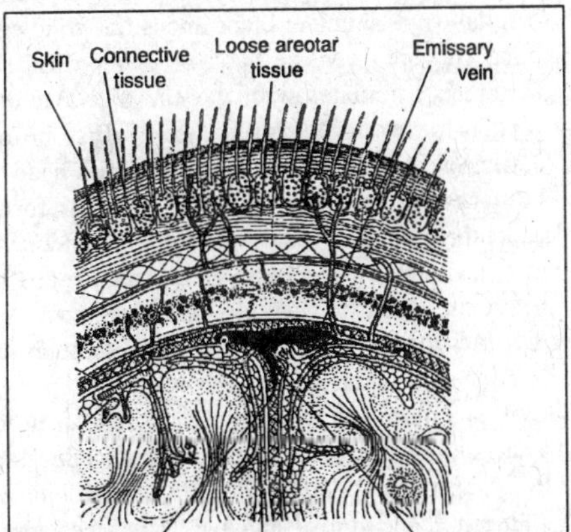

underlying sheet of muscle. This muscle is loosely attached to the skull. Scalp is richly supplied with blood vessels. It is affected by a variety of skin disorders. Dandruff may lead to loss of hair.

Scalp vein set It is a readymade properly sterilised tube with thin needle fixed at end used for fluid therapy in small children. Scalp vein is usually utilised. Movement of limbs does not dislodge it.

Scalpel It is a surgical knife for cutting tissues. Mostly steel blades are used but in sophisticated scalpels, diamond or ruby blades are used.

SCAN Scientific content analysis.

Scan speed The speed at which the detecting system traverses the organ being scanned.

Scanner Something that scans; a scintiscanner.

Scaphoid It is one of the small bones of wrist. It is the outermost bone of thumb side in the proximal row of carpals. It is exposed to fracture as a result of fall on an outstretched hand. Treatment consists of immobilising the wrist in a cast. Untreated scaphoid may not heal and necrosis may develop. In some cases persistent pain may start resulting in restrictions of movements.

Scaphoid pad Resilient dome-shaped material placed at the junction of the inner sole and medial quarter of the shoe, with the apex located between the navicular tuberosity and the sustentaculum tali of the calcaneus; intended to support the longitudinal arch.

Scapula The flat triangular bone of shoulder girdle. It is known as shoulder blade and is flat, triangular bone situated over the back of upper ribs. The acromian articulates with the end of clavicle to form a acromioclavicular joint. Just below acromion is glenoid cavity into which head of humerus fits to form shoulder joint. It forms attachment point of many muscles and tendons of arm, neck, chest and back. Being surrounded by heavy muscles it is generally not fractured.

Scapular line A vertical line passing through the inferior angle of scapula.

Scar It is a mark left on damaged tissue after it has healed. Even on internal wounds scar may develop. Body repairs a wound by forming a tough, fibrous collagen at the site of damage. When cut edges are nearby, healing takes place by narrow pale scar. If edges are left apart scar is extensive. Infected scar is a large unsightly scar. Some people have family tendency to develop large scar. Keloid is a large, irregularly-shaped scar that continues to grow in size as the body continues to produce extra collagen.

Scar formation Replacement of damaged cells with fibrous tissue.

Scarf sign A test to assess infant maturity. The infant's arms are drawn across the neck and as far across the opposite shoulder as possible. In the premature infant there is less resistance and greater draping or scarf effect; the elbow will reach near or across the midline. In the full-term infant, the elbow will not reach the midline.

Scarpa's fascia Membranous part of superficial fascia of lower abdomen.

Scarpa's triangle Femoral triangle.

Scattergram A graph which illustrates the extent to which two series of paired measurements are correlated.

SCFE Abbreviation for slipped capital femoral epiphysis.

Schedule of reinforcement An established procedure of sequence for reinforcing operant behaviour. Thus, in a lever-pressing situation, every displacement of the lever may bring a pellet of food (continuous reinforcement); the pellet may come every five seconds, regardless of how many displacements occur earlier (fixed interval schedule); the pellet may come at every tenth displacement (fixed ratio schedule); the pellet may appear on an average of every five seconds (variable interval schedule): or the pellet may appear on an average of every tenth displacement (variable ratio schedule)

Scheffe test A multiple-comparison procedure.

Schick test The test includes an intradermal injection of standard test dose of purified diphtheria toxin, with a control test, and the result is read in 24 and 48 hours. In a positive test there is no reaction in control site but erythema and oedema occur on the test site, reaching their maximum in 48 hours and then fade. A positive test indicates susceptibility to diphtheria, and a negative indicates resistance to diphtheria.

Schirmer's test A test measuring tear secretion. It is accomplished by using 35 x 5 m.m. strip of filter

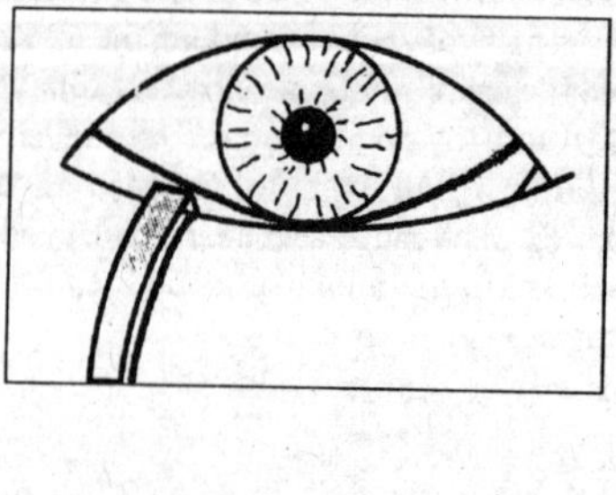

paper. More than 25 m.m of wetting would indicate excessive tear secretion.

Schizont A multinucleated cell undergoing schizogony, prior to cytoplasmic division.

Schizophrenia Person develops disturbance in thinking, emotional reaction and behaviour. These are known as 'split personality'. Disorder should not be confused with multiple personality. Onset is between 15 and 25 years of age. Inheritance has been shown to play a role in its cause.

Certain forms of temporal lobe epilepsy, tumours and encephalitis may also relate it. It may begin insidiously. Person becomes slow, more withdrawn and introverted and losing his drive. Person may suffer from delusions.

Delusions may take a form that one is god or superman. Auditory confusions occur in schizophrenia. Most schizophrenics also suffer from a variety of thoughts in the form of thought disorder which impair concentration or clear muddled and disappointed speech. The treatment includes antipsychotic drugs and long acting depot injections.

Schizophrenia in pregnancy Patient's thoughts become strange and disorderly. Florid symptoms rarely occur more during puerperium. She shows neglect towards the child being preoccupied with bizzre changes of thought and is oblivious to her child's crying or discomfort.

Schizophrenic disorder Literally, "splitting of the mind or of the personality." A form of psychosis characterised by extreme withdrawal from reality. Since it involves marked mental deterioration (dementia) and often appears relatively early in life (adolescence or early adulthood), it originally was given the name dementia praecox. Four common types: catatonic, disorganised, pranoid, undifferentiated.

Schizothymia On cattell sixteen personality factor questionnaire. High scores indicates withdrawn, internally preoccupied, precise and skeptical. Low scores are labelled as cyclothymic.

Schlemm, canal Sinus venosus sclerae.

Schmidt's syndrome A syndrome characterised by Addison's disease, chronic lymphocytic thyroiditis, and perhaps diabetes mellitus.

Schneider nail A four flanged self broaching intermedullary nail for fracture of femoral shaft.

School phobia A Youngester's specific irrational fear of a school related stimulus that immediately provokes avoidance.

School refusal behaviour Substantial child motivated, refusal to attend school.

School stress Unusual distress during school days that leads to others to not to attend school.

Schuffner's dots Fine granules distributed throughout erythrocytes infected with *Plasmodium vivax*.

Schultz-Charlton reaction In this an intradermal injection of scarlet fever antitoxin or convalescent humans serum in an area of scarlet fever rash produces blanching around the site of injection in 8 to 12 hours. This reaction may be needed for the confirmation of the diagnosis of scarlet fever.

Schwabach test The essence of this test is comparison of patients hearing of tuning fork on the mastoid bone with that of examiner's. It is called absolute because background noise is eliminated by masking the meatus of ear under test. The test is only of value when the level of bone conduction of examiner is known. The patient's ear is masked by pressing the tragus firmly into the ear with the finger and the fork is then placed on mastoid bone. If the patient assents to a sensation of hearing the fork is transferred to the examiner's mastoid. The examiner having heard the fork himself replaces it on patient's mastoid and subsequently on his or her own until the fork is no longer heard by one of the participant. If the patient ceases to hear the fork before the examiner the test is recorded 'absolute bone conduction reduced.' This test is conductive.

Schwachman Diamond Syndrome Metaphyseal chondrodysplasia with malabsorption and neutropenia.

Schwann cell Neuroglial cell forming myelin sheaths around axons in the peripheral nervous system.

Schwann cells Large nucleated cells that form myelin.

Schwann sheath It is a sheath of flattened cells. Each cell is called a Schwann cell which is derived from neural crest cell. The Schwann sheath is surrounded by a basement membrane. The basement membrane together with plasma membrane of Schwann cell constitutes 'neurlemmal sheath.' Between Schwann sheath and axon is called periaxonal space which allows ionic diffusion.

Schwann, cells Neurilemma cells.

Schwartz test Two fingers of left hand are placed over or just below the saphenous opening and with the right middle finger the most prominent part of the varicosity is tapped—a thrill like impulse will be felt by fingers at the saphenous vein opening particularly in severe cases.

Sciatic nerve The major nerve of the leg that arises from the sacral plexus. It is formed by confluences of fourth, fifth lumbar and first, second and third sacral roots.

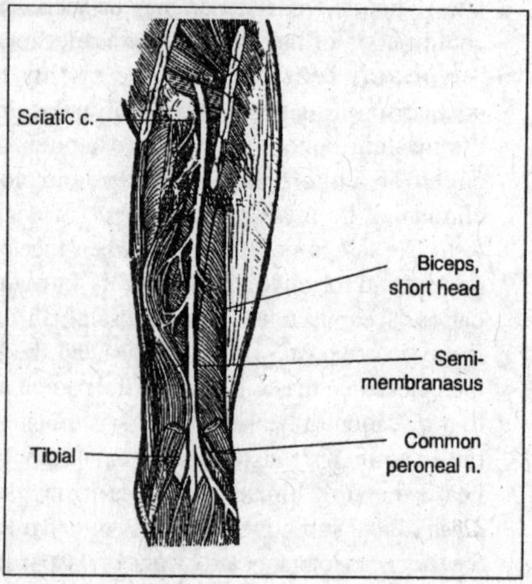

Sciatica Sciatic nerve is the primary nerve of leg and largest in body. It is a branch of sacral plexus in the pelvis and is formed from several lumbar and sacral spinal nerves. From sacral plexus it passes below the sacroiliac joint. Sciatic nerve divides into two main branches called tibial nerve and common peroneal nerve. The upper part of it supplies the hip joint, thigh muscles and skin on the back of thigh. Lower part the tibial and peroneal nerves supply knee and ankle joints. Sciatica is the pain that radiates along the sciatica nerve extending from buttock down the leg to foot. Main cause is prolapsed intervertebral disc or due to pressure from abscess or tumour. Treatment depends on cause. Symptomatic relief may be got from non-steroidal anti-inflammatory drugs (NSAIDs).

Science Body of knowledge unique to a particular subject.

Scientific content analysis A method designed to detect deception in written reports using procedures of content analysis.

Scientist A person in the practice and theory of one of the scientific disciplines to university graduate or postgraduate level, and who is actively engaged in research or analysis in an area related to his training.

Scintigram A graphic recording of the distribution of a radioactive tracer in a part of body. It is produced by recording the flashes of light given off by a scintillator as it is struck by radiation at different intensities.

Scintigraphy A diagnostic procedure in which a radionuclide is injected intravenously, and a photographic recording of its distribution is made.

Scirrhous Pertaining to or of the nature of a hard cancer.

Scissors These are used to cut the tissue and so depending on the type of tissue to be cut, one uses

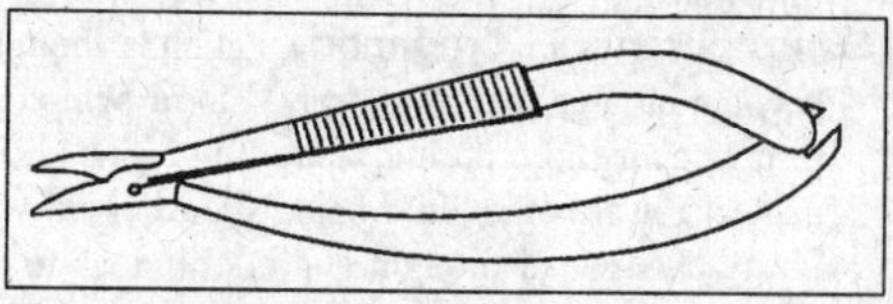

the scissors accordingly. These are also available with or without spring action, straight or curved blades, blunt end or fine sharp ends.

Sclera It is a white outer coat of eye visible through the transparent conjunctiva. It is formed of collagen which is protective. Inflammation of it, i.e. scleritis often responds well to corticosteroid eyedrops. In severe cases these drugs may increase the risk of perforation. It forms the posterior five sixth of eyeball. It is fibrous and protective. Its anterior portion is known as white of an eyeball. It is about 1 mm thick in its posterior part and becomes thin anteriorly. It is very thin (0.3 mm) at the bite of insertion of extraocular muscles.

Scleral venous sinus A circular venous sinus located at the junction of the sclera and the cornea through which aqueous humor drains from the anterior chamber of the eyeball into the blood.

Scleritis Inflammation of sclera is known as scleritis. it is associated with collagen diseases in more than

50 % cases. Tuberculosis. sarcoidosis, leprosy and herpes zoster can cause it. There will be localised congestion with watering and discomfort. There is pain and tenderness. Nodule is away from limbus, conjuctiva over nodule moves freely.

Sclerocornea It is a congenital scarring and vascularisation of the peripheral cornea without any signs of inflammation.

Scleroderma It is a skin disease that occurs in circumscribed as well as in diffuse forms. In circumscribed form it develops as one or more red or ivory coloured smooth, hard patches on skin. The condition is benign and does not present oral manifestation. Diffuse type generally develops in females and is a serious disease in which skin becomes red, oedematous and then undergoes atrophy and shrinkage. Oral manifestation develops in jaws, mucous membrane and tongue. There becomes widening of periodontal space. Oral mucous membrane atrophies and becomes fixed with underlying structures. Tongue may become hard and painful. There may be difficulty in deglutition and mastication. In skin lesions there is atrophy of skin appendages.

Sclerosing chronic osteomyelitis The mandible is affected more and premolar and molar are usual sites. Teeth may or may not be present in affected area. Affected area is enlarged. Person may feel repeated episodes of pain around jaws while some lesions may be asymptomatic. Disease is extensive but self-limiting. If lesion is near the crest of an edentulous ridge person may develop ulceration and sequestration. Multiple, well-defined or diffuse, dense radiopacities may be surrounded by radiolucencies. Jaw lesions have a cotton wool or pagetold appearance. Because the cause is not known, antibiotics and cortisone are of little value.

Sclerosing peritonitis It may result due to long-term use of beta-blocker practolol. The visceral peritoneum is thickened and small bowel becomes encased in the thickened membrane. There will be vomiting, weight loss and signs of small bowel obstruction. Altered bowel motility reults in malabsorption. Some patients may have skin rashes resembling psoriasis, deafness due to serious otitis media, pleural fibrosis and effusions.

Sclerosis tuberous The classic triad includes mental retardation, infantile spasm and hypopigmented macules. Intracranial calcifications are round, radiopaque areas located along lateral ventricular surface and in superficial cortex.

Sclerotic bone A well-defined focal opacity seen below the apices of vital noncarious teeth.

Sclerotomal pain A deep, diffuse, aching, ill defined pain arising from deep somatic tissue.

Scolex The holdfast organ of tapeworms.

Scoliosis In it spine is bent to one side. Thoracic or lumbar regions are mostly affected. Scoliosis usually starts in childhood. Spine may become 'S'-shaped even because spine curves toward the opposite side of the body to compensate. It may develop due to congenital abnormality of vertebrae. Occasionally a spinal injury and disc prolapse causes temporary scoliois.

Minor scoliosis does not require any treatment, but progressive disease may require surgical intervention.

Scoop method Technique for threading the needle of a syringe into the cap without touching the cap itself.

Scope of practice The knowledge base and practice parameters of a profession.

Scopolamine It is derived from *Hyosynamus niger*. It is a better drying agent than atropine. It was used to produce amnesia in labour. It crosses the brain barrier, its action is similar to atropine. It is a depressant of CNS causing drowsiness, sleep and amnesia in some patients. It decreases the intensity and duration of analgesia produced by opiates, pethidine and methadone. It is a mild respiratory stimulant while its action on iris, salivary, sweat and bronchial glands is stronger than atropine. It has a beneficial effect on motion sickness. Action on heart, intestine and bronchioles is weaker than that of atropine. Adult dose is 0.3 to 0.6 mg parenterally.

Scored tablet Tablet with a groove in its center.

Scoring In implant dentistry, the creation of an indentation on the ridge crest to record the position of a planned osteotomy directly upon the bone.

Scorpion bite Red scorpion is smaller and more poisonous. Venom can be haemolytic or neurotoxic. About 25% victims develop only severe pain at the site. In most cases pain grows within hours of bite. In rest of 75% person may develop vomiting, profuse sweating, cold extremities and mydriasis.

Hypertension and pulmonary oedema develop within 2 to 24 hours. Myocarditis may develop in severe cases.

Scotch cast A trademark for a synthetic fiberglass casting material.

Scotoma Small blind spot in the visual field caused by a small lesion, an epileptic focus, or migraines of the visual cortex.

Scotoma-perimetery Size and location of a scotoma caused by localised retinal lesion on perimetery is determined entirely by the size and location of lesion. Scotoma is an island of blindness surrounded by vision.

Scotty dog appearance Lachapele noted that the diagonal X-rays of the spondylotic crack had the

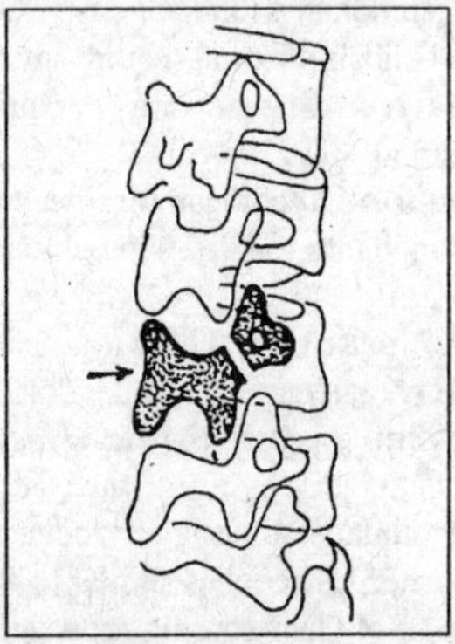

appearance of scotty dog. The transverse process corresponds to the mouth of the dog, the superior process to the ears, inferior articular process to the feet. The neck is the intervertebral joint and the body is the spinous process.

Scratch reflex A reflex by which the hind limb removes a stimulus from the surface of the body.

Scratch, film Appears as a radiopaque line on a film; results when the emulsion of a film is removed from its base by a sharp object.

Screen memory A consciously tolerable memory which serves as a cover for an associated memory that would be emotionally painful if recalled.

Screening The process of identifying a subgroup of people who are at high probability of having asymptomatic dixease or who have a risk factor that puts them at high risk for developing a disease or becoming injured. Screening takes place in a community setting and is applied to a community population, such as students in a school or workers in an industry.

Screening palpation Digital examination of a muscle to determine the absence or presence of palpable bands and tender trigger points using flat or pincer palpation.

Scrofula It is the tuberculosis of the lymph nodes in neck and generally forms local abscess. Antituberculous treatment is advised.

Scrofuloderma It runs a chronic course secondary to the existing tuberculosis in the body and involves the lymph nodes. Specially cervical group, bone or joints are involved. Lesion presents as purplish induration on skin of the overlying affected lymph nodes usually on neck and groins. It appears as dermal nodule or swelling which after months softens and ruptures to discharge purulent exudate. It may lead to formation of sinus or ulcer. Ulcer has irregualr, undermined edges and formation of granulation tissue. Lesions produce thin atrophic scars on healing.

Scrotum It is a pouch that hangs below the penis and contains the testes. The scrotum consists of outer thin, widely wrinkled skin. Swelling of scrotum may be due to inguinal hernia, hydrocele or haemocele.

Scrub Rinse your forearms and hands under the running water. Remember to run the water from

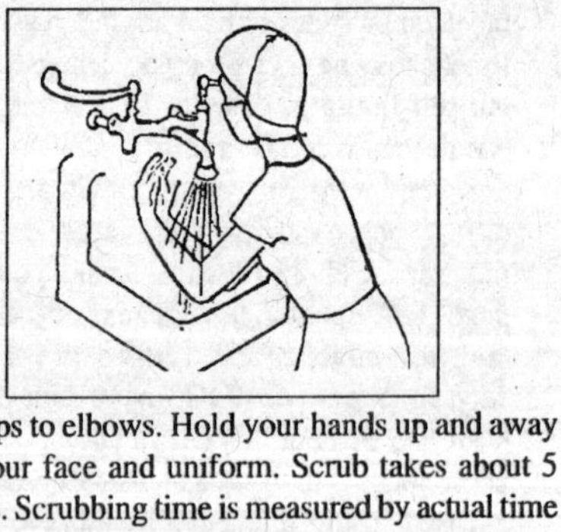

fingertips to elbows. Hold your hands up and away from your face and uniform. Scrub takes about 5 minutes. Scrubbing time is measured by actual time in brushing not rinsing time.

SE Single ended, as a dental instrument with only one working end.

Sea snake bite Sea snake bite is most toxic. These are pinhead-sized puncture wounds usually 1 to 8 in number without much of local pain. Venom produces paralysis which is of ascending type.

Speech becomes slurred with ptosis and ophthalmoplegia. Bulbar involvement may lead to respiratory failure. Full recovery from myotoxic effects can take several months.

Searman rank correlation test A test that is analogous to the pearson correlation coefficient but is used for ranked data.

Seasmoditis A local inflammation of seasamoid usually at the head of the metatarsal.

Sebaceous adenoma It is a benign tumour arising from sebaceous gland. Histologically, simple hyperplasia of the cells occur. Clinically it is a solid swellling may be single or multiple occurring in frontal region or in the region of nose and cheek. When occurring in scalp it may be associated with some lesions in brain.

Sebaceous cyst It is a fat containing cyst on skin. It is caused by blockage of duct of sebaceous gland. Gland itself swells up. It develops on any part which has hair. It has to be removed surgically.

Sebaceous gland These are minute glands in the skin secreting sebum. Sebum is lubricating substance. Sebaceous gland directly opens in skin. Scalp, face and anus are having numerous glands. Palms and soles are devoid of it.

Seborrhoea It is the excessive secretion of sebaceous gland. Sebum is composed of fats and waxes. It lubricates the skin and sebum protects the skin from bacteria and fungi. Excessive secretion of sebum causing increased oiliness of face and greasy scalp. Exact cause is uncertain. Its production is related to androgen level. It may result in acne vulgaris. In adult age it subsides automatically.

Seborrhoeic keratosis It is a senile, benign, pigmented epidermal hyperplasia. Histopathologically, it gives discrete lesion with hyperkeratosis and irregular acanthosis. The condition spontaneously gives rise to raised sit up on skin surface type nodular growth or plaque with warty or flat surface covered by loosely attached greasy crust. It has well demarcated edges. It is asymptomatic and does not require any treatment.

Sebum An oily waterproofing secretion of sebaceous glands.

Sooificity The probability that, given the absence of a disease, a normal test result excludes the disease.

Second lumbar root Compression Standing for some time causes pain in back radiating to front of thigh as far as knee. Sitting down abolishes it.

Second messenger A molecule or ion whose concentration within a target cell is increased by the action of a regulatory compound (e.g., a hormone or neurotransmitter). It stimulates the metabolism of that target cell in a way that it mediates the intracellular effects of that regulatory compound.

Second molars Seventh tooth from the midline in each quadrant of the permanent dentition.

Second Opinion The administration and evaluation of a patient before surgery specially amputation by another surgeon.

Second stage of labour It is the stage of expulsion of fetus. It begins from full dilatation of the cervix and ends with the birth of baby.

Secondary Second or inferior in order of time, place, or importance.

Secondary amenorrhoea A condition characterised by cessation of menstruation for 3-6 months in a female who has previously menstruated.

Secondary appraisal Where the person estimates the degree to which they have the personal resources to cope with the demands of some particular event.

Secondary bond Bonds, such as van der waals forces and hydrogen bonds, that usually are weaker and less stable than primary chemical bonds.

Secondary bone callus In the next stage of healing of fracture immature bone of primary callus is gradually removed and replaced by mature lamellated bone. This stage is referred as formation of secondary callus. It is not as exuberant as primary. It is radiopaque and X-ray taken at this stage shows healed fracture. In final stage of fracture healing secondary callus is remodelled.

Secondary bronchi The initial divisions off the primary bronchi; the lobar bronchi; three from the right primary bronchus; two from the left primary bronchus.

Secondary care Health services to which primary caregivers refers patients for consultation and additional testing.

Secondary carrier Company insuring the dependent employee when the patient is the spouse or dependent child of the employee covered by the primary carrier.

Secondary consistency State to which a dental material is mixed that allows the material to be thick, rolled, or doughy before placement in increments into the prepared tooth.

Secondary contracted kidney There will be diminution of large amount of albumin which was present in early stage. Volume of urine rises, specific gravity falls and urea content is reduced. Oedema disappears as diurnal quantity of urine increases. BP rises progressively. In terminal stages renal failure and urinary volume falls and uraemic symptoms ensue.

Secondary data Collected for one study and later reanalyzed for another study, usually to test new research hypotheses.

Secondary decay Decay that forms at the site of an existing restoration.

Secondary dressing A dressing used to cover or hold primary dressings in place.

Secondary gain The external gain derived from any illness, such as personal attention and service, monetary gains, disability benefits, and release from unpleasant responsibility.

Secondary gigantism Excessive growth secondary to disorder of adrenal, pineal, gonadal or pituitary gland.

Secondary habitual aborters Those aborters who have carried a pregnancy to viability sometime are known as, secondary habitual aborters.

Secondary hypoadrenalism Subnormal secretion of cortisol by the adrenal glands.

Secondary hypotonic inertia This is where uterus has been contracting adequately and than contractions become inefficient later in labour. Causes include cephalo pelvic disproportion, rigid cervix, malpresentation and oversedation.

Secondary illness Disorder that develops from a preexisting condition.

Secondary infertility An existing condition of infertility but with at least one prior conception having been documented.

Secondary infusion Administration of a diluted intravenous drug at the same time a solution is infusing, or intermitently with an infusing solution.

Secondary motives Acquired motives; drives not directly related to physiological conditions. For example, the desire for an auto or a fashionable dress.

Secondary prevention Early detectin to stop or reduce the effects of a disease or illness.

Secondary prevention of cardiovascular disease Program components aimed at reducing risk of illness and death after coronary artery disease diagnosis as well as improving function and quality of life.

Secondary process In psychoanalytic theory, mental activity and thinking characteristic of the ego and influenced by the demands of the environment. Characterised by organisation, system-atisation, intellectualisation, and similar processes leading to logical thought and action in adult life.

Secondary pseudomyxoma peritonei There may be involvement of peritoneum by spread from adenocarcinoma with ascites. Peritoneum may be involved by a mucin secreting cystadenocarcinoma of ovary or large bowel. Peritoneal cavity may be filled with mucus material lying free or as encysted masses. Rarely curvilinear calcification is seen on abdominal X-rays. Abdomen will be distended. Surgical evacuation is the result.

Secondary reinforcer A learned reinforcer. Reinforcement through something which, while it does not satisfy a biological need directly, has been associated with this need satisfaction. Thus, a sound associated with food may come to have reward value in itself and serve as a secondary reinforcer. Other secondary reinforcers include the receipt of praise, a trophy, or a high grade.

Secondary sex characteristic A characteristic of the male or female body that develops at puberty under the influence of sex hormones but is not directly involved in sexual reproduction; examples are distribution of body hair, voice pitch, body shape, and muscle development.

Secondary structure The residue-by residue information of the back bone of a polymer.

Secondary uterine intertia A state of uterine exhaustion where the fault has developed following an initial strong contraction without any obstructive element. It is a hypotonic dysfunction in the active phase of labour.

Secondary visual cortex Visual cortical areas outside of the striate cortex; often called extrastriate cortex.

Second-generation antidepressant An antidepressant that is thought to be more selective then a first generation antidepressant in its action on serotonin reuptake transporters.

Second-intention healing Reparative process when wound edges are widely separated.

Secretin It is the hormone secreted by duodenum as partly digested food enters it. It stimulates the secretion of other enzymes also.

Secretin test In this test the bicarbonate concentration and amylase of duodenal aspirates are measured following intravenous administration of secretin so as to test the pancreatic exocrine function.

A diminished pancreatic exocrine function is seen in chronic pancreatitis.

Secretory diarrhoea Secretory diarrhoea persists when there is total fasting and is usually of large volume. In secretory diarrhoea the concentrations of sodium and potassium when added together and doubled will approximate to the plasmaosmolality of 290 mosmol/l. In some patients it may be associated with IgA deficiency even without infection.

Sedation It is given to calm down a person. It relieves anxiety and controls aggressive behaviour. It is used as premedication resulting in relaxation before an operation.

Sedative A drug that allays activity, excitement, apprehension.

Sedative enema This is given for sedative purpose and at times to relieve pain in case of diarrhoea and dysentery. Enema solution is used of 200 CC of fine starch at body temperature with 1 to 2 CC of tincture opium. Opium reduces seretions and peristalsis and relieves pain and local irritation. Other solution used can be a mixture of potassium bromide or chloral hydrate with normal saline. Rectum is made free of faecal matter before giving it.

Sedatives Drugs which have a calming quietening effect and in large doses induce sleep.

Sedimentation rate The rate at which erythrocyte settle out of unclotted blood in one hour.

Seduction In seduction the woman is said to have been persuaded to enter into sexual relationship by an unconditional promise of future marriage otherwise she would not have consented to have intercourse. Only male is indicted for this offence, the female is not an accomplice but a victim.

See-ability Ergonomic positioning of the dental equipment, patient, and dental health team to enable the dental team to see the site of operation without undue stress on any of the parties involved.

Seesaw respiration Infant's chest falls when the abdomen rises and vice-versa. It is a sign of respiratory difficulty.

Segmental antinociception Relief of pain at segmental level, e.g. by rubbing the sore spot.

Segmental fracture A fracture consisting of more than one fracture line at different levels in the same bone which creates several fracture fragments.

Segmental instability An abnormal response to applied loads characterized by motion in motor segment beyond normal constraints.

Segmentation Refers to animals that can be divided into a number of parts that are similar; also refers to idea that many animals, including vertebrates, are composed of similarly organized body segments.

Segments Any of the parts into which a body naturally separates or is divided, either actually or by an imaginary line; the oral cavity is divided into six segments, two anterior and four posterior.

Segond fracture A capsular avulsion fracture at the margin of lateral tibial plateau in association with anterior cruciate ligament.

Seizure It is the sudden episode of uncontrolled electrical activity in the brain. If abnormal activity remains confined to one area person may experience tingling or twitching of a small part of body. Seizures may be caused by head injury, infection, cerebrovascular accident, brain tumour or alcohol.

Seizure precautions Measures that protect the client from injury during a seizure.

Seizure-febrile These are convulsions, twitching or jerking of limbs with loss of conciousness occurring in a child after sudden rise of temperature. These are caused by disturbance in normal electric activity in the brain but in most cases there is no underlying cause.

Some children may lose consciousness and their arms/legs twitch uncontrollably for a few minutes.

After regaining consciousness child may be drowsy. So Crocin should be given and fever should be kept under control. There remains no after ill effects.

Selection bias The inadvertent selection of a non-representative sample of subjects or observations. A classic example is a 1936 Literary Digest poll which predicted Landon's election over Roosevelt because telephone directories were used as basis for selecting respondents.

Selective absorption Act of selectively absorbing, reflecting, or transmitting electromagnetic radiation depending on structure, atomic number, density, and thickness.

Selective permeability The property of a membrane by which it permits the passage of certain substances but restricts the passage of others.

Selective reduction The procedure of removing or aborting unwanted fetuses in multiple pregnancies.

Selective serotonin reuptake blocker A drug that selectively blocks the reuptake of serotonin into the terminal.

Selectivity The ability of a drug to interact with specific receptors on the target tissue and not with other receptors or other tissues.

Selenium A nonmetallic chemical element having the symbol Se; a micronutrient required by all life forms, as well as a potent toxicant when it is present at high concentrations in ecosystems.

Self attitude Feeling of personal worth ranging from grandiosity to self loathing.

Self catheterization In case of chronic retention of urine male or female both can be trained to pass catheter.

Self centered lies Lies told to benefit oneself.

Self concept Ones mental representation of self.

Self concious emotions Emotions that can only appear after the young infant has formed a central neural representation of him.

Self-curing A chemical polymerization or setting reaction that occurs through a chemical activation when two specific component systems are mixed; this is contrasted to materials cured by the application of heat or light energy; also called "auto-cure"

Self disclosure Refers to verbally revealing about oneself. A particular coping strategy related to the expression of thoughts and feelings about upsetting event.

Self efficacy That part of optimism related to a belief in one's ability to do the behaviors necessary to achieve some desired outcome. Beliefs about personal abilities and characteristics which guide responses to situations.

Self employment To work for oneself rather than another.

Self esteem Firm feelings and beliefs about ones own worth as a person. Personal value that an individual places on himself.

Self limited disease A disease by its very nature will run a limited and definite course.

Self-actualisation The postulated fifth and last level in Maslow's hierarchy of human motivation; the motivation to realise one's potential, whatever it may be, to the fullest, regardless of the rewards involved; doing what one is best-suited to do or intended to do.

The term is controversial because it is said to lack a precise definition.

Self-care contract Contract developed independent of a health professional. The contract is between two individuals for the purpose of improving a health behavior.

Selfcatheterization The ability of individuals to insert a urinary catheter into their urinary meatus.

Self-concept The individual as represented in his or her own awareness and in the setting of those things with which he or she identifies. The ego and its external involvements.

Self-efficacy The perception or judgement of one's ability to perform a certain action successfully or to control one's circumstances.

Self-esteem The evaluative part of the self-concept; one's feeling of self-worth.

Self-examination, breast Breast cancers are discovered accidentally when a woman finds a lump in her breast. Because an early detection may prolong life.

Woman should examine her breasts each month after menstruation to locate a lump if any, standing in front of a mirror in bathroom. Technique of palpation is shown in figures.

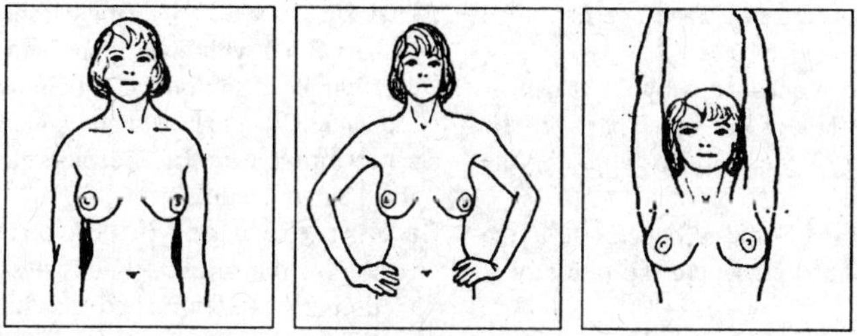

Looking

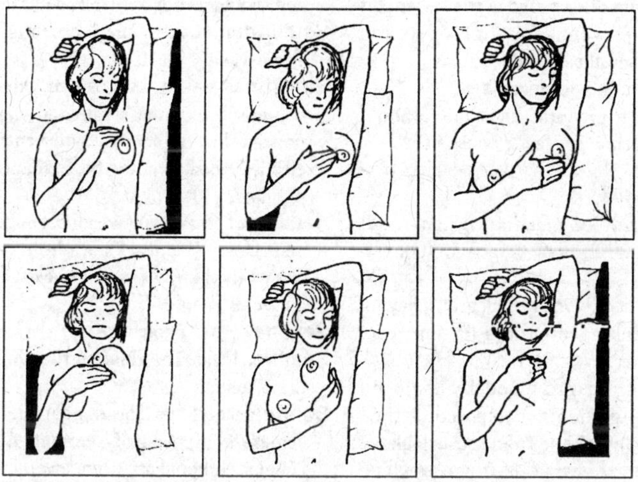

Feeling

Self-fulfilling prophecy A distortion of an event or situation that eventually leads an individual to behave as he or she is expected to behave by others in his or her social setting.

Self-image The self as the individual pictures or imagines it.

Self-mobilizing Techniques whereby the patient is taught to apply joint mobilization techniques to his own restricted joints, using proper gliding techniques.

Self-perception A psychological process whereby individuals infer the nature of their attitudes and beliefs by observing their own behavior.

Self-retaining catheter Self-retaining catheter is introduced through urethral meatus to bladder in conditions where continuous evacuation of bladder content is required. It may be required in bladder for longer time. Foley's catheter is used for this purpose. Indications are collapse of bladder, neurogenic bladder after prostate operation, for incontinence of urine and for recurrent retention of urine. Foley's catheter is introduced as an

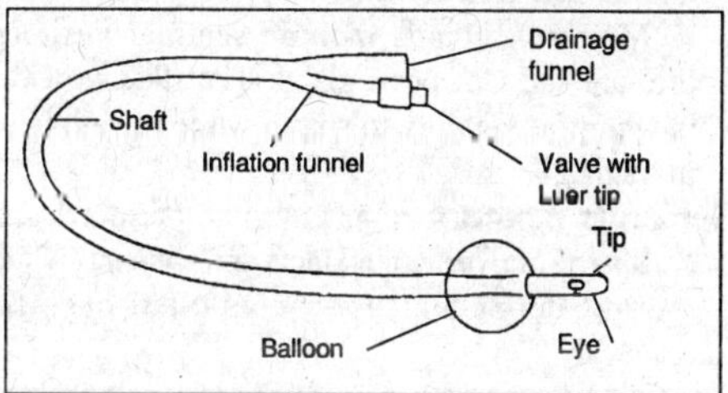

ordinary cather. After it has gone to bladder 5 to 30 CC of water is injected by a sterile syringe. The injected water inflates a balloon-like bulb which does not permit slipping out of catheter. When removal of catheter is required never forget to remove the injected water by a syringe first, then remove the catheter gently.

Self-stretching Techniques whereby the patient is taught to stretch a joint of soft tissue passively by using another part of the body for applying the stretch force.

Sella turcica The saddle-shaped depression in the inner surface of the skull where the pituitary is located.

Sellick's method A technique in which pressure is applied to the ring of cartilage at the lower part of the larynx to prevent aspiration of gastric contents during anaesthesia induction.

Semantic Having to do with meaning.

Semantic memory General knowledge about words and their meanings, facts, concepts.

Semantic retrieval Retrieving the meaning of a word from memory stores.

Semantics The study of meaning in language; includes the relationships of language, thought, and behavior.

Semelparity The fact of being semelparous; having only a single breeding season in a lifetime; e.g., certain invertebrates.

Semen It is the fluid produced by male on ejaculation. Major portion is composed of fluid from seminal vesicles, a fluid from prostate gland. Secretion of seminal vesicle is fructose which produces the sperm to remain mobile. Production of it depends on sex hormone– testosterone. Semen analysis is done in case of infertility.

Normal semen contains 20 million to 200 million sperm per ml. Sperm may be less in number, not motile or deformed. The male sex glands secrete it. Male sex glands include seminal vesicles, prostate and Cowper's gland. The fluid provides medium for viability to sperm while travelling up in vagina.

Sementic memory A general fund of knowledge, consisting of overlearned facts and concepts which are not dependent upon contexual cues for retrieval.

Semicircular canal One of three canals in each temporal bone; involved in the detection of motion.

Semicircular canals Located in the inner ear; contains a specialized receptor call crista ampullaris that geneates a nerve impulse on movement of the head.

Semicircular ducts The membranous semicircular canals filled with endolymph and floating in the perilymph of the bony semicircular canals; they contain cristae that mediate dynamic equilibrium.

Semicricular canals Receptors in the middle ear for head movements.

Semi-Fowler's position A position of labour whereby the client's knees are flexed on the abdomen, hands grasped just below the knees during the onset of a contraction, and the head and shoulders possibly raised in a 45-degree angle.

Semilunar cusps The crescentic leaflets of the aortic valve.

Semilunar valve One of two valves in the heart composed of three semilunar-shaped cusps that prevent flow of blood into the ventricles following ejection; located at the beginning of the aorta and pulmonary trunk.

Semilunar valves Valves located between the two ventricular chambers and the large arteries that carry blood away from the heart; valves found in the veins.

Seminal Fluid Semen

Seminal fluid The fluid surrounding the sperm in the ejaclulate.

Seminal plasma The nongamete component of semen, composed of secreted fluid, cells, and cellular components from several male accessory sex glands.

Seminal relating To semen or its ejaculation.

Seminal vesicle One of two glandular structures that empties into the ejaculatory ducts; its secretion is one of the components of semen.

Seminal vesiculitis It accompanies prostatitis. Symptoms are similar to prostatitis. It is the cause of persistent pyuria following prostectomy. It may

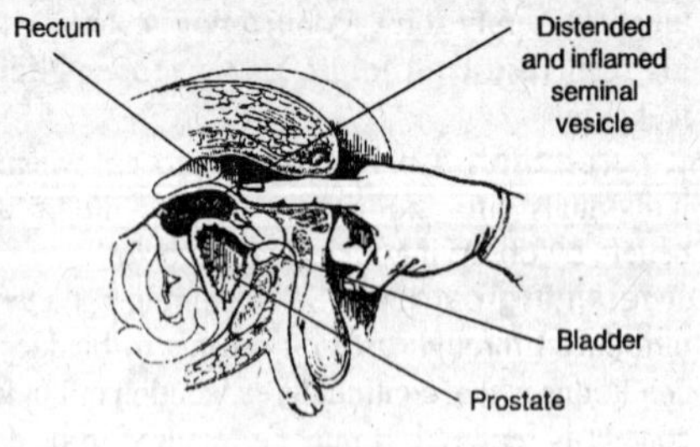

Palpation of seminal vesicle

be accompanied by prostatitis and posterior urethritis. There will be pain in groin and lower abdomen referred to testicles. Low backache is frequent complaint and sometimes blood appears in seminal fluid. Seminal vesiculogram helps.

Seminiferous tubule Tubule in the testis in which sperm cells develop. These are fine convoluted

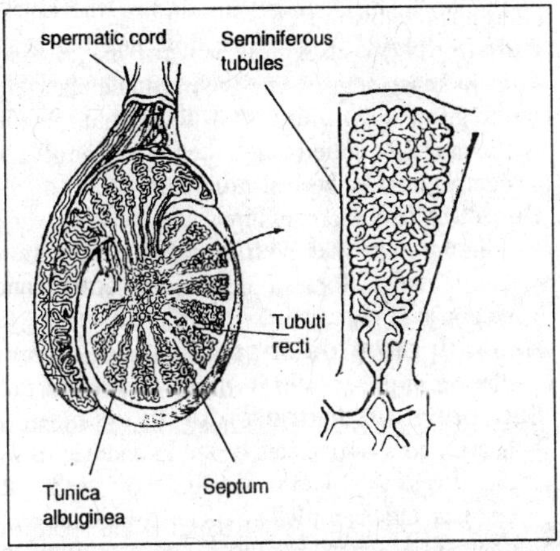

tubes that comprise the main constituent of secreting seminal fluid. There are two vesicles one at the top of each testis. In tubules sperms are formed.

Semipermeable membrane A membrane with pores of a size that permits the passage of solvent and some solute molecules while restricting the passage of other solute molecules.

Senescence Process or condition of growing old; physiologic ageing not necessarily related to chronologic age.

Sengastaken-blake more tube It is a double cuffed gastric tube designed to compress gastrooesophageal varices to control bleeding.

Senile Of or pertaining to old age; characteristic of old age.

Senile kyphosis It is due to loss of height of anterior discs and osteophyte formation.

Senile macular degeneration Senile macular degeneration is age related and is one of the main causes of blindness. It is a bilateral disease. On ophthalmoscope there are small discrete yellowish white spots at the posterior pole of eye. These spots are known as drusen or colloid bodies. It manifests as ring of fine pigment spots at fovea. It is due to obliterative sclerosis of the underlying choriocapillaries. There is gradual loss of vision. There is no treatment available.

Senile nuclear cataract In it there is sclerosis of lens nucleus and cortical fibres remain transparent. With the passage of time the nucleus of lens becomes diffusely cloudy. The cloudiness spreads gradually towards the cortex until entire lens is occupied by lens nucleus. Occasionally the lens nucleus becomess dark brown or dusky red or even black. This change in colour is due to deposition of melanin. Clinically, there is iris shadow and grey pupil. On ophthalmoscopy fundus gives a hazy appearance. There is progressive myopia due to increased refractive index of lens nucleus. If myopia is corrected patient improves his or her visual acuity. It is advisable to remove lens without waiting for maturity.

Senile Osteoporosis Osteoporosis in aged.

Senile retinoschisis It is splitting of sensory retina into 2 layers, outer and inner. The splitting occurs at the outer plexiform layer and less commonly at the level of nerve fibre layers. It is prevalent in young and hypermetropes. It progresses circumferentially and involves the entire periphery of fundus. Retinal breaks in the inner or outer layers of retinoschisis often lead to retinal detachment.

Senile tremor Benign essential tremor, often mistaken for a sign of Parkinson's disease..

Senile vaginitis As a result of oestrogen deficiency vaginal epithelium becomes thin and atrophic. Glycogen content and acidity of vagina are lowered. A purulent and often slightly blood-stained discharge is evident. Vagina is inflamed, tender and skin is excoriated. Frequency of urine and dysuria are common. There may be patchy granular vaginitis in which there develops red spots which bleed easily. As treatment oestrogen improves the resistance of the vaginal epithelium, raise the glucose content and lower vaginal pH.

Senility It is the reduction of mental capability during old age. After the age of 65 most of the persons suffer from impaired memory and some loss of concentration. There is increased risk of dementia and confusion.

Sensate focus A therapeutic approach to sexual dysfunction which emphasises the aim of providing pleasure for a partner. The partners guide one another in pleasurable activities, without demands for any specific sexual performance.

Sensation It is the faculty by which information about external environment and internal state of body is collected and appreciated. Information is collected by millions of microscopic structures throughout the body. Receptors are attuned to a particular stimulus. They send external signals whenever fired or excited. Some receptors are the terminals of long nerve cell fibres. These have different pathways. Special senses include vision, hearing, taste, and smell. An awareness of feeling due to stimulation of one of senses.

Sense, of taste There are four essential sensations of taste, sweet, bitter, sour and saltish. Nasal allergic reactions, acids, or metallic salts can alter

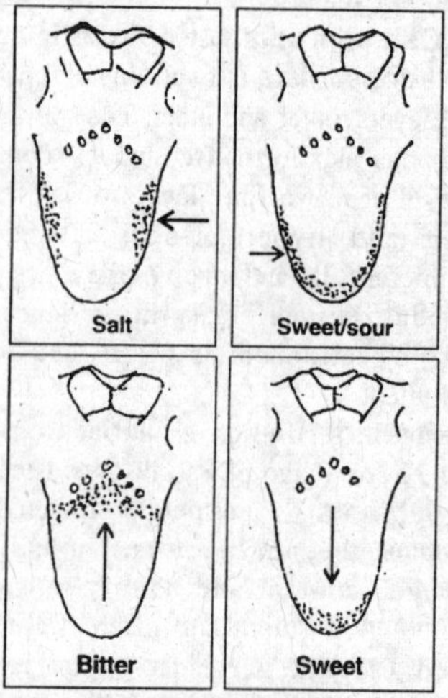

the mucosa and impair the sense of taste. In the adults the sense of taste is localised in dorsal portion of tongue as well as tongue borders, soft palate and velipalatine structures.

Sensibility The conscious appreciation and precise interpretation of sensation.

Sensitisation When an antigen reacts with fixed antibodies the reaction either destroys the cell or leads to release of histamine or histamine-like substances. These substances produce a variety of untoward substances, i.e. increased permeability of blood vessel walls, i.e. angioneurotic oedema, skin rash and spasm of smooth muscles. The phenomenon in which second dose of an antigen reacts with fixed antibodies and produces altered tissue reaction is called hypersensitivity. Antigen is called allergen and person who on second contact shows an allergic response is a sensitised individual.

Sensitivity The percentage of individuals with a particular diagnosis who are correctly identified as positive by a test.

Sensitivity group A group in which members strive to increase self-awareness and understanding of the group's dynamics, as distinct from treatments designed to ameliorate identified, individual, egodystonic emotional problems.

Sensitization A process by which the response to a stimulus increases with repeated presentation of that stimulus; for example, increased behavioral response to the same dose of a drug.

Sensorineural deafness Deafness caused by disease of the cochlea or of the cochlear nerve.

Sensorineural deafness due to diseases The hearing loss of diabetes is due to damage to small blood vessels affecting structures diffusely within cochlea. Otic capsule in Paget's disease may cause deafness, stapedial ankylosis produces conductive loss like that of otosclerosis, collagen diseases like DLE. Rheumatoid arthritis may also result in deafness.

Sensorineural defness Deafness caused bydisease of the cochlea of of the cochlear nerve.

Sensory Pertaining to or subserving sensation.

Sensory aids Devices to increase the efficiency of receiving sensory stimuli, e.g., hearing aids or eyeglasses.

Sensory aphasia Sensory speech with numerous uncorrected paraphasias including jargon and severe disturbed sentence structure.

Sensory area A region of the cerebral cortex concerned with the interpretation of sensory impulses.

Sensory block Loss of sensation caused by regional anesthesia.

Sensory competition An explanation for cortical sensory plasticity.

Sensory cortex It shows the layout of cells according to areas that they recieve information from large area is involved in sensation of lip hence they are very erotic too.

Sensory deficit A lack or deficiency in one of the senses.

Sensory deprivation An experimental setup in which a subject is allowed only restricted sensory input; subjects generally do not like deprivation and may even display hallucinations.

Sensory distribution of hand Hand is supplied by radial, median and ulnar nerve.

Sensory extinction Failure to report sensory stimuli from one region if another region is stimulated simultaneously, even though when the region in question is stimulated by itself, the stimulus is correctly reported.

Sensory information Information gained from sight, taste, touch, smell and hearing.

Sensory intensification In drug usage, the experience of perceiving colours as more saturated, shapes as more distinct than normal. Under this condition, variations in stimulation are more noticeable than usual.

Sensory memory The persistence of a sensory impression for less than a second; it allows the information to be processed further.

Sensory message Impression conveyed by an afferent nerve to a sensory nerve center.

Sensory modality A distinct mode of sensation, e.g. touch vs pain.

Sensory nerve A collection of nerve fibers that carries sensory information from sensory receptors into the spinal cord and brain.

Sensory nerve fibers, type I Myelinated sensory nerve fibers with a diameter of 12-22 micrometers and a conduction velocity of 65-130 m per second. They are the most rapidly conducting of the peripheral sensory nerve fibers. The synonym is type Aa fibers.

Sensory nerve fibers, type II Myelinated sensory nerve fibers with a diameter of 5-15 micrometers and a conduction velocity of 20-90 m per second. The synonyms is type Ab or Ac fibers.

Sensory nerve fibers, type III Myelinated sensory nerve fibers with a diameter of 2-10 micrometers and a conduction velocity of 12-45 m per second. Some nociceptive signals are carried by such fibers. A synonym is type Ad fibers.

Sensory nerve fibers, type IV Unmyelinated sensory nerve fibers with a diameter of 0.2-1.5 micrometers and a conduction velocity of 0.2-2.0 m per second. Some nociceptive signals are carried by such fibers. A synonym is type C fibers.

Sensory neuron A neuron that carries information from sensory receptors of sensory organs into the nervous system. Neurons that transmit impulses to the spinal cord and brain from all parts of the body.

Sensory overload A condition in which a person receives an excessive or intolerable amount of sensory stimuli.

Sensory Processing The ability to interpret sensory signals.

Sensory projection areas Areas of the brain most specifically involved in the mediation of sensory experience. For example, the occipital lobes are related primarily to visual experience, the temporal lobes to auditory experience, and the parietal lobes to the various skin and muscle senses.

Sensory register The first of three postulated stages in human memory, the memory which consists only of the residual stimulation in the sensory systems. After direct stimulation ceases, sensory memory is only momentary.

Sensory unit A cutaneous nerve fiber together with all of its sensory terminals.

Sensory-motor period Approximately, the period from birth to 18 months of age, during which time the infant's thinking apparently is limited largely to sensory and motor responses. The basic intellectual achievement at this stage, according to Piaget, is gaining the idea of object permanence, meaning that objects which are not in one's direct sensory awareness can continue to exist and can be thought about in their absence.

Separation anxiety The fear and apprehension noted in infants when removed from the mother (or surrogate mother) or when approached by strangers. Most marked from sixth to tenth month. In later life, similar reactions may be caused by separation from significant persons or familiar surroundings.

Separation-in-dividuation Psychologic awareness of one's separateness. In the separation-in-dividuation stage, the child begins to perceive himself as distinct from the mother and develops a sense of individual identity and an image of the self as object. Mahler described four subphases of the process : differentiation, practicing, rapprochment (active approach toward the mother, replacing the relative obliviousness to her that prevailed during the practicing period), and separation-in-dividuation proper (awareness of discrete identity, separateness, and individuality).

Separator Instrument or device used to wedge teeth apart.

Sepcific heat This is defined as the amount of energy required to raise the temperature of 1gm. of water by 1°C.

Sepsis It is an infection of a wound or body tissues with bacteria that leads to the formation of pus. If bacteria that form toxins are present in the blood in large numbers and are multiplying rapidly the condition is called septicaemia. Person becomes suddenly seriously ill with a high fever, chill, rapid breathing and cloudy consciousness. It becomes a life-threatening condition.

Sepsis scores Index of severity of sepsis. Score is assigned to local infection, pyrexia, systemic response and laboratory results.

Septal defect An opening in the septum (interatrial or interventricular) between the left and right sides of the heart.

Septal rage A rage attack thought to originate in the spetal nuclei.

Septate Divided by a septum.

Septation A mode of cell envelope invagination during division; it involves the ingrowth of the cell envelope forming a T-like structure.

Septic abortions It is complicated by infection of uterus and its contents. Septic abortion becomes serious when it follows infected induced abortion. There will be fever, hypotension and vaginal discharge. Suprapubic pain results from virulent infection. Cervix may be open or closed.

Septic discitis It is due to tuberculosis or pyogenic infection. There is soft tissue abscess formation and bulging of parasternal lines in A.P. view.

Septic Obstetric shock Gram negative coliform bacilli are commonly associated with septic shock. Esch, Coli is the most common cause of septic shock. Grampositive cocci e.g. streptococci and staphylococci also produce shock with their lethal exotoxins. Earliest sign appear with shaking chills followed by fever.

Septic shock It is a highly dangerous condition in which there is tissue damage and a dramatic drop in blood pressure as a result of septicaemia. In most of cases damage occurs in kidneys, lungs and heart. It is more common in patients who are admitted as patients of diabetes mellitus, cancer or liver cirrhosis. Symptoms include cold hands and feets, often with cyanosis due to slowed blood flow, weak and rapid pulse flow and low blood pressure. There may be vomiting and diarrhoea. Poor output of kidneys is seen in oliguria. It requires immediate treatment according to focus of infection and rapid fluid replacement. Survival rate is less than 50 per cent.

Septicemia The presence of pathogenic organisms or their toxins in the blood along with signs of clinical infection.

Septomarginal trabecula The anteroinferior boundary between the inflow and outflow tracts of the right ventricle near the apex.

Septoplasty Plastic reconstruction of the nasal septum.

Septum Interdental the portion of the alveolar, process extending between the roots of adjacent teeth.

Septum pellucidum 'Transparent partition' separating the frontal horns of the lateral ventricles.

Septum primum The crescent-shaped membrane arising from the dorsocephalic wall of the primitive atrium that initiates the partitioning of the atrium into two chambers; the ends of the septum eventually fuse with the dorsal endocardial cushions of the atrioventricular canal.

Septum secundum The crescent-shaped membrane arising from the ventrocranial wall of the atrium on the right side of the septum primum; the ends of the septum reach dorsally toward the sinus venosus.

Sequele A morbid condition following or occurring as a consequence of another condition or event.

Sequential treatment The use of two or more chemical or physical methods in succession to develop a latent fingerprint.

Sequestration This is the term used in medicine to a necrotic tissue being separated. The term is generally used in case of osteomyelitis in which case a part of bone dies and becomes separated from healthy bone.

Sequestrectomy The surgical removal of sequestrum.

Sequlae Consequences or effects.

Serial Extraction of selected primary teeth over a period of years often ending with removal of the first premolar teeth to relieve crowding of the dental arches during eruption of the lateral incisors, canines, and premolars.

Serial casts The sequential application of casts for the progressive correction of deformity.

Serial study A type of clinical trial in which a series of patients with similar treatment plans is evaluated over time.

Series infusion An IV of compatible or identical solutions may be hung in stand. The second bottle

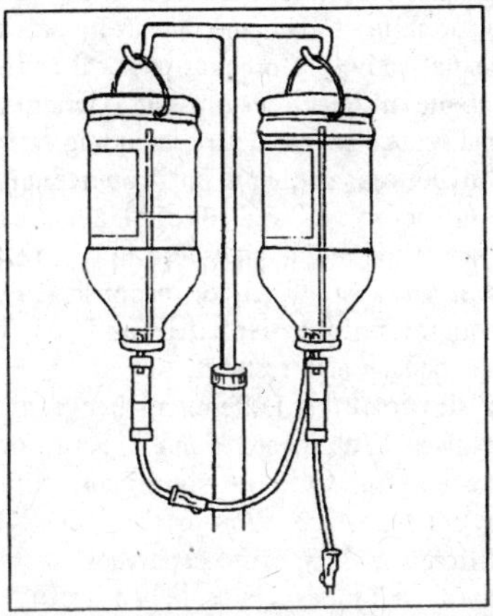

is attached to the air inlet of first bottle and fluid flows into it so that the distal bottle empties first.

Serogroup Bacteria of the same species with different antigenic determinants on the cell surface.

Serology Branch of medicine dealing e\with serum and blood products.

Seropositive Serologically positive.

Serosa Outermost covering of the digestive tract; composed of the parietal pleura in the abdominla cavity.

Serosanguineous Composed of serum and blood.

Serotonin An amine found in platelets that induces vasoconstriction; functions as a neurotransmitter at some neural endings.

Serotonin syndrome There develops impaired mental state, increased muscle activity and autonomic instability due to excessive 5 HT activity in brain stem and spinal cord.

Serotype The antigenic character that distinguishes a subdivision of a species from other strains.

Serous cavities Hollow spaces filled with serum or a substance having a watery consistency.

Serous cells Bronchial epithelial cells that secrete mucus.

Serous drainage Leaking plasma.

Serous labyrinthitis Spontaneous nausea, vomiting and vertigo occurring in a subject known to have suppurative otitis media is indicative of spread of inflammation to within bony labyrinth. If the inflammation has advanced to the stage of pus production it is known as suppurative labyrinthitis. If only to a stage of hyperaemia and increased permeability it is called serous labyrinthitis. Suppuration in labyrinth results in permanent loss of function. The patient who had symptoms of labyrinthitis but at the end of illness retains some normal vestibular and auditory function has had serous labyrinthitis.

Serous membrane Thin sheet consisting of epithelium and connective tissue that lines cavities not opening to the outside of the body; does not contain glands but does secrete serous fluid.

Serous pericardium The inner sac of the pericardial sac consisting of a visceral layer and a parietal layer.

Serrated Having a sawlike edge.

Serratus anterior It arises by fleshy slips from outer surface of upper nine ribs. Its nerve supply is from C_5 C_6 C_7. It is the principal muscle involved in pushing and punching. It stabilises scapula during abduction of arm.

Serratus anterior muscle An accessory inspiratory muscle from the outer surfaces of the upper eight or nine ribs to attach along the costal aspect of the medial border of the scapula.

Sertoli cell Cell in the wall of the seminiferous tubules to which spermatogonia and spermatids are attached.

Sertoli cell-only testis A condition in which Sertoli cells are the only cellular element in the seminiferous tubule.

Sertoli-germ cell ratio A ratio that is fixed for a species and appears to result from the fixed capability of Sertoli cells to support germ cells.

Serum It is a clear fluid that separates from blood when it clots. It does not contain blood cells or the protein in blood. It does not contain salt or glucose. Serum prepared from the blood of a person who has been infected with microorganism usually contains antibodies that can protect against that organism if same serum is injected into someone else. This procedure is used for passive immunisation.

Serum sickness It is the reaction to the infusion of antiserum. It takes place when body's production of antibodies is too slow to cope. Symptoms may be of allergy syndrome.

Service An action performed for another person that results in a specific outcome.

Service competency The ability of a worker to meet defined job performance standards.

Service delivery The process of getting health care services to the people who need them.

Sesamoid Resembling sesame seed.

Sesamoid bones Many sesamoid bones are present in normal foot. Mostly these are asymptomatic.

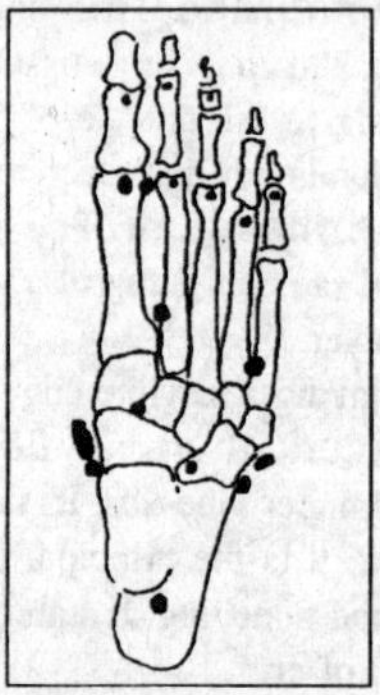

An unusually large accessory navicular bone may cause pain due to local pressure. Sometimes surgical excision may be needed.

Sesamoiditis It is described an inflammatory condition of the tissues surrounding the sesamoids. The athlete most prone to medical sesamoid pathology is the one with a rigid cavus foot, tight Achilles tendon.

Session objectives The desired outcomes of a specific treatment session; mini goals or objectives that are steps or building blocks toward short-term objectives.

Set point A natural level that the body reguylates or defends.

Sever's disease An apophysitis of the calcaneus in which increased density and fragmentation of apophysis is seen on X-Ray.

Sex Biological maleness or femaleness, determined by genetic endowment and hormones.

Sex chromosomes These are pair of chromosomes which determine gender of a child. There are four other chromosomes. In women sex chromosomes are called X-chromosomes. In man one sex chromosome is X and another is Y. Thus normal sex chromosome complement for women is XX and for men XY. Full female sex characteristics develop only in presence of a second X-chromosome Addition of Y-chromosome converts the female to the male pattern.

Sex desire, inhibition This is lack of sexual desire or of ability to become physically aroused during sexual activity. Common physical causes include fatigue, ill health, vaginismus. Certain drugs also can reduce sexual desire including sleeping pills, antidepressant, and antihypertensives. Oral contraceptives and alcohol also result in it. Depression and anxiety also lowers performance. Woman is rarely frigid, responsible is partner's poor technique. Hostility and fear of sexual inadequacy also result it.

Sex differences Differences between males and females. With regard to intelligence, for example, there seems to be no significant differences in overall ability, though there may be slight differences in specific capacities, such as verbal ability and mathematics. When sex differences do exist, it is difficult to determine whether they may be due to cultural influences or inborn characteristics.

Sex drive It is the primary instinctual urge for sexual gratification. It reaches its peak in late teens in males and mid-30's among females. In contrast to animals the human sex drive is less seasonal, less dependent upon an oestrous cycle, more varied in expression and aroused by a wide range of stimuli.

Sex education It helps young people to understand what masculinity is to boys and men, feminity to girls and women and the male-female relationship.

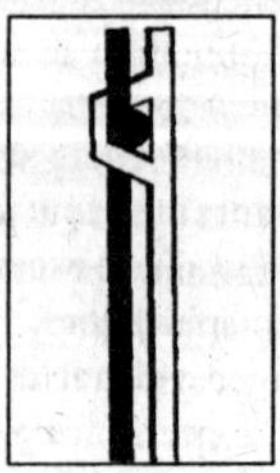

It explains not only the facts of reproduction but also the development of proper attitude towards sexuality.

Sex formation The sex of zygote is determined at the time of fertilization by the type of spermatozoon X or Y which fertilizes ovum. If the male contributes its 'X' chromosome to the female germ cell, the new individual now having XX chromosomes becomes female. If on the other hand Y part of spermatozoon makes union with female germ cell, the individual possessing XY becomes a male. The 'Y' chromosome is the most useful determinent. Fertilization takes place at ampullary end of fallopian tube.

Sex hormones These are hormones which control development of primary and secondary sexual characteristics and regulate various sex-related functions in the body. These functions are menstrual cycle and production of egg or sperm. Responsible hormones are androgen, oestrogen and progesterone.

Sex maniac This is an individual who is preoccupied with sexual satisfaction and sexual exploits. He has history of seducing a maximum number of men or women as well or more malignant behaviour such as murder and violent physical assault.

Sex skin Labia minora of the sexually excited woman becomes progressively more pink and red during the plateau phase of sexual response cycle. If erotic stimulation continues, labia become more swollen and engorged with blood; orgasm is usually inevitable.

Sex steroids These are produced in gonads and to a lesser degree in the adrenal cortex. Estradiol and testosterone play major roles in female-male reproduction.

Sex stimulants Every body is very keen to improve his/her sex performance and hence several drugs have been tried labelled as sex stimulants. Rhino horn has earned a reputation of an aphrodisiac because of its phallic shape. Spanish fly found in southern Europe is another so-called aphrodisiac. When taken it dilates the blood vessels of the penis but can irritate and inflame the intestinal tract.

Sex therapy A short term therapy aimed at relief of the sexual symptom, which uses systematically structured sexual experience with conjoint therapeutic sessions. It is designed to modify immediate obstacles to sexual functioning, although intrapsychic and transactional conflicts are also dealt with to some extent.

Sexism Prejudice against a person because of their sex. Generally applied to expectation that women are not as qualified or competent as men.

Sex-linked inheritance trait An inheritance trait in which the gene is carried on the X-chromosome and is expressed in the male offspring (males do not possess another X chromosome to offset the effects of the X chromosome that carries the gene.)

Sexologist A specialist in the area of human sexuality; one engaged in sex research or particularly learned in the physiological, behavioural, or psychoemotional aspects of sexuality.

Sex-specific behavior A behavior shown exclusively by members of one sex and largely dictated by physical factors, e.g., suckling in female mammals.

Sexual aberrations Any deviations from normal or typical sexual behaviour such as sexual sadism, sexual masochism, fetishism, etc.

Sexual abuse Sexual exploitation involving physical contact between a child and another person.

Sexual addiction There exists an excessive, repetitive sexual activity resembling addiction to alcohol or drugs in providing relief from feelings of anxiety or worthlessness. Sex becomes compulsion to these addicts.

Sexual advances Any deliberate attempt to arouse sexual interest or sexual response in the opposite sex. Sexual advances vary widely and include indirect approaches such as smiling, winking, firmly holding hand, etc.

Sexual affinity This is a strong sexual attraction between two individuals of opposite sex.

Sexual apathy It is a negative attitude towards sexual relations, ranging from indifference to listlessness to active repulsion. Apathy is often based on distasteful or painful experiences, and monotonous and unimaginative approach of the partner.

Sexual dimorphism Process whereby gonadal hormones act on the brain to produce a distinctly female of male brain.

Sexual ecstasy Sexual ecstasy is the peak of pleasure, excitement and euphoria experienced at the moment of orgasm.

Sexual exploitation It is taking advantage of another person for sexual purposes either as a source of financial gain or for person gratification, for example using her/him for pornographic films, or as a mole.

Sexual expression The ability to recognize, communicate, and perform desired sexual activities.

Sexual favours These are sexual privileges, including intercourse and other such activities, granted by women either free or sometimes for remuneration.

Sexual flush It is the rushing of blood during sexual excitement, specially in women. Flushing begins with rash-like discolouration of the lower chest and spreads to breasts, rest of the chest, neck, reaching a peak during the late plateau phase.

Sexual frustration It is thwarting of sexual impulse by such internal forces as parental admonitions, the demand of religion, confinement to prison, rigid social rules or lack of opportunity to meet members of the opposite sex.

Sexual harassment Unwelcome sexual advances, requests for sexual favors, and other verbal or physical conduct of a sexual nature.

Sexual imprinting A form of imprinting by which an individual learns to identify members of its own species and used later as the basis for selecting sexual partners.

Sexual instinct In Freud's theory, the innate tendency toward pleasure seeking, particularly through achieving sexual aims and objects.

Sexual intercourse The insertion of the erect penis of a male into the vagina of a female. Also called coitus.

Sexual maturation The sexual maturation and secretion of sex steroids are regulated by the hypothalamicpituitarygonadal axis. Sex steroids exert a negative feedback on hypothalamus. Production of gonadotropins which stimulates sexual maturation and secretion of gonadal hormones such as oestrogens in females and androgens in males are increased.

Sexual misconduct Any behavior that is sexually oriented in the professional setting.

Sexual organs The reproductive structure of human bodies. Although generally include only 'males (penis, testes, scrotum, chest hair) and females (vagina, ovaries, uterus, breasts), one in every 2,000 live births is "intersexed." These infants are born with a mixture of female and male traits. Most are then surgically "assigned" to one sex.

Sexual orientation A pattern in an individual of persistent and consistent sexual and romantic attraction, either to the opposite sex, to one's own sex, or to both.

Sexual permissiveness It advocates that sexual activity should be as free as possible from restrictions on regulations including orogenital sex, homosexuality, etc.

Sexual psychopath It is an individual with antisocial personality who commits repeated sexual aggression, child molestations, etc.

Sexual response It is a reaction to sexual stimulation such as fondling or kissing, causing vaginal lubrication and erection of nipples. In males most obvious reaction is erection of penis.

Sexual tension It is a condition of restlessness and strain resulting from an acute desire or need for sexual gratification and release, and is usually relieved after orgasm.

Sexual terms Libido is sexual desire, i.e. lust. Patency is the ability to maintain an erection of sufficient rigidity so that the vagina can be penetrated. Priapism is the erection that will not go away and may develop in early days of spinal injury. Emission is the discharge of semen at external urethral orifice. Ejaculation is emission of semen accompanied by brief series of rhythmic movements of pelvic floor. Orgasm is a pleasurable feeling of sexual crisis.

Sexuality The complex of emotions, attitudes, preferences, and behaviours related to the individual's expression of the sexual self and eroticism. Components of sexuality include the individual's genetic, hormonal, gonadal, and morphologic sex, gender identity, sex role, and sexual partner preference.

Sexually dimorphic Traits that differ between men and women.

Sexually transmitted disease (STD) Anybody can become infected with STD when having vaginal or anal intercourse with an infected person.

STDs are a group of communicable diseases transmitted through sexual contact. Usual

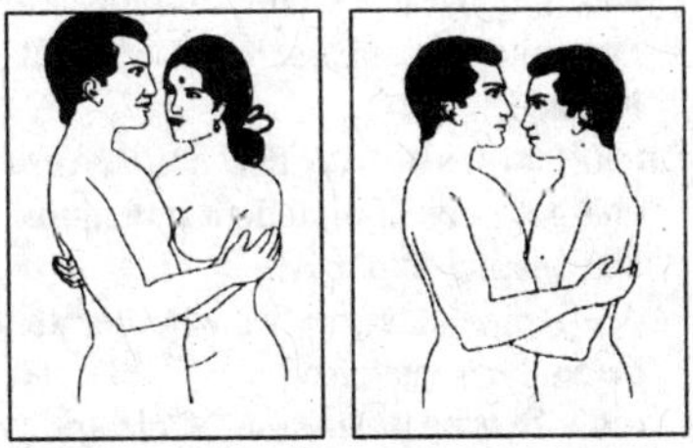

symptoms are discharge from penis/vagina with sores/ulcers on or near sex organs. There will be itching in the groin and burning pain when having sex or passing urine. STD increases the risk of getting AIDS.

SGOT Abbreviation for Serum Glutamic Oxaloacetic Transaminase.

SGPT Abbreviation of Serum Glutamic Pyruvic Transaminase.

Shade selection Tooth color selection. The determination of the color hue, brilliance, saturation, translucency of the artificial tooth or set of teeth for a given patient.

Shaft Long portion of a needle or bone.

Shaft of the rib The central portion of the rib.

Shake test The foam stability test to measure precisely the L/S ratio in the fetus. It is relatively simple and quick. The test depends on the ability of the surfactant in the amniotic fluid when mixed with ethanol to generate stable foam at the air-liquid interface.

Shaken baby syndrome Refers to an injury to the brain of an infant that results from vigorous shaking. It is a form of physical abuse.

Shaking Shaking is a single or double handed technique in which a significant rhythmic shaking movement or temor is conveyed to the tissues by the hand or finger tips.

Shank Portion of the instrument that unites the shaft or handle with the working point or blade.

Shape memory alloy Alloys of nickel and titanium used in orthodontics that have the property of reverting to an original shape simply by being heated to a certain temperature.

Shaping Reinforcement of responses in the patient's repertoire that increasingly approximate sought-after behaviour.

Shared environment Environmental influences that are shared by two or more individuals.

Sharp dissection The surgical separation of tissues by means of sharp edge of a scalpel.

Shaw It is a discharge of blood-stained mucus. It is secreted abundantly during labour, the slight haemorrhage comes from the lower uterine segment. Here beginning of dilatation causes a little separation of membrane.

Shear A process in which parallel bodies, layers, or surfaces move against each other in such a way as to remain parallel, but with deformation or displacement in a direction parallel to themselves.

Shear rate A measure of the speed at which intermediate fluid layers move with respect of each other. The unit of measure is the reciprocal second.

Shear stress A measure of the force per unit area required to produce shearing action. The unit of measure is dynes/cm2.

Shearing Force exerted against the surface and layers of the skin as tissues slide in oppoiste but parallel directions.

Shearing strength Maximum stress an object can withstand before fracture when a shearing force is applied.

Sheath A structurally well defined, usually laminated, extracellular polysaccharide covering, escpecially such a layer in filamentous cyanobacteria.

Sheehan's syndrome It occurs in adult women due to pituitary necrosis following postpartum haemorrhage and is characterised by flabby facial appearance with thinning of eyebrows, increased susceptibility to cold, low basal metabolic rate, and low urinary 17-ketosteroids.

Sheet graft A skin graft that is taken from the donor site and placed directly over the burn wound. It provides 1:1 coverage.

Sheet padding A glazed cotton bandage used for padding under a cast.

Sheet wadding Stretchable sheets of cotton padding used to cover skin befor a cast is applied.

Shelf life The amount of time a material cab be stored before experiencing a significant change in handling characteristics or mechanical properties that causes it to be clinically useless.

Shell temperature Warmth at the skin surface.

Shiatsu An acupressure and meridian-focused bodywork system from Japan.

Shielding Any material or obstruction that absorbs radiation protecting person from its effect.

Shin splints Commonly used term for a syndrome of exercise induced leg pain.

Shingles An eruptive rash, usually in a girdle-like distribution on the trunk of the body, resulting from infection with varicellazoster virus.

Shistosomiasis It is also known as Bilharziasis S. hematobium, S. mansoni and S. Japonicum. These are sexually dimorphic. Female is longer and more slender than male and is held in gynaecophoric canal permitting almost continuous mating. Male consist 5-9 testes.

Shivering Involuntary trembling of entire body caused by rapid contraction and relaxation of muscles. Shivering is a normal response to cold and also occurs with rigors and fever. When body becomes cold, temperature sensitive nerve cells in hypothalamus act as a thermostat initiating shivering reflex. Shivering causes muscles to contract and generating heat. Shivering during rigors and fever is caused by release of certain substances by white blood cells.

Shock Reduced blood pressure is a major factor in causing physiological shock. It is accompained to severe injury or illness. In it either blood volume is reduced or vessels are widened or a combination of both. It is made worse by pain and anxiety. There will be rapid, shallow breathing, cold clammy skin, weak pulse, dizziness and fainting. First aid includes arrest of bleeding and replacement of fluids or blood. Oxygen therapy is to be given.

Shock absorption The dampening of applied force.

Shock anaphylactic Reaction to penicillin are most common and fatal. Reaction can occur in patients who have never been given the drug before although majority are seen in patients who have been sensitised by previous treatment. There is no reliable way by which patients liable to develop generalised reaction can be identified. Even subcutaneous test may give misleading results. Treatment includes adrenaline 1:1000 1 CC subcutaneously immediately. Inj. decadron 2 CC IM Inj. Avil 2 CC IM. Oxygen inhalation may be given.

Shock in toxaemia Preeclamptic toxemia of pregnancy is characterised by vaso spams with sodium and water retention. Eclampsia is an acute condition of vaso spasm leading to cellular anoxia and damage to essential organs. Hemorrhage in the ventricles, subarachnoid area and basal ganglia is noted.

Shock sensitivity The ability of an explosive charge to be initiated to detonation by another deteonating explosive.

A special category is whether the explode is detonator sensitive.

Shock therapy The use of electricity to produce sudden and severe disturbance in nervous system as a means of treating mental disease specially depression. Mechanism of action is not known. ECT is in common use. Insulin coma therapy has been discontinued.

Short arc extension exercise Active or active-resisted extension of a joint through the final degrees of its range of motion; most often applied to the knee from 35 degrees flexion to full extension.

Short leg Anatomical, pathological, or functional leg deficiency leading to dysfunction.

Short leg gait A limp produced by a shortened lower extremity.

Short stature Lower than average body height.

Short term satiety Satiety that lasts for a few minutes to several hours after a single meal.

Shortening Any loss of length of body part.

Shortness Tightness; denotes a slight to moderate decrease in musclelength; movement in the direction of elongating the muscles is limited.

Short-term goals Outcomes that can be met in a few days to a week.

Short-term memory A memory system of limited capacity that uses rehearsal processes either to retain current memories or to pass them on to long-term memory.

Shoulder dystocia Head is born but shoulder is not descending and child's face gets more and more blue and cannot completely be freed from perineum. It may be a large child to a diabetic mother. Some babies may have broad shoulder. A thick neck and large head should give rise to suspicion of shoulder dystocia. Caesarian section may be needed.

Shoulder joint A synovial joint, where the humerus articulates with the scapula.

Shoulder presentation A serious complication of birth in which the infant lies crosswise in the uterus instead of longitudinally. The risk of perinatal mortality is reduced by a caesarean delivery.

Shoulder spica cast A body jacket or cast enclosing the trunk, shoulder and part of upper extremity.

Shoulder, tendinitis Tendons are tough, rope-like fibres that connect muscles to bones. Injury or overuse can cause pain, tenderness and inflammation in the tendons or the tissues

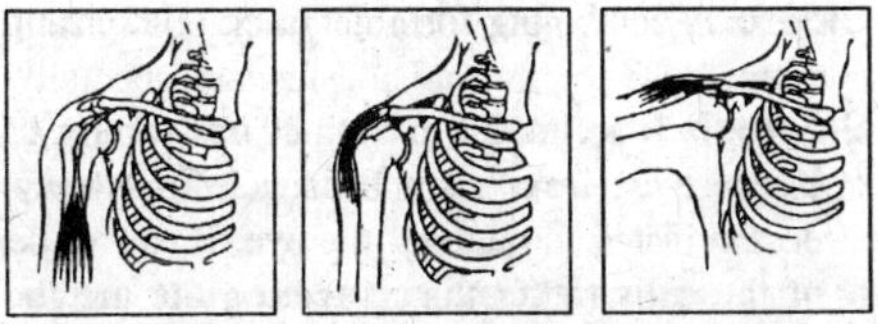

surrounding them is known as tendinitis. It can be related to job, sports or household activities which require repeated twisting or rapid joint movement. Shoulder and ankle joints are prone to it. Warm up before exercise helps in preventing it.

Shoulder-hand syndrome The syndrome gives rise to pain and tenderness of the shoulder, pain and swelling and weakness of the hand with evidence of trophic changes, and limitation of movement of the joints.

Show It is a discharge of blood-stained mucus. It is secreted abundantly during labour, the slight haemorrhage comes from the lower uterine segment. Here beginning of dilatation causes a little separation of membrane.

Shroud A dress or garment for the dead; winding sheet.

Shunt It is the tube introduced surgically into the body for occurring as congenital deformity. It diverts fluid from one duct to another.

Shy-Drager syndrome There is severe loss of cells from the intermediolateral cell column of the spinal cord, the origin of sympathetic and parasympathetic outflow. In addition to Parkinsonian features, impotence is a common feature and patient fails to sweat in response to thermal challenge. Important sign is of low BP. There will be marked bradykinesia and rigidity. These people do not respond to L-dopa.

Sialadenitis It is an inflammation of the salivary glands. Bacterial sialadenitis occurs in children and presents with recurrent, acute, painful enlargement of the involved gland. Overlying skin may be red and milking the gland will yield a purulent discharge. Pain and swelling are not related to eating.

Treatment consists of heat application, pain relieving drugs and antibiotics. Microscopic sections of bacterial sialadenitis show oedema and infiltration of ducts. Obstructive sialadenitis is more common and is associated with salivary stones. In it gland is also inflamed. Glands are submaxillary to be involved. Clinical examination may reveal presence of stone in excretory duct. X-ray may confirm it.

After radiopaque material irregular pattern of duct can be demonstrated. The interstitial tissue of gland lobules shows oedema and infiltration by plasma cells, neutrophils and lymphocytes. There may be atrophy of acini. Surgical excision is often necessary.

Sialadenosis It is usually painless but may even be painful swelling of both parotid glands which may be intermittent or persist for just a few days. Saliva may be normal in quantity and consistency or salivary viscosity may increase leading to dry mouth.

Sialytransferase An enzyme that transfers sialic acid to a glycoconjugate.

Sibling Brother or sister.

Sibling rivalary Feelings of jealousy and fear of replacement when a young child share potential parentral attention with a new born infant.

Sibson's fascia Suprapleural membrane.

Sicard sign A diagnostic marker in sciatica.

Sick role An identity adopted by an individual as a patient that specifies a set of expected behaviours, usually dependent.

Sick sinus syndrome It may be caused by arteriosclerosis with or without hypertension, rheumatic disease, thyrotoxicosis or so. This is due to abnormal pacemaker function of SA node or defective conduction.

From time to time there may be bradycardia followed by tachycardia. Bradycardia is due to sinus bradycardia.

Tachycardia is due to paroxysmal supraventricular tachycardia. There may be syncope, chest pain or palpitation.

Sickle Scaler with two curved or straight blades, triangular in cross section, and a pointed tip. Used to debridge supragingival deposits.

Sickle cell anaemia It is characterised by distorted or sickle-shaped erythrocyte. Sickling of cell is due to abnormal type of haemoglobin.

These cells are destroyed in spleen, liver and bone marrow. It results in haemolytic anaemia. Oral mucosa becomes pallor. X-ray changes in jaw are more prominent.

Jaw shows osteoporosis and coarse trabecular pattern. The radiolucent areas are specially prominent between the apices of teeth and inferior border of mandible. There may be loss of alveolar bone height and prominence of lamina dura.

Sickle cell syndrome There is an evidence that in some pathological conditions the integrity of the cell membrane is diminished and intracellular metabolic processes are disturbed. Sodium pump mechanism becomes inefficient and water with sodium passes into cells with resultant fall of serum sodium.

Hyponatraemia occurs without loss of total body sodium. Potassium ions leak out of cells.

Treatment includes administration of insulin and glucose.

Sickle scaler Hook shaped instrument to remove calculus.

Sickness of radiation It is a disorder caused by overexposure to radioactivity related to exposure of duration. High doses in short duration may prove fatal.

Low doses cause nausea, loss of hair, leucopenia and anaemia. It may affect fertility and some patients may even develop leukaemia.

Sicle cell trait When only one defective fene is inherited and only a small amount of hemoglobin that is less soluble than usual is produced.

Side effect It is an undesired effect of drug. It may be mild or severe. It may be produced if drug is used beyond its desired period.

Sometime side effects may be unrelated to dose quantity and its duration. If side effects are in form of rash, jaundice and swelling of face, drug should be discontinued.

Side to side grip It requires adduction of two fingers usually the index or middle finger. It is a weak grip.

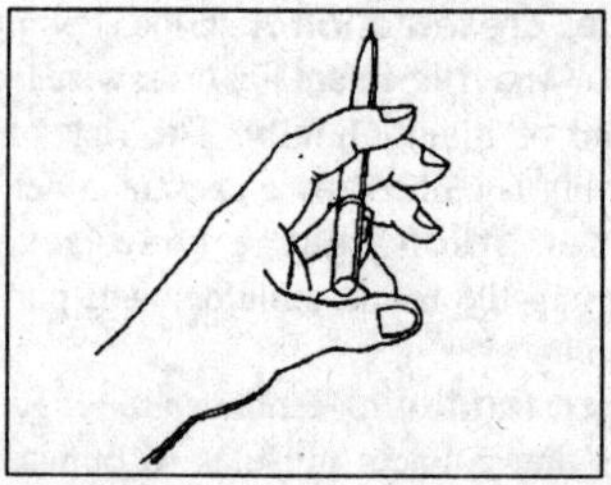

Side-lying The position in which the patient is lying on his or her side.

Sidero A combining form denoting relationship to iron.

Siderosis It occurs due to retained iron foreign body in eye even from a small particle. Iron may be desseminated throughout the eye. It causes death of the cells rather than affecting the metabolic activity. There develops a gradual diminution of visual acuity due to changes in cornea, lens and retina. There is concentric contraction of the visual fields due to degeneration of retina. Patient complains of dim vision. Ultimate fate of any eye is complete blindness.

Siegel's pneumatic speculum Speculum has a lensed window which can be fitted into ear canal to make an airtight chamber. Rubber bulb is

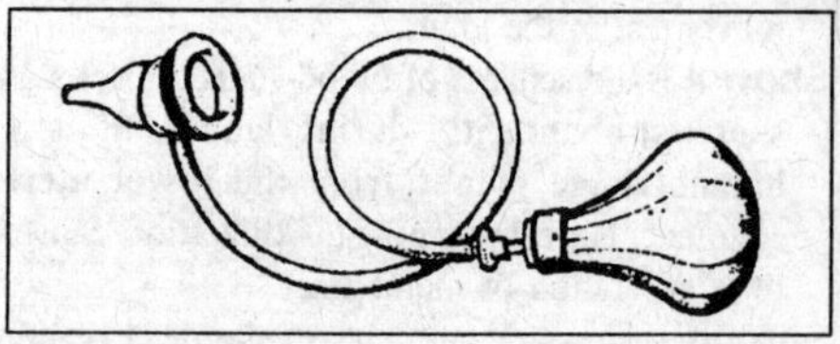

attached to speculum which can be used to apply suction or pressure on drum. It is used to see the magnified view of small perforation, to see mobility of tympanic membrane. Through it, medicine can be introduced into middle ear.

Sigmoid colon S-shaped segment of a large intestine that terminates in the rectum.

Sigmoid flush It is a technique used in patients with severe diverticular disease in sigmoid colon. At the end of a standard double contrast barium enema the sigmoid colon is filled with dilute barium suspension. This improves detection of lesion.

Sigmoidoscopy Various forms of sigmoidoscopes are available. For general outpatient use a narrow bore, 25-cm instrument is useful for it is easily managed with the patient in the left lateral position. The lubricated, warmed sigmoidoscope is gently introduced into rectum. As soon as rectum is reached obturator is removed and further passage of instrument is carried out under direct vision following lumen of bowel till rectosigmoid junction is reached at a distance between 13 and 15 cm from anus.

Any suspicious lesion should be biopsied properly. When ulcerative proctitis or colitis is present, mucosa is inflamed, friable and bleeds easily when swabbed.

Sign Indication of an abnormality, related to disease or dysfunction, that is evident to the examiner, i.e., objective evidence.

Sign of life A breath, a cry, a pulsation of the umbilical cord, or any spontaneous movement at the time of birth.

Sign test A nonparametric signifincance test for use with continuous, ordinal, or dichotomous data. The sign test is used to determine sheather or not, on average, one group experienced a better outcome on significantly more variables than another group.

Signal anxiety Attenuated anxiety that functions as an early warning system for the ego. It derives from the normal capacity to anticipate a potentially dangerous situation and react to it by deploying emergency defences before it becomes intense. Signal anxiety may progress to a full-fledged anxiety attack or even to a panic state if the early warning is not heeded or if available defences prove insufficient. A situation becomes traumatic when the influx of stimuli is too great for the psyche to master or discharge.

Signal learning In the two-factor view of conditioning, the learning of the meaning of stimuli through the process of classical conditioning. Individuals make positive or negative evaluations based on past experiences.

Signal transduction A term that refers to the whole process of getting a chemical signal (such as a hormone or neurotransmitter) to the inside of a cell; in a way, signal transduction is really "signal translation" by the cell.

Significance In statistics a relationship between two groups of observations.

Significance level The degree of likelihood that research results are attributable to chance.

Significant differences When statistical tests show that a given difference is not likely to have occurred by chance. In many behavioural studies, the likelihood of an event occurring less frequently than 1 in 20 times ($p<.05$) is considered the minimal acceptable significance level.

The determination that a given difference between two groups is significant can merely serve to identify the likelihood that it was not a chance event.

Systematic factors not considered by the investigator can sometimes be responsible for significant differences.

Signs Objective data; information that is observable and measurable.

Signs of colporrhexis Shock develops slowly, uterine vessels are torn. In heavy intraperitoneal or retroperitoneal bleeding grave shock will develop.

In slow hemorrhages, thrombosis and cellulitis are after results. The diagnosis is only made at laparotomy or at delivery.

Silane A molecule with silicon-oxygen groups at one end and methacrylate groups at the other, enabling it to couple or link ceramic materials (i.e., composite fillers and porcelain) to polymer resins.

Silence Intentionally withholding verbal comments.

Silent ischemia A condition of inadequate blood circulation to the myocardium without the typical accompanying signs or symptoms.

Silent mutation A mutation in a gene that causes no detectable change in the biological characteristics of the gene product.

Silhouette sign A radiographic finding demonstrated when the normal line of demarcation between two structures is partially or completely obliterated used to localized lesions within the lung fields.

Silicate cement A dental material made by mixing a fluoride- containing silicate glass powder with a phosphoric acid liquid; used as a restorative material before dental composites.

Silicone Impression material.

Silicone septum Silicone partition that covers the part chamber housed in the metal or plastic body of the implanted infusion port.

Silicophosphate It is a combination of zinc phosphate and silicate cement. It is less irritant, less translucent and less soluble than silicate.

Silicosis A type of pneumoconiosis that results from occupational exposure to or inhalation of silica dust; characterized by slow, progressive fibrosis of the lungs.

Silver It is white, malleable and best known conductor of heat and electricity. It melts at 960.5°C, below the melting point of gold as well as copper.

Pure silver is not used because of the black sulphide formation on the metal in mouth. Silver points serve as a root cannal filling material in endodontics. Silver is a readily alloyed with gold to be used for dental purposes. In dental gold alloys the silver is important in developing white colour when combined with platinum and palladium.

Silver point Filling for root canal in endotonic work when canals are small.

Sim's position A position of labour in which the woman lies on her left side with her left leg extended and her right knee flexed at her side and up against the abdomen or with both knees flexed.

Simmon's procedure A technique for anterior cervical disectomy.

Simmonds syndrome It is due to lesion of anterior pituitary gland due to infarct, injury or haemorrhage. Clinically there will be weight loss and hypotension, dry skin, brittle nails and amenorrhoea. Sella will be enlarged and delayed fusion of epiphysis.

Simple carbohydrates Monosaccharides and disaccharides.

Simple cell disease A genetic disorder in which red blood cells are curved or "sick-led".

Simple diffusion A passive process in which there is a net movement of molecules or ions from a region of high concentration to a region of low concentration until equilibrium is reached.

Simple febrile convulsions The most common cause of seizures during early childhood is simple febrile convulsions. Convulsions are associated with fever and infection. Convulsions are not related to the degree of elevation of fever. Fits occur within first 24 hours and convulsions are generalised, never focal. There is no residual weakness.

Simple goitre In this thyroid gland becomes increased in size due to diffuse overgrowth of glandular tissue caused by excessive secretion of thyrotropic hormone of anterior pituitary. Condition is due to lack of iodine in the water. There may be interference of absorption of iodine from the bowel. Excess of calcium and deficiency of vitamin A can add fuel to fire.

Simple kidney cyst It is commonly encountered, single or multiple cysts of cortex lined by cuboidal epithelium usually 2 to 5 cm in diameter. These have smooth walls with clear serous fluid. Person develops flank pain and irregular contour.

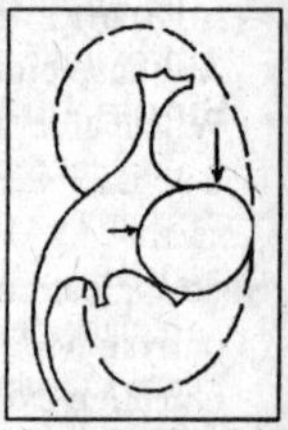

Simple mask Device for administering oxygen that fits over the nose and mouth.

Simple melancholia There is lack of interest, loss of feeling for others and inability to concentrate. It consists of misery, sleeplessness, self-approach and inability to continue at work. This form is common in the overworked, much worried and in menopausal women. Suicidal preoccupations are usual.

Simple protein A protein yielding only amino acids on hydrolysis.

Sims' speculum It requires an assistance to hold the speculum. Patient is put in lithotomy position with hips at edge of table so that speculum may be held in position by assistant. It is used in retracting

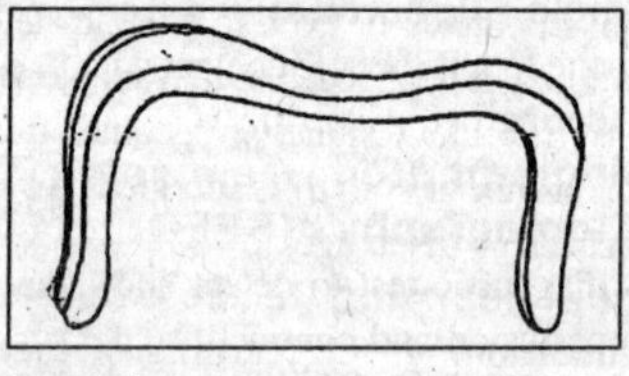

the posterior wall during dilatation and curettage, and for taking biopsy. It is useful in routine speculum examination and outdoor cauterisation and erosion of cervix.

Simulated nosebleed This occurs when bleeding source is extrinsic to the nose and the blood merely drains or is removed through the nose as in haemoptysis, injury to the internal carotid artery, bleeding oesophageal varices or bronchial neoplasm.

Simultagnosia Impairment in body scheme; a lack of awareness of the body structure and the relationship of body parts of oneself or of others.

Simz' position Lying on the left side with the chest leaning forward, the right knee bent toward the head, the right arm forward, and the left arm extended behind the body.

Singh index X-Ray material used for grading osteoporosis based on trabecular pattern of proximal femur.

Single blind In research, any method used to prevent the subject from knowing what treatment, such as a drug, he or she has received.

Single lung transplantation Surgical replacement of one lung with a donor lung using a posterolateral thoracotomy.

Single parent Custodial parent when there is not foreseeable contact with the other spouse.

Single photo emission computed tomography (SPECT) It is a method for reconstructing cross-sectional images of radiotracer distribution in an organ. Perfusion SPECT of brain provides functional information to diagnose and manage stroke, dementia, epilepsy, and cerebral degeneration.

SPECT imaging of infarct is more accurate. SPECT is very useful in differentiating Alzheimer's disease from multi-infarct dementia. Postictal SPECT can identify epileptic foci as reasons of increased activity with a sensitivity of 70 to 90 per cent.

Single Support Time The time (in seconds) that one foot is the sole contact with the support surface during one gait cycle.

Single-photon emission computed tomography (SPECT) A noninvasive diagnostic test to detect and quantify myocardial perfusion and contractility defects.

Sinoatrial (SA) node The heart's pacemaker; where the impulse conduction of the heart normally starts; located in the wall of the right atrium near the opening of the superior vena cava.

Sinoatrial A region of the right atrium near the junction with the venae cava composed of specialised cardiac cells; site of the cardiac pacemaker.

Sinography The injection of contrast medium into sinus for taking X-Ray.

Sinter The process of heating a densely packed powder (i.e., porcelain) to a temperature just below its melting point, causing the edges partially to melt and fuse the individual particles together.

Sintering To transform into a solid mass of desired density or cause attachments between separate parts by heating without melting.

Sinus It is a slendrical cavity within a bone. Term is also used for an abnormal often infected tract. It also means a wide channel which contains blood.

Sinus block Failure of an impulse, generated in the sinoatrial node, to get out of the sinoatrial node.

Sinus bradycardia A slow heart rate less than 60 beats per minute that has its origin in the sinoatrial node.

Sinus cavity Bony cavity in body of maxilla.

Sinus Cavity, recess, or hollow space.

Sinus of the larynx A fusiform recess between the vestibular and vocal folds.

Sinus tarsi syndrome It is defined as synovitis and arthritis of subtalar joint after ankle sprain.

Sinus tract The channel through which a sinus cavity communicates with the external surface.

Sinus venosus The dilatation of the heart tuber inferior to the atrium that is formed by the proximal portions of the veins.

Sinus, piriform Piriform recess.

Sinusitis It is the inflammation of membrane lining facial sinuses due to infection. Infection generally spreads to the sinuses from nose, as a complication

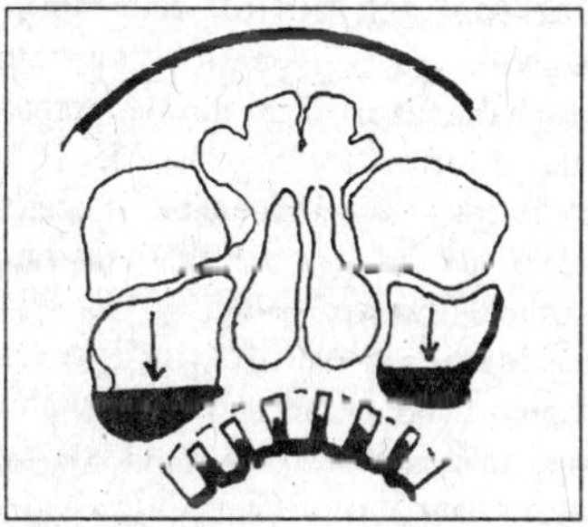

of common cold. Infection may arise from an abscess in upper tooth. It gives feeling of tension and fullness in affected area. It may cause throbbing pain, fever, stuffy nose and loss of smell. Antibiotics are useful. Decongestent drops combat the infection. Steam inhalation moistens the secretions.

Sinusoid A blood channel in certain organs that is lined by reticuloendothelium.

Sipple's syndrome A condition of multiple endocrine neoplasia characterised by phaeochromocytoma, hyperparathyroidism, and medullary carcinoma of the thyroid.

Site of insulin injection Insulin is given subcutaneously either in thigh, abdomen and posterior of arm.

Site-directed mutagenesis A set of methods used to create specific alterations in the sequence of a gene.

Site-specific recombination A type of genetic recombination that occurs only at specific sequences.

Sitting posture If sitting posture is not straight and person keeps his neck bent while writing, reading or typing, may develop cervical spondylitis soon.

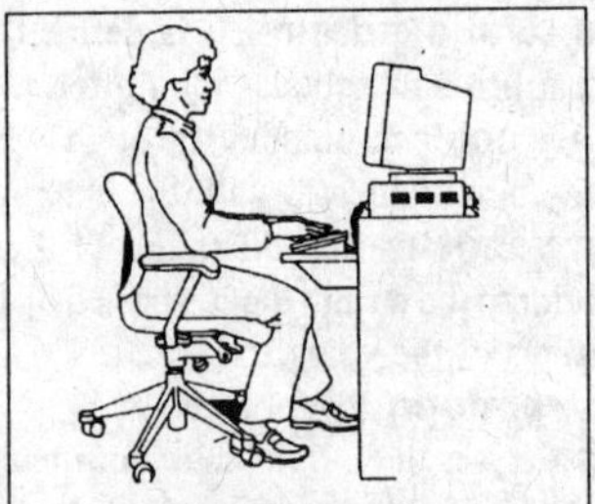

Proper sitting posture

Situational attribution Ascribing a person's behaviour to a given situation, rather than to personal traits or disposition. External rather than internal factors are emphasised.

Situational crisis Unanticipated even that poses a threat to an individuals psychosocial or psychological well being.

Situational or nonnormative transitions Unpredictable events such as changes in personal relationships, roles, and status; the environment, physical and mental capabilities, and possessions. These may occur at any time.

Situational test A test situation in which a candidate is observed as he or she reacts to a daily task or to a sample of the job or role to be filled.

Sitz bath The sitz bath is a method of applying water to the mid-portion of the body, especially to the perineum and the areas adjacent to it.

Six minute walk test A valid submaximal exercise test useful for assessing exercise tolerance in patients with pulmonary disease or congestive heart failure.

Size constancy The tendency for an object to be seen as maintaining its absolute size despite changes in the size of the retinal images.

Skeletal muscle Also known as voluntary muscle; muscles under willed or voluntary control.

Skeletal traction Pull exerted directly on the skeletal system by attaching wires, pins, or tongs into or through a bone.

Skeleton On vertebrates the bony framework of body.

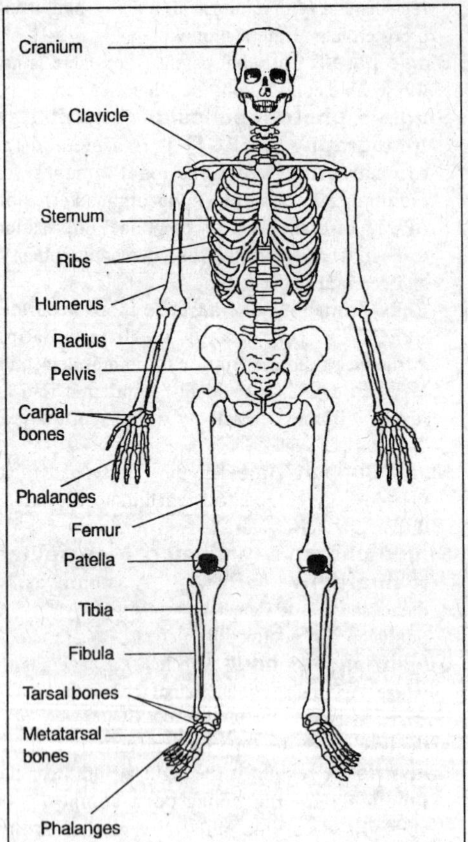

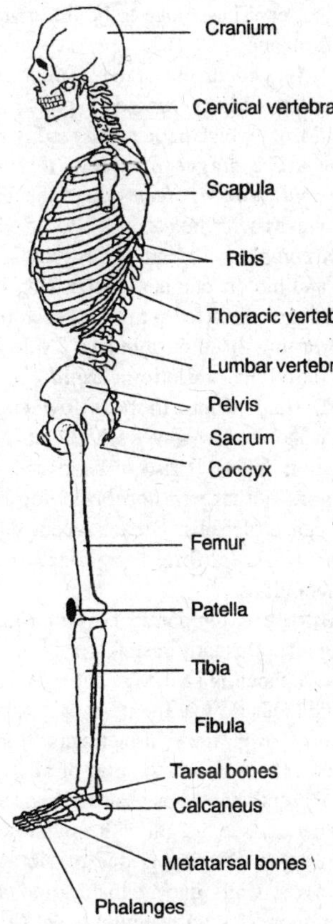

Skene's ducts or glands Paraurethral ducts of glands.

Skene's gland One of the two glands just within the meatus of female urethra regarded as homologue of prostate gland in male.

Skepticism Doubt in the absence of conclusive evidence.

Skewness Horizontal distortin of a frequency distribution, so that one tail of the plot is longer and contains more observations that the other.

Skiameter An instrument measuring the intensity of X-Rays.

Skill Highly coordinated movement that allows for investigation and interaction with the physical and social environment.

Skilled nursing facility Nursing home that provides 24 hour nursing care under the direction of a registered nurse.

Skin It is the protective structure to protect internal organs. It consists of thin outer layer of epidermis and a thicker layer the dermis. Beneath the dermis is the subcutaneous tissue which contains fat. Hair and nails are extension of skin. These contain keratin.

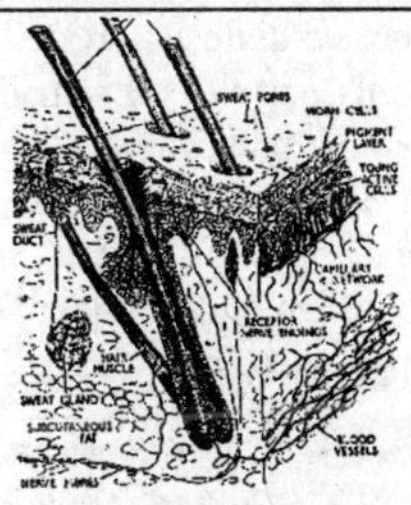

Structure of skin

Outermost part of epidermis is composed of dead cells which form a tough, horny, protective coating. These dead cells are replaced. Dermis is composed of a connective tissue. It also contains blood vessels, nerves and lymph vessels. It is a very sensory organ containing many cells that are sensitive to touch, temperature, pain and pressure. It helps in keeping body temperature constant. When body is hot, skin perspires and blood vessels dilate to dissipate heat. When it is cold the blood vessels in skin constrict, which conserves the body's heat. Epidermis contains a unique fatty substance that makes the skin waterproof.

Skin allergy Large number of substances can provoke an allergic reaction through direct contact with the skin of a susceptible person. Contact allergic dermatitis consists of red, itchy patches which may blister or form crusts. Certain adhesives, jewellery, cosmetics can cause it. In contact urticaria red, itchy, raised areas may develop within a few minutes. Many drugs can cause skin eruptions. Atopic eczema is an itchy skin condition most common in children.

Skin barrier An artificial layer of skin, made of plastic or vinyllike material, applied to skin before application of tape or ostomy drainage bags. Protects skin from chronic irritation.

Skin flap A full thickness mass of flap of tissue containing epidermis, dermis and subcutaneous tissue.

Skin patches Drugs that are bonded to an adhesive bandage.

Skin Rolling In skin rolling, the skin and subcutaneous tissues are rolled over the deeper structures. it is usually performed quite slowly and taking performed quite slowly and taking care not to pinch the tissues and cause pain.

Skin tear Shallow brak in the skin.

Skin traction Pulling effect on the skeletal system by applying devices to the skin.

Skull Skull consists eight bones which are strong enough to protect brain.

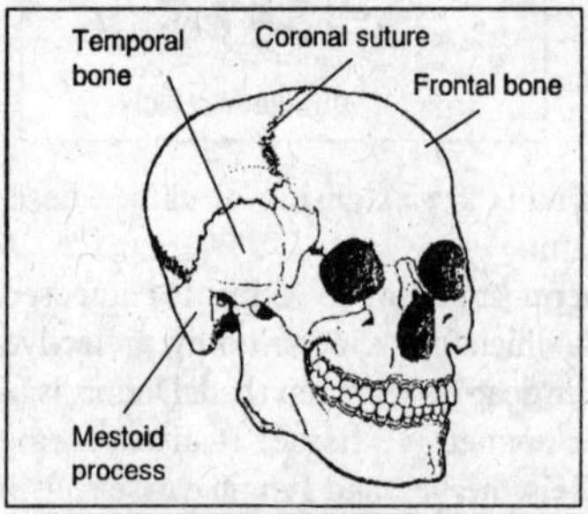

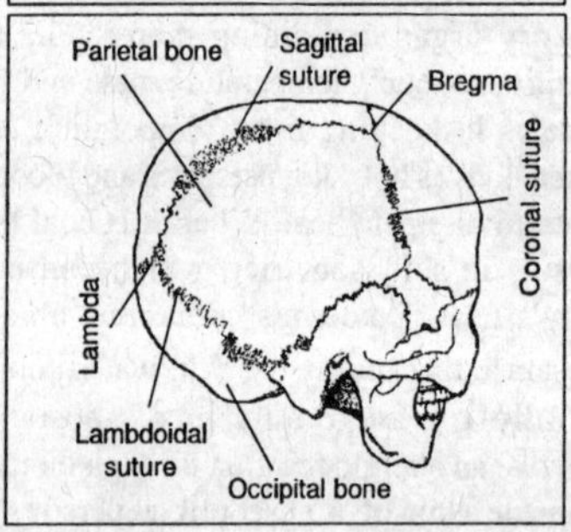

Skyline view In X-Ray a tangential view of patella.

Slander Character attack that is uttered in the presence of others.

Slapping A form of tapotement that uses a flat hand.

SLE (Systemic lupus erythematosus) It is a disease with multiorgan involvement. The most common sites of lesions are buccal mucosa, lips and palate. Oral complaints include burning mouth, xerostomia or soreness. Many lesions are called vasculitis. Lip lesions appear with a central atrophic area with small white dots with radiating white striae. There is occasional ulceration of central area. These have to be differentiated from lichen planus.

Sleep It is a recurrent state of unconsciousness associated with decreased response to external stimuli from which patient can readily be aroused. There are 2 stages of sleep. *Non-rapid eye movement (NREM) sleep* where the EEG shows slow waves with bursts of 12 to 14 Hz spindles and K complexes. Heart and respiration rates are slow and motor tone is reduced. Non-REM sleep has 4 stages of 60 to 90 minutes each followed by REM lasting 30 to 60 minutes. Cycle is repeated with individual variation. *Rapid eye movement (REM) sleep* where there is low voltage EEG pattern shows slow waves with bursts of muscular relaxation. There is rise in heart and respiration rate and increase in cerebral blood flow and tumescence of penis. Dreams occur during REM sleep. It is inhibited by barbiturates and amphetamines.

Sleep apnea A temporary cessation of breathing during sleep, usually lasting for several seconds. Central apnoea is said to occur when there is no detectable air flow at the nose or mouth. There is failure of respiratory movements. Sometimes it may be caused by obstruction of airflow through nose or mouth known as obstructive apnoea. These are generally overweight with small lower jaw and large tongue. Snoring is due to vibration of lax pharyngeal walls during inspiration. Increasing snores increases with depth of REM sleep and increasing pharyngeal obstruction.

Sleep apnea/hypopnea syndrome Sleep disorder in which the sleeper stops breathing or the breathing slows for 10 seconds or longer, five or more times per hour.

Sleep diary Daily account of sleeping and waking activities.

Sleep disorder A chronic disorder involving sleep.

Sleep EEG An electroencephalogram taken during sleep.

Sleep paralysis It is a complete flaccid paralysis with atonia and may develop at sleep onset or on first walking. Sensory input such as light touch from another person will abort paralytic attack. It may be accompanied with hallucination. Repeated attacks of sleep paralysis may occur as a familial disorder. Twenty five mg of clomipramine may prevent such paralysis.

Sleep rituals Habitual activities performed before retiring.

Sleep terror disorder Condition occurring in stage 4 sleep manifested by panic, confusion, and poor recall for the event.

Sleep walking More complex motor behaviour may occur during sleep in which young children up to 12 get out of their bed. They may sit on bed or wander around their bedroom, Child does not respond to vocal command because he or she is disoriented and confused, sleep walking occurs in deep stage of NREM sleep.

Sleeping drugs or pills These are drugs used in insomnia. These include benzodiazepine drugs, barbiturate drugs, antihistamines, anti- depressants and chloral hydrate. Sleeping drugs should be taken in smallest effective dose for shortest period of time. Certain drugs have hangover effect with alcohol and may be proved hazardous and risky. They may produce tolerance and drug dependence.

Sleeping sickness A disease caused by *Trypanosoma brucei rhodesiense* and *T.b. gambiense* in Africa.

Sleeplessness It is necssary to ensure adequate sleep. Patient develops nights filled with wakeful, anxious preoccupations. Daily massage and exercise will build up muscular tone to have sound sleep.

Sleep-wake cycle disturbance Condition that results from a sleep schedule that involves daytime sleeping.

Slice fracture Unstable fracture dislocation of the lumbar spine produced by flexion and rotation injury.

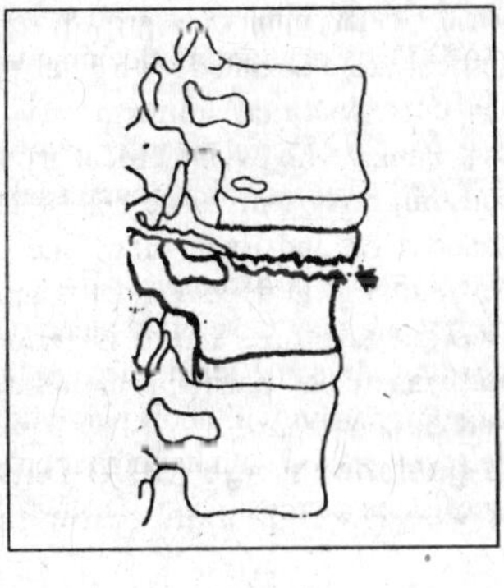

Sliding filament mechanism Mechanism by which actin and myosin myofilaments slide over one another during muscle contraction.

Sliding friction Mechanism consisting of solid structures that resist motion by moving against each other, such as a clamp on the knee bolt.

Sliding-filament mechanism The explanation of how thick and thin filaments slide relative to one another during striated muscle contraction to decrease sarcomere length.

Sling It is a device to immobilise, support or elevate an upper limb. It is generally made of triangular

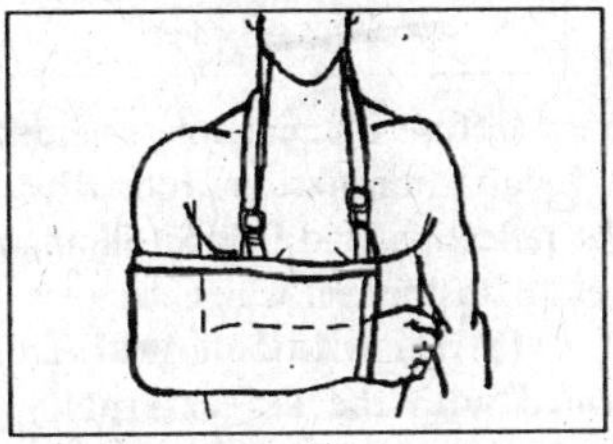

bandage. An elevation sling is used in first aid to hold the hand in a well-raised position to control bleeding or to prevent movement of arm and shoulder or when clavicle is broken.

Sling & Swathe Immobilization of upper extremity in which forearm is suspended in a sling and secured to anterior chest wall by swathe wrapped around trunk.

Slip angle It is the degree of forward tilting of vertebral body at the level of slipping.

Slipped epiphysis It occurs in upper femoral epiphysis and resembles like a pathological

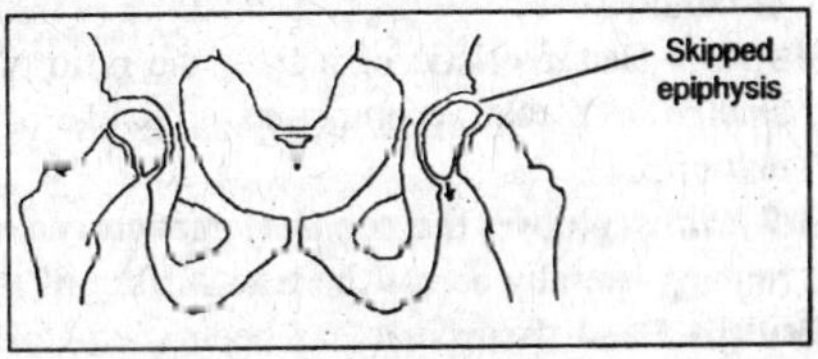

fracture, Young boy will complain of pain which is worse on any weight bearing activity. There will be loss of internal rotation.

Slit lamp examination The slit lamp is the most useful instrument for examination of cornea. Basically slit lamp consists of an illuminating system which can be adjusted to height, width, angle and a movable binocular microscope. Both of these can be aligned to provide simultaneous illumination and magnification of the area to be seen. There are six methods of examination with

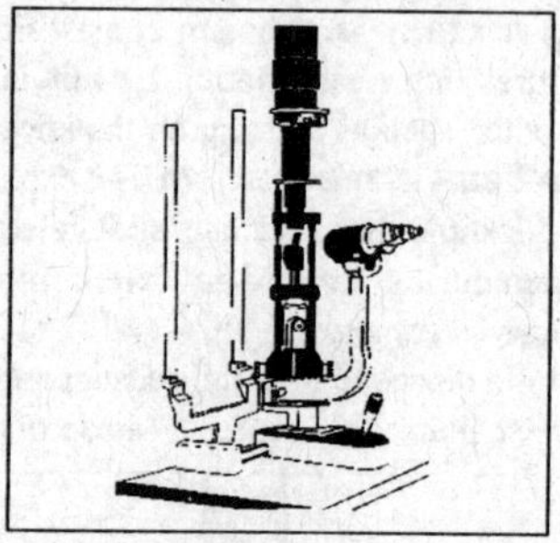

slit lamp : diffuse illumination, sclerotic scatter, direct focal illumination, retroillumination, specular reflection, and indirect illumination.

Sliva ejector Instrument which suctions saliva.

Slocum external rotation test This test is performed with the leg externally rotated. Anteromedial rotatory instability is indicated if the

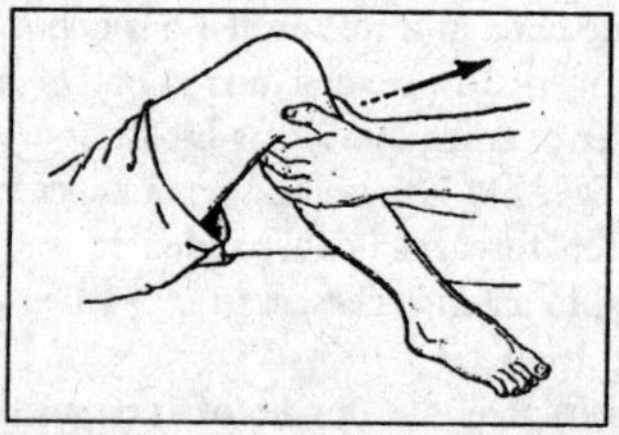

majority of anterior translation occurs on the medial side or the amount of anterior translation remains the same or increases, indicating anteromedial instability.

Slope A characteristic of a line; the ratio of the change in Y that accompanies a change of one unit of X.

Slot Narrow grooves that connect larger groves, often running laterally across the tead surface of a tire.

Slough Dead tissue that has been shed from its source. Menstruation is also the shedding of mucous membrane of uterus. It also occurs as a part of healing process of ulcers and wounds.

Slow learner A student able to profit from normal classroom instruction, providing that the material is presented at a somewhat slower than normal rate. This student is not considered mentally retarded.

Slow sand filtration A technique for purifying water by filtering it throug a large bed of packed sand, on which an organic layer forms and assists in the filtration process.

Slow speed hand piece Hand piece holding cutting and polishing instrument rotating at the speed of 100,000 to 500,000 rpm.

Slow wave sleep Sleep characterised by EEG waves of duration slower than 4H2 and high amplitude.

Slowly adapting receptor A body sensory receptor that responds as long as a sensory stimulus is on the body.

Slow-wave sleep Stages of sleep in which the electroencephalogram displays slow waves; also called NREM (nonrapid eye movement) sleep.

SLR Straight leg raising.

Sludge-gall bladder Sludge refers to gall bladder mucin with entrapment of particulate matter nucleated from bile. It develops when gall bladder emptying is slow and incomplete and progresses to stone formation in majority of cases.

Small cardiac vein A vein that receives blood from the back of the right atrium and ventricle; runs between the right atrium and ventricle in the coronary sulcus.

Small flat pelvis It may be a feature of sub-clinical rickets. Disproportion at the brim occurs due to increased forward projection of sacral promontory making AP diameter unlikely small.

Small for gestational age (SGA) Pertaining to a neonate weighing below the 10th percentile or standard deviations below the normal for the gestation age.

Small-for-date babies Babies small-for-gestational age below 10th percentile may show symmetrical or asymmetrical growth retardation. Symmetrical are associated with fetal pathology such as chromosomal abnormality or fetal infection. Babies with asymmetrical growth show long and thin body with large heads. They lack subcutaneous fat and liver, lungs and heart are smaller. Neurological development is mature and brain weight is more. There is reduction in placental transfer of nutrients including amino acids and carbohydrates.

Small-for-gestational age (SGA) Pertaining to infants whose weight falls below the tenth percentile for their gestational age. These infants have experienced growth retardation during the prenatal period and may be born close to term but weigh less than 2500 g.

Smear layer A layer of debris containing mineral and protein loosely adhered to the underlying dentin tooth structure and produced after the dentin has been abraded by a dental instrument, such as a burr.

Smears These are used to prepare organisms or tissues for microscopic examination. This is a

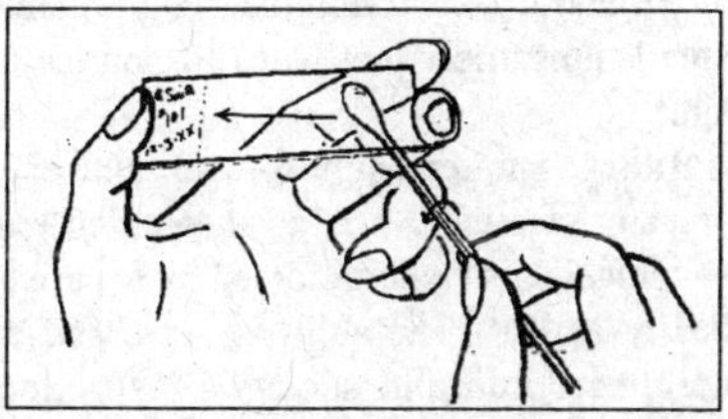

small amount of specimen material spread on a clean glass slide. It should neither be too thick nor too thin. These are made of blood, CSF, sputum, exudate, gastric content, cervical content, etc. to be examined under microscope.

Smegma The cheesy secretion of sebaceous glands, especially that found under the penile foreskin.

Smell In insomnia there is loss of smell. Abnormal smell perception is dysosmia. It may be accompanied with disturbance of taste. Common cold, rhinitis and cigarette smoking also cause anosmia. In atrophic rhinitis mucous membrane thickens distorting the olfactory nerve endings and some degree of permanent anosmia. The olfactory nerve can be torn in a head injury.

Smelling acuity Ability to smell and identify odors.

Smith's fracture This is due to a fall on back of hand or a direct blow to the dorsum of the hand.

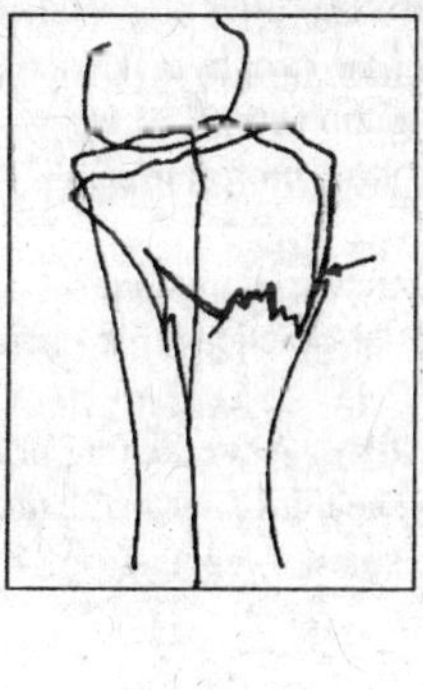

The distal fragment is displaced ventrally with radial deviation of hand giving a garden spade deformity.

Smoke inhalation There may be visible fire or smoke. Person may burn or develop difficulty in

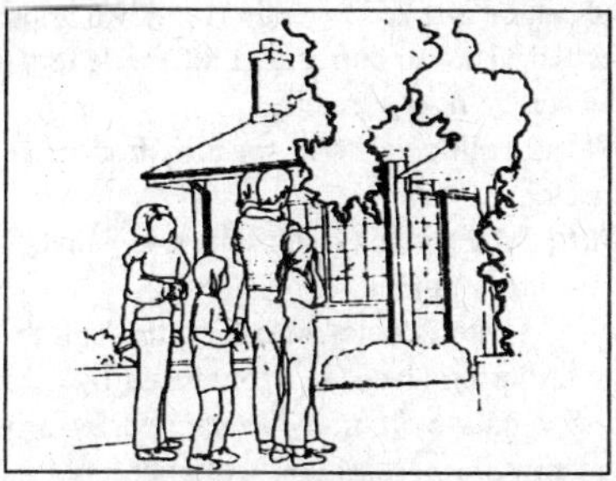

breathing. One should come out of immediate danger and into fresh air. Start cardiopulmonary resuscitatiion (CPR) if person is not breathing.

Smokeless powder Frequently used propellant powder containing mainly nitrocellulose (Single base) or both nitrocellulose and nitroglycerine (double base).

Smooth muscle Muscle that are not under conscious control; also known as involuntary or visceral; forms the walls of blood vessels and hollow organs.

Snake bite True venomous snakes are true vipers and pit vipers, make two distinct puncture wounds in skin. There is burning pain at the site of bite. The venom may prevent blood from clotting, causing bleeding from site of bite. There may be blood coming from mouth and in urine. Internal bleeding lowers down the BP. While a bite from coral snake usually causes little pain or swelling. Venom primarily affects nervous system. Serious sequences include drooping eyelids, slurred speech and double vision, victim becomes drowsy and delirious and may have convulsions. If not treated respiratory paralysis causes death. Antivenom helps the patient.

Snapping hip It is a condition seen in ballet dancers and refers to a snapping noise in the hip region. Condition resolves with rest.

Sneezing This is an involuntary, compulsive expulsion of air through the nose and mouth due to irritation of upper respiratory tract. Common cold and allergic rhinitis may lead it.

Snellen eye chart Tool for assessing far vision.

Snellen's chart It is the most commonly used method to measure visual acuity during vision test. In it there are rows of letters of standard decreasing size set at a distance of 20 feet. One eye is covered and patient is asked to read as far down as possible. Normal vision requires that all the letters of that row can be read correctly.

Sniffer A colloquial term for a hydrocarbon vapor detector.

Sniffing Taking in toxic substances by inhaling them through the nose.

Snoring There is noisy breathing through the open mouth during sleep. It is produced by vibrations of soft palate. It may be caused by anything hindering the respiration. Common cold, allergic rhinitis or enlarged adenoids may result it. Snoring alternates with sleep apnoea.

Snow blindness It generally develops in mountaineers who are exposed to bright sunlight which is reflected from snow at high altitude in clear weather. It is the ultraviolet rays causing damage to eye. Early symptoms are photophobia, feeling of foreign body sensation. There may be lacrimation, blepharospasm and intense pain in eye. There develops conjunctival congestion, chemosis and oedema of corneal epithelium. Fluorescein staining may show partial or complete staining of cornea due to desquamation. Antibiotic eye oinment will help.

Soak A soak is the direct immersion of a body part in a warm water or in a medicated solution. These are generally employed to clean burns, to apply

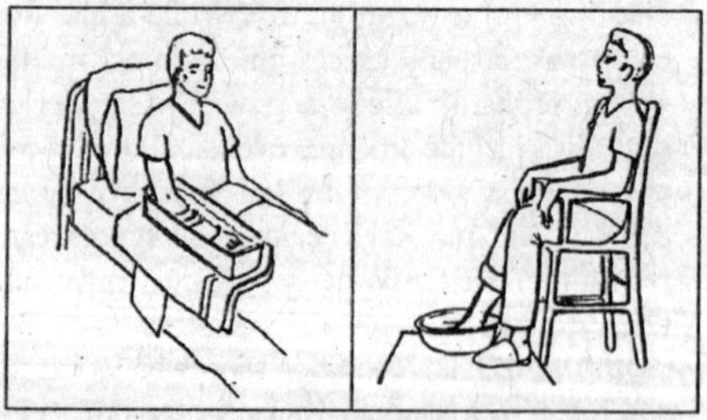

medication to an infected area to increase circulation. The soak temperature should be 105°F to 110°F and body part is gradually immersed. The warmth of soak causes the skin in pink colour and warm to touch.

SOAP charting Documentation style more likely to be used in a problemoriented record.

Soap, total fatty matter Every soap contains some percentage of total fatty matter (TFM) and quality of any soap is judged by its TFM contents. High TFM means high production cost.

Grade I quality bathing soaps contains TFM more than 76%, grade II 70% and grade III 60% at lest. Glycerine is a good emollient and moisturiser. Considering all above factors Dewdern soap is best to its cost. Popular soap Skinsect L&E contains lanolin and excellent emollient and vitamin E, a natural moisturizer that helps to nourish tone of skin.

Sociability The tendency to seek and enjoy the company of others. It is an innate and temperamental which is then reinforced by experience.

Social adaption The ability to live and express oneself according to society's restrictions and cultural demands.

Social anomie Lack of social rules and orientation in a social group often associated with feelings of anxiety and helplessness.

Social breakdown syndrome The concept that some psychiatric symptomatology is a result of treatment conditions and inadequate facilities and not a part of the primary illness. Factors bringing about the condition are social labelling, learning the role of the chronically sick, atrophy of work and social skills, and identification with the sick.

Social capital Patterns of co-operative social exchange in neighbourhood and community life characterised by mutual commitment and trust.

Social class A large group of people with relatively similar incomes, amount of wealth, life conditions, life chances, and lifestyles. Synonymous terms are "socioeconomic status" and "social status."

Social cognition The area of social psychology concerned with how people make sense of social events, including the actions of other.

Social competence Comfort in public, able to get along.

Social culture Refers to dominant set of symbolic codes and material practices that characterises a group.

Social disintegration A weakening of social ties.

Social distance The third zone in the measurement of interpersonal space, ranging from 4 to 12 feet.

often occur at this distance.

Friendly conversations and business conferences often occur at this distance.

Social epidemiology The scientific study of social factors in relation to occurence and distribution of disease.

Social expressivity Verbal speaking skill and the ability to engage others in conversation.

Social facilitation Occurs whenever the individual in a group situation exceeds his or her characteristic performance level when working alone. It does not necessarily mean that the person is more efficient in the group situation, for he or she may have increased output but may make more mistakes.

Social fathers Men who are socioculturally generative by caring for the growth of younger adults or contributing to the well being and continuity of the larger community.

Social health The ability to interact with people in an acceptable manner and to sustain relationship with family member, friends and colleagues.

Social identity theory A theory maintaining that people are motivated to create and maintain a positive identity in terms of qualities and, especially, group memberships.

Social learning theory A view which stresses that learning occurs through interacting with and especially by observing others. Also called observational learning. The observed person serves as a model and the learner is prompted to imitate that person, especially when the model's behaviour results in favourable consequences, called reinforcement.

Social phobia A condition characterized by fear of the possible scrutiny or criticism of others.

Social psychobiology The study of interactions between social, psychological and biological process.

Social psychology The study of individual's responsiveness to one another, especially at the human level. An area of psychology emphasising the study of groups and group interactions.

Social referencing Using the behaviour of others as a guide for social behaviour.

Social resources Social factors that operate as stress moderators such as emotional support and assistance from family members and friends.

Social role Set of expectations or norms directed toward people who hold important social problems.

Social sensitivity Ability to decode verbal communication and knowledge of social norms.

Social smile A smile response to another's face, a developmental milestone of 2 months.

Social space Distance of 4 to 12 feet.

Social status Placement of a particular animals within a social hierachy with subordinate animals deferring to the wishes of more dominant animals.

Social stress Stress arising from interactions with others or the perception of others attitude.

Social support The amount of help actually received, satisfaction with that help, and the person's network providing that help. Help received may be in the form of instrumental or physical aid, information, emotional support, or the appraisal of one's role performance.

Socialisation The process by which an individual gradually becomes integrated into the noun and value system of a society. The ability to interact with people in appropriate contextual and cultural ways.

Socio environmental risk factors Degree of ecological and interpersonal destruction and intensity of exposure to morbidity.

Sociocultural identification Introjection of socially meaningful behavioral pattern through significant person.

Sociogram A graphic representation of the results obtained with a sociometric questionnaire, showing interactions between group members in terms of acceptance and/or rejection.

Sodium It regulates body water along with potassium. It is responsible of nerve conduction and contraction of muscles. Body contains about 55 gm of sodium. The level in blood is maintained by kidneys.

Practically all foods being cooked contain salt (sodium chloride). Main dietary source of sodium are processed food, cheese, bread, cereals and prickles. So its deficiency is rare. Average consumption is 1 to 7 gm per day. Excessive use of diuretic, excessive sweatings, kidney orders may result its deficiency. Deficiency symptoms include tiredness, weakness, muscle cramps and dizziness. Excessive consumption of sodium results in hypertension.

Sodium bicarbonate Antacid is used to combat indigestion and other stomach disorders because of its alkaline properties. High doses may cause stomach upset or alkalosis.

Sodium citrate Non particulate antacid widely used pre operatively to increase gastric pH in patients at risk of aspiration of gastric content.

Sodium depletion It usually occurs when salt is lost but fluid intake is normal as in vomiting and diarrhoea. Symptoms include lassitude, apathy, weakness, anorexia, vomiting with peripheral circulatory failure. Amount of urine is normal. There will be disturbance of acid-base balance if the loss of chloride and sodium ion is disproportionate. With continued loss of gastric juice there is hypochloraemia with production of alkalosis. One point eight percent IV saline helps the patients.

Sodium nitroprusside Its action is direct one on smooth muscle of blood vessels to produce relaxation and hence vasodilatation. There is greater effect on arteries than veins, cardiac output is maintained. Moderate tachycardia is frequent. Renal blood is increased while cerebral blood flow is maintained. Maximum safe dose is 1.5 mg/kg. Response is seen within 30 seconds. It is used during neurosurgery.

Sodium pump An active transport pump located in the plasma membrane that transports sodium ions out of the cell and potassium ions into the cell at the expense of cellular ATP. If functions to keep the ionic concentrations of these elements at physiological levels.

Sodium retention This may occur with water retention as in oedema or as sodium retention alone. It may be due to excessive intake as in overinfusion, excessive oral intake or use of sodium containing medicine in children. there may be inability to excrete as is seen in Cushing's syndrome, excessive steroid therapy or some neurological syndromes. Effects of sodium retention are mild oedema, confusion, apathy, leading to coma. Witholding of sodium and giving of chlorothiazide is helpful.

Sodium valporate It is an anticonvulsant drug used in epilepsy. It may be enhancing GABA. Half life is 15 hours and is rapidly absorbed orally.

Sodium-potassium pump A system of coupled ion pumps that actively transports sodium ions out of a cell and potassium ions into the cell at the same time—found in all living cells.

Sodomy Anal sex is sometimes disapproved of and is illegal in many countries. There is nothing physically and psychologically wrong with anal sex except of aesthetic sense. Without lubrication there may be severe discomfort. It should be done with candom on. Incidence of HIV positivity is higher in case practicing anal sex. This is especially true in male homosexuals.

Soft copy Electronic record.

Soft corn A painful hyper keratosis lesion that occurs between the toes.

Soft diet Soft diet means easily digestible solid diet having minimum residue. During convalescence, after liquid diet patient is put on soft diet before starting normal diet. Soft diet includes suji, boiled, gruel, oat meal, mashed potato, apple mashed, custard and ice-cream.

Soft disk A discarded term applied to an intervertebral disk disorder caused by herniation of soft disk material such as nucleus pulposus.

Soft liner An elastic, resilient polymer containing plasticizers that is attached to the tissue- bearing surface of a denture base to improve the fit and comfort of the denture.

Soft tissue integrity The maintenance of anatomical and physiological normality of the interstitial tissue and the skin.

Soft tissue opacity A well-defined radiopacity located in soft tissue and viewed on a radiograph; a salivary stone or calcified lymph node appears as a soft tissue opacity.

Soft tissues of pelvic floor Levator ani muscles slope forwards, downwards and incwards. During the process of labour these muscles, ligaments stretch and dilate to allow the fetus to pass through the bony pelvis.

Soft water Water has been filtered to replace some of the minerals with sodium.

Software piracy Illegal copying of copyrighted software.

Solar dermatitis Sunburn results from overexposure of skin to sunlight or ultraviolet light. It can also result due to hypersensitivity. Histopathologically skin shows intense hyperaemia and varying degree of oedema and may even blister formation. Resolution occurs with desquamation and increase in pigmentation. Patches of erythema may become rough and scaly and finally keratosis may develop. Lesions are bilateral and symmetrical. Affected person may complain of local burning, feeling of warmth, itching, pain and tenderness.

Solder The metallic material and procedure used to join two metal parts; solder is melted and flowed into a small space between the metal parts, joining them through the formation of a metallic bond on cooing.

Sole nerve supply Damage of medial branch could be anaesthetic to 2/3 rd of sole while lateral branch will anaesthetise lateral 1/3rd of sole and the short 4-5th toe flexors and adductors weak or paralysed.

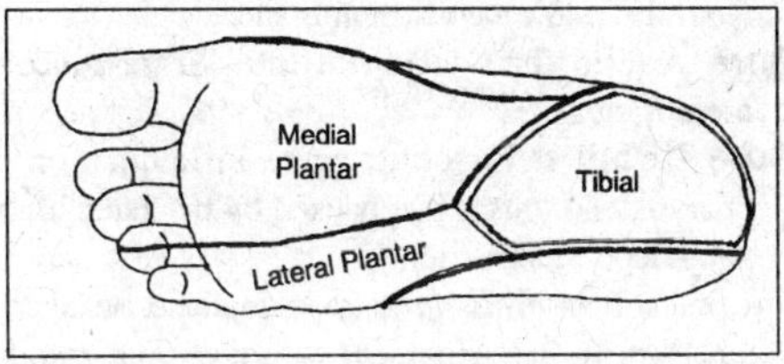

Soleal line A line on the upper third of posterior surface of tibia.

Solid ankle-foot orthosis Plastic ankle-foot orthosis that has a posterior shell continuous with an insert. The shell extends anteriorly beyond the malleoli.

Solidarity Strong shared group identity that leads to promotion of that group and its causes. Class solidarity would include working for unions to secure or to better the life of those within the working class.

Solitary rectal ulcer Pathogenesis is unknown but it probably arises from trauma and ischaemia associated with recurrent prolapsing of rectal mucosa into antral canal. Ulcer is almost always on anterior or anterolateral rectal wall about 5 to 10 cm above the anal verge. Ulcer is flat and fibrotic. Patients present with blood and mucus per rectum, tenesmus and pain in rectum, perineum and sacrum. Stool softeners and bulking agents are useful.

Solubility Capability of being dissolved.

Soluble dietary fibers Dietary fibers that dissolve in fluids.

Solute A substance dissolved in another substance.

Solution Homogeneous mixture formed when a solute dissolves in a solvent (liquid).

Solution learning Learning how to respond to various conditions in the environment, chiefly through operant conditioning.
Responses determined through the principle of reinforcement.

Solvent The liquid in which another substance (the solute) is disolved to form a solution.

Soma The whole body of an organism excluding reproductive cells.

Somaesthetic Consciously perceived body sensations.

Somatic Implies body wall as distinct from viscera.

Somatic cell division Type of cell division in which a single parent cell duplicates it self to produce two identical daughter cells; consists of mitosis and cytokinesis.

Somatic cells Body cells others than gamets or germ cells.

Somatic death Death may be defined as complete and persistent cessation of circulation and respiration. In somatic death there is complete stoppage of actions of heart, lungs and brain. Molecular death means death of an individual cells of tissues of body which takes 3 to 4 hours in human being.

Somatic dysfunction Impaired or altered function of related components of the somatic (body framework) system; skeletal, arthrodial, and myofascial structures and related vascular, lymphatic, and neural elements.

Somatic dyspnea Difficulty in breathing or air hunger related to the vertebra subluxation complex or other somatic dysfunction.

Somatic motor A type of motor (efferent) neuron of the peripheral nervous system that innervates skeletal muscle.

Somatic nervous system The portion of the peripheral nervous system consisting of somatic sensory (afferent) neurons and somatic motor (efferent) neurons.

Somatic pain Discomfort genearted from deeper connective tissue.

Somatic protein Skeletal muscle protein.

Somatic protein stores Proteins in skeletal muscle.

Somatization disorder A psychiatric disorder in which the patient has so many somatic complaints but no underlying medical pathology found.

Somatogenic Produced by activity, reaction, and change originating in the musculoskeletal system.

Somatomedins A group of small polypeptides believed to be produced in the lecer in response to growth hormone stimulation and to mediate the actions of growth hormone on the skeleton and other tissues.

Somatostatin A polypeptide produced in the hypothalamus that acts to inhibit the secretion of growth hormone from the anterior pituitary.

Somatostatinoma Somatostatin inhibits the release and tissue action of most of the gastrointestinal hormones, in particular both insulin and glucagon. These are slow growing but mostly malignant. Clinical features include steatorrhoea, impairment of glucose tolerance, cholelithiasis and hypochlorhydria.

Somatotopic Containing a body map.

Somatotropic hormone Growth hormone; an anabolic hormone secreted by the anterior pituitary that stimulates skeletal growth and protein synthesis in many organs.

Somatovisceral reflex Alteration in the tone of smooth or cardiac muscle or glandular activity in response to a somatic stimulus. The provocative somatic stimulus can result from injury to or dysfunction of somatic structures, including subluxation. Under such circumstances they may create a disturbance of visceral tone. A synonym is somatoautonomic reflex.

Some premedication sedative may be given at the level of second rib. After the procedure seal the puncture site by tincture benzoin. Apply sterile gauze and adhesive plaster.

Somesthetic Somatic sensory, e.g. s. cortex.

Somi cervical brace A metal and metal rigid brace requires careful adjustment and fitting. Firm occipital and submental supporting plates are rigidly held by a removal bar to a chest plate. The chest plate is held firmly to the chest by over the shoulder and under the arm straps. This brace provides excellent stabilisation to lower cervical spine.

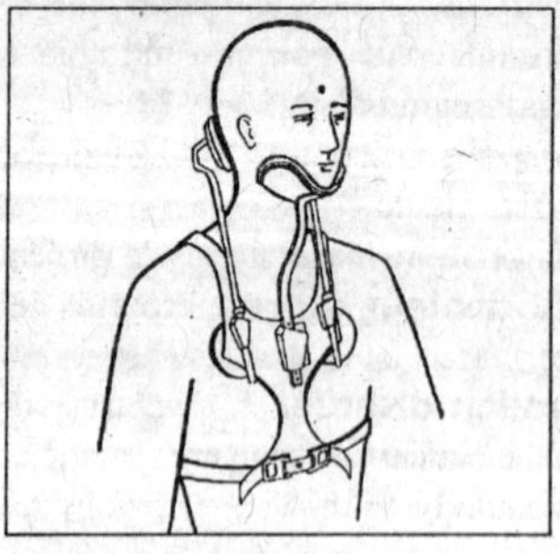

Somnambulism the scientific term for sleepwalking; formerly a term for hypnosis.

Sonohysterography A procedure in which the uterine cavity is filled with a saline solution and evaluated by transvaginal ultrasound.

Sorders Dried crusts around the mouth containing mucus, microorganisms, and epithelial cells shed from the oral mucous membrane.

Sore A term for a lesion of the skin or mucous membrane.

Sore throat It is due to acute inflammation of pharynx and tonsil. It is caused by betahaemolytic streptococcal infection.

Clinical features include fever, malaise, headache, and sore throat. Hoarseness, cough and rhinitis are common in viral infection, cervical lymph nodes are enlarged and illness is more acute with rigor. Tonsil becomes swollen and covered with exudate.

Sorption The process by which an object or material takes up a solvent by diffusion of the solvent into its structure; a common example is water sorption of polymers.

Sound attenuation Dampening of sound by contraction of stapedius or tensor tympani.

Sound field The peripheral field of sound perception by one ear.

Sound of korotkoff The sounds heard when pressure measurements are taken. These sounds are produced by the turbulent flow of blood through an artery that has been partially constricted by a pressure cuff.

Source credibility In mass media communication, the degree of confidence held by the audience with respect to the communicator. A credible source is perceived to be highly reliable and therefore most important in the audience's acceptance of the communication.

Source evidence Evidence whose origin is known.

Source-oriented records Records organized according to the source of information.

Space Chamber that is attached to an inhaler.

Space maintainer A fixed or removable appliance used to replace missing primary teeth to prevent drifting of surrounding teeth until eruption of permanent teeth.

Spacer Material used between two surfaces to allow or the placement of another material. Commonly used as a nonasbestos liner between a dentulous or edentulous model prior to fabricating a custom acrylic impression tray. The spacer allows room for placement of final impression material.

Spadix The male reproductive organ in molluscs, used for sexual arousal in females.

Spalding's sign It is an evidence of intra uterine fetal death. There is gross overlapping of the bones of the vault of the skull due to shrinkage of the brain substance. It becomes evident after 7 days of death and other radiological signs include intrafetal gas, bubbles of gas in the great vessels and heart of fetus. There becomes hyperflexion of spine, collapse of thoracic cage and fetus may adopt transverse lie, very low in the lower pole of uterus.

Sparganosis Infection with plerocercoid larvae.

Spasm An involuntary muscle contraction.

Spasmodic angina The pain is sudden, not in proportion to exertion, severe and often associated with a feeling of impending death. It is due to coronary spasm accentuated by emotions and exertion. There is an acute pain radiating down after meals in cold weather. Face becomes expression of pain. Pallor and sweating are present. Sense of suffocation, bodily discomfort, constriction of chest and end of impending dissolution is extreme. Attack lasts for a few minutes. Heart shows some enlargement. BP is raised. Mainly attacks are accompanied by a profuse flow of urine. Pain is relieved by nitroglycerine.

Spasmodic cough An involuntary, uncontrollable sudden explosive forcing of air through the glottis.

Spasmodic croup It occurs in children between the ages of 1 and 3 years. Child wakes up suddenly in early hours of morning with brassy cough and noisy breathing. Symptoms improve within few hours. Illness may recur but course is generally benign. Cause is unknown.

Spasmodic torticollis It is a term that refers to a disease entity consisting of spontaneous onset of painful contractions of various muscles around cervical spine. Cause is unknown. Spasm may be bilateral. These spasm tend to hold the head toward affected side and are uncontrollable. These patients have strong psychoneurotic tendencies.

Spasmus nutans The benign condition appears in first year and disappears in second year. It is characterised by irregular flexion movements and habitual tilting of head with marked nystagmus in one eye. Brain tumour of third ventricle may also have similar features.

Spastic Clonus or rapid series of rhythmic contractions during quick stretch of a muscle as a result of abnormally increased tension.

Spastic diplegia A form of cerebral palsy involving corticospinal fibers destined for lower limb motor neurons.

Spastic entropion It is a condition of rolling inwards of the lid margin. Spastic entropion is limited to lowered lid in old and debilitated person who lacks orbital fat. Skin of lid is redundant. Spastic entropion occurs due to spasm of orbicularis muscles associated with degeneration of palpebral connective tissue.

Degeneration of Muller's muscle which is lower lid retractor also plays a part. Degeneration of the interior lid aponeurosis also plays a role in it. Lashes rub against the cornea and conjunctiva. There is irritation, conjunctival congestion of lower bulbar conjunctiva and epiphora. Superficial erosions or opacities may be seen on lower margin of cornea.

Spasticity It results from damage to motor areas of cerebrum characterised by increased muscle tone. Strong exaggerated muscle contractions are common and in some cases muscles will continue to contract. Lower limb involvement results in hip flexion with thigh pulling towards midline. Flexion at knee will be there. Scissoring gait may develop with imbalance.

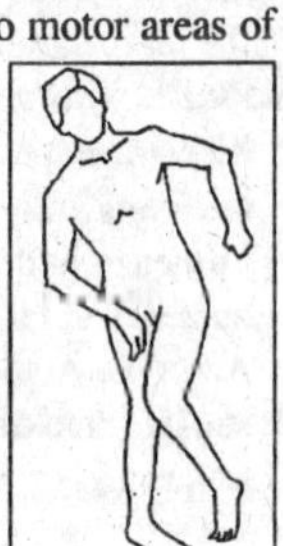

Spatial orientation Is the ability to relate to the position, direction or movement of objects or points in space.

Spatial relations Ability to determine the relationship of one object to another in space.

Spatial relations deficit The inability to perceive the relationship of one object in space to another object or to oneself.

Spawn A large number of eggs released into water for hatching by fishes, amphibians, mollucs, and other such animals.

Speaker profiling A classification task performed mostly by phoneticians, where a recording of the voice of a perpetrator is the only lead in a case.

Speaker recognition Any process that use some features of the speech signal to determine if a particular person is the speaker of a given utterance.

Speaker recognition by listening (SRL) SRL involves the study of how human listners associate a particular voice with a particular individual or group, and indeed to what extent such a task can be performed.

Specialty A branch of dentistry in which the professional is specially qualified after having completed an advanced program of study and having met specified criteria.

Speciation The fact of organisms being divided into different species, or the processes by which this takes place.

Species A category of biological classification ranking just below genus; in the wildlife forensic sense; the biological classification level at which a group of like plants or animals, capable of reproducing with each other, is typically protected by wildlife laws.

Specific heat The amount of energy needed to raise the temperature of 1 g of a pure substance by 1°C.

Specific immunity The ability of the system of discriminate between different antigens. The antigens may be significantly different, e.g., influenza and poliomyelitis viruses; or they may be very similar, e.g., human blood group substances A and B. Also, specificity.

Specific rates Rates calculated for specific subgroups of the population; contrast with *crude rates*.

Specific rotation The rotation, in degrees, of the plane of plane-polarized light by an optically active compound at 25°C, with a specified concentration and light path.

Specificity The percentage of individuals without a particular diagnosis who are correctly identified as negative by a test.

Specimens Samples of tissue or body fluids.

Speckled corneal dystrophy It leads to dot-like, sometimes circular, sometimes areolar opacities in the corneal stroma. This is a benign, non-progressive dystrophy with small opacifications in entire stroma. These are best seen in retroillumination. It is asymptomatic and does not decrease visual acuity. The deposits consist of acid mucopolysaccharides and lipids in the kerotocytes.

Speculum A short, funnel-like tube for examining canals, such as the nasal canal and the vaginal canal.

Speech disturbance Any disorder of verbal communication that is not due to faulty innervation of speech muscles or organs of articulation. The term includes many language and learning disabilities.

Speech production Speech production is composed of two basic mechnanical functions; phonation and articulation.

Speech therapy It is a long-term therapy to improve speech disorder. It depends on study of phonation. Therapist develops a confidence.

Speed Rate of application i.e. fast, slow and varied.

SPEM Smooth-pursuit eye movements.

Sperm bank Sperms can be stored for a while in sperm bank. Cattle breeders usually use sperm

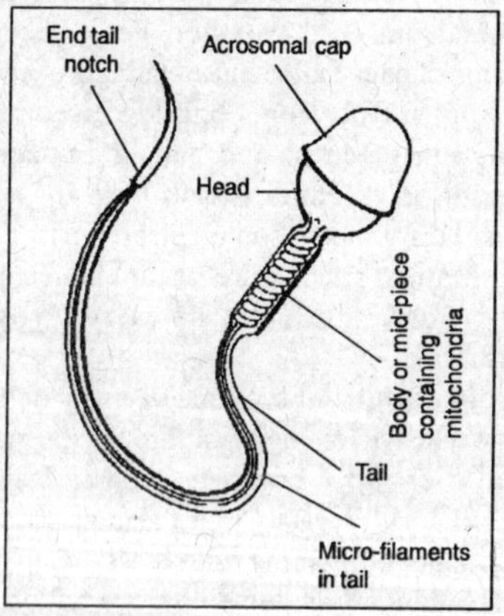

banks. A complete ejaculation of semen is collected and stored at an extemely low temperature. Properly frozen sperms can be kept for 4 to 5 years. This can be used by some infertile women by artificial insemination.

Sperm capsule The rigid, sclerotized covering that often encases a sperm packet.

Sperm cell A mature male gamete. Also termed spermatozoon.

Sperm droplet A naked, unpackaged droplet of spermatozoa and accessory fluids.

Sperm incorporation The physical incorporation of the sperm into the egg cytoplasm.

Sperm maturation The process occurring in the epididymis during which immature spermatozoa produced in the testis gain the potential to fertilize eggs.

Sperm migration The movement of sperm from the point of insemination to the site of fertilization.

Sperm packet Spermatozoa and accessory fluids packaged in a flexible membranous covering.

Sperm speed Human spermatozoan moves on an average rate of 1.5 millimetres per minute, i.e. 1 inch per 15 minute. It reaches fallopian tube within

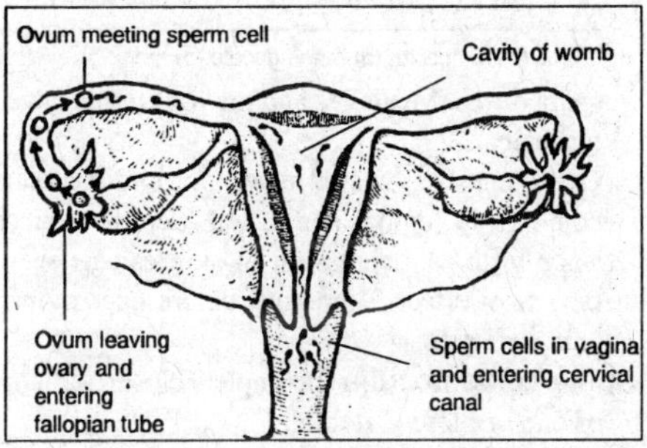

a few hours. Of the 300 million spermatozoa in a single male ejaculation, it is believed that no more than a few thousand survive. Within vagina sperm survives for 2 days.

Sperm wash An artificial insemination technique involving the removal of seminal plasma by centrifugation of semen diluted with culture medium followed by resuspension of the sperm in culture medium.

Spermatic cord The Structure formed by the pampiniform plexus and the coils of the internal spermatic artery between the inguinal canal and the testis.

Spermatid The haploid germinal cell arising from meiotic divisions of spermatocytes, which differentiates, within the seminiferous epithelium, into a spermatozoon. The resulting daughter cells from the primary spermatocyte undergoing meiosis; these cells have only half the genetic material and half the chromosomes of other body cells.

Spermatocyst A unit of spermatogenesis present in anamniote testis.

Spermatocyte A developing sperm cell in one of two stages. A primary spermatocyte develops from a spermatogonium and subsequently divides into two secondary spermatocytes. Each spermatocyte divides into two spermatids.

Spermatogonia Sperm precursor cells.

Spermatogonium The undivided male germ cell that develops in the seminiferous tubes. Each will eventually develop into four spermatozoa.

Spermatozoa Sperm cells (singular; spermatozoon).

Spermatozoon A mature male germ cell; the mobile microscopic sexual element that resembles in shape an elongated tadpole.

Spermia A suffix referring to sperm or semen.

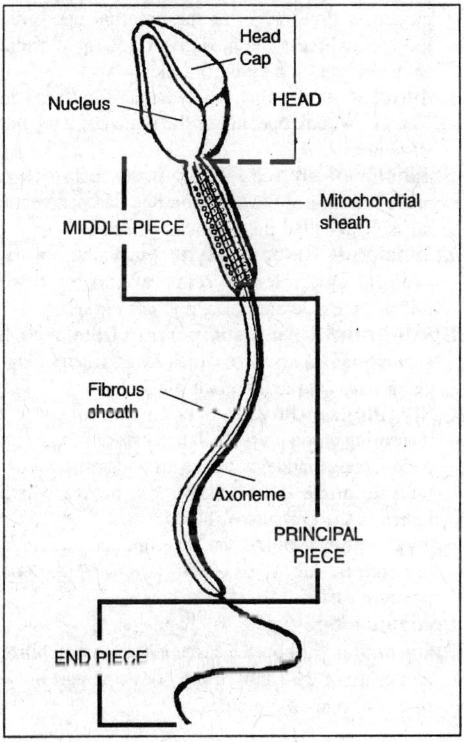

Spermicidal cream These are not effective when used alone. Some couples find it aesthetically unpleasant, causing too much lubrication, feeling unpleasant to touch or taste.

Spermicide A substance or agent that acts to kill sperm; i.e., for the purpose of contraception.

Spermination The release of spermatozoa from the seminiferous tubules; the counterpart to ovulation in the female.

Spermiogenesis The maturation of spermatids into sperm.

Spermiophagy The phagocytic ingestion of spermatozoa.

Sphenoid bone Irregular, wedge-shaped bone located at the base of the skull in front of the temporal bone and the basilar portion of the occipital bone. Sphenoid body is more or less cuboidal and hollowed out interiorly to form the sphenoidal air sinuses. Extending from the body laterally are two great wings and two lesser wings. Projecting below the body are two pterygoid processes. The lateral surfaces of the pterygoid processes give origin to the external pterygoid muscles, whereas the medial surfaces give origin to the internal pterygoid muscles.

Sphincter A circular muscle that functions to constrict a body opening or the lumen of a tubular structure.

Sphincter of ampulla The muscular constriction at the opening of the common bile and pancreatic ducts; also called the sphincter of Oddi.

Sphincter-detrusor dyssynergia Failure of the urethral sphincter to relax at the onset of micturition; a feature of spinal cord injury.

Sphingolipid An amphiphathic lipid with a sphingosine backbone to which are attached a long-chain fatty acid and a polar alcohol.

Sphygmomanometer It is an instrument for measuring blood pressure. It consists of a cuff with an inflatable bladder wrapped around arm, a rubber bulb to inflate the bladder and a device which indicates the pressure of blood.

Sphygmomanometry The determination of blood pressure by means of auscultation and a blood pressure cuff.

Spica bandage Figure 'S" bandage.

Spica cast An orthopedic cast applied to immobilize part or all of the trunk of the body and part or all of one or more extremities.

Spigelion hernia The hernia protrudes through the linea semilunaris along the lateral border of rectus muscle at the level of arcuate line. It appears as a small, tender swelling to one side of the lower abdomen wall along the lateral margin of rectus muscle. Operation is the treatment of choice.

Spillan scot syndrome There may be incomplete bilateral deafness, tinnitus, numbness and tingling in legs and abnormal tendon reflexes. There will be greatly reduced vision, specially near vision, relative or absolute central or paracentral scotomas.

Spina bifida There is failure of fusion between the neural arches only. So the spinous process will be divided into two leaving a bony gap giving rise to

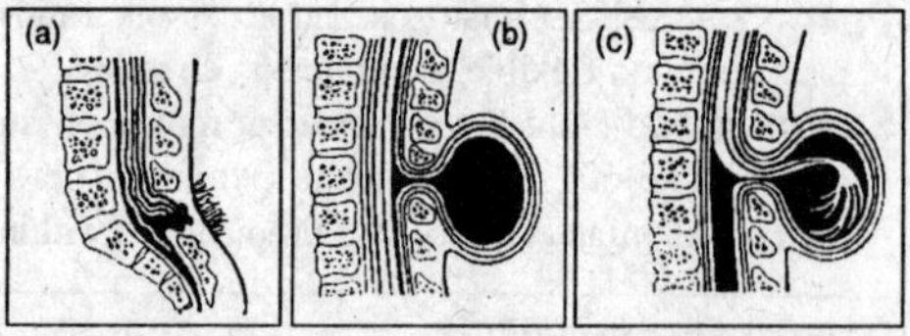

(a) Spina bifida occulta (b) meningocele (c) meningomyelocele

spina bifida. Meninges and nervous tissue develop normally.

Overlying skin remains intact. Deformity is usually common in lumbar and sacral area. It is present since birth. A depression in skin can be seen at the site of effect. There may be presence of tuft of hair over defect.

Spina bifida occulta Incomplete closure of lamina of one or more vertebra.

Spinabifida cystica with myelomeningocele The myelomeningocele contains spinal cord. The surface resembles a big ulcer with constant oozing. There may be associated hydyrocephalus. It can be surgically repaired and should be done with in 12 hours of birth.

Spinal anaesthesia It is a method of blocking pain sensations, before they reach the central nervous system by injecting an anaesthetic into CSF in spinal canal. The procedure is done by inserting a delicate needle between two vertebrae in lower part of spine. Because the nerves emerge from spinal cord and are bathed in CSF, they absorb anaesthetic agent. After it certain patients may develop headache.

It is similar to epidural anesthesia except that it is given directly into subarachnoid space.

Spinal arachnoiditis It may develope as a complication of disc surgery. The pain is very severe burning type, affects the back and one or both legs, is relieved by rest but is not readily relieved by analgesics.

Spinal cavity The space inside the spinal column through which the spinal cord passes.

Spinal cord It is a cylinder of nerve tissue about 18 inches long, thickness of a finger running down the central canal in spine. Actually it is a downward extension of brain. At the core of spinal cord is a region with a butterfly-shaped cross-

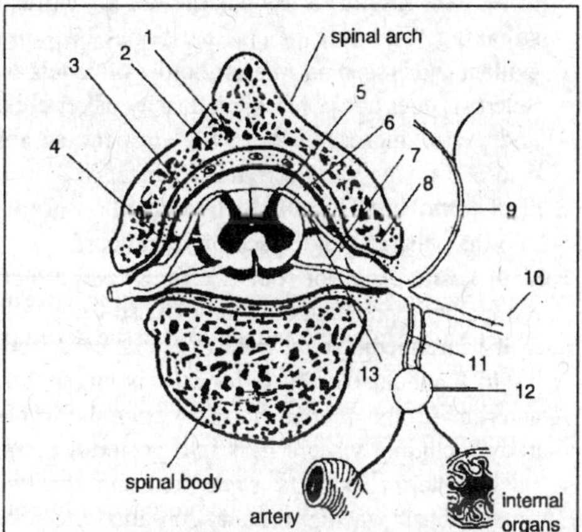

1. periosteium 2. epidural cavity 3. dura mater & arachnoid 4. subarachnoid space 5. spinal cord 6. dorsal root 7. ventral root 8. spinal ganglion 9. posterior ramus 10. anterior ramus 11. symapathetic communicans 12. sympathetic trunk ganglion 13. dentate ligament

section called grey matter. It contains the cell bodies of neurons. Some of nerve cells are motor neurons. Surrounding the grey matter are areas of white matter consisting bundles of nerve cell axons. Sprouting from the spinal cord on each side at two regular intervals are two nerve bundles : the spinal nerve roots which contain the fibres of motor and sensory nerve cells. Whole of spinal cord is bathed in CSF and surounded by protective sheath a continuation of meninges that protects the brain. Pressure on cord can affect movement and sensations. Injury can lead to a variety of pattern of paralysis and loss of sensation which are usually permanent because nerve cells and fibres within cord do not regenerate at all.

Spinal cord injury This is caused by traction on the arms in vertex deliveries or traction on the legs in breech extraction. Sometimes there may be complete cord injury when the flaccid paralysis is bilateral.

Spinal cord syndromes The spinal cord may be compressed by what is known as extramedullary lesion that takes up space in spinal cord. Such lesions may be extruded disc material and

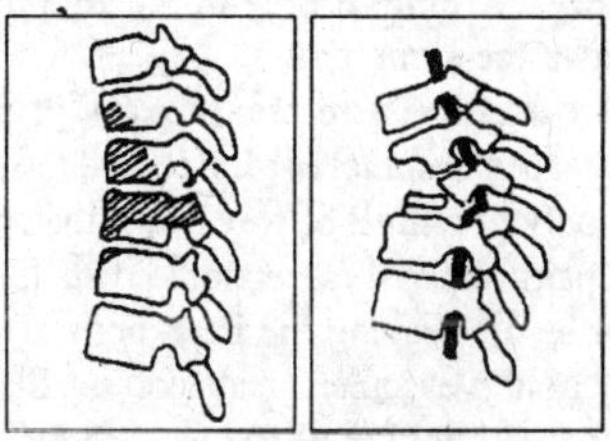

spondylotic bars. Lesions within spinal cord are known as intramedullary lesions such as astrocytoma. Severe spinal trauma causes haemorrhage within and compression and distortion from outside the spinal cord. There will be interruption of some sensory and motor functions below the level of lesion.

Spinal cord trauma It is usually caused by fracture and displacement of vertebra. Spinal cord may be crushed, overstretched, partially crushed, overstretched or completely transected. Resulting movement disorder is quadriplegia. High quadriceps who have injuries between C1 and C4 rarely survive because of respiratory depression. Damage at T1-T2 results in 'rocking horse' pattern. Lower cord damage below S1 results primarily in bowel and bladder incontinence and sexual impotence. Initially, victim experiences spinal shock in which a flaccid paralysis occurs.

Spinal fusion Surgical immobilization of adjacent vertebrae.

Spinal index A method of assecessing the size of lumbar spinal canal on plain X-Ray.

Spinal injury There may be damage to spine and even to spinal cord resulting in loss of sensation and muscle weakness or paralysis. Injury may be longitudinal compression, hinging and shearing. Damage to vertebra and ligaments usually causes severe pain and swelling of affected area. Damage to the spinal cord results in loss of sensation and/

or motor function. Damage below neck causes paraplegia while in cervical area results in quadriplegia. Pressure on spinal cord may result in muscle weakness, pain, tingling or burning sensation. Surgical repair of damaged nerve tracts in spinal cord is not possible. Recovery is usually complete when spinal cord has not been damaged although there may be some residual pain and stiffness. When there is pressure on spinal cord, surgery to remove the source of pressure can improve the symptoms.

Spinal nerves There are 31 pairs of nerves that connect to the spinal cord. Because the spinal cord runs only two-third of way down the canal lowest nine pairs showed travel some distance down the canal before leaving the back-bone. They form a spray of nerves called cauda equina. Spinal nerves consist of bundles of axons, i.e. long fibres of individual neurons i.e. nerve cells. Some of these fibres carry information from sensory receptors in the skin, muscles and elsewhere towards spinal cord. Other motor fibres carry information from spinal cord to muscles and glands. Damage, degeneration from diabetes, vitamin deficiency and poisoning can lead to neurological symptoms such as pain, numbness or twitching.

Spinal neural tube defect There are 3 main defects (a) Meningocele is herniation of the meninges, unaccompanied by the spinal cord. (b) Meningomyelocele is herniation of the meninges and spinal cord. (c) Myelocele is herniation of the spinal cord, without any protective covering. (d) Spina bifida occulta. There is a defect in the neural tube, but the skin is intact and the meninges and spinal cord are not herniated. It may be marked by a dimple in the skin or a tuft of hair.

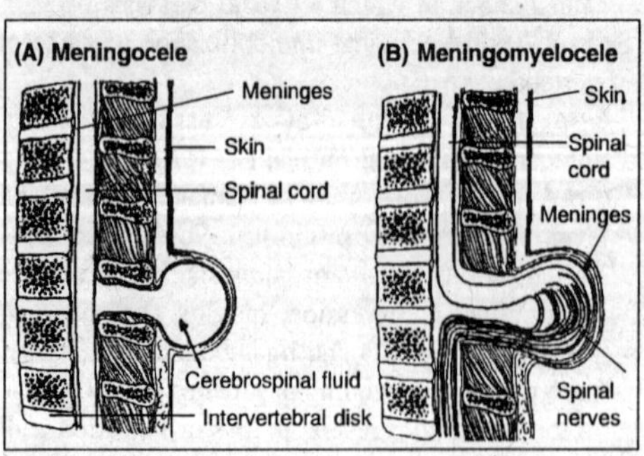

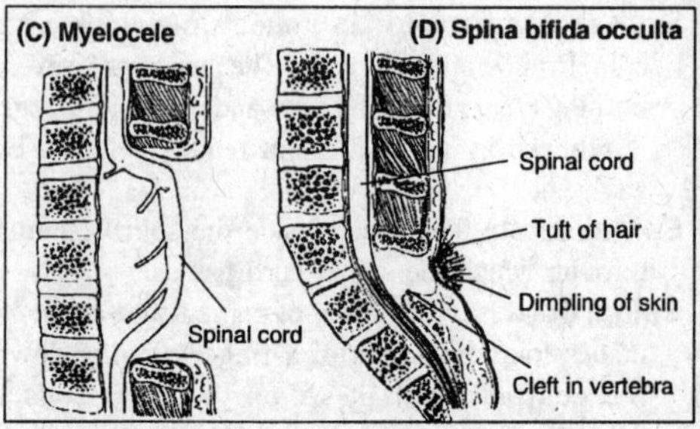

Spinal osteoporosis Resorption of horizontal trabeculae results in the appearance of vertical streaking. Thinning of cortical bones becomes evident and is seen on anterior border of vertebrae. Sclerosis does not increase but density of vertebral end plates increases. Vertebral trabeculae are resorbed giving picture frame appearance.

Spinal puncture The introduction of hollow needle into the subarachnoid space of spinal cord.

Spinal roots Anterior root is efferent and motor. Sympathetic preganglionic axons arise from cells in the intermediolateral horn of spinal cord from T_1 to L_2 inclusive. Posterior root is larger than anterior. All the afferent impulses from the whole body including viscera pass into posterior roots. Each posterior root has a ganglion and conveys fibres of pain, tactile, thermal sensation, deep or muscle sensation from bones, joints, tendon and afferents from viscera and vasodilator fibres.

Spinal segment The spinal cord is divided into segments by pairs of spinal nerves which arise from

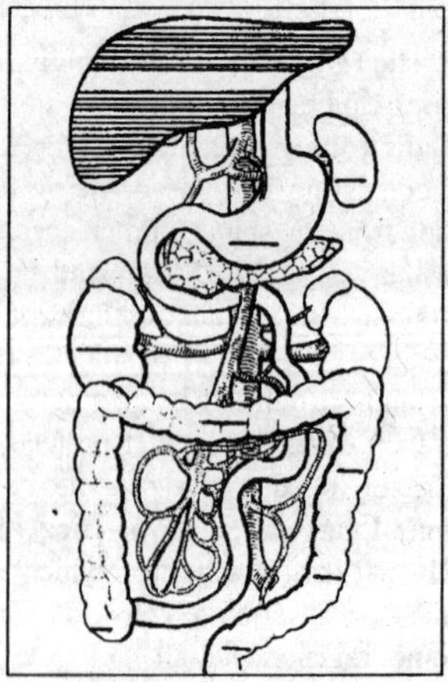

it. These pairs are 31 in number and are cervical 8, thoracic 12, lumbar 5, sacral 5, and coccygeal 1.

Spinal segments-abdominal viscera The spinal segments that receive afferent input from abdominal viscera are in general the same as those that contain the visceral efferent neurons.

Spinal shock This occurs immediately following the injury with abolition of volutary power, sensation and all reflex activity below the level of lesion. Recovery usually occurs after 24 hours of injury starting at distal cord. If recovery does not start within 48 hours prognosis becomes bad. Ankle jerks return within weeks. In case of spinal concussion there may develop neurological deficit.

Spinal stenosis It can be diagnosed on conventional films. The anteroposterior diameter measured from the posterior surface of the vertebral body to a line drawn through the base of the superior process of the spinous process should not be less than 15 m.m.

Spinal tap Procedure that involves insertion of a needle between lumbar vertebrae in the spine but below the spinal cord itself.

Spinal tracts The white columns of the spinal cord that provide two-way conduction paths to and from the brain; ascending tract carries information to the brain, whereas descending tracts conduct impulses from the brain.

Spindle cells Sensory receptors in the belly of the muscle that detect stretch.

Spindle fiber A network of tubules formed in the cytoplasm between the centrioles as they are moving away from each other.

Spine It is the column of bones and cartilage extending from base of skull to pelvis. It encloses and protect spinal cord. There are 33 roughly cylindrical bones called vertebrae. Each pair is connected by a joint called facet joint. This joint stabilises the vertebral column and allows movement in it.

Between two vertebrae lies a disc-shaped pad of tough fibrous cartilage. Peripheral nerves branch off from the spinal cord to every part of body, their roots passing between the vertebrae. Vertebrae are bound together with two long thick ligaments running the length of whole spine and by smaller ligaments between each vertebrae. In normal spine cervical sections curve forward, the thoracic sections backward, lumbar sections forward and pelvic sections backward.

Spine of tibia Tibial eminence.

Spinn barkeit Clear, slippery, stretchy quality of cervical mucous during ovulation.

Spinocerebellar Refers to all parts of the cerebellum rostral to the primary fissure; corresponds to the region of distribution of the spinocerebellar tracts.

Spinothalamic tracts Sensory (ascending) tracts that convey information up the spinal cord to the thalamus for sensations of pain, temperature, crude touch, and deep pressure.

Spinous process A sharp projection of bone or a ridge of bone, such as on the scapula.

Spiral blade angle The angle formed by the cutting edge of the blade and the long axis of the bur.

Spiral organ The functional unit of hearing consisting of a basilar membrane supporting receptor hair cells and a tectorial membrane within the endolymph of the cochlear duct; also known as the organ of Corti.

Spiritual health The cultural beliefs that give purpose to human existence. This belief may be found through faith in the teachings of organised religions in an understanding of nature or science or in an acceptance of humanization of life.

Spiritual well-being A sense of a inner peace, compassion for others, reverence for life, gratitude, and appreciation of both unity and diversity; It includes the conviction that there is a purpose and meaning in life, a relationship with God, and realistic views of adversity and loss.

Spirituality Generally encompasses a sense of relation of connectedness within oneself, others, nature, and God, or a higher power, that draws one beyond one-self.

Spirogrma A tracing or graphic representation of the depth and rapidity of respiratory movements.

Spirometer Gasometer used for measuring the volume of respiratory gases; usually consisting of a counterbalanced cylindrical bell sealed by dipping into a circular trough of water.

Spirometry Process of making pulmonary measurements with a spirometer.

Spironolactones Diuretic drugs that act as an alsosterone antagonist.

Splanchnic 'Visceral'.

Splayfoot Transverse spreading of the forefoot.

Spleen It is an organ situated in left upper quadrant which removes and destroys worn-out red blood cells and helps fight infection. It is covered with a capsule from which many fibrous bands run to give spleen a sponge-like structure. The spaces between bands are filled with lymphocytes and phagocytes and RBCs. It is richly blood supplied. It controls the quality of circulating red blood cells. It removes out all RBCs in 120 days after these have been produced in bone marrow. The other role of spleen is to help fight infection by producing some of antibodies, phagocytes and lymphocytes. In fetus spleen produces RBCs and after birth this function is being taken over by bone marrow. Still it is not very essential organ and if removed its function is being taken over by other lymphatic system. Spleen enlarges in malaria, tuberculosis, leukaemia, typhoid and haemolytic anaemia.

Splenenctomy It is indicated in rupture, torsion or extensive infarction, most cases of acholuric jaundice, splenic anaemia and thrombocytopenic purpura. It may be useful in abscess, tumour and single cyst of spleen. Persistent attacks of perisplenitis not responding to medical treatment favours surgery.

Splenic flexure Where the descending colon turns downward on the left side of the abdomen.

Splenium Refers to posterior end of corpus callosum.

Splenomegaly Enlargement of the spleen.

Splint It is a device to immobilise part of body. This may be made of wood, acrylic, plaster of Paris, aluminium or a rolled magazine even. It is used as a first aid measure to prevent movement of a fractured limb, finger injury, inflammation of tendon and rheumatoid arthritis.

Splinter skill A trained or learned skill that is acquired in a manner inconsistent with, or incapable of being integrated with, skills the individual already possesses.

Splinting Ligating, tying, or joining of periodontally involved teeth to one another to stabilize and immobilize the teeth, thus preventing them from begin adversely affected by occlusal forces. Splinting includes acrylic resin bite guards, orthodontic band splints, wire ligation, provisional splints, and fixed prostheses.

Splinting mallet deformity The finger is fully extended and dorsal joint does not extend. Splinting is done with an aluminium finger splint in slightly hypextended position.

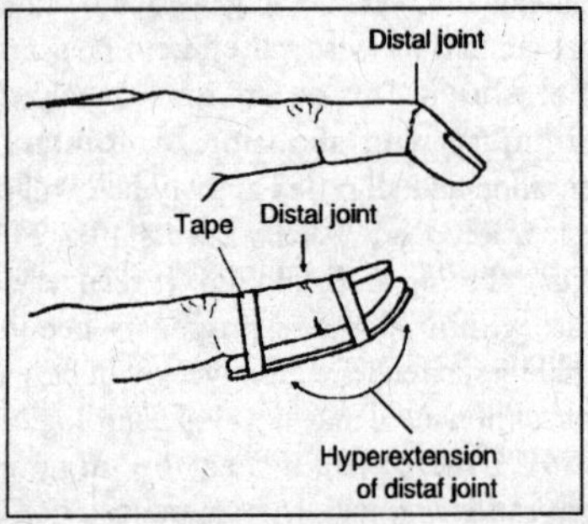

Split brain A condition in which the cerebral hemispheres are surgically disconnected by severing the corpus callosum and anterior commissure.

Split-brain technique A method or research, sometimes modified for use in therapy, where the corpus callosum is severed, leaving the two hemispheres connected essentially at subcortical levels only. When the optic chiasma is also severed, visual information presented to one eye is limited to one hemisphere, as well. Split-fitter technique in research, assigning the offspring of a litter to different experimental and control groups, thus providing animals of comparable heredity for each group of subjects when the mammalian stock from which the animals come is inbred.

Spondylarthrosis Arthrosis of the synovial joints of the spine.

Spondylitis An inflammatory disease of spine.

Spondylolisthesis There is slipping of above vertebra over lower one mostly common in lower lumbar vertebra. It generally develops due to

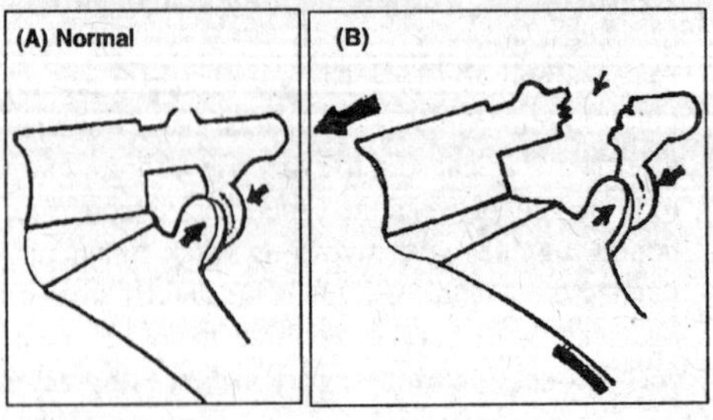

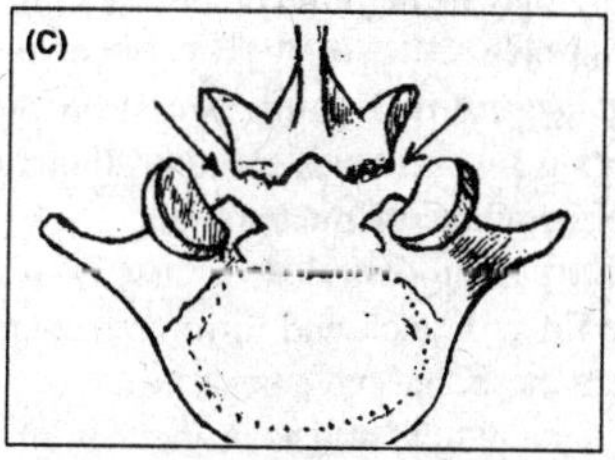

spondylolysis or to osteoarthritis. It results pain, while standing it becomes worst. Cervical spondylolisthesis may be caused by neck injury, rheumatoid arthritis or congenital abnormality of cervical spine. Main symptoms remain pain and stiffness in neck, numbness or weakness in sufferer's hands or arm. X-ray helps in diagnosis. Cervical collar and physical therapy help the person.

Spondylopathy Any disease of vertebrae.

Spondyloptosis One factor in agenesis is that the facet joints between L_5 and S_1 do not hook on to each other. This predisposes to spondyloptosis and

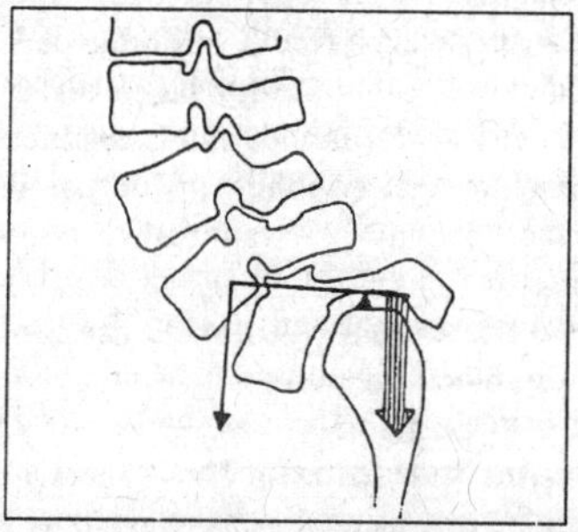

one notes that in this lesion the pars interarticularis is not broken but greatly elongated. There develops a hump back deformity with body of L_5 on its anterior slope. There is a tree lumbosacral kyphosis.

Spondylotherapy Therapeutic application of percussion or concussion over the vertebrae to elicit reflex responses at the levels of neuromeric innervation to the organ being influenced.

Sponge holding forceps It has oval-shaped tips which may or may not be serrated. It is used to hold the sponges to swab the cavities, i.e. vagina. It does not traumatise the part it holds. It becomes handy to hold cervix in suction or evacuation operation.

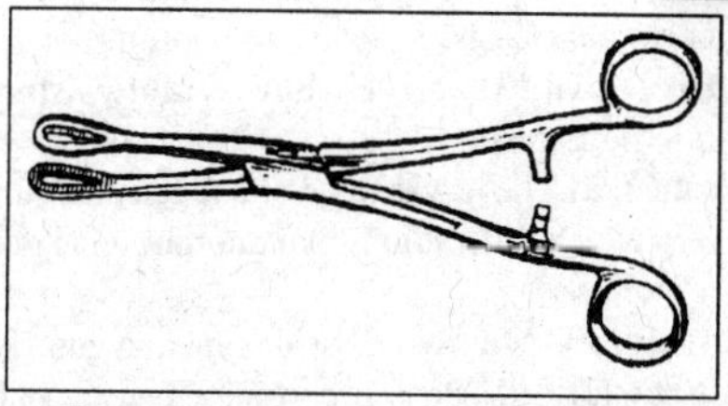

Spongy bone Porous bone in the end of the long bone, may be filled with marrow.

Spongy bone tissue Bone tissue that consists of an irregular latticework of thin plates of bone called trabeculae; spaces between trabeculae of some bones are filled with red bone marrow; found inside short, flat, and irregular bones and in the epiphyses (ends) of long bones.

Spontaneity Acting without effort or premediation; driven by internal forces.

Spontaneous abortion It is defined as interruption of pregnancy before the 28th week of gestation, the fetus is capable of independent existance after this period.

Spontaneous fracture A fracture occuring with little or no apparent trauma.

Spontaneous inversion of uterus There may be atony of uterus with fundal inversion with placenta attached. Sharp rise of intra-abdominal pressure may initiate it. Short cord or cord around the neck may start it. There may be severe hemorrhage.

Spontaneous pneumothorax It is the accumulation of air in pleural space. It may be due to trauma, rupture of subpleural emphysematous bulla. In closed type lung is automatically sealed due to fibrin clot or collapse of lung. In fistulous type communication occurs between bronchus and pleural sac. Here collapsed lung cannot re-expand. Onset is sudden during bouts of coughing.

Spontaneous remission In psychiatry, disappearance of symptoms without formal treatment.

Causes for their disappearance are assumed to exist but these are not yet knows.

Spontaneous uterine rupture Commonest cause of spontaneous uterine rupture is prolonged obstructed labour, impacted shoulder presentation, brow presentation and cephalopelvic disproportion.

Sporadic Describing a disease that occurs on an occasional basis.

Spore An inactive but viable state of microorganisms.

Sporocyst The larval stage of a digenetic trematode into which miracidium metamorphoses, usually in a mullusc.

Sporogony Multiple divisions of a zygote.

Sporotrichosis It is a chronic mycotic but self-limiting granulomatous infection caused by dimorphic fungus found in decaying vegetables and plant debris. It gives rise to chronic inflammation and granulomas that undergoes necrosis and results in formation of deep abscesses, sinuses and ulceration. There will be a small, nontender, movable, hard, subcutaneous nodule at the site of inoculation Lesion slowly enlarges in size. Ulcer intermittently discharges exudate. Inhalation of fungus gives rise to mild form of pneumonia.

Sporulation The process by which quiescent spores are formed from vegetatively growing bacteria, a response to nutrient depletion or stress.

Spot color test Qualitative microchemical analysis that is carried out in a drop of solution and results in the formation of colored products of the reaction of the substance under investigation with a particular reagent. The color obtained varies depending on the conditions of the analysis and the composition of the test material.

Spot Koplick Oral lesions of measles called Koplick's spots do not consist of vesicles. It consists of a few or a cluster of white or yellow white pin-point papules on an inflamed, red background on buccal mucosa. Under microscope one sees necrosis of epithelial cells and dense neutrophilic infiltration. German measles is not associated with Koplick's spot.

Sprain It is the result of tearing, stretching of ligament of a joint. Fibrous capsule that encloses the joint may be damaged. Ankle is mostly affected generally due to overgrowing the outside of foot so that complete weight is placed on the ankle. It causes painful swelling.

Movement increases the pain. X-ray is done to exclude the possibility of fracture. Treatment with ice-packs for 48 hours and anti-inflammatory drugs help the person. Only in very severe cases surgery may be required otherwise immobilisatio[n] of joint helps.

Spring ligament The plantar calcaneonavicular or spring ligament ties together the anterior and posterior pillars of medial arch.

Sprouting A process that occurs when remainin[g] nerve fibers branch and form new connections t[o] replace those that have been lost.

Sprue A small tube of wax or metal used to connec[t] a wax pattern to a crucible former, thus providin[g] a channel for molten metal to flow through durin[g] the casting process.

Spur Projection body as from a bone.

Spurling's test Clinical evaluation of cervica[l] radiculopathy.

Spurring The developing of spur.

Sputum It is the material produced by the cells lining respiratory tract. Sputum is released from glands in the walls of bronchi. Production of sputum increases by infection, or by an allergic reaction, and inhalation of smoke. Bacterial infection usually causes yellow or green sputum, an allergic reaction usually produces colourless sputum, and pulmonary oedema results in frothy, pink sputum. Blood-stained sputum may be caused by cancer and pulmonary tuberculosis. It is commonly called phlegm, mucus coughed up out of bronchial passages. It may be examined to diagnose the disease.

Spygmomanometer A device used to directly measure blood pressure.

Squamous Scalelike.

Squamous metaplasia The transformation of glandular or mucosal epithelium into stratified squamous epithelium.

Squamous suture The immovable joint between the temporal bone and the sphenoid bone.

Squatting In case of Fallot's tetralogy patient assumes a squatting posture after exercise in order to get relief from breathlessness. Squatting improves arterial oxygen saturation by increasing systemic vascular resistance thereby decreasing right to left shunt. It increases pulmonary blod flow. It traps desaturated blood in lower extremity.

Squeeze kneading In this technique, the tissues are pressed upward and lifted away from the underlying tissues, squeezed gently and then allowed to relax. The squeezing is produced by a "lumbrical" action of the fingers, the tissues being squeezed between the palm and the fingers.

Squeeze technique It is a method of treating premature ejaculation, preferably under the guidance of a sex therapist. The female partner stimulates erection, then squeezes or pinches the head of man's penis with her fingers as soon as he signals that ejaculation is about to take place. Repetition of this brings delay in ejaculation. This method is employed to treat premature ejeculation.

S-R psychology Focusing research upon stimulus-response relationships. Concerned with behaviour which is relatively independent of the conditions of individual organisms.

Stabile Not moving, stationary, resistant; opposite of labile.

Stabilisation The process of making something firm and steady.

Stabilised retinal image An image which, by use of special projector, always matches the eye movements and therefore presents unchanging stimulation to the retina. Eventually, the eye ceases to be responsive to this image.

Stability The ability to maintain a steady position in a weight-bearing, antigravity posture.

Stabilization Holding the body in a fixed position during joint movement, lengthening, and stretching.

Stabilizing boot orthosis Ankle-foot orthosis that includes an inner plastic foot plate and shell that maintains the foot in plantarflexion. The plastic component is worn in a flat-bottomed boot. This orthosis is intended for clients with paraplegia.

Stable angina This is a classical angina pectoris which is provoked by effort or exercise, relieved by rest or by taking nitroglycerine. ECG shows ST segment depression.

Stable v.s. unstable The degree to which people blame the cause of bad events on factors that are long lasting and relatively permanent or on factors that are more temporary and changeable.

Stages of eclampsia (I) Eyes become fixed with a sudden turning of head on one side. It is followed by rolloing of eyes and twitching of hands/face. Pupils are dilated. (II) In tonic stage patient becomes rigid, and arched. Face is distorted with clenched fists and legs are inverted. Patient is cyanosed and respiration stops; stage lasts for 15 to 20 seconds. (III) In clonic stage jaw begins to open and close violently and tongue may be bitten. Whole body assumes jerky movements. Froth tinged with blood are expelled from mouth (IV) Stage of coma is final.

Stagnation Inactivity; self-absorption.

Stainless steel Steel containing at least 12% chromium that forms a protective oxide coating keeping it frm corroding in aqueous environments such as the mouth.

Stainless steel crown Preformed steel crown used for the restoration of badly broken down primary teeth and first permanent molars.

Stalking A pattern of repeated harassing or threatening behaviour including following a woman, appearing at her home or office, making phone call or leaving written messages even in absence of serious harm.

Stance Time The stance time is the time (in seconds) that one foot is in contact with the support surface.

Standard care Level of care that can be expected of a professional.

Standard deviation The square root of the variance; expressed in the units of the original measure. A methematical measure of the dispersion or spread of scores clustered about the mean. In any distribution which approximates the normal curve in form, about 65% of the measurement will lie within one SD of the mean, and about 95% will lie within two SDs of the mean.

Standard error (SE) The standard deviation (SD) of a population of sample means, rather than of individual observations. The SE is calculated as the observed SD divided by teh square rood of N.

Standard error of measurement A measure of absolute reliability; represents the standard deviation of measurement errors.

Standard error of the mean The standard deviation of the sampling distribution.

Standard of care Predetermined level of care that is acceptable to the community of professionals.

Standard precautions Measures for reducing the risk of microorganism transmission from both recognized and unrecognized sources of infection.

Standardised procedures Clear and objective methods for the administration, scoring, and evaluation of a test.

Standardized mortality ration (SMR) The observed total events in the study groupk divided by the expected number of events based on the standard population rates applied to the study group. The constant multiplier for this measure is 100.

Standardized rates Crude rates that have been modified so as to allow for valid comparisons of rates. Standardization is usually necessary to correct for differing age distributions in different populations.

Standards for care Policies that ensures quality patient care.

Standing order One that is carried out until it is cancelled by the physician or until the prescribed number of doses have been given.

Standing tolerance The ability to stand for a given period of time.

Stapes The third of the three middle ear bones; attached to the oval window; the stirrup.

Staph A short from of staphylococcus, a category of bacteria that can infect the skin and other organs, sometimes seriously.

Staphylococcus Spherical or ovoid 0.8 to 1.0 micrometre. It is non-motile. It is gram positive, arranged in grape-like clusters in pairs, small groups or in short chain in liquid medium. It grows on ordinary culture media and may produce pigment. Strains vary to produce haemolysin and coagulase.

Staples Stainless steel wire used to close a surgical wound.

Stappling Any procedure that uses a bone staple for internal fixation.

Starch It plays in chlorophyll-containing plants the same role as glycogen does in animals. Starch is more complex than glycogen and is a mixture of two substances, amylase and amylopectin. Raw starch is insoluble in cold water due to resistance of outer cellulose layer of granule. When this layer is ruptured by heating in water, starch becomes soluble.

Starling's forces The force tending to move or retard a substance across a membrane as the result of the differences between hydrostatic and oncotic pressures.

Starling's hypothesis The idea that net filtration through a capillary is proportional to the transmembrane hydrostatic oncotic pressu difference.

Starling's law of the heart Force of contractio of cardiac muscle is a function of the length of i muscle fibres at the end of diastole; the great the degree of filling of the heart (the greater th venous return), the greater the force of contractio of the cardiac muscle.

Startle reflex The reflex which is present at bir till 4th month characterized by symmetric drawing up of legs and grasping of arms i response to a sudden jarring.

Startle response Generalized muscle twitch i response to sudden loud noise.

Startpoint The position on DNA that correspond to the first base transcribed into RNA.

Start-up costs The initial expenses involved i starting a business.

Starvation It is lack of necessary supply of flui and food for the maintenance of life. But if wate is taken regularly without food person may surviv from 20 to 30 days. After 4 to 5 days depletion o fat starts. An environmental condition in whic bacteria donot grow at all due to the lack of a essential nutrient.

Starvation promoters Promoters that ar selectively switched on during starvation or semi starvation conditions. Their sequences ar recognized by starvation specific RNA polymerases.

Starvation protein A protein whose level goes u in starving bacteria or that is uniquely synthesize in starving bacteria.

Stasis Stoppage of flow.

Stat order An order to be carried out immediately

State board of dentistry Group of individual responsible for the implementation of dental laws and rules within a state.

Static equilibrium The maintenance of posture in response to changes in the orientation of the body, mainly the head, relative to the ground.

Static labyrinth The utricle and saccule.

Static posturography Study of postural responses on an unstable platform.

Static-dynamic control The ability to shift weight onto one side and free the opposite limb for non-weight-bearing dynamic activities.

Statistic A characteristic of a sample; used to estimate population parameters.

Statistical inference The process of using a limited sample of data to infer something about a larger population of potentially obtainable data which has not been observed.

Statistical regression effect Same as Regression toward the mean.

Statistical significance A result is statistically signigicant whenever a significance test produces a P value less than the preset value of alpha, which is conventionally 0.05. The implication of statistical significance at an alpha of 0.05 is that chance would produce such a difference between comparison groups no more often than 5 times out of 100.This is taken to mean that chance is not responsible for the outcome.

Statistics The analysis of numerical data. Also, analyses pertaining to a sample, rather than a population.

Status asthmaticus Severe, prolonged asthma.

Status epilepticus It is defined as serial of seizures without recovery of full consciousness between them and long periods of hypoxia leading to cardiorespiratory problems. Status epilepticus may be the first manifestation of epilepsy.

Statute of limitations Designated amount of time within which a person can file a lawsuit.

Statutory law Law enacted by a legislative body; such a law must conform to state and federal constitutions.

Statutory rape Consensual sexual activity between a child who is below the age of consent and an adult. Activity usually involves sexual penetration.

Steady state A nonequilibrium state of a system through which matter is flowing and in which all components remain at a constant concentration.

Steatorrhea Stools with an abnormally high fat content.

Steeppage gait The high stepping walk seen in patients with a foot drop. There is footdrop during entire cycle.

Stein broker scale A four stage grading system for X-Ray evaluation of rheumatoid arthritis.

Stein-Leventhal syndrome The syndrome is manifested by menstrual abnormalities, hirsutism, infertility, obestity, hirsutism, and palpable enlargement of the ovaries.

Stellate cell A star-shaped neuron found in the central nervous system.

Stem cell A cell of embryonic origin that is able to develop along any cell pathway to differentiate ultimately into a pluripotential cell, then a progenitor cell, and then into a specific type of fully developed cell.

Stenosed valve A valve that has its opening narrowed or partially closed.

Stensen, canal Incisive canal.

Stensens's ducts The ducts of the parotid gland as they enter the mouth.

Stent A thin cylinder of crushed metal, inserted into the diseased artery, that has tiny, stainless steel scaffolds designed to reduce the chance that the artery will reclose after angioplasty.

Step Consists of two dimensions; a distance step length and step time; two steps comprise a stride.

Step duration The time (in seconds) between contraletral foot contracts.

Step length The distance (in centimeters) between heel strikes of conrralateral feet; normal range is 37.5 to 50 cm.

Step test Submaximal fitness test involving a timed stepping activity.

Step time The number of seconds between consecutive right and left foot contacts; both right and left step times should be measured.

Stepdown units Units for patients who were once in critical condition but have recovered sufficiently to require less intensive nursing care.

Stepping reflex The reflex, which is present at birth but disappears within 2 months, that causes infants to make little stepping or prancing movements when they are held upright with their feet touching a surface. Also known as dancing reflex.

Stereochemical theory A view of smell which assumes that the experience of an odour is based on the fit or congruence of various gas molecules with variously shaped "sockets" in the olfactory receptors. A rancid odour, for example, contains molecules of a specific shape, and they fit into a receptor socket of that shape.

Stereognosis The sense by which the form of objects is perceived, such as the ability to judge the shape of an object pressed against the skin.

Stereopsis Three-dimensional vision.

Stereotype A general description applied to all members of a given group or race without regard to individual differences. It may be a concomitant of prejudice.

Stereotypes Repetitive and often unusual motor movements.

Sterile Not able to reproduce; unable to produce offspring.

Sterile field A specified area, such as within a tray or a sterile drape. that is considered free from microorganisms.

Sterile gloves Sterile gloves are worn to avoid contaminating sterile supplies. Nowadays disposable gloves are available.

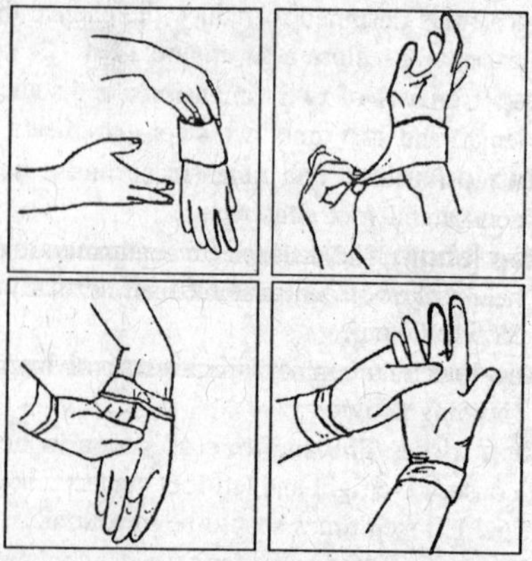

Sterile soak It is an application of moist heat over skin surface by immersing the part specially an extremity in hot water or medicated solution. It promotes drainage and reduces swelling. It applies medication in skin diseases and increased blood circulation to aid prevention of infection. It prevents cold injury like chilblain or frostbite by increasing circulation.

Sterile technique Practices that avoid contaminating microbe free items.

Sterilisation It is the term which refers the complete destruction and living of organisms or any procedure which renders a person unable to reproduce. Elimination of microorganisms is vitally important in preventing the spread of infection. It can be achieved by physical or chemical means such as boiling, steaming or autoclaving, irradiation with ultraviolet rays or using antiseptic or disinfectants. Liquids can also be sterilised by passing them through extremely fine filters which trap the microorganisms.

Sterilisation, female It is a permanent method of contraception in which fallopian tubes are sealed when families do not plan to have more children or when pregnancy may cause threat to woman's life. It can be done using laparoscopy or surgeon can work directly through a small incision just below naevus known as mini-laparotomy.

Sterility Infertility implies apparent failure of couple to conceive and sterility indicates absolute inability to conceive for one reason or other. Physiological sterility is present before puberty and after menopause. Physiological sterility during pregnancy is due to inhibition of ovulation. Total inability to concieve.

Sterilization Act or process of rendering sterile; the process of freeing from germ life.

Sternal angle The angle formed between manubrium and body of sternum.

Sternal line A vertical line corresponding to the lateral margin of sternum.

Sternal puncture It is done to remove some amount of red marrow from sternum by means of a sternal puncture needle.

Sternoclavicualr joint The direct point of attachment between the bones of the upper extremity and the axial skeleton.

Sternoclavicular Pertaining to joint between the sternum and clavicle.

Sternocleidomastoid "Strap" muscle located on the anterior aspect of the neck.

Sternocleidomastoid muscle An accessary inspiratory muscle that arises by two heads sternal and clavicular that unite to extend obliquely upward and laterally across the neck to the mastoid process.

Sternocostal The surface of the heart in contact with the sternum and ribs.

Sternotomy A surgical incision through the sternum.

Sternum Breastbone.

Steroid hormones Lipidsoluble hormones that pass intact through the cell membrane of the target cell and influence cell activity by acting on specific genes.

Steroid myopathy Muscle weakness predominantly proximal muscles secondary to long-term use to steroids.

Steroidogenic Relating to or involved in the synthesis of steroid hormones.

Steroids, anabolic It has an anabolic effect similar to testosterone and other sex hormones. These build tissues, promote muscle recovery, and helps strengthen bones. These help in anaemia and treat postmenopausal osteoporosis. These are widely abused by athletes. Side effects include acne, oedema, liver and adrenal gland damage, infertility and virilisation in women.

Sterols A class of lipids containing the steroid nucleus.

Steromicroscope A microscope consisting of two compound microscopes which are aimed at slightly different areas of an object.

Steropsis Three-dimensional vision.

Sterotoxic surgery These are brain operations done by inserting delicate instruments through surgically created hole in skull and guiding them using X-rays or CT scanning. It is used in pituitary gland tumour. In it either pituitary gland is cut or radioactive implant is inserted into the gland. It is used for brain biopsy and destruction of areas of brain to treat disabling neurological disorder. It is done under local/general anaesthesia. Area to be treated is located by CT and best position to insert instrument is calculated mathematically. Skull is entered by means of a burr hole and angle of frame is adjusted to hold and guide a hollow tube at the correct angle. Required instrument is then inserted through the tube and operation is done.

Stertor Snoring sound produced when patients are unable to cough up secretions from the trachea or bronchi.

Stertorous breathing Noisy ventilation.

Stethoscope The stethoscope was invented by Laennec in the 17th century as an aid in hearning the breath and heart sounds in the chest. The stethoscope comes in many forms and is used to enhance the listening of all sounds produced by human body. Principal use of it is for measuring blood pressure and listening heart and lung sound. It makes the sound clearer and louder.

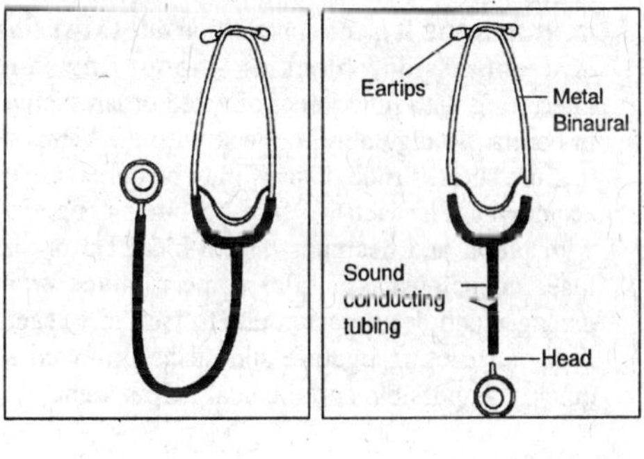

Stevens-Johnson syndrome A condition associated with erythematous-bullous eruptions of the skin, particulary of the genital area, blisters or erosions of the mucous membrane, fever and varying degree of constitutional symptoms.

Stiff neck It is called wry neck due to spasm of neck muscles. It is first noticed after waking. It may be due to ligament sprain or subluxation. It can also result due to disk prolapse or by a whiplash injury in cervical spine. It may result with headache, fever, photophobia and pain while bending the neck.

Stiffness Measure of resistance offered to external loads by a specimen or structure as it deforms.

Stigma Derived from the Christian tradition, stigmata refers to the blood on the palms and feet of Christ when nailed to the cross. A stigma is a social marker that labels people negatively as a deviant. Stigma may be about race, physical disability, sex and sexual orientation.

Still birth rate It is defined as the number of fetuses born dead after the 28th week of pregnancy per 1000 total births.

Stillbirth Same as Late fetal death.

Still-Chauffard syndrome It is characterised by arthritis of cervical spine, cutaneous pigmentation especially of the cheeks, anaemia, leucopenia, lymphadenopathy, and splenomegaly.

Stimulant These are the substances which stimulate the action of part of body. Amphematines are stimulants.

Stimulant drugs These increase nerve activity in brain by initiating the release of norepinephrine from nerve endings. There are two types of stimulants : *nerve stimulants* which reduce drowsiness and increase alertness by their action on alertness by their action on reticular activating system in brain, and *respiratory stimulants* which act on respiratory centre in brain. Nerve stimulants are given to treat narcolepsy. These also suppress appetite. These are generally abused because these prevent fatigue, increase alertness. Side effects include shaking, nervousness, sleeping problems, hallucinations, paranoid delusions and drug dependence.

Stimulation Excitation that activates the sensory nerves.

Stimulus Agent that causes a change in the activity of a structure.

Stimulus-induced analgesia Analgesia induced by electrical stimulation of the periaqueductal gray matter.

Stippled A term used to describe healthy gingiva; refers to the texture of an orange peel.

Stippling Rough surface texture.

Stipulate Where the parties to a lawsuit agree to a particular statement of facts and dispense with the need to produce evidence to formally prove those facts.

Stock supply Drugs kept in a nursing unit for use in an emergency.

Stockholm syndrome A syndrome in which hostages identify with, and have sympathy for, their captors on whom they are dependent for survical. Not uncommonly seen in terrorist-hostage situations.

Stokes-Adams syndrome It is a condition of complete ventricular asystole or standstill in a case of partial heart block. It is a complication of complete heart block. There will be headache, fainting attacks, unconsciousness and convulsions. If asystole is prolonged for more than 2 minutes death becomes inevitable. Pulse may be very slow 10 to 20 per minutes.

Stoma An opening, such as the opening creased in a colostomy procedure.

Stomach An expansion of the digestive tract between the esophagus and small intestine.

Stomach tube with funnel This is a plain thick-bore stomach wash tube having a funnel at the mouth end. There is one big opening at the lower and, This is used in food or drug poisoning case. Cleaning fluid is poured through the funnel and by a jug holding upright. The contents are drained out when the funnel is lowered below the level of stomach.

Stomach wash–poisoning Keep the witness or relative as an evidence being medicolegal case. Plain water or $KMnO_4$ water may be used. Remove first stomach content in clean sterilised bottle with proper labelling for medicolegal examination of poison. Then introduce $KMnO_4$ solution, later on continue flushing of stomach till the colour of $KMnO_4$ returns to its original colour. Leave 200 ml of $KMnO_4$ in stomach to neutralise any poison left.

Stomatitis Inflammation of the soft tissues of the oral cavity resulting from mechanical, chemical, thermal, viral, radiation, or allergic causes or as a secondary manifestation of a systemic disease; aphthous stomatitis refers to common cancer sore or recurrent ulcers of the mouth that appear to be a manifestation of recurrent herpes simplex.

Stool Waste eliminated from the colon.

Stopcock A value that controls the flow of fluid or air through a tube.

Storage granule A membrane-coated structure that contains a number of vesicles containing a neurotransmitter.

Strabismus congergent Deviating eye turns inward.

Strabismus divergent Strabismus in which deviating eye turns outward

Straight A colloquial term for heterosexual people.

Straight catheter Urine drainage tube that is inserted but not left in place.

Strain The dimensional change produced in a material or object in response to the imposition of a force; a change in length per initial length (i.e., mm/mm) stated as a percent change in dimension.

Strain hardening The process by which a metal becomes harder and more difficult to deform as a result of being strained beyond its maximum flexibility.

Strangulated hernia The infant is irritable and fretful. Pain is severe and patient has vomiting. He or she refuses feeds and respiratory rate is increased.

Strangulations It is the constriction due to twisting or compression, blocking blood flow and interfering with function of affected organ such as in hernia. Strangulation of neck with the hands or ligature such as rope or scarf may be deliberate or accidental. The victim's face becomes congested with blood and becomes purple blue. He or she loses consciousness. After some minutes brain damages and death occurs due to lack of oxygen. Any constricting ligature should be removed as quickly as possible and medical help sought.

Strapping It is an application of adhesive tape to apply on the part of body to exert pressure and hold the structure in position specially used in rib fracture. It is used to reduce pain and swelling caused by soft tissue injury such as muscle tears and sprains. It may be applied to a joint to prevent recurrence.

Strategic Actions International acts performed by a person directed toward solving identity and existential problems.

Strategic disclosure Disclosure that is meant to achieve social or interpersonal goals.

Stratified Arranged in layers, or strata.

Stratified allocation Assignment of patients to different risk groups on the basis of variables such as the severity of disease (e.g., stage of cancer) and age.

Stratified epithelium It is composed of more than 3-4 layers of cells. Cells nearest the surface are always flattened while the deepest are polyhedral. Deep cells are soft and multiply by karyokinesis. These are distributed in epidermis and covers anterior surface of cornea. It lines part of urethra and lines vagina. It protects against friction and injury.

Stratum A layer.

Stratum basal The deepest layer of the epidermis; consists of columnar cells that undergo mitotic divisions.

Stratum basalis The superficial layer of the endometrium (next to the myometrium) that is maintained during menstruation and gesation, and that produces a new stratum functional is following menstruation or parturition.

Stratum corneum The most superficial layer of the epidermis; consists of dead, squamous cornified cells that have undergone keratinisation.

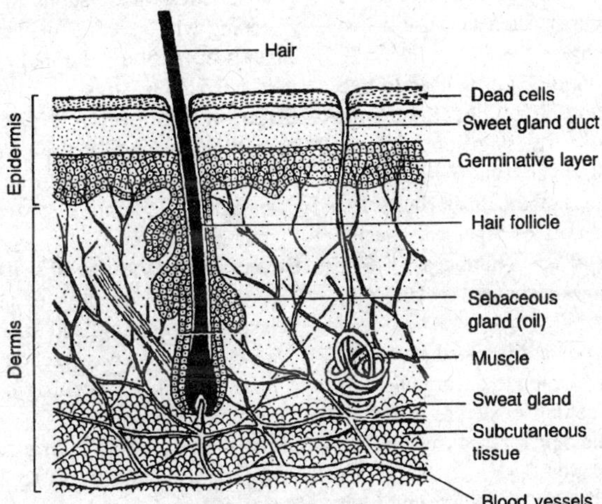

Stratum corneum

cholesterol esters, fatty acid and methyl steroids. The deposits are usually flat but may be raised and polypoid. It is known as cholesterolosis also and does not cause any symptoms.

Strength of association The degree to which variation in one variable explains variation in another. The greater the strength of association between variables, the more completely variation in one predicts variation in the other.

Strength training Contracting muscles against resistance to enhance muscle hypertrophy.

Stratum functionalis The deep layer of the endometrium (next to the uterine cavity) that is shed during menstruation, and that forms the maternal portion of the placenta during gestation.

Stratum germinativum The innermost of the tightly paced epithelial cells of the epidermis; cells in this layer are able to reproduce themselves.

Straw berry gall bladder It refers to pathologic change in gall bladder and cystic duct wall consisting of submucosal macrophages filled with

Strep throat It is an infection cause by *Streptococcus* group specially in children. Bacteria cause a few or no symptoms but symptoms may be sore throat, fever, malaise and enlarged lymph glands. Bacteria can be grown after throat swab. Penicillin and allied group of drugs effectively treat it. Untreated patients may develop glomerulonephritis and rheumatic fever.

Streptococcus It is a genus of spherical bacteria which tend to group together in strings or chain. These may cause bacterial endocarditis, pneumonia and scarlet fever and allergic reaction. One type causes sore throat. These respond to antibiotics.

Streptokinase It is a thrombolytic drug used to dissolve blood clots in myocardial infarction and pulmonary embolism. It is most effective in dissolving newly developed clots. Streptokinase will limit the amount of damage if given early. It may be given under supervision because it may cause excessive bleeding.

Streptomycin It is an antibiotic drug used to treat a number of uncommon inflections. Sometimes along with penicillin it is given to treat endocarditis. It was discovered in 1940 and was very effective drug against tuberculosis. Side effect includes damage of nerves of inner ear causing dizziness and ringing of ear. Numbness of face and tingling of hands, headache and malaise may develop.

Stress A psychological process initiated by events that threaten, harm or challenge an organism or that exceed available coping resources. Stress is characterized by psychological responses that are directed towards adaptation.

Stress carrier An individual who attracts high levels of stressors but more passively than the stress generator. It is more common in patient of depression and anxiety.

Stress echocardiography Two-dimensional echocardiographic studies during immediately after exercise to evaluate ishcemia-induced wall motion abnormalities noninvasively.

Stress electrocardiogram Test of electrical conduction through the heart during maximal activity.

Stress fracture It is a fracture that occurs as a result of repetitive trauma of bone. Common site is

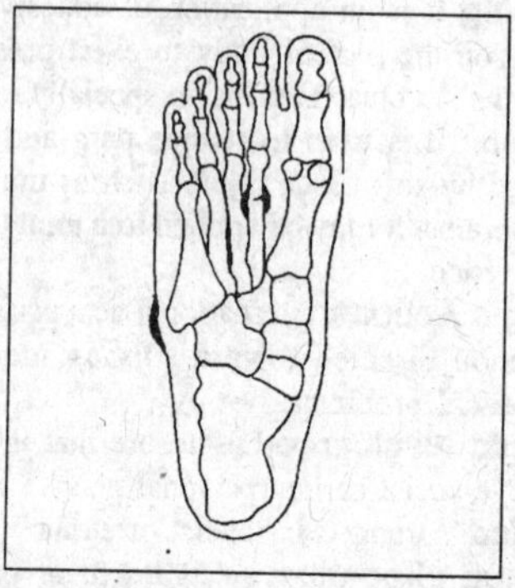

metatarsal bone in foot, neck of femur and skin of tibia. Main symptoms are pain and tenderness at the fracture site. X-ray helps in diagnosis. Treatment includes rest of part.

Stress generator An individual tendency to bring about stressful situations for others through poor coping with practical matters.

Stress hormone A hormone, such as cortisol, that is activated by stress.

Stress incontinence in pregnancy If occurs in multiparas due to laxity of pelvic floor muscles. There is dribbling of urine during coughing or sneezing. Reparative surgery may be done 3-6 months later on.

Stress incontinence of urine It is very common. A very small quantity of urine is passed while laughing, coughing and sneezing or while lifting a weight. It may be psychological too. A few may have genuine neurological lesions such as disseminated sclerosis.

Stress induced anorexia Decreased food ingestion secondary to a severe stressor interoceptive.

Stress induced eating Eating induced in response to an external stressor.

Stress management approach A set of diverse techniques for reducing psychosexual activation.

Stress management training A range of techniques with the overall aim of training people to recognise and cope with psychological stress.

Stress proteins A family of molecules produced by cells and organism under stress.

Stress response It is an interlinked set of reflexes basically designed to preserve life during injury and illness. The afferent side of these reflexes is frequently neural, e.g. pain sensation, and afferent side frequently endocrine. The response is immediate secretion of catecholamines, adrenaline and noradrenaline which generate fear and fight reaction. Pupils dilate, cardiac rate and output increases. Blood flow is diverted to muscles and muscle tone increases. Other endocrine changes include, aldosterone secretion causing retention of sodium. Antidiuretic chormone (ADH) secretion causes retention of water. Insulin secretion makes glucose available for energy. Steroids, renin, growth hormones are liberated.

Stress Urinary Incontinence This is manifested by urine loss during physical activities that increase intra-abdominal pressure. This increased abdominal pressure causes an increase in intravesicle pressure, which exceeds resistance, in the absence of detrusor contractions. A major factor in stress urinary incontinence is hypermobility or downward displacement of the urethra during exertion. It may also be due to the relaxation of pelvic floor muscles during the stressful events.

Stressor A demand placed on the family that produces, or has the potential of producing, changes in the family system.

Stressors Any internal perceptions or external stimuli that demand a change in the body.

Stretch To elongate; increase in length; The implied meaning is that it is not beyond the normal length of the muscle.

Stretch receptor Receptor in the walls of blood vessels, airways, or organs that monitors the amount of stretching.

Stretch reflex It is also known as extensor reflex. Knee jerk is an example. It is an important postural reflex. It is elicited by tapping the patellar tendon. This causes the sensory endings in neuromuscular spindles to be stimulated.

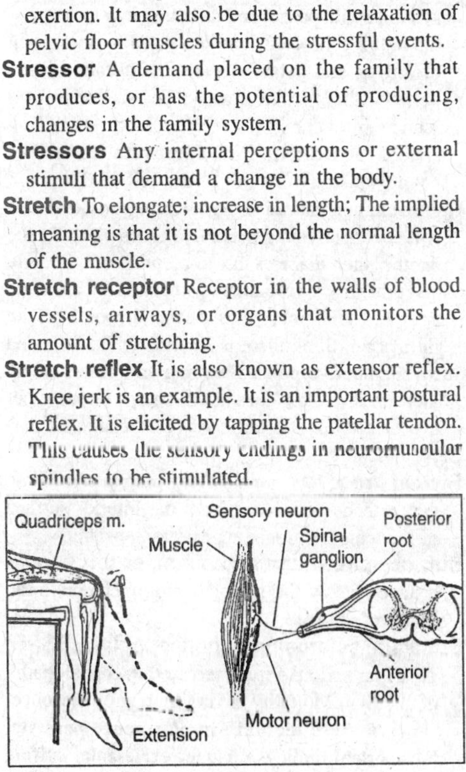

Stretch weakness Weakness that results from muscles remaining in an elongated condition, however slight, beyond the neutral physiological rest position, but not beyond the normal range of muscle length.

Stretcher It is a litter carrying an ill-patient who cannot walk. It consists of two long poles with

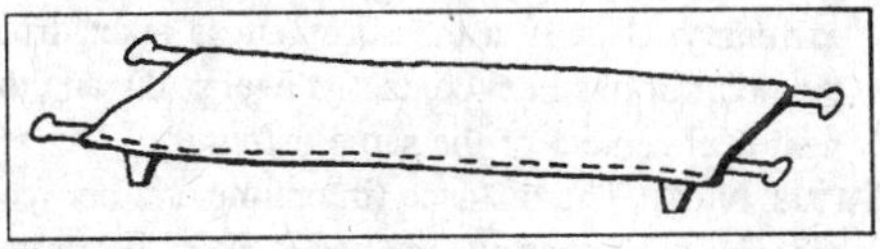

canvas slung between. It is carried by 2 persons. Nowadays beautiful aluminium made folding stretchers are available.

Stretching Separation of the origin and insertion of a muscle of attachments of fascia or ligaments by applying constant pressure at a right angle to the fiber of the muscle or fascia.

Stretching passive A type of mobility exercise in which manual, mechanical, or postional stretch is applied to soft tissue, and which the force is applied apposite to the direction of shortening.

Stretching, active A type of mobility exercise in which there is reflex inhibition and subsequent elongation of muscles, using neurologic principles to reduce tension and lengthen the contractile elements within muscles.

Stria Narrow band, e.g. stria terminalis originating in the amygdala.

Striae gravidarum Elongated streaks of red or pink often found on the abdomen and breasts of a pregnant woman; stretch marks.

Strial distenase It appears in second trimester. These are thin atrophic pink or purple linear bands found on abdomen, breasts and thighs. Striae are permanent but the pinkish colour fades.

Striate area (area 17) It is known as visuosensory area also. It occupies the walls of post-calcarine sulcus in front. Visual area is formed by interlacing dendrites of large stellate cells. It is the cortical receiving centre for visual impressions. This area recognises colour, size, form, illumination and transparency.

Striate cortex The primary visual cortex in the occipital lobe; it has a striped appearance when stained, which gives it this name.

Striatum Refers to caudate nucleus and putamen taken together.

Stricture Narrowed lumen.

Stride Consists of two dimensions; a distance stride length and a time stride time.

Stride Duration The time (in seconds) between ipsilateral foot contracts.

Stride length The linear distance between two consecutive foot contacts of the same lower extremity. Usually a measurement is taken from the point of one heel contact at heel strike and the next heel contact of the same extremity.

Stride Width The distance (in entimeters) between the midline of contralateral heel strikes; the normal range is 7.5 to 15 cm.

Stridor A high-pitched inspiratory or expiratory sound created by an obstruction to air flow, especially an obstruction occurring in the trachea or larynx.

Stringiness Palpable tissue texture abnormality characterized by fine or string-like myofascial structures.

Stripping the membranes The manual separation of chorioamniotic membranes from the lower uterine segment.

Strobila In tapeworms, a chain of segments formed by budding.

Strobilization The formation of a strobila by a tapeworm.

Stroboscopy To enable the collection of data for a series of time instants, one photograph may be produced with multiple exposures on it.

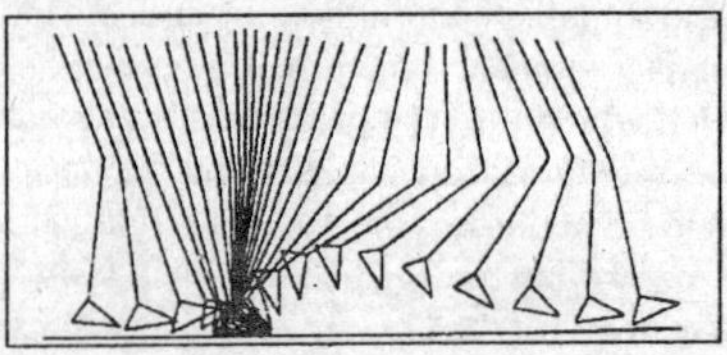

Stroboscopy involves a subject walking in front of a still camera taking multiple exposures. This produces the whole motion as one picture as a stick diagram, with the position of the limbs shown at equal time intervals.

Stroke A sudden and severe attack.

Stroke volume The volume of blood ejected from either the right or left ventricle during each heart beat.

Stroma The space and aqueous solution enclosed with the inner membrane of a chloroplast.

Stromal keratitis Inflammation of the deep layers of the cornea of the eye.

Structural bowing Involves actual bowing of the bones of the lower extremities; genu varum.

Structure of conflict Conflict of interest, the incompatibility of needs, desire or preferences.

Structured interview Oral administration of a written questionnaire without deviation from the wordings of the questionnaire.

Structured item In a questionnaire or inventory, test item which requests a highly specific answer. For example, the subject may be asked: "How many times do you use profanity each day?"

Strut chordae The specialized variants of rough zone chordae of the anterior leaflet of the mitral valve; leaflet chordae.

Strut volume The amount of blood ejected from the ventricles with each systolic contraction.

Stuttering It is a defect in speech characterised by hesitation. There is spasmodic repetition of some syllables with pauses and difficulty in pronouncing the initial consonants and is caused by the spasm of lingual and palatal muscles. It usually begins between the ages of 2 and 5 years. The parents who remind the child of his or her stumbling speech or ridicule him aggravate his or her emotional stress. So child loses self-confidence.

Stye Common causative organism is staphylococci. If it occurs in young person, in crops one after the another then diabetes has to be ruled out. In early stage of any stye patient complains of an acute pain and tenderness at a particular point on the lid margin. Soon there is oedema of lid followed by suppurative point. Swelling and abscess may increase if abscess does not discharge or pus is not evacuated. Pain subsides soon on evacuation of pus.

Stylet Metal guidewire.

Styloid process A pointed long projection of bone that extends downward from the inferior surface of the temporal bone; appears radiopaque.

Sub occipito bregmetic diameter It is 9.5 cms distance below the occipital protruberance to the center of sincipit.

Subacute sclerosing panencephalitis (SSPE) This is a serious virus-mediated encephalopathy of children. Mortality is very high and whosoever survive intellectual impairment persists. Postmortem findings include perivascular cuffing with lymphocytes and plasma cells. Gliosis is prominent. Those who develop SSPE are likely to have had measles at an early date. Cases follow immunisation with measles vaccine. The initial features are behavioural disturbances or a decline in school performance. The child is subsequently affected by myoclonic jerks, seizures, dysarthria and spastic weakness of limbs. Person becomes mute and rigid before death. Measles antibodies are present in high titre in blood and CSF. CSF contains high concentration of IgG.

Subacute sensorimotor polyneuropathy Patient first notices unpleasant sensations in the tips of toes or soles of foot. Sensations may be pricking, sore or burning. Abnormal sensations may spread to feet and involve toetips. Distal muscles may waste. Tendon reflex may become depressed. Discrimination between two points may be impaired. There is loss of perception of vibration. Pinprick may be felt less. Sense of joint position is lost.

Subarachnoid Between the arachnoid and pia matter, which are membrane layers of the brain.

Subarachnoid haemorrhage Most common cause is burst haemorrhage of aneurysm. Bleeding takes place in between arachnoid and pia mater. Space also contains cerebrospinal fluid which mixes with blood. It may occur without any head injury. An attack may cause immediate loss of consciousness or a sudden headache often followed by consciousness. Even if conscious, person may develop photophobia, nausea, vomiting and drowsiness. Treatment includes general life support and in certain cases angiomas can be surgically removed, blocked off or obliterated after a few days.

Subarachnoid space The fluid-filled space below the arachnoid layer covering the brain and spinal cord; contains cerebrospinal fluid.

Subchondral Below the cartilage.

Subclavian steel syndrome The syndrome presents with headache, dizziness, weakness in the arm, pain at rest, paraesthesia, periodic attacks of chocking sensation, diminished pulse on the affected arm, unequal blood pressure in two arms, and central nervous system involvement.

Subclinical Without clinical manifestations; said of early stages of a disease.

Subclinical hypothyroidism Conditions characterized by normal levels of circulating T4 and T3 but elevated levels of TSH. There is also an enhanced TSH response to TRH.

Subcoerulear nucleus One of the areas of the brainstem producing the paralysis of REM sleep.

Subcorneal pustular dermatosis It is a rare condition of superficial pustular dermatosis. Pathological changes show pustules just beneath the stratum corneum. It gives rise to superficial pustular blisters on the erythematous skin. The lesions appear on lower abdomen and are arranged in annular and serpiginous pattern. The pustules show sterile pus. Diagnosis is on clinical grounds.

Subcortical myoclonus There is generalised jerk. These may or may not be a cortical EEG correlate. First myoclonic response in muscles innervated by lower brainstem nuclei may precede the cortical discharge. It suggests that origin of events lies in brainstem reticular formation.

Subcultures Unique cultural groups that coexist within the dominant culture.

Subcutaneous Under the skin; same tissue as the hypodermis.

Subcutaneous injection By this method drug reaches blood stream by way of absorption from local site. Usually not more than 2 ml of drug is given by subcutaneous route. This route is

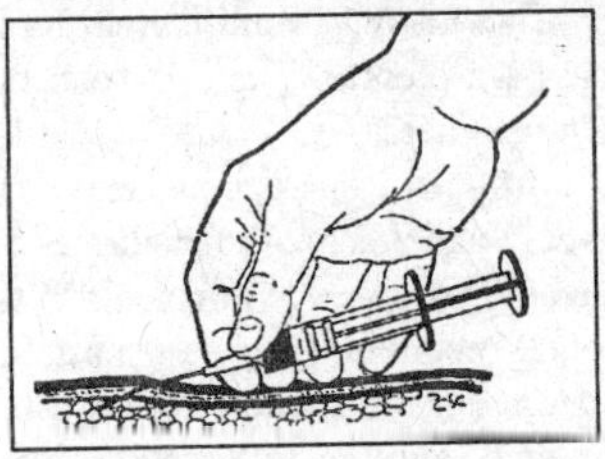

preferred when oral route is contra-indicated and rapid action is required. All hypodermic injections should be given in an upward direction towards head because this correspond to flow of lymph in lymphatic channel through which drug is carried to blood stream. It should not be given over joint. Insulin is given this way only.

Subcutaneous lipoma It is painless, soft, solid swelling. The lobules can be seen and felt on the surface and at the edge of the lump. Overlying skin is free. Edge is well defined and may have a series of irregular curves corresponding to each lobule. Edge of the swelling slips under the examining finger. Cutaneous dimples appear on the surface. Repeated trauma may result in necrosis, haemorrhage and calcification.

Subcutaneous tissue Tissue below the layers of skin; made up of loose connective tissue and fat.

Subcutaneous layer A continuous sheet of areolar connective tissue and adipose tissue between the dermis of the skin and the deep fascia of the muscle. Also called the superficial fascia.

Subdivision The largest phylogenetic grouping within a division. This grouping canbe considered analogous to a phylum, and includes one or more orders.

Subdural abscess It is often secondary to sinus or mastoid infection. The organisms spreading via the diploic veins without necessarily involving the vault. Once in subdural space the infection spreads rapidly. It results in thrombotic occlusion of many cortical veins. Progress is grave because it is difficult to eradicate pus. Residual neurological deficits are common in survivors.

Subdural effusion Subdural effusions are often associated with bilateral meningitis. These are small and regress spontaneously. Large effusion may produce increased intracranial pressure. Clinical features are non-specific. Subdural space enlarges. Convulsions, vomiting, irritability and drowsiness are present. There is persistent fever and heart size increases.

Subdural empyema Pus is collected in the space between dura and arachnoid membrane. Mostly it is unilateral. This space is infected due to spread from frontal, ethmoidal sinuses, mastoids, brain abscess or osteomyelitis. There develops high fever, headache and vomiting followed by mental and meningeal signs. Focal neurological signs appear depending up on area of pus collection and include convulsion, hemipareasis or aphasia. Papilloedema is present in many patients.

Subdural haematoma Extra-vasated subdural blood results from tears in the superficial veins or venous sinus or brain contusions. The blood spreads over cerebral hemispheres. There may be associated parenchymal tissue damage on third day. SDH have an initial lucid interval with subsequent neurological deterioration. 40% patient do not become unconscious to start with. Motor dysfunction and pupillary dilatations are characteristic. Peneal shift is not seen.

Subdural haemorrhage There is bleeding into space between dura mater, the tough outer layer of meninges and the arachnoid. The trapped blood forms a haematoma. Common cause is torn veins following a blow.

Bleeding occurs slowly and it may take weeks before the haematoma enlarges. Symptoms tend to fluctuate and consist of headache, episodes of confusion, drowsiness and one-sided weakness. CT scanning is a better tool to diagnose it.

Subendocardial infarction Injury to the subendocardium and adjacent tissue; nontransmural.

Subepithelial fibrosis Fibrosis occurring beneath the epithelium.

Subfalcal herniation Displacement of brain tissue beneath the flax cerebri.

Subgingival Below the gingival margin.

Subhyoid bursal cyst It is the accumulation of infllammatory fluid giving rise to cystic swelling of subhyoid bursa.

The subhyoid bursa is situated over the thyroid membrane below the hyoid hone slightly posterior to its lower border.

There is history of painful onset with features of mild inflammation. It moves with deglutition but there is no protrusion of tongue. It is cystic in feel. Transillumination test is negative. Complete excision is the treatment.

Subiculum Refers to transitional zone between six layered parahippocampal gyrus and three-layered hippocampus.

Subject An individual who participates in an experiment and whose responses are the dependent variables of the experiment.

Subjective data Information that only the patient feels and can describe.

Subjective fatigue A need for rest which is caused by psychological factors, not physical ones; usually caused by repetition of the same behaviour. The fatigue is said to be subjective when a different response can be performed readily using the same muscles.

Subjectivity A condition known only to the individual concerned; not directly observable by other; private. A pain is subjective; the person's behaviour response to pain is objective.

Sublethal Of an injury or condition, significantly damaging but not fatal.

Sublethal injury The temporary loss in a microorganism to tolerance for specific conditions.

Sublimation A process whereby a material changes from the solid to vapor phase without going through a liquid phase. A defence mechanism, operating unconsciously, by which instinctual drives, consciously unacceptable, are diverted into personally and socially acceptable channels.

Subliminal infection An infection in which the virus multiplies in the originally infected cell but is unable to spread to adjacent cells.

Sublingual Under the tongue, referring to a parenteral route of a drug administration; also subglossal or hypoglossal.

Sublingual adminstration Placing of a drug under the tongue to dissolve and to be absorbed through mucous membrane.

Sublingual application Placement of a drug under the tongue.

Sublingual calculus Calcium deposited on the tooth structure and found apical to the gingival margin. These are more darker and denser than supragingival calculus.

Sublingual gland One of a pair of salivary glands situated in the floor of the mouth deep to the lingual frenulum, with a duct that opens into the floor of the mouth.

Sublingual route A few specific drugs like amylnitrate or nitroglycerine are usually administrated under tongue to produce its effect in case of heart patients with anginal and ischaemic pain.

Sublingual sulcus Groove under tongue.

Subluxation A complex of functional and/or structural and/or pathologic articular changes that compromise neural integrity and may influence organ system function and general health.

Submandibular calculi Patient complains of pain and swelling at the submandibular region, beneath and in front of angle of jaw aggravated by food specially sucking of lemon. The gland gets tense and tender. At first attacks are transient and gland quickly resumes its normal size but in course of time it increases permanently. A stone impacted in duct may produce referred pain in the tongue due to irritation of lingual nerve as it hooks around submandibular duct. Shape is oval or flattened and overlying skin is usually normal and freely mobile over the swollen gland. Gland can be moved from side to side. Glands becomes less mobile. X-ray will show radiopaque shadow. Excision of the swelling is the choice of treatment.

Submandibular fossa A depressed area of bone along the lingual surface of the mandible; appears radiolucent.

Submandibular gland It is a mixed mucus and serous in type, consists of large superficial part

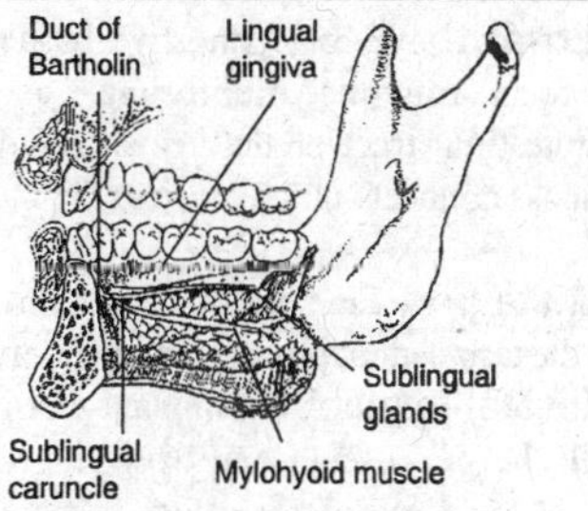

Submandibular and sublingual glands

and a small deep part which are continuous with one another round the free posterior margin of mylohoid muscle.

Submandibular nodes These lie near or in the submandibular gland between mandible and myelohyoid muscle. Afferent vessels come from lips, cheeks, anterior part of scalp, eyelids and side of tongue. On their infection, glands become enlarged.

Submandibular shadow An artefact seen on a panoramic film; appears as an area of increased radiolucency below the mandibular posterior teeth.

Submaxillary caruncle The orifice of sublingual duct that opens into mouth on a small papilla.

Submaximal fitness test Exercise test that does not stress a person to exhaustion.

Submaximal treadmill testing An exercise protocol with the endpoint being less than the maximal potential.

Submento bragmetic diameter It is 9.5 cms measuring from below of chin to the surface of bregma. This diameter is presented during face presentation.

Submento vertical diameter It is 11.5 cm extending from the point where the chin joins the neck to the highest point on vertex.

Submerged tooth One which is below the line of occlusion and may be ankylosed, intrusion, infraocclusion.

Submersion A healing protocol in which an endosteal implant is placed within bone and covered with gingiva, with no portion protruding, allowing for afunctional healing to promote the osteointegrated mode of tissue integration.

Submersion injury Injury resulting from a near-drowning incident. Injury may appear even up to 48 hours.

Submucosa A layer of connective tissue located deep to a mucous membrane, as in the gastrointestinal tract or the urinary bladder; the submucosa connects the mucosa to the muscularis layer.

Subordinate part Element of movement without which the task cannot proceed safely or efficiently.

Subperiosteal implant An implant that is placed beneath the periosteum and overlying the bony cortex at the time of insertion, to be sheathed ultimately by dense fibrous connective tissue contiguous with the outer layer of the periosteum to function in the periosteal mode of tissue integration.

Subscribe Person, usually the employee, who represents the family unit in relation to the prepayment plan. Other family members are dependents.

Substance abuse Use of a drug for the psychological and behavioral changes that it produces aside from its therapeutic effects.

Substance dependence Desire for a drug manifested by frequent use of the drug.

Substantia Substantia gelatinosa of the spinal gray matter.

Substitution A defence mechanism, operating unconsciously, by which an unattainable or unacceptable goal, emotion, or object is replaced by one that is more attainable or acceptable.

Substitution mutation A mutation caused by the replacement of one base by another.

Substraction radiography Use of a computer to compare a series of radiographs or printed images of an area and indicate differences between them.

Substrate In enzymatic reactions, the molecules that combine with the amino acids lining the active sites of an enzyme and are converted to products by catalysis of the enzyme.

Subtle energies Weak electrical fields that surround and run through the body.

Subtotal Incomplete.

Succedaneous Referring to teeth that replace the deciduous teeth after they have been shed.

Succenturiate placenta It is an anomally in which one or more small accessory lobes of placenta develop in the membranes at a distance from the main placenta. A sucenturiate lobe.

Success criteria Condition established by a study protocol for the evaluation of a procedure as a sucess.

Succint Brief but complete.

Suck To draw usually liquids into the mouth by movements of the tongue and lips, creating a suction or a partial vacume.

Sucking The reflex in infants to suck anything that comes in contact with their lips. It seems to be a great need for the first 2 months of life, is present while sleeping, and need not be nutritive.

Suckle To draw liquids into the mouth by a forward and backward movement of the tongue as is done during breastfeeding.

Suckling Giving or taking nourishment from breast.

Suck-swallow-breath synchrony A skill used continuously throughout life that allows an individual to breath while simultaneously and unconsciously sucking in and swallowing food, drink, or saliva; a skill whose disruption can interfere profoundly with development.

Sucrose Crystaline disaccharide carbohydrate found in many plants, mainly sugar cane, sugar beet, and maple, and used widely as a sweetener, preservative, and in the manufacture of plastics and cellulose.

Suctioning Technique for removing liquid secretions with a catheter.

Suction catheter Thin plastic or rubber tubing used to remove secretions.

Sudden cardiac death Death within 1 hour of the onset or cardiac symptoms; the primary cause being the cardiac arrest.

Sudden death When obviously healthy person dies suddenly. The most common cause is cardiac rrest. Elderly people may be having coronary eart disease. It may happen in people suffering rom myocarditis or as a result of stroke. Regular heck-up gives a warning of the underlying lisease.

dden infant death syndrome (SIDS) Jnexpected and unexplained death of an apparently well, or virtually well, infant; death usually occurs during sleep.

dden vestibular failure It may result due to skull fracture or viral infection. Syndrome can follow sudden occlusion of anterior vestibular artery. Other causes include multiple sclerosis, varicella zoster infection, brainstem encephalitis and diabetic neuropathy. There will be sudden onset of vertigo, nausea and vomiting followed by gradual recovery of balance. Nystagmus may develop.

dden weight gain in toxemia pregnancy It may be the first warning sign in many cases. Weight gain of 1 kg in a week gives suspicion. More than this is attributed to abnormal fluid retention and is known as fulminating type of toxaemia pregnancy.

doriferous gland An exocrine gland in the dermis or subcutaneous layer that produces perspiration. Also called a sweat gland.

et Hard fat around kidneys.

ffer A substance that can help a solution to resist or counter act changes in free acid or alkali.

ffering State of severe distress associated with events that threaten the intactness of the person. The state may or may not be associated with pain.

fficient cause Precedes a disease and has the following relationship with it. If the cause is present, the disease will always occur.

uffix A word element placed at the end of a root word to change the meaning of the word.

uffocation It is due to prevention of passage of air in and out of lungs. Person may become unconscious. It may develop due to choking.

ugar alcohols Nutritive sweeteners related to carbohydrates by which provide 4 kcalories per gram; includes sorbitol, mannitol, and xylitol.

ugar free Saccharin is nonnutritive sweetner without calories. Aspartum has same calories as sugar but only a small quantity is required to provide desired sweetness.

Suggestibility Uncritical compliance or acceptance of an idea, belief, or attribute. The degree to which a person's attitude or opinions are easily swayed by the expressed opinions of others.

Suggestion The process of influencing a patient to accept an idea, belief, or attitude suggested by the therapist.

Suicide It is taking one's own life. It is a cry to get help. These are all frustrated and emotional people. It is a cowardice act to end one's own life.

Suicide gesture A suicide attempt that is taken primarily to get attention rather than to actually end ones life.

Suicide inhibitor A relatively inert molecule that is transformed for an enzyme, at its active site, into a reactive substance that irreversibly inactivates the enzyme.

Suicide threat A statement of behaviour that usually occurs prior to overt suicidal activity.

Suit Civil court proceeding where one person seeks damages or other legal remedies from another.

Sulcular fluid Crevivular fluid; characteristic fluid in the gingival sulcus that is similar but not identical to tissue fluid.

Sulcus A groove on the surface of the brain between gyri.

Sulcus temperature gauge Device that electronically measures and records the temperature of the sulcular fluid.

Sulkowitch test In this test when Sulkowitch reagent containing solution of distilled water with oxalic acid, glacial acetic acid and ammonium oxalate is added to urine, it produces milky precipitate of calcium oxalate if the urine contains calcium. The test is done to determine urinary calcium as in hypoparathyroidism.

Summarization Reworking a lengthy in teraction or discussion into a few brief sentences.

Summation The addition of the excitatory and inhibitory effects of many stimuli applied to a neuron.

The increased strength of muscle contraction that results when stimuli follow one another in rapid succession.

Summation effect The normal blending together of the various densities of the soft tissues that overlie one another in a radiograph.

Sump tube One that contains a double lumen.

Sun protection factor There are three types of ultraviolet rays : *UV-A rays* have longer wavelengths. These can penetrate deep into layers of your skin gradually destroying the elasticity and causing premature ageing. While *UV-B rays* are shorter sun rays known as burning rays. These are dangerous to unprotected skin and can alter the structure of skin cells and may even cause cancer. *UV-C rays* are absorbed before it ever reaches us by the earth's own sunscreen, the ozone layer in upper atmosphere. Sun protection factor ranges from 2 to 20+. The number denotes the amount of time. You can stay in the sun without burning while bearing sun screen. Fair skin needs more protection from sun. Nowadays Shalaks pharmaceuticals have produced reliable tube UV AVO 25+UV/UV Dew SPF 15+ for fair skin and UV dew SPF 10+ for dark skin to be applied before going in sun.

Sunburn Persons who burn easily should use a preparation with Sun protection factor (SPF) 15 to 20. It will reduce or prevent tanning as well as burn. Lower lip receives a substantial dose of UV but may be neglected when sunscreen is applied. Sunscreen can cause allergic dermatitis. Severe case is helped by hydrocortisone.

Sundown syndrome Onset of disorientation as the sun sets.

Sunrise syndrome Early-morning confusion.

Super fecundation It is the fertilization of two different ova by sperm from different fathers within a short period of one another.

Super fetation It is the fertilization and imbedding of a second ovum in the uterus already occupied by one in the process of development. After 12 weeks superfetation is not possible.

Superantigen Any of a number of soluble proteins that are secreted by bacteria and bind to the major histocompatibility complex of T lymphocytes. This stimulates a massive antigen-independent proliferation of T lymphocytes.

Superfecundation It is the fertilisation of two ova at same period of ovulation by two separate acts of coitus committed at short intervals. Both ova do not always develop to maturity. One fetus may die and be retained until the labour that expels the other.

Superfetation It is the impregnation of an ovum belonging to subsequent period of ovulation after the ovum discharged from a previous ovulati has been developing for a month or more. This not possible after 3 months of pregnancy.

Superficial Toward or on the surface.

Superficial burn A burn injury that extends o through the epidermis.

Superficial fascia A continuous sheet of fibr connective tissue between the dermis of the s and the deep fascia of the muscles. Also cal subcutaneous layer.

Superficial palmar arch It is formed by branch of ulnar and radial artery supplying the palm. Pa is very vascular.

Superficial pressure Pressure that remains on t skin.

Superficial stroking It is usually slow and gen but firm enough for the patient to be conscious the passage of the hand throughout the moveme when given in this manner, the stroke is extreme relaxing for the patient.

Superinfection The subsequent infection of a viru infected host by a second virus.

Superior In a direction above or higher than specified point.

Superior foramina of the incisive canal Tv tiny openings in bone located on the floor of t nasal cavity; appears radiolucent.

Superior laryngeal neuralgia Patient presen with unilateral, paroxysmal, stabbing pain in t region of larynx, radiating to the side of neck. Ent site of superior laryngeal nerve in the thyrohyo membrane is very tender.

Superior mesentric artery It arises from anteri aspect of abdominal aorta a short distance belo the celiac artery at the level of L_1. Superi mesentric vein lies to the right of the artery.

Superior olivary complex A group of audito nuclei in the medulla concerned especially wi the location of the sources of sounds.

Superior pulmonary veins The veins that retur blood from the left upper, right upper, and midd lobes of the lungs to the left atrium.

Superior rectus forceps It is used to hold th superior rectus muscle to pass a suture so that th

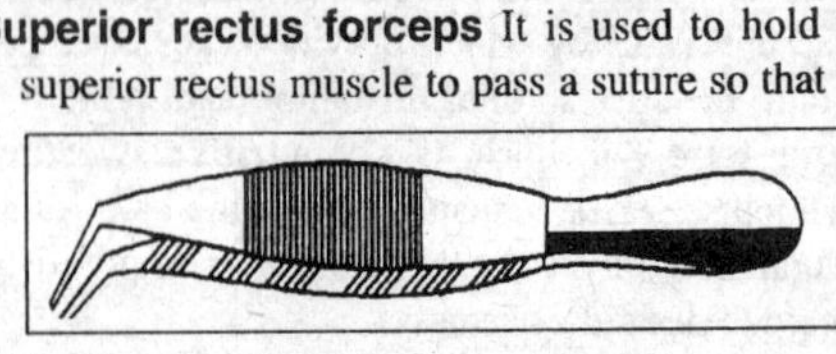

eye can be made to look downwards during surgery for cataract and glaucoma. Any tooth forceps can be used for this purpose, if this forceps is not available.

Superior thoracic aperture syndrome This is a condition characterised by pain, paraesthesia and muscular wasting of upper extremity due to some pathology at thoracic outlet due to cervical rib. There may be angulation of or compression of the artery and or of the first thoracic nerve. Patient may complain of pain or tingling and numbness along the ulnar side of hand and forearm. Pain becomes worst on carrying a heavy weight. In addition to sensory disturbances there may be performing fine actions and later wasting of small muscles of hand.

Vasomotor disturbances include coldness of fingers, periodic changes in skin colour, cyanosis, excessive sweating and trophic changes with ulceration. Rarely there may be gangrene of tips of fingers.

Superior vena cava Receives blood from the head, neck and upper limbs and empties into the right atrium of the heart. One of two large veins returning deoxygenated blood to the right atrium.

Superior vena cava syndrome It consists of oedema and engorgement of the vessels of the face, neck and arm, puffiness of the face, cough, dyspnoea, and flashing of the head and neck.

Superior vesical arteries The remains of the proximal portions of the umbilical arteries of the fetus; supplies the superior portion of the bladder.

Supernumerary tooth Extra tooth; one which is in excess of the normal number.

Superoxide radical Oxygen free radical which causes cell damage.

Supinate To turn the palm of the hand upward; opposite of pronate.

Supination To place something on its back rotation of the forearm so that the anterior surface is anterior, starting in the anatomical position.

Supine Position of the body lying on the back with the face up.

Supine hypotensive syndrome A condition in which the blood pressure is lowered and bradycardia occurs when the pregnant woman is in the supine position. Caused by compression of the inferior vena cava by the pregnant uterus.

Supine position Position in which the person lies on the back.

Supplemental groove Small groove on the occlusal surface of tooth.

Supplementary speech area A region on the dorsal surface of the left frontal lobe that takes part in the production of speech.

Supportive psychotherapy A type of psychotherapy that aims to reinforce a patient's defences and help suppress disturbing psychologic material. Supportive psychotherapy utilises such measures as inspiration, reassurance, suggestion, persuasion, counselling, and re-education. It avoids probing the patient's emotional conflicts in depth.

Suppositious child This is a false child, not conceived but claimed by a women as her own. A woman may substitute a living one for a dead child. She may feign pregnancy and produce a false child after a faked delivery.

This is done for extorting money or for the purpose of claiming property.

Suppository A solid form of medication inserted into a body cavity e.g., the rectum or vagina. The drug is absorbed after it dissolves in the cavity.

Suppository, contraceptive A suppository containing a spermicide that is inserted in the vagina prior to intercourse for purposes of contraception.

Suppression The conscious effort to control and conceal unacceptable impulses, thoughts, feelings, or acts.

Suppression of lactation Important indication for suppression of milk is stillbirth. Stilboestrol 5 mg thrice daily for 2 days is followed by lower doses for 3 days. Administration of oestrogen is not recommended.

Suppressor T cell A subpopulation of T lymphocytes that acts of inhibit the production of antibodies against specific antigens by B lymphocytes.

Suppressor mutation A mutation that totally or partially restores a function lost by a primary mutation; located at a site different from the site of the primary mutation.

Suppuration The formation of pus.

Suprabony pocket Pocket with base above the level of the alveolar crest.

Suprachiasmatic nucleus A nucleus, located just above the optic chiasm, that is the main pacemaker of circadian rhythms.

Supraclavicular Area above the clavicle.

Supracondylar fracture This is the most common injury in children. There is side to side mobility of the lower fragment with crepitus. Shortening of

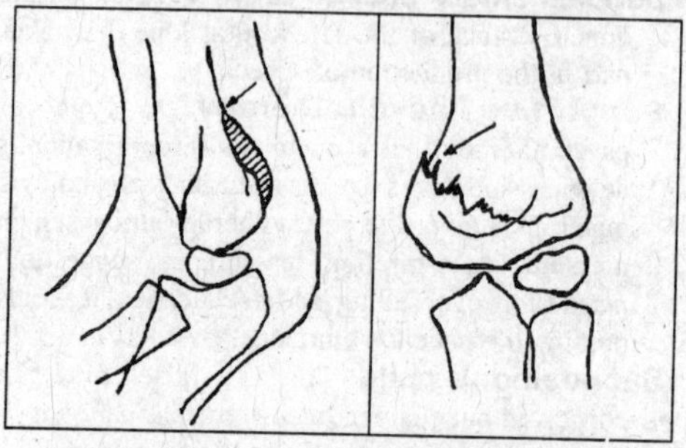

arm can be measured. Complications include cubitus valgus or varus and limitation of movement of elbow joint, Volkmann's ischaemic contracture and injury to ulnar or radial nerve.

Supragingival Above the gingival margin.

Supraorbital margin The upper margin of the orbit.

Suprapubic catheterisation This is a procedure of introduction of catheter into urinary bladder through an incision made above symphysis pubis to relieve aute retention of urine when ordinary method of urethral catheterisation with rubber catheter has failed.

Supraspinal antinociception Pain suppression by pathways descending to the posterior horn gray matter from the brainstem.

Supraspinatous tendinitis When pain occurs on active abduction after 30° but disappears after 70 degrees.

Supraspinatus bursitis Pain associated with bursitis is often relieved by supporting the elbow with the opposite hand.

Suprasternal notch Notch in the proximal end of sternum.

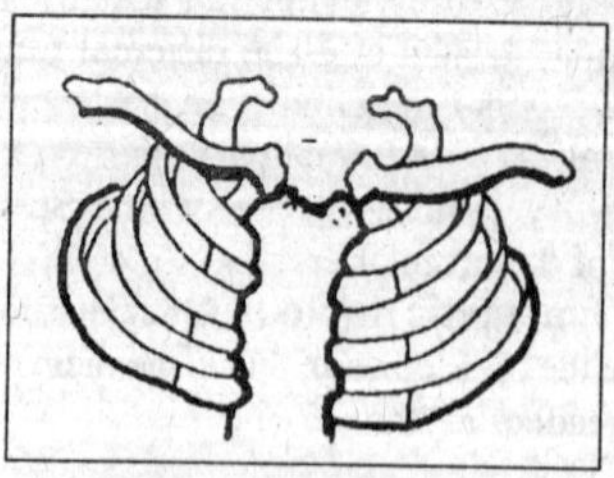

Supratentorial tumours These develop w seizures and hemispheres. Rarely ataxia may caused. Vomiting, headache and papilloedema relatively late features. Tumours of deep structu such as basal ganglion, thymus or ventricu system are not associated with seizures.

Supraventricular crest The boundary between posteroanterior inflow tract and the antero-super outflow tract of the right ventricle.

Surface anatomy The division of anato concerned with the structures that can be identifi from the outside of the body.

Surface anatomy face Landmarks of face a nasolabial groove, philtrum and labioment groove to be identified. These land marks may altered in facial paralysis and space occupyi lesions.

Surface energy The energy of a surface th determines how well it will be wetted by a liqui

Surface pit A hole or cavity in a material or tissu a tiny depression.

Surface tension The force that results from th interactions of the pressures tending to collaps the alveoli and those tending to expand them.

Surface traits Personality characteristics which ar readily apparent, such as sociability or shyness.

Surfactant A mixture of the secretions of the lung and air passages that reduces the surface tensio of pulmonary fluids and thus contributes to the elastic properties of lung tissue.

Surfactant replacement therapy An artificial surface-active agent sometimes given to an infant via endotracheal intubation.

Surgery Treatment of disease, injury, or deformity by the use of manual or automatic instruments; remaining parts or tissue by cutting.

Surgical anesthesia It consists of four planes.

Plane I

- Loss of conjuctival reflex
- Swallowing and vomiting depressed
- Pupils normal
- Lacrimation increased

Plane II

- Until onset of intercostal paralysis
- Shallow breathing
- Loss of corneal reflex
- Lacrimation increasing
- Pupils becoming larger

Plane III

- Shallow breathing
- Light reflex depressed
- Laryngeal reflex depressed
- Lacrimation depressed

Plane IV

- Until diaphragms paralysed
- Carinal reflex diminished.

Surgical asepsis Measures that render supplies and equipment totally free of microorganisms.

Surgical diathermy It is a radiofrequency power oscillation with a patient in circuit producing intense heat at the small electrode. Spark gap sets give 350 kHz coagulation and 450 kHz cutting power. It uses electrical apparatus which may cause explosions, burns or electrocution or may interfere with pacemaker.

Surgical fomentation This is a fomentation to broken part of skin like over an open wound. Purpose of it is to accelerate the process of suppuration, to promote better drainage, reduce swelling, congestion, pain and muscle spasm.

Surgical history Previous abdominal operation such as appendisectomy or caesarian section.

Surgical neck humerus It is a narrowed area of proximal humeral neck. Mostly fracture occurs here.

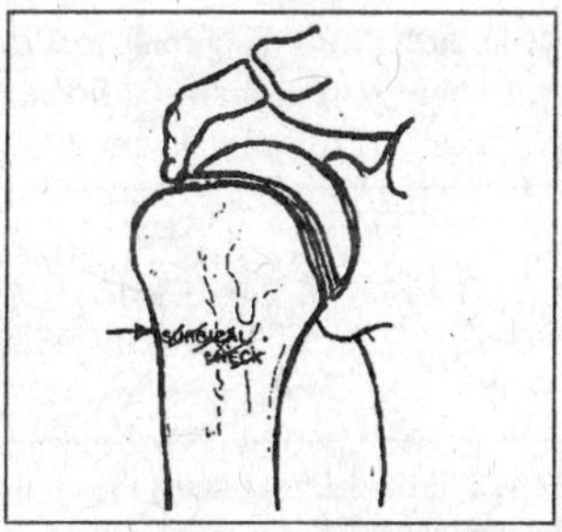

Surgical phase Portion of periodontal treatment in which surgery of the periodontal soft tissue and alveolar bone is completed.

Surgical scrub Process of removing as many microorganisms as possible from the hands and arms by mechanical washing and chemical antisepsis.

Surgical waiting area Roomwhoro fumily and friends await information about the surgical patient.

Surrogate Temporary substitute or stand in acting of behalf of another. Surrogate mother may have children by the husband of an infertile wife and hand over the baby at birth for them to bring up as their own.

Surrogate motherhood The contractual hiring of a woman to bear another couple's child. Either the father's sperm impregnates the surrogate or the surrogate is implanted with the genetic parent's embryo.

Survey A research method based on self reported informatiton from participants rather than on observations or measurements taken by researchers.

Surveying Process of studying the parallelism or lack of parallelism of the teeth and associated structures to determine a path for the placement of a restoration with the least interference and most stability.

Survivor A person who has lived through a trauma.

Survivor Action A legal cause of brought on behalf of a dead person to recover losses sustained by the deceased during his or her lifetime.

Susceptibility Lack of resistance of a body to the deleterious or other effects of an agent such as a pathogen.

Susceptible host One whose biologic defense mechanisms are weakened in some way.

Suspect A person who may be a possible offender, a hypothetical offender. Not a synonym for 'offender' or code for 'we think this is the offender'.

Suspend To delay or to bring to stop temporarily.

Suspension A technique that is used to free a body part from the resistance of friction by suspending the part in a sling attached to a rope that is fixed either above the center of gravity or above the axis.

Suspensory ligament 1. A portion of the peritoneum that extends laterally from the surface of the ovary to the wall of the pelvic cavity. 2. A ligament that supports an organs or body part, such as that supporting the lens of the eye.

Sustained (constant) fever Consistently elevated temperature with little or no fluctuation.

Sustained release Drug that dissolves at timed intervals.

Sustained release medication Medication taken in a single dose but designed to dissolve slowly releasing medication into blood. Time usually taken is 12-24 hours.

Sustained traction It is also applied continuously but usually for no longer than 45 minutes, because of short duration relatively longer forces can be applied.

Sustentacular cells specialized cells within the testes that supply nutrients to developing spermatozoa; also called Sertoli cells or nurse cells.

Sutural bone A small bone positioned within a suture of certain cranial bones; also called a wormian cells.

Suture An immovable joint that represents a line of union between adjoining bones of the skull; appears radiolucent.

Suture forceps These forceps have one and two teeth, available in different sizes of teeth to suit

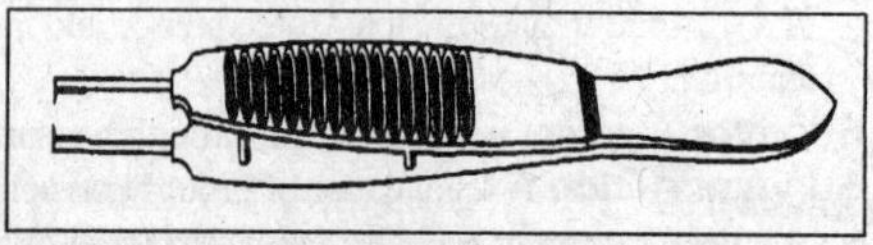

the requirement of the tissue to be held by the suture forceps for the suturing. Usually 0.5 mm or 1 mm size teeth suture forceps is used.

Sutures Commonly known as stitches used in sewing up a wound. It is used for the fibrous junctions of many of bones of skull which form only after birth.

Sutures skull It is composed of bones forming the base, the face and vault. Bones of base and in the face are firm and incompressible whereas the skull bones of vault are soft cartilaginous plates joined at their edges by fibrous tissue. These fibrous joints are called sutures which allows for considerable moulding or even overlaping of bony plates during labour.

Suturing It is the procedure of closing of a surgical incision or a wound by sutures to promote healing. A variety of sterile material is used as sutures, including catgut, linen, silk, or synthetic fibre and stainless steel wire. Catgut are absorbable. Deep incisions or wounds may need to be sutured at

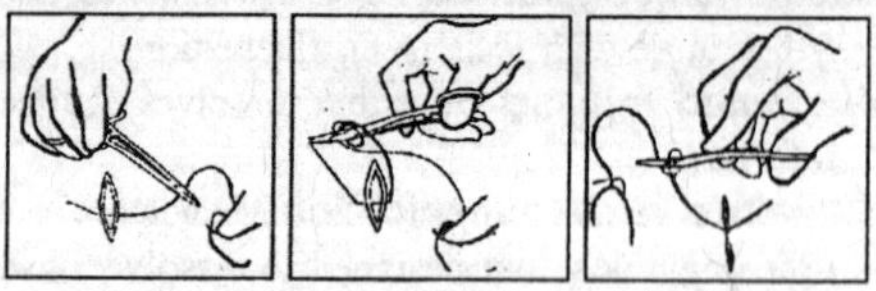

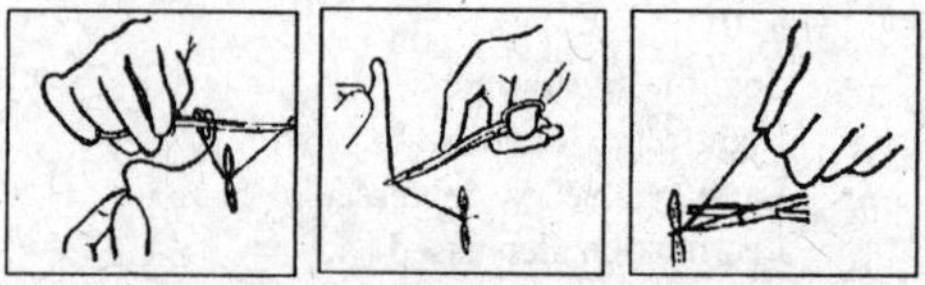

several levels to achieve full closure throughout the depth of tissue. Internal sutures made of absorbable material are left in place permanently. Skin sutures are removed painlessly.

Swab It is a pad of absorbent material used in surgery or to obtain a sample of bacteria from an infected patient. Commonly it is a surgical sponge usually a folded piece of cotton gauze held in clamp. It is used to apply cleansing and antiseptic solutions to the skin before incision is made. Bacteriological swab consists of a twist of cotton at the end of thin stick that is sealed in a container and sterilised.

Swallowing It is the process by which food or liquid is conveyed from mouth to the stomach, once food has been well chewed and mixed with saliva it is pushed back into pharynx. Rest of swallowing act is involuntary. Entry of food into the pharynx causes epiglottis to close over the larynx. Swallowing of difficulty may be due to lack of saliva and oesophageal spasm. Pressure on the outside of oesophagus may obstruct the passage of food.

Swan-neck deformity A chronic mallet deformity leading to hyperextension of the proximal interphalangeal (PIP) joint as a result of changed

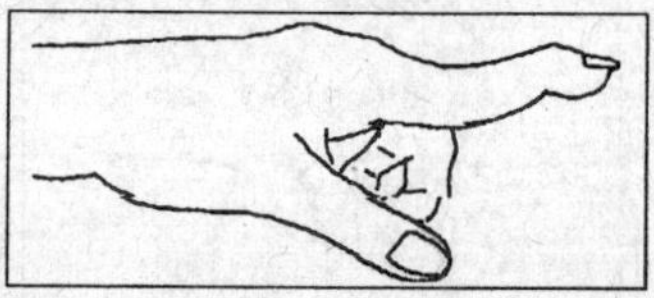

line of pull of the lateral bands, the combination of two deformities is known as swan-neck's deformity. Splinting is rarely effective.

Swayback posture A posterior shift of the upper trunk (flexion of the thoracic spine on the lumbar spine) and an anterior shift of the pelvis (extension of the hip) result in a swayback posture. Decreased lumbar lordosis (flattened spine), posterior tilt of the pelvis, and increased kyphosis of the thoracic spine are also present.

Sweat Transparent, watery liquid released by glands in the skin that eliminates ammonia and uric acid and helps to maintain body temperature; also known as perspiration.

Sweat gland Usually means a secretory organ that produces a watery secretion called sweat that is released onto the surface of the skin; some sweat glands, however, produce an organic secretion.

Sweat retention syndrome The syndrome represents miliaria with severe systemic symptoms due to blockage of the sweat gland ducts, and collapse.

Swing phase The phase of gait during which the reference limb is not in contact with the supporting surface.

Swing time The number of seconds during the gait cycle that one foot is off the ground. Swing time should be measured separately for right and left extremities.

Swinging It involves legally married couples during intercourse and various types of erotic behaviour with other legally married couples. This is characterised more by sexual activity than emotional and personal interaction or intellectual sharing, business or carrier ties. Swing is a couple activity while open marriage consists of independent relationship formed by each partner.

Switch sequences Highly conserved repetitive sequences which mediate class switching in the immunoglobulin heavy chain gene locus.

Sydenham's chorea Childhood disease associated with rheumatic fever. The disease is self-limiting, and recovery is usually complete; characterized by involuntary, abrupt, jerky, extraneous movements and disturbances of balance and gait; impairments of speech but memory may be apparent.

Syllable A unit of speech whose central phoneme is a vowel, which may stand alone or be surrounded by one or more consonants; for example, I, in, me, men.

Symbiosis A mutually reinforcing relationship between two persons who are dependent on each other; a normal characteristic of the relationship between the mother and infant child.

Symbiotic Any intimate relationship between two species.

Symbiotic psychosis A condition seen in two-to-four-year-old children with an abnormal relationship to a mothering figure. The psychosis is characterised by intense separation anxiety, severe regression, giving up of useful speech, and autism.

Symbiotic relationship An overprotective, often enmeshed relationship between a parent and child.

Symblepharon It is a condition in which palpebral conjunctiva gets adherent to the bulbar conjunctiva. In anterior symblepharon lid margin gets adherent to the bulbar conjunctiva. In posterior symblepharon, there is adhesion in the fornix. While in total symblepharon there is adhesion of palpebral conjunctiva to the bulbar conjunctiva. It is caused by chemical burn, ulceration in membranous conjunctiva or injury. Patient complains of double image and is unable to close the lids properly because it is adherent.

Symbolic information In the structure-of-intellect model, information which appears in symbolic form, such as numbers, letters, words, and so forth. This information is part of the contents dimension.

Symbolic model In social learning theory, someone who emits a certain behaviour yet is not actually present. Symbolic models typically include the characters in television, radio, and stories.

Symbolisation A general mechanism in all human thinking by which some mental representation comes to stand for some other thing, class of things, or attribute of something. This mechanism underlies dream formation and some symptoms, such as conversion reactions, obsessions, and compulsions. The link between the latent meaning of the symptom and the symbol is usually unconscious.

Syme's amputation Amputation at the supramalleolar level, in which all foot bones are

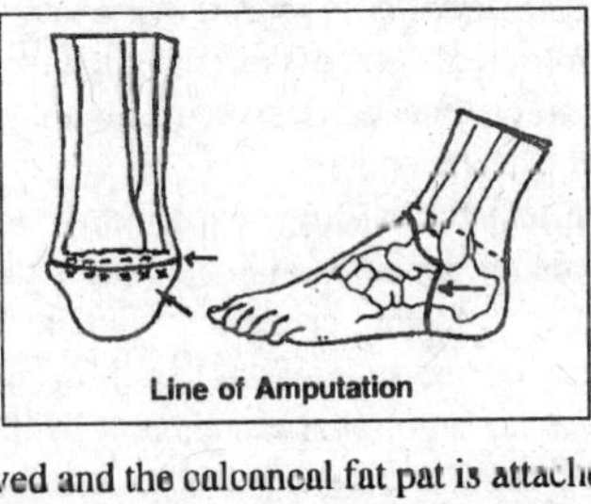

Line of Amputation

removed and the calcaneal fat pat is attached to the anterior skin flap to cushion the distal end of the limb.

Symmetric Evenly balanced or uniformly developed.

Sympathectomy A severing of the sympathetic nervous system at either the cervical or lumbar ganglion. The area can also be blocked for a short time with drugs.

Sympathetic Responsice to emotional state.

Sympathetic division The division of the autonomic system which plays a predominant role in emotion and which functions in opposition to the parasympathetic system. When the sympathetic system assumes control, secretion of adrenalin is accelerated, heart beat is accelerated, and stomach secretions are inhibited.

Sympathetic nervous system It is a part of autonomic nervous system which respond to meet emergencies such as it speeds heart beat raising blood pressure. It cools the skin by sweating, it dilates bronchi of the lungs to have more oxygen. The release of extra glucose to meet energy requirement in need is also a part of it.

Sympathetic postganglionic neurons Dendrites and cell bodies are in sympathetic ganglia and axons travel to a variety of visceral effectors.

Sympathetic tone The basal rate of activity of the sympathetic nervous system.

Sympathetic trunk ganglion A cluster of cell bodies of postganglionic sympathetic neurons lateral to the vertebral column, close to the body of a certebra column., close to the body of a vertebra. These ganglia extend inferiorly through the neck, thorax, and abdomen to the coccyx on both sides of the vertebral column and are connected to one another to form a chain on each side of the vertebral column.

Sympathoadrenal system An anatomical and physiological unit of adrenal medulla and the sympathetic nervous system, synthesized and stored catecholamines.

Sympatholytic A drug that inhibits adrenergic receptors of the autonomic nervous system.

Sympathy A feeling or capacity for sharing in the interests or concerns of another. May arise when there is no emotional attachment to the person toward whom one is sympathetic, since the feelings of the sympathetic person remain essentially internal.

Symphalangism Heriditory ankylosis of proximal interphalangeal joints. Fusion of carpal and tarsal bones also occur in this autosomal dominant disorder.

Symphysis Line of fusion of the lateral halves of the anterior portion of the mandible at the midline. Present only in fetal life. The mandibular symphysis is a large joint of the suture type, with intramembranous ossification.

Symport Process by which two substances, often Na^+ and another substance, move in the same direction across a cell membrane. Also called co-transport.

Symporter A membrane transporter protein catalyzing movement of the coupling ion in the same direction as the substrate molecule.

Symptom It is an abnormal feature of body which patient complains to the doctors such as cough, pain, headache, loss of vision, etc. While sign is a feature which doctor elicits on examination such as tenderness, murmur, etc. With the help of sign and symptoms putting together doctor reaches to a diagnosis of the illness.

Symptom substitution The appearance of a new symptom as a replacement for one which has been removed through treatment. The outcome has been a source of debate among therapists of different orientations.

Symptomatic treatment It relieves symptoms but not curing the root cause of them. For example in caries tooth pain killer gives relief of pain but does not cure caries.

Symptoms Subjective data; that which only the patient can identify.

Synapse It is the junctional region where one neuron ends another begins. The nerve cells are linked together into chains. Anatomical path is interrupted at the synapse but physiological. Changes are transmitted from one neuron to another. A block or resistance always occurs at synapse. Transmission of nerve impulses in one direction and never in the reverse direction. Synapses have a distributing, focussing and commutator action.

Synapsis The portion of the recombinational process that positions homologous molecules of DNA to bring them into alignment.

Synaptic cleft The narrow gap that separates the axon terminal of one neuron from another neuron or muscle fiber (cell), across which a neurotransmitter diffuses to affect the postsynaptic cell.

Synaptic end bulb Expanded distal end of an axon terminal that contains synaptic knob.

Synaptic knob A tiny bulge at the end of a terminal branch of a presynaptic neuron's axon that contains vesicles with neurotransmitters.

Synaptic vesicle An organelle consisting of a membrane structure containing chemical neuotransmitters.

Synarthrosis A joint in which fibrous connective tissue joins bones and holds them together tightly; commonly called sutures. Synchysis and syneresis are two most common degenerative changes in vitreous gel. In synchysis there is liquefaction of vitreous gel which may be total or partial. In syneresis there is contraction of vitreous gel which separates its liquid from solid component of gel. Synchysis senilis is an age-related phenomenon of vitreous gel caused by alteration of its micromolecular structure. The liquefaction of vitreous acts as a predisposing factor for posterior vitreous detachment. In partial synchysis there is formation of cavity or lacuna in the posterior vitreous. This lacuna appears as empty space on slit-lamp examination.

Synchondrosis A cartilaginous joint in which the articulating bones are separated by hyaline cartilage.

Synchysis scintillans It is characterised by numerous white or yellow cholesterol crystals in the vitreous. The vitreous is fluid. These crystals move freely in the vitreous and later settle down in lower part of fluid vitreous. These are asymptomatic and do not affect the vision. These are usually bilateral and are easily seen by a torch light or slit lamp.

Syncope Swooning or fainting; temporary suspension of consciousness caused by cerebral ischemia.

Syndesmophyte Osseous excrescence or bony outgrowth from a ligament. Usually projecting vertically in the spine.

Syndesmosis A slightly movable joint in which articulating bones are united by fibrous connective tissue.

Syndrome It is a group of symptoms constituting particular disorder. Such as irritable bowel syndrome is characterised by intermittent pain, abdominal swelling, irregular bowel movements, mucus in faeces, etc.

Syndrome diagnosis Cluster of problems that are present due to an event or situation.

Syndrome X The occurence of angina like symptoms in the absence of atherosclerotic disease of ischemia.

Syndrome, burning mouth There is painful burning sensation of tongue, lips and other oral mucosal surfaces. Idiopathic cases presenting as burning, painful or itching sensation are located in oral mucosa with or without involving tongue. Women outnumber males. Tongue temperature lowers down. Pain intensity is that of toothache. Some relief of symptoms one can get from use of topical analgesics such as 0.5 per cent Benadryl alone or mixed with 0.5 per cent dyclone. Clinical trials of oestrogen and progesterone have been encouraging.

Synergies Stereotyped, primitive movement patterns associated with the presence of spasticity.

Synergist A muscle that assists the prime mover by reducing undesired action or unnecessary movement.

Synergistic Acting jointly; enhancing the effect of another drug, force, or agent.

Synergistic massage Massage structured to affect one body system primarily. This approach usually is used for lymphatic and circulation enhancement massage.

Synergistic reaction An undesired reaction that occurs when one drug potentiates the effect of another.

Synergy Is present when the impact that two or more factors have on an individual or population is greater than the sum of the separate effects of each factor.

Synesthesia Ability to perceive a stimulus of one sense as a sensation of a different sense, as when sound produces a sensation of color.

Syngamy The fusion of gametes (ovum and sperm) initiating fertilization.

Synkineticptosis It is congenital and unilateral. On asking the patient to move the jaw laterally right and left or open and shut the mouth, the affected drooping lid shoots upwards with movement of the jaw. It is due to abnormal nervous connection in the central nervous system between the nerve supply to the levator muscle and associated muscles. It can be treated by excision of levator muscle on both sides.

Synovial Lubricating fluid of the joints.

Synovial cavity The space between the articulating bones of a diarthrotic joint, filled with synovial fluid. Also called a joint cavity.

Synovial fluid It is a clear, viscid alkaline fluid in joint cavities, bursae, etc. Its chief function is lubrication of the rubbing surfaces of moving joints. In composition it resembles plasma except a lower concentration of protein. It contains a mucus-like substance, synovin of unknown nature.

Synovial joint Freely movable joint.

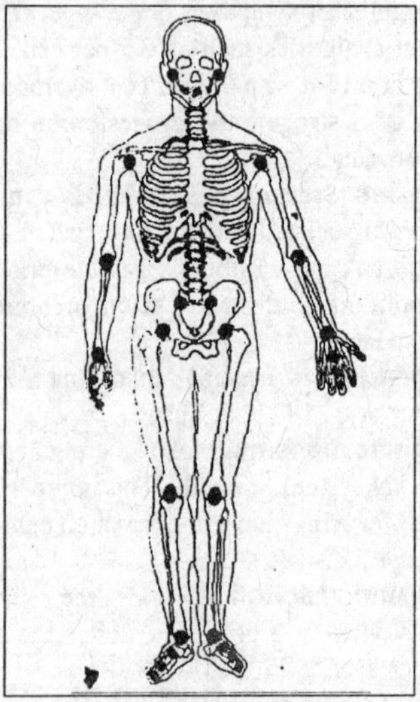

Synovial membrane Connective tissue membrane lining the spaces between bones and joints that secretes synovial fluid.

Synovial membrane The deeper of the two layer of the articular capsule of a synovial joint, composed of areolar connective tissue that secretes synovial fluid into the synovial (joint) cavity.

Synovitis Inflammation of the synovium.

Synovium Tissue lining synovial joints, tendon shealths, and bursa. In the joint it produces fluid to lubricate the joint and is the part of the joint that becomes inflammed in inflammatory joint disease.

Syntax The way in which words are put together, following the rules of grammar, to form phrases, clauses, or sentences; proposed to be a unique characteristic of human language.

Syntaxic mode The mode of perception that forms whole, logical, coherent pictures of reality that can be validated by others.

Synthases Enzymes that catalyze condensation reactions in which no nucleoside triphosphate is required as an energy source.

Synthesis reaction The combination of atoms, ions, or molecules to form a new and larger molecule.

Syntocinon rupture Syntocinon or pitocin I.V. drip is now liberally used for induction of labour and to stimulate uterine contraction in hypotonic uterine inertia. Fundal rupture is common.

Syntrophic Providing nutritional requirements for each other.

Syringes Different variety of syringes are available of glass and plastic. Plastic ones are presterilised disposal ones, while glass ones can be utilised again and again after proper sterilisation by boiling for 20 minutes. These are used for calculated amount of drug to be injected or drawing blood. Insulin syringes are thin finely calibrated in units to give hypodermic insulin.

Syringomyelia It is characterised by gliosis and cavitation (syrinx) of the upper portion of spinal cord or medulla. It is believed to be a congenital

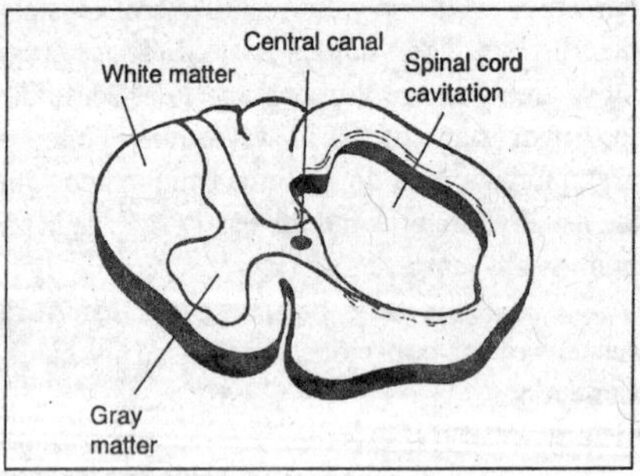

abnormality associated often with cervical rib, kyphosis, and spina bifida. The cavity usually extends transversely across the cord into dorsal areas. It may invade ventral horns. There may be loss of pain and temperature sensation at the level of lesion while intact sensation remains above and below it. As the cavity spreads to involve motor cells the hands and arms become atrophic and weak when lateral tracts are involved spasticity may develop.

System A group of organs that have a common function.

System consultation Consultation that addresses the needs of a large system or agency.

Systematic desensitisation A behaviour therapy procedure widely used to modify behaviours associated with phobias. The procedure involves the construction of a hierarchy of anxiety producing stimuli by the subject, and gradual presentation of the stimuli until they no longer produce anxiety.

Systemic Affecting or involving the entire organism; i.e, the whole system.

Systemic anatomy The anatomic study of particular systems of the body; such as the skeletal, muscular, nervous, cardiovascular, or urinary systems.

Systemic assessment Organised method of collecting data.

Systemic circulation Blood flow from the left ventricle to all parts of the body and back to the right atrium.

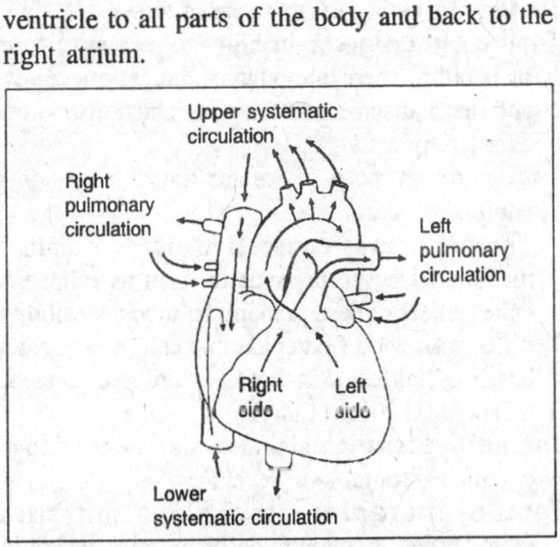

Systemic desensitisation A technique used in behavior therapy to eliminate specific fears by requiring the patient to imagine different

Systemic factors Generalized biologic factors that are implicated in the causation, modification, and perpetuation of a disease entity. Within the oral cavity, the actions of the systemic factors are modified by interaction with local factors.

Systemic infection An infection that pervades the host tissue and sometimes the whole organism.

Systemic therapy Therapy that is given to a patient to treat the whole body.

Systemic vascular resistance All the vascular resistance offered by systemic blood vessels. Also called total peripheral resistance.

Systems In general, groups of related elements. In the history of psychology, a way of ordering the facts so that they have meaning in relation to one another.

A theoretical model which embraces as many relevant facts as possible and serves as a framework for obtaining new information. The various schools or models of psychology, such as behaviourism, psychoanalysis, humanistic psychology, and cognitive psychology, are designed to systematise psychological knowledge and point the way for further research. therefore, they are called systems or models of psychology. In the structure-of-intellect model, this term refers to an outcome in the products dimension.

Systems model A step by step model of treatment planning; the solution to each problem is dependent on information obtained in the preceding step.

Systems youth Youth who live in or leave foster care of institutional settings.

Systole Contraction of the heart chambers during which blood leaves the chambers; usually refers to ventricular contraction.

Systolic dysfunction The impaired contraction of the ventricles during systole that produces an inefficient expulsion of blood.

Systolic murmur A periodic sound occurring during the systolic phase of the cardiac cycle and heard during auscultation of the heart; usually attributable to mitral or tricuspid regurgitation or to aortic or pulmonary obstruction.

Systolic pressure The higher blood pressure measurement, reflects pressure within the arterial system during the period of ventricular contraction.

T

T cells A small circulating lymphocyte produced in the bone marrow that mediates cellular immune responses.

T wave Deflection on an electrocardiogram that occurs with repolarization of the ventricles.

T4 syndrome Pain or numbness in the hand and/ or forearm in a glove-like distribution associated with upper thoracic subluxation in general and subluxation of the T3-4 or T4-5 motion segments in particular. Concomitant symptoms may include headache, chest pain, and interscapular pain of stiffness. Risk factors include a forward posture of the head and disturbed tone in the muscles of the shoulder girdle. Patients suffering from this disorder are often dismissed as hysterics because of the glove-like distribution of symptoms.

Tabanid flues These are large, stouty built and brightly coloured. Strong fliers attack viciously,

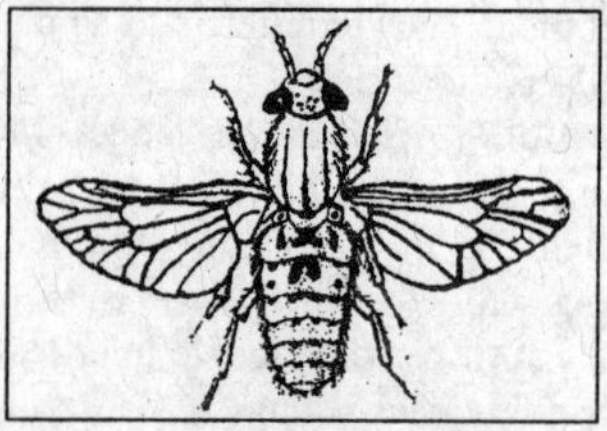

only adult females are blood feeders and have mouthparts adopted for cutting and piercing. These may cause anthrax and tularemia.

Tabes dorsalis Tabes means wasting specially of dorsal roots. There is mild leptomeningeal thickening over the roots and dorsal column. It begins 10 to 12 years after the primary infection. There will be early lightening pain in legs. Autonomic reflexes are impaired so that impotence and postural hypotension results. It is generally associated with optic atrophy, nerve deafness and partial oculomotor palsies with ptosis. Iris les pigmentation and appears atrophied.

Table top test A useful clinical guide to the timining of surgery for Duputren's contracture. Ask the patient to place his or her hand flat on the table top. Test is positive if he is not able to do.

Tachyarrhythmia Rapid irregular heart beat.

Tachycardia It is a heart rate over 100 beats per minute. It may occur during exercise. Tachycardia at rest may be caused by fever, hyperthyroidism and coronary heart disease. Types of tachycardia include atrial fibrillation and sinus tachycardia. Symptoms of tachycardia may include palpitations, breathlessness and light headedness.

Tachykinins It is a group of neuropeptides involved in cardiovascular, respiratory, endocrine and behavioral response.

Tachyphea Condition characterized by respiratory rate greater than 20 breaths per minute.

Tachyphylaxis Term usually referring to tolerance that develops quickly.

Tachyzoite A form of merozoite in Taxoplasma, found in parastrophorous vacuoles of vertebrate hosts.

Tackler's exostosis A bony mass resulting from traumatic myositis.

Tactile Pertaining to the sense of touch.

Tactile agnosia The inability to recognize forms by bandling them, although tactile, proprioceptive, and thermal sensations may be intact; also known as astereognosis.

Tactile corpuscle These are found in certain of papillae of skin.

The perineural connective tissue sheath of medullated nerve expands to form an ellipsoidal enlargement. These respond to touch sensibility.

Tactile disk Modified epidermal cell in the stratum basale of hairless skin that functions as a cutaneous receptor for discriminative.

Tactile system Pertaining to the sense of touch obtained through skin receptors.

Tactile therapies It employs soft tissue mobilization, manipulation of muscles and riding other restrictions in an effort to decrease constraints due to stress and its resulting pain.

Tadoro's tendon A tendonous structure extending from the right fibrous trigone of the heart toward the valve of the inferior vena cava.

Taenia coli One of three flat bands of thickened, longitudinal smooth muscle running the length of the large intestine.

Tail pinch eating Eating induced in rodents and cats by gently pinching their tail.

Talectomy Surgical removal of all or part of talus.

Talfa dressing Sterile, nonadherent wound dressing.

Talion law or principle A primitive, unrealistic belief, usually unconscious, conforming to the Biblical injunction of an "eye for an eye and a tooth for a tooth." In psychoanalysis, the concept and fear that all injury, actual or intended, will be punished in kind.

Talipes equinovarus The typical club foot. Its elements are equinus or plantar flexion of the foot at the ankle, varus or inversion deformity of the heel and forefoot adduction.

Tamponade Compression of the heart as the result of fluid accumulating within the pericardial sac.

Tandem Romberg sign A toe the line test for presence of ataxia.

Tandem walking A pattern of walking during which the heel of one foot approximates the toes of the other foot.

Tannin A water-soluble phenolic compound having the property to combining with proteins, cellulose, gelatin, and pectin to form an insoluble complex.

Tapetum Refers to sheet of callosal fibers above the lateral ventricles.

Tapeworm It is a parasitic worm that may infect intestine. The larvae are consumed in undercooked contaminated beef, pork or fish. Tapeworms have a hooked head attached to the intestinal wall with a flat, segmented body dangling beneath. Eggs form in segments are broken and pass out of body. It may cause abdominal pain. Despite their size beef, pork and fish tapeworms rarely cause symptoms except mild abdominal discomfort or diarrhoea. Stool examination is diagnostic. Cysticercosis is treated with drugs such as praziquantel.

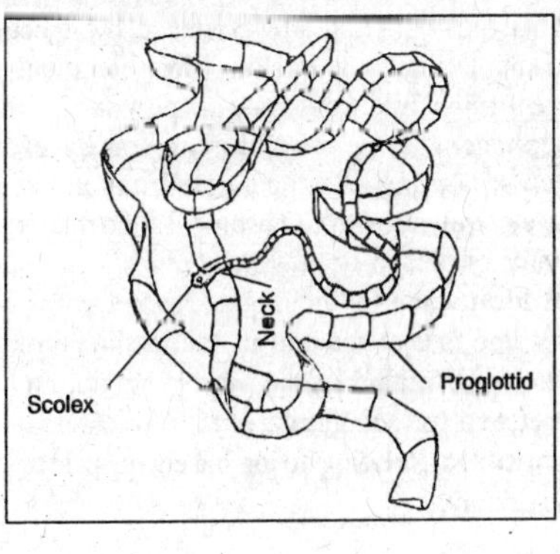

Taping of thumb It allows an athlete to continue playing without jeopardising a mild sprain and to play after surgery. First the metacarpophalangeal

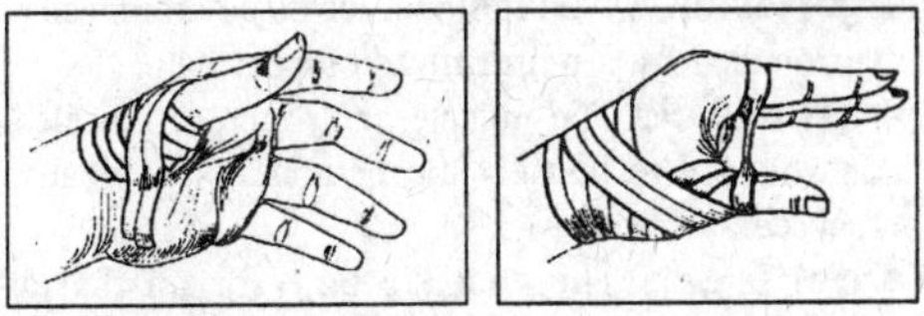

joint is stabilised with the tape and then index finger is taped to his thumb holding the thumb adducted and preventing abduction of matacarpophalangeal joint. Alternatively elastic tape is used to hold the thumb adducted.

Tapotement Percussion.

Tapotement Springy blows to the body at a fast rate to create rhythmic compression of the tissue; also callsed *percussion.*

Tapping A type of tapotement that uses the fingertips.

Tappotement Striking the belly of a muscle with the hypothenar edge of the open hand in rapid sucession to increase its tone and arterial perfusion.

Tar The conglomerate of some 5000, chemical components of tobacco smoke excluding nicotine and gases.

Tarasoff decision A California court decision which essentially imposes a duty on the therapist to warn the appropriate person or persons when he becomes aware that his patient may present a risk of harm to a specific person or persons.

Tardive dyskinesia Literally, "late-appearing abnormal movements", a variable complex of choreiform or athetoid movements developing in patients exposed to antipsychotic drugs. Typical movements include tongue-writhing or protrusion, chewing, lip-puckering, choreiform finger movements, toe and ankle movements, leg jiggling, or movements of neck, trunk, and pelvis. These movements may be either mild or severe and may occur singly or in many combinations and permutations.

Tardy Median Nerve Palsy Carpal Tunnel Syndrome.

Target amplification A nucleic acid amplification procedure in which many copies of the nucleic acid target are made.

Target cell A cell whose activity is affected by a particular hormone.

Target heart rate Goal for heart rate during exercise.

Target lesion A well-defined, localised radiopacity surrounded by a uniform radiolucent halo.

Target muscle The muscle or groups of muscles on which the response of the methods is specifically focused.

Target organ The specific body organ that a particular hormone affects.

Target organ cell Organ or cell acted on by a particular hormone and responding to it.

Target site A site at which a transposition event occurs or has occurred.

Target tissue Tissue on which a hormone acts.

Tarnish Deterioration that involves only the surface and whose end result is usually discolouration is called tarnish.

Tarsal gland An oil-secreting gland that opens on the exposed edge of each eyelid; also called a meibomian gland.

Tarsal tunnel syndrome It presents with pain in or around ankle joint due to entrapment and compression of the posterior tibial nerve and the pain is relieved by rest.

Tarsals Seven bones of the heel and back part of the foot; the calcaneus is the largest.

Tarsals bones The seven bones of the ankle. Also called tarsals.

Tarsometatarsal dislocation Dislocation at this joint may be with and without fracture.

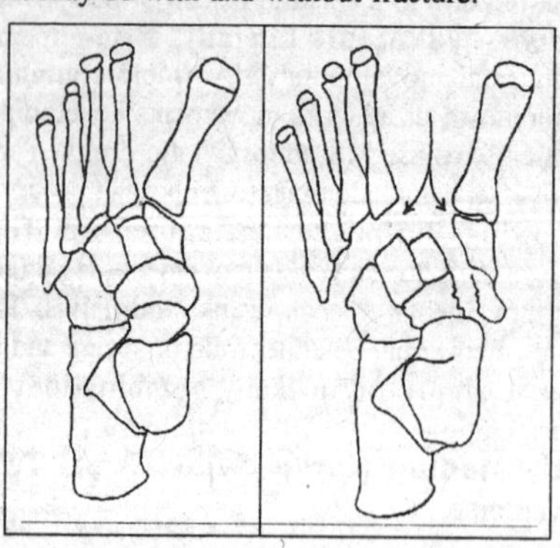

Tarsus The region of the foot containing the seven tarsal bones.

Tartar Hardened plaque.

Task-oriented touch Personal contact that is required when performing nursing procedures.

Taste Alone taste is a relatively crude sense able to distinguish only between sweet, salty, sour and bitter. But different grades of tastes can be discriminated with the sense of smell. Because of this only when sense of smell is diminished then

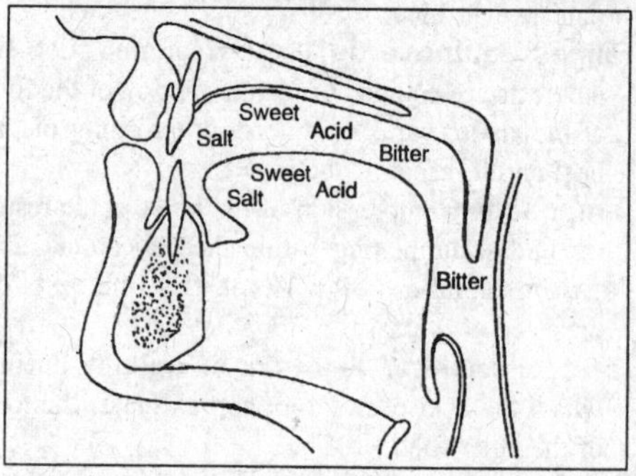

sense of taste also goes down in case of common cold. Dry mouth can cause loss of taste. Complete or partial loss of taste may result from damage to tastebuds due to stomatitis. Loss of taste may also be caused by damage to the cranial nerves. Nerve damage may be caused by head injury. Disturbance of taste may occur in some psychiatric disorder.

Taste bud Sensory structure that is found mostly on the tongue and functions as a taste receptor. These develop early in fetal life by about 14 weeks of intrauterine life. Man has 9000 taste buds most of which are on the tongue and situated on the papillae on its dorsum.

Tattoo marks These are produced by injection of insoluble pigments in skin. Most commonly used are Indian ink, soot or gun powder. Although permanent, these may be removed by excision, burns, pouring of concentrated mineral acids or by electrolysis with CO_2 snow. Tattoo marks reflect status of person or may have one's own name.

Taut Firm when fully elongated; not slack. Muscles become taut at the end of the available range or motion permitted by the muscle length, i.e., when stretched to their limit.

Taxonomic Relating to or based on principles of taxonomy.

Taxonomy The branch of biology concerned with naming and classifying the diverse forms of life.

Tay sach's disease A hereditary metabolic disorder with degeneration of brain cells and a red spot on each retina, eventually dementia, blindness, paralysis and death. An inherited birth defect that appears 4 to 6 months after birth and results in retardation, physical changes, and death at about age 5; caused by the loss of genes that encode the enzyme necessary for breaking down certain fatty substances.

Taylor orthosis Thoracolumbosacral flexion extension control orthosis.

T-Bandage It can be made from two strips of gauge or bandage, one folded at right angles over the middle of the other. It is convenient for retaining dressings on the perineum.

T-cane A cane whose handle sits at a right angle to the shaft, resembling the letter T.

T-cell determinants Portion of protein that provides all the residues required for recognition within a major histocompatability complex context by T-Cell receptor.

T-cells In fetus immature lymphocytes develop in yolk sac, liver and bone marrow. From there they pass through the thymus and become the T-lymphocytes or go through GIT to become B-lymphocyte. In the blood 80 per cent are T-lymphocyte and rest are B- lymphocytes. T-cells are responsible for cellular defence of organism.

T-dependent antigen An antigen which requires helper T cells in order to elicit an antibody response.

Team nursing Pattern in which nursing personnel divide the patients into groups and complete their care together.

Tear film It consists of three layers. Superficial lipid layer is a nonmolecular layer derived from the secretions of meibomian glands and help to retard the evaporation of middle aqueous layer. Middle aqueous layer derives the secretions of lacrimal and accessory lacrimal glands. While deep mucinous layer is composed of mucin, a glycoprotein and overlies the corneal and conjunctival epithelial cells. Mucin is derived from secretions of globlet cells.

Tear fluid It is a mixture of secretion from lacrimal and accessory lacrimal glands, the goblet cells and meibomian glands. The lacrimal glands, the orbital and palpebral portion secrete about 95% of aqueous component of tear fluid. Main functions of tear fluid are to keep the cornea as a smooth optical surface.

It keeps well the surface of cornea and conjunctival epithelium. Tears inhibit growth of microorganisms. Tears are isotonic fluid, slightly alkaline and consist of water, potassium, chloride, sodium, urea, glucose, lysozyme, globulin and albumin. Tear production starts after 3 to 4 weeks of birth of a child.

Technetium 99m A radioactive perfusion agent; used for diagnostic purposes in the cardiac muscles/coronary arteries.

Technician A person who is skilled in the practice of an area of science. A technician may be a university graduate, but is distinguished from a scientist by the fact that less theoretical under standing and often greater practical skill is expected in the technician. A technician can carry out scientific analysis, but cannot validate the analytical process used unless supervised by the scientist.

Technician, dental laboratory A technician who performs any type of dental laboratory procedure not requiring the presence of a patient.

Technique The method of a procedure. Methods of therapeutic massage that provide sensory stimulation or mechanical change of the soft tissue of the body.

Tectopulvinar system A system consisting of projections from the retina to the superior colliculus to the pulvinar (thalamus) to the parietal and temporal visual areas.

Tectorial membrane Membrane attached to the spiral lamina and extending over the hair cells; hair of the hair cells have their tips embedded in the membrane.

Tectum The roof of, or area above the ventricle of, the midbrain; its functions are sensory.

Teeth brushing It is a special type of brush to clean teeth, remove plaque and food particles. Fluoride paste is more useful. For effective brushing it should have easily gripped handle and soft, rounded ends or polished bristles.

Size and shape must allow every tooth to be reached. Toothbrush should be rinsed after every use. Interspace brushes are useful to clean around bridges and fixed orthodontic appliances.

Teething It is a period when a baby cuts his or her first set of teeth. Primary teeth usually begin to erupt at about six or seven months. On an average, first set of teeth is complete soon after the second birthday. During teething baby becomes irritable, fretful and crys more than usual. There will be dribbling of saliva and baby tends to chew anything he or she can hold. The gum may become red and swollen and erupting teeth can be felt through the gum as a hard lump. It does not result in high temperature and simple dose of Crocin may help.

Tegmentum The floor of, or area below the ventricle of, the midbrain; it has motor functions.

Tegretol It is structurally related to imipramine. It is the drug of choice in trigeminal neuralgia. Half-life is 20 to 35 hours after few weeks of therapy. Cimetidine and valproate inhibit its metabolism. Dose is 600 to 1200 mg daily in divided doses. Adverse effects include reversible blurring of vision, diplopia and dizziness. It results in osteomalacia due to enhanced metabolism of vitamin D.

Tegument The syncytium that covers the surface of trematodes and cestodes.

Tela choroidia Membranous web', consisting the embryonic cerebral hemispheres.

Telegraphic utterances Word combinations which convey the essential elements of a message while omitting nonessential elements; frequent among children in the early stages of language acquisition.

Telencephalon The anterior portion of the forebrain, constituting the cerebral hemispheres and related parts.

Teleodendrion A division of an axon.

Teleology Ethical theory based on final outcomes.

Telepathy An aspect of extrasensory perception in which someone allegedly is able to know another person's thoughts without any of the traditional sensory modalities.

Telophase The final stage of mitosis in which the daughter nuclei become established.

Temegesic It is a synthetic analgesic of high potency and long action. It exhibits both agonist and antagonist actions. It is 35 times as potent as morphine and half as potent as fentanyl. Duration of action is upto 10 hours. 200 microgram can be given sublingually in postoperative pain. Not reversed by naloxone but respiratory depression may be treated by doxapram.

Temperament A person's characteristic modes of emotional response, such as sociability. Such tendencies are to some extent innate and subsequently modified by experience.

Temperate In Lab. context, a bacteriophage that can either infect and lyse a host with the production of further phages in an infectious cycle, or enter the lysogenic state and be stably herited as part of the host genome.

Temperate phage A phage whose DNA may be incorporated into the host-cell genome without being expressed; as distinct from a virulent phase, which destroys the host cell.

Temperature The normal body temperature is 98.6°F (37°C). Exercise, sleep, eating and drinking may bring change in temperature. It is lowest in early morning and higher at 6 pm. Body temperature is maintained within normal limits by hypothalamus. It acts as a thermostat. When temperature falls the hypothalamus sends nerve impulses to stimulate shivering. When body temperature rises hypothalamus stimulates sweating. Certain patterns of fever are specific for specific diseases.

Temperature profile in warm and cold About 1% difference exist between the core and peripheral temperature but in cold temperature it may extend to 10°C between periphery and trunk.

Temperature translation Conversion of tympanic temperature into an oral, rectal, or core temperature.

Template A macromolecular mold or pattern for the synthesis of an informational macromolecule.

Template Pattern or mold A curved or flat plate used as an aid in setting teeth.

Temple Fay He recommends that cerebral palsied be taught motion accorfing to its development in evolution. He regards ontogenic development (in man) as a recapitulation of phylogenetic development. Based on these ideas, he developed progressive pattern movements which consist of five stages :-

Stage 1 Prone lying :- Head and trunk rotation from side to side.

Stage 2 Homolateral stage.

Stage 3 Contralanted stage. Stage 4 Bear walk or elephant walk. Stage 5 Normal walking pattern.

Temporal Indicating the temple; the temple of the head is so named because it is there that the hair first begins turning white, indicating the passage of time.

Temporal arteritis It is the disease of elderly persons in which walls of arteries which pass over the temples over scalp becomes inflamed. Vessels become narrowed and blood flow then is reduced. Cause is not known fully but is often associated with polymyalgia rheumatica. Most common symptom is headache. Temporal artery may be prominent and scalp may be tender. Person may develop low fever, poor appetite and lethargy. There may be partial loss of vision. Disease responds to corticosteroids.

Temporal bone Lateral bone of the skull composed of squamous and mastoid portions.

Temporal lobe It includes centres for hearing, smell, memory and speech. Centre for hearing is areas 41 to 42 close to figure of Sylvius. The centre for memory is within uncus around the hippocampus.

A dreamy state can result from temporal lobe epilepsy. Person may experience unpleasant smell. The centre for smell is within uncus on the medial surface of temporal lobe.

Temporal lobe epilepsy It is a form of epilepsy in which an abnormal electrical discharge in the brain is confined to temporal lobe. There is an area of damage within one of temporal lobe. Damage may be caused by birth injury, brain tumour, brain abscess or stroke. Person feels partial loss of awareness to total surrounding. Person may have unpleasant hallucination of smell or taste. Person may perform task without remembering after attack. Attack may last for hours. Treatment consists of an operation to remove the part of lobe containing the irritating focus.

Temporal lobe, lesions These often produce seizures. Dominant temporal lobe lesion will produce aphasia if it extends posteriorly beyond the anterior 6 cm. Changes in mood and potency may also be associated. Bilateral temporal lobe damaged results in gross defect of recent memory so much so that patient may forget his or her own name. In animals it may produce aggression and hypersexuality but in humans it results in impairment of libido and potency.

Temporal regulation The depression of enzyme synthesis that occurs as a batch culture enters the stationary phase.

Temporal summation Graded potentials that occur at approximately the same time on a membrane are added together (summate).

Temporary (provisional) prosthesis Device consisting of a socket designed to accept full weight bearing, attached to a pylon and foot. Unlike a permanent prosthesis, the temporary one may not be cosmetically finished. For the above-knee prosthesis, the pylon usually is surmounted by a knee unit.

Temporary denture A denture to serve a very short time in a temporary or emergency situation.

Temporary filling Dressing should be protected from saliva by a 3-4 m.m. thick layer of sealing material i.e. zinc sulphate. If there is risk of fracture dual filling may be done. Outer one for occlusal function and aesthetic reason.

Temporary glycosuria It may arise in many conditions in which carbohydrate metabolism is deranged. It is of no consequence. There may be temporarily diminution of sugar tolerance particularly with septic infections. Chronic alcoholism, Graves' disease and head injury or after heavy meal in obese may result it. Emotions and fatigue may also precipitate glycosuria.

Temporomandibular joint (TMJ) syndrome There is dental malocclusion, overaction of jaw joint followed by development of loose joint due to absorption of meniscus, condyles and bone. Clinically there may be severe neuralgia, headache, full ear sensation with reduced hearing, tinnitus and facial pain.

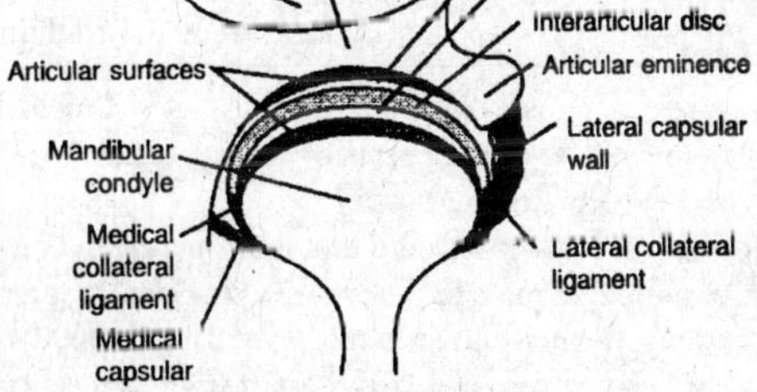

TM Joint—Coronal section

Tenacious Adhesive, sticky.

Tendencies Analysis Also named differential crime analysis. Specific crime analysis form. Study of the variation with time of crime data, of relationship between crime data, and of other relevant data representing the evolution of a criminal phenomenon.

Tendinosis It is suggested by an antalgic gait, weakness when attempting to perform a single heel rise, local thickening of part, warmth and tenderness.

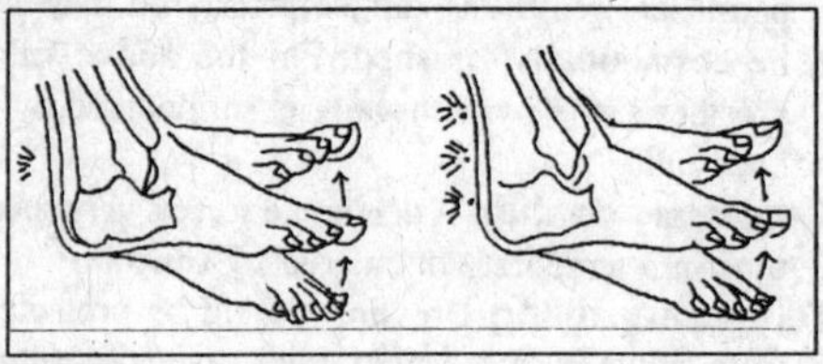

Tendinous inscription One of the bands of connective tissue crossing the rectus abdominis muscle subdividing it and attaching it to adjacent connective tissue.

Tendocalcaneus The tendon is about 15 cm long and is formed by union of tendons of

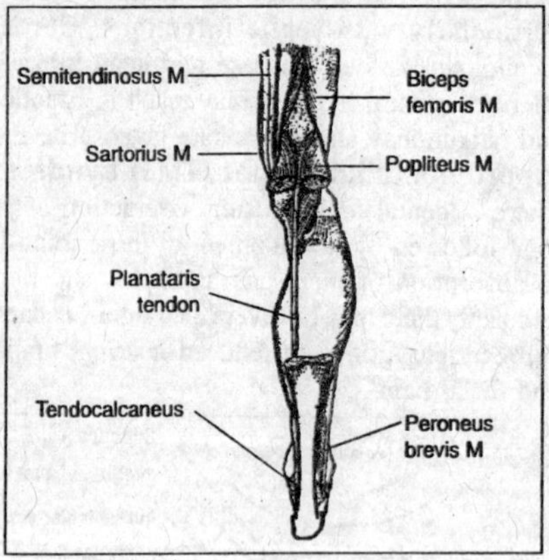

gastrocnemius, soleus and plantaris. It is attached to the middle of the posterior surface of calcaneus and is separated by bursa.

Tendon It is a fibrous cord that joins muscle to bone or muscle to muscle. These are cylindrical and are strong, flexible and inelastic. Squeezing the tendon hard causes pain and stretching it triggers a reflex contraction. Inflammation of a tendon is usually

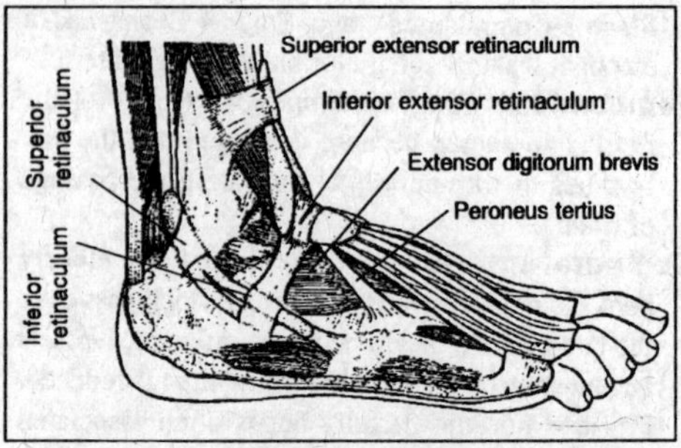

caused by an injury. Symptoms include pain, tenderness and restricted movements.

Tendon action of muscle If you rest your elbow on table and flex your wrist your fingers will open. If you hyperextend your wrist your fingers have a tendency to close.

If tendons are little tight, opening and closing will be more prounced known as tendon action of muscle or tenodesis.

Tendon health Tube-shaped structure lined with synovial membrane that encloses certain tendons.

Tendon of the infundibulum A fibrous band connecting aortic and pulmonary annuli.

Tendon organ A proprioceptive receptor, sensitive to changes in muscle tension and force of contraction, found chiefly near the junctions of tendons and muscles. Also called a Golgi tendon organ.

Tendon sheath Tube-shaped structure lined with synovial membrane that encloses certain tendons.

Tendonitis Inflammation of a tendon.

Tendons Cords of fibrous connective tissue that connect a muscle to a bone to allow for joint movement.

Tenesmus It is a feeling of incomplete emptying of bowel. Even after straining it is not completely emptied. It may be caused in dysentery, ulcerative colitis or polyps of rectum.

Tenia solium It is known as pork tape worm. Adult worm usually measures 180-400 cm and contains 800-900 proglottids. One small scolex measuring about 1 m.m. in diameter is armed with two circles of 22-32 rostellar hooks. The testes are scattered throughout the medullary region of proglottid. The mature proglottid is squarish in outline and has a common genital pore situated on lateral edge in mid center.

Teniae coli The segmented, longitudinal smooth muscle layer of the colon.

Tennis elbow It is the condition caused by inflammation around the epicondyle on the outer side of elbow. It results in pain and tenderness. Pain becomes worst while lifting heavy weight. It is caused by overuse of muscle. Rest to the part, ice-packs and anti-inflammatory drugs help the person.

TENS Transcutaneous electrical nerve stimulation.

Tensile strength 1. Resistance to a pulling force. 2. The amount of stress a material is able to withstand when being pulled lengthwise before permanent deformation results.

Tension fracture It is known as traction fracture when bone fibres fail at right angles to the direction of tensile force applied.

Tension pneumothorax The air within the pleural cavity as the result of a communication between the lung and the pleural space in which a valve effect exists; air enters the pleural space or inspiration but is trapped during expiration.

Tentaculum It has a single tooth and it pierces only at one point with minimal bleeding. It can hold anterior lip of cervix transversely.

Tentorium Tentorium cerebelli.

Tentorium cerebelli A extension of dura mater that forms a partition between the cerebral hemispheres and the cerebellum and covers the carebellum.

Tenure A permanent position of appointment in an academic setting.

Teolophase Last stage of mitosis in which the cell divides.

Tepid Moderately warm to the touch.

Teratogen Anything that causes the development of abnormal structures in an embryo and results in a severely deformed fetus.

Teratogenesis The production of fetal abnormalities by some agent or process.

Teratogenic Any drug or process which may cause serious deformity in fetus in pregnant woman such as rubella infection and X-rays.

Teratoma A neoplasm composed of multiple tissues, including tissues not normally found in the organ in which it arises.

Teratospermia A condition in which most ejaculated sperms are structurallly abnormal.

Term birth A birth that occurs between the 38th to 42nd weeks of gestation.

Terminal disinfection Measures used to clean the patient environment after discharge.

Terminal hair The most obvious of the three types of hair found on the mature human body. Terminal hair include scalp, pubic, beard, axillary, eyebrow, eyelash and nasal hair. The majority of the remainder of the human body is covered by vellus hair. In addition, there are intermediate hair between these two types.

Terminal illness An incurable condition that will lead to a person's death within a short time.

Terminal nerve A cranial nerve that may mediate information on pheromones.

Terminal plateau A flat place at the end of a learning curve indicating no further improvement in performance. This plateau presumably represents a physiological limit in the organism; the individual simply cannot perform the task any more rapidly or successfully.

Terminal stance The phase from the end of mid stance to the point of heel off (just before the contralateral limb strikes the ground).

Terminal swing Invloves the slowing of swing limb just prior to its contact with the support surface.

Terminating phase Ending of a nurse-patient relationship when there is mutual agreement that the patient's immediate health problems have improved.

Termination factors Protein factors of the cytosol required in releasing a completed polypeptide chain from a ribosome; also known as release factors.

Termination sequence A DNA sequence that appears at the end of a transcriptional unit and signals the end of transcription.

Tertiary adrenal insufficiency State of hypocortisolism due to pathological process that involves the hypothalamus.

Tertiary care Health services provided at hospitals or medical centers that offer specialists and complex technology.

Tertiary intention A type of wound healing: delayed or secondary closure, such as a draining abdominal wound

Tertiary medical center Hospital that has most or all of the latest technology and usually participates actively in medical education and even in clinical research.

Tertiary prevention Occurs after a disorder to minimize further complications or to assist in the restotation of health.

Tertiary prevention Programs that intervene directly with patients to reduce the duration of their cancer as a patient.

Tertiary structure The three-dimensional conformation of a polymer in its native folded state.

Test A procedure for obtaining measurements to be interpreted according to a standard; e.g., a muscle length, muscle strength, range of motion, or alignment test.

Test movement A movement of the part in a specified direction and through a specified arc or motion.

Test position The position in which the part is placed by the examiner and held by the patient.

Test Sample Analyzed to provide scientific information that will assist in reaching conclusions or establishing facts concerning an acident.

Test tube baby It is the result of fertilisation of human ovum outside the body of the prospective mother. Later on implantation of fertilised of ovum in uterus leads to normal pregnancy.

Testes Male gonads that produce the male sex cells or sperm.

Testicle The male reproductive gland.

Testicond Having the testes retained within the abdominal cavity, a characteristic of various mammals.

Testicular Relating to involving or affecting the testes i.e. male reproductive glands.

Testicular feminisation syndrome It is characterised by absent axillary and pubic hair, short vagina, absent or rudimentary uterus, and testes in the labial folds or inguinal canal in women with normal external genitalia and well-developed breasts.

Testimony Statements made at a hearing or trial by a witness under oath.

Testing This threat to internal validity is realized when repeated testing itself is likely to result in changes in the dependent variable.

Testing a hypothesis In research gathering information for one view or another; attempting to obtain information in support of a particular viewpoint.

Testis The testes are formed within abdomen near the kidneys. In response to hormones produced by mother and produced in testicles, the testes gradually descend through the inguinal canal.

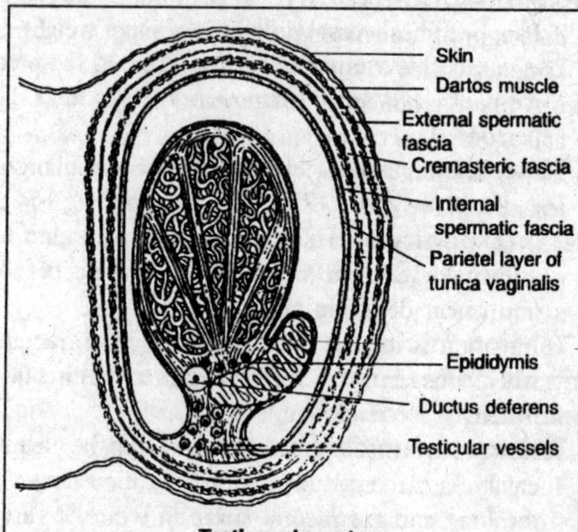

Testis and scrotum

Each testis has seminiferous tubules, delicate coiled tubes producing sperms. Seminiferous tubules lead to epididymis via vas deferens. Epididymis matures newly formed sperms. Interstitial cells between the seminiferous tubules produce the male sex hormone testosterone. Each testis is protected by a tough, fibrous capsule the tunica albuginea.

Testis, cancer It is not very common. It occurs in middle-aged person. These are of two types, seminomas and teratomas. Seminomas are made up of single cells while teratomas consist of several different types of cells. Testis becomes firm and painless. Orchidectomy may be sufficient to cure testicular cancer in early stage. Radiation therapy is followed along with anticancer drugs.

Testis, torsion Twisting of the spermatic cord causing acute, severe pain and swelling of testis. Unless treated within a few hours, the testis is damaged permanently and sperm production ceases. Testical pain develops acutely accompanied by abdominal pain. Testis becomes swollen and very tender and scrotal skin becomes discoloured. Ultrasound studies help. Treatment is by surgery. Even if one testis is removed the other is usually capable of maintaining fertility.

Testosterone It is an androgen hormone and stimulates bone and muscle growth and sexual development. It is produced by testes and in small amount by ovaries. It is used to treat infertility. In puberty it may cause over rapid sexual development.

Test-retest reliability A common way of determining consistency, by administering the same test twice to the same persons.

Tests These are medical procedures which are key and essential part of diagnosis specially when signs and symptoms are not clear cut. There are many tests available.

Tetanic contraction It is sustained muscle contraction caused by repetitive electrical stimulation of a motor nerve. About 25 Hz stimulation is required.

Tetanic contraction Sustained contraction.

Tetanus Disease results from effects of neurotoxin produced by infection of *Clostridium tetani.* Incubation period includes 5 days to 2 to 3 months. Toxin tetanospasmin is bound to neuronal membranes. First clinical feature is trismus, lock jaw and retraction of mouth. Pain and stiffness in paraspinal and abdominal muscles follow. Paraspinal muscle spasm may be very severe. There is no ventilation during spasm and is the cause of death. There may be profuse sweating, excessive salivary and pharyngeal secretions and hypotension.

Tetanus neonatorum It is caused by gram-positive, non-capsulated, anaerobic spore forming bacilli *Clostridium tetani*. Symptoms appear by 5 to 15 days after birth. Excessive unexplained crying followed by refusal of feeds and apathy are the common initial symptoms. Mouth is kept slightly open due to pull and spasm of neck. Feeding becomes painful. Lock jaw or reflex trismus is followed by spasm of limbs. There is generalised rigidity followed by spasm of limbs. Constipation persists.

Tetany Hyperexcitability of neurons and muscle fibers caused by hypocalcemia and characterized by intermittent or continuous tonic.

Tethering, of spinal cord In some persons conus medullaris is placed abnormally low, tethered by a short and thickened filum terminale. There may be intraspinal lipoma or cyst. Diastematomyelia or hydromyelia may also occur. Neurological abnormalities associated with tethered cord include asymmetrical muscle weakness in legs. There may be trophic ulceration of feet and neurogenic bladder.

Tetra-acetic acid This is a better anticoagulant than oxalate. It is available as salts in solid form. It acts by chelating calcium and preserves cellular morphology. It is used for blood collection for counts, ESR and PCV estimations. For blood chemistry it is not used.

Tetracyclines These have a broad range of antimicrobial activity. These are bacteriostatic. These are partially absorbed from alimentary tract. These are excreted mainly unchanged in urine and should be avoided in renal disease. These are active against gram-positive and gram-negative bacteria. These are selectively taken up in teeth and growing bones of fetus and children due to their chelating properties and calcium phosphate. This causes dental enamel hypoplasia with pitting, cusp malformation, yellow or brown pigmentation and increased susceptibility to caries. After the fourteenth week of pregnancy and in first few months even short course may be damaging. Dairy products reduce absorption to a degree but antacids and iron preparations do so much more.

Tetraiodothyronine (T4) One of the thyroid hormones that contains four iodine atoms, also called thyroxine.

Tetraplegia Synonymous with quadriplegia.

Tetraplegia Four-paralysis'. Synonymous with quadriplegia.

Tetrapod These are four legged sticks which gives greater stability. These are used where patient has particularly poor balance or lacks confidence. The size of base between the legs can vary and selection will depend on how much extra stability patient needs

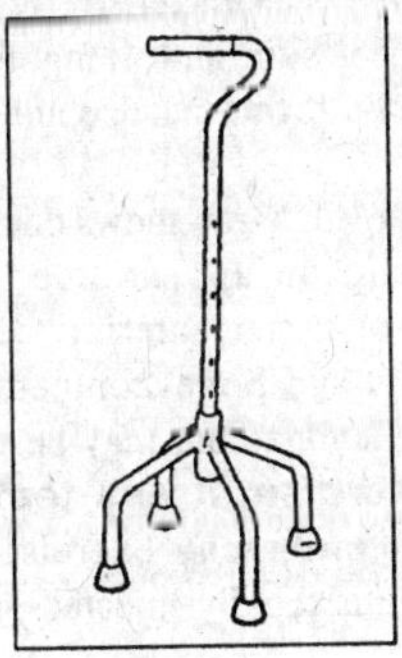

Tetrodotoxin Toxin obtained from fish which selectively blocks sodium channels.

Texture gradient In the visual perception of space, a cue to distance based on the haziness of details due to atmospheric interference. Objects at a distance appear hazier and less distinct than nearby objects.

Thalamic pain syndrome It is a continuous pain on the side, contralateral side to thalamic lesion which affect the orofacial area and can cause sensory and motor abnormalities. Pain may be aching or burning. The disease is usually a complication of CVA, neoplasm and multiple sclerosis. X-ray may reveal diffuse bony changes in affected area. Narcotic agents have been successful.

Thalamic sensory syndrome Continuous, unpleasant sensation on the hemiplegic side.

Thalamic syndrome Vascular lesion of the thalamus resulting in sensory disturbances and partial or complete paralysis of one side of the body, associated with severe, boring-type pain. Sensory stimuli may produce an exaggerated, prolonged, and/or painful response.

Thalamus It is like an antichamber through which all sensory data pass through before reaching the cerebral cortex. It is about 2.5 cm in length and is more or less egg-shaped. Laterally it is covered by a sheet of white matter. It plays an important subcortical correlation or relay station. Thalamus transmits the cerebellar fibres to the cortex of frontal lobe and it is by this means that the cerebellum guides and controls the cerebral cortex. Essential organ of thalamus is the centre for recognition of crude forms of sensibility such as pain and temperature.

Thalasaemia It is characterised by anaemia, yellow colouration of skin and mongoloid appearance. There may be fever, malaise and enlargement of spleen.

Head is enlarged. X-ray shows thickening of diploe and hair end on appearance. There will be protrusion of upper anterior teeth. Jaw shows osteoporosis and honeycombed appearance of trabeculae. Lamina dura may be thin.

Thallium exercise stress test Radionuclear perfusion scintigraphy exercise test in which thallium 201 is rapidly injected into the blood at near maximal exercise; either treadmill or bicycle ergometer protocols may be used.

Thallium imaging Myocardial perfusion imaging uses thallium 20%. It is a radioactive cation that is useful because it behaves as a potassium analogue. Following IV of $^{201}T_1$ rapidly leaves the vascular compartment and enters the cells in proportion to initial blood flow. About 4% of dose enters the myocardium temporarily. Small accumulation shows the heart in relief against the low surrounding background of lung activity. Since positron-emission tomography (PET) is not available easily stress thallium remains the best modality to look for reversible ischaemia. Thallium imaging is more informative than stress test about coronary circulation after CABG and angioplasty.

Thanatology The medicolegal study of the dying process and death.

Thanatophobia Fear of death and whatever has become associated with death.

The 'four Ps' Four factors that determine the success of spontaneous labour are (i) pelvis (ii) power of uterine contraction (iii) position of presenting part of fetus and (iv) position of mother during labour and delivery.

Thebesian valve Valve of coronary sinus.

Thebesian veins A number of minute veins arising in the walls of the heart, most emptying directly into the atria, but a few ending in the ventricles; smallest cardiac veins.

Theca A protective case or covering; e.g., the total cell wall composed of cellulose plates in dinoflagellates.

Thelarche Enlargement of breast is the earliest indication of onset of puberty. Development occurrs in 5 stages : (*i*) increased vascularisation of areola and nipple, (*ii*) palpable nodule of mammary tissue enlarges to form mammary bud—diameter of areola increases, (*iii*) breast and areola enlarge further, (*iv*) areola and nipple form a secondary mound, which is slightly raised above the level of breast, and (*v*) in fully mature breast only nipple projects and areola recedes to conform to the general contour of breast.

Thelectomy Surgical removal of the nipples.

Themoregulation Ability to control temperature within acceptable range.

Thenar Thenar eminence of thumb.

Theophylline A xanthine, closely related to caffeine; found in tea leaves.

Theory A set of statements that tentatively describe, explain, or predict relationships between concepts. They are selected and organized as abstract representations of phenomenon.

Theory of mind Our understanding that other people have separate mental states and see the world from their point of view which differs from our own. Young children do not have this theory of mind and can't imagine that someone else is experiencing different feelings or thoughts.

Therapeutic Any treatment considered necessary to return the patient to a preclinical status or establish a stationary status.

Therapeutic abortion When evacuation of the uterus is carried out by a registered medical practioner as treatment in the interest of mother's health and life.

Therapeutic baths Baths performed for other than hygiene purposes.

Therapeutic community A term of British origin, now widely used, for a specially structured mental hospital that encourages patients to function within the range of social norms.

Therapeutic exercise Activity performed by people with health risks or those being treated for a health problem.

Therapeutic index The numerical ratio of the concentration of a substance that will achieve a desired effect in 50% of the patients, andthe concentration that produces unacceptable toxicity in 50% of the patients. Book containing details of medicines.

Therapeutic range Range or levels of the drug in the blood that will produce a desired effect without causing toxic effects.

Therapeutic touch A method of pain relief based on the folk-healing practice known as laying on of bands, whereby healers place themselves in a meditative state, hold their hands just above the client, and transfer their energy to the client to relieve pain or other problems.

Therapeutic ultrasonics In order to transmit ultrasonic energy to the tissues it is necessary to provide a couplant. Virtually no transmission occurs through air. Ultrasonic energy is absorbed by air-bubbles so degassed water is best used. Inflammatory skin lesions or open wounds are avoided. Couplant is placed on skin to be treated and the treatment head which is then pressed upon the skin before the output is turned on.

Therapeutic verbal communication Using words and gesturs to accomplish a particular objective.

Therapeutic window The well-defined range of blood levels associated with optimal clinical response to antidepressant drugs, such as nortriptyline. Levels above or below that range are associated with a poor response.

Therapy The treatment of disease.

Theriogenology The diagnosis, treatment, and prevention of reproductive diseases in animals.

Thermal burn Skin injury caused by flames, hot liquids, or steam.

Thermal conductivity A property characterizing the rate at which heat is transferred through a material

Thermal strain Any deviation of body temperature induced by sustained thermal stress that cannot be fully compensated by temperature regulation..

Thermal stratification The zonal separation of a body of water maintained by density gradients based on water temperature.

Thermanalgesia Inability to perceive heat.

Thermanesthesia Inability to perceive sensations of heat and cold.

Thermatome Area of cutaneous vasomotor disturbance most commonly related to dysfunction at a particular nerve root level. Thermatomes often overlap with dermatomes but do not have identical boundaries.

Thermesthesia Ability to perceive heat and cold sensations, temperature sensibility.

Thermhyperesthesia Increased sensitivity to temperature.

Thermhyposthesia Decreased temperature sensibility.

Thermic effect of food An increase of cellular activity when food is eaten.

Therminization The procedure of exposing microrganisms to a relatively mild thermal process e.g. 63°C.

Thermictor Temperature sensor.

Thermoacidophilic Growing optimally in conditions of both extreme heat and extreme acid.

Thermocautery Cauterization by a heated wire or point.

Thermocoagulation Coagulation of tissues by means of high frequency currents.

Thermodilution method A means of determining the cardiac output; a cold bolus of saline is injected into the right atrium via the proximal lumen of a flow-directed, thermal-sensitive catheter; the resultant temperature change is sensed by a thermistor near the tip of the catheter located in the pulmonary artery.

Thermoduric Describing the ability of a microorganism to survive pasteurization.

Thermoeffector An organ and its function that affect heat balance in a controlled manner as part of process of temperature regulation.

Thermogenesis The production of heat in the body by metabolic oxidation of food substrates.

Thermographic imaging It is the process of an image of temperature distribution by sensing and imaging the distribution as a function of wavelength depends directly on temperature. The peak of emitted spectrum ranges from about 2 mm for every hot objects (>1000°k) to about 15 mm for objects near 0°C.

Thermometer It is an instrument used to measure temperature. It contains a glass capillary tube sealed at one end and mercury- filled bulb at the another.

When bulb is kept in mouth, mercury expands and temperature is indicated by level of mercury. There is small kink in the capillary tube just above the bulb to prevent the mercury from moving down the tube. Clinical thermometer may be calibrated in centigrade or fahrenheit.

Thermophile Literally, heat lover; an organism that grows optimally at temperatures between 50 and 80°C. Organisms that prefer temperatures higher than 37°C and have constitutive heat resistance.

Thermophilic Growing optimally at temperatures between 50 and 80°C.

Thermoplastic The ability to be reversibly transformed from a glassy,brittle solid to a softened moldable plastic by heating beyond a certain temperature.

Thermoplastic impression material Thermoplastic solids can be transformed from a hard, solid material into a softened moldable material by heating. Process can be reversed by cooling to room temperature.

Thermoplastics Plastics that will soften repeatedly at high temperature and rehardens at lower temperature.

Thermoprotectant A molecule that plays an active role in thermotolerance by protecting proteins and perhaps other cellular components from the damaging effects of elevated temperatures.

Thermoreceptor Receptor that detects changes in temperature.

Thermoregulation The regulation of heat, such as the body heat of a warm-blooded animal.

Thermosensitive neurons Peripheral sensory neurons having sensory receptors activated by heat.

Theta rhythm Slow-wave temporal lobe rhythm associated with the septohippocampal cholinergic pathway.

Thiamine deficiency It is found in cereals, nuts and yeast. Its deficiency results in beri beri. Beri beri is of two types, *wet form* is characterised by conjestion, oedema and enlargement of right side of heart : *Dry form* leades to degenerative changes in nerves leading to polyneuritis. Oral manifestations consist of oedema of tongue, pain and loss of papillae.

Thiamine pyrophosphate The active coenzyme form of vitamin B_1; involved in aldehyde transfer reactions.

Thick blood smear This is required for detection of malarial parasite and microfilaria. Here a large drop is taken at the centre of slide and not at the end as in thin smear. Then by means of corner of another slide, the drop is spread over an area of an inch on the slide.

Thickened pleura It may be caused by recurrent dry pleurisy, following a chronic empyema, a persistent pleural effusion or haemothorax. When pleura is thickened there will be diminished movement over chest, dullness on percussion and diminished vocal fremitus or resonance.

Thigh The proximal portion of the lower extremity between the hip and the knee in which the femur is located.

Thiol Any of a group of organic compounds resembling alcohols, but with the oxygen of the hydroxyl group replaced by sulfur.

Thiopental It is a very short-acting barbiturate which when administered I.V. as a single dose, rapidly induces hypnosis and anaesthesia without analegesia. Half-life is 9 minutes. Thiopentone, in a single dose usually exerts its cerebral depressant effect within 30 seconds and it persists for 4 to 7 minutes.

Anaesthesia is introduced rapidly, presently and without excitement. Disadvantage is of short muscular relaxation for any practical value. It requires prolonged anaesthesia and slow recovery period. It should not be given in severe cardiac cases and obstructive respiratory diseases. It requires experienced anaesthetist.

Third degree atrioventricular block The pathologic loss of conduction through the atrioventricular junctional tissues; atrioventricular dissociation in which atrial or sinus foci elicit depolarization of the atria, while an idioventricular focus stimulates the ventricles.

Third ear Literally, listening with "the third ear", i.e. the utilisation of intuition, sensitivity, and awareness of subliminal cues to interpret clinical observations of patients in therapy.

Third heart sound It is a low-pitched filling sound resulting from distension and vibration of ventricular wall and papillary muscles. It is normal in high cardiac output states.

After the age of 40, third sound indicates ventricular decompensation and AV value regurgitation. Left sided S_3 is better heard with bell piece in cardiac apex during expiration in left lateral position. Right sided S_3 is better heard in lower left sternal border during inspiration.

Third heart sound (S3) A weak, low-pitched sound occurring in early diastole, soon after the second heart sound; believed to be caused by vibrations of the poorly compliant ventricular wall as it is distended during filling.

Third lumbar root Compression The root pain occupies the upper buttock, whole front thigh and knee spreading down the front inner side of knee. Flexion is of full range.

Third molars Eighth tooth from the midline in each quadrant of the permanent dentition.

Third stage of labour This stage begins with the birth of the baby and ends with the delivery of placenta.

Third ventricle A narrow cavity between the right and left halves of the thalamus and between the lateral ventricles that contains cerebrospinal fluid.

Third-intention healing Reparative process when a wound is widely separated and later brought together with some type of closure material.

Third-spacing Movement of intravascular fluid to nonvascular fluid compartments, where its becomes trapped and useless.

Thirst It is a desire to drink. It is the process by which amount of water in the body is controlled. Thirst is increased by the concentration of salt and sugar in blood. As concentrated blood passes through the hypothalamus in the brain, special nerve receptors are stimulated inducing the sensation of thirst. Thirst is stimulated if volume of blood decreases as a result of sweating, vomiting, diarrhoea, bleeding or burns. Strong need to drink develops in case of dehydration and in diabetes.

Thirst center A cluster of neurons in the hypothal amus that is sensitive to the osmotic pressure of extracellular fluid and brings about the sensation of thirst.

Thomas heel Heel designed by Hugh Owen Thomas in which the anterior margin is curved, such that its medial border extends anteriorly, usually with a slight medial wedge; intended to support flexible pes valgus.

Thomas test This test is applied to measure hip deformity, with the patient lying supine. The good hip is flexed fully ensuring that the lumbar lordosis

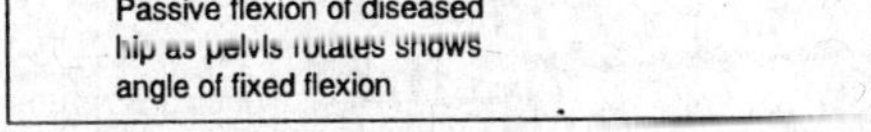

is flattened. If the affected hip rises from the couch this indicates the presence of fixed flexion deformity and angle may be measured. The rotation hip ranging 30 to 90 degree indicates a flexion deformity of 30 degree and a hip that flexes to 90 degree.

Thoracic Pertaining to the chest region.

Thoracic cavity Superior portion of the ventral body cavity that contains two pleural cavities, the mediastinum, and the pericardial cavity.

Thoracic duct It is a major vessel of lymphatic system which collects lymph from lower limb and left side of the body. It channels to blood through vein.

Thoracic inlet The upper margin of the thorax; formed by the first thoracic vertebra posteriorly, the superior border of the manubrium anteriorly, and the first ribs laterally.

Thoracic outlet The lower margin of the thorax; formed by the twelfth thoracic vertebra posteriorly, the seventh through tenth costal cartilages anteriorly, and the eleventh and twelfth ribs laterally.

Thoracic scoliosis A lateral curvature of spine with an apex T2 to T11.

Thoraco lumbar curvature Any spinal curvature that has its apex at T12 or L_1.

Thoracocentesis It is the procedure of removal of fluid from pleural cavity puncturing through chest wall. It helps in relieving pain, breathlessness and provide comfort from heavy pressure on chest. Patient is allowed to sit up and lean forward. Puncture area is usually midaxillary line or below scapula. Watch the signs of shock. Measure the fluid and level for laboratory investigations.

Thoracolumbar corset This is a fabric corset with adjustable lacing and classic components to permit snugness of fit. It is reinforced by straps to increase

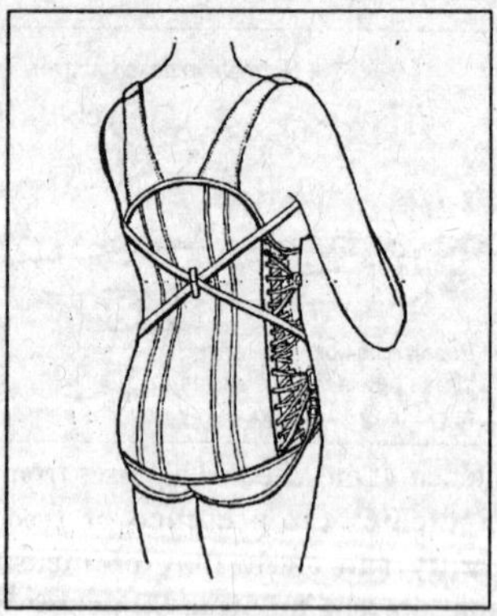

rigidity. This corset extends from beneath the lower curve of the buttocks to the midscapular area and is held in place superiorly by shoulder straps. It is useful in generalised osteoporosis.

Thorax The chest; the upper part of the trunk between the neck and the abdomen.

Thornsen's disease Myotonia congenita.

Thought disorder A disturbance of speech, communication, or content of thought, such as delusions, ideas of reference, poverty of thought, flight of ideas, perseveration, loosening of associations, etc. A thought disorder can be caused by a functional emotional disorder or an organic condition. A formal thought disorder is a disturbance in the form of thought rather than the content of thought, e.g. loosening of associations.

Thready pulse Fine and barely perceptible pulse; easily obliterated.

Threatened abortion Haemorrhage may occur during early pregnancy without leading to dilatation of the cervix. It is possible that slight detachment of some part of ovum or of the decidua itself may be healed and gestation may continue. Haemorrhage must therefore never be regarded as a certain indication of abortion unless it is accompanied by pain and dilatation of internal os. By suitable treatment process can often be arrested and abortion averted.

Threatened uterus rupture In threatened rupture following prolonged obstructed labour the lower segment is found stretched, elongated and tender with retracted upper segment. Fetal distress is present. At the height of intense uterine contraction the patient complains of sharp shooting pain within the lower abdomen. Patient may cry. External or internal bleeding may continue. Shock may develop.

Three point gait A walk in which two crutches or one cane and the affected leg advances together followed by unaffected leg.

Three-quarter crown Cast restoration that covers most of the clinical crown, commonly with the exception of the buccal surface, and fits over the prepared tooth.

Threshold The point at which an experience just barely occurs. A stimulus of threshold strength is one which, if it were weaker, would have no typical effect. A more specific term is absolute threshold. The terminal threshold is the upper limit of sensitivity; the point beyond which further increases in intensity have no typical effect. "Typical effect" in these definitions means no change in the type of experience being studied. If increasing the intensity of light stimulation brings pain, that is not a visual effect, hence not typical for this kind of stimulation. Limen is a synonym for threshold.

Threshold dose The highest dosage level of a toxic substance at which the incidence of harm or damage is not statistically greater than that of a neutral control substance.

Threshold exposure The minimum exposure that will produce a detectable degree of any given effect.

Threshold level The level below which the body can adapt to an adverse exposure successfully and with little or no harm resulting. There is such a threshold level for most chemical and physical agents and even for most chemical and physical agents and even for most microbes.

Threshold potential The membrane voltage that must be reached to trigger an action potential.

Threshold stimulus Any stimulus strong enough to initiate an action potential or activate a sensory receptor.

Thrill It is a temporary switching on of body as a response of high emotion. It results due to sudden release of adrenaline.

Thrombin The active enzyme formed from prothrombin that acts to convert fibrinogen to fibrin during formation of a blood clot.

Thrombocyte A blood platelet formed from a fragmented megakaryocyte. Play a role in blood clotting.

Thrombocytopenia A decrease in circulating platelets.

Thromboembolism An embolism from a venous thrombus.

Thrombolysis The dissolving of a thrombus.

Thrombolytic agent Chemical substance injected into the body to dissolve blood clots and restore circulation; mechanism of action is direct or indirect activation of plasminogen; examples include tissue plasminogen activator (t-PA), streptokinase, and urokinase.

Thrombophlebitis A condition in which inflammation of the wall of a vein has preceded the formation of a thrombus.

Thromboplastin A substance produced in the blood, plays a role in the coagulation process.

Thrombosis It is a formation of blood clot within an intact blood vessel. Thrombus formation is abnormal if it occurs when vessel wall has not been cut or injured. Thrombus within artery may grow and block the artery, blood supply to legs, kidneys, retina and other organs causing severe damage. Angio and venography helps in diagnosis. Venous thrombosis may also cause pain and swelling. Treatment includes anticoagulant drugs or thrombolytic drugs which help in dissolving thrombus. Antibiotics and anti- inflammatory drugs are useful.

Thrombus A blood clot formed by platelet aggregation and conversion of soluble fibrinogen to an insoluble mesh of polymerised fibrin.

Thromocytopenia An abnormally small number of platelets in the blood.

Throttling It means compression of neck by means of fingers. A slight compression is sufficient to cause complete closure of glottis as it forces the base of the tongue upwards and backwards against the posterior pharyngeal wall causing complete occlusion of air passage. In some cases superior laryngeal branch of vagus is injured which inhibits respiration. Victims of throttling are children, female or weak individuals.

Thrush Also called moniliasis.

Thrust Sudden manual application of a controlled directional force upon a suitable part of the patient, the delivery of which effects an adjustment.

Thudichum's nasal speculum It is used to examine anterior part of nasal cavity. Speculum is closed and gently introduced in patient's nostril. The spring is allowed to open a little to observe the floor of nasal cavity, nasal septum and lateral wall of nasal cavity.

Thumb contribution Thumb contribute in powergrip, precision, pinch grip and lateral or key pinch grip.

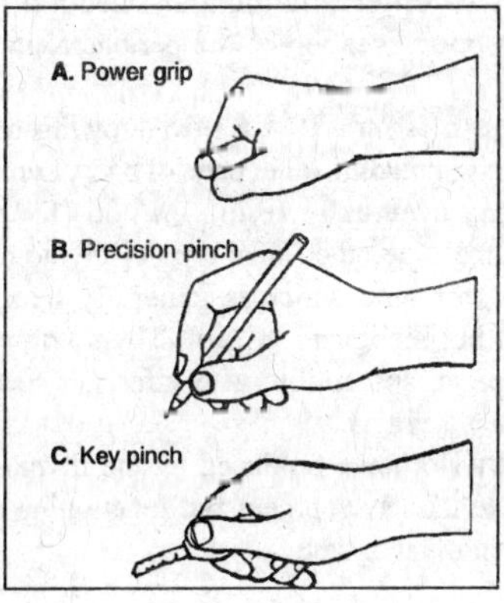

Thumb Effleurage Thumb effleurage is another form of deep stroking massage. As it is applied with only one or two digits it makes it possible for the pressure to be concentrated on small areas of muscle tissue, and it is also of particular use where the muscles lie flat to the above.

Thumb friction Forward and backward strokes are applied in the same manner as in the fingertip friction movement.

Thumb Pad Kneading Basic circular kneading strokes are performed with the pads of one or both thumbs, usually working side by side. This technique is expevially useful along fusiform muscles. It is also very useful for the treatment of very small areas in the hand, foot, and face.

Thumb sucking It indicates that a pleasurable sensation is derived by the child from this self-stimulation. This is a manifestation of feeling of insecurity. It has little effect on tooth alignment.

Thurston Holland Fragment Triangular metaphyseal fragment of bone that remains attached to epiphysis.

Thygeson's disease In Thygeson's superficial punctate keratitis, grey, superficial, round or oval sometimes stellate or irregular epithelial changes occur. These are transiently filiform occurring in varying members. Disease is usually bilateral. Corneal lesions may disappear and recur in other areas. There may be photophobia and foreign body sensation.

Thylakoid Closed cisterna, or disc, formed by the pigment-bearing internal membranes of chloroplasts.

Thymocyte An immature T cell undergoing the process of differentiation and selection in the thymus prior to export to the peripheral immune system.

Thymoma It is rare. It is a slow growing tumour that rarely spreads to other parts of body. Lymphoid thymoma eventually results in non-Hodgkin's lymphoma. The other main type of thymoma is a thymic teratoma which is generally benign in women but malignant in men. Thymoma results in increased susceptibility to infection specially myasthenia gravis.

Thymosin Hormone produced by the thymus that is vital to the development and functioning of the body's immune system.

Thymulin Hormone produced into thymus. Its activity decreases in association with zinc deficiency.

Thymus Bilobed lymphatic organ located in the inferior neck and superior mediastinum; involved with the maturation of T-cells. It is a gland which forms part of immune system. It is situated in the upper part of chest behind sternum. It consists of two lobes that join in front of trachea. The gland gradually enlarges until puberty when it begins to shrink. Lymphoid and epithelial tissues are replaced by fat. Function of thymus is to cause lymphocytes to become T-cells. Abnormal enlargement of the thymus sometimes occurs in myasthenia gravis, acromegaly, thyrotoxicosis and Addison's disease.

Thymus gland Endocrine gland located in the mediastinum; vital part of the body's immune system.

Thyroid-stimulating hormone (TSH) yoo-layting HOR-mone) A tropic hormone secreted by the anterior pituitary gland that stimulates the thyroid gland to increase its secretion of thyroid hormone.

Thyroglobulin (TGB) A large glycoprotein molecule produced by follicle cells of the thyroid gland in which iodine is combined with tyrosine to from thyroid hormones.

Thyroglossal cyst of duct Thyroglossal duct is blind epithelial duct that ascends from tongue to the location of thyroid gland. After differentiation of thyroid gland the duct degenerates but certain epithelial remnants are left in wake. These may undergo cystic degeneration giving rise thyroglossal cyst.

Thyroid cancer It is not very common. It is noticed as a single, firm nodule in the neck which is industinguishable from benign mass. If there are several nodules chances are of being benign. Cancerous tumours grow slowly but spreads to lymph glands early. Advanced cancers are usually hard and irregularly shaped and firmly attached to adjacent structures. Symptoms develop when tumour presses structures in neck including severe hoarseness or loss of voice and difficulty in swallowing. Treatment is surgical removal.

Thyroid cartilage Largest laryngeal cartilage; forms the laryngeal prominence of Adam's apple.

Thyroid crisis It is the major complication of thyrotoxicosis. It usually follows thyroid surgery in severe cases with sepsis. Onset is acute with tachycardia, restlessness, fever, hypotension, delirium and often coma. Antithyroid medication is to be given on priority.

Thyroid follicle One of many small spheres with walls consisting of cuboidal epithelial cells in the thyroid gland, and which is filled with proteins to which thyroid hormones are attached until they are secreted.

Thyroid gland Endocrine gland located inferior to the larynx and consisting of two lobes connected by a narrow band; secretes the thyroid hormones.

Thyroid gland, lingual Generally thyroid gland develops as an endothermal down growth from foramen caecum. Part or all of this thyroid may

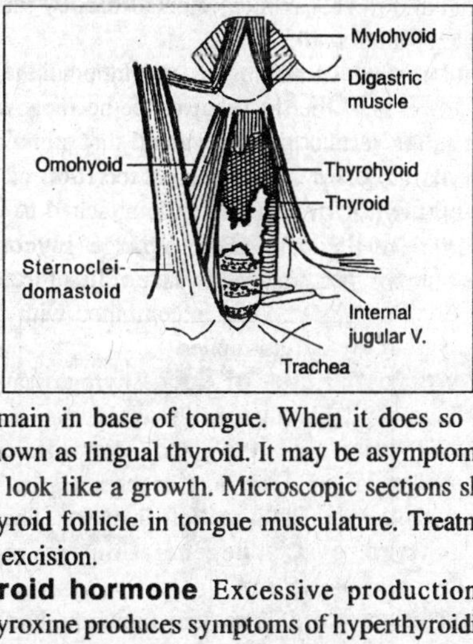

remain in base of tongue. When it does so it is known as lingual thyroid. It may be asymptomatic or look like a growth. Microscopic sections show thyroid follicle in tongue musculature. Treatment is excision.

Thyroid hormone Excessive production of thyroxine produces symptoms of hyperthyroidism. Primary function of thyroxine is to stimulate cellular metabolism and growth. In children it may result in premature eruptions of teeth. In adults it results in mandible and maxilla. If thyroxine level is reduced there will be retardation in growth. In childhood cretinism may develop. Head appears large for small stature. Skin becomes coarse, hair become brittle and blood pressure is lowered. In hyperthyroidism myxoedema may develop. It results in fatigue, low BP, coarse oedematous skin and retarded mental process. Oral manifestations consist of thickened lips and enlarged tongue.

Thyroid in pregnancy Physiological enlargement of thyroid is noted in early pregnancy. Increased vascularity and hyperplasia of glandular tissue were causes of thyroid enlargement. B.M.R. increases by 25%.

Thyroid scanning Radionuclide scanning is the method available for location, anatomy and function of thyroid gland. Radioisotope usually contains a tiny dose of technetium or radioiodine and images are recorded on gamma camera. The scan also shows the amount of radioisotope taken up by gland. Radionuclide can suggest whether it is benign or malignant. Ultrasound scanning is of more limited use because it shows whether a goitre is solid, cystic or mixture of the two.

Thyroid stimulating hormone It is also known as thyrotropin. This hormone is secreted by pituitary and acts on thyroid cells to stimulate the production of T4 and T3.

Thyroidectomy Surgical removal or destruction of the thyroid gland, or inactivation by chemical means.

Thyroiditis It is the inflammation of thyroid gland. Most common form is Hashimoto's thyroiditis resulting in hypothyroidism. In subacute thyroiditis thyroid becomes tender and painful. Pain may be referred to jaw and ears. There may be fever and weight loss. Corticosteroids help in reducing inflammation.

Thyrotoxic exophthalmos Exophthalmos is due to fatty infiltration of extracellular muscle. There are all signs of thyrotoxicosis like tachycardia, muscular tremors and raised basal metabolism. Proptosis is the main feature. Person develops a 'stare look' and when person is asked to look down the upper lid lags behind or does not move at all. There develops diminished frequency of blinking with incomplete closure of lids. Power of convergence is also reduced.

Thyrotoxic myopathy Weakness and wasting of muscles around shoulder girdle are common in acute thyrotoxicosis. Bulbar and external ocular muscles are also sometimes involved. Muscle biopsy shows fibres containing central nuclei and fibre atrophy. There may be focal collections of lymphocytes.

Thyrotoxicosis Toxic condition as a result of hyperactivity of the thyroid gland.

Thyrotropic exophthalmos It occurs in any state of thyroid activity but usually in the state of hypothyroidism often following a thyroidectomy. The exophthalmos is due to oedema, lymphocytic infiltration and fibrosis of orbital contents. Main presenting ophthalmic features are proptosis of one or both eyes. Proptosis is irreducible, marked and may result in exposure keratitis. There is marked restriction of eye movements.

Thyroxine It is a standard practice to give thyroxine in a dose of 0.1 to 0.2 mg daily to suppress endogenous thyroid-stimulating hormone (TSH) production. Failure of suppression to a level of less than 0.1 ml/litre may indicate an inadequate dose of thyroxine. Thyroid hormone replacement is necessary after total thyroidectomy. Thyroid hormone that stimulates cellular metabolism.

TIA Transient ischemic attack.

Tibia It is the inner and thicker bone of lower leg also called the shinbone and is easily felt anteriorly.

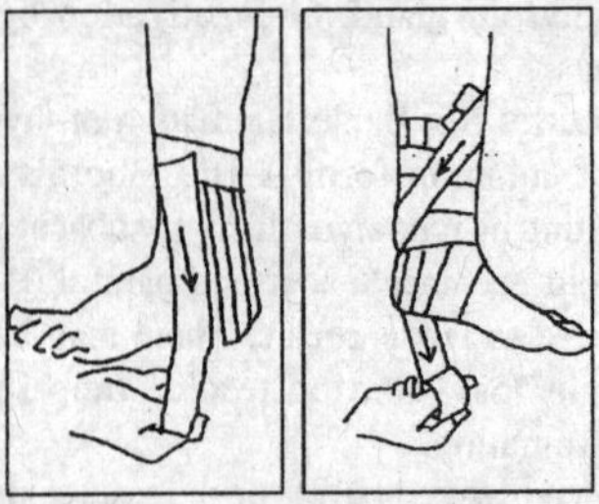

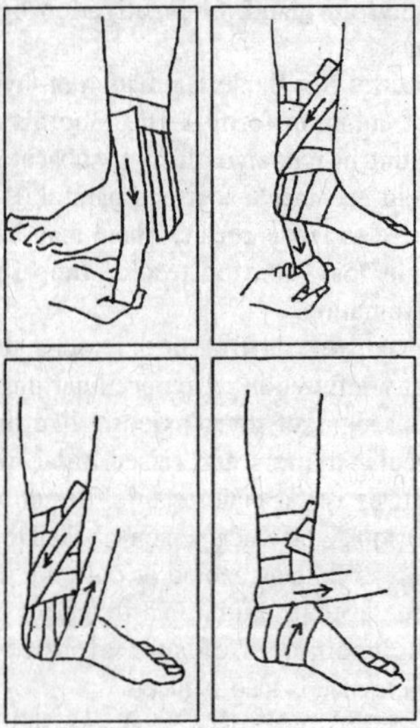

It is the most commonly fractured bone due to direct blow. Prolonged running or walking on hard ground may cause a stress fracture of tibia.

Tibial external (lateral) torsion External rotatory angulation of the tibia results in this position; up to 15° of external torsion is considered normal.

Tibial internal (medial) torsion Internal rotatory angulation of the tibia.

Tibial nerve Common site of damage of tibial nerve is at lower end ot if behind the inner ankle bone. Result may be partial or complete anesthesia of entire sole of foot, and weakness or paralysis of all short plantar foot muscles.

Tibial plateau fracture Majority of these fracture involve the lateral tibial plateau. Mechanism of injury is due to twisting or valgus force.

Tibial spine fracture Any fracture through the tibial eminence or tibial spine.

Tibial torsion Is a deformity in which the horizontal plane of the tibia is rotated medially or laterally beyond the normal range. The deformity may be medial (internal) or lateral (external). Medial tibial torsion is common in toddler. Lateral tibial torsion is generally seen in later childhood or adolesclence. Surgical correction by osteotomy of tibia may be required if TFA is more medial than 10° or more lateral than + 40°.

Tibial varum A frontal plane angulation of the distal third of the tibia in relation to the floor during standing results in tibial varum.

Tibialis anterior Dorsiflexor of the foot.

Tibialis anterior muscle It is attached to lateral surface of tibia and adjacent part of interosseous membrane. It is attached to base of first metatarsal.

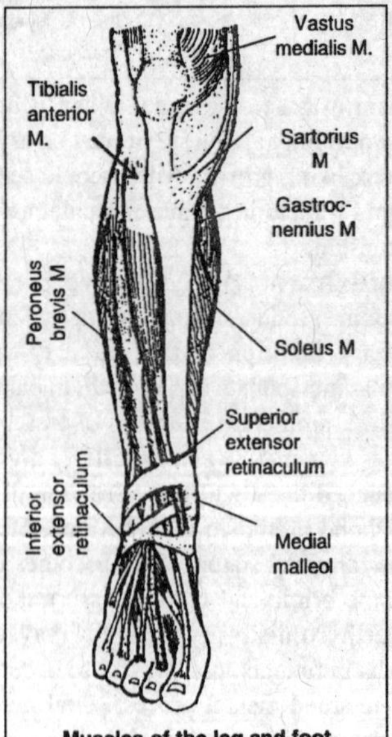

Muscles of the leg and foot

It is supplied by deep peroneal nerve. Its actions are dorsiflexion and inversion of foot and maintenance of medial longitudinal arch.

Tic An involuntary purposeless movement of muscle, which usually occurs under emotional stress; a twiching, especially of facial muscles.

Tic disorder A mental disorder characterized by tics.

Ticks These may be hard or soft ticks. In soft ticks, the mouth parts are completely concealed by soft body. Hard ticks contains hard, shiny shields. Soft ticks hide in cracks, animal burrows while hard ticks live on their host gorging on blood.

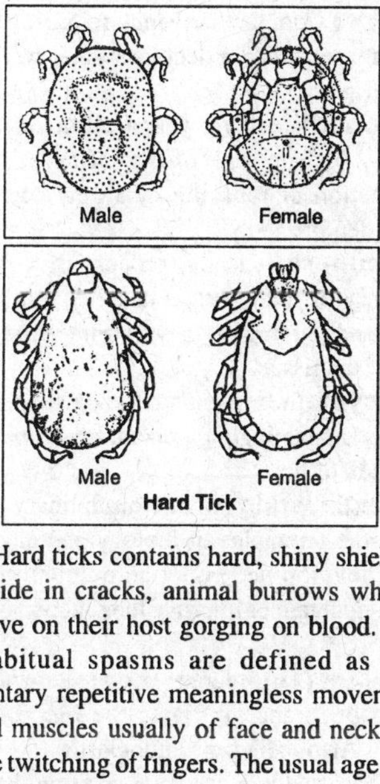

Hard Tick

Tics Habitual spasms are defined as sudden involuntary repetitive meaningless movements of striated muscles usually of face and neck. It may include twitching of fingers. The usual age of onset is after 6 years.

Tidal volume Amount, in ml, of air inhaled with each breath. Spontaneous tidal volume is 5 to 10 ml/kg body weight.

Tidaling Rhythmic rise and fall of water in a chest tube drainage system.

Tietze's syndrome It results in chest pain made worst by movement of arms and trunk. It is caused by inflammation of one or several rib cartilages where they join the sternum. Symptoms may persist for several months. Nonsteroidal (NSAIDs) anti-inflammatory drugs are useful.

Tightness Shortness; denotes a slight to moderate decrease in muscle length; movement in the direction of lengthening the muscle is limited.

Tillaux fracture An avulsion fracture of anterolateral articular surface of distal tibia due to pull of tibiofibular ligament.

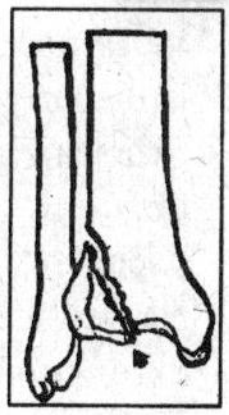

Time This threat to external validity is realized when the results of a study are applicable to limited time frames.

Timolol It is a beta-blocker drug to treat hypertension and angina pectoris. This drug is also given after myocardial infarction to prevent further damage to heart muscle. In liquid form it is used in glaucoma of eye.

Timolol maleate eyedrops It is available in the form of 0.25 and 0.5 per cent eyedrops. It is instilled only twice a day irrespective of the intraocular pressure (IOP) gravity. It takes about 3 weeks for the drug to show its effect on reducing the IOP. It may cause bradycardia. It reduces the IOP by decreasing the formation of aqueous humour.

Tincture An alcoholic solution of a drug or other chemical substance.

Tincture iodine Iodine is a stable, solid but marketed one are usually liquid and in ointment form. One application is sufficient as an disinfectant. If skin is painted with strong solution of iodine there may be burning and pricking sensation all over followed by rashes. It may be used as local analgesic and counterirritant in joint pain, sprain and muscular stiffness. A compound of 12% iodine, 2% potassium iodide in 90% methylated spirit is powerful, rapid skin disinfectant. Alcoholic solution is too irritant for use on broken skin and aqueous solution.

T-independent antigen An antigen which is able to elicit an antibody response in the absence of T cells.

Tine test A skin test for tuberculosis using multiple puncture.

Tinea barbae It develops on the bearded area. It presents with localised boggy swelling with or without abscesses. Lesions show loss of beard hair. In others lesions appear as patch of scaling with inflammations and itching. Lesions are generally unilateral. Follicular opening may express pus.

Tinea corporis It generally involves the exposed skin of face, neck and hands. It affects waist area in females. Lesion develops as circular or irregularly shaped round patches of varying sizes. Size varies from 1 to 8 to 10 cm. These have well-defined, raised and active margins of papulovesicles and healing hyperpigmented scaly centres. Lesions spread to periphery with direct extension. There develops intense itching. Inflammation is usually present. Topical corticosteroids are useful.

Tinea cruris It affects the groins and upper part of inner thighs. The lesions spread to the genitalia, pubic, perineal skin and later to buttocks and trunk. It develops as sharply marginated erythematous macules and annular plaques with clear centres. There are active raised margins spreading at periphery. Follicular pustules may be present. It results in intense itching, worse at night. Heat and swelling enchance the disease.

Tinea pedis It is known as athlete's foot and presents with scaling and fissuring on the fourth interdigital toeweb. There may be varying degrees of inflammation. Later on interdigital spaces of foot with white sodden areas may become eroded or may show marked scaling and fissuring. Lesion may extend to lateral margins. Condition is generally asymptomatic.

Tinel's sign In carpal tunnel syndrome percussion produces a positive median nerve. Tinel's sign, i.e. tingling in the area percussed with radiating distally to the median innervated digits. According to this sign, in trauma of foot and ankle and in nerve compression when the affected nerve is tapped, it gives rise to tingling, "needle pricking" sensation or pain.

Tinidazole It is similar to metronidazole but has longer 13 hours of half-life. The longer duration of action of tinidazole makes it advantageous in giardiasis, trichomoniasis and acute ulcerative gingivitis. In acute ulcerative gingivitis 2 gm by mouth in a single dose is effective.

Tinnitus It is ringing, buzzing, whistling, hissing or other noise heard in silent environment. There is some element of hearing loss. Tolerance of tinnitus varies considerably from one person to another. Some may find it most untolerable. It is an unformed auditory hallucinations of sound. It is usually of whistling or pulsating nature accompanied with sensorineural deafness. Tinnitus may be associated with depression. Pharmacological treatment is ineffective.

Tinted denture A denture base that simulates the colouring and shading of a natural oral tissue.

Tip Part of a syringe to which the needle is attached.

Tissue A group of similar cells and their intercellular substance joined together to perform a specific function.

Tissue conditioner A rubbery material used on the tissue bearing surface of the denture to cushion the gingiva from the hard denture base; temporary material used when a denture wearer has severely irritated gums.

Tissue conditioning Preparation of soft oral tissues, by the use of soft liners, prior to construction or rebasing of a new complete or partial denture.

Tissue culture It is the process of growing in laboratory of living tissue taken from a donor or patient and put in growth environment to generate more of the tissue.

Tissue cyst In certain protozoa, a protective structure containing the asexual bradyzoites in the intermediate host.

Tissue engineering An interdisciplinary field that applies the principles of biology and engineering to the development of viable substitutes that restore, maintain or improve the function of human tissues.

Tissue factor (TF) A factor, or collection of factors, whose appearance initiates the blood clothing process. Also called thromboplastin.

Tissue fluid A dilute saltwater solution that bathes every cell in the body.

Tissue hormone Prostaglandins; produced in a tissue and diffuses only a short distance to act on cells within the tissue.

Tissue ischemia Decreased blood supply to body tissues.

Tissue plasminogen activator An enzyme that dissolves small blood clots by initiating a process that converts plasminogen to plasmin, which degrade the fibrin to a clot.

Tissue repair Substitution of viable cells for damaged or dead cells by regeneration or replacement.

Tissue typing A procedure used to identify tissue compatibility before an organ transplant.

Titer Measure of the relative 'strength' of an antibody or antiserum, usually given as the highest dilution which is still operationally detectable in, for example, an agglutination assay.

Titration A means of adjusting a drug's dosage by repeatedly increasing or decreasing the dose administered until the desired effect is achieved or the undesired effect is eliminated.

Titration curve A plot of the pH versus the equivalents of base added during titration of an acid.

TM joint, septic arthritis It results from blood-borne bacterial infection or trauma. Gonococcus is the primary causative agent.

There will be a severe pain on movement and an inability to occlude the teeth. Redness over joint develops. Large, tender cervical nodes are observed. Serious sequelae include ankylosis and facial asymmetry. Treatment includes antibiotics and surgical drainage.

TMJ arthropathy There develops unilateral attacks of pain in the periauricular area over the TMJ or in the ear. Malocclusion and occlusal dysfunction. Radiograph shows set back condyle.

Tobacco Dried leaves of nicotiona tobacum. During its combustion 1600 compounds are given off.

Tobacco smoking There is a direct link between lung cancer and smoking. Pipe and cigar smoking have higher risk of cancer of oral cavity. Tobacco chewers have risk of causing carcinoma of cheek. In mild smokers it results in chronic bronchitis and emphysema. Smoking results in atherosclerosis and peripheral vascular diseases. It raises your blood pressure. It may cause painful neuropathy.

Babies born to smoking mother are lighter in weight. Passive smokers also suffer. Nicotine is the substance that causes addiction to tobacco. Tar in tobacco produces chronic irritation to respiratory system carbon monoxide passes from the lungs into blood stream where it easily combines with haemoglobin and interfering with oxygenation of tissues.

Tocolytic A drug that inhibits uterine contractions.

Tocotrienoles Vitamin E like substance present in food such as barley and palm oil.

Toe Tip end of instrument blade.

Toe Out The angulation of the long axis of the foot (in degree) to the line of walking progression; the normal range is upto 15 degree.

Token economy A system involving the application of the principles and procedures of operant conditioning to the management of a social setting such as a ward, classroom, or halfway house. Tokens are given contingent on completion of specified activities and are exchangeable for goods or privileges desired by the patient.

Tolbutamide Half-life is eight hours. It is rapidly metabolised by oxidation in liver. It is the preferred sulphonylurea in the presence of impaired renal function. It activates receptors on the 'b' cells of the pancreatic islets to release stored insulin in response to glucose. These do not increase insulin formation. These appear to enhance insulin action on liver. These cause hypoglycaemia in normal subjects as well as in diabetics.

Tolerance The specific absence of an immune response to an antigen. Lymphocytes which have receptors for self antigen are eliminated by the tolerance mechanism.

Tolosa-Hunt syndrome Initial symptoms are deep aching and constant orbital pain. It is severe and may awaken the patient from sleep. Pain is accompanied by diplopia and paraesthesia. Neurological symptoms include ophthalmoplegia and pupillary abnormalities. Symptoms respond to cortisone although symptoms reappear.

Tomography The recording of internal body images in a particular plane by using an X-ray source.

Tone It is a resistance to passive stretch. Denervated muscles are floppy or hypotonic and can be stretched further than usual. When large groups of muscles are affected by lower motor neuron lesions such as in plexus lesion affected limb is called flail.

Tongue It is a muscular, flexible organ which occupies the floor of mouth. It is composed of mass of muscles covered by mucous membrane. Muscles are attached to hyoid bone. Minute nodules on anterior surface gives it a rough texture. Between papillae at the side and base of tongue are tastebuds. Tongue is not only a taste organ but it breaks down food and is used in swallowing and speech. Large bulky tongue is seen in Down's syndrome, cretinism and acromegaly. Smooth tongue is a feature of pernicious anaemia. It may be coated in certain fevers and under certain conditions. Tongue can be a site for mouth ulcer and leucoplakia. The upper surface is known as anterior part and posterior part is known as dorsum. Dorsum surface is covered by fairly thick, non-keratinised, stratified epithelium covered with different types of papillae. Posterior third of dorsum of tongue has irregular surface due to nodules of lymphatic tissue. On anterior part, deep lingual vein can be seen passing towards apex. The lingual frenulum is a vertical midline between tongue and floor of mouth.

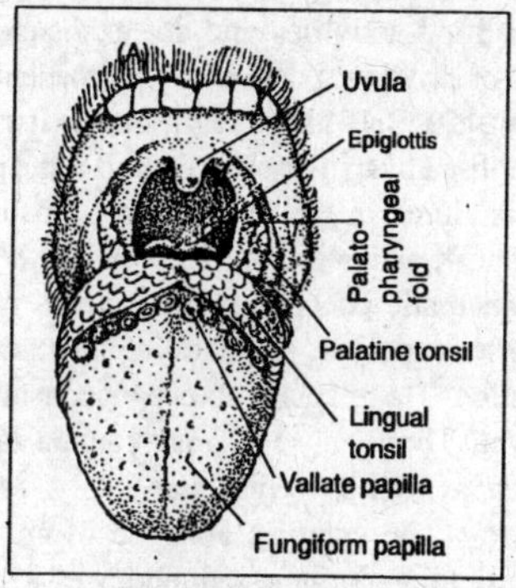

Upper surface of tongue

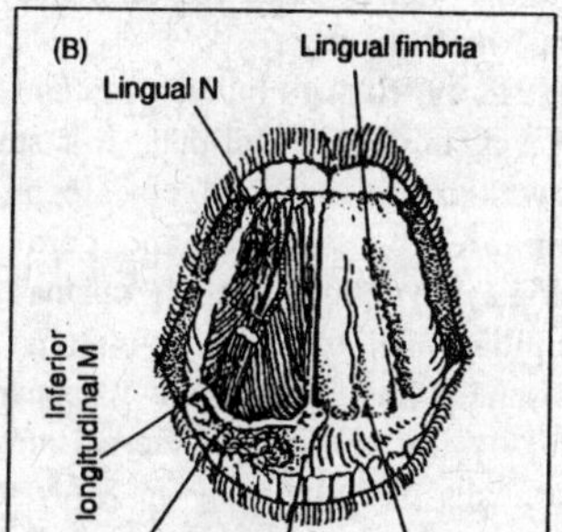

(A) Inferior surface of tongue

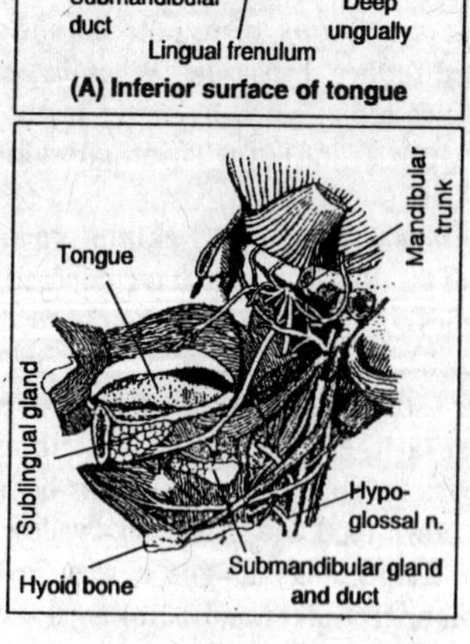

Tongue carcinoma Carcinoma of tongue occurs in posterior two-third and on lateral borders. In anterior third it is rare. It metastasises early and 40 per cent show regional lymph node metastases. In 75 per cent cases cervical lymph glands of same side enlarges. Only one-third number of patients survive for two years.

Tongue depressor It has handle and a depressing part. Holding part gives a good grip and is used to examine oropharynx. Patient opens his mouth and

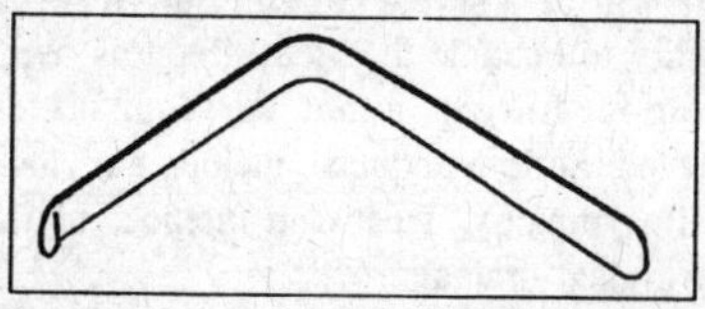

two-third of tongue is depressed with this spatula. At the same time patient is asked to say aa-aa-ah. By doing so palate moves up allowing a good view of orapharynx. It is useful to examine palatine tonsil, pillars and soft palate.

Tongue thrust A movement in which the tongue extends outside the lips, interferes with swallowing, and causes food to be pushed outside the mouth; often seen in individuals with cerebral palsy or Down syndrome.

Tonguethrust reflex An immature form of swallowing in which the tongue is projected forward instead of retracted during swallowing.

Tongue-tie A condition in which the attachment of thin ridge of tissue in the middle of the base of the tongue (the frenulum linguae) extends far forward causing a concavity at the tip of the tongue on its upper surface. Also called lingua frenata.

Tonic accommodation In patients with Adie's syndrome there may be a change in pupillary reaction along with tonic course lasting 3 to 15 seconds when accommodating associated with constriction of the pupil for near vision or when relaxing accommodation associated with dilatation of pupil for distance vision.

Tonic contraction Special type of skeletal muscle contraction used to maintain posture.

Tonic holding Stability control of postural extensor muscles holding in the shortened range of motion.

Tonic lumbar reflex Rotation of the upper trunk toward the affected side produces flexion of the upper limb and extension of the lower limb. Rotation towards the sound side produces the opposite response.

Tonic motor neuron Motor neuron innervating a squad of slow, oxidative-glycolytic muscle fibers.

Tonic neck reflex The tendency of infants while lying on the their backs to turn their heads to one side and extend the arm and leg on that side, flexing the arm and leg on the other side.

Tonic seizures There is tonic contraction of muscle with altered consciousness but no clonic phase. These are more likely to occur during NREM sleep with day drowsiness. These are of 3 types : axial, axorhizomelic and global. *Axial* variety is marked by wide opening of eyes and mouth. In *axorhizomelic* variety there is involvement of proximal muscles too. In *global* form head is extended, upper limbs are thrown out. Lower limbs are extended.

Tonic vibration reflex A sustained contraction of muscle in response to a vibratory stimulus.

Tonic-clonic convulsions Convulsions characteristic of temporal lobe epilepsy.

Tonic-clonic seizures Epileptic spasms of tonic muscular contractions, and clonic contraction and relaxation of muscles.

Tonicity A measure of the concentration of impermeable solute particles in a solution relative to cytosol. When cells are bathed in an isotonic solution, they neither shrink nor swell.

Tonsil These are pair of oval masses at the back of throat. These are made of lymphoid tissue and form part of lymphatic system. These are important part of defence against infection. Tonsils gradually enlarge from birth, reach their maximum size at about 7 and after 12 years it shrinks. Tonsillitis is a common infection of childhood resulting in fever and difficulty in swallowing. Child may have headache, earache, enlarged and tender glands in neck. Antibiotics are useful.

Tonsil holding forceps Its fenestrated tip does not have a cutting edge and it has a simple joint. Fenestrated tip gives a good grip and is used to hold tonsil during dissection.

Tonsillar dissector It has a sharp dissecting end and a blunt retracting end. Sharp end is used to divide the mucosa to expose the capsule while retracting end is used to follow up the exposed capsule.

Tonsillar tuberculosis Symptoms include painless swelling of palatine tonsil with peritonsillar oedema. Flat ulceration or deep tissue defects in tonsillar area is seen. Lymph nodes are enlarged but are not painful. Tumour-like enlargement of tonsil is uncommon.

Tonsillectomy Surgical procedure used to remove the tonsils.

Tonsilloadenoidectomy Combined tonsillectomy and adenoidectomy.

Tonsillolith A concretion or calculus in a tonsil.

Tonsils Masses of lymphoid tissue; protect against bacteria; three types: palatine tonsils; located on each side of the throat; pharyngeal tonsils (adenoids), near the posterior opening of the nasal cavity; and lingual tonsils, near the base of the tongue.

Tonus The slight, continuous contraction of muscle, which in skeletal muscle aids in the maintenance of posture and the return of blood to the heart.

Too evulsion Displacement of tooth from its alveolar housing.

Tooth Each tooth has two portions, crown and root portions. Crown is covered with enamel while root is covered with cementum. Crown and root join at the cementoenamel junction. Each tooth has four tissues. Enamel, cementum and dentin are hard tissues while pulp is a soft tissue. The root portion of tooth may be single as found in anterior teeth and some of premolars. In molars one finds bifurcation or trifurcation dividing the root portion into two or more extensions of roots are found. The root portion of tooth is firmly fixed in the bony process of jaw. The portion of jaw serving support for teeth is called alveolar process. The bone of tooth pocket is called alveolus. Crown portion is never covered by bone tissue once it is fully erupted.

Tooth cavity Hole in a tooth.

Tooth eruption The combination of movements of a tooth both before and after the emergence of its crown into the oral cavity, which serves to bring the tooth and maintain occlusion with the tooth or teeth of the opposing arch.

Tooth extraction with forceps Patient is seated comfortably in the chair with head rest adjusted to fit the nap of neck and support the head. After local anaesthesia, forceps is then picked up in correct

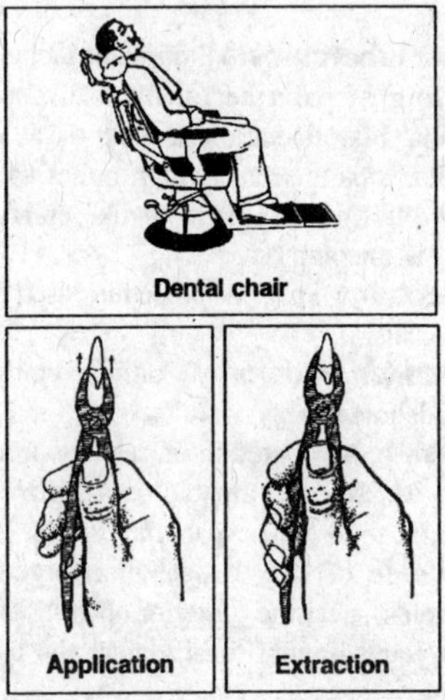

position. Control the opening of forceps/blades during their application to root. When tooth is gripped firmly with force it is being taken out.

Toothache It may be felt as a dull throb or as a sharp twinge. Early dental caries results in mild toothache while eating sweet or very hot or very cold. Deep decay causes sharp, stabbing pain which is often worse while lying down. It becomes difficult to locate the exact tooth by patient. Periapical periodontitis may develop localised pain during biting or chewing. In dental abscess pain is severe and often continuous. Gum around tooth becomes swollen and tender. Sinusitis also results in referred toothache. Antibiotics and anti-inflammatory drugs are useful.

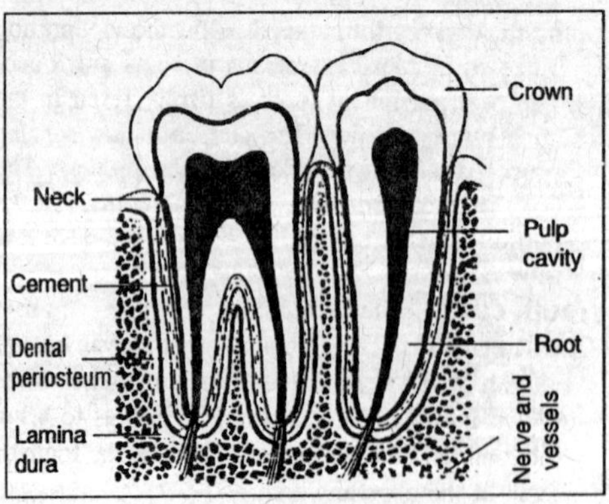

Topagnosia Loss of ability to localize site of tactile sensations.

Tophaceous Gritty or sandy.

Topical Pertaining to a particular surface area of skin or mucous membrane.

Topical agents Pertaining to a drug or treatment applied to the surface part of the body.

Topical anaesthesia A form of local anaesthesia, whereby free nerve endings in accessible structures are rendered incapable of stimulation by application of an anaesthetic drug directly to the surface of the area.

Topical route Drug administration to the skin or muscous membranes.

Topographic disorientation Difficulty in understanding and remembering the relationship of one place to another.

Topographical disorientation Difficulty in understanding and remembering the relationship of one place to another.

Topography The detailed description and analysis of the features of an anatomic region or of a special part.

Torn cartilage A tearing of an articular disk (meniscus) in the knee.

Torque (moment of force) The turning of rotational effect produced by the application of a force. Torque is calculated by multiplying the force by the perpendicular distance from the point of application of the force and the axis of rotation.

Torsion Motion or state where one end of a part is turned about a longitudinal axis while the opposite end is held fast or turned to the opposite direction.

Torsion dystonia The movements of dystonia are slow and carried out against the resistance of antagonist muscles. They are forced and often have a rotatory component.

Torsion of gravid uterus Some rotation of gravid uterus to the right is a normal event. Occasionally uterus undergoes ninety degree rotation. In early pregnancy, condition resembles ectopic pregnancy and in advanced pregnancy condition may be mistaken for concealed accidental hemorrhage.

Tort Litigation in which one person asserts that an injury, which may be physical, emotional, or financial, occurred as a consequence of another's actions or failure to act.

Torus Bulging projection of bone; mandibularis torus is a bony enlargement unilaterally or bilaterally on the lingual aspect of the mandible in the canine-premolar region of a small percentage of people; palatinus torus appears in the midline of the hard palate in about one fifth of the people.

Total allergy syndrome It is a very rare condition in which patient develops allergy to most of the allergents. The condition starts as a gradual allergy to few known allergens. Then allergy goes on increasing. Life becomes difficult.

Total body water during pregnancy Water accumulated up to 30 weeks pregnancy without generalised edema is accounted by water content of product of conception and growth of maternal organs. Excess of water gain with generalised edema reaches 5 litres more than 0.4 gm/100 ml. There is no significant retention of sodium, more than 12 gm.

Total lung capacity The sum of tidal volume, inspiratory reserve volume, expiratory reserve volume, and residual volume; about 6000 mL in an average adult.

Total metabolic rate (TMR) Total amount of energy used by the body per day.

Total parenteral nutrition Hypertonic solution of nutrients designed to meet almost all the caloric and nutritional needs of patients.

Total peripheral resistance The force opposing the flow of blood in the systemic circulatory bed; derived by devising the mean arterial pressure by cardiac output.

Total quality improvement Process of promoting care that reflects established agency standards.

Total variation Equal to the sum of the squared deviations from the mean. It is usually called the total sum of squares but is sometimes referred to simplay as the sum of squares.

Totally dependent The most extreme condition of retardation. Persons in this classification require custodial care for personal needs and survival.

Touch It is a sense by which size, shape, surface texture, temperature can be ascertained by physical contact. Most receptors are in non-hairy areas such as lips and fingertips. Signals from touch receptors pass via sensory nerves to spinal cord then to thalamus and on to the sensory cortex. Fingertips are good at touch discrimination but relatively insensitive to pain. Blind people develops better touch sense.

Toughening/hardening The reaction to repeated exposure to stimuli that elicit arousal responses.

Toughness The ability of a material to absorb energy without breaking; depicted as the total area under the stress-strain diagram.

Touraine-Solente-Gole syndrome It is characterised by thickened and widened soft tissue of the terminal phalanx, periosteal lesions and hypertrophy of long bones, thick bracelet-like band on the wrist in males appearing at or after puberty, sterility and increased thickness of epidermis with hypoplasia or sebaceous and sweat glands.

Tourette's syndrome Involuntary exclamations associated with anterior cingulate cortex dysfunction.

Tourniquet It is a device placed around limb to compress blood vessels. In common practice it is used at mild humerus to locate vein for an IV

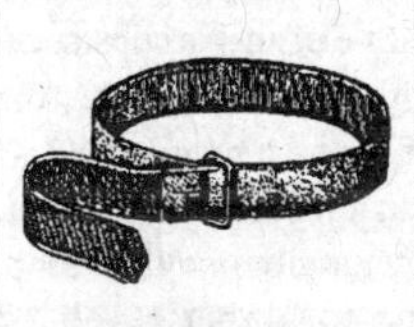
Tourniquet

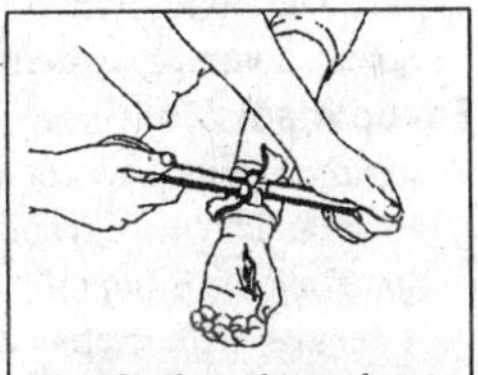
Application of tourniquet

injection or withdrawal of blood. An inflatable tourniquet is used in BP instrument. In first aid, these are used to control bleeding, but are risky because leaving tourniquet for long may cause gangrene.

Tourniquet test In this test increased capillary fragility produces numerous tiny haemorrhages when a tourniquet is applied on the arm. It is seen in vitamin C deficiency.

Towel bath Technique for bathing in which a single large towel is used to cover and wash a patient.

Toxemia The clinical syndrome caused by toxic substances in the blood.

Toxic effect Harmful effects.

Toxic neuropathy It may result from pharmaceutical, occupational, biological and environmental agents. In acute arsenic poisoning, the symptoms of neuropathy may be delaved for 4 to 8 weeks. In chronic arsenic poisoning neuropathy develops more slowly. Sensory symptoms like pain and paraesthesia dominate in initial phase followed by motor weakness. Lead neuropathy causes weakness of extensor muscles of fingers and wrist.

Toxicant A poison, especially one of man-made origin.

Toxicity Degree of virulence of a toxic microbe or of a poison; the capacity of a drug to damage body tissue or seriously impair body functions.

Toxicology The study of organisms, substances, and agents that can induce disease or otherwise damage biological systems.

Toxin Any substance or agent capable of harming living organisms, specifically, a microbial organism, product, or component that causes injury or disease in multicellular organisms, including humans and animals.

Toxin weapon Any poisonous substance, whatever its origin or method of production, which can be produced by a living organism, or any poisonous isomer, homolog, or derivative of such a substance.

Toxocariasis Infection with *Toxocara canis*, the common round-worm of dog is manifested as visceral larva migrans in children with pica. Sometimes eosinophilic meningitis may develop. It results in epilepsy due to higher levels of antibodies.

Toxoid It is a chemically treated toxin which is no more toxic but retains the capacity to form antibodies. Toxoids can be used as vaccines.

Toxoids Inactivated or altered bacterial exotoxins, such as diphtheria vaccine and tetanus vaccine.

Toxoplasmosis *Toxoplasma gondii* is an intracellular protozoan parasite. Several sexual stages of parasite cycle take place in cats. When oocytes are ingested by host, they form trophozoites persisting for life. Consumption of undercooked meat, ingestion of sporulated cysts, result it. It is most common parasitic infection in AIDS patients. It presents with headache, confusion, focal neurological signs and seizures. Toxoplasma IgG antibody is found in serum of most patients. Brain biopsy confirms the diagnosis.

T-Piece Device the fits securely onto a tracheostomy tube of endotracheal tube.

TPR Temperature, pulse, and respiration.

Trabecula Irregular latticework of thin plate of spongy bone. Fibrous cord of connective tissue serving as supporting fiber by forming a septum extending into an organ from its wall or capsule.

Trabeculae Needle like threads of spongy bone that surround a network of spaces.

Trabeculae carneae Irregular muscular ridges or bundles of variable thickness, lining the walls of the ventricles.

Trabecular bone A type of mature bone composed of three diamensional lattice work of osseus plates and columns.

Trace elements These are necessary in diet in trace amounts.

Trace minerals Essential nutrient minerals required daily in amounts less than or equal to 20 mg.

Trachea It starts immediately below the larynx and runs down to divide into two main bronchi. It consists of fibrous and elastic tissue and smooth muscle. It also contains 20 rings of cartilage which keep the trachea open and does not allow to be compressed easily. The mucus and other cells bear minute, hair like cilia. Mucus helps trapping tiny particles in inhaled air. Cilia moves upwards to throw particles out. Inflammation of it results in tracheitis associated with bronchitis. Symptoms produced are painful breathing and harsh cough. Rarely a congenital malformation occurs in which it is communicated to oesophagus resulting in tracheooesophageal fistula. Length of trachea is 10 to 11 cm. It commences at the level of 6th

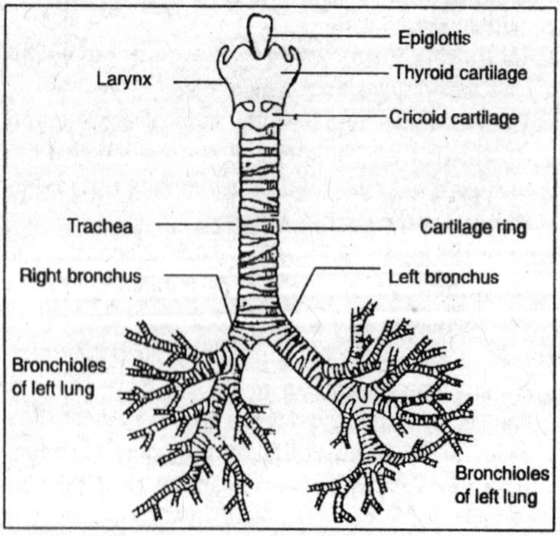

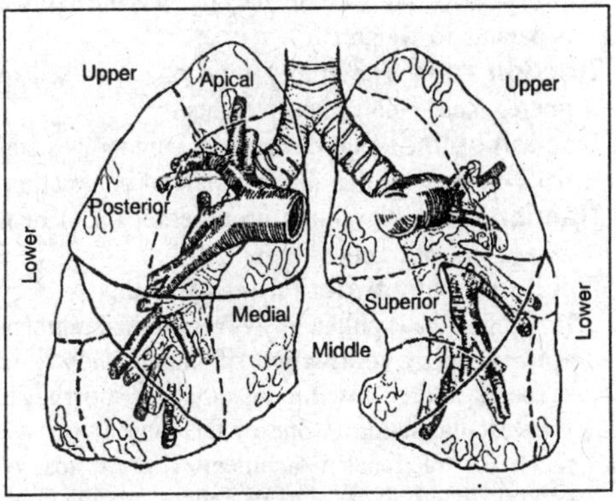

cervical vertebra and ends by dividing into two bronchi at carina at the level of 5th thoracic vertebra. Anteriorly it corresponds to angle of Louis. Diameter is about 1.5 to 2 cm. High tracheal bifurfaction and deformity may cause problems during intubation. Tracheostomy should be done below first tracheal ring to avoid stenosis. Upper two-third is supplied by inferior thyroid artery and lower one-third of it by bronchial artery. Trachea is known as wind pipe and measures about 11.5 cm in length and is about 2.5 cm in diameter. It has rings of cartilages to prevent it collapsing. It passes through the neck in front of oesophagus branching into two bronchi. The right bronchus is 2.5 cm long and left bronchus 5 cm long. Bronchi branch into bronchioles with no cartilage and have clusters of thin walled air sacs–alveoli.

Tracheal suctioning Suctioning of secretions following a tracheostomy is of importance in maintaining a patent airway. Patients lose their ability to cough effectively because they are unable to develop a high endobronchial pressure behind the closed glottis. Frequent suctioning may be required. Suction should not extend beyond 6 to 8 seconds and one should not poke the catheter in and out because it may injure the tracheal mucosa.

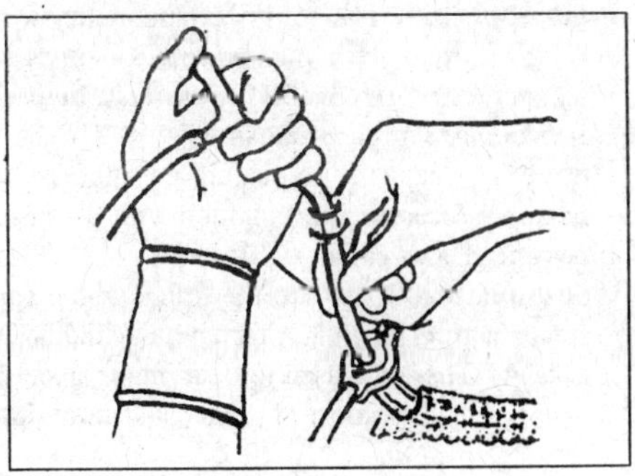

Tracheitis Inflammation of the mucosal lining of the trachea.

Tracheomalacia It may be caused by space occupying lesions adjacent to trachea over a long period. Dyspnoea of gradual onset develops and is accompanied by inspiratory and expiratory stridor. Tracheomalacia is a dystrophic condition of tracheal cartilage caused by pressure atrophy, nutritional deficit and trauma.

Tracheopathica osteoplastica It develops possible foreign body sensation in trachea. Many cases may not show any features. Pathy formation of hard bony and cartilaginous deposits in trachea wall may be the causative factor.

Tracheosophageal fistula A congenital abnormality in which the trachea and esophagus freely communicate; frequently associated with esophageal atresia; may also be acquired in later life.

Tracheostomy Creation of an opening into the trachea through the neck (below the cricoid cartilage), with insertion of a tube, to facilitate passage of air or evacuation of secretions.

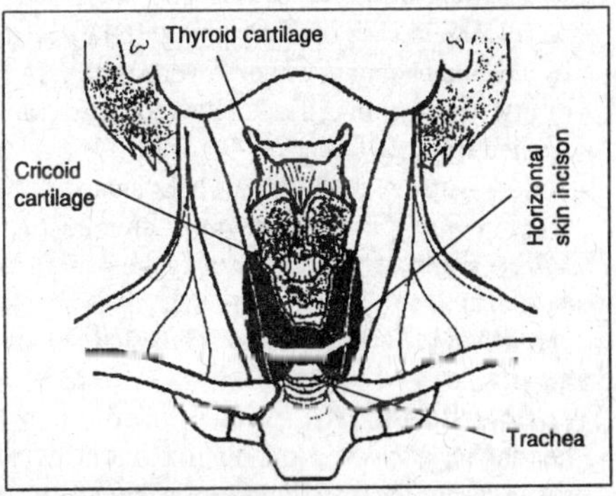

Tracheostomy collar Device that delivers oxygen near an artificial opening in the neck.

Tracheostomy tube Curved, hollow plastic tube in the trachea.

Tracheotomy Surgical operation to provide an artificial opening into the trachea.

Trachoma Living under unhygienic condition helps its spread. It is caused by Bedsonian organisms belonging to psittacosis lymphogranuloma group. There develop irritation, photophobia and lacrimation. Child blinks his or her eyes more often. The abnormal blinking gives him relief from irritation due to follicles in lids and mild corneal involvement. One feels tired after reading for a short period. Follicles are the main lesion and may assume the size of 0.5 mm in diameter. These involves upper fornix commonly, often forming a row along the upper margin in tarsus. Trachomatous infiltration spreads deeply into subepithelial tissues of palpebral conjunctiva and may even the tarsal plate. Star-shaped scar develops later on.

Tracking Smooth visual pursuit of a moving object.

Tract Nerve tract; a bundle of neuron cell processes (axons) in the central nervous system, usually sharing a common function.

Traction It is a procedure in which part of body is placed under tension to correct the alignment of two adjoining structures specially bones. Fracture of femur is generally treated this way. Traction is also used to align and immobilise unstable fracture of cervical spine.

In it upper end of fractured bone is kept immobilised while the lower end is pulled in a straight line away by putting weights and pulleys. It is pulling outwards. It is gently steady pulling on fracture in case of overlapping. It may be done by attaching hanging weights over a pulley. In case of delivery also in difficult labour, traction can be applied through forceps.

Traction boot A foam rubber boot shaped to fit a forearm or leg, used for a type of skin traction.

Traction By Inversion It requires the patient to be held in an inerted position by the ankles and other part of the lower extremities. The traction force is gravity.

Traction headache Term is used when the headache is caused by displacement of pain sensitive intracranial blood vessels and traction of dura. It is often associated with brain tumour. With brain tumours there will be headache, vomiting and papilloedema.

Traction in water It requires the patient to be suspended vertically in the water with a floating ring around the chest while the weights are attached to the ankles.

Traction knot The rope tie that connects the traction apparatus to weights.

Traction rope The sturdy rope of cord used to interconnect pulleys and weights.

Traction splint Metal device that immobilizes and pulls on muscles that are in a state of contraction.

Traction spur Any bony protuberant on or near attachment of fascia to bone.

Tractional retinal detachment In this sensory layer of retina is pulled away from retinal pigment epithelium by contraction of bands, mostly in diabetes and following vitreous haemorrhage. Neovascularisation is one of the most important factor for tractional detachment. There is loss of central visual acuity and peripheral visual field. There are no floaters and photopsia. On ophthalmoscopy proliferative fibrovascular membranes are found.

Trade name Name used by the pharmaceutical company for the drug it sells.

Traditional Sustaining, inherited, conventional cultural patterns.

Traditional time Time based on two 12-hour revolutions on a clock.

Trainable The middle classification of the mentally retarded. Judged unable to profit from traditional classroom education, even at a slower rate, the trainable child instead is assisted in the development of self-help skills, including personal care and hygiene and limited tasks in the home.

Training effect Heart rate and consequently pulse rate become consistently lower than average with regular exercise.

Trait A relatively constant aspect, characteristic or dimension of behaviour. Usually applied to personality and exemplified by such terms as introversion, dominance, sociability, persistence, and honesty.

Trait approach The study of personality which focuses upon personal disposition or traits; techniques of personality assessment involving inventories and questionnaires.

Trance The capacity to sustain an attentive and intensely focussed concentration with diminished peripheral awareness.

Tranquillisers These are the drugs which calm, soothe and relax without taking away intellectual capacity. These are used to treat minor anxiety to major psychosis. Most of these cause drowsiness.

Transabdominal tube Tube placed through the abdominal wall.

Transactional analysis A method of group therapy emphasising interpersonal actions. Participants arrange activities in pairs or small groups, while other members analyse and interpret these events. The focus is upon detecting undesirable elements in interpersonal communication.

Transamination The transfer of an amino group from an amino acid to an alpha-keto acid, forming a new keto acid and a new amino acid without the appearance of free ammonia.

Transaxial Directed at right angles to the long axis of body or part.

Transcendent religion A religion that teaches techniques to transcend or transform the reality of senses or that denies the existence or importance of mundane reality.

Transcendental meditation A form of meditation which attempts to alter the individual's awareness of reality.

One technique includes the repetition of a special sound, which provides a focus for the individual's attention and thus excludes elements in the external environment.

In this way, the individual can concentrate more completely on his or her own inner experience and perception of reality.

Transcervical fracture A fracture through neck of femur.

Transcondylar fracture Transverse fracture through the condyles of bone.

Transcortin A high affinity binder for cortisol and cortisone made by liver that reversibly binds corticosteroids in the circulation.

Transcription When the double stranded DNA molecules unwind and form mRNA.

The transcription of disputed utterances consists in converting spoken language into written language.

Transcriptional Pertaining to process of synthesizing RNA from DNA template.

Transcultural nursing Providing nursing care in the context of another's culture.

Transcutaneous electrical nerve stimulation Medically prescribed pain management technique that delivers bursts of electricity to the skin and underlying nerves.

Transdermal Refers to form of medication that is applied to the skin's sufrace and is absorbed across the dermal or outer skin layer.

Transdermal application Method of applying a drug on the skin and allowing it to become passively absorbed.

Transdermal medication Drug delivered by patch on skin; a mode for slow release over extended time.

Transducer Instrument that receives and transmits biophysical energy.

Transduction Conversion of sensory stimuli into trains of nerve impulses.

Transection A cross-sectional cut.

Transesophageal echocardiography It gives a good view of much of the heart and is being used preoperatively and in I.C.U. to monitor left ventricular function.

Trans-fatty acids Fatty acids with unusual bouble-bond structures caused by hydrogenated unsaturated oils.

Transfectant Carrying genetic material introduced by experimental genetic techniques.

Transfemoral Above-knee

Transfer of patient (1) Discharging a patient from one unit or agency and immediately admitting him or her to another; (2) moving a patient from place to place.

Transfer summary Written review of the patient's previous care.

Transference The unconscious assignment to others of feelings and attitudes that were originally associated with important figures (parents, siblings, etc.) in one's early life.

The transference relationship follows the pattern of its prototype. The psychiatrist utilises this phenomenon as a therapeutic tool to help the patient understand emotional problems and their origins. In the patient-physician relationship, the transference may be negative (hostile) or positive (affectionate).

Transformer An electrical device that increases or reduces the voltage of an alternating current by mutual induction between primary and secondary coils or windings.

Transfusion It is a closely matched replacement blood, plasma or saline solutions into patient's blood stream with a desired speed.

Transgender Different than transsexual, transgendered people feel more comfortable displaying or living in the gender that is different than their sex. For example, a woman who wears men's suits or a man who wears makeup and female dresses. Transgendered people are not necessarily gay; a transgendered man may still desire women.

Transgeneration From one generation to another.

Transgenic over expression The excessive production of foreign protein in cells and tissues of an organism that has made transgenic by introduction of foreign DNA into its genome.

Transient global amnesia Patient although alert and communicative is amnesic for much of his or her life until the incident and is unable to lay down new memories during the attack. Consciousness is not disturbed, as patient comes out of episode. Usually gradually it becomes clear that he or she is totally amnesic for the events of previous few hours. Patient may develop epileptic seizure.

Transient Incontinence Is seen in state of delirium, urinary tract infections, atrophic urethritis or vaginitis, side effects of sedative hypnotics, diurectics, anticholingeric drug, calcium channel blockers etc. Severe depression, endocrine imbalance, restricted mobility and stool impaction etc.

Transient microorganisms Pathogens picked up during brief contact with contaminated reservoirs.

Transient tachypnoea of newborn It is a benign self-limiting disease occurring usually in term neonates and is due to delayed clearance of lung field. These have tachypnoea and minimal respiratory distress. Prognosis is good.

Transillumination The use of light to examine anterior teeth for the presence of caries.

Transition A base pair substitution mutation that substitutes a purine for a purine or a pyrimidine for a pyrimidine.

Transition state An activated form of a molecule in which the molecule has undergone a partial chemical reaction; the highest point on the reaction coordinate.

Transitional cell carcinoma Tumour frequently occurs at the base of tongue in oropharynx. It appears as a small red raspberry like velvety lesion that may show erosion but in which deep ulceration of squamous cell carcinoma is present. It metastasises early. It is radiosensitive so both surgical excision and radiation therapy are used in its treatment. Prognosis is poor.

Transitional epithelium Type of epithelial tissue that forms membranes capable of stretching without braking, as in the urinary bladder; cells in this type of tissue can stretch from roughly columnar out to flattened (squamous) and back without damage.

Transitional milk Breast milk that appears between secretion of colostrum and mature milk.

Transitional movements Movements between positions, i.e., sit to kneel, kneel to stand.

Translation Motion of a rigid body in which a straight line in the body always remains parallel to itself.

Translational control The regulation of a protein's synthesis by regulation the rate of its translation on the ribosome.

Translational repressor A repressor that binds to an mRNA, blocking translational.

Translocation Attachment of all or part of a chromosome to another chromosome.

Transmissible Capable of being carried across from one person to another.

Transmission The passing of some form of radiation, such as light, through an object.

Transmission-based precautions Measures for controlling the spread of infectious agents from patients known to be or suspected of being infected with highly transmissable or epidemiologically important pathogens.

Transmitter substance A chemical material which is responsible for making the synaptic connection. It is discharged from the presynaptic neuron into synaptic space, where it acts upon the membrane of another fibre, causing it to become activated. A different substance, when discharged into synaptic space, is presumed to cause inhibition, causing the receiving membrane to become more resistant to firing.

Transneuronal atrophy Atrophic neuronal degeneration passing from one neuron to another, in either an orthograde or a retrograde manner.

Transosteal implant 1. A dental implant that completely passes through the alveolar ridge bucco/labio-lingually. 2. A dental implant that completely passes through the parasymphseal region of the mandible, from the inferior border through the alveolar crest.

Transphenoidal surgery Surgical procedure of choice to remove pituitary tumors.

Transplacental Crossing the placenta, especially the exchange of hormones, nutrients, waste products, and drugs between the mother and fetus.

Transplant Tissue removed from one part of the body and placed at a different site.

Transplantation Implanting a tissue or organ that has been taken from another part of the same body or from another person.

Transport protein A protein that catalyzes the movement of a molecule across the plasma membrane.

Transposition of the great vessels A congenital cardiac anomaly in which the aorta originates from the right ventricle rather than the left, and the pulmonary artery originates from the left ventricle rather than the right.

Transpulmonary pressure The pressure difference across the wall of the lung, equal to the difference between intrapulmonary pressure and intrapleural pressure.

Transsexual A disturbance of gender identity in which the person feels a life-long discomfort with his or her own sex and a compelling desire to be of the opposite sex. People who have undergone some form of physical change, hormones, surgery, or both to achieve a body to suit the gender they prefer.

Transsulfuration pathway An intrahepatic intermediary amino acid metabolic pathway.

Transtibial Below-knee.

Transtracheal catheter Hollow tube inserted in the trachea to deliver oxygen

Transudate The material that passes through a membrane as a result of a difference in hydrostatic pressures on either side of the membrane.

Transudate ascites In ascites fluid is usually generally distributed throughout the peritoneal cavity but occasionally loculi are demarcated by inflammatory adhesions.

In transudate ascites fluid is of pale yellow colour of low protein content less than 25 gm/L and often with a few cellular constituents. This type of ascites is seen where hypoproteinaemia or increased portal pressure is there such as cirrhosis or chronic heart failure.

Transurethral catheterization It is used in urinary retention, neurogenic bladder, monitoring of urinary output, retrograde irrigation of bladder and sterile urinary sampling.

Transvaginal ultrasound Ultrasound in which a transducer is placed within vagina to visualise the pelvic structure.

Transverse fissure The prominent cleft that horizontally separates the cerebrum from the cerebellum.

Transverse friction The fingers are spread out and short strokes are applied, forward and backward, with the fingertips. Pressure is regulated throughout the treatment, commencing gently and progressively increasing.

Transverse plane A horizontal plane, dividing the body into upper (Cranial) and lower (Caudal) portions.

Transverse ridge 1. Elevation or prominence formed by the union of two traingular ridges crossing transversely the occlusal surface of lower premolars obuccal and lingual ridge cusps). 2. Ridge found on maxillary molar running from buccal to lingual.

Transverse section A cut made at right angles to the long axis of an organ.

Transverse sinus A cul-de-sac formed by the epicardial covering of the aorta and the pulmonary trunk.

Transverse tubules (T tubules) Small, cylindrical invaginations of the sarcolemma of striated muscle fibers (cells) that conduct muscle action potentials towards the center of the muscle fiber.

Transversion A type of base pair substitution mutation that substitutes a purine for a pyrimidine or a pyrimidine for a purine.

Transversus abdominis The innermost layer of the anteriolateral abdominal wall.

Trapeze bar Overhead bar on a bed, which the patient can grab.

Trapezium The carpal bone of the wrist that forms the saddle joint that allows the opposition of the thumb. Back muscle, shaped like a trapezium (a four-sided) geometric figure where not two sides are parallel), that rotates the scapula.

Trapezius Triangular muscle in the back that elevates the shoulder and extends the head backwards.

Trapezius muscle It is a large, diamond-shaped muscle that extend from back of skull to lower part of thoracic spine. It is broadest at shoulders attached to scapula and to the outer part of clavicle. It is attached by ligaments to vertebra. It helps in supporting neck and spine. It is involved in movements of arm.

Trapezoid Collection of second-order auditory fibers in the pons.

Trauma An injury, either a physical wound or psychic disorder, caused by an external agent or force, such as a physical blow or emotional shock[the agent or force that causes the injury.

Trauma center A hospital that is especially equipped to care for severely injured patient.

Traumatic asphyxia Common examples are severe compression of chest, crushing by vehicles or machine. Asphyxial changes are confined to the head, neck and shoulders. There is well-marked demarcation between neck and chest and skin below this line is normal. Discolouration disappears in 10 to 14 days.

Traumatic dementia It may result due to closed head injury. In addition to defects in cognitive function irritability and social disinhibition are important factors.

There is an evidence of an amyloid deposition. Repeated trauma is sustained by boxers. Impairment of memory is accompanied by dysarthria, unsteadiness and extrapyramidal syndrome. Even repeated minor cranial injuries may result in loss of intellect and memory.

Traumatic grief A disordered psychic or behavioral state resulting due to mental and emotional stress.

Traumatic hysteria After a few days of accident patient develops hysterical symptoms. Mentally patient becomes introspective with a profound conviction of seriousness of his or her complaint. Person becomes sleepless and irritable and anxieties are increased. Practically all kinds of hysterical movements are met. Pains of all kinds are complained off.

Traumatic occlusion Bite with such poor distribution of forces in one or more areas that injury to the periodontium results.

Traumatic retrograde amnesia A retrograde amnesia resulting from a concussive blow to the head. Most of the affected memory is recovered.

Traumatic shock Severe mechanical trauma, loss of blood and overexcitation of nervous system of CNS contribute its occurrence. Three degrees of shock are distinguished. *First degree* is a state of compensation, pallor and weakness, pulse rate 90 to 100 and maximal blood pressure above 100 mm Hg. *Second degree* shock is a state of partial compensation including pallor, anxiety, cold sweats and nausea. Pulse rate is 120 to 140 weak and barely countable. Systolic BP remains 70 to 80 mm Hg. *Third degree* shock is a state of decompensation. General state becomes grave. There develops marked weakness and pallor, cold sweat and vomiting. Pulse becomes 120 to 160/ minute and BP drops below 70 mm Hg.

Traumatic stressor The occurence of an event that invoIes actual or threatened death or serious injury or threat to physical integrity of one self or family member as either the victim or as a witness.

Traveller's diarrhoea Usually it lasts a few days. Commonly there are symptoms of fever, colicky abdominal pain, nausea and vomiting. Most cases seem to be due to toxin producing varieties of *E. coli*. The incubation is short, often 2 or 3 days but sometimes 2 or 3 weeks. Precautions advised include the avoidance of eating raw fruit, raw vegetables or unwashed salads. Personal hygiene should be maintained. Prophylactice antibacterial drugs are not of much use.

Trcheal stenosis Narrowing of the trachea that occurs as a result of scarring.

Treadmill stress test A test that measures heart rate and blood pressure response to clinically controlled active exercise on a treadmill with a moving belt, a machine on which one walks while staying at one place.

Treatment The management and care of a patient for the purpose of curing a disease or disorder.

Treatment plan Sequence of procedures planned for the treatment of a patient.

Treatment planning Preparing an intervention plan that addresses a client's identified need.

Trefoil bandage It can be used to cover the side of face or an ear or to support an injured jaw. Two or three turns of the end are passed round the head.

The bandage is passed obliquely behind head and brought out on the other side under the lower jaw. Several vertical spirals are then made over the top of head. After several circular turns around the head it is secured.

Treitz, muscle or ligament Suspensory muscle of duodenum.

Tremetode The phyllum platyhelminths include various dorsoventrally flattened animals known as flat worms. These are bilaterally symmetrical and lack abdominal cavity.

Tremor These are involuntary, rhythmic movement of hands, feet, jaw, tongue or head. It is caused by rapidly alternating contractions and relaxation of muscles. Temoporary tremors develop during excitement, fear and at heightened emotions. Fine movements may be hereditary. Coarse tremors 4-5 per second present at rest and reduced during movement is seen in Parkinson's disease. Intention tremor worse on movement is a sign of cerebellum disease.

Tre known as immersion foot. Virtually there is a death of surface skin on the foot caused by longterm exposure to freezing water. In severe cases gangrene may develop.

Trend Related to data analysis of single-system reasearch designs; describes whether the direction of change during a study phase is upward or downward.

Trendelenburg position This position is used while doing operation over pelvic organs to displace intestines into upper abdomen. It is used for patients under shock and to check bleeding from lower limbs. In this patient lies on back with head lowered and body on inclined plane and hips higher than the head. Knees are flexed over adjustable lower section of table.

Trendelenburg sign The patient may be asked to walk on his heels to strength of the dorsoflexors of the foot. With a positive test when patient is standing on one leg, the buttocks away from the affected muscle will fall. This may be related to an S_1 nerve root lesion or hip disease.

Trendenlenburg position

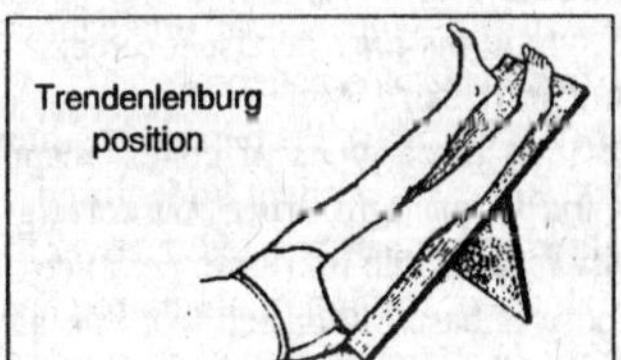

Trendenlenburg test Patient lies down and limb is elevated above the level of heart to allow the varicose veins to empty. Then the thumb is placed firmly over saphenous opening. Keeping the firm pressure over saphenous opening patient is asked to stand up quickly. The pressure is not released but maintained for about one minute. If there is gradual filling of veins from below, indicates incompetency of leg perforating veins allowing retrograde flow. Now pressure is released and if there is quick filling from above it indicates that there is incompetency of valves at the saphenofemoral junction.

Treponema pallidum The causative agent of syphilis. It is extremely similar, possibly identical, to the organisms that cause endemic syphilis, yaws, and pinta.

TRH test TSH is measured 15 minutes interval for 90 minutes after administration of TRH. In hypothyroidism TSH response to TRH is exaggerated.

Triacylglycerol An ester of glycerol with three molecules of fatty acid; also called a triglyceride or neutral fat.

Triage The screening and classification of patients to determine the priority of their need.

Trial of labour An attempted labor to determine whether the fetal head can pass through the pelvis with adequate contractions.

Trial point radiograph Intermediate radiograph for determining the placement of a master cone.

Trial-and-error The apparently random, haphazard, hit-or-miss exploratory activity which often precedes the acquisition of new adjustments. It may be overt, as exemplified in a rat's running here and there in a maze, or covert, as when one thinks of this and then that way of coping with a situation.

Triangular bandage These are convenient for supporting an arm in certain illnesses and injuries. Such a bandage can be made from square of any

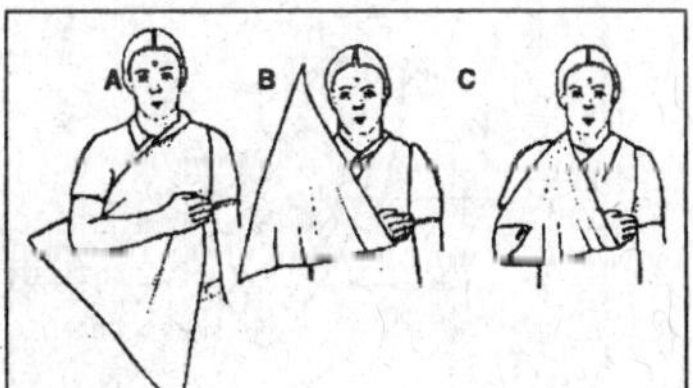

material by folding it diagonally. It is most useful to be used as arm sling otherwise triangular bandage can be used for any part.

Triangular ridge Elevation or prominence on the occlusal surface of posterior teeth that extends from the point of a cusp to the approximate center of the crown.

Triceps brachii A three-headed muscle in the posterior arm that extends the forearm.

Trichinosis Disease caused by eating raw cooked pork due to trichinella spiralis.

Trichlorethylene It is a colourless liquid used in anaesthesia. Specific gravity is 1.47. Boiling point is high 87 °C and saturated vapour pressure at 20°C is 60 mm Hg. It should not be used to produce deep anaesthesia due to side effects. It is a potent nerve poison and may produce paralysis of cranial nerves or even death. Fifth and seventh nerves are mostly involved. It is useful for the production of analgesia without loss of consciousness. It maintains cardiovascular stability. Tachypnoea is due to peripheral action in the lung. It is a good analgesic, useful supplement of nitrous oxide. There is relative lack of irritation of upper respiratory tract.

Tricholoroethane It is a colourless, pleasant smelling liquid which is highly volatile. It is used as metal cleaner. It has a low toxicity. Most cases of intoxication may produce excitement, diplopia, hallucinations, ataxia and dizziness. If exposure continues CNS depression leads to respiratory depression. Sudden death may develop due to cardiac arrhythmias. Occasionally it may produce myocardial damage.

Trichomonas Trichomonas tenax and T. vaginalis possess four free anterior flagella while T. hominis has five free flagella.

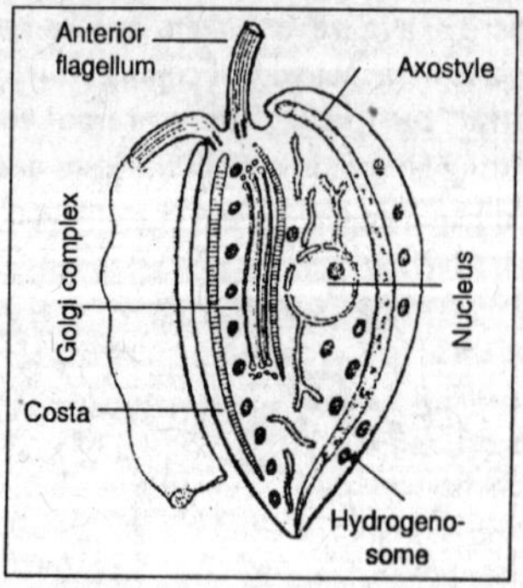

Trichomonas vaginalis Woman who complains of pruritus vulvae harbours this organism. It is mostly found in child bearing period. It is actively motile, slightly larger than a leucocyte and is anaerobic. Man harbours it in urethra and prostate. The vaginal

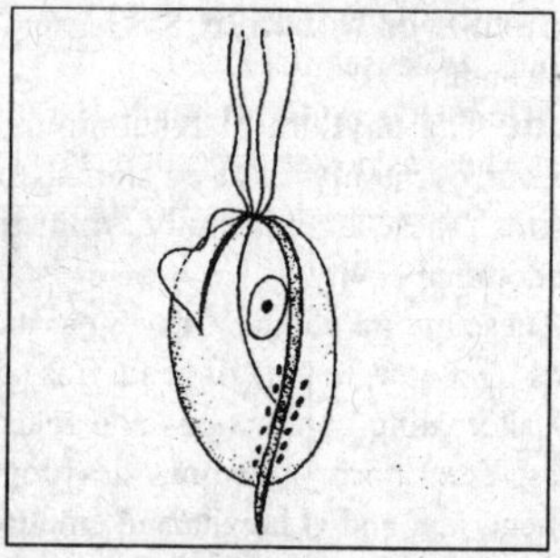

discharge is profuse, thin, creamy or slightly green in colour. It is frothy and irritating. There is itching and inflammation of vulva. There may be small punctate strawberry spots on vaginal vault and erosion of cervix. There may be dysuria and frequency and low-grade urethritis. This organism is generally mixed with *E. coli.* Metronidazole is effective.

Trichomoniasis urogenitalis It is a disorder that produces vaginitis and vaginal discharge in women and urethritis in men and is caused by *Trichomonas vaginalis*. Transmission is through sexual intercourse. Women appear to be more susceptible to the infection than men. It is a pear-shaped organism with 3 to 5 flagella. The infection is normally limited to the vulva, vagina and cervix in women and urethra, seminal vesicles and prostate in men. Woman may complain of green or yellow frothy vaginal discharge having unpleasant odour. There may be redness and oedema of vulva and vagina. There develops burning and itching of vulva and skin of inner thighs. Patient may complain of dyspareunia, dysurea and frequency of micturition. Inguinal lymph nodes may be enlarged and tender. If not treated symptoms may persist for years.

Trichromatic theory A view of color vision which assumes that three types of cones, responsive to short, medium, and long wavelengths, are primarily responsible for our experience of colour. The theory is based upon the fact that any colour can be obtained by an appropriate mixture of blue, green, and red wavelengths.

Trichuriasis It is known as whipworm. In humans it is contracted by eating food contaminated with worm's egg. These hatch and colonise the large intestine. Eggs of next generation are passed through anus. It causes itching.

Trichuris trichiura Anterior body is long and cylindrical where as posterior portion is widen and

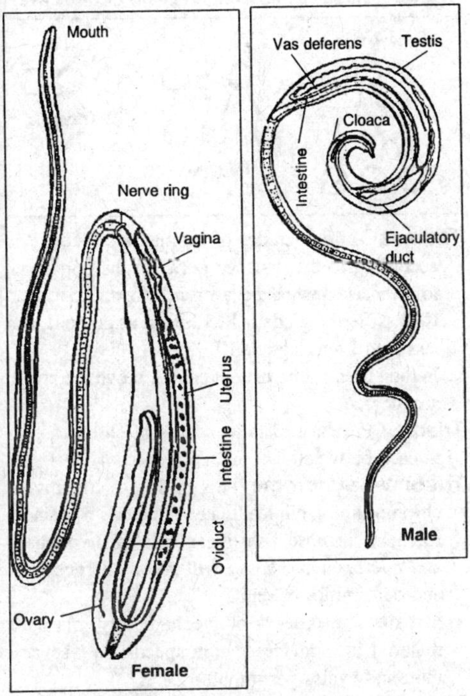

thickened known as 'whipworm'. Males are smaller than females. Chronic infection causes pain lower abdomen, weight loss and anemia.

Tricuspid valve The valve located between the right atrium and ventricle.

Trifurcation Division into three parts or branches, as the three roots of a maxillary first molar.

Trigeminal nerve Fifth cranial nerve; a mixed motor and sensory nerve connected with the pons through three roots motor, proprioceptive, and large sensory, the latter root expanding into the trigeminal ganglion, from which arise the opthalmic, massentric, and mandibular divisions.

Trigeminal nerve ganglion-herpes Herpes may involve the sensory neurons in the trigeminal nerve ganglion. Oral vesicles are formed preceded by toothache or pain in area for last 2-3 days. Vesicles rupture and leave painful ulcers but heal in a few days without scars. Lesions may be seen on cheek, soft palate, buccal mucosa and tongue.

Trigeminal neuralgia In it an episode of severe, stabbing pain affecting the cheek, lips, gums or chin on one side of face. Pain is brief lasting for a few seconds. During pain person cannot do anything. Attacks occur in bouts which may last for weeks and cause is not known. The pain nearly always starts from one trigger point on the face and can be brought by touching the face, washing, shaving, drinking or even talking. Carbamazepine suppresses the pain in most sufferers but resistance to drugs occur. If drug treatment fails surgical options are available.

Trigeminal pulse Three regular pulse beats followed by a pause.

Trigger area An area of local nerve facilitation; pressure on the trigger point resutls in hypertonicity of a muscle bundle and referred pain patterns.

Trigger finger It results when a thickened segment of a finger flexor tendon has to pass through a narrowed segment of its tendon sheath. It occurs

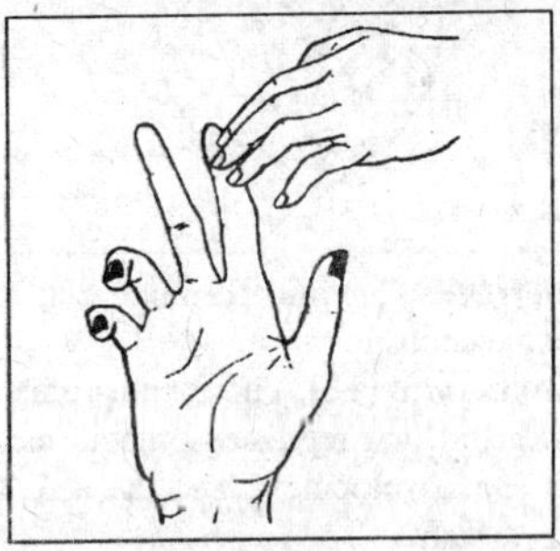

in patients with rheumatoid arthritis. Flexion of finger may require more effort than usual and extension is attempted. This proceeds up to a certain point, then greater force has to be applied.

Trigger points Palpable band or nodule within the muscle or connective tissue that refers pain and other phenomena, elicits a local twitch response when pressed, and is generally hypersensitive.

Trigger thumb The thenar and hypothenar eminences are palpated for discomfort or trigger points. Also palmar fascia is palpated for

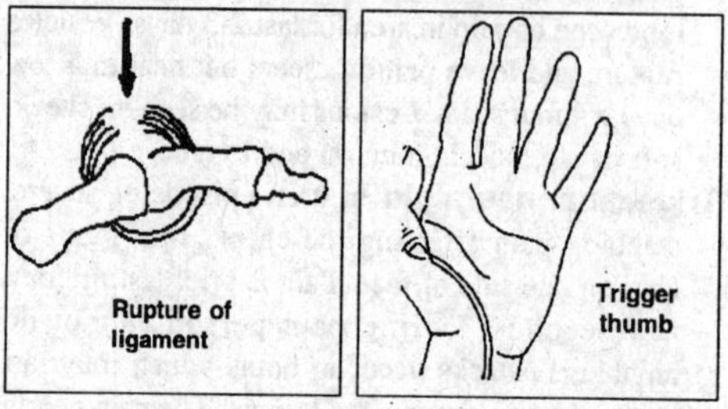

tenderness or mass. A tender nodule in the area of palmar crease with patient complaining of digit catching with movement may suggest flexor tenosynovitis or what is commonly known as trigger thumb.

Trigone It is a triangular area at the base of the bladder between the two ureteral orifices above and laterally and internal urethral orifice below and centrally.

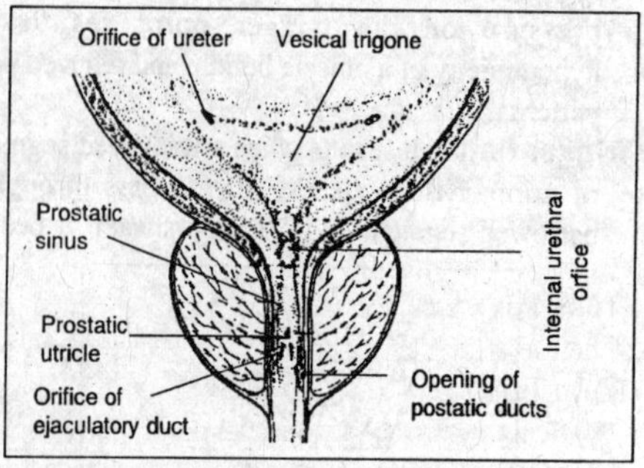

Triiodothyronin Thyroid hormone that stimulates cellular metabolism.

Triiodothyronine (T3) A hormone produced by the thyroid gland that regulates organic metabolism, growth and development, and the activity of the nervous system.

Trimester A period of 3 months.

Trimethoprim It is antimicrobial of considerable efficacy of its own. It is active against many gram-positive and gram-negative aerobic organisms. Drug is rapidly and effectively absorbed. It is effective against urinary and respiratory tract infection. Side effects include skin rash and nausea.

Triose A simple sugar with a backbone containing three carbon atoms.

Triple angle Refers to three angles of a shank of a dental instrument; commonly found in a hoe or scaler.

Triple marker screening Analysis of maternal serum for abnormal levels of alpha-fetoprotein, human chorionic gonadotropin and estriols that may predict chromosomal abnormalities of fetus.

Triple response The line-flare-wheal response to a sharp stroke to the skin, involving an axon reflex.

Triplets These can be from one, two or three ova.

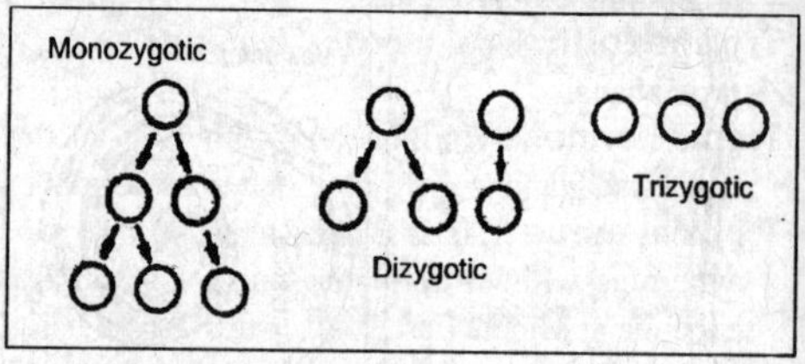

Trismus Various grades of trismus are recognised according to the distance between the upper and lower incisors when the jaw is fully open 2.5 to 4 cm is classified as grade I, 1 to 2.5 cm as grade II, and less than 1 cm as grade III.

In total trismus the patient cannot move the jaw to any degree.

Trisomy Presence of three copies of chromosomes in each body cell.

Trisomy-I syndrome This is due to trisómy of chromosome-I, clinical features include prominent forehead and nose, fish-like mouth, nail hypoplasia and micrognathia, X-ray will show microcephaly and deformities of digits.

Triturate The process of mechanically mixing a material in a device at high speeds (i.e., several thousand cycles per minute)

Trochal larva A larva with cilia arranged in distinct bands.

Trochanter A broad, prominent process on the proximolateral portion of the femur.

Trochlea A pulley-shaped structure.

Trolard, vein Superior anastomotic vein of cerebrum.

Trophic 'Nourishing.

Trophic nerve function The function of nerves related to nutrition and growth. Trophic substances produced by nerves have been found to be essential for the maintenance of proper tissue structure and function.

Trophic ulcers These develop due to an impairment of nutrition of tissues which depends on adequate blood supply and also a properly functioning nerve supply. Ischaemia and anaesthesia will cause these ulcer. Neuropathic ulcers due to anaesthesia, diabetes, neuritis are called perforating ulcers.

Trophoblast The peripheral cells of the blastocyst, which attach the fertilised ovum to the uterine wall and become the placenta and the membranes around the embryo/fetus.

Trophozoite The motile, feeding stage of protozoans.

Tropic hormone Hormone that stimulates another endocrine gland to grow and secrete its hormones.

Tropical sprue This is a persistent malabsorption syndrome without definable cause. Condition is endemic in Middle East. It is regarded as infective. Major early features are diarrhoea, abdominal distension and anorexia. Abdominal discomfort occurs in many patients and nausea and vomiting in a few.

In acute condition there may be fever and blood and mucus in stool raising the suspicion of dysentery. In chronic stage vitamin B_{12} deficiency may be severe and can lead to neurological manifestations. Symptoms may be persistent and there are often partial remissions.

Tropical ulcer It is an acute or chronic ulcer resulting from anaerobic bacteroids. These bacteria are normal inhabitors of upper respiratory tracts. Initially a small abraded or ulcerated area appears on the part exposed to trauma. It later changes to a bulla and then ruptures to form a deep, circular ulcer usually solitary with undermined edges. Ulcer is covered with foul smelling pus or thick, dirty crusts and peeling of crusts leads to bleeding. Lymph glands do not enlarge.

Tropism An unlearned orienting movement of the whole organism which causes it to move toward or away from the stimulus. Examples are a moth flying into the flame (positive phototropism) and a cockroach running away from light (negative phototropism)

Tropomyosin A filamentous protein that attaches to actin in the thin myofilaments and that acts, together with another protein called troponin, to inhibit and regulate the attachment of myosin cross bridges to actin.

True aneurysm An aneurysm is defined as a localised dilated sac filled with blood in direct communication with the lumen of an artery. True aneurysm is due to actual dilatation of an artery, either symmetrical or eccentric.

In fusiform expansion of the entire circumference of the arterial wall in long axis of an artery occurs. Saccular aneurysm is an extension of a part of the circumference of the arterial wall.

True chordae A fibrous collagenous cord spanning the gap between the papillary muscles and the valve leaflets.

True leg length discrepancy This is the measurable difference in the overall length of the two legs from anterior superior iliac spine (ASIS) to the medial malleolus.

True ribs The first seven ribs on either side of the thorax whose cartilages articulate directly with the sternum.

Truncal ataxia Inability to maintain the upright position; a feature of midline cerebellar disease.

Truncal ridges The spiral epithelial outgrowths the walls of the truncus arteriosus that combine with the bulbar ridges to form the aorticopulmonary septum.

Truncus arteriosus The primitive ascending aorta that opens from both ventricles in early stages of fetal development.

Truss It is a tight support for hernia. In consists of a belt to which strapping and pad are attached.

Truth telling Ethical principle proposing that all patients have the right to receive complete and accurate information.

Try in Preliminary insertion of a removable denture wax-up (trial denture), or of a partial denture casting or of a finished restoration to determine factors such as fit, esthetics, and maxillomandibular relation.

Trypanosomiasis *Trypanosoma brucei* and *gambiense* cause sleeping sickness. The flagellated parasite is transmitted by a bite from infected tsetse fly. Transmission is from human to human. Changes in behaviour and a propensity to sleep during the day are early manifestations. Trypanosomes can be shown in CSF. Melarsoprol is effective in treating encephalopathy but relapses occur.

Trypomastigote It exhibits various degrees of polymorphism. A hemoglagellate form with an elongated undulating membrane and kinetoplast located posterior to the nucleus.

Trypsin An enzyme released from the pancreas that digests proteins.

Trypsinogen The inactive form of trypsin.

T-tests Tests that compare differenes between two means.

Ttracheostomy collar Curced oxygen delivery device with an adjustable neck strap that fits around the tracheostomy.

Tubal abortion It occurs in 8-10 weeks of pregnancy. Bleeding is caused by placental separation. It is moderate in complete tubal abortion. Mild abdominal distension with pyrexia, tenderness, indefinite pelvic mass and uterus is displaced upwards.

Tubal ligation A sterilization procedure in which the uterine (Fallopian) tubes are tied and cut.

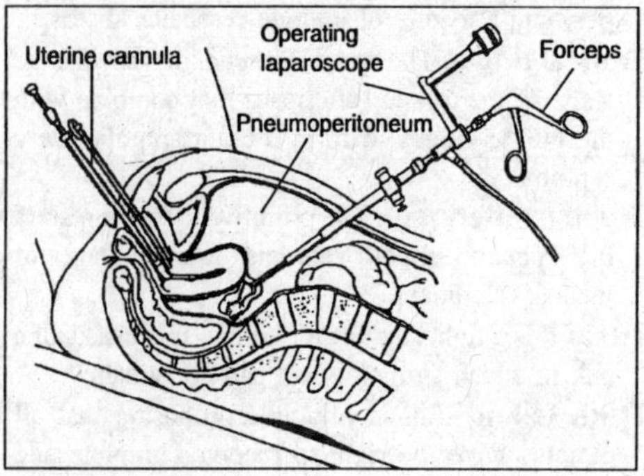

Tubal pregnancy It is more prevalent where gonococcal infection is present. Ampulla is the commonest site of implantation. Tubal gestation product may continue to grow and remain intact within the fallopian tube so long blood supply is adequate. But rarely pregnancy goes beyond 3-4 weeks.

Tubal rupture It occurs from the narrow isthmus at about 4 to 6 weeks of conception or from the, interstitial pregnancy at 12 weeks. Rupture may take place due to erosion of tube-wall and sudden increase in presence in the intervillous space.

Tube feeding It may be oral or nasal. It is used in comatose patient, paralysis of soft palate of pharyngeal muscles, after oral operation, in premature infants and in insane persons. Tube should go to stomach, when second mark comes to the opening of nostrils,it is assumed that tube is in stomach. When person is unable to swallow liquid diet is given by gastric tube. Eggs and powdered milk have the highest biological degree of utilisation and surpass other natural proteins for tube feeding. Various artificial food of different composition are available. Complications include pharyngeal and oesophageal ulceration, reflux oesophagitis, cross-infection and diarrhoea.

Tubectomy It is the operation in which fallopian tubes are ligated with or without cutting. This prevents the sperms from meeting the ovum so that conception cannot take place. Operation can be done just after delivery.

Tubercle A small rounded nodule or elevation on the surface of the skin, bone, or other tissue.

Tubercle of the rib The junction of the neck and the shaft of the rib; an articular portion of tubercle articulates with transverse process of the inferiormost vertebra to which the head is connected.

Tubercular meningitis It is spreading where HIV infection is widespread. *Mycobacterium tuberculosis* does not gain access to the nervous system. Tuberculous meningitis may not develop when other organs are affected. One or two meningeal tubercle may develop. Meningeal tubercle is called Rich focus. The gelatinous meningitis is particularly prominent in the anterior basal cistern. General malaise, headache, irritability appear within 2 to 6 weeks. Low-grade fever and meningeal irritation develop. Papilloedema develops in untreated cases.

Tuberculin syringe Syringe that holds 1 mL of fluid and is calibrated in 0.01-mL increments.

Tuberculin test Purified protein derivatives (PPD) in different tuberculin unit (TU), first being 1 TU and the next 5 TU, is administered by intradermal or multiple puncture method on the skin of the forearm. A positive reaction produces a palpable induration of over 10 mm in diameter, a negative of less than 5 mm in diameter, and a doubtful of between 5 and 10 mm in diameter, after 48 hours. A positive reaction indicates past or present tuberculous infection and the person is grouped as being in risk, but a negative indicates absence of tuberculous infection and the person does not belong to the risk group, and a doubtful may indicate presence of recent infection or of non-tuberculous infection. The test is done for diagnosis and for susceptibility to tuberculosis.

Tuberculoma These are granu-lomatous lesions with varying degrees of central necrosis within brain and spinal cord. When it reaches a sufficient size it may produce seizures. A tuberculoma less than 2 cm will resolve on treatment. Larger lesions will require excision. Lesion may coexist with tuberculous meningitis.

Tuberculosis It is caused by *Mycobacterium tuberculosis*. In early 19th century it was a killing disease, before invention of streptomycin. Infection is passed from person to person in air-borne

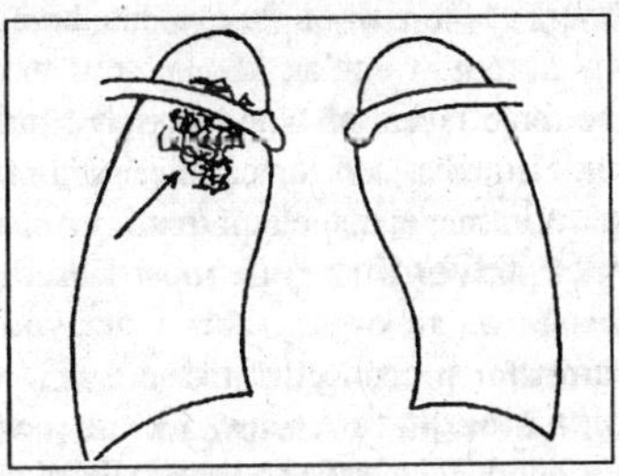

droplets. X-ray chest and blood tests are helpful. Sputum staining may reveal AFB bacilli. A strongly positive test result may indicate an active infection. Rifampicin/streptomycin, isoniazid (INH), pyrazinamide combination is most effective.

Tuberculosis and pregnancy There is no increased incidence of spontaneous abortion. If treated well child born will be normal.

Tuberculosis of conjunctiva Tuberculosis of conjunctiva occurs in young person. It is an exogenous rare infection. Clinically there is an ulceration of conjunctiva. Primary lesion is an acute process and heels quickly. Secondary lesion is chronic and ulcer takes a long time to heal with enlargement of preauricular glands. Scraping and cauterisation is done with diathermy.

Tuberculosis of placenta It is rare and is seen with generalised TB only. The tuberculous deposits are found either in decidua, upon chorionic epithelium or in villi. Caseation is frequently found in these deposits. In case of acute TB miliary deposits may be seen in fetal portion of placenta.

Tuberculous endosalpingitis In it tube becomes enlarged, thickened and tortuous. Patient may develop fever and abdominal pain. Caseation in the wall of tube and collection of cheesy material in the lumen may form a pyosalpinx if both ends of fallopian tube are sealed by fibrosis.

Tuberculous exosalpingitis There is tuberculous pelvic peritonitis and may be direct extension from adjacent organs. Peritoneal surface is studded with miliary tubercles. It is known as frozen pelvis.

Tuberculous laryngitis Inter-laryngeal manifestations are diverse. Hoarseness and cough increase over a period of month. Pain supervenes and may radiate to ears. Reddish brown submucous nodules may be seen. Ulcerating mucosal tuberculosis is a common form. Deep crater-like soft tissue ulcers are seen. There will be greasy coating. Hoarseness increasing pain may be severe. Dysphagia may develop.

Tuberculous lymphadenitis Mostly it affects upper deep cervical and mesenteric nodes, less frequently the axillary and very rarely the inguinal group. In the first stage, the nodes become simply enlarged without matting as there is no periadenitis. This may remain for long time. In the second stage, the enlarged nodes become matted to each other. In third stage, caseation takes place in the interior forming a cold abscess. Sinus may be formed.

Tuberculous lymphadenopathy It is a painless swelling of various groups of cervical lymph nodes, sometimes may be bilateral. Patients are of younger age group and lesion may be solitary, multiple, small or large. Gland biopsy is diagnostic.

Tuberculous paraplegia Spinal cord may be affected by direct pressure from tuberculous pus and granulation material or by a displaced sequestrated disc. On occasion a whole vertebral body may sequestrate and protrude backwards or there may be a pathological dislocation of spine.

Tuberculous peritonitis It may present with abdominal distension due to ascites. It is more common in alcoholics and with evidence of tuberculous infection elsewhere. Patient complains of lassitude, weight loss, pyrexia and abdominal distension. Abdomen may have doughy feel and one or several masses may be palpable. Examination of ascitic fluid shows characteristics of an exudate, high protein with lymphocytes and endothelial cells. Laparoscopy is helpful as peritoneal lining and that over viscera is studded with tubercles. Biopsy yields typical caseating granulomata.

Tuberosity Lump on a bone, usually larger than tubercle.

Tuberous xanthoma It is associated with types II a and III hyper-lipoproteinaemia. Tuberous xanthoma presents with flat or rounded, multiple, yellow or brown, infiltrated tumour-like growth anywhere on skin specially over bony prominences of hands, elbows and knees. These do not give rise to any symptoms.

Tubo-ovarian abscess Inflammation and abscess formation involving the ovary and the Fallopian tube.

Tuboplasty Surgery on a tubular body; e.g., the Fallopian tube, most commonly to restore tubal patency or reduce scarring to promote fertility.

Tubular necrosis Cell death in the tubule cells in the kidney.

Tubular reabsorption The movement of filtrate from renal tubules back into block in response to the body's specific needs.

Tubular secretion Movement of materials, by means of active transport, from the blood into the filtrate of a nephron.

Tubulodermoid It is a cystic swelling from the non-obliterated portion of a congenital ectodermal duct or tube. The swelling is due to distension caused by the accumulation of secretion of the lining epithelium of patent segment of duct. Thyroglossal cyst is the most common. Post anal dermoid is remnant of neuroenteric canal. Ependymal cyst in the brain is the remnant of neuroectoderm.

Tukey test A multiple-comparison procedure.

Tularemia A bacterial disease of humans transmitted by tabanid files and for which rabbits often serve as reservoir hosts.

Tumor grade The level of aggressiveness of a tumor.

Tumor marker A specific and easily accessible protein that can be used for the evaluation and management of a certain malignancy.

Tumor necrosis factor Also known as cachectin.

Tumor Suppressor gene A gene whose product is normally involved in the negative regulation of cellular growth and division, thus, inhibiting cancerous growth. The loss of function of a tumor suprressor gene, usually due to mutation, contributes to abnormal growth and transformation.

Tumour It is a new growth of cells which are harmful. It is new growth and not inflammatory swelling. These can be benign or malignant. Both benign and malignant tumours are due to excessive replication of cells. This may occur either as a result of diminished restraint of cell replication or of increased stimulus to cell reproduction. Benign tumour grows by expansion and does not invade body tissue while a malignant tumour grows by invasion of surrounding tissue and can spread by metastasis.

Tunic A layer or coat; one of the three enveloping layers of the wall of the eye; the three tunics are : the fibrous, vascular, and nervous tunics; one of the three layers of blood vessels : tunica intima, tunica media, and tunica adventitia (externa).

Tunica Intima endothelium that lines blood vessels.

Tunica adventitia Outermost fibrous coat of a vessel or an organ that is derived from the surrounding connective tissue.

Tunica albuginea A tough, whitish membrane that surrounds each testis and enters the gland to divide it into lobules.

Tunica externa The superficial coat of an artery or vein, composed mostly of elastic and collagen fibers. Also called the adventitia.

Tunica interna The deep coat of an artery or vein, consisting of a lining of endothelium, basement membrane, and internal elastic lamina. Also called the tunica intima.

Tunica intima Innermost layer of a blood or lymphatic vessel; consists of endothelium and a small amount of connective tissue.

Tunica media The muscular middle layer found in blood vessels; the tunica media of arteries is more muscular than that of veins.

Tuning fork It is a simple instrument used for testing the auditory status of patient. Tuning fork with a frequency of 512 vibrations per minute is the ideal instrument for this purpose. Tuning fork should be

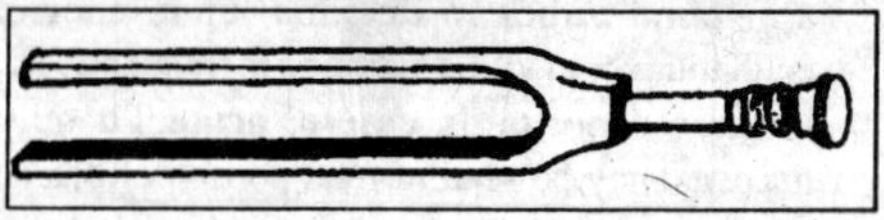

struck on rubber pad or at knee. It is used in Rinne's test. Weber's test and absolute bone conduction test.

Tunnel, carpal Carpal canal.

Turbinate Conchea

Turbo-inhaler Propeller-driven device used to instill medication into the airways.

Turbulence This is an irregular movement of water molecules. Within a hydrotherapy pool, turbulence may be created by an underwater douche which is

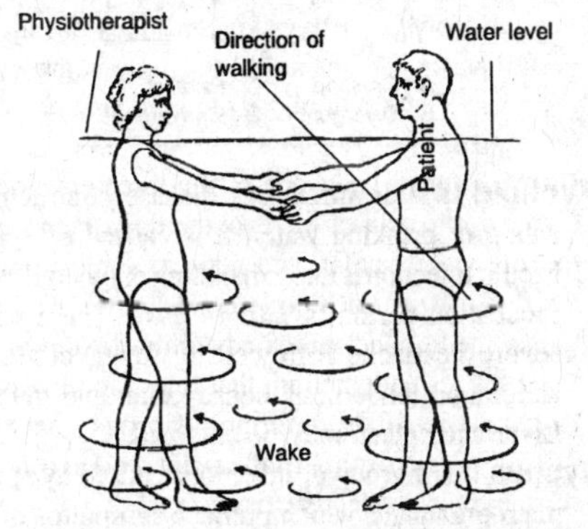

The application of turbulence with the physiotherapist and the patient walking through the water

a jet of water from hose pipe. The douche is used to apply a pressure on tissues and may be moved around a painful area. Patient reports dramatic pain relief. Turbulence may be produced by physiotherapist moving through the water. If patient cannot move physiotherapist can move around the patient.

Turbulent flow Oscillations create uneven flow.

Turf toe Acute hyperdorsiflexion injuries to the first MTP joint occur as the toes are pressed down into

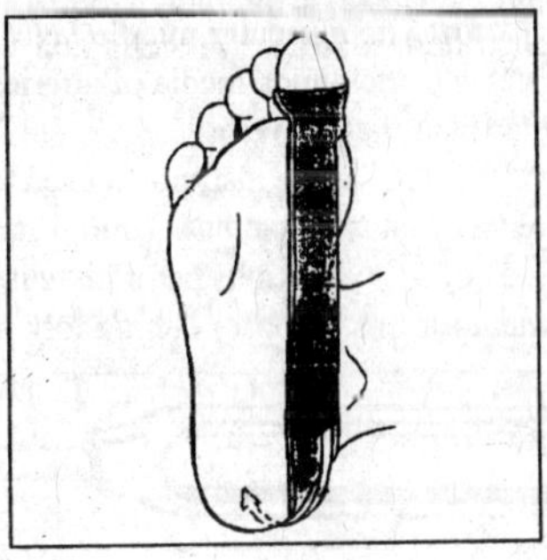

an unyielding surface just prior to toe-off. This force causes hyperflexion of MTP. Repeated trauma, sudden acceleration under high loads against unyielding astroturf are the usual mechanisms of injury. Turf toe taping prevents excessive hyperextension.

Turgor Normal tension of a cell; swelling; distention; elastic condition of skin.

Turner's syndrome A chromosomal anomaly associated with dwarfism, gonadal dysgenesis, infantile sexual development, webbed neck, lymphangiectatic oedema of the hands and feet, and mental and physical retardation.

Turpentine stupes Turpentine is obtained from distillation of crude oleoresin of various species of pines. Oil of turpentine has counterirritating action in addition of volatile oil. When fomentation is used for counterirritation purpose, it is known as stupe.

Twave deflection on an electrocardiogram that occurs with repolarization of the ventricles.

Twenty-four-hour specimen Collection of all the urine produced in a full 24 hour period.

Twin concordance The degree to which two twins are identical on a trait.

Twin research A powerful method of investigating the relative degree of phenotypic variance that can be attributed to genetic factors and to transmissible and nontransmissible environmental factors.

For example, the dissimilarities between monozygotic twins are compared with the behavioural variations occurring in non-twin siblings or dizygotic twins.

Twins There will be two babies out of one pregnancy. These are of two types. *Monozygotic* when a single ova divides into two. These are identical in shape and size. Such twins share the same placenta. They are of same sex and look alike.

Twins from two ova are called *dizygotic* or binovular twins. Ova may be released from the same ovary or from different ovaries. Each dizygotic twin has its own placenta. These look quiet different and may or may not be of different sexes.

Twist drill In certain root form osteotomy preparation protocols, a drill used to widen a preliminary osteotomy.

Twitch A quick, jery response to a single stimulus.

Twitch contraction Brief contraction of all muscle fibers in a motor unit triggered by a single action potential in its motor neuron.

Two-point discrimination Ability to detect that the skin is being touched by two pointed objects at once.

Tylose An abnormal outgrowth of xylem parenchyma cells that balloons into the xylem vessel lumen, restricting the flow of water.

Tympanic Drumlike.

Tympanic membrane Cellular membrane that covers the inner opening of the external auditory meatus and separates the middle and external ears; vibrates in response to sound waves; the eardrum.

Tympanosclerosis Morphological changes include swelling of collagen fibres and hyaline degeneration with subsequent calcium deposition. Tympanic membrane is scarred and thickened and contains calcium deposits and possibly atrophic areas. A whitish material may be seen through membrane. Conductive hearing loss may develop.

Tympany A low-pitched, drumlike resonance produced by percussing the chest wall or other hollow structure.

Type A behaviour Complex of behaviors and emotions defined by excessive striving competitiveness, hostility and impatience.

Type A personality A temperament characterised by excessive drive, competitiveness, a sense of time urgency, impatience, unrealistic ambition, and need for control. Believed to be associated with a high incidence of coronary artery disease.

Type B personality A temperament characterised by a relaxed, easy-going demeanor; less time-bound and competitive than the type A personality.

Type I error Error that occurs when data lead one to conclude that somethhing is false when in reality it is true. Type II error is also called beta error and false-negative error.

Type II cutaneous mechanoreceptor A receptor embedded deeply in the dermis and deeper tissues that detects stretching of skin. Also called a Ruffini corpuscle.

Types of obstetrics forceps These may be grouped in four groups. Branches either cross in the shape of X, diverge in shape of V, are parallel or convergent towards the toes of blades.

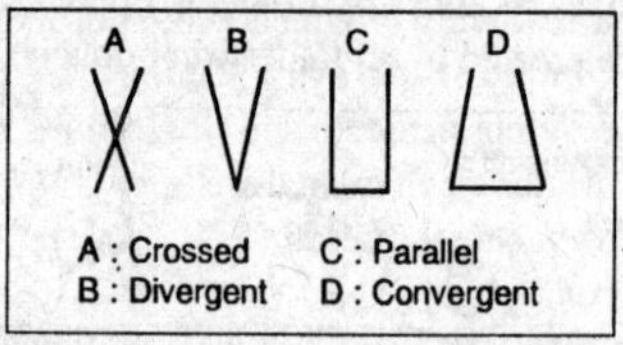

Typhoid It is an infectious disease contracted by eating or drinking water. It is caused by typhoid bacilli. Infection is due to handling of typhoid carrier. Incubation period is 7 to 14 days. There will be severe headache followed by fever, confusion, abdominal tenderness, constipation and delirium. Liver and spleen may be enlarged.

Typhus It is a group of infections caused by specific microorganisms which produce symptoms of very high temperature, severe headache, rash, shock and delirium. Infective organism is carried by rat fleas, ticks and mites.

Tyramine A sympathomimetic amine that acts by displacing stored transmitter from adrenergic axonal terminals; a constituent of many foods such as flat beans, cheese, red wine, etc. which are forbidden when using monoamine oxidase (MAD) inhibitors because of hypertensive crisis.

Tzanck test The test shows altered epithelial cells and disruption of intercellular connections in the smear from the base of the bulla or of vesicle scraping. It is seen in pemphigus and also in herpes simplex, herpes zoster, varicella and vaccinia.

U

UCR Usual, customary, and reasonable fee.

Ulcer It is an open discontinuation on the skin or on mucous membrane. Ulcer may be shallow or deep. It is usually inflamed and painful. Skin ulcers are common on legs. Mucous membrane ulcer develops in mouth and GIT. Skin as well as mucous membrane of genitalia can also be affected in case of Venereal disease (VD). Corneal ulcers are also common.

Ulcer edge There are different types of ulcer edge. Punched-out edge follows death and loss of whole thickness of skin without much attempt by body to repair it. Slopping edge indicates that ulcer is shallow and epithelium is growing in from the edge in an attempt to heal it. This sign is found in venous ulcers. Undermined edge affects the subcutaneous tissues or deeper tissues more than skin or superficial tissues found in tuberculous and amoebic ulcer. Everted edge of the ulcer is growing quickly and spilling out of ulcer to overlap normal skin found in squamous cell carcinoma. Rolled-out or beaded ulcer is found in basal cell cancer.

Ulcer healing drugs These are the drugs used in healing and preventing peptic ulcer specially. Histamine-2 receptor antagonist works by blocking the effects of histamine. It reduces the secretion of acid in the stomach and thus promotes healing. Such drugs are famotidine and ranitidine, other group of drugs such as sucralfate are believed to form a protective layer over ulcer. Antacids are also effective.

Ulcer, aphthous It is a chronic inflammatory disease charac-terised by repeated episodes of oval or round ulceration of oral mucosa specially on lips, cheeks and soft palate. Lesions are 2-20 mm in diameter and are painful. They start with burning pain lasting for 1-2 days followed by appearance of small white area or red raised papule on mucosa. These expand in size and then become necrosed. Its incidence appears to decrease with age. Microscopically, non-ulcerative stage shows non-nuclear and lymphocytic infiltration. After ulceration the lesion shows polymorphonuclear leucocytes, oedema and fibroblastic proliferation. Treatment is symptomatic only. Tetracycline has been used for oral rinse as well as four times daily orally. Corticosteroids have also been used.

Ulcer, Mikulicz's This occurs on salivary gland and is considered a more severe form of aphthous ulcer. It begins as small, smooth, painful red nodule which ulcerate soon. These are crater like, larger and deeper which heal more slowly. Lesions may heal in 3 to 6 weeks but leave scar. Treatment is symptomatic only.

Ulcerative colitis It is characterised by inflammation and ulcertion of colon with bloody diarrhoea and occasional remission and excerbations. It may be autoimmune phenomenon. It starts in rectal mucosa which becomes inflamed and roughened. Mucosa bleeds easily to trauma and multiple small ulcers and exudates are seen. The disease spreads proximally upto caecum. In severe cases patient is very ill, temperature is high and toxaemia is present. Tongue is dry with tachycardia.

There may be loose motion with blood, pus and mucus. Patient becomes anaemic and exhausted. History of intolerance of dairy products may be present. Liver is palpable, soft and tender. There may develop dehydration and electrolyte imbalance. Electrolyte shows anaemia, leucocytosis and high ESR. Proctoscopy shows small superficial ulcer which bleeds easily. Barium enema shows loss of haustration with multiple ulcers.

Ulcerative secondary tuberculous enteritis Here dose and virulence of organism are more and host resistance is less therefore necrosis, caseation and ulceration of intestine is seen. Onset is gradual and abdominal pain is an important sign and is felt diffusely over abdomen. It is cramping and colicky in nature and partially removed after vomiting. Some may develop symptoms of intestinal obstruction, i.e. distension of abdomen, increased borborygmi. Abdominal shape becomes bloated, visible and small peristalsis noted.

Ulna It is longer of two bones of forearm. It is on inner side parallel to radius. Upper end of ulna articulates with radius. Fracture of ulna typically occurs across the shaft or at olecranon process. Putting plaster helps in healing.

Ulnar drift Abnormal ulnar deviation of the fingers at the metacarpophalangeal joints.

Ulnar nerve It is the main nerve of the arm running down its full length into the hand. It is a branch of brachial plexus and controls the movement of thumb and fingers. It carries sensation from fifth and half of fourth finger. Osteoarthritis or fracture of humerus may cause persistent pain, numbness and muscle weakness supplied by ulnar nerve.

Ulnar nerve compression There develops pins and needle sensations running down the ulnar aspect of the forearm into ring and little finger

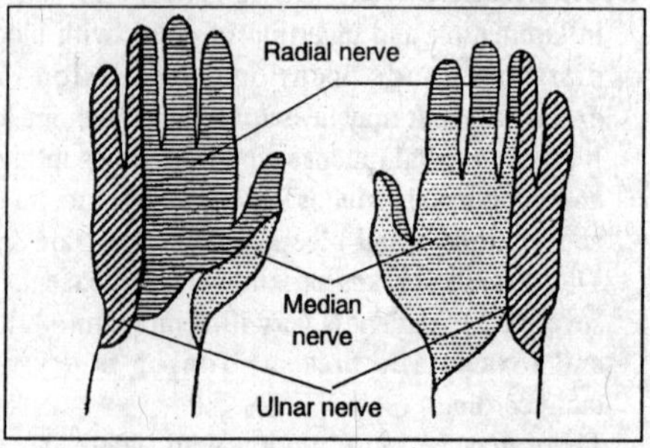

after striking the elbow. Previous elbow fracture or recurrent trauma and increased carrying angle may predispose it. There may be wasting of web between thumb and index finger. Occasionally sensory impairment splits middle finger.

Ultimate strength The maximum stress a material can withstand without fracturing what is referred to as a material's "strength"

Ultrasonic cleaner Open bath of cleaning solution vibrated at a very high frequency.

Ultrasonography Soft tissue examination that uses sound waves in ranges beyond human hearing.

Ultrasound Ultrasound used in medicine is typically in the frequency range of 1 to 15 million Hertz. It was first used in 1950s. Ultrasound waves pass readily through soft tissues and fluids making it useful in examining fluid-filled organs such as gall bladder and uterus. It is a very useful tool to examine fetus. It can help knowing the welfare of

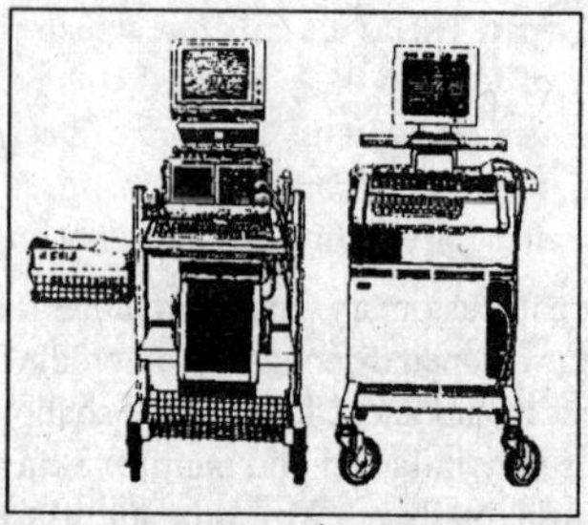

fetus and measuring different parameters. It helps in monitoring the progress of fetus. It is very helpful in knowing liver and gall bladder pathologies.

Ultraviolet light Long wavelength ultraviolet light is often termed UVA, intermediate wavelength ultraviolet light is designated UVB and short wavelength is called UVC. Ultraviolet light occurs naturally in sunlight but most of it is absorbed by the ozone layer of atmosphere. UVA reaching to earth is helpful in production of Vitamin D in the skin. A mercury-vapour lamp can also be used to produce ultraviolet rays artificially.

Ultraviolet radiation Ability of sunlight to kill bacteria is due to ultraviolet rays it contains. Most of these rays are screened by glass and foggy atmosphere. UV rays becomes more effective with short wavelength as steriliser. Gram-positive bacteria show slightly higher resistance to ultraviolet radiation than gram-negative. Spores are highly resistant.

Umbilical adenoma It is a pathological condition arising from patent distal segment of vitellointestinal duct.

The mucosa of the patent duct prolapses through the umbilicus and gives rise to a soft pink tumour which looks like a raspberry, hence it is known as raspberry tumour. It usually develops only in infancy.

There is a soft fleshy mass, pinkish in colour. Mass may be pedunculated or sessile.

There may be discharge from umbilicus. Intestinal obstruction may occur. If a ligature is tied around its base, in a few days the polypus drops off. If there is recurrence umbilectomy may be done.

Umbilical artery Two small arteries that carry oxygen-poor blood from the developing fetus to the placenta.

Umbilical cord This is the structure which connects the body of fetus to the placenta. Along it passes the fetal vessels which vascularise the growing chorion. These are branches from internal iliac arteries. when fully formed it contains ventral stalk, umbilical blood vessels, the allantois, the vitelline duct and the obliterated extraembryonic coelom. In early embryo it is thick and short. About the 3rd month of gestation four vessels are found in cord, 2 arteries and 2 veins. At term its length varies from 5 to 60 inches and average being 18 to 24 inches. Vessels are always twisted. Arteries encircling veins from left to right.

Umbilical granuloma It is a chronic infection of the umbilical cord after severance and tying off of it. When the infection continues for weeks and becomes florid, excess granulation tissue is formed which prevents the raw area from becoming epithelialised. The baby presents with a pouting umbilicus surmounted by a bright red moist mass of granulation tissue. Mass is friable and bleeds on touch. One application of silver nitrate stick followed by dry dressing usually destroys the umbilical granuloma. Recurrence is common.

Umbilical hernia It is a swelling, soft in nature at the umbilicus caused by protrusion of abdominal contents. These are common in newborns and develop when baby cries. At the age of two these generally disappear. If infection supercedes there may be a discharge. After the age of six if it persists, surgery is the remedy.

Umbilical vein Vein in the umbilical cord of the fetus by which the fetus receives nourishment from the maternal system; becomes the round ligament of the liver in the adult.

Umbilicus The point at which the umbilical cord attaches to the fetal abdomen, or the umbilical cord itself.

Uncal herniation Displacement of the uncus through the tentorial notch.

Uncertain APH This includes bleeding from marginal placental sinus. The bleeding may be due to local causes such as ectopic columnar epithelium, cervical polyps.

Uncertainity A state characterised by embiguity or lack of information to a particular situation or outcome. Uncertainity is often experienced as stressful and unpleasant.

Unclotted blood after death A sudden death may result in reduced amount of clotting. Blood is fluid in certain cases of septicaemia, in CO poisoning, death due to asphyxia and hypofibrinogenaemia and in retained placenta.

Unconditional acceptance In the person-centred approach to therapy, acceptance by the counsellor without regard to the way in which the other person feels or thinks or behaves. It includes an attitude of caring and valuing the person as a person, regardless of expressions of anxiety, disappointment, confusion, love, and so forth.

Unconditional positive regard The attempt by a therapist to convey to a client that he or she genuinely cares for the client.

Unconditioned response An original or inborn response, such as salivation stimulated by food in the mouth, withdrawal from an injurious stimulus, or contraction of the pupil to light. Ordinarily reflex in character. In classical conditioning, it is elicited by the unconditioned stimulus.

Unconscious That part of the mind or mental functioning of which the contents is only rarely subject to awareness. It is a repository for data that have never been conscious (primary repression) or that may have become conscious briefly and later repressed (secondary repression).

Unconscious motivation Urges, such as fears, hopes and desires, of which the individual is not aware, presumed to be repressed.

Unconsciousness It is an abnormal loss of awareness resulting from a reduced level of activity of reticular formation in brainstem. Unconsciousness may be brief as in fainting or deep and

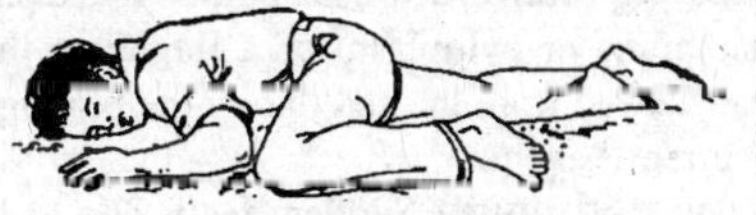

Position of unconsciousness

prolonged as in coma. After head injury a brief transient state of unconsciousness i.e. concussion develops.

Uncontrollable reinforcer A reinforcer whose probability is same whether an emitted response is present or absent.

Undercut An area like the cervical portion of a tooth that curves under and has a tendency to lock a material within it making the material difficult to remove.

Underdeveloped A light film that results from inadequate exposure time, kilovoltage, milliamperage, or a combination of these factors.

Underfeeding It results in sleepless nights by excessive crying and prevents weight gain. Child develops constipation. There may be loose stools too with passage of flatus. In such cases additional feed with artificial milk may be given.

Undermining Condition of a wound in which the loss of underlying tissues is greater than the loss of the skin.

Underwater seal drain Normally there is negative pressure in pleural space between lungs and chest wall. Fluid or air enters causing positive pressure and thereby collapse of lung. Under such condition one underwater seal drain is given immediately to remove fluid or air and allow restoring of function of lung.

At no time bottle must be lifted at same level or above patient level. In such mistake, by gravity water from bottle will get into pleural cavity causing fatal consequences.

Undescended testis A testis that is retained in the abdomen or the inguinal canal.

Undifferentiated type A form of schizophrenia characterised by diverse symptoms found in other types or by symptoms not readily classified.

Undoing A defence mechanism, operating unconsciously, in which something unacceptable and already done is symbolically acted out in reverse, usually repetitiously, in the hope of relieving anxiety.

Undulating membrane That portion of the plasma membrane or cytoplasm of a flagellate that is drawn away from the cell during the beating of a recurrent flagellum.

Unexpected death Sudden death due to heart attack is becoming common. Thrombosis of one of larger coronary arteries causes instantaneous death. Aortic stenosis myocardial degeneration, left ventricle failure and sudden heart block are causes in elderly person. Poison of hydrocyanic acid acts very rapidly, acting less quickly is cocaine and volatile/non-volatile narcotics.

Unexposed film A film that has not been exposed to the X-ray beam; appears clear.

Unfilled acrylic An esthetic dental restorative material made from polymethylmethacrylate, which preceded dental composites.

Unilateral One sided.

Unilocular A term used to describe a radiolucent lesion that exhibits one compartment.

Unimodal sensory cortex Primary somatic sensory, visual or auditory cortex.

Unintentional tort Situation that results in an injury, although the person responsible did not mean to cause harm.

Uninvolved stance time The length of time (up to 30 seconds) that an individual can stand in the parallel bars while bearing weight on the uninvolved lower extremity (involved extremity is raised off the supporting surface).

Unit dose Self-contained packet that holds one tablet or capsule.

Unit of observation The source of data in a medical study. The unit is usually a study participant.

Unitary animal An animal that does not undergo asexual reproduction, with a single ramet per genet.

Unitdose system System of drug distribution is which a portable cart containing a drawer each client's medications is prepared by the pharmacy with a 24hour supply of medications.

Universal donor A person with blood type O who is able to donate blood to people with other blood types in emergency blood transfusions.

Universal Goniometer It is an instrument used in clinical practive to measure the range of motion of joints. It is made of metal or transparent plastic. It consists of a central protractor portion on which are mounted two arms of varying lengths. The protractor protion may be either a full circle or half circle, both of which have one degree intervals. A straight line runs from the 0 degree to 180 degree mark on protractor. One of the two arms of Goniometer is an extension of the protractor (stationary arm), while the other arm is riveted to, and can move independently of , the protractor (moving arm). The central rivet, which attaches the moving arm to protractor, functions as the axis of the Goniometer.

Universal numbering system Numbering system used to code or identify teeth by using numbers and letters.

Universal precautions Combination of devices and techniques used to protect patients and dental health care workers from infectious diseases.

Universal precautions Procedures developed by the Centers for Disease Control and Prevention (CDC) to prevent the spread of contagious diseases.

Universal recipient A person with blood type AB who can receive blood of any type in emergency transfusions.

Universal system In this system each permenant tooth is given a number from 1 to 32. The mandibular right number is 32. The primary teeth are indicated in the same sequence, using capital letters A to T.

Unoccupied bed Changing the linen when the bed is empty.

Unrefined grains Grains prepared for consumption containing all edible protions of kernels.

Unrestrained eaters Individuals who are not unduely concerned with their weight or shape and dont attempt to control it.

Unsaturated fat Fatty acids that come from vegetables, nuts or seeds. Lipids that are missing some hydrogen.

Unsaturated zone In a body of water, the region that spans the area located just beneath the surface and directly above the water table.

Unstable angina It is of recent origin. Pain may occur at rest or at night more frequent and very often leads to myocardial infarction. It is of longer duration and lasts 15 minutes or more and may improve with nitrates. ECG shows ST changes stimulating subendocardial injury. Coronary artery shows significant obstruction.

Upper airway The mouth, throat, and larynx,

Upper and lower body obesity In men fatty tissue is distributed in upper segment of body. Normal waist hip ratio is 0.7, a person with upper body obesity has a ratio of 0.85 or higher.

Upper motor neuron signs Physical signs indicating presence of upper motor neuron disorder.

Upper motor neuron syndrome It is synonymous with a disorder of pyramidal function. If pyramidal syndrome develops due to lesion in internal capsule then hemiparesis results and if it results due to compression of lateral cortical spinal tracts then spastic paraparesis occurs.

Upregulation Increase in the number of membrane receptors.

Upright patient position It is a comfortable position for patient to prevent complications with the support of pillows at back upto head, patient sits on bed with leg stretched in front and hands at sides.

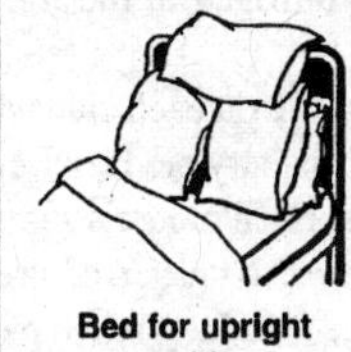

Bed for upright position

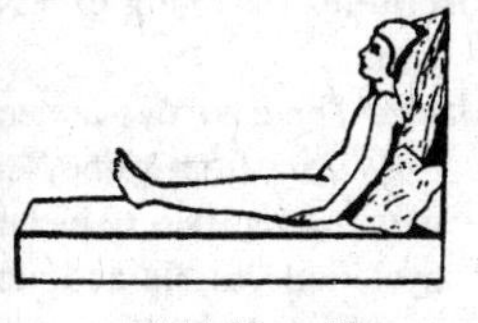

Upright position

Upright tilt testing In upright position there is venous pooling of blood in legs and hypotension due to decreased venous return. This is neglected by reflex tachycardia and stimulation or renin angiostensin system. Upright or tilt table position along with graded isoproferenol infusion result in higher rates of provocation of vasovagal syncope.

Urachal cyst It is a rare pathological condition arising from the patent central portion of the urachus with the umbilical and vesicle ends obliterated. It also gives rise to intraabdominal swelling. The patient presents with a small immobile swelling in the hypogastrium deep to umbilicus. Patient presents small immobile swelling in the hypogastrium deep to umbilicus. Treatment includes excision of the cyst.

Urea It is a waste product of breakdown of proteins and main nitrogen content of urine. Proteins in intestines form amino acids which are carried to liver through blood. In liver excess of amino acids are converted into urea and are thrown out through kidneys. In normal course blood urea level is 25-40 mg/100 gm of blood. Normal kidneys are able to throw it out but if kidney fails uraemia may develop.

Urea cycle A metabolic pathway in vertebrates, for the synthesis of urea from amino groups and carbon dioxide; occurs in the liver.

Urease The enzyme which converts urea into ammonia and CO_2.

Uremia High levels of nitrogen containing waste products in the blood; also referred to as uremic poisoning.

Uremic syndrome The symptoms of renal failure e.g., water retention and edema, acidosis, excessive concentrations of urinary retention products.

Uremic toxicity A buildup of toxic waste products in the blood; symptoms include anorexia, nausea, metallic taste in the mouth, irritability, confusion, lethargy, restlessness, and pruritus.

Ureotelic Excreting excess nitrogen in the form of urea.

Ureter There are two ureters one on each side which carry urine from kidneys to urinary bladder. Length of ureters is 10 to 12 inches. Each ureter is supplied by blood vessels and nerves. Number of ureters may be more, congenitally. If kidney stone passes in ureter and there it stucks may cause severe pain resulting in renal colic. Ureteritis may be developed due to ascending infection.

Ureteric catheterisation This is done sometime to remove small ureteric stone. Small stones may pass out with sufficient urination.

Ureteric colic It is a severe pain experienced in loin, flank, groin and testicular-labial areas. Ureteric pain is phasic, waxing over 20 to 30 minutes and waning for longer periods in between. Exacerbations may be severe and are accompanied by cold sweats, nausea, vomiting and restlessness. Radiopaque calculus is causative factor. Concomitant slight haematuria is usual.

Ureterostomy An ostomy site in which one or both ureters are surgically brought to the abdominal surface for the excretion of urine.

Uretheral sphincter Voluntary muscle at the neck of the bladder that relaxes to allow micturition.

Urethra It is the tube by which urine is passed out from bladder. In females it is short and opens in front of vagina. In males urethra is much longer. Urethritis may develop due to infection, minor injury and inflammation followed by scarring. Gonococcal infection may result in urethral stricture. Male urethra may be damaged in accident.

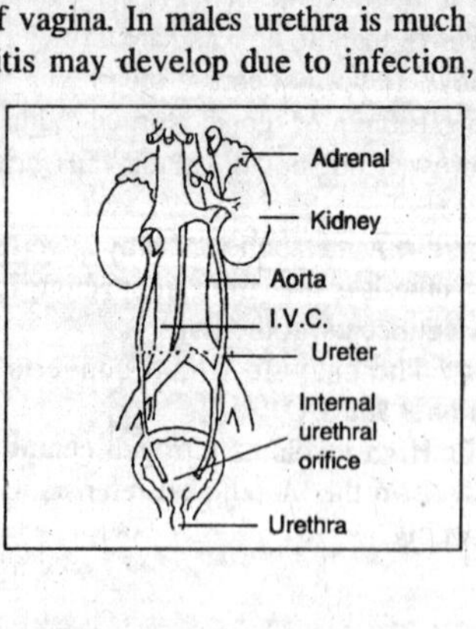

Urethra, anterior Spongy, or spongy and membranous, part of male urethra.

Urethral Relating to or involving the urethra.

Urethral catheterisation It is done to empty bladder when patient cannot pass urine or to provide continuous drainage. It helps in getting a sterile sample of urine directly from bladder or after certain operation over bladder, urethra or prostate. It can be done during paralysis of bladder in lower motor neurone type of paralysis.

Urethral meatus The opening to the canal for the discharge of urine.

Urethral stricture In it urethra becomes narrowed and even may be shortened due to scar formation. After injury or persistent urethritis may cause it. Gonorrhoea may also result it. Person may feel difficulty in passing urine or during ejaculation. It may result in urinary tract infection too. It may be treated by urethral dilatation. It may be done in local anaesthesia.

Urethritis It is the inflammation of urethra, certain bacteria and yeast may also result it. Bacteria from skin or urethra may also result in urethritis. It causes a burning sensation and pain while passing urine.

Urine may be blood stained. It may result in scar formation and stricture may be developed. Pencillin or uroflox are effective drugs.

Urge Incontinence Its symptoms include the involuntary loss of moderate to large volume of urine associated with an abrupt and strong desire to void. It may be caused due to unstable bladder (detrusor instability), Detrusor hyperreflexia, Detrusor hyperactivity with impaired bladder contractility (DHIC) and urethral instability.

Urge incontinence of urine Patient must pass urine at a moment's notice and unless patient is quick she is unable to control her bladder and may pass a few drops before reaching to lavatory. Amount of urine passed in urgency incontinence is always considerable while in stress incontinence it is minimal.

Urgency Strong feeling that urine must be eliminated quickly.

Uric acid It is a waste product of breakdown of nucleic acid. A small amount of uric acid is always produced by digestion of food which is excreted by kidney. Normal blood level is 4 to 7 mg%. High level of uric acid may develop gout. It may be the result of kidney disease, leukaemia, haemolytic anaemia etc.

Urinal Cylindrical container for collecting urine.

Urinalysis The physical, chemical, and microscopic analysis or examination of urine.

Urinary bladder It occupies anterior part of pelvic cavity behind symphysis pubis. It can accomodate 4-5 liters of urine. Distended bladder may be mistaken for full time pregnancy.

Urinary diversion Procedure in which one or both ureters are surgically implanted elsewhere.

Urinary elimination Process of releasing excess fluid and metabolic wastes.

Urinary frequency in pregnancy Often during first 3 months of pregnancy the growing uterus places increased pressure on bladder. Urinary frequency usually will improve as uterus rises out of pelvis by second trimester. Finally when head engages near time of delivery it puts pressure on bladder increasing frequency of urine.

Urinary meatus External opening of the urethra.

Urinary retention Condition in which urine is produced but is not released from the bladder.

Urinary Stress Test It is a simple test and can be used for women with stress incontinence. It also acts as a feedback and demonstrates improved pelvic floor function. It should be done on empty bladder. Ask the patient to perform five jumping jacks. After thirty minutes, repeat the jumping jacks, At the end of one hour asks the patient to perform 10 jumping jacks while coughing during the last five jumps.

Urinary suppression Failure of the kidneys to produce sufficient urine.

Urinary system System responsible for excreting liquid waste from the body.

Urinary tract infection It is an infection anywhere in urinary tract. It includes cystitis, pyelonephritis and urethritis caused by bacterial infection. Sexually transmitted diseases like gonorrhoea may also cause urethritis. Because females are having short urethra, chances of infection are more. Urethritis causes burning sensation, abdominal

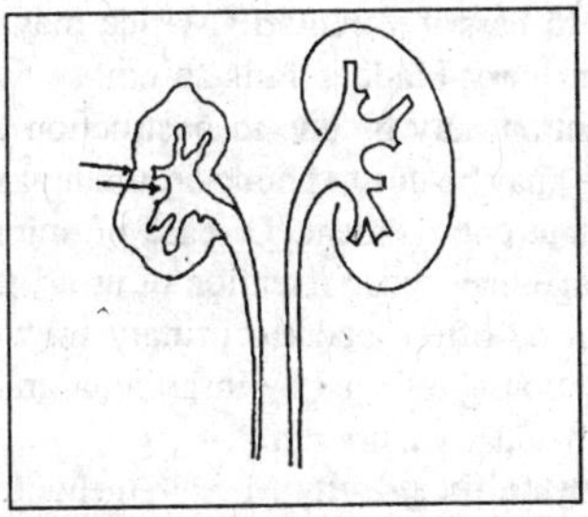

pain, haematuria and general malaise. Urethritis can lead to scarring of urethra. Infection can be diagnosed by culture of few drops of urine. Antibiotics are drug of choice.

Urination Passage of urine from the body; emptying of the bladder.

Urination, frequent Most people pass urine 4-6 times daily and hardly anyone require it to pass during night hours. Often the cause is cystitis due to infection. Consumption of lot of water may help such persons. Anxiety is another cause in increasing frequency. Other causes include enlarged prostate gland in old age, bladder tumour, renal failure, etc. Treatment is always of underlying cause.

Urination, painful Pain during passing of urine is known as dysuria. Pain is of burning or scalding quality. While stranguary is a strong desire to continue passing of urine. Most common cause of dysuria is cystitis especially in women while bladder tumour and calculus may also result it. Urethritis due to gonococcal infection may also cause it. Highly concen-trated urine during summer may also cause burning in micturition.

Urine It is the pale yellow watery fluid having ammonical smell excreted from kidney. It is produced by the filtration of blood through kidneys. Urine carries out waste products from body. Kidney passes about 1 to 4 pints of urine per day. A high intake of fluid increases the amount of urine produced. Urine examination helps in diagnosis of wide variety of conditions from kidney diseases to diabetes and pregnancy. Urine is normally sterile. Smell of stale urine is due to the action of bacteria which causes release of ammonia. Colour of urine is due to substance urochrome.

Urine retention It is inability to empty the bladder fully. When retention is complete person is not able to pass it voluntarily. Urine may be passed but urinary bladder fails to empty completely. Retention may be due to obstruction of flow of urine, may be due to phimosis, urethral stricture or prostate enlargement. Disease of spinal cord or damage may cause retention of urine. Incomplete retention often leads to urinary tract infection. Retention is relieved by inserting a drainage tube into bladder via urethra.

Urine specific gravity Measurement of the degree of concentration of the urine.

Urinoma These are circumscribed usually perirenally located collection of urine. Surgical and other traumas are possible causes. Extravasation of urine into fatty tissues leads to local lipolysis which is completed after about 5 days. About 10 to 12 days a membrane forms around the urine collection and becomes thicker.

Urinometer An instrument that measures the specific gravity (thinness or thickness) of urine.

Urogenital system A collective term for the urinary and reproductive organs and their associated structures, especially in an organism in which the ducts of these system are fused and release their products through the same pore.

Urogenital triangle The region of the pelvic floor containing the external genitalia.

Urokinase It is a thrombolytic drug derived from human urine or from a tissue culture of human kidney. It is given to dissolve blood clot who had recent myocardial infarction. It limits the damage of heart if given early. It should be given under supervision of a specialist doctor because it may lead to excessive bleeding.

Urology The specialized branch of medicine that deals with the structure, function, and diseases of the male and female urinary systems and the male reproductive system.

Urostomy Urinary diversion that discharges urine from an opening on the abdomen.

Urticaria It is a skin condition in which itchy wheals are developed. Wheals vary considerably in size and large ones may fail to form irregular raised patches. These are more common on limbs and trunk. Wheals last for several hours. Angio-oedema is a more severe form. Exact cause is not known except that it is an allergic disorder in which histamine is released. Application of Calamine lotion and antihistamine drugs help. In severe cases corticosteroid drugs may be given.

Urticaria pigmentosa, childhood type It is the lesion soon after birth or during first year of life. Condition gives rise to hyperpigmented macular, papular or nodular eruption. There may be bullae formation. Scratching makes the lesion to become red, swollen and enlarged resulting urticarial wheals. Fresh lesions appear in crops. Condition is benign and disease subside without recurrence.

Urticaria, wheals It is a skin condition in which itchy wheals are developed. Wheals vary considerably in size and large ones may fail to form irregular raised patches. These are more common on limbs and trunk. Wheals last for several hours. Angio-oedema is a more severe form. Exact cause is not known except that it is an allergic disorder in which histamine is released. Application of Calamine lotion and antihistamine drugs help. In severe cases corticosteroid drugs may be given.

Useful test A test that provides information of value for determining the proper course of treatment. One of the criteria for muscle length and strength tests.

Uteral leiomyomas These are benign and accunt for 98% of all myometrial tumors. These are multiple. These may be submucosal, intramural or subserosal.

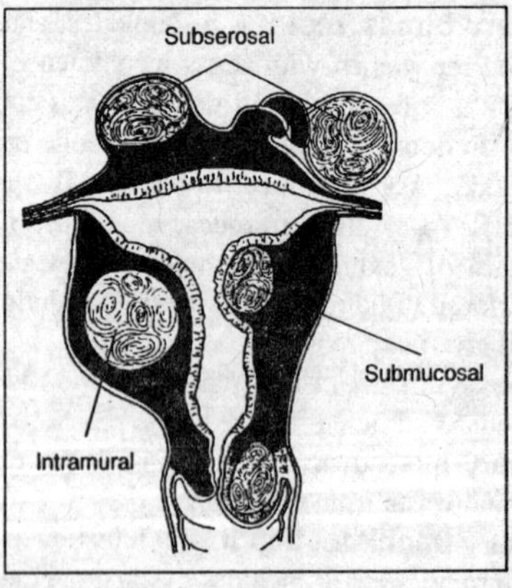

Uterine atony An ongoing inability of the uterus to maintain its muscular tone in the postpartum state, usually resulting in hemorrhage.

Uterine cancer The term uterine cancer refers to cancer of endometrium. It generally develops in

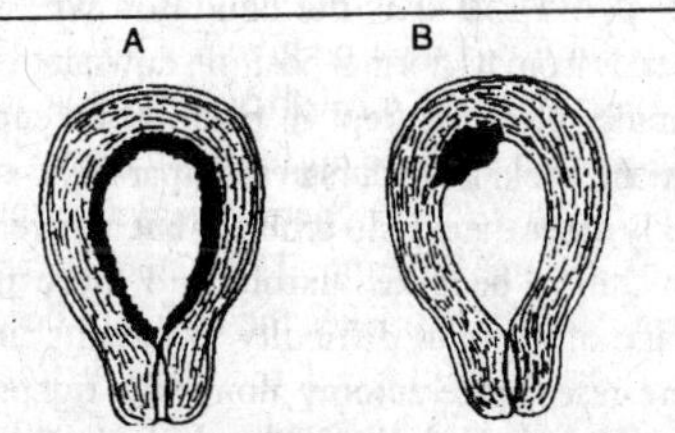

A : Diffuse carcinoma
B : Localised tumor involving myometrium

women who have an excess of oestrogen in their system and specially when progesterone hormones are low. It is more common who had no children. Use of birth control tablets lowers the risk. In young women symptom may be heavy periods, bleeding between periods or bleeding after sexual intercourse. Hysterectomy followed by radiation therapy is the choice of treatment.

Uterine change in pregnancy At eight weeks size of uterus felt is equivalent to hen's egg. At ten weeks size becomes of an orange. Tip of cervix is like tip of lips while of non pregnant is that of tip of nose. At 12 weeks uterus comes just above the level of pelvic rim.

Uterine contraction Uterine contraction during first stage of normal labour. Low resting tone, good amplitutude lasting for 50-70 seconds every 3-5

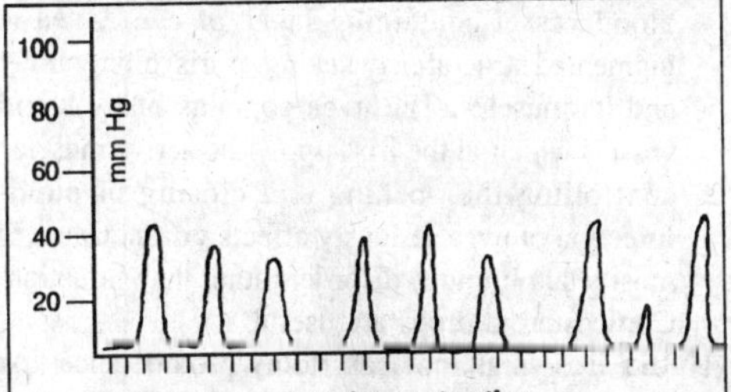

Normal uterine contraction

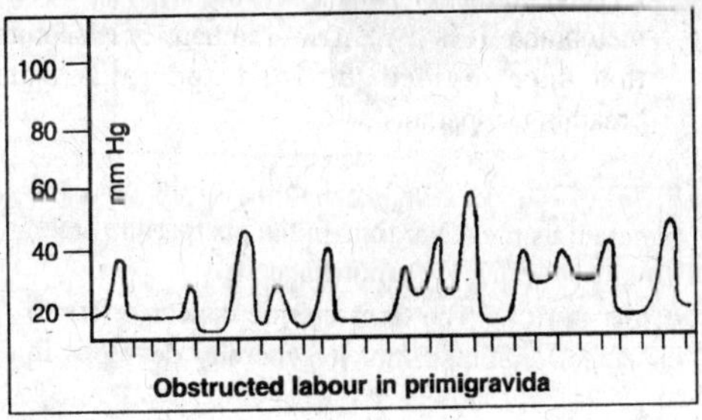

Obstructed labour in primigravida

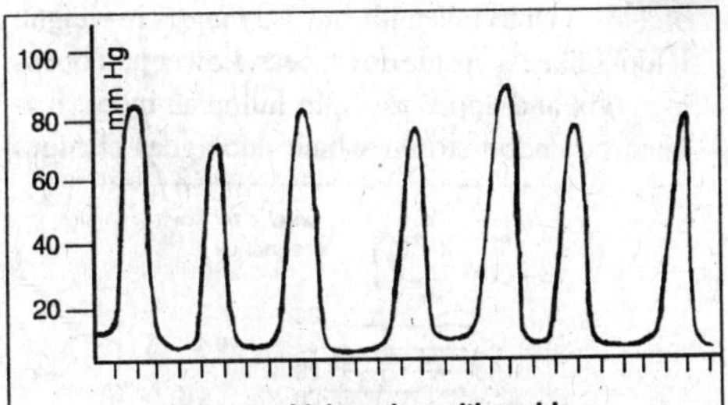

Obstructed labour in multigravida

minutes. While uterine contractions during obstructed labour in primigravida during first stage of labor have high resting tone, poor amplitude, irregular time while in multigravida regular contractions are with high amplitude..

Uterine inversion Turning of uterus inside out after birth of fetus.

Uterine orgasm It does not involve vulval contractions but is expressed by a special type of breathing. Woman at peak goes under a series of gasping and then stops breathing for a moment. She may utter joy in words or in sounds. It is followed by a feeling of relaxation and sexual satisfaction.

Uterine rupture A tear in the wall of the uterus.

Uterine sound It is a graduated metallic stuff of about 12" long. The distal end is curved at 60° and is 2" long. Tip of the instrument is blunt. It is used to access the size and direction of uterus, to locate tumour, polyp, placenta or an intrauterine copper device (IUCD). It may be used cautiously for correction of mobile retroverted uterus. In suspected pregnancy it should be used.

Uteroglobin In some animals, the major protein in the uterine fluid at the time of implantation.

Uterotubal insufflation A proce-dure used in Rubin's test involving the introduction of carbon dioxide into the uterus by way of a cannula. If one or both tubes are patent, the carbon dioxide flows through the uterus and tubes into the peritoneal cavity. When the patient sits up, the carbon dioxide rises to the diaphragm, causing pain in the shoulder referred there by way of the phrenic nerve.

Uterus It is a hollow muscular organ of female reproductive system. In it generally fertilised ovum gets embedded. It lies in pelvis behind the bladder and in front of bowel. In non-pregnant ladies, it is of 3 to 4 inches in length and 2-3 ounces in weight. It looks like an upside down pear. Lower part opens in cervix and upper part into fallopian tubes. It is lined by endometrium which undergoes changes

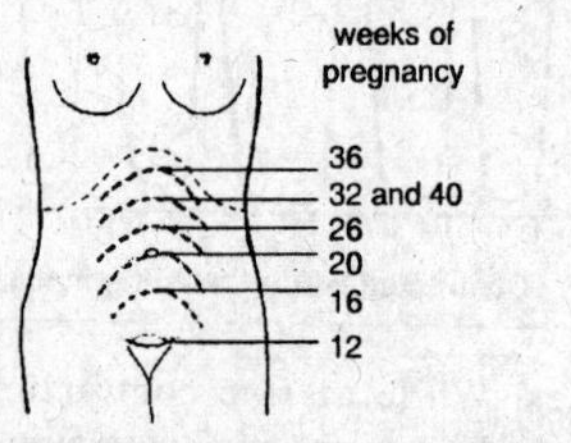

Height of uterus during pregnancy

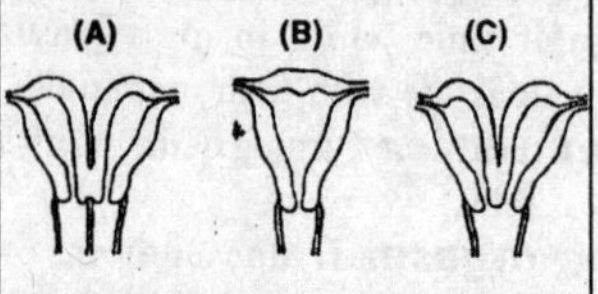

(A) Ulnervs didelphys with double vagina
(B) Uterus arcuatus
(C) Uterus bicornis

during menstrual cycle. It is build up by hormones and when hormone support is withdrawn at the end of menstrual cycle the blood supply to endometrium is cut off and endometrium is thrown out in the form of menstrual cycle. In different weeks of pregnancy size of uterus increases accordingly and becomes palpable per abdomen.

Uterus Couvelaire A severe uterine condition seen in some cases of placental separation, when coagulation is impaired and there is extensive bleeding into the uterine muscle, causing a blue discoloration.

Uterus in 3rd stage of labour Soon after alternate contractions and retractions the uterine fundus reaches the level of the umbilicus. The uterus assumes a globular shape and relaxation.

Uterus in tubal pregnancy Uterus under influence of hormones associated with muscular hypertrophy, increased vascularity and decidual reaction.

Uterus prolapse It is the condition when uterus descends from its normal position down into vagina. Normally uterus is kept in position by supported ligament. Prolapse occurs in multipara who is obese. In early cases there is no problem but in severe cases even uterus become visible and there may be leakage of urine or difficulty in passing urine. In severe cases hysterectomy along with tightening of support ligaments is done otherwise plastic pessary may be inserted which requires periodic changing.

Utilatarian theory Ethical theory holding that the right course of action is one that produces the greater good.

Utility The moral principle that we should act to bring about the greatest benefit and the least harm.

Utilization management Same as managed care.

Utricle The large of the two divisions of the membranous labyrinth located inside the vestibule of the inner ear, containing a receptor organ for static equilibrium.

Utrine contraction Uterine contractions begin during early weeks of pregnancy and occur at intervals of 5-10 minutes through out pregnancy. Contractions may be palpated during later months by placing the hand on the abdomen and during bimanual examination. Contractions held in accomodating growing fetus.

Uvea It is the coloured part of the eye and middle blood vessel containing layer of eye. Uvea is pigmented structure consisting of iris, ciliary body and its muscles. The uvea contains many blood vessels which in the iris supply the active muscles controlling the opening and closing of pupil. Infection of uvea seriously affects vision. Cause is mostly autoimmune disorder rather than infection. Corticosteroid drops are useful.

Uvula It is small, conical, fleshy protuberance that hangs from the middle of lower edge of soft palate. It is composed of muscle and is covered by mucous membrane. It is a vestigial remnant of a septum that once divided the food apparatus from breathing apparatus.

V

Vaccination It is an active immunization in which dead or weakened micro-organisms are introduced into the body. These micro-organisms sensitise the immune system and if next time enter the body are destroyed by already produced antibodies. While in passive immunisation the ready-made antibodies are given by injection to provide short-term immunity. It should be differentiated from passive natural immunity, which the baby recieves from the mother.

Vaccine It is the preparation which is given against an infectious disease. It sensitises the body's immune system to a particular disease causing bacteria or virus. Next time if the same causing agent invades the body, the sensitised immune system quickly produces antibodies which destroy the agent itself or the toxin produced. Live attenuated organisms are organisms which have been rendered harmless as in case of mumps, measles and rubella. Salk vaccine contains killed virus. Vaccines are given in upper arm. Oral polio is given as drops on tongue. Some vaccines require several doses while others require only one dose. Duration of vaccine also varies.

Vacum aspiration with metal suction curette Tubular metal suction cannulae with a rounded tip of 8, 10, 12 and 14 m.m. diameter corresponding to the duration of pregnancy. After I.V. syntocinon and ergometrine 0.25 I.V. suction curette of a suitable size is then passed through the cervix. Aspiration curette is connected with aspiration vacuum bottles.

Vacumm investing Investing of a pattern within a vacumm to form a mould.

Vacuole Small spaces of cavities within the cytoplasm of a cell.

Vacutainer tube A glass tube with a rubber stopper; air has been removed to create a vacuum.

Vacuum aspiration A method used for first-trimester abortions in which the contents of the uterus are removed by applying a vacuum through a hollow curette or cannula inserted into the uterus.

Vacuum Curettage Removal of the uterine contents by application of a vacuum through a hollow curet or cannular into the uterus.

Vacuum extractor It is a traction apparatus to aid extraction of fetus by a suction cup applied to scalp. Usually 3 sizes of cups are available. Cup may be detached from scalp if the pull is not used at right angles to cup.

Vagina It is the muscular passage forming part of female reproductive system. It connects cervix with external genitalia. It is 2.5 to 4 inches long. The

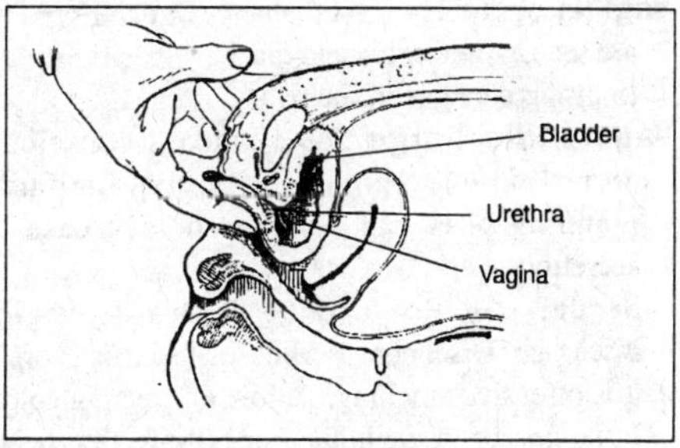

muscular walls have ridges on inner surface and are richly supplied with blood vessels. It is a receptacle of male organ, brings sperm closer to the ova for fertilisation and provides outlet for menstruation as well as baby to come through.

Vaginal acidity Vaginal acidity is due to lactic acid. The pH value is 5.7 in newborn and reaches 6 to 8 in children and comes down to 4 at puberty. During pregnancy pH is usually 4. After menopause pH rises to 7. As the acidity of vagina falls and pH rises normally nonresident pathogens are able to thrive.

Vaginal bleeding Blood may come from uterus, cervix or vagina itself. From puberty to menopause menstruation occurs regularly at intervals. Other causes of bleeding are endometritis, endo-metrial cancer, cervical erosion or cancer cervix. Any bleeding other than menstruation should be investigated seriously, because polyp, fibroid or growth will require surgery to be done.

Vaginal bleeding in placenta previa There is sudden, painless, causeless and recurrent vaginal bleeding. It may occur during sleep and in majority of cases bleeding is plainless as placenta separates with painless rhythmic Braxton Hick's contraction. Fresh bouts of bleeding occur during each uterine contraction in labour. Bleeding is recurrent due to separation of fresh areas of placenta. Bleeding is always revealed.

Vaginal carcinoma

Stage I - Carcinoma limited to vaginal wall

Stage II - Carcinoma has involved the sub-vaginal tissue but has not extended to pelvic wall.

Stage III - Carcinoma has extended to lateral pelvic wall

Stage IV- Carcinoma has extended to involve adjacent organs.

Stage O - Intraepithelial carcinoma

Vaginal cycle The cyclic changes in cell type that are seen in the vagina and that have been correlated to cyclic changes in the ovary.

Vaginal discharge Some mucous secretion is normal during reproductive years. The family planning pills can increase or decrease the secretions.

Sexual stimulation also increases vaginal discharge. Discharge is abnormal if it is more, if it is offensive smelling, yellow or green in colour. It may occur in vaginitis. Fungal infection results in white, thick discharge. *Trichomonas vaginalis* require profuse and highly offensive discharge. Treatment depends on cause. Generally systematic antibiotics and vaginal tablets are useful.

Vaginal douche It is the process of introduction of plain or medicated water or normal saline into vaginal cavity for cleaning purpose and allowing the fluid to come out.

It is done to remove irritating discharge from vaginal cavity. It is useful to disinfect and deodourise the mucous membrane, to relieve pain and congestion. Plain sterile water or normal saline can be used.

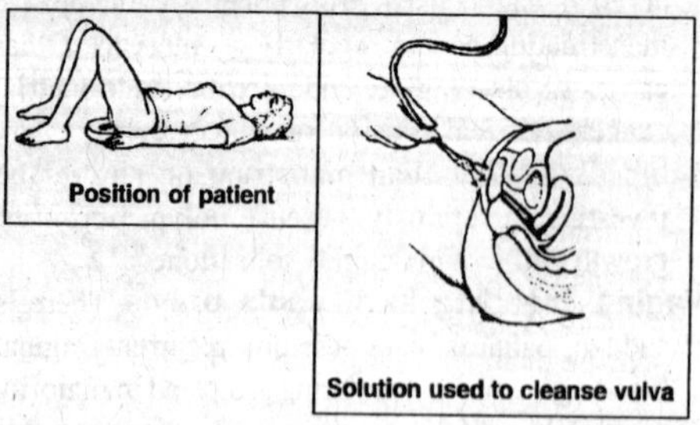

Position of patient

Solution used to cleanse vulva

Vaginal hernia It is also known as complete or scrotal hernia. Here the processus vaginalis is patent throughout. Hence the sac is continuous with the tunica vaginalis of the testis. The hernia descends down to bottom of the scrotum covering the testis in front and at the sides so that testis cannot be felt separately before reduction of hernia.

Vaginal hydrocele Here the fluid collects between visceral and parietal layers of the tunica vaginalis of the testis. It gives rise to a scrotal swelling. Hydrocele fluid is amber or straw coloured. It contains water, inorganic salts, traces of albumin and fibrinogen. Fluid does not clot unless it comes in contact with blood. Patient presents with scrotal swelling. There may be pain or discomfort in secondary hydrocele. Swelling may be unilateral or bilateral. Swelling is confined in scrotum. One can get the upper border of swelling. Fluctuation is positive. Swelling may be tense if fluid is more. Swelling is not reducible.

Vaginal itching Pruritus vulvae is intense irritation and tickling in vagina or in external genital area. Low oestrogen level after menopause also results in itching. Treatment includes antibiotics and antifungal drugs or hormones.

Vaginal spermicide A physical barrier to sperm penetration that also exerts a chemical action on the sperm.

Vaginismus It is a hyperaesthesia which leads to spasm of sphincter of vagina during attempted coitus or while doing PV examination. In primary vaginismus there is no organic lesion while in secondary vaginismus there is painful lesion nearby genital tract such as urethral carbuncle and vulvitis. Typical vaginismus always has a psychoneurotic basis. History of mental trauma can be traced out. There may be subconscious fear of sexual intercourse. It has to be differentiated from frigidity. Extramarital sex, guilt complex may be associated factor.

Vaginitis It is the inflammation of vagina. It may be caused by infection, allergic reaction and hormone deficiency. Most of vaginal infection causes irritation and vaginal discharge. It may be caused by spermicidal creams, barrier, contraceptives and soaps. Atrophic vaginitis may develop after menopause. Vaginitis is treated by antibiotic and antifungal drugs.

Vaginosis An infection of the vagina caused by Gardnerella vaginalis. Vaginosis is characterized by an increase of vaginal discharge that is typically thin, gray white, homogeneous and has a fishy odor particularly after intercourse and during menstruation.

Vagus The tenth cranial nerve—the major parasympathetic nerve in the body, whose path is traced through most thoracic and abdominal organs. It emerges from medulla oblongata and passes through neck, chest to abdomen. It releases the chemical acetylcholine. It causes narrowing of bronchi and slowing of heart rate. Vagus nerve branches to the larynx and trachea thus involves in swallowing, coughing, sneezing and speech quality. Its overactivity produces peptic ulcer.

Valence The combining capacity of an atom; the number of deficit or extra electrons in the outermost electron shell of an atom.

Valgus Bent outward twisted; denoting a deformity in which the angulation is away from the midline of the body, as in talipes valgus.

Valid test One that measures, quantitatively and qualitively.

Validate To make certain that the information collected during assessment is accurate.

Validity A test is said to be valid or to have validity when it actually does what it has been designed to do, such as predicting an individual's success in school or in a vocation. It is valid to the degree that test scores correlate with criteria of success.

Valine An essential amino acid.

Vallecula 'Little valley' between the cerebellar hemispheres.

Valproate It acts by inhibiting the enzyme responsible for breakdown of inhibitory neurotransmitter GABA. 90 per cent of it bound to plasma albumin. It does not induce drug metabolising enzymes. Minor sideeffect includes nausea but on continuous use may result in liver failure.

Valsalva's maneuver Attempt to forcibly exhale with the glottis, nose, and mouth closed. It causes increased intrathoracic pressure, slowing of the pulse, decreased return of blood to the heart, and increased venous pressure, and increases the likelihood of dangerous arrhythmias in cardiac patients.Contraction of the muscles of the abdomen, chest wall, and diaphragm in a forced expiratory effort against the closed glottis.

Valsalva, sinus Aortic sinus.

Values A measure of worth or efficiency; an ideal, custom, or institution of a society toward which the members of the groups have an affective emotional connection.

Valve of the foramen ovale A fold of tissue from the margin of the foramen ovale that projects into the left atrium of the fetus; at birth, left atrial blood pressure increases and closes the valve.

Valve of the inferior vena cava A crescent shaped fold attached to the left ventral aspect of the orifice of the inferior vena cava. the remnant of the upper part of the right venous valve of the fetus; eustachian valve.

Valvular insufficiency The inadequate closure of one of the valves of the heart, allowing regurgitant flow of blood through the closed valve.

Valvular stenosis The narrowing of a valvular orifice.

Valvuloplasty The surgical reconstruction of a deformed valve or valve leaflet to relieve an incompetence or stenosis.

Valvulotomy A surgical incision through a stenosed valve or valve leaflet to relieve an obstruction.

Van Buchem's syndrome It is characterised by overgrowth, distortion of mandible, facial palsy, and increased serum alkaline phosphatase.

Vancomycin It acts on multiplying organisms by inhibiting cell wall formation at a site different from b-lactam antibacterials. It is bactericidal against most strains.

It is poorly absorbed from gut. It is a drug of choice for antibiotic associated pseudo-membranous colitis. It may cause auditory damage. Tinnitus and deafness improve the moment drug is stopped. It is nephrotoxic too.

Vapour Matter in gaseous form below its critical temperature. As liquid vaporises heat is required and as vapour condenses an equal amount of heat is produced.

Variability, measures of The degree to which individuals, or measurements in a frequency distribution, differ from the average. The standard deviation is a measure of variability.

Variable A changeable aspect of a situation which can be manipulated or measured, as in the case of independent and dependent variables in any experiment.

Variable (V) gene segments Genes that rearrange together with D (diversity) and J (joining) gene segments in order to encode the variable region amono acid sequences of immunoglobulins and T cell receptors.

Variable friction Mechanism that applies greater friction at early and late swing; may be incorporated in sliding, hydraulic, or pneumatic friction mechanisms.

Variable region Part of an antibody that combines with an antigen; responsible for the specificity of the antibody.

Variance Conceptually, the average of the squaed deviations about the mean. The population variance is found by dividing the sum of the squared deviations by the number within the sample; the sample variance is found by dividing the sum of squared deviations by n-1.

Variant angina Atypcial angina.

Variant angina pectoris Pain is typical but may occur without any provocation. It often recurs in cyclic fashion with waxing and waning and even may have a fixed time each day. ECG shows ST elevation. Nifedepine is best suited.

Varicella Same as Chickenpox.

Varicella zoster Chickenpox; herpes zoster virus.

Varicocele Enlarged tortuous veins which surround the testis. In most cases it affects left testis. It develops due to failure of testicular valves. It is

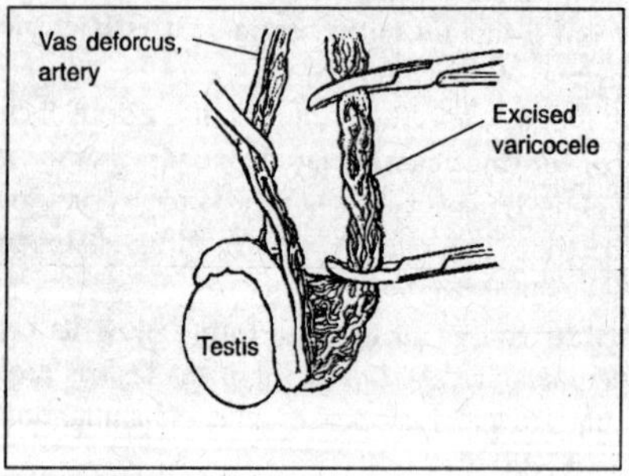

not serious but may cause discomfort in scrotum. Athletic support and tight underpants are helpful. Sometimes surgery may even be needed.

Varicose bronchiectasis The tortuous dilation of the bronchial or bronchiolar airways.

Varicose veins These are twisted, distended superficial veins. Valves in the veins prevent blood from draining back down the legs under the force of gravity. In old age and otherwise in some persons these become defective resulting in pooling of blood in superficial veins. Veins become swollen and distorted. Obesity, long hours of standing in job, pregnancy may result it. Back of the calf is the most common site. In some people it may not cause any symptoms but some may develop severe pain made worst by prolonged standing. Persons feel happy sitting keeping the legs at high level. In severe cases skin becomes thin, hard, scaly and even ulcer may develop. Wearing of elastic support stockings, sitting with feets up helps the patients. Some may require surgery known as stripping.

Varicosities Swollen, distended, and knotted veins, usually in the subcutaneous tissues of the leg.

Varicosities of vulva It may be relieved by placing a pillow under the buttocks and elevating the hips for frequent rest periods.

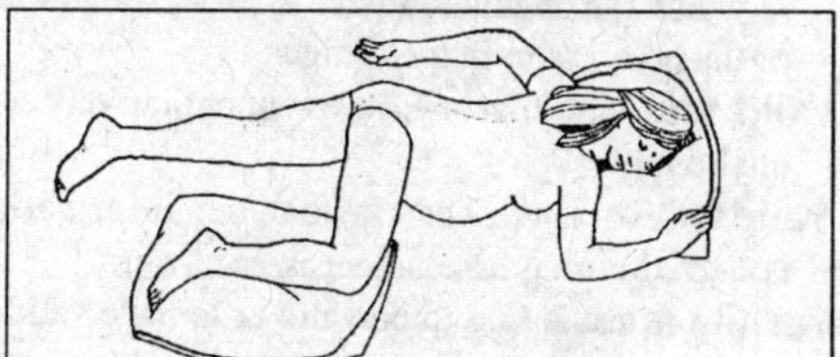

Sim's position

Varicosity The abnormal, chronic swelling and twisting of a vein.

Variola Another term for smallpox, deriving from the Latin word for “pock” and “pustule”.

Variolation The introduction into the skin of pustular or scab material containing smallpox virus.

Varix Distended vein that has bulged enough to elevate the overlying mucosa.

Varnish It is a lining material when it is coated into the walls and floor of a cavity preparation before an amalgam is placed. These are liquid composed of resins or polymers suspended in solvent.

Vas deferens It is a narrow tube which carries and stores sperms released from testis. At the base of bladder it connects to a tube from spinal seminal vesicles to form ejaculatory duct. Duct passes to prostate. Sperm and seminal fluid passes through

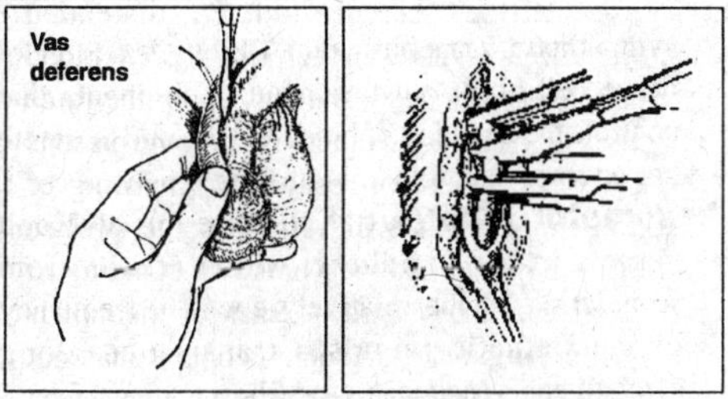

this duct during ejeculation. Vas deferens is about two feet long.

Vasa efferentia testis Ductuli efferentes.

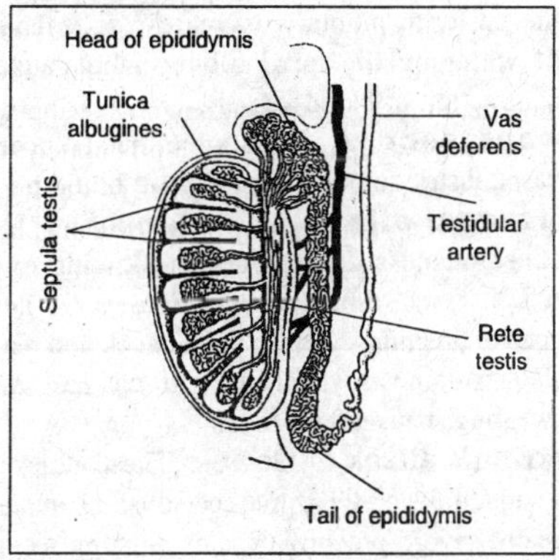

Vasa previa The blood vessels of the umbilical cord, usually presented in front of the fetal head during labor.

Vasa recta Extensions of the efferent arteriole of a juxtamedullary nephron that run alongside the loop of the nephron (Henle) in the medullary region of the kidney).

Vasa vasorum Tiny blood vessles that form a network through the tunica of larger blood vessles to supply the nutrients.

Vascular access devices Devices such as needles, cannulas, or catheters, which allow direct access to the circulatory system.

Vascular changes in pregnancy High levels of estrogen are responsible for proliferation of blood vessels and congestion. Vasomotor instability may produce pallor, flushing, and mottling of skin in response to temperature changes. Increased fragility of capillaries are common in late pregnancy. Scattered petechie are seen in lower legs. Spider angiomata are found on face.

Vascular dementia Cerebrovascular disease is the common cause of dementia. Single brain lesion does not lead to dementia but may affect mental function. Angular gyrus lesions due to left middle cerebral artery disease can be mistaken for Alzheimer's disease. Acute confusional states are well documented . Posterior cerebral artery lesions apart from visual defect may produce severe amnesia specially when lesions are bilateral. Subcortical infarcts like thalamic infarct even when unilateral can lead to disturbances of attention, memory, language and abstract thinking.

Vascular disease of decidua basalis There is an etiologic role of vascular disease of the decidua basalis. Spasm of spiral arterioles is followed by dilatation and flooding into choriodecidual space with resultant separation of placenta.

Vascular markings The shadows produced on a radiographic image of the chest by the pulmonary vasculature.

Vascular spasm Contraction of the smooth muscle in the wall of damaged blood vessel to prevent blood loss.

Vascular tunic The middle layer of the eyeball, composed of the choroid, ciliary body, and iris.

Vasculitis It is the inflammation of blood vessels. It leads to damage to the linning of vessel with narrowing or blockage. Tissues supplied by vessels may become ischaemic. Causative antigens may be virus. Vasculitis is the basic disease process in number of diseases known as periarteritis nodosa, erythema nodosum, serum sickness, Burger's disease etc.

Vasectomy It involves blocking of passage of sperm by cutting and tying the cut ends. The man continues to ejaculate but semen does not contain sperm which are reabsorbed in testes. It is a safe and 100 per cent effective technique. Nowadays

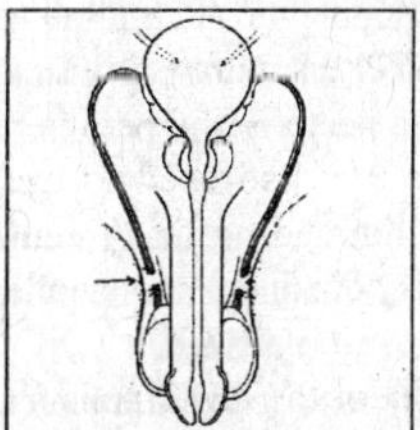

Vasectomy (front view)

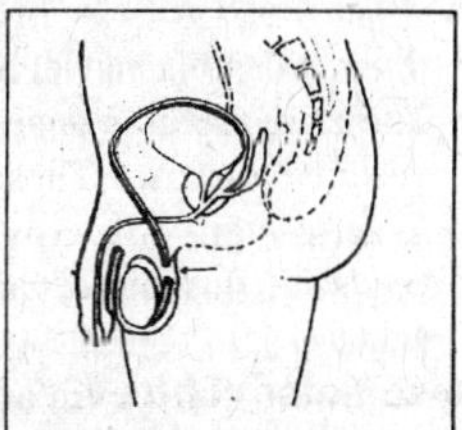

Vasectomy (side view)

vasectomy is done in such a way that the cut ends may be reanastomatised if child is needed. It is done under local anaesthesia on OPD basis. Most men return to work next day. Just after vasectomy man may remain fertile until the sperm already present either die or are being ejaculated. In rare case vasectomy fails because the cut parts of vas deferens reunite.

Vasoactive amines Substances including histamine and 5-hydroxytrypatamine which increase vascular permeability and smooth muscle contraction.

Vasocongestion In sexual activity, engorgement of the blood vessels serving the relevant areas, occurring through dilation of the blood vessels. The other major physiological reaction in sexual activity is myotonia.

Vasoconstriction It is narrowing of blood vessel in response to cold to reduce heat loss. It also results due to fall in BP. Decongestant drugs also cause it.

Vasoconstrictor Vasopressor, an agent that causes a rise in blood pressure by constricting the blood vessles. In local areas it causes constriction of the arterioles and capillaries.

Vasodepressor syncope Most of young persons once in life experience it. It occurs in upright position evidenced by pallor, sweating, mydriasis, hypotension and brady-cardia. It occurs in the environment of emotional stress and fear. Warning signs include perspiration, pallor, visual blurring or epigastric discomfort. Vasovagal syncope is often used interchangeably with vasodepressor syncope but the former is secondary.

Vasodilatation It is widening of blood vessels causing increased blood flow. It generally happens under the skin in response to hot season and increases heat loss from body. Vasodilator drugs widen blood vessels. These include ACE inhibitor drugs, calcium channel blockers, nitrate drugs etc. These are useful in angina pectoris and peripheral vascular disease. These are also used to treat hypertension. All vasodilator drugs may cause headache, flushing of face, dizziness and swollen ankles.

Vasomotor centre An area of the lower pons and upper medulla oblongata that continually transmits a low frequency of nerve impulses to the sympathetic vasoconstrictor fibres. A cluster of nerve cell bodies in the medulla oblongata that controls the diameter of blood vessels and therefore has an important role in regulating blood pressure.

Vasomotor tone Partial constriction of blood vessels in the periphery, which results from stimulation by the relatively constant frequency of sympathetic impulses transmitted along sympathetic vasoconstrictor fibres.

Vasopressin A peptide hormone also known as antidiuretic formed by neurons in the hypothalamus and released by nerve endings in the posterior pituitary, increases the reabsorption of water by the renal tubules and causes the contraction of blood vessels.

Vasopressor A substance that produces vasoconstriction or an increase in blood pressure.

Vasovagal attack It is a temporary loss of consciousness due to sudden slowing of heart attack. Over stimulation of vagus nerve helps to control breathing. Severe pain, shock and fear may also result in vasovagal attack. It may precede with sweating, nausea and dizziness.

Vasovagal attack of Gowers These attacks have a sudden onset, there may be sense of impending death, severe precordial pain radiating to arm or tingling of arms. Marked pallor and bradycardia are striking signs and patient becomes faint.

Vasovagal syncope It occurs when the vagus is reflexly stimulated by lesion in its area of supply. Vagally induced sinus bradycardia, sinus arrest or AV block are responsible for the syncopal attack.

Vastus Wide; of great size.

Vastus lateralis site Injection area in the outer thigh.

Vater, ampulla Hepatopancreatic ampulla.

Vaulting position Arching part of the body, often the back.

Vectis The purpose of vectis is to deliver the lens whenever there is any subluxation or dislocation of lens during surgery.

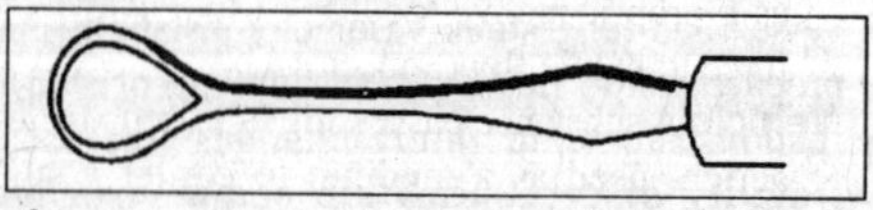

Vector Any agent, most commonly an arthropod, that actively transmits a disease-producing organism.

Vectorial capacity A mathematical form that expresses the malaria transmission risk, or, in other words, the 'receptivity' to malaria of a defined area.

Vegan A complete vegetarian who does not eat any animal products. Persons who rely exclusively on plant sources for protein.

Vegetarian One whose diet is lacto-ovo vegetarian, lacto vegetarian, or vegan.

Vegetarianism We need not to eat meat and fish products to maintain health as long as nutrients from vegetarian food meets our requirement. Vegetarians should select proteins from different

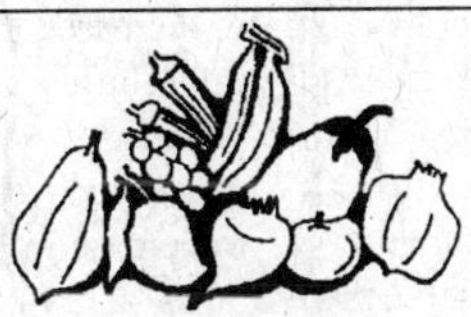

Vegetarian diet

foods so that in combination all amino acids may be consumed. Milk and milk products are rich in calcium and are having class one proteins. Advantages of vegetarians are manyfold. They consume high fever diet. High fibre diets protect from cancer of intestine and diverticular disease. Vegetarians have less risk of coronary artery disease, high blood pressure and insulin-dependent diabetes.

Vegetative cell A nonstarved actively growing bacterial cell.

Vegetative growth Exponential growth that usually occurs by simple binary cell division and produces two identical progeny cells.

Veginal Cone Retention Vaginal cones are useful to teach pelvic floor muscle excercises. The cones of varying weight come in a set of five. The shape and volume of the cones is equal but weight from 20 to 70 gms. The cones are made of plastic and stainless steel with a nylon string attached to the tapered end to permit easy removal. The cone acts as a proprioceptive feedback as well as resisting force to pelvic floor muscles.

Vehicle A substance possessing little or no medicinal action, used as a medium to confer a suitable consistency or form to a drug.

Vein It is a vessel that returns blood towards heart. These carry deoxyge-nated blood. Blood is collected by venules. Venules form to join veins. Walls of veins consist of smooth inner lining, a muscular middle layer and a fibrous outer covering.

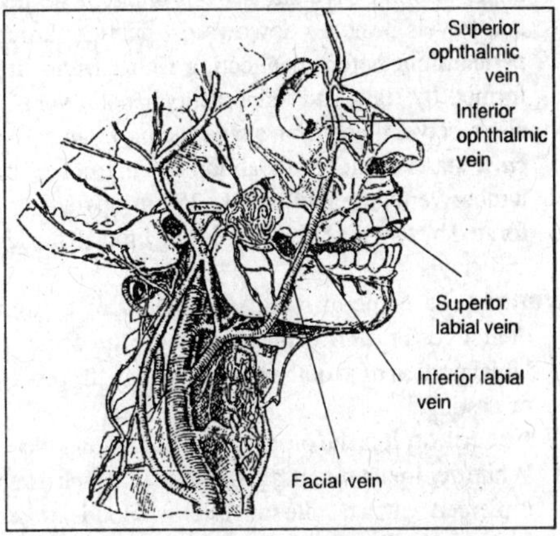

BP in veins is lower than arteries. Walls of veins are thinner, less elastic, less muscular and weaker. Veins when empty collapse while arteries do not. Veins have valves which allow blood to flow in the direction of heart only.

Vein lumen Central opening through which blood flows in a vein.

Velamentous placenta Blood vessels course unprotected for long distance through the membranes to insert into the margin of the placenta.

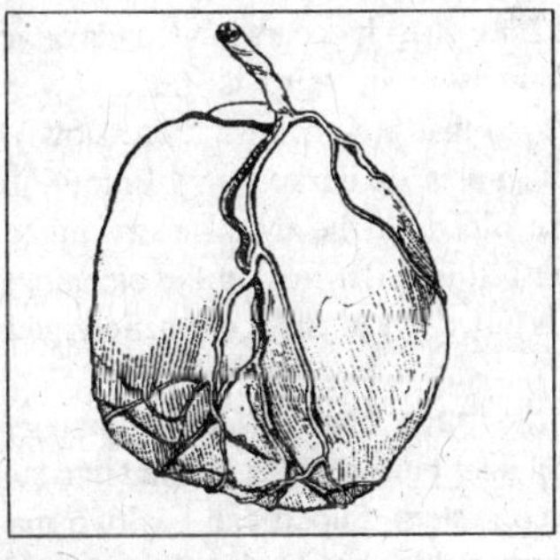

Velar Sounds formed with the back of the tongue on or near the soft palate. Velar sounds are referred to as gutteral.

Vellus Soft, fine hair covering all parts of the body except the palms, soles, and areas where other types of hair are normally found.

Velocity A measure of a body's motion in a given direction.

Vena cava There are two venae, superior and inferior. *Superior vena* cava starts from breast bone level and travels 3 inches downwards, passing through pericardium before connecting right atrium. It is formed by right and left brachochepalic veins. It also receives blood from azygos veins. *Inferior vena cava* starts from lower abdomen in front of 5th lumbar vertebrae and travels 25 cm upward. It is formed by two iliac veins receiving blood from legs and pelvis

Veneer An esthetic metal- porcelain or ceramic dental restoration cemented on to the facial or labial portion of a tooth usually through the process of casting.

Venesection It is the process of withdrawing blood. While veni-puncture is a procedure in which a vein is pierced with a needle to withdraw blood or inject fluid specially in forearm. A suitable vein is selected.

For intravenous infusion also same vein is selected. After the required amount of fluid is pushed or withdrawn then needle or cannula is removed. Slight bruising may develop if venipuncture has taken place.

Venipuncture Accessing the venous system by piercing a vein with a needle.

Venography Test to assess for severity of venous insufficiency prior to any surgical intervention.

Venous Pertaining to the veins.

Venous bleeding It occurs in wounds of veins. The blood pressure in veins is much lower than in arteries so that blood flows more slowly in even stream and is of dark cherry colour. But with profuse bleeding the main artery must also be compressed in order to stop the bleeding. Venous blood is moved by muscle contractions and sucking action of heart.

Venous drainage breast Venous drainage follows arterical distribuiton and is divided into superficial and deep system. Superficial has two main types transverse and longitudinal and there are 3 groups of veins to consider deep drainage system.

Venous drainage-Superficial leg The surperficial veins drain the subcutaneous tissues through two main longitudinal channels, the great and small saphenous vein.

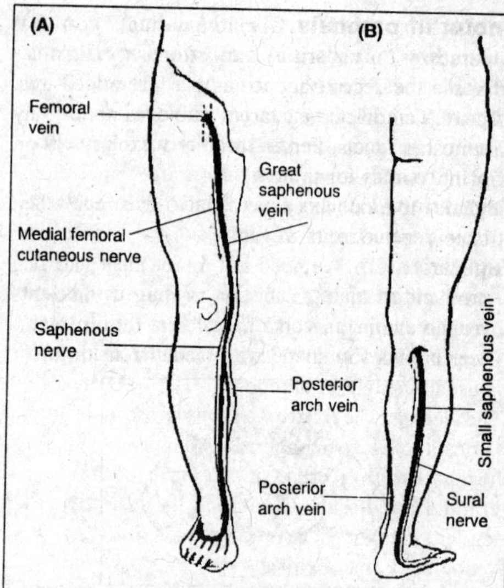

Veins of lower limb

Venous filling time test An assessment of the efficiency of arterial blood flow through capillaries and into veins.

Venous hum In children auscultation at the base of neck just above clavicle and lateral to sternocleidomastoid muscle often reveals a venous hum. It can be intensified by asking patient to inspire deeply. It can be obliterated by lightly compressing vein.

Venous pressure Venous pressure depends on venous tone and blood volume and can easily be measured by simple water manometer. Central venous pressure in the great veins is normally 2 to 8 mm Hg and peripheral venous pressure is 8 mm Hg higher than this. CVP is raised by Trendenlenburg tilt, fluid infusions, coughing, vomiting, straining and heart failure. It is lowered by sitting and standing upright. Hypovolaemia, tachycardia and reduction of venous tone by unconsciousness reduce venous pressure. The central venous pressure is a measure of competence of right heart and ability of right ventricle to deal with venous return.

Venous return Volume of blood returning to the heart.

Venous stasis Stoppage or diminution of the flow of blood in the veins.

Venous thrombosis Obesity, old age, certain operations, myocardial infarctions, malignant disease, oral contraceptives are predisposing factors. One important factor in the formation of haemostatic plugs and in thrombosis is defective fibrinolytic system. Prevention after operation includes reduction of coagulability of blood and frequent movements of limbs and toes and early ambulation.

Venous ulcer of leg Duration is long if it occurs over the medial aspects of the lower third of leg. Ulcer is ovoid in shape with irregular margin. It is usually single in number.
The ulcer may be fixed to the bone due to associated periostitis. Ulcer may be at healing stage when it has a slopping edge and a base of healthy granulation tissue. Ulcer may be painful and tender. Peripheral arterial pulses are normal. Venography may help.

Ventilation (1) Movement of air in an out of the lungs; (2) movement of air in the environment.

Ventilation Resperatory process by which gasses are moved into and out of the lungs.

Ventilation perfusion mismatching An inequality between the amount of air breathed per unit of time and the amount of blood pumped through the pulmonary vasculature per unit of time; normally a ratio of about 0.8.

Ventilators Mechanical devices for delivering ventilation to the lungs.

Ventilatory failure A mechanical inadequacy of the respiratory musculature to move air into and out of the lungs; inability of the lungs to adequately exchange carbon dioxide (Pa_{co2} in excess of 50 mm Hg); pulmonary insufficiency.

Ventilatory reserve The difference between the amount of air normally breathed i.e. tidal volume and that which can be maximally breathed.

Ventilatory threshold A measurement determined during exercise testing using a metabolic cart; the level of exercise at which there is a nonlinear increase in the ventilation in relation to oxygen uptakes; also considered to be estimated upper limit of aerobic exercise.

Ventral Pertains to the lower or underneath portion of the body opposite of dorsal.

Ventral root Motor root of a spinal nerve.

Ventral surface The anterior surface of the body.

Ventricle A cavity; in the brain, one of four cavities filled with cerebrospinal fluid; one of two chambers of the heart that pump blood into arteries; there is a left and right ventricle.

Ventricular ejection phase The portion of the cardiac cycle in which blood is driven out of the ventricles.

Ventricular end-diastolic volume The volume of blood in the heart ventricles at the end of diastole; just prior to being ejected.

Ventricular fibrillation (VF) A life-threatening arrhythmia originating from an ectopic focus in the ventricles that results in a twitching of individual fibrils, resulting in a lack of cardiac output.

Ventricular gallop The triple cadence of heart sounds heart on auscultation and characterized by an audible sound (third heart sound) occurring in early diastole in addition to the normal first and second heart sounds; protodiastolic gallop; "lub-dub-dub".

Ventricular hemorrhage Bleeding within the ventricles of the brain.

Ventricular septal defec In it blood from left ventricle goes to right ventricle. Thus left ventricle and right ventricle including left atrium enlarge.

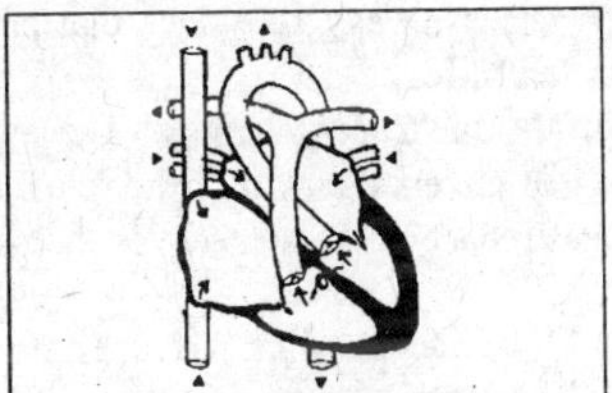

V.S.D.

It may remain symptomless till 3rd decade. Later on symptoms include breath-lessness, fatigue and cardiac failure. A halo systolic murmur over the left sternal edge with accentuated S_1 is heard. A middiastolic murmur over mitral area may be heard.

Ventricular tachycardia A life threatening arrhythmia originating from an ectopic focus in the ventricles; ventricular depolarization at a rate in excess of 100 times per minute.

Ventrogluteal site Injection area in the hip.

Venturi mask A supplemental oxygen delivery device that can be adjusted to deliver a specific fraction of inspired oxygen at relatively high flow rates.

Venule Small blood vessels the collect blood from the capillaries and join to form veins.

Verapamil A calcium channel blocking agent.

Verbal In words; expressed orally.

Verbal apraxia Impairment of volitional articulatory movement secondary to cortical, dominant hemisphere lesion. It is manifested in imprecise and awkward articulation.

Verbal communication Communication that uses words.

Verbal paraphrasia In Wernicke's aphasia, the use of words of allied meaning.

Vergence Convergence of gaze for close-up viewing.

Verification Demonstrating the truth of something; in research, the confirmation of a particular finding, usually by a repetition of the same or a similar investigation with the same result.

Vermicle The infective stage, analogous to a sporozoite, of *Babesia* transmited by ticks.

Vermiform appendix A tubular structure attached to the cecum composed of lymphatic tissue.

Vermillion zone Red area of lips.

Vermis Segmented appearance of the vermis of the cerebellum.

Vernix A cheesy, waxy substance that protects the skin in fetal life.

Vernix caseosa "Cheesy varnish." The layer of fatty matter that covers the skin of the fetus. Epithelial cells and sebaceous matter, cover the skin of the fetus.

Verruca It is a plantar wart. Verrucas are naturally subject to great pressure on walking and standing. When becomes callused causes pain. These are contagious. Treatment is by freezing, cauterisation and surgery.

Verrucosu carcinoma It is a low grade neoplasm. There is white, warty appearance forming a well circumscribed mass raised above the level of surrounding mucosa. It is associated with the habit of sniff dipping. It is slow growing and spreads laterally than deeply. It can be excised easily if not very extensive.

Version The act of turning; specifically, a turning of the fetus in the uterus so as to change the presenting part and bring it into more favourable position for delivery. Turning the fetus from one presentation to another before birth usually from breech to cephalic.

Vertebra These are weight bearing and being many in number facilitate body movements. Cervical vertebrae are seven in number, are relatively small and support the weight of head weighing 5 kg. Thoracic vertebrae are 12 in number and serve for

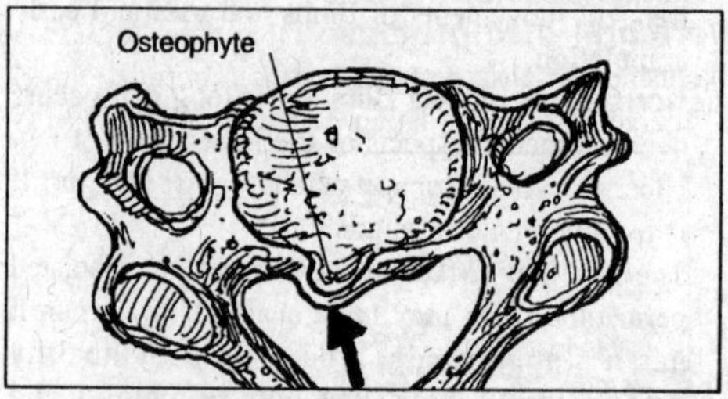

the attachment of rib. There are five lumbar vertebrae. In addition to weight bearing they withstand enormous leverages. Last lumbar vertebra joins the pelvis at sacrum. Sacrum has five pieces having a small convexity in front to shape the pelvis which contains rectum, genital organs and bladder. Convexity serves to accommodate baby's head. The tail or coccyx attached to lower end of sacrum has three or four segments and is normally only about 1" long.

Vertebral canal The tubelike cavity extending through the vertebral column that contains the spinal cord; also called the spinal canal.

Vertebral disc In between two vertebrae there is a disc. It varies in thickness gradually becoming thicker from the neck through the thoracic area to lumbar area. Lowest disc may be slightly thinner. Each disc has a soft centre having the consistency of firm jelly known as nucleus pulposus and it

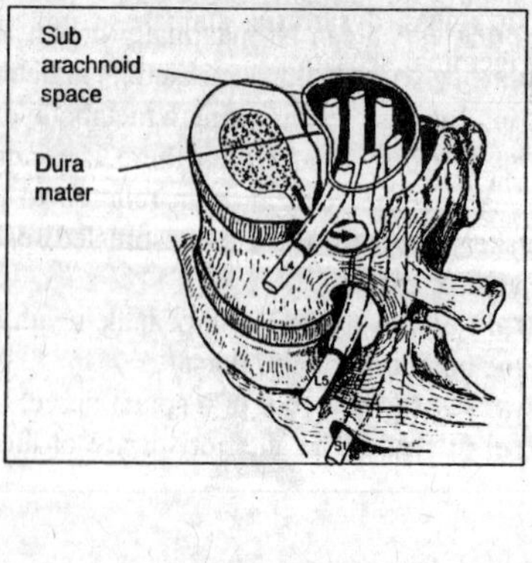

gradually merges with fibres known as annulus fibrosus and these form ring around the nucleus. Annulus has several layers like onion. Discs are insensitive structures because these have no nerve endings. There are 23 discs in the spine and they form one-quarter of spinal column. Average length of spine is 60 cm.

Vertebral disc prolapse Disc acts both as a cushion to absorb shock and as a buffer to keep the vertebra apart. The pressure within the disc is

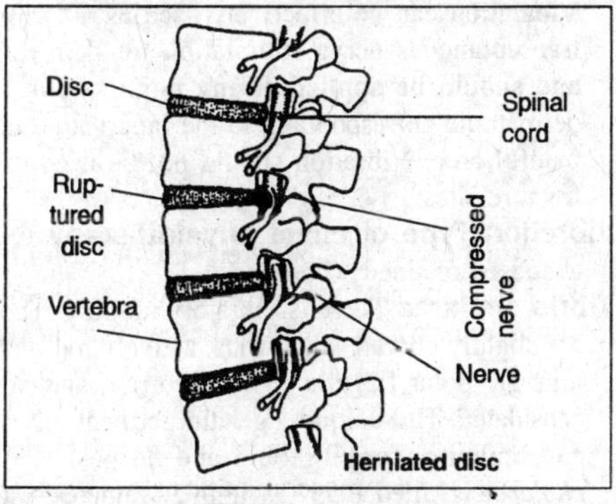

100 pounds per square inch. The load bearing capacity is high. Young weightlifter can lift 374 pounds. In a degenerating disc only minimal pressure is needed to displace it. Displaced disc can put pressure on spinal nerves to cause severe pain.

Vertebrobasilar insufficiency The foramen transversaria offers two vertebral arteries protection from compression during physiological movements and external trauma. But when osteophytes grow these impinge on vertebral artery impending blood flow and producing vertebrobasilar insufficiency. Common symptoms are dizziness, dysarthria, ataxia and impairment of trigeminal sensation.

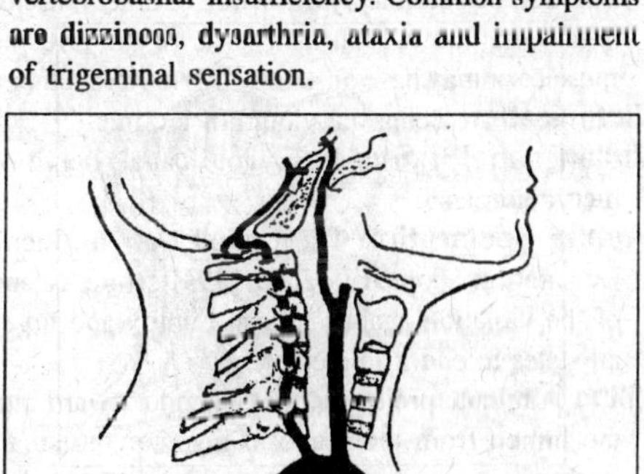

Vertex It is the area bounded infront by anterior fontanelle, behind by posterior fontanelle. The vertex presents when head is well flexed.

Vertex presentation When the head is well flexed found in 94 percent of cases.

Vertical angulation The angulation of the positioning indicating device (cone) in a vertical (head-to-toe) direction.

Vertical bone loss Bone loss that occurs in a plane not parallel to the cemento-enamel junction of adjacent teeth (also called angular bone loss).

Vertical diffusion A dynamic that occurs when one family member initiates a health behavior change and thereby influences another family member to make a similar change.

Vertical dimension Length of the face as determined by the amount of separation of the jaws.

Vertical disorientation A distorted perception of the upright position.

Vertical resistance Resistance conferred by the action of a single gene exerting a major effect expressed as immunity or hypersensitivity.

Vertical transmission The transmission of microorganisms from a parent insect to its offspring.

Vertigo A sensation of rotation or whirling movement; dizziness. It is a feeling of being spinned either horizontally or vertically. It results from a disturbance of the semicircular canals in the inner ear. The attacks are accompanied by severe vomiting, tinnitus and nystagmus. Elderly people with atherosclerosis often suffer from it. It may also have a psychological aspect. Antihistamine and anticholi-nergic drugs help the person.

Verumontanum Colliculus seminalis.

Very low density lipoproteins (VLDL) One of the major classes of lipoproteins, containing high concentrations of triglycerides and moderate concentrations of cholesterol and phospholipids; has a density between 1.006 and 1.019.

Very-low-calorie diets (VLCD) Usually defined as diets containing 800 kcalories a day or less.

Vesicant A drug capable of causing tissue necrosis when extravasated.

Vesicular mole It is a disease of young chorionic villi, It is characterised by formation of immense numbers of irregular clusters and chains of cysts.

These cysts vary in sizes. It may be seen even at third week of pregnancy. As a rule contour of ovum is completely lost and a mass of vesicles is formed. The formation of vesicles may be so abundant to produce a mass weighing 4 to 5 pounds. The cystic villi are closely packed together. Vesicles themselves are oval or globular grape-like bodies, pale yellowish or milky white in colour. Vesicles may be arranged in chains or in clusters. No cause is known. Treatment consists of evacuation of uterus.

Vestibular folds The supporting folds of tissue for the vocal folds within the larynx, also called the oval window.

Vestibular membrane The membrane that separates the cochlear duct from the scala vestibuli.

Vestibular nerve A division of the vestibulocochlear nerve, the eighth cranial nerve.

Vestibular nystagmus Nystagmus resulting from vestibular disorder.

Vestibule Located in the inner ear; the portion adjacent to the oval window between the semicricular canals and the cochlea.

Vestibulocochlear nerve It is an eighth cranial nerve. It carries sensory impulses from the inner ear to the brain. It has two parts : vestibular nerve and cochlear nerve. The vestibular nerve carries sensory impulses from semicircular canals in inner ear while cochlear nerve carries sensory impulses from cochlea. Its damage may cause tinnitus.

Viable Capable of living; able to survive outside of the womb.

Viable child It is one who is capable of an independent existence apart from its mother. Earliest viable age recorded is 174 days while average age is 210 days.

Vial Glass or plastic container of parenteral medication with a self-sealing rubber stopper.

Vibration Vibration is a single or double handed technique in which a fine shaking movement or

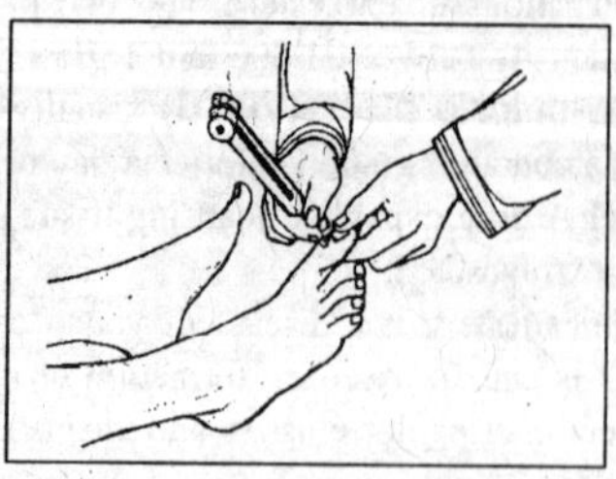

tremor is conveyed to the tissues by the hand or finger tips.

Vibration sense A test of posterior column function, using a tuning fork placed on a bone, e.g. shaft of tibia.

Vibration therapy Simple inexpensive massage vibrators can be used for facilitations of muscle activity or pain relief. Mechanical vibration of muscle tendon using a frequency of more than 50 Hz produces muscle strengthening and endurance. Vibaration can be effectively used as a form of transcutaneous nerve stimulation for pain relief and should be applied at any point within the dermatome corresponding to the innervation of a painful area. Vibration should not be used over fracture sites.

Vibration Type of chest physiotherapy Used to loosed retained secretions.

Vibrio cholerae There is vibratory motility. These are slightly curved, small rods, actively motile by a single polar flagellum, non-sporing, and non-capsulated. These liquefy gelatin, ferment glucose and mannitol forming acid and no gas. *Vibrio cholerae* is killed at 55°C within 20 minutes. Eltor tends to be more resistant than V. *cholerae* to most antibiotics. It produces rice watery stools and dehydration.

Vibroacoustic stimulation test Use of sound stimulation to elicit fetal movement and fetal heart rate.

Vicarious learning Learning: without direct experience, either by observing or by receiving verbal information.

Vicarious motion Also known as 'trick action' or trick movement. When muscles are weak or paralyzed the movements they normally perform may still be possible by the action of other muscles which may be normal synergists of the affected muscles or may have an action different from them.

Victimization Being the victim of a crime.

Vidian canal, nerve Peterygoid canal, nerve of pterygoid canal.

Vienna declaration The United Nations Viena Declaration adopted in June 1993 torture as one of the violation against human dignity and urges all states to end it immediately.

Villus A minute projection that extend outward into the lumen from the mucosal layer of the small intestine.

Violence Seriously injurious, aggressive behaviour, typically having some larger social significance.

Viral arthritis Rubella and mumps may result in arthritis. It may develop after 2 weeks of rubella vaccine. It presents with bilateral and symmetrical polyarthritis. Lymph glands are enlarged. Transient synovitis involving hip joints is often seen in small children who usually recover in 1 to 2 weeks. Arthritis may occur with rubella and mumps. It begins a few days after the development of or 2 weeks after rubella vaccination. It presents with bilateral symmetrical polyarthritis similar to rheumatoid arthritis, Lymphadeno-pathy is often present. In chickenpox also transient polyarthritis may develop.

Viral load Number or viral copies.

Viral Vector A viral DNA altered so that it can act as a vector for recombinant DNA.

Virginity Hymen is a thin membrane which particularly closes the mouth of vagina. Generally when young girl has her first intercourse the hymen is stretched and may rupture to bleed. But on the day of honeymoon if she does not bleed it does not mean that girl has lost her virginity enjoying sex in the past.

Due to some injury and during games hymen may rupture. So it is a myth that an intact hymen means that girl is virgin because on repeated intercourse also hymen may remain intact.

Virulence Pathogenicity denotes the ability of microorganism to cause disease while virulence induces the concept of degree. Virulence of organisms may be attenuated or exhalted. Attenuation can be achieved by repeated cultivation or by presence of antiseptic. Attenuation decreases the virulence of organism but retains the antigenic character.

Virulence is measured in terms of number of microorganism or microgram of toxin necessary to kill a given host when administered. It is usually expressed as LD50 which is to kill 50% of susceptible animals.

Virulence factor A protein or other molecule, or an inherent property, that contributes to the ability of a pathogen to cause disease.

Virulent Having the property of virulence; capable of causing disease when introduced into a susceptible host.

Virus A self-replicating, infectious, nucleic acid-protein complex that requires an intact host cell for its replication, its genome is either DNA or RNA.

Virus receptor A protein on the outer surface of a cell that serves as a site for adsorption of the virus to the cell and facilitates entry into the cytoplasm.

Virus replication The synthesis of new virus particles, including both replication of the genome and assembly of virus particles.

Viruses Viruses are the smallest infective agent. Their sole activity is to invade the cells of other organisms. Outside living cells these are wholly inert. They are incapable of activities typical of life. They parasitise all recognised life forms—mammals, insects, plants and even bacteria. The nucleic acid at the core is called genome. It consists of string of genes that contain coded instructions. Depending on type of virus the nucleic acid may be either DNA in which there are two strands of nucleic acid or RNA consisting of single strand. HIV is an RNA virus. Virus can enter in body by all routes, Adenovirus causes respiratory and eye infections. Paramyxovirus causes mumps, measles and rubella. Rabdovirus results in rabies. Viruses possess genetic material which when it is within the host cell, behaves as part of cell and they also exist in an extracellular form which is the product of host cell under the genetic control of virus itself. Viruses can reproduce only when they are within their host cells. They have no ribosomes and are devoid of enzymes to generate high energy bonds. They have no mitochondria. The virus lacks biosynthesis enzymes.

Viscera The organs within the abdominal or thoracic cavities.

Visceral Pertaining to the viscera or to the covering of an organ.

Visceral effectors Organs of the ventral body cavity that respond to neural stimulation, including cardiac muscle, smooth muscle, and glandular epithelium.

Visceral fat Fat that is within the abdominal cavity.

Visceral Larval migrans Migration of second-stage larvae of nematodes in the internal organs of unnatural hosts.

Visceral pain Discomfort arising from internal organs.

Visceral pericardium The pericardium that covers the heart.

Visceral peritoneum That part of the serous membrane in the abdominal cavity covering the surface of some abdominal organs.

Visceral pleura The deep layer of the serous membrane that covers the lungs.

Visceral portion Serous membrane that covers the surface of organs found in the body cavity.

Visceral protein malnutrition Same as Kwashiorkor.

Visceral protein stores Proteins contained in the internal organs.

Visceral reactions Stomach contractions, secretion of adrenalin, and other responses of the organs of the body cavity. Visceral reactions underlie such experiences as nausea and butterflies" in the stomach.

Visceroceptor A sensory receptor located within body organs that responds to information concerning the internal environment.

Viscerosomatic reflex Altered tone of musculoskeletal structures in response to stimuli originating in visceral tissues. Referred visceral pain is one possible consequence of such a reflex.

Viscosity The physical property of a liquid that is characterised by the degree of friction between its component molecules; determines the case with which the liquid will flow. Stickiness; ability of a fluid to resist change in shape or arrangement during flow.

Viscous Sticky or gummy; having a high degree of viscosity or resistance to flow; thick.

Vision It involves eye and brain. When light rays reach the eye most of focusing is done by cornea. However, eye itself does fine focussing by changing the curvature of lens. These two systems provide sufficient optical power to form an image on retina. The light sensitive rods and cones in retina convert image into nerve impulses and pass to brain through optic nerve. Colour sensitive cones are more in centre than in periphery.

Vision tests Most vision tests are of visual acuity. Refraction tests are done to discover patient's refractive error. Power of accommodation may be measured by correcting any refractive error with glasses and then determining the nearest distance at which very small point can be read.

Vision, loss of It may affect one or both eyes. It can cause partial or complete blindness, suddenly or slowly. *Progressive loss* of visual acuity is common with advancing age as a developing process of cataract. Other causes are macular degeneration, diabetes mellitus and glaucoma. *Sudden loss* of vision may be caused by optical or neurological disorders. Severe uveitis, vitreous haemorrhage, retinal detach-ment and retinal haemorrhage may reduce vision suddenly. Optic neuritis can cause loss of vision.

Visual acuity Ability to see both far and near.

Visual acuity for distance It is recorded by using Snellen's test type. Snellen's type each letter is at an angle of 5 minutes at the nodal point at a given distance, the largest letter at 60 metres and letters

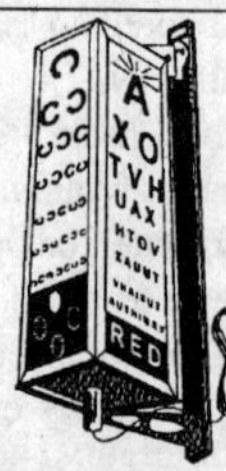

Testing drum distance vision

in subsequent lines at 36, 24, 18, 12, 9 and 6 metres. For convenience patient is kept fixed at 6 metres. Each eye is tested separately. Normal visual acuity is 6/6 meaning the patient is able to read from 6 meters which is normal. Visual acuity of 6/18 means that patient is able to read at 6 metres which he or she should have read from the distance of 18 metres.

Visual acuity for near vision For near vision the near test types are used. The patient is asked to hold the test card in his or her hand at a distance at which he or she normally keeps his or her books while reading or writing. It is normally at 14 inches.

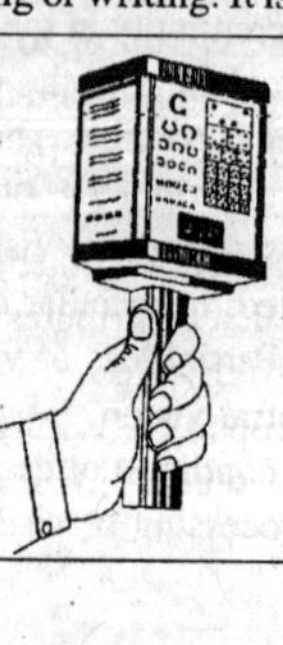
Near vision chart

Note the line which he or she is able to read. Normally the near vision should be corrected to N5, on the chart. If he or she is unable to read the test type marked N5, add convex lens until the test type N5 becomes clear with comfortable reading. It is always better to slightly undercorrect than to over correct for the near vision. This is for the patients having normal distance visual acuity without glasses. If the patient is using distance glasses, then test him or her for the near vision with his distance correction in the trial frame.

Visual analog pain scale (VAS) The VAS and a - 0 (least pain) to 10 (worst pain) scale are used to assess pain intensity. It can be administred in several forms as below :

Worst No Pain Pain

Worst No Pain Severe
Moderate Mild Pain
Worst No Pain 20 19 18 17 16 15 14 13 12 11 10 9 8 7 6 5 4 3 2 1 0 Pain

Visual closure The ability to identify forms or objects from incomplete presentations..

Visual coding The study of individual brain cells to determine the ways in which visual symbols are translated or collated in the brain. This research has shown that single cells are responsive to specific visual features, rather than responsive to any visual stimulus.

Visual disturbance in toxemia pregnancy It is from blindness to blurred vision. There may be retinal arteriolar spasm and ischemia of retinal detachment. Ratio of venous to arteriolar diameter becomes 2 :1 instead of 3 :2. Papilledema may occur.

Visual dyslexia The lack of ability to translate observed written or printed language into meaningful terms.

Visual field examination Assessment of peripheral vision and continuity in the visual field.

Visual field tests Visual field is the total area in which visual perception is possible. The visual field normally extends left and right 90° on either side. Above and below it is restricted. Visual fields of both eyes are concealed. In macular degeneration central vision is lost. Partial loss of visual field is less obvious than central vision

Visual impairment A condition of deceased visual acuity or impaired processing of visual input.

Visual learning Learning through what is seen.

Visual object agnosia The inability to recognize familiar objects despite normal function of the eyes and optic tracts.

Visual perception Perception obtained through the sense of vision.

Visual tracking Following targets with smooth eye movements.

Visuopsychic area (area 18-19) It sourrounds the visuosensory area except in its anterior part. It is concerned with the correlation of visual impressions and their association with past experience, leading to recognition and identification of objects. It is also responsible for effecting determination of distance and proper orientation of objects in space. Here again visual, tactile and to a lesser extent auditory impressions are correlated and synthesised to give proper visual perception and appreciation. In lesions of area 18 and 19 written or printed words are not appreciated. Stimulation of area 19 causes visual hallucinations, constriction of pupil and conjugate deviation of eyes to opposite sides.

Vital capacity The sum of the inspiratory reserve, tidal, and expiratory reserve volumes; it is the maximum amount of air that can be exhaled following a maximum inhalation.

Vital exhaustion Unusal fatigue and loss of energy, increased irritability and feelings of demoralization.

Vital reaction The 'flush' which surrounds a skin injury sustained during life due to dilatation of small vessels. An injury inflicted after death when circulation has ceased produces no such reaction.

Vital sense Feelings of physical well being including energy, clarity, sense of illness and speed of thought.

Vital sign Vital signs indicate that person is still alive. These include chest movements by breathing, the presence of pulse at neck or wrist, and constriction of the pupil, i.e. reflex when it is exposed to bright light. If all signs are absent doctor gives a certificate of death.

Vital signs Signs necessary to life that include temperature (T), pulse (P), respiratory rate (RR), and blood pressure (BP).

Vitalism The historic concept that all living organisms possess a "life-force" or "vital principle"

which accounts for the distinct properties of life, beyond the chemical and physical organization of the organism.

Vitamin This is essential for normal functioning of body. These are generally not manufactured by body. These are ACDEK and vitamin B complex group. These are required in small amount. These can be categorised into water soluble vitamins B and C and vitamin EDEK as fat soluble.

Vitamin B_{12} deficiency It leads to two major syndromes first is impaired DNA synthesis and is expressed most clearly in rapidly dividing cells. Deficiency results in megaloblastic anaemia, glossitis and hypospermia. Second is neurological syndrome and may affect peripheral nervous system resulting in distal neuropathy. B_{12} deficiency may cause neuropsychiatric problem of an old age.

Vitamin toxicity If fat soluble vitamins A & D are used for long in higher doses may cause toxicity while water soluble vitamins dont do.

Vitamin, fat soluble Vitamins ADEK are absorbed with fats from intestine into blood and stored in fatty tissue. These are not excreted in urine. Body reserves may last for several years so daily consumption is not necessary. Deficiency of a fat soluble vitamin is usually due to a disorder in fat absorption from intestine.

Vitamin, water soluble Being water soluble these vitamins are stored in body for a short period. Extra vitamins than required by body are excreted in urine. These are to be consumed daily.

Vitamin-A It is required for bone growth, normal growth, normal vision and cell structure. Rich sources of vitamin A are liver, milk, green leafy vegetables. Yellow coloured fruits such as mango, papaya are rich source of it. Its deficiency is rare in well-to-do families but is common in poor children where it may result in poor night vision, keratomalacia and even loss of vision. Skin may become rough and dry with loss of appetite. Prolonged excessive use of vitamin A may result in headache, tiredness, nausea and loss of appetite.

Vitamin-C It is an ascorbic acid needed for various enzymes and production of neurotransmitters. Principal sources are fresh fruits and vegetables. Daily requirement is 40 mg. Mild deficiency may cause weakness, pains, swollen gums and nose bleed. Excessive consumption for years may result in diarrhoea, cramps and kidney stones.

Vitamin-D The richest source of vitamin D is fortified milk and egg yolk. Body requires only small amount of it. Deficiency may develop in those who are deprived of sun light. Other causes may be liver and kidney disorder and some genetic defects. Prolonged use of phenytoin may also result in its deficiency. Long-term deficiency may lead to low levels of calcium and phosphate which result in softening of bones. Condition is known as rickets. Excessive consumption may result in abnormal calcium deposits in soft tissue, kidney, blood vessels and may result in retarded growth.

Vitamin-E Chemically it is known as tocopherol. It is essential for normal cell structure to maintain certain enzymes and for the formation of blood cells. Principal sources are vegetable oils, nuts, meat, cereals specially wheat. Balanced diet provides all the needed quantity of vitamin E. It is known as antisterility vitamin also.

Vitamin-K It is essential for formation of substance in liver which promotes blood clotting. Principal sources are cabbage, broccoli, vegetable oils and egg yolks. Prolonged treatment with antibiotics may result in its deficiency. Deficiency may lead to nosebleed, seeping of blood from wounds and gums.

Vitamins Chemical substances that are necessary in minute amounts for normal growth, maintenance of health, and functioning of the body.

Vitiligo These are white patches devoid of melanin. Patches may expand and may on occasion disappear automatically. There is no reliable treatment. It is a feeling of being spinned either horizontally or vertically. It results from a disturbance of the semicircular canals in the inner ear. The attacks are accompanied by severe vomiting, tinnitus and nystagmus.

Vitreous The vitreous is a transparent, colourless and avascular gel of semisolid consistency. It fills posterior two-third of volume of eyeball behind the lens. It takes the shape of wall of eyeball. It has a saucer-shaped depression in front for accommodating the lens. The vitreous is firmly attached anteriorly in a ring of 3 mm width. The hyaloid canal runs through the central region of vitreous.

Vitreous abscess It is a severe inflammation of vitreous and the adjacent structures. Inflammation does not extend beyond sclera. It is usually unilateral inflammation of ocular cavity. The most common causative organism is *Bacillus subtilis*. The vitreous is a very good culture media for organisms to grow and multiply rapidly as the vitreous is avascular with no natural defence mechanisms. There will be pain, redness of eye with marked circumciliary congestion. Visual acuity is diminished. Slit-lamp biomicroscopy shows hazy vitreous with cells. Cornea appears dull due to oedema of corneal endothelium.

Vitreous floaters Patient complains of seeing various types of dark spots floating or moving before the eyes like a fly or mosquito. It may appear as fine or thick regular or irregular dark spots. It may also appear like a thread, worm or cotton wool. The opacity is seen when eye is moving and even when it is stationary. A sudden appearance of large number of floaters should arouse suspicion for an acute vitreous detachment.

Vitreous haemorrhage A common cause of vitreous haemorr-hage is diabetic neuropathy. Any bleeding into vitreous humour is likely to affect vision, a major haemorrhage into centre of the gel. Large haemorrhage may persist for months.

Vitreous humor The jellylike fluid found in the eye, posterior to the lens. It fills the area between the crystalline lens and the retina. It consists entirely of water. It may pull retina, cause tear or detachment. Vitreous humour shrinks with age and may develop floatters.

Vocal abuse It results in hoarseness following exertion, more pronounced in the evening. Frequent throat clearing becomes habit. It may result in hyperfunctional dysfunction.

Vocal cords These are two fibrous tissue sheet in larynx which are responsible for voice production. Cords are attached to thyroid cartilage. True vocal cords are the cord which vibrate and make sound while false cords are folds in the larynx that have nothing to do with sound production.

Most of the time vocal cords lie apart forming a V-shaped opening called glottis. Vocal sounds are produced when vocal cords are tight. Alteration in the tension of cord produces sound of different pitch.

Vocal fold One of the ligaments that extends from the posterior surface of the thyroid cartilage to the paired cartilages of the larynx; the superior pair are the false vocal folds and the inferior pair are the true vocal folds.

Vocal ligament A continuation of the cricothyroid ligament.

Vocal nodules Main symptoms include hoarsensess, vocal cord disuse, diplophonia and foreign body sensation. Vocal nodules in singers limit the ability to sing softly or reach higher notes. It is caused by demands that exceeds vocal capacity.

Vocal polyp Usually there is severe hoarseness with atrophic episodes. With pedunculated lesions the voice may be essentially normal at low volume. There develops feeling of dryness in the throat. The polyp may be sessile or pedunculated and may arise from upper surface.

Vocal tract That part of the speech mechanism above the level of the vocal folds capable of modifying speech sounds generated by the vocal folds, including the pharyngeal, oral, and nasal cavities.

Vocational Trade, profession or occupation.

Vocational rehabilitation Training, following disease or injury, for an occupation or profession, taking into account the special physical or mental capabilities of the patient.

Voice, loss of Disturbance of working or vocal cords may cause partial loss of voice known as dysphonia. Temporary loss of voice may be caused by straining of muscles of larynx. Inflammation of vocal cords in laryngitis disturbs speech. Persistent or recurrent dysphonia may be due to polyps. In hypothyroidism thickening of vocal cords may result. Total loss of voice is having psychological element.

Voiced sounds Sounds produced with simultaneous vibration of the vocal folds; includes all vowels, semivowels, diphthongs, and voiced consonants.

Voiceless sounds Sounds produced without vibration of the vocal folds.

Voiceprint The term 'voiceprint' is supposed to describe spectrograms of human speech, but it is in fact a fallacious analogy to fingerprints; the acceptable term is voicegram.

Void An absence of stains in an otherwise continuous bloodstain pattern.

Voided specimen Freshly urinated sample of urine.

Voiding Emptying of the bladder.

Voiding reflex Spontaneous relaxation of the urinary sphincter in response to physical stimulation.

Volar In forearm, anterior, in hand, palmar.

Volar splint Splint can be fabricated to adjust wrist and metacarpophalangeal position in extensor tendon injuries.

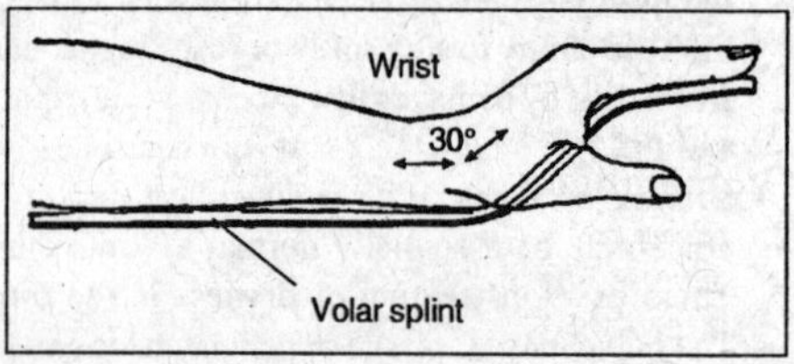

Volatile Tending to evaporate readily.

Volatile fatty acids Short-chain fatty acids that are major products of microbial fermentation in the gut.

Volesselum forceps It is used to hold anterior lip of cervix where it is not friable. It also helps in introducing laminaria tent. Having sharp teeth it provides firm grip. It is useful in holding anterior or posterior lip of cervix in D & C, and cauterisation of cervix.

Volition The act of the power of willing.

Volkman's contracture In it the wrist and fingers become parmanently fixed in a bent position. It occurs due to ischaemia in forearm muscles which result due to damage of brachial artery.

It generally happens in mid humerus fracture. Initially fingers become cold, numb, white and blue.

Finger movements are weak and painful. Physical therapy and injection of vasodilator drug in artery may help.

Voltage The potential or electro-motive force of an electric charge, expressed in volts.

Voltage-gated channel An ion channel in the plasma membrane. It is composed of integral proteins; functions like a gate to permit or restrict the movement of ions across the membrane in response to changes in membrane voltage.

Volume of lochia It is assessed by the method of peripad saturation depending on the amount.

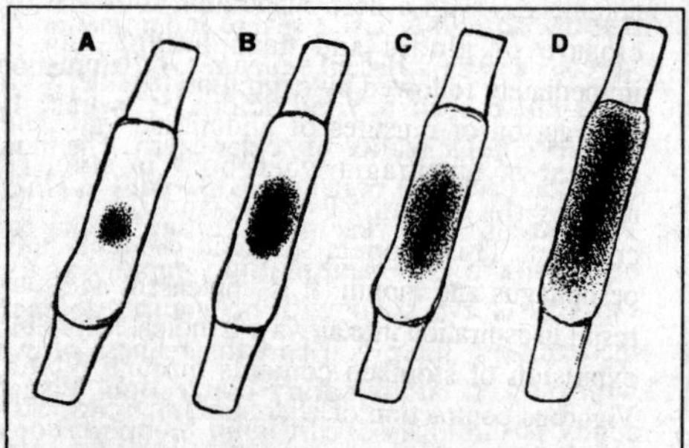

A : Scant amount : Body less than 1-inch stain
B : Light amount : Less than 4-inch stain on period.
C : Moderate amount : Less than 6-inch stain on period.
D : Heavy amount : Saturated period within 1 hour.

Volume transmission Nonsynaptic release of neuropeptides into the extracellular space.

Volume-control set Chamber in intravenous tubing that holds a portion from a larger volume of intravenous solution.

Volumetric controller Electronic infusion device that instills intravenous solutions by gravity.

Volunteer bias Individuals who volunteer for some procedures are not generally representative of the total population. Self-selected patients who seek out treatment based upon newspaper publicity, for example, are likely to do significantly better than random patients who are simply offered the treatment.

Vomer The flat bone that forms the inferior and posterior part of the nasal septum.

Vomiting It is an involuntary forcible expulsion of stomach content orally. It happens when brain centre is activated. Centre can be triggered by chemo-receptor trigger zone. Then diaphragm presses stomach and contents are pushed up. It generally happens after overeating and alcohol consumption or after general anaesthesia. Peptic ulcer, acute appendicitis, gastroenteritis and food poisoning result in vomiting. Balancing mechanism within inner ear such as Meniere's disease and acute labyrinthitis or while moving may result in vomiting. Psychological emotional problems may be a cause of vomiting. It is the expulsion through the mouth of material from the alimentary tract by muscular action. The act of vomiting is preceded by salivation, rapid breathing, sweating, tachycardia and discomfort. Vomiting commences with a deep inspiration followed by closure of glottis and nasopharynx and is immediately followed by expiration together with contraction of muscles of abdominal wall and descent of diaphragm when body of stomach relaxes the antrum. Pylorus and duodenum contract. This propels stomach contents into oesophagus and mouth. It is unpleasant and may result in aspiration into airway. It indicates forcible expulsion of stomach contents through mouth. Vigorous contraction of abdominal muscles takes place.

Vomiting, in pregnancy It develops in first trimester of preg-nancy. In some it may continue throughout pregnancy. It is due to change in hormones. Vomiting occurs most frequently in early morning often after waking up.

Vomiting, of blood It is known as haematemesis. It is bleeding from digestive system. Vomiting of blood from lung is known as haemoptysis. Common causes of haematemesis include oesophageal varices, peptic ulcer, oesophageal pathologies, gastritis, cancer of stomach etc. Vomited blood may be dark red, brown, black resembling coffee ground. Endoscopy is the best investigation to do.

Vomitus Substance that is vomited.

Von Braun's sign It is a clear longitudinal groove, dividing the corpus uteri into 2 parts of different

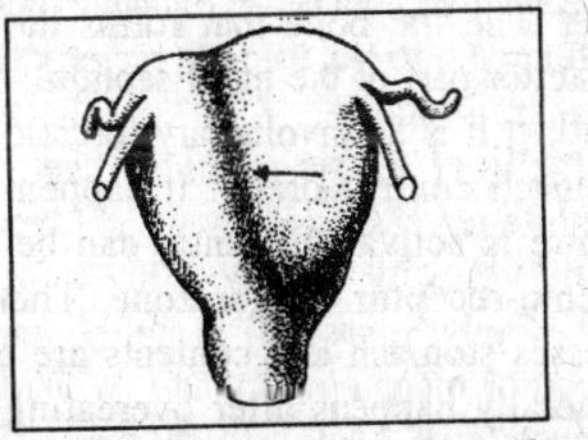

size and consistency. It can be detected at about 5 weeks. Later in pregnancy uterine symmetery is restored.

Von Hippel-Lindau disease It is an abnormal dominant disorder characterised by a predisposition to a wide variety of tumours, specially haemangioblastoma of cerebellum, spinal cord and retina. The cerebellar tumours can usually be excised.

Von Willebrand's disease It is transmitted most commonly as an autosomal dominant disorder with spontaneous bleeding from wounds and menorrhagia. Patients have a compound defect involving platelet function and coagulation pathway.

Voyeurism It is an invasion of privacy. It is the circle drawn by people around themselves and what they do in which activity they participate. Uninvited strangers to see is the reflection of low esteem in which they hold women.

Vtreous humor The transparent gel that occupies the space between the lens and retina of the eyeball.

Vulcanite A hard rubber prepared by vulcanising. India rubber with sulphur, formerly used for making removable dentures.

Vulnerability The lack of personal and social resources thereby increasing the risk of greater adverse impact of stressful conditions.

Vulnerable factors Enduring abnormalities that predispose an individual to the onset or recurrence of illness.

Vulva It is the external visible part of female genitalia. It comprises the clitoris and labia a fold of skin. Itching, various skin disorders such as dermatitis, genital warts and vulvitis may develop.

Vulval hematoma A very large accumulation of blood in the paravaginal and vulval tissue extending downwards to labia majora giving purple/black colour known as vulval hematoma. Rupture, laceration or tear of rich perivaginal venous or arterial plexus is the source of blood. Gradually increasing purple or black glistening swelling in the labium majora with pain and tenderness is a characteristic feature. Shock may be treated.

Vulval varicosities First appearing in second and third months of gestation and persistently enlarging to terms. It is generally associated with varicosities of lower limbs. Elastic support to maintain varicosities is necessary.

Vulvar Relating to or affecting the vulva.

Vulvitis It is the inflammation of vulva. Cause may include candidiasis genital herpes and warts. It may be the result of changes in vulval skin specially after menopause. There may be red or white patches.

V-wave The rise in the atrial pressure curve near the end of ventricular contraction that results from the gradual accumulation of blood in the atria while the atrioventricular valves are closed during ventricular contraction.

W

Waardenburg syndrome An autosomal dominant inheritance characterised by pigmentary disturbances including partial albinism and white forelock, unilateral deafness, fused thick eyebrows, broad nasal root, and laterally displaced medial canthi.

Wada test With the help of this localisation of area of language is confirmed as may be necessary prior to temporal lobe surgery by the intracarotid injection of a small dose of amylobarbitone. If a carefully calculated dose of drug is injected into the internal carotid artery supplying the hemisphere in which language is located there will be a temporary arrest of language without impairment of consciousness.

Waldenstroem's syndrome It presents with petechial eruptions on the body, anaemia, frequent epistaxis, visual disturbances, perhaps dryness of the mouth and eye, lymphadenopathy, and splenohepatomegaly.

Waldeyer's ring Lymphatic ring in the pharynx.

Walk-a-mile test Fitness test that measures the time it takes a person to walk a mile.

Walking The manner in which a person walks is known as gait. It depends on shape, size and posture. It reflects an individual's personality. Walking is controlled by nerve signals from motor cortex and signals from basal ganglion and cerebellum. Signals are sent from spinal cord to nerve cells and from there are carried by nerve fibres to the muscles. Abnormal gait may be caused by muscle weakness, by abnormalities of skeleton or by joint stiffness causing immobility in lower limbs or spinal column. In parkinsonism there develops difficulty of starting to walk. Steps are short and shuffling with the feet barely clearing the ground. Person may fall unless he or she is assisted.

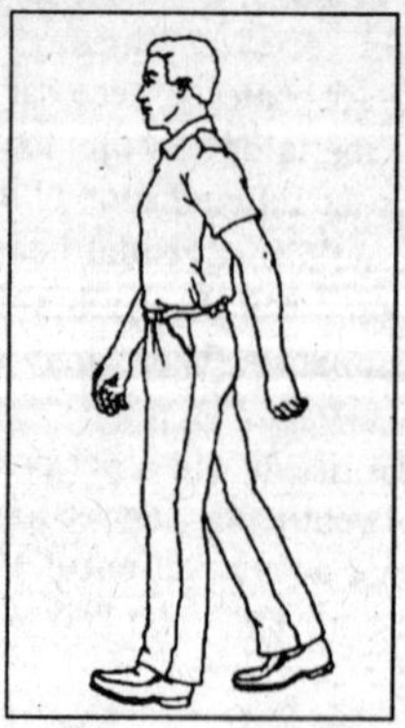

Walking belt Leather device with handles that enables the nurse to help a client walk.

Walking frames This gives a large amount of support as they have a very wide base and thus stable. These can be used in younger age group

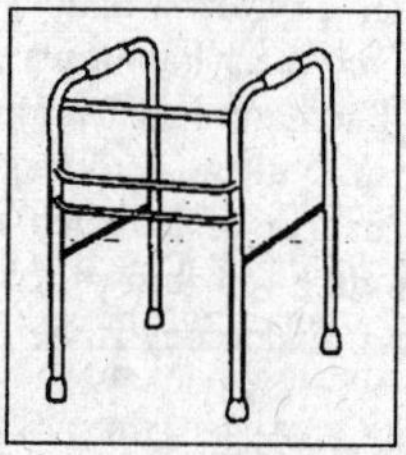

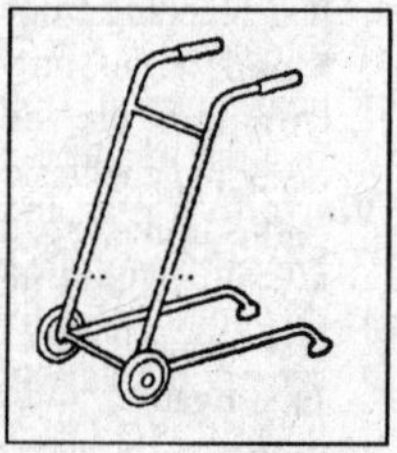

when higher levels of supports are required, when the patient with a total hip arthroplasty. In children these are used with neurological or muscles skeletal dysfunction. Rigid, folding, reciprocal and rollator types are available.

Walking heel Plastic or rubber heel placed in the sole of a leg cast to allow weight bearing.

Walking velocity The rate of linear forward motion of the body; measured in either centimeters per second or meters per minute. Walking velocity = distance/time. Also, velocity may affect cadence, step, stride length and foot angle, as well as other gait variables.

Wallerian degeneration When a nerve is cut transversely, the part of nerve distal to the point of section, i.e. distal part rapidly undergoes certain changes known as wallerian or secondary degeneration.

Change commences in the first hour after section and becomes complete by third day when nerve fibre loses excitability to stimuli and ceases to conduct impulses.

Walsham's forceps Tip of this forceps is beaked. It is used in impacted nasal bone fracture. After disimpaction the bones are realigned using the forceps. Reduction is maintained by nasal Leukoplast.

Wandering macrophage Phagocytic cell that develops from a monocyte, leaves the blood, and migrates to infected tissues.

Wandering pacemaker An abnormal cardiac rhythm in which the site of controlling focus of depolarization shifts from depolarization to depolarization, usually between the sinus and atrioventricular nodes.

Wandering rash It is characterised by one or more irregular areas of desquamation on the tongue. Cause of it is not known but may be allergic one. The bald spots are surrounded with normal papillae. These heal but new areas appear in another part of tongue. The bald spots on the tongue may change size and shape within two hour's period. Condition may be associated with fissured tongue.

Warfarin It is an anticogulant drug used to treat and prevent abnormal blood clotting. It is used to treat thrombosis, ischaemic attacks and after heart surgery but its action starts after many days while heparin is a faster acting than warfarin but may result in abnormal bleeding.

Warm caloric test A test of kinetic labyrinthine function.

Warm caloric test A test of kinetic labyrinthine function.

Warm Up The warm up period involves activities that incease the preparedness of the neuromuscular and articular system activity. The cool down involves some light aerobic activity that will supply blood, oxygen and nutrients to the area that has been used and remove waste products from those areas. It also involves stretching exercises to restore the muscle (lengths) spindle bias to more appropriate levels of activity as well as provide a stimulus for functional healing following any inflammatory process, should any micro traumas have occurred.

Warthin's tumour It consists of 4 per cent of all salivary gland tumours between the age of 40 and 60 years. Majority of patients affect parotid gland but tumour may arise in submaxillary gland. Gross specimen are encapsulated and cut surfaces show cystic spaces which exude thick mucus seen under microscope. Excision is the treatment of choice.

Warts It is a benign condition of epithelial outgrowth produced by human papilloma virus. Infection spreads through direct or indirect contact. Genitalia may be involved due to sexual intercourse. The condition produces capillaries acanthiosis with marked hyperkeratosis and cellular infiltration in dermis. Common warts are sharply demarcated, small, brown or skin coloured, round or oval papules or nodules. On the scalp wart may assume the shape of cauliflower. Lesions grow slowly and become dirty and irregular in surface. Filliform warts present as thread-like projections. Plantar warts develop usually on pressure points of the soles and on the palms as flat corn-like warty growth. They are deeply embedded in dermis. Warts are painful and tender on touch. Warts reappear on the same site.

Water It is the most common chemical in the human body. About 99 per cent of molecules in body are water. Woman or man weighing 60 kg is having 48 kg of water. It is essential for life. In it only all metabolic reactions take place. Plasma carries water to all parts of body. Water is lost from the body in urine, sweat, faeces and as water vapour it is breathed out. It depends on physical activity and external temperature. The minimum daily urinary output to remove waste products is 0.5 litres although normal output is about 1.5 litres. In some diseases such as heart failure and oedema there is accumulation of water. Excess of salt results in water retention.

Water borne infection Water can be a source of infection. It may contain virus, infective bacteria or parasitic organisms. It may cause diarrhoea, typhoid fever, cholera, amoebiasis and worm infestations. Adequate and effective safe water supply minimises these diseases. If nothing water should be sterilised before drinking by boiling for 10 minutes. It kills infective organisms.

Water diuresis Diuresis occurring about 15 minutes after intake of large volume of hypotonic fluid.

Water intoxication It is caused by excessive water retention of brain resulting in headache, dizziness, nausea, confusion and in some cases may result in seizures. Renal failure, liver cirrhosis, severe heart failure and diseases of adrenal glands may result it.

Water soluble Dissolves in water; in nutrition refers to a group of vitamins classified according to their method of metabolism.

Water soluble vitamins These are B complex group and vitamin C.

Waterhammer pulse Strong, jerky pulse of short duration that suddenly collapses.

Watermarking Originally a faint design seen in paper when held against a strong light to identify the maker or the design. It is more widely used as a term indicating a marking introduced within an object to identify that object and among other things to make forgery difficult. The term has been adopted and extended to cover 'electronic watermarking'. Electronic water-marking is defined as the introduction into an image of an identication code. This can be hidden in the image data by encryption. Electronic water-marking is an extra level of security.

Water-seal chest tube drainage Technique for evacuating air or blood from the pleural cavity.

Water-soluble vitamins Vitamins present and carried in body water; B complex and vitamin C.

Wating syndrome An involunatry weight loss of > 10% in 1 month with the presence of either chronic diarrhea, weakness, or fecer for more than 30 days in the absence of a concurrent illness or condition.

Wave summation The increased strength of muscle contraction that results when stimuli follow one another in rapid succession.

Wavelength The length of a single cycle of ultrasound wave. It determines the resolution of the scanner. The distance between two corresponding positions in a wave, as from crest to crest.

Wax bath It is one type of heat treatment in which liquid hot wax is applied to part of body with the aim of relieving pain and stiffness of an injured joint. It is more useful in rheumatoid arthritis. Temperature is kept 120 to 130°F. Wax is solidified on the part within a few seconds. Again hand is put in wax, till a thick layer solidifies. After 20 minutes the wax is peeled off and exercise is done.

Wax out Elimination of undesirable undercut area on a cast to be used in the fabrication of a removable denture.

Wax pattern A replica of a dental restoration fabricated in wax; used to fashion a permanent metallic (or ceramic) restoration through the process of casting.

Waxes Waxes used in dentistry may be composed of natural and synthetic waxes, gums, fatty acids and synthetic resins and pigments of various types. Most mineral waxes have their chief constituents as hydrocarbons ranging from 17 to over 44 carbon atoms. Hydrocarbons in plant waxes are saturated alkanes from 19 to 31 carbon atoms. Waxes used in dentistry contain molecules having a range of molecular weight that affect the melting and flow properties of waxes.

Weak pulse Fine and barely perceptible pulse; easily obliterated.

Weakness It is the most easily understood disorder of motor function and occurs in upper motor neuron syndrome too. The pattern of upper motor neuron weakness is characteristic. In upper limb first muscles to be affected by advancing pyramidal lesions are triceps and extensors of fingers. In lower limb first affected muscles are flexors of hip, dorsiflexors and evertors of foot. Power of extensors of knee and plantar flexors of foot are well preserved.

Wean To progressively discontinue artificial ventilation and develop independent breathing.

Weaning The termination of nursing behavior; specifically, the change of diet for domestic animals from milk to solid feed.

Wear It is a complex phenomenon that occurs when two surfaces are brought in direct contact or into indirect contact with a third body acting between then.

Web space The area between the thumb and index finger that needs to be wide open in a drawing or writing grasp for the fingertips to use sensory feedback to gauge pressure accurately.

Weber test It is a tuning fork test of hearing. Tuning fork is set into light vibration and placed in the midline of skull.

Patient is asked to indicate on which side the sound is better heard. In sensorineural deafness sound is heard better in the normal ear as might be expected. In conductive deafness the sound is referred to the deaf ear.

Weber-Christian syndrome The syndrome includes recurrent malaise and fever, non-suppurative inflammatory subcutaneous nodules in the trunk and extremities, and subcutaneous atrophy at the sites of the nodules.

Webril Stretchable cotton material applied over the skin to protect from plaster irritation.

Wechsler scales Individual intelligence tests originally developed by David Wechsler. These include tests for preschoolers, children, and adults. Each is characterised by a series of subtests assessing different mental abilities.

Wegener's granulomatosis It is a systemic granulomatous vasculitis affecting upper and lower respiratory tract with or without associated glomerulonephritis. Nervous system may be involved by direct spread of granulomatous lesions from paranasal sinuses or by vasculitis. Disease responds to cyclophosphamide.

Wegener's syndrome Aetiology is not known and develops in fourth decade of life. There will be weight loss, multiple arthritis, features of neuritis, carditis, headache and weakness.

Wegener's vitreoretinal degeneration There is dim vision with floaters. Slit-lamp examination of vitreous shows empty spaces. Ophthalmoscopy shows peripheral pigmentary degeneration and choroidal sclerosis with atrophy. Refraction is myopic, ECG is abnormal. It is complicated by formation of cataract and retinal detachment.

Weight Force exerted on a body by the gravity of the earth.

Weight bearing Loading part or all of the body onto the arms or legs or distributing the body weight through all extremities occurs on the legs and feet in the standing position and on the knees in a kneeling position.

Weight bearing points of foot When the foot is weight bearing on the ground it rests on three places, calcaeum posteriorly, head of first metatarsal anteromedially and head of fifth metatarsal anterolaterally. These points form a triangle.

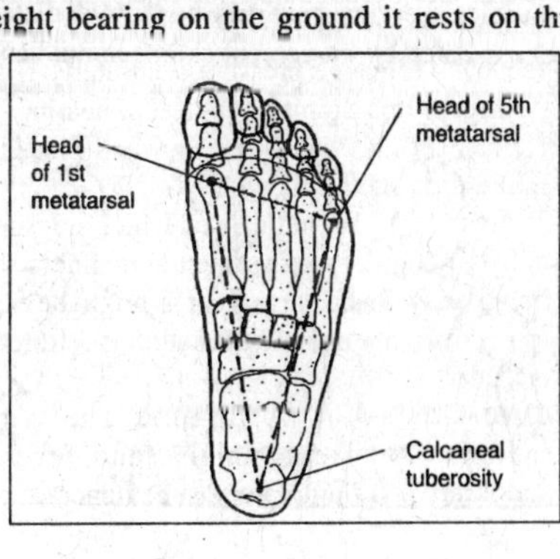

Weight gain in pregnancy The average weight gain during first 20 weeks is 2 kg and during next 20 weeks about 9 kg. Any weight above 0.5 kg per week after fourth month of gestation should be considered abnormal. Increase in blood volume is 1.3 kg, extracellular fluid gain 1.1 kg and fat storage in subcutaneous tissue is 2.7 kg.

Weight loss When calorie expenditure is more than consumption loss of weight may occur. It may be desirable while dieting or due to disease where there is decrease in appetite like jaundice. Gasteroenteritis may result in loss of weight. The disorders like cancer, tuberculosis and hyperthyroidism, untreated diabetes mellitus also results in weight loss. Unexplained weight loss may be a sign of disease and should be investigated by a physician.

Weight proportion of body The percentage of total body weight depend on body part, foot 1.8%, below knee 6%, above knee 13% hand 1%, below elbow 3%

Weight-shifting Movement away from the body's upright center of gravity; used to elecit righting and equilibrium reactions that restore or maintain upright postures.

Wellness The efficient balance of body, mind, and spirit, all working in a harmonious way to provide quality of life.

Werdnig-Hoffman's disease It is characterised by marked hypotonia. There will be fasiculations of tongue.

Child is alert. Feeding behaviour and cry are poor. Deep tendon reflexes are absent. Muscle biopsy shows neurogenic type of atrophy.

Werner's syndrome It presents with scleroderma, atrophy of the skin and subcutaneous tissue, bilateral juvenile cataract, premature greying and loss of hair, and endocrine disturbances.

Wernicke's aphasia There is lesion involving posterior superior temporal gyrus, speech is fluent but contains few substantives. Grammatical constructions appear normal.

However, semantic and phonemic confusions are common and muddled phonemes are strung together to make unknown meaningless words. Comprehension is impaired.

Wernicke-Korsakoff syndrome This is the malnutrition due to alcohol dependence or in cancer. It is due to deficiency of thiamine and vitamin B complex. Wernicke's encephalopathy develops suddenly and produces various abnormal eye movements, ataxia, slowness and confusion Sufferer may develop signs of neuropathy such as loss of sensations, pin and needle sensations. There are impaired reflexes. Unconsciousness may lead to coma and death if not treated. Korsakoff's psychosis may develop severe loss of memory, apathy and disorientation. Recent memory is affected more than old memory. It is a medical emergency. It may become irreversible.

Wet beriberi Thiamin deficiency with edema affecting cardiac function by weakening of heart muscle and vascular system.

Wet dressings and lotions Water is the most important component. Wet dressings are generally used to cleanse, cool and relieve pruritus in acutely inflamed lesions. It is applied when there is much exudation and on hairy areas. Sodium chloride solution 0.9 per cent or solutions of astringent and aluminium acetate lotion are often used.

Wettability Measure of the affinity of a liquid for a solid as indicating by spreading of a drop.

Wetting The interaction between a fluid adhesive and a substrate that determines the extent of the contact between the two; good wetting is essential for adhesion ; water "balling up" on a wax surface is an example of poor wetting.

Wetting agent A surface-active agent that forms a monomolecular layer over the pulmonary alveolar surfaces.

WFOT World Federation of Occupational Therapists.

Wharton's duct Submandibular duct.

Wheal An acute circumscribed transitory area of edema of the skin; an urticarial lesion.

Wheel chair It is a life line for invalid paraplegics. A good sitting environment is more critical for full-time wheelchair user. Person with limited trunk strength will have trouble maintaining the lumbar lordosis much less actively moving into it. There should be solid back with cushion supporting posture of patient. Different types of mechanised wheelchairs are available nowadays. Well-chosen wheelchair may considerably reduce handicap by increasing mobility in and outside the home. Unsuitable wheelchair may increase the problem

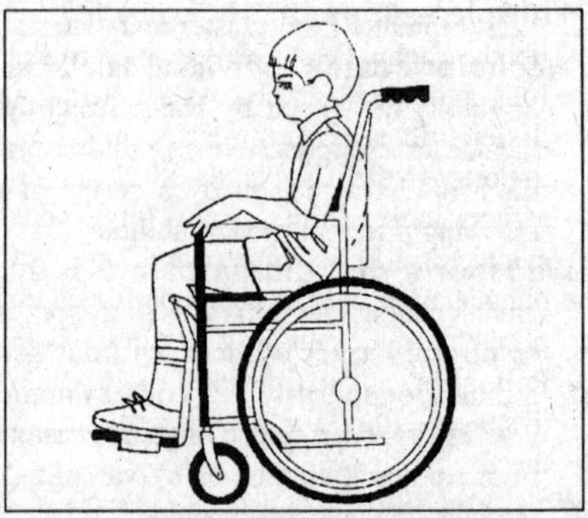

of a person. It can be used for indoor or outdoor or both. It can be collapsing to be kept in car and may be manual or electric. Whether the arm should be removable to allow sideways transfers, one should have a complete survey and knowledge before having it.

Wheeze The high-pitched sound made by air passing through narrowed tracheobronchial airways.

Wheezing It refers to high-pitched whistling sounds audible without auscultation. It is more common in first decade of life. Partial obstruction of bronchi and bronchioles leading to narrowing produces wheezing.

Whey The fluid from the precipitated protein while forming curd. It contains little fat and little protein.

Whiplash injury Rear end collisions account for about 20% of all vehicle accidents. As trunk is moved forwards the inertial mass of head results in a forced hyperextension strain of ligaments and muscles. Cervical pain may be of immediate onset, exacerbated by movement and occipital headache.

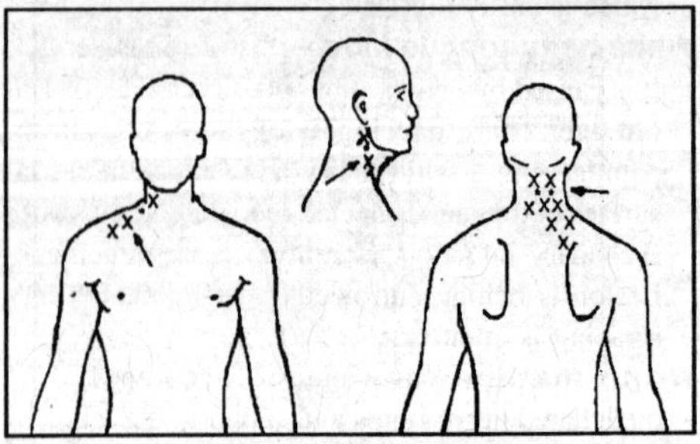

Cervical pain and limitations of cervical movements may persist for months. X-ray does not help. Supportive soft collar is useful.

Whipple's disease It is called intestinal lipodystrophy. Person develops diarrhoea, weight loss and steatorrhoea. Abdominal pain and distension are common. Arthritis occurs in majority, which is usually mild, migratory and affects larger joints. Joints involved may be symmetrical or asymmetrical. There will be skin pigmentation over exposed parts without buccal pigmentation. Clubbing of finger is common. Pulmonary manifestations include cough and dyspnoea. Rarely cardiac involvement may be there.

Whirlpool bath It is a deep cylinder of stainless steel or ceramics in which the temperature of water an degree of agiation can be controlled.

Whispered pectoriloquy An auscultatory technique; the whispered voice is transmitted through the lungs and chest wall in the same manner as the normal voice; it indicates an increase in the density of the underlying lung tissue.

Whistle-blowing Reporting incompetent or unethical practices.

White coat hypertension Blood pressure that is elevated when measured in the clinic by a physician or a nurse but normal when measured in other situations.

White collagen fibres The principal constituent to the insoluble protein collagen. The protein is characterised by forming gelatin when it is boiled with water for a few hours. Collagen and gelatin are practically free from cystine, tryptophan and tyrosine and are rich in glycine. Collagen although insoluble is attached in the stomach, giving gelatin which is easily digested.

White hairy tongue Mostly it is of fungus origin. It is caused by dehydration, poor oral hygiene and old age. There develops elongation of filiform papillae and a white hairy appearance of dorsal surface of tongue. Collected food debris may cause secondary infection. Condition is asymptomatic. Lesion is benign and needs no treatment. Daily scraping is curative.

White matter White matter is composed of medullated nerve fibres and supporting glial cells. Three types of fibres are available : transverse fibres, projection fibres and association fibres. *Transverse fibres* connect two cerebral hemispheres making up the corpus callosum. Anterior commissure connects the two olfactory bulbs while the hippocampal commissure joins the 2 hippocampi. *Projection fibres* connect the cerbral conrtex with lower portion of brain and spinal cord. The *short association* fibres connect adjacent gyri while the *long association fibres* connect widely separated areas.

Whitecoat hypertension Condition in wihch the blood pressure is elevated when taken by a health care worker but is normal at other times.

Whitlow It is an abscess of fingertip. Toe tip may also be involved. It causes finger to swell and become extremely painful and sensitive to touch and pressure. It may be caused by herpes virus or bacteria. It may be treated by suitable antibiotic, if not it has to be excised and drained. Rarely if not treated may result in osteomyelitis.

WHO World Health Organization.

Whole grain products Food items made using unrefined grains.

Whole versus part learning An issue in educational practice, concerned with the mastery of a task by focusing on the whole or upon its separate parts. The answer to this question depends upon the nature of the task and the learner's prior experience. In most cases a flexible plan seems best, perhaps starting with the whole and then dealing with the specific parts, as necessary.

Whooping cough Same as Pertussis.

Width of walking base The linear distance between one foot and the opposite foot; measured in centimeters or meters.

Wilooxon matched-pairs signed-ranks test A nonparametric significance test used to compare paired, ordinal data. It is analogous to the paired t-test for continuous data.

Wilcoxon rank sum test The nonparametric version of the independent 't' test; synonymous with Mann-Whitney test.

Wilcoxon signed rank test The onoparametric version of the paired 't' test.

Wild rice An american grass bearing a grain used for food. It is high in protein, phosphorus and potasium.

Wild yeasts A term for yeasts that are present in the brewing process that were not introduced purposely nor tolerated for a specific purpose during brewing.

Wilms' tumour It is a nephroblastoma which occurs in children. It is highly malignant tumour. It occurs prior to the age of four. Ten per cent are bilateral.

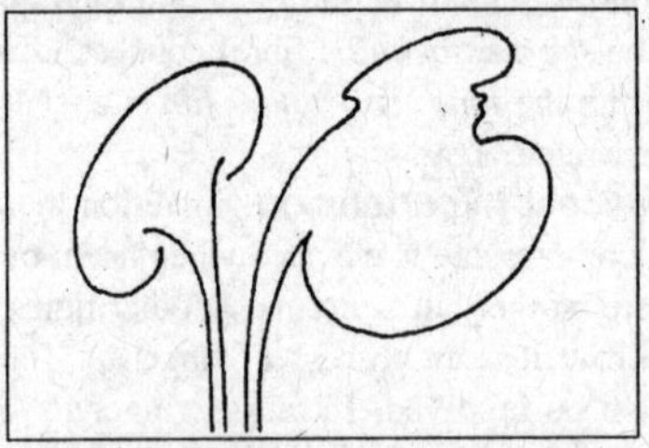

It may be congenital arising from embryonal cells. Parents notice palpable mass. There may not be a pain but haematuria may develop. Child may develop hypertension and may be relieved after nephrectomy. Treatment includes nephrectomy and chemotherapy.

Wilson's disease This is a rare disorder of copper metabolism inherited on an autosomal recessive basis, the gene lying on chromosome 13. Basic lesion is a hepatic defect in biliary copper excretion, leading to copper deposition in liver and cirrhosis with recurrent jaundice. Neurological disabilities include dysarthria, clumsiness, dystonic postures, tremors, intellectual retardation and disturbance of gait. Speech sound becomes strained. Automatic swallowing of saliva may fail and patient may drool. There is atrophy and softening of basal ganglion. Liver may show fatty infiltratioin. Disease responds to penicillamine.

Wind It is also known as flatulence. It is presence of air and other gases in alimentary canal. When wind is passed out through mouth it is known as belching.

Windblown position Positioning of the lower extremities to the side with one limb adducted and the other abdueted.

Window Square cut from a cast.

Windowing Cutting a small area of a cast to permit inspection of the tissues below.

Winged/wingless clamps Metal clamps placed on a tooth to stabilize a rubber dam in the mouth. Wing glamps have lateral extensions capable of holding the dam; wingless clamps require the dam be placed on the tooth before attaching the clamp since there are no projections to attach the dam.

Winslow, foramen Epiploic foramen.

Winterbottom's sign The sign represents presence of enlarged, rubbery, painless, lymph nodes, particularly of the posterior cervical group. It is seen in African try-panosomiasis.

Wipe Pattern A bloodstain pattern created when an object moves through an existing stain, removing and/or altering its appearance.

Wire edge Fine light burr, roughness left on a instrument blade as a result of sharpening.

Wirsung, duct Pancreatic chief duct.

Wisdom Having good judgement based on accumulated knowledge.

Wisdom teeth These are four large molar teeth that erupt at the back of each jaw after puberty. Sometimes these are known as third molars and erupt between the age of 17 and 21. These on occasion may not erupt. Each wisdom tooth has strong root and bulky crown with many cusps. It has extensive grinding surface. Some may develop these very late. Physical symptoms include nervous agitation, loss of sense of wellbeing, sweating and tremors.

Witches' milk A milky fluid secreted from the breast of the newborn.

With minimal excavation of tooth Application of it is followed by sealing the entire occlusive surface. It is typically used in premolars and molars.

Withdrawal The practice of retracting the penis from the vagina in intercourse prior to ejaculation, used as a method of contraception. Also, withdrawal reflex in which whole of limb extends by application of painful stimulus.

Withdrawal design A family of single-system designs characterized by implementation and withdrawal of treatment over the course of the study; known generically as A-B-A designs.

Withdrawal reflex Reflex restraction of a limb in response to a noxious stimulus; includes the flexor reflex.

Withdrawal state, alcoholism Those who drink heavily refer to morning shakes, irritability and feeling of anxiety which is relieved by another drink. If person resists drinking, tremors decline slowly over 12 hours. In case of chronic alcohol poisoning on withdrawal person may feel delirium tremens.

After 2 to 3 days of restlessness and agitation person develops vivid auditory and visual hallucinations. Consciousness may be clouded. Sedation with diazepam 40 to 50 mg/day orally may be successfully given. Atenolol is also useful in reducing tachycardia and anxiety in delirium tremens.

Withdrawal symptoms Symptoms that occur when a person suddenly stops taking drugs.

Withdrawal syndrome It is an unpleasant experience when a person stops a drug on which he or she is dependent like alcohol or smoking. In general any drug which relieves pain and causes euphoria can develop dependence and withdrawal symptoms.

In case of alcohol withdrawal symptoms start 6 to 12 hours after last drink and last for 4 to 7 days. Common symptoms are trembling of hands and tongue, sweating, anxiety and abdominal cramps to vomiting.

These symptoms may be frightening and to get relief person may restart drinking.

Within functional limits (WFL) A term used to indicate that an individual has the necessary muscle strength, muscle tone, and range of motion to perform daily living activities, play activities, and work and productive activities independently.

Within normal limits (WNL) A term used to designate that performance within the performance components is normal for an individual.

Within-groups mean square Same as Within-groups variance.

Within-groups variance Measurement based on the variation within each group.

Within-subject design An experimental plan in which each subject receives each level of the independent variable.

Wobble The relatively loose base pairing between the base at the 3' end of a codon and the complementary base at the 5' end of the anticodon.

Wolf syndrome It is a disorder which results from partial deletion of short arm of chromosome-4. Clinical features include mental retardation, hypotonia, cleft lip and coloboma. There may be fused ribs, fused vertebra, club feet and cleft palate.

Wolff's law A bone, normal or abnormal, develops the structure most suited to resist the forces acting on it. Bone is laid along the lines of resistant strains.

Wolffian duct One of a pair of embryonic ducts draining the mesonephros; the Wolffian ducts regress in females but are the precursor of the internal accessory reproductive organs in the male.

Wollfian body and duct Mesonephros and mesonephric duct.

Wood's screw maneuver It is performed with pressure applied to the anterior aspect of shoulder.

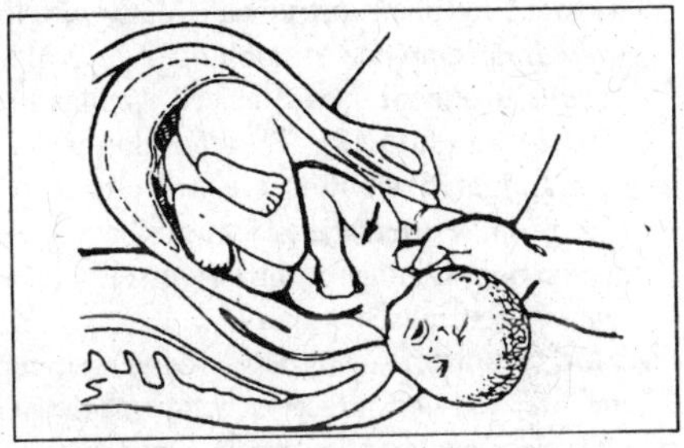

This abducts the shoulder while producing the rotation. It does not allow much of reduction in shoulder diameter.

Word recognition An early stage in language learning, usually occurring before the end of the first year, at which time the infant learns to distinguish the meaning of certain sounds in its language.

The emphasis is upon the early receptive, not expressive, use of the language. This stage is followed by the first use of words.

Working memory Holding relevant memories briefly in mind while performing a task.

Working myocytes The cardiac muscle cells that compose the bulk of the heart; to be distinguished from conducting myocytes.

Working phase Period during which the nurse and patient plan the patient's care and put the plan into action.

Working range Similar to maximum flexibility; in orthodontics the extent to which a wire can efficiently move teeth before needing reactivation.

Working through Exploration of a problem by patient and therapist until a satisfactory solution has been found or until a symptom has been traced to its unconscious sources.

Working time The time available to dental personnel for practical use of a setting material after it has been mixed.

Wound It is a breech of skin and/or underlying tissues caused by an accident, act of violence or surgery. These may be open or closed wounds. These are of many types :

Incised wound is an injury in which skin is cleanly cut; An *abrasion* is where surface is scraped away; *Laceration* in which skin is torn as in animal bite; *Contusion* in which the underlying tissues are damaged by blunt instrument; Many *penetrating wounds* develop due to stabbing or by bullets. As regards treatment, clean incised wounds may be closed by suturing if wounds are fresh. Contaminated wounds are not closed due to infection. Penetrating wounds will require exploration. Damage to blood vessels and nerves requires specialised surgery.

Wound infection Any type of wound is susceptible for infection and infection delays healing. Even after clean and aseptic surgery 5 per cent of cases during followup dressing develop infection which may even spread systematically. Antibiotics are therefore given as preventive measure even up to five days. Signs of infection in a wound are redness, swelling, warmth, pain and pus. Pus is usually accompanied by tender dark swelling. Pus should be cultured for sensitivity test. An abscess should be drained surgically.

Woven Bone Bony tissue found in the embryo, young children, early healing, and in various pathologic conditions, in which the bone fails to show the oriented arrangement of collagen fibers characteristic of lamellated bone.

Wrigley's Forceps This is a short curved forceps possessing a generous cephalic curve and an addea pelvic curve. It is made of stainless steel, is light. It is also shorter than long curved forceps as the handle and blades are shorter in length.

Wringing Wringing is a manipulation in which the tissues are lifted with both hands and compressed alternately between the fingers and thumb of opposite hands.

Wrinkle It is a furrow in the skin. It is a natural process developed during ageing or after severe prolonged illness. Wrinkles are most obvious on face and other exposed parts. Premature deep wrinkle may be caused by over exposure to sunlight or due to malnutrition. Vitamin A and vitamin E are supposed to be helpful.

Wrinkles and stretch marks The interwoven collagen fibres of reticular layer provide considerable tensile strength, and extensive array of elastic fibres enable the dermis to stretch and recoil repeatedly during normal movements. The water content also helps to maintain its flexibility and resilience, properties known as skin turgor. Dehydration causes a temporary decline in skin flexibility. Age, hormones and ultraviolet radiation permanently reduce the amount of elastin in dermis, producing wrinkles and sagging skin. After delivery abdominal skin wrinkles and creases creating a network of stretch marks. Stretch marks may be considered normal during periods of active such as adolescents.

Wrisberg, cartilage Cuneiform cartilage.

Wrist drop Wrist drops down so that back of hand cannot be brought horizontal. This causes weakness

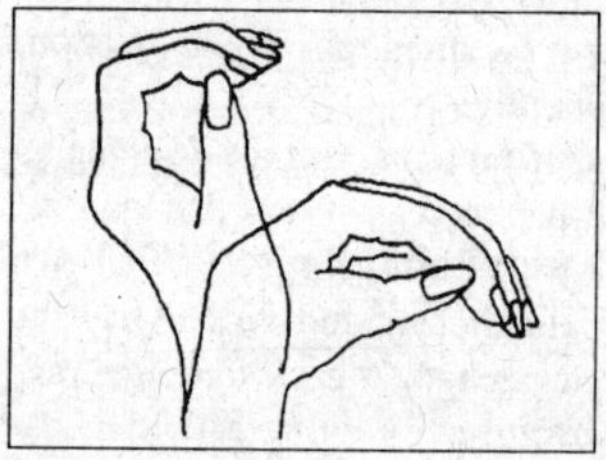

of grip because hand muscles cannot function efficiently. It is caused due to injury of radial nerve. Treatment involves holding the wrist straight with the help of simple splint. If damage is permanent treatment is arthrodesis.

Wrist It is the joint between hand and arm. It consists of eight bones arranged in two rows. The scaphoid, lunate, triquetral and pisiform bones which

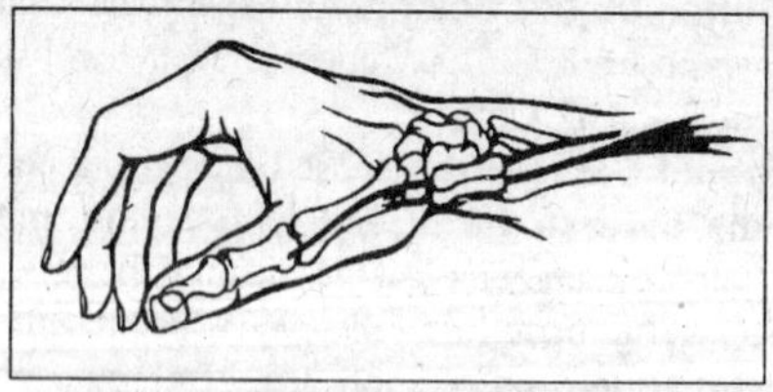

articulate with the radius and ulna and trapezium, trapezoid, capitate and hamate which are connected to the bones of palm that is metacarpals. Wrist injuries may limit movements due to scaphoid bone which often fails to heal and results in avascular necrosis. While in Colles fracture the lower end of radius is fractured and the wrist is displaced backward. Pressure on median nerve as it passes through the carpal tunnel causes numbness, tingling and pain in thumb, index and middle fingers. Radial nerve damage leads to wrist drop. Treatment involves holding the wrist drop.

Writer's cramp This is an occupationally induced dystonia. In it attempt to write is inhibited by dystonic posturing of hand and arm. The pen is gripped tightly. The hand can be successfully used for other purposes. No drug has been proved effective. It is probable that sustained muscular contraction and electrolyte imbalance are contributory factors. Some of such cramps would respond to night time dose of quinine (300 mg H.S.)

Written authorization Consent given in writing specifically empowering someone to do or assume a duty for another.

Wrongful death A legal cause of action brought by the relatives of a person who has died to recover the relatives losses, such as the loss of economic support.

Wuchereria bancrofti It is a thread-like worm with both sexes coiled which can only be separated with difficulty. The male worm is coiled with corkscrew-like tails while the anterior end tapers ending in swelling in female worm. The worm in humans mature in or near lymphatics and lymph nodes. The female produces large number of motile larvae. Many patients may remain asymptomatic. Episodes of fever with or without inflammation of the lymphatics and lymph nodes come and go. There may also be chills, headache, malaise and urticaria. Inflammation of spermatic cord and development of orchitis and epididymitis is common. Abscess may be formed at the site of lymphatic inflammation. Later, interference with normal lymphatic flow may produce hydrocele and lymphatic varices and elephantiasis in both sexes. Microfilaria may be seen in peripheral blood. Diethylcarbamazine (Hetrazan) 9 to 12 mg per kg of body weight daily in divided doses orally. The course may be repeated once or twice after 4 to 6 weeks treatment free intervals.

X

Xanthelasma It is a form of hyperlipidaemia due to abnormalities in lipid metabolism resulting in elevated levels of cholesterol and triglycerides. It affects the elderly person and gives rise to soft, flat, slightly elevated, round or oval, yellowish plaques on eyelids near inner canthus. Lesions may be multiple and symmetrical in distribution. It is a symmetrical butterfly-shaped slowly growing. It is produced by the accumulation of fat containing foam cells. It is more commonly seen in diabetic patients. It is more commonly seen in whites than non-whites and its presence indicates underlying coronary artery disease, hypertension or a definite predisposition.

Xanthoma It is a yellow deposit of fatty material in the skin often on elbow and buttocks indicating lipid disorder. It may deposit on internal organs and brain. It is commonly seen on eyelid. It is seen in atherosclerosis. Treatment aims to lower body cholesterol level.

Xenobiotic Foreign to life; desribing a synthetic product not formed by natural biosynthetic processes; i.e., a manufactured substance.

Xenodiagnosis Diagnostic technique in which researchers identify a disease by infecting a laboratory animals and assessing its symptoms.

Xenogeneic Genetic differences between species.

Xenogenic Graft Also xenograft, beterograft, beterolgou graft. Grafting material harvested from a species different from that of the recipient.

Xenograft A tissue or organ graft between individuals of different species.

Xenophobia Fear of outsiders.

Xenotransplantation Transplantation of an organ from a different species (e.g., pig organs).

Xeroderma pigmentosa It is a rare familial disorder inherited as an autosomal recessive trait develops due to defect in repair of ultraviolet light damaged DNA. There is hyperkeratosis and marked acanthosis of rete malpighian. It presents with mild erythema and gross freckle-like macules usually worse on face, neck and exposed hands and arms. The freckles generally coalesce together. Later condition gives rise to pigmented macular lesions with atrophic patches, continued exposure to sunlight may lead to epidermal scarring and even epidermal malignancies. It may develop aggressively and may prove fatal.

Xerosis It is a dry lustreless condition of conjunctiva. It occurs in two groups. Due to vitamin 'A' deficiency triangular white patches on cornea develops. It is covered by a dried foam, not being wetted by tears known as Bitot's spot. Due to trachoma, burns resulting cicatricial degeneration of conjunctiva lead to decreased secretion of mucus.

Xerostomia Actually it is not a disease but it is a sign of impaired function of the salivary gland. Mumps may produce temporary xerostomia. But diseases like Mikulicz's disease or Sjogren's syndromes produce irreversible disease. Radiation to head and neck results in atrophy of salivary glands and dry mouth. Ganglion blocking agents may also result it. In mild form patient may be asymptomatic and mucosa appears normal. In severe cases, it may result in dry mouth and burning syndrome. Patches of mucosa will develop atrophic. In severe xerostomia, erosion and ulceration of inflamed mucosa will occur.

Xiphisternum It is known as xiphoid process, the small, leaf-shaped projections which constitute lower three parts of sternum.

Xiphoid process The lower segment of the sternum.

Xiphoid Sword-shaped. The inferior portion of the sternum is the xiphoid process.

X-linkage Mode of genetic transmission in which a tract or gene is linked to the X-chromosome. Has been implicated in some cases of bipolar disorder.

X-linked recessive inheritance In it mother is a carrier. Statistically, 50% male offspring are affected and 50% of female offspring are carriers.

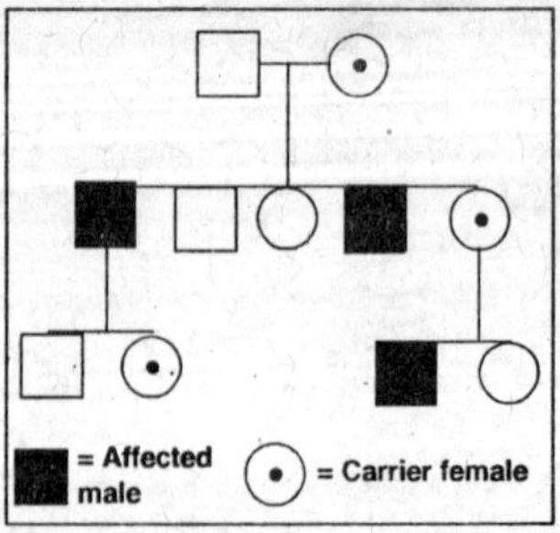

X-ray These were discovered in 1896 by Wilhelm Conard Roentgen. These can be used to produce images of bones, organs and soft tissues. Bones are dense and contain calcium, they absorb X-rays well. These are harmful to body.

X-ray crystallography The analysis of x-ray diffraction patterns of a crystalline compound, used to determine the molecule's three-dimensional structure. It is a pivotal technique in determining molecular structure. Insulin and secretin were among the first few chemicals whose structures were determined using this technique.

XXY syndrome It is a chromosomal disorder which results from genotype with 47 chromosomes, 44 autosomes and XXY sex chromosomes. Clinically there will be growth acceleration in early and mid childhood, myopia, hypogonadism and neuromuscular incoordination. Bones of cranium and limbs become thick.

Xylem Tube-like cells of the plant conductive tissue that carry water and minerals from the roots to other parts of the plant and also provide structural strength.

Y

Yang The portion of the whole realm of function of the body, mind, and spirit in Eastern thought that corresponds with sympathetic autonomic nervous system functions. It is a chinese assumption like vat, Pita and kaph of Ayurveda of India.

Yates' correction A correction factor sometimes used chisquare tests in which the expected frequency in several cells is very small.

Yates correction for continuity An adjustment to the chisquare value rcommended when counts in the contingency table are small, because the binomial distribution is discontinuous.

Yawning It is an involuntary act usually associated with drowsiness and boredom. It is accompanied by increase in heart rate, slight constriction of blood capillaries and watering of eyes. It is caused by raised levels of CO_2 and aim of yawning is to reduce CO_2 and to raise oxygen. It is infections and its mechanism is unknown.

Yaws A fly-transmitted disease that is caused by the spirochete *Treponema.*

Years Lived with Disability In public health, a measurement of the number of years lived with a disability of known severity and duration.

Years of Life Lost In public health, a measurement of the number of years of life lost due to premature death. Defined as a death occurring before the age to which the dying person could have expected to survive.

Yeast A single-celled fungus that reproduces by budding or fission.

Yeild point 1. Place on the stress-strain curve marked permanent deformation occurs; it is just beyond the proportional limit. 2. The point where permanent deformation starts in a metal.

Yellow colouration of mucosa Jaundice or icterus makes yellow discolouration of conjunctiva and sclera. The discolouration is produced by an increase in blood level of bilirubin. Jaundice appears when serum bilirubin exceeds 2 to 3 mg. Haemolysis is the most common cause of excessive production of bilirubin. It is a feature of number of diseases, i.e. sickle cell anaemia, polycythaemia, etc. Reduced excretion of conjugated bilirubin is found in cases of hepatocellular injuries such as viral hepatitis. Physical manifestation of jaundice is yellow tinge of eyes, skin and oral mucous membrane.

Yellow fever A viral disease transmitted by the mosquito Aedes aegypti.

Yellow marrow Specialized lipid storage tissue, within bone cavities.

Yellow nail syndrome It is a familial disorder transmitted genetically. Clinically, there are yellow coloured nails and lymphatic oedema. Nail growth ceases with thickening of nails and increased convexity followed by loss of nails. There may be non-specific pleural effusion. Multiple papillomas may be seen over lips. Along with mental retardation nails are atrophic, brittle and dystrophic. Patient will have prominent chin and small skull.

Yergason's ring Resisted supination of arm when elbow is flexed causes pain with bicipital tendinitis.

Yerkes-Dodson law The principle that moderate levels of arousal tend to yield optimal performance.

Yield strength The amount of deforming force, or stress, just above the elastic limit, at which point a substance begins to exhibit plastic deformation.

Yin The portion of the whole realm of function of the body, mind, and spirit in Estern thought that corresponds with parasympathetic autonomic nervous system functions.

Yoga A series of exercises aimed at controlling one's body and mind. Most of the various types involve intense concentration on some specific form of stimulation. It involves, centering, onself through physical stretches and psychological focussing and awareness.

Yogurt It is a concentrated milk in which for fermentation lactic acid is used. Soured and fermented milk contains all vitamins and nutrients as that of milk.

Yolk protein Proteins stored in the eggs of oviparous and ovoviviparous vertebrates, and utilized during embryonic development.

Yolk sac In humans, involved with the production of blood cells in the developing embryo.

Yolk sac tumour It is the most common testicular neoplasm in infants and young children. Pure form presents as infiltrate, homogeneous, yellow white mucinous lesions. Microscopically they are composed of cuboidal neoplastic cells arranged in a lace-like network. Solid areas and papillae may also be seen.

Y-shaped infusion set In this two bottles can be hung in a parallel line using 'Y' type of administration set. Hence one can switch from one solution to another by simply adjusting the clamps on the tubing. This method is simply employed to administer normal saline solution and whole blood.

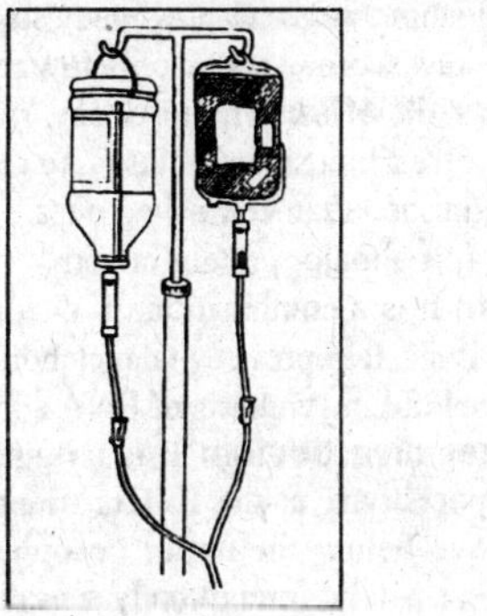

Z

Z score A deviation score divided by the standard deviation; indicates how many standard deviations the raw score is above or below the mean.

Zeigarnik effect The tendency, when one is ego-involved in a series of tasks, to recall more of the unfinished than completed ones.

Zein It is a major protein in corn.

Zemin It is a combination of Vitamin E, vitamin C and zinc. It improves vital metabolic functions. Zinc is helpful in synthesis of RNA and DNA.

Zenker diverticulum It is an outpouching of the hypopharynx at the Killian triangle immediately above below the upper oesophageal sphincter. There will be foreign body sensation, scratchiness or fullness during and after eating. Larger diverticula cause constant fullness and a sensation, of food sticking in the throat. They also cause frothy saliva, oral fetor, cough and regurgitation. It commonly presents with dysphagia.

Zinc It is essential for normal growth, development of reproductive systems and normal function of prostate gland. It helps in healing of wounds. Rich sources are lean meat, whole grain bread and cereals. Dried beans also contain lot of zinc. Unprocessed foods contain good amount of it. So deficiency develops when intestinal absorption is impaired like malabsorption. Symptoms include impairment of taste and loss of appetite. Hair may also be thinned out and lost. Its deficiency impairs child's growth. Excess of it interferes with absorption of iron and copper and can develop nausea and vomiting.

Zinc finger A specialized protein motif involved in DNA recognition by some DNA-binding proteins; characterized by a single atom of zinc coordinated to four Lys residues or to two His and two Lys residues.

Zinc oxide It is a mild astringent and have soothing effect. It is used to treat painful, itchy or moist skin. It makes creams thicker to be used easily.

Zinc oxide eugenol A material made by mixing zinc oxide powder with eugenol liquid used in dentistry as a cement, base temporary restorative, impression material and the like.

Zinc oxide eugenol impression paste It is used as an impression material as well as peridontal dressing cavity base, temporary cement and temporary restorative material. Chemical composition for each application is the same.

Zincolak capsule Zinc is necessary in the synthesis of serum proteins. Its deficiency leads to delay in healing of wounds and ulcers.

Zinc helps in acne vulgaris and improves taste perception.

Zinn, annulus Annulus tendineus communis.

Zollinger-Ellison syndrome It is rare. There develops severe and recurrent peptic ulcers in stomach. It is caused usually by pancreatic condition which often goes undiagnosed. But high levels of gastrin are sufficient to confirm the diagnosis. Tumour is slow growing in origin. Total gastrectomy is necessary.

Zona fasciculata Middle zone of the adrenal cortex that secretes glucocorticoids.

Zona glomerulosa Outer zone of the adrenal cortex that secretes mineralocorticoids.

Zona pellucida Clear glycoprotein layer between a secondary ooccyte and the surrounding granulosa cells of the corona radiata.

Zona reticularis Inner zone of the adrenal cortex that secretes small amounts of sex hormones.

Zone alveolar Bony socket in which the tooth is held in mandible and maxilla.

Zonular cataract It is an opaque area around the embryonic nucleus. The opaque area is sharply demarcated and lens within and around the opaque zone is clear. In some cases there may be linear opacities from the opaque zone running towards the equator.

It has a genetic origin with strong hereditary tendency. Deficiency of vitamin D appears as a potent factor. The incisors and canines show erosion and transverse lines across them. Infant is not able to see and there is an abnormal movement of eyes.

Zoonosis Any disease of animals that can be transmitted to humans.

Zoonotic Describing a human disease that derives from a nonhuman infection, especially a disease transmitted to people from vertebrate animals.

Zoospore A free-living and flagellated reproductive structure of fungi.

Zoster Infection with varicella-zoster virus which leads to skin lesion on the trunk following the distribution of the sensory nerves; commonly called shingles.

Zoster ophthalmicus It will lead to neuralgia, unilateral pain as well as vesicles and oedema in the skin area supplied by first branch of trigeminal nerve. It may involve nose. There may be acellular serous iritis with secondary glaucoma.

Zoster oticus Onset is with intense neuralgic form of ear pain involving areas supplied by specific nerves. Rapid formation of clustered vesicles on an erythematous base. It is present only for a few days involving auricle and/or the external ear canal. Fever may develop.

Zovirax (acyclovir) It inhibits viral DNA synthesis. Taken orally about 20 per cent is absorbed from the gut which is sufficient to treat some systemic infections. It is effective in skin infections including genital herpes when new lesions are forming. In ointment form it is used against ocular keratitis. Drug is excreted in urine.

***Z*-score** A deviation score divided by the standard deviation; indicates how many standard deviations the raw score is above or below the mean.

Zsigmondy palmer Tooth numbering system involving a grid which indicates four quadrants.

Z-tests Significance tests used to compare differences between proportions.

Z-track Causing a needle track, or pathway, in the shape of a "Z".

Z-track technique Injection method that prevents medication from leaking outside the muscle.

Zuckerkandl, organs Paired chromaffin-cell bodies on the aorta near origin of inferior mesenteric artery.

Zwitterion A dipolar ion, with spatially separated positive and negative charges.

Zygoma The cheek bone; appears as a diffuse radiopaque band posterior to the zygomatic process of the maxilla (also called the zygomatic or malar bone).

Zygomatic Referring to the zygomatic, or cheek bone; the zygomatic arch is a bony arch created by the junction of the zygomatic and temporal bones.

Zygomatic arch Zygomatic process of the temporal bone. Bowlike prominence created at the side of the head by temporal process of the zygoma uniting with the zygomatic process of the temporal bone.

Zygomatic bone Malar; quadrangular bone on each side of the face that unites the frontal and superior maxillary bones with the zygomatic process of the temporal bone.

It forms the cheek prominence, a portion of the lateral wall and floor of the orbit, and parts of the temporal fossa and infratemporal fossa.

Zygomatic process of the maxilla A bony projection of the maxilla that articulates with the zygoma; appears as a J-or U-shaped radiopacity on a maxillary molar periapical film.

Zygomaticus Muscle that elevates the corners of the mouth and lips; also known as the smiling muscle.

Zygomaticus muscle A muscle originating on the zygomatic, or cheek, bone; the zygomatic arch is a bony arch created by the junction of the zygomatic and temporal bones.

Zygote It is produced when sperm fertilises an ovum. It contains all the genetic material for a new person, half from sperm and half from ova. It measures 0.1 mm. After about a week it implants into uterus.

Zygote intrafallopian transfer (ZIFT) An assisted reproductive procedure in which eggs are retrieved, fertilized in vitro, and transferred to the fallopian tube at the pronuclear stage prior to cell division. ZIFT is used when proof of fertilization is essential in situations such as severe male factor infertility or immunologic infertility.

Zymogen The inactive form of a protein in a cell, converted to an active enzyme after being secreted by the cell. Inactive enzymes that becomes active when part of their structure is removed by action of another enzyme of some other means.

Section-2
General Information

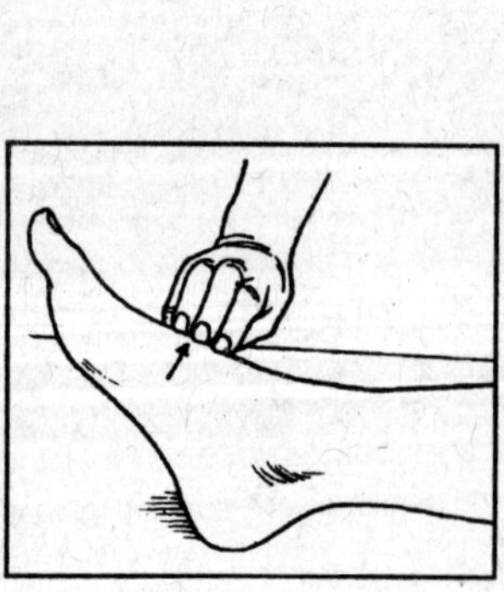 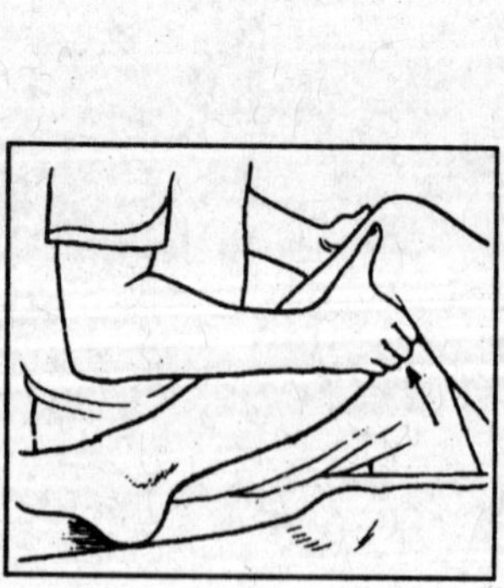 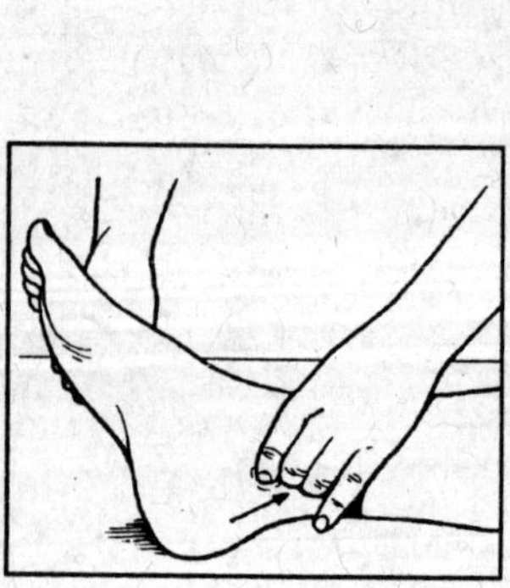

CONTENTS

ABBREVIATIONS (Nuclear Medicine)

Accuracy Probability that a test will yield the correct diagnosis.
ACEI Angiotensin-converting enzyme inhibitors
AD Alzheimer's dementia.
ADHD Attention deficit hyperactivity disorder
Anion Electro negative ion, element or molecule.
Antisense In molecular genetics; Strand of DNA having set of nucleotides complementary to the sense strand.
Apoptosis Programmed cell death, suicidal pathway of cell stored in the genes.
Aptamer Novel nucleic acid-binding species
BGO Bismuth germanate.
Cation Electro positive ion, element or molecule.
Chelate Chemical compound that sequesters and firmly binds a metallic ion into a ring, thus shielding the chemical effects of the metal.
Chemotaxis Orientation of a cell along a chemical gradient, or movement in the direction of the gradient.
Compartmental analysis Method of analyzing the data, in which the organ or system under study is represented a set of compartments, e.g. intra-vascular, extra-cellular fluid (ECF), intra-cellular, and excretion compartments.
DAS Dynamic antral scintigraphy.
Deconvolution analysis Mathematical technique to reconstruct a function at time T from measurements at a later time.
DLBD diffuse Lewy body disease.
Dose, exposed Amount of radiaton emitted to the organ or system or body under study, expressed in Coulombs/kilogram int he current SI system, or mR (milli Roentgen) in the old system : 1 Roentgen = $2.58.10^{-4}$ Coulombs/kilogram.
Eluate Product of elution, i.e. separation by washing, such as freeing an enzyme from its absorbent.
EOB End of bombardment, i.e, of the target in a cyclotron.
Epitope Antigenic determinant.
ER Estrogen receptor in breast cancer.
ETT Esophageal transit time, in gastro-enterology; or exercise treadmill test in cardiology.
Oncogenesis The formation of cancer cells.
OSEM Ordered subsets maximum-likelihood expectation-maximization; iterative reconstruciton algorithm.
PCR Polymerase chain reaction.
PET Positron emission tomography; the term ET for emission tomography, combining both SPECT and PET, has not been generally accepted.
Pgp P-glycoprotein.
PIOPED Prospective Investigation of Pulmonary Embolish Diagnosis.
Plasmid An automously replicating DNA molecule.
PMT Photomultiplies tube.
PNA Polypeptide nucleic acid.
PPV Positive predicitive value; likehood that a positive test result indicates presence of disease.
PR Progesterone receptor of tumors.
PTCA Percutaneous transluminal coronary angioplasty.
Radiolysis Decomposition of a radio-labeled compound by the raditation emitted by its own radioactive nuclide.
Radionuclide Radio-active element; formerly isotope.
Radiopharmaceutical Biological compound or pharmaceutical labeled with a radioactive element to trace its pathway; used for diagnositc or therapeutic purposes.
RASON Radiolabeled antisense oligodeoxynucleotide.

RBF Renal Blood Flow.
RCBF Regional cerebral blood flow.
RCMR-Xx Regional cerebral metabolic rate of substance Xx.
Rebinning Regrouping of data, for faster processing by computer algorithms.
ROI Region of interest.
Scintillator Substance that emits light after interaction with high-energy photons.
Sensitivity Probability that a test will detect presence of disease.
Specificity Probability that a test will determine absence of disease.
SPECT Single photon emission computed tomography.
SPM Statistical parametric mapping.
SPN Solitary pulmonary nodule.
SUV Standardized uptake value; ratio of measured activity in a certain area to the expected activity if the radioactivity were homogeneously distributed through the body.
TCA cycle Tricarboxylic acid cycle.
TER Tubular extraction rate.
Transduction Transfer of DNA via a bacteriophage to another cell, thereby changing the constitution of the second organism, also called genetic recombination.
Transfection Artificial infecton of cells by nucleic acid isolated from virus or bacteriophage, resulting in production of mature virus or phage particles.
Transgenic animal Animal in which every cell carries a specific new or altered gene of interest.
TTNA Trans-thoracic needle aspiration.
USP United States Pharmacopoeia.
YSO Yttrium oxy-orthosilicate; high-energy scintillator.
FBP Filtered back-projection reconstruction algorithm for tomography.
FNA Fine-needle aspiration.
FWHM Full width at half maximum.
FWTM Full width at one tenth of the maximum.
Genome The full set of genes of an individual.
GFR Glomerular filtration rate.
Glucose Clamp method to keep serum glucose within a specific range by infusing insulin and glucose stimultaneously; originally developed for arterial glucose levels (invasive), but in most PET centers applied to keep venous glucose levels constant in myocardial metabolism studies.
GLUT Glucose transporter: subtypes are indicated with an ARabic numeral.
Glycolysis Breaking down of sugars into simpler compounds; specifically, the metabolic degradation path of glucose.
Glycoprotein Conjugated protein, having protein (s) with a carbohydrate group.
HAMA Human anti-mouse antibody.
HPLC High-pressure liquid chromatography.
HSSTR Human somatostatin receptor.
HVIPR Human vasoactive intestinal peptide receptor.
Hydrophilic Having affinity for water.
Hygroscopic Material that attract water or water vapors.
IBD Inflammatory bowel disease.
ICAM Intercullar adhesion molecule.
K_a Association constant of a chemcial reaction, e.g. binding of an agonist or antibody to its receptor on the cell membrane.
K_d Dissociation constant of a chemical reaction.
KeV Killo electron Volt: energy an electron accumulates after acceleration over 1000 Volts.

Ligan Molecule or compound active in biological processes, usually a small molecule that binds specifically to a larger one, e.g. antibody binding to an antigen, hormone or neurotransmitter binding to a receptor, substrate binding to an enzyme.
Lipophilic Having affinity for fat.
LSO Cerium-activated lutetium oxy-orthosilicate; high energy scintillator.
LVEF Left ventricular ejection fraction.
MDR Multidrug resistance.
Micturition Voiding of bladder.
MIRD Medical internal radiation dose.
MLEM Maximum-likelihood expectation-maximization.
MoAB, MAB monoclonal antibody.
MSA Multi-system atrophy.
Normoxic Having normal oxygen tension.
NPV Negative predictive value, likelihood that a negative test result indicates absence of disease.
NSCLC Non-small-cell lung cancer.
OCD Obsessive compulsive disorder.
Oncogene Gene with properties for inducing cancer.
Accelerator A machine to accelerate charged particles linearly or in circular paths by means of an electromagnetic field. The accelerated particles such as a -particles, protons, deuterons, and heavy ions posses high energies and can cause nuclear reactions in target atoms by irradiation.
Accuracy A term used indicate how close a measurement of a quantity is to its true value.
Annihilation radiation g-Radiations of 511 keV energy emitted at 180° after a b^{+}-particle is annihilated by combining with an electron in matter.
Atomic mass unit (amu) By definition, one twelfth of the mass of 12/6 C, equal to 1.66×10^{-24} G or 931 MeV.
Atomic number (Z) The number of protons in the nucleus of an atom.
Attenuation A process by which the intensity of radiation is reduced by absorption and/or scattering during its passage through matter.
Attenuation coefficient The fraction of g-ray energy attenuated, absorbed plus scattered per unit length of an absorber (Linear attenuation coefficient, m) or per gram of an absorber mass attenuation coefficient, m_m.
Auger electron An electron ejected from an energy shell, instead of a characteristic x-ray emission, carrying the energy equal to that of the x-ray minus its binding energy.
Average life (t) See Mean life.
Avogadro's number The number of molecules in 1 g. mole of any substance or the number of atoms in 1 gm atom of any element. It is equal to 6.02×10^{23}.
Becquerel (Bq) A unit of radioactivity. One becquerel is equal to 1 disintegration per second.
Binding energy The energy to bind two entities together. In a nucleus, it is the energy needed to separate a nucleon completely from other nucleons in the nucleus. In a chemical bond, it is the energy necessary to separate two binding partners an infinite distance.
Biological half-life (T_b) The time by which one half of an administered dosage of a substance is eliminated by biological processes such as urinary and fecal excretions.
Bremsstrahlung g-Ray photons produced by deceleration of charged particles near the nucleus of an absorber atom.
Carrier A stable element that is added in detectable quantities to a radio-nuclide of the same element, usually to facilitate chemical processing of the radionuclide.
Carrier-free A term used to indicate the absence of any stable atoms in a radionuclide sample.
Collimator A device to confine a beam of radiation within a specific field of view. Collimators may be converging, pinhole, diverging, and parallel hole types.

Collimator efficiency The number of photons passing through the collimator for each unit of activity present in a source.

Collimator resolution A component of spatial resolution of an imaging system contributed by the collimator. It is also called geometric resolution.

Committed dose equivalent (H_T, 50) The dose equivalent to organs or tissues of reference (T) that will be received from an intake of radioactive material by an individual during the 50-year period following intake.

Compton scattering In this process, a g-ray transfers only a partial amount of energy to an outer orbital electron of an absorber, and the photon itself is deflected with less energy.

Cross section (s) The probability of occurrence of a nuclear reaction or the formation of a radionuclide in a nuclear reaction. It is expressed in a unit termed barn; 1 barn = 10^{-24} cm^2.

Curie (Ci) A unit of activity. A curie is defined as 3.7 x 10^{10} disintegrations per second.

Dead time The period of time that a counter remains insensitive to count the next after an event.

Decay constant (l) The fraction of atoms of a radioactive element decaying per unit time. It is expressed as l = 0.693 /t½, where t½ is the half-life of the radionuclide.

Deep-dose equivalent (H_d) Dose equivalent at a tissue depth of 1 cm (1000 mg/cm^2) resulting from external whole-body exposure.

Dosimetry The calculation or measurement of radiation absorbed doses.

Effective half-life (Te) Time required for an initial administered dose to be reduced to one half as a result of both physical decay and biological elemination of a radionuclide. It is given by $T_e = (T_p \times T_b) (T_p + T_b)$; where T_e is the effective half-life, and T_p and T_b are the physical and biological half-lifes, respectively.

Electron (e^-) A negatively charged particle rotating around the atomic nucleus. It has a charge of 4.8 x 10^{-10} electrostatic units and a mass of 9.1 x 10^{-28} g, equivalent to 0.511 MeV, or equal to 1/1836 of the mass of a proton.

Electron capture (EC) A mode of decay of a proton-rich radionuclide in which an orbital electron is captured by the nucleus, accompanied by emission of a neutrino and characteristic x-rays or Auger electons.

Electron volt (eV) The kinetic energy gained by an electron when accelerated through a potential difference of 1 V.

Energy resolution Capability of a detecting system to separate two g- rays-ray peaks of different energies. It is given by the full width at half maximum (FWHM) of a given photopeak.

Erg The unit of energy or work done by a force of 1 dyne through a distance of 1 cm.

Fission (f) A nuclear process by which a nucleus divides into two nearly equal smaller nuclei, along with the emission of two to three neutrons.

Free radical A highly reactive chemical species that has one or more unpaired electrons.

Generator, radionuclide A device in which a short-lived daughter is separated chemically and periodically from a long-lived parent absorbed on absorbent material. For example, ^{99m}Tc is separated from ^{99}Mo from the Moly generator with saline.

Gray (Gy) The unit of absorbed radiation dose in SI units. One gray s equal to 100 rad

Half-life (t½) A unique characteristic of a radionuclide, defined by the time during which an initial activity of a radionuclide is reduced to one half. It is related to the decay constant l by t½ = 0.693/l .

Half-value layer (HVL) The thickness of an absorbing material required to reduce the intensity or exposure of a radiation beam to one half of the initial value when placed in the path of the beam.

Internal conversion An alternative mode to g-ray decay in which nuclear excitation energy is transferred to an orbital electron, which is then ejected from the orbit.

Intrinsic efficiency The number of radiations detected divided by the number of radiations striking the detector.

Intrinsic resolution A component of the spatial resolution of an imaging system that is contributed by the detector and associated electronics and depends on the photon energy, detector thickness, and the number of PM tubes.

Ion An atom or group of atoms with a positive charge cation or a negative charge anion.

Isobars Nuclides having the same mass number, that is, the same total number of neutrons and protons. Examples are 57/26 Fe and 57/27 Co.

Isomeric transition (IT) Decay of the excited state of an isomer of a nuclide to a lower excited state or the ground state.

Isomers Nuclides having the same atomic and mass numbers but differing in energy and spin of the nuclei. For example, ^{99} Tc and ^{99m} Tc are isomers.

Isotones Nuclides have the same number of neutrons in the nucleus. For example, 131/53 and 132/54 Xe are isotones.

Isotopes Nuclides having the same automatic number, that is, the same number of protons in the nucleus. Examples are 14/6C and 12/6C.

LD 50/30 A quantity of a substance that, when administered or applied to a group of any living species, kills 50% of the group in 30 days.

Linear energy transfer (LET) Energy deposited by radiation per unit length of the matter through which the radiation passes. Its usual unit is kev/mm.

Mass defect The difference between the mass of the nucleus and the combined masses of individual nucleons of the nucleus of a nuclide.

Mass (A) The total number of protons and neutrons in a nucleus of a nuclide.

Mean life (t) The average expected lifetime of a group of radionuclides before disintegration. It is related to the half-life and decay constant by t =1/l = 1.44½.

Metastable state (m). An excited state of a nuclide that decays to a lower excited or the ground state by isomeric transition with a measurable half-life.

Modulation transfter function A quantitative value of the spatial resolution of an imaging system.

No carrier added (NCA) A term used to characterize the state of a radioactive material to which no stable **isotope** of the compound has been added purposely.

Nucleon A common term for neutrons or protons in the nucleus of a nuclide.

Organ, critical The organ that is functionally essential for the body and recieves the highest radiation dose after administration of radioactivity.

Organ, target The organ intended to be imaged and expected to receive the greatest concentration of administered radioactivity.

Pair production g-Rays with energy greater than 1.02 MeV interact with the nucleus of an absorber atom, and a positron and an electron are produced at the expense of the photon.

Photoelectric effect A process in which a g-ray, while passing through an absorber, transfers all its energy to an orbital electron, primarily the K-shell electron of an absorber, and the photoelectron is ejected from the shell.

Photofraction The fraction of all detected g-rays that contributes to the photopeak.

Precision A term used to indicate the reproducibility of the measurement of a quantity when measurements are made repeatedly.

Quality factor (QF) A factor dependent on linear energy transfer that is multiplied by absorbed doses to calculate the dose equivalents in rem. It is used in radiation protection to take into account the relative radiation damage caused by different radiations. It is 1 for x-, g-, and b-rays and 10 for neutrons and protons

Rad The unit of radiation-absorbed dose. One rad is equal to 100 ergs of radiation energy depo ed per gram of any matter, or 10^{-2} J/kg of any matter.

Radiation weighting factor (Wr) A factor that depends on the types of radiation and is used to convert rad to rem in radiation protection. Rem = rad x Wr.

Range The straight line distance traversed by a charged particle in an absorber.

Relative biologic effectiveness (RBD) A factor used to calculate the dose equivalent in rem from rad. It is defined as the ratio of the amount of a standard radiation that causes certain biological damage to the amount of radiation in question that causes the same biological damage.

Roentgen The quantity of x- or g-radiations that produces one electrostatic unit of positive or negative charge in 1 cm^3 of air at 0°C and 760-mm Hg pressure. It is equal to 2.58 x 10^{-4} C/kg air.
Roentgen equivalent man (rem) A dose equivalent defined by the absorbed dose (rad) times the relative biological effectiveness or quality factor of the radiation in question.
Scintillation scanning or imaging Recording of the distribution of radio-activity in the body or a section of the body by the use of a NaI (TI) detector to form an image.
Scintigraphy A photographic recording of the distribution of radioacitivity in an area of interest in the body by the use of a gamma camera.
Sensitivitiy The number of counts per unit time detected by an imaging device for each unit of activity present in a source. It is expressed in cps/mCi.
Shallow-dose equivalent (Hs) Dose equivalent at a tissue depth of 0.007 cm (7mg/cm^2) from external exposure to the skin.
Sievert (Sv) The SI unit of dose equivalent and equal to 100 rem.
Spatial resolution A measure of the ability of an imaging device to faithfully reproduce the image of an object. It is given by the modulation transfer function i.e. MTF and is determined by the Fourier transform of the line spread function.
Specific activity The amount of radioactivity per unit mass of a radionuclide or labeled compound.
Specific ionization The number of primary and secondary ion pairs produced by an incident radiation per unit path length in an absorber.
Thermal neutron Neutrons of thermal energy 0.025 eV.
Tissue weighting factor (W_T) The weighting factor of an organ or tissue is the proportion or risk of stochastic effects resulting from irradiation of that organ or tissue to the total risk of stochastic effects.

APGAR SCORING CHART (Newborn)

Sign	*0*	*1*	*2*
Heart rate	Absent	Slow (below 100)	Over 100
Respiratory effort	Absent	Weak cry, hypoventilation	Good strong cry
Muscle tone	Limp extremities	Some flexion	Well flexed
Reflex response			
(i) Response to catheter in nostril (tested after oropharynx is clear)	No response	Grimace	Cough or sneeze
(ii) Tangential foot slap	No response	Grimace	Cry and withdrawal of foot
Colour	Blue, pale	Body, pink, Extremities blue	Completely pink

APPEARANCE OF OTHER POINTS OF OSSIFICATION

1st year	Heads of humerus, femur, and tibia
2nd year	Lower ends of radius, tibia, and fibula
3rd year	Patella
4th year	Upper end of fibula, great trochanter of femur (4-5)
5th year	Lower end of fibula. Greater tubercle of humerus.
6th year	Head of radius. Lower end of ulna.
8th-10 years	Rami of ischium and pubis, olecranon.
10th-11th years	Trochlea of humerus. Lesser trochanter of femur.
12th-14th years	External condyle of humerus.
14th-16th years	Acromion, iliac crest, lesser trochanter.
17th-18th years	Tuber ischii (17 in female, 10 in male). Inner clavicle 20-21.

APPEARANCE OF POINTS OF OSSIFICATION

	Food	*Hand*
5th-6th month, intra-uterine	Calcaneus (body)	Whole hand cartilaginous during intrauterine life
7th ,, ,,	Talus	
9th ,, ,,	Cuboid	
1st year, extra-uterine	External	Capitate and hamate
2nd ,, ,,	cuneiform (1-2)	First four metacarpal heads
3rd ,, ,,	Internal cuneiform Tarsal navicular	Triquetral (2-3)
4th ,, ,,	Mid cuneiform	Lunate (4-5)
5th ,, ,,	Scaphoid (4-5)	Trapezium (5-6) Carpal navicular
6th ,, ,,		Scaphoid (6-7)
8th ,, ,,		Trapezoid (6-7)
10th ,, ,,	Calcaneus (epiphysis) (0-10)	m. (10-11)[1]

DENTITION TABLE

Milk Teeth

The first dentition begins at the sixth or seventh month and is complete by about second year.

Central incisors	—	Lower, 6th month
	—	Upeer, 7th month
Lateral incisors	—	Upper, 9th month
	—	Lower, 10th month
First molar	—	12 month
Canines	—	18 month
Second molars	—	2 years

In fully primary dentition there are 20 teeth, 10 in each jaw.

Permanent Teeth

First molar	—	6.5 years
Lower central incisors	—	7 years
Upper central incisors	—	8 years
Lateral incisors	—	9 years
First bicuspid	—	10 years
Second bicuspid	—	11 years
Canines	—	12 years

Second molars (wisdom) 17 to 25 years or any later date. The full permanent dentition comprises 32 teeth, i.e. 16 in each jaw.

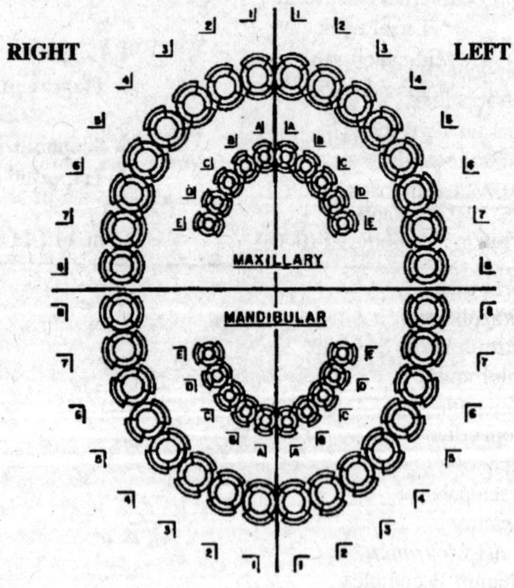

Drugs that may harm the child who is on breast feeding

Agent	*Adverse feeding*
Phenobarbital	Drowsiness, rickets, rash, methaemoglobinaemia
Diazepam	Drowsiness, rise in serum bilirubin
Laxatives	Loose motion
Penicillin	Rash
Narcotics	Withdrawal symptoms
Theophylline	Irritability
Sulphas	Drug rash, haemolysis
Oral contraceptives	Failure to thrive, gynaecomastia

Drugs that discolour the stools

Iron
Bismuth
Lead
Aspirin
Activated charcoal
Anticoagulants
Vanquin
Aluminium hydroxide

Drugs which may cause photosensitivity

Photoallergy
- Sulphonamide
- Tetracyclines
- Antihistaminics
- PABA

Phototoxicity
- Sulphonamides
- Tetracyclines
- Coal tar derivatives
- Nalidixic acid
- Antibacterial soaps

Drugs that discolour the urine

Rust yellow or brownish
- Furazolidone
- Nitrofurantoin
- Chloroquine
- Primaquine
- Mepacrine
- Alcohol
- Arsenicals
- Mercury

Yellow or green discolouration
- Vitamin B complex
- Vitamin C

- Methylene blue

Pink to red brown

- Phenothiazines
- Haemolysis producing drugs
- Haematuria producing drugs

Magenta to purple orange

- Phenoiphthalein
- Brown to black discolouration
- Resorcinol
- Methylene blue
- Furoxone
- Furadantin
- Aniline dyes

Blue discolouration

- Methylene blue

Drugs excreted in Breast Milk

Analgesics	• Morphine • Codeine • Heroin • Aspirin • Phenacetin
Antibiotics	• Chloramphenicol • Isonex • Neomycin • PAS • Streptomycin • Sulphonamides • Tetracycline
Antihistaminics	• Benadryl group and other (cough syrups)
Barbiturates and sedatives	• Luminal (Phenytoin) • Gardinal (Phenobarbitone) • Bromides
Laxatives	• Rhubarb • Senna • Cascara
Vitamin	• Practically all
Miscellaneous	• Nicotine • Corticosteroids • Alcohol • Ether • Oral contraceptives • Ephedrine

---

Drugs which are nephrotoxic (toxic to kidneys)

Gentamicin
Kanamycin
Tetracycline
Neomycin

Nalidixic acid
Rifampicin
Mercurials
Trimethadone
Griseofulvin
Viomycin

Drugs that may cause hepatotoxicity (toxic to liver)

Mepacrine
Chlorpromazine
Tetracycline
Isonex (isoniazid)
Paracetamol
Nalidixic acid
Ethambutol
Erythromycin esolate
Griseofulvin

Drugs that may cause hiccup

Short-acting barbiturates
Muscle relaxant
Diezepam

EFFECTS OF DRUGS

Drugs that are known teratogens and have adverse fetal effects during pregnancy

Drug	*Adverse fetal effects*
A. In the first trimester	
Alcohol (chronic)	Fetal alcohol syndrome
Cytotoxic drug	Greatest risk with alkylating agents and anti-metabolities.
Lithium	Cardiovascular anomalies
Phenytoin	Fetal phenytoin syndrome
Synthetic progestogens	Virilization of female fetus
Thalidomide	Phocomelia
Valproate	Neural tube defects
Warfarin	Limb defects, optic atrophy, deafness
B. In the second and third trimester	
Alcohol (large chronic dose)	Fetal alcohol syndrome
Analgesics	
Aspirin Closure of ductus	
Indomethacin	Closure of ductus
Narcotic analgesics	Respiratory depression and withdrawal syndrome
Antibiotics	
Streptomycin	Auditory and vestibular nerve damage
Chloramphenicol	'Grey' syndrome, vascular collapse
Tetracycline	Discolouring of primary and secondary dentition
Sulphonamide	Neonatal jaundice, kernicterus
Dapsone	Neonatal haemolysis
Anticoagulant drugs	
Warfarin	Neonatal haemorrhage
Anticonvulsive drugs	
Barbiturates	Prolonged depressant effects
Antihypertensive drugs	
Diazoxide	Fetal distress and impaired carbohydrate metabolism
Propranolol	Hyperglycaemia
Anti-psychotics	
Tricyclic antidepressants	Neonatal irritability, fits
Benzodiazepines	Hypotonia/hypothermia
Anti-thyroid drugs	
Iodides	Neonatal goitre and hypothyroidism
Diuretics	
Thiazides	Fetal hyponatraemia, hypokalaemia, thrombocytopenia
Hormones	
Progestogens	May produce virilisation of the female fetus

Drugs that are commonly contraindicated in lactating mothers

Drug	*Adverse effects to the neonates*
Chloramphenicol	Haemolytic anaemia
Cimetidine	Suppresses gastric acidity CNS stimulant
Cytotoxic agents (cyclophosphamide, amethopterin)	Immune suppression
Ergotamine	Vomiting, diarrhoea, convulsion
Lithium	Lethargy, hypotonia, poor feeding
Tetracycline	Possible brown staining of teeth
Phenindione	Bleeding tendency

Causes of neonatal hypoglycaemia

1. Depleted stores of glycogen : low birthweight or small-for-date, infants, hypoxia, respiratory distress syndrome, difficult delivery, hypothermia.
2. Endocrine disorders
   (a) hyperinsulinism : maternal diabetes, erythroblastosis, Beckwith-Wiedmann syndrome, pancreatic b-cell abnormalities (islet cell tumour, functional b-cell hyperplasia, nesidioblastosis)
   (b) Panhypopituitarism
   (c) Isolated growth hormone deficiency
   (d) Adrenal insufficiency : cortisol deficiency, maternal steroid therapy, adrenal haemorrhage, adrenogenital syndrome, corticosteroid unresponsiveness.
   (e) Hypothyroidism
   (f) Glucagon deficiency
3. Inborn errors of metabolism
   (a) Carbohydrate metabolism : galactosaemia, glycogen storage disease and fructosaemia
   (b) Amino acid metabolism : maple syrup urine disease, methylmalonic acidaemia, tyrosinosis
   (c) Fatty acid metabolism : acyl CoA dehydrogenase deficiency
4. Iatrogenic
   (a) Abrupt cessation of hypertonic glucose infusion
   (b) Following exchange transfusion
5. Miscellaneous
   (a) CNS abnormalities
   (b) Chronic diarrhoea
   (c) Sepsis
   (d) Liver disease
   (e) Hyperviscosity
   (f) Maternal drugs, e.g. propranolol, tolbutamide, tocolytic agents.

Drugs that are contraindicated during breastfeeding

Drugs	*Reported sign or symptom in infant or effect on lactation*
Bromocriptine	Suppresses lactation
cyclophosphamide	Possible immune suppression; unknown effect on growth or association with carcinogenesis; neutropenia
Cyclosporine	Possible immune suppression; unknown effect on growth or association with carcinogenesis
Doxorubicin	Possible immune suppression; unknown effect on growth or association with carcinogenesis
Ergotamine	Vomiting, diarrhoea, convulsions (doses used in migraine medications)
Lithium	1/3 to 1/2 therapeutic blood concentration in infants
Methotrexate	Possible immune suppression; unknown effect on growth or association with carcinogenesis; neutropenia.
Phenindione	Anticoagulant; increased prothrombin and partial thromboplastin time in one infant (not used in USA)

Drugs of abuse that are contraindicated during breastfeeding

Drugs	*Effects*
Amphetamine	Irritability, poor sleep pattern
Cocaine	Cocaine intoxication
Heroin	Withdrawal symptoms (i.e. shakiness)
Marijuana	Only one report in literature; no effect mentioned
Nicotine (smoking)	Shock, vomiting, diarrhoea, rapid heart rate, restlessness; decreased milk production
Phencyclidine (PCP)	Potent hallucinogen

Radiopharmaccuticals that require temporary cessation of breastfeeding

Drugs	Recommendation alteration in breastfeeding pattern
Gallium-67 (^{67}Ga)	Radioactivity in milk present for 2 wks
Indium-111 (^{111}In)	Small amount present at 20 hr
Iodine-125 (^{125}I)	Risk of thyroid cancer; radioactivity in milk present for 12 days
Iodine-131 (^{131}I)	Radioactivity in milk present 2 to 14 days depending on study
Radioactive sodium	Radioactivity in milk present 96 hr
Technetium-99m (^{99m}Tc), ^{99m}Tc macroaggregates, $^{99m}TcO_4$	Radioactivity in milk present 15 hr to 3 days

Anti-infectious factors in human milk

Factor	Functions
Bifidus factor	Stimulates growth of bifidomacreria, which antagonises the surviyal of enterobacteria.
Secretory IgA (sIgA), IgM, IgE, IgD, and IgG	Act against bacterial invasion of the mucosa and/or colonisation of the gut (show bacterial and viral neutralising capacity; activate alternative complement pathway)
Antistaphylococcus factor	Inhibits systemic staphylococcal infection
Lactoferrin	Binds iron and inhibits bacterial multiplication
Lactoferrin	Binds iron and inhibits bacterial multiplication
Lactoperoxidase	Kills streptococci and enteric bacteria
Complement (C3, C1)	Promotes opsonisation (the rendering of bacteria and other cells susceptible to phagocytosis)
Interferon	Inhibits intracellular viral replication
Lysozyme	Lyses bacteria through destruction of the cell wall
B_{12}-binding protein	Renders vitamin B_{12} unavailable for bacterial growth
Lymphocytes	Synthesise secretory IgA; may have other roles
Macrophages	Synthesise complement, lactoferrin, lysozyme, and other factors; carry out phagocytosis and probably other functions.

FORAMINA OF THE SKULL AND THEIR CONTENTS

Foramen	*Location on skull*	*Location on bone*	*Contents*
Anterior ethmoidal	Medial wall of orbit	Fronto-ethmoidal suture	Anterior ethmoidal nerve and vessels
Carotid canal	Middle cranial fossa	Petrous portion of temporal bone	Internal carotid artery and associated sympathetic plexus
Caecum	Anterior cranial fossa	Between the base of the frontal crest and crista galli	Emissary veins
Condyloid	Posterior cranial fossa	In condylar fossa just behind the condyle	Emissary veins
Hiatus of the facial canal	Middle cranial fossa	Petrous portion of temporal, lateral to trigeminal impression	Greater petrosal nerve
Greater palatine	Anterior base of the skull	Between the palatomaxillary suture; lingual to the third molar	Greater palatine vessels and nerve
Hypoglossal canal	Posterior cranial fossa	Directly above the anterior aspect of the occipital condyle	Cranial nerve XII, meningeal branch of the ascending pharyngeal artery
Incisive	Palatal midline	Opens into the incisive fossa just behind the interdental septum between the two central incisors	Nasopalatine nerves and descending septal arteries
Incisive canal	Palatal midline	Opens into the incisive foramen	Descending septal artery and nasopalatine nerve

Contd.

Foramen	*Location on skull*	*Location on bone*	*Contents*
Inferior orbital fissure	Orbit	Between lateral wall and floor of orbit	Maxillary division of cranial nerve V; zygomatic nerve; infraorbital vessels and veins to the pterygoid plexus, ophthalmic vein
Infraorbital	Inferior to rim of orbit	Inferior to rim of orbit, lateral to nasal aperture, above canine fossa	Infraorbital vessels and nerve
Internal auditory meatus	Posterior cranial fossa	Posterior aspect of the petrous portion of temporal	Cranial nerves VII and VIII, nervus intermedius and internal auditory vessels
Jugular	Posterior cranial fossa	Lateral to the foramen magnum, medial to the styloid process	Cranial nerves IX, X, and XI, inferior petrosal and transverse sinuses; meningeal arteries, jugular bulb of internal jugular vein
Lacerum	Middle cranial fossa	Medial to the apex of the petrous part of the temporal, lateral to basilar part of occipital	Covered by cartilaginous plate which is pierced by meningeal arteries and emissary veins
Lesser palatine	Palate (posterior part)	Pyramidal process of palatine	Lesser palatine vessels and nerves
Magnum	Posterior cranial fossa	Posterior to the clivus	Medulla oblongata and associated meninges, spinal roots of cranial nerve XI, vertebral arteries; anterior and posterior spinal arteries, postganglionic sympathetic fibres

Contd.

Foramen	*Location on skull*	*Location on bone*	*Contents*
Mandibular	Medial surface of the mandible	Medial surface of ramus, inferior to lingula	Inferior alveolar vessels and nerve
Mastoid	Posterior external surface	Above and behind the mastoid process, near temporo-occipital stature	Emissary veins
Mental	Anterior surface of mandible	Inferior to interproximal region between first and second premolar	Mental nerve and vessels
Nasolacrimal canal	Anteromedial aspect of orbit	Region of articulation between the frontal process of the maxilla and the lacrimal bone	Nasolacrimal duct
Olfactory	Anterior cranial fossa	Cribriform plate of ethmoid surrounding the crista galli	Olfactory nerves
Optic	Middle cranial fossa	Apex of the orbit; between the two roots of the lesser wing of the sphenoid	Optic nerve, ophthalmic artery and associated postganglionic sympathetic fibres, central artery of retina
Ovale	Middle cranial fossa	Greater wing	Mandibular division of cranial nerve V; accessory meningeal artery, sometimes the lesser petrosal nerve
Parietal	Anterior to lambda on either side of the sagittal suture	On superior aspect near the sagittal sture	Emissary vein to superior sagittal sinus; sometimes a branch of the occipital artery
Pharyngeal canal	External base of skull, medial to medial pterygoid plate	Between the vaginal process of the sphenoid and the sphenoidal process of the palatine	Pharyngeal nerve, pharyngeal artery

Contd.

Foramen	*Location on skull*	*Location on bone*	*Contents*
Posterior ethmoidal	Medial wall of orbit	Fronto-ethmoidal suture, posterior to the anterior ethmoidal foramen	Posterior ethmoidal nerve and vessels [when present]
Posterior superior alveolar	Anterior to the pterygomaxillary fissure	Infratemporal surface and maxillary tuberosity	Posterior superior alveolar nerves and vessels
Pterygoid canal [Vidian canal]	Extends from foramen lacerum to pterygopalatine fossa	Body of sphenoid just above the pterygoid processes	Nerve and vessels of the pterygoid canal (vidian nerve and vessel)
Rotundum	Middle cranial fossa	Greater wing	Maxillary branch of the trigeminal
Sphenopalatine	Medial wall of pterygopalatine fossa	Between sphenoidal and orbital processes	Pterygopalatine nerves and vessels
Spinosum	Middle canial	Spine of the sphenoid	Middle meningeal branch of mandibular division of cranial nerve V
Stylomastoid	Between styloid and mastoid processes	Posterior to the base of the styloid process	Facial nerve, stylomastoid vessels
Superior orbitual fissure	Posterior superior aspect of orbit	Between roof and lateral wall, lateral to apex	Cranial nerves III, IV, VI or ophthalmic division of V, sympathetic fibres; branches of middle meningeal artery; recurrent branch of lacrimal artery; superior ophthalmic vein
Supraorbital	Superior rim of orbit	Below superciliary arch	Supraorbital nerve and vessels
Zygomaticofacial	Lateral to the inferolateral angle of the orbital rim	Malar surface, above the origin of zygomaticus major muscle	Zygomaticofacial nerve and vessels
Zygomaticoorbital	Anterior floor of orbit	Orbital surface	Zygomaticofacial an zygomatico-temporal nerves and vessels
Zygomaticotemporal	Temporal fossa	Temporal surface	Zygomaticotemporal nerves and vessels

GENERAL MEASURES

Measures of weight (mass) in metric system

1 Kilogram (kg)	=	1000 gram (g or g)
1 gram	=	1000 milligram (mg)
1 milligram (10-3 g)	=	1000 microgram (mcg)
1 microgram (10-6 g)	=	1000 nanogram (ng)
1 nanogram (10-9 g)	=	1000 picogram (pg)
1 picogram (10-12 g)	=	1000 femtograms (fg)

Measures of capacity (volume) in metric system

1 litre (I)	=	1000 millilitres (ml)

Measures of weight (mass) in imperial system

1 pound (Ib)	=	1 ounce (oz) = 7000 grain
1 ounce	=	437.5 grains (gr)

Measures of capacity (volume) in imperial system

1 quart	=	2 pints (pt or 0)
1 pint	=	20 fluid-ounces (fl oz)
1 pound	=	16 fluid-ounces
1 fluid ounce	=	8 fluid drachms (fl dr)
1 fluid drachm	=	60 minims (min)

Domestic weights and measures

Domestic measure	*Imperial*	*Metric equivalent*
1 drop	= 1 minim	= 1/20 ml
1 teaspoonful	= 1 fl dr	= 4 ml
1 dessert spoonful	= 2 fl dr	= 8 ml
1 table spoonful	= 4 fl dr	= 15 ml
1 wine glassful	= 2 fl oz	= 60 ml
1 teacupful	= 6 fl oz	= 180 ml
1 tumbleful	= 8 fl oz	= 240 ml

Relation between Metric and Imperial system

1 kilogram	=	2.2046 pounds
1 gram	=	15.432 grains (15 gr approx)
1 pound	=	453.59 grams
1 ounce	=	28.35 grams (30 G approx)
1 grain	=	65 milligrams (60 mg approx)
1 litre	=	1 quart (approx)
1 litre	=	1.7598 pint
1 millilitre	=	15 to 20 minims
1 fluid ounce	=	30 ml (approx)

HISTORY OF MEDICINE

1. Penicillin was discovered by Alexander Fleming in 1920. The accidental contamination of the culture plates in Fleming's laboratory by the mould led to the discovery of penicillin. It was introduced into clinicial medicine in 1941 by Florey, Chain and their associates.
2. Streptomycin was discovered in 1944 by Prof. Selman Waksman of Rutger University from the soil micro-organisms *Streptomyces griseus,* for which he was awarded the Nobel prize in 1952.
3. Chlortetracycline was isolated from a culture of *Streptomyces aureofacieus* by Subba Rao and Duggar in 1948. It was followed by the discovery of Oxytetracycline isolated from *Streptomyces rimosus* by Finlay and his associates in 1950.
4. In 1882 Robert Koch discovered the tubercle bacillus.
5. In 1895 Roentgen discovered X-rays.
6. In 1907 Von Pirquet discovered the tuberculin test. BCG vaccine was evolved by the French scientist Calmette and Guerin in 1921. In India BCG vaccine was introduced in 1949.
7. In 1880, Laveran, a French army surgeon discovered the malarial parasite in Algiers, North Africa. In 1891 Romanowski developed a new method of staining blood films. In 1894 Manson hypothesised that mosquitoes transmitted malarial. In 1897, Ronald Ross in Secundarabad found malaria parasites of man growing as cysts, i.e. oocysts on the stomach wall of Anopheles mosquito which has fed on a malaria patient.
8. In 1939 Paul Muller discovered the insecticidal properties of DDT. Venezuela was the first country to launch an eradication programme against malaria in 1945.
9. In 1709 Clark in Cochin gave the name 'Malabar legs'. In 1866 Wucherer in Brazil found microfilaria in chylous urine. In 1872, Lewis working in Calcutta found microfilaria in peripheral blood. In 1876 Bancroft in Australia discovered the adult female. In 1940, Rao and Maplestone discovered the adult of *B. malayi* in India.
10. Negri bodies were first described by Negri in Italy in 1903 in the cytoplasm of brain cells. It is diagnostic of rabies.
11. In 1873 Hansen of Norway discovered *Mycobacterium leprae.*
    In 1941 Sulphones were used against it.
12. In 1916 Japanese worker K.Mitsuda described the intradermal test to classify leprosy and to find out the prognosis.
13. Charaka (200 AD) the most popular name in Ayurvedic medicine was a court physician to Buddhist king Kaniska. Based on the teachings of Atreya, Charaka compiled his famous treatise on medicine, 'Charaka Samhita'.
14. Susruta of Benaras compiled his surgical knowledge in his classic 'Susruta Samhita' between 800 BC and 400 AD. Early Indians set fractures, performed amputations, excised tumours and repaired hernias.
15. Homeopathy which was propounded by Samuel Hahnemann (1755-1843) of Germany, gained foothold in India during 1810 and 1839.
16. Egyptian medicine dates from 2000 BC. The best known medical manuscript is the Ebers Papyrus (1500 BC) which was found with mummy on the banks of Nile. It contains 800 prescriptions with 700 drugs.
17. An early leader in Greek medicine was Aesculapius (1200 BC) whose daughter Hygiea was worshipped as a goddess of health.

18. Hippocrates (460-370 BC) is described as father of medicine. He studied and classified diseases. His famous oath is the basis of medical ethics of today. His book Airs, Water and Places is considered a treatise on social medicine. He was born in Greece.
19. Medical man of Rome (25 BC-50 BC) was Celsus who gave us the cardinal signs of inflammation.
20. Another Roman medical scientist Galen (130-205 A.D.) was a pioneer of experimental medicine. He noted that diseases were due to three factors : (i) predisposing factors, (ii) exciting factors, and (iii) environmental factor, a truly modern fact. He was a medical dictator of his own time.
21. Arabs developed Unani system of medicine. Two arab physicians Rhazes (865-923) who differentiated between smallpox and measles and Avicenna (980-1037) who was the first to describe guineaworm.
22. Medicine was revived by Paracelsus (1490-1541) who publicly burnt the works of Galen and attacked superstitions and dogma in medicine.
23. Fracastorious (1843-1553) enunciated the 'Theory of contagion' and explained the cause of epidemics. He became the founder of epidemiology.
24. Vasallus (1514-1564) did lot of dissection on human body and demonstrated some of Galen's error.
25. Pare (1517-1590) revived surgery and became and father of modern surgery.
26. Fracastorius of Verona (1546) in his book on contagious disease pointed out that the agent of communicable disease was contagium vivum. He told that infection itself consists of minute particles, too small to be seen by naked eye. He further defined infection and expressed that infectious diseases were transmitted per contactum, by direct contact, per fonitem by fomites or inanimate objects.
27. Francesco Redi (1688) conclusively proved that 'Life comes from life by observing that maggots appeared in decomposing meat where flies laid eggs. Athanasius Kircher (1602-1680) a monk was first to make direct microscopic study of bacteria in 1658, using simple microscope of low magnification. The magnification of his microscope was only 32 times.
28. The fundamental observation in bacteriology started with the invention of microscope by Antony Van Leeuwenhock (1602-1680). He was Dutch and he produced magnification of 40 to 300. He was the first and the greatest of all microbiologist who discovered bacteria and spirochaetes in the mouth and intestines.

29(a) Louis Pasteur (1822-95) is known as father of microbiology. He devised various methods of sterilisation, namely by steam steriliser (100°C), autoclave (120°C) or hot air oven (160°C) by direct flamming or by short exposure to high temperature followed by rapid cooling.

The last technique of sterilisation is known as pasteurisation. In 1817 he worked on the investigation of anthrax. In 1881 he prepared anthrax vaccine from attenuated anthrax bacillus.

He achieved monumental fame by his method of immuni-sation against rabies. The results were encouraging and in 1888. Pasteur Institute was established in Paris for mass antirabic treatment.

29(b) Robert Kock is called the father of modern bacteriology. In East Germany he prepared dried bacterial film and stained them with aniline dyes for the study of their morphology. Kock discovered old tuberculin in 1890-1901 but it was not universally accepted for the treatment of tuberculosis.

He studied cases of cholera in the Medical College, Calcutta and in July 1884 in Berlin conference, he announced the discovery of cholera causative organism.

30. In 1881 Klebs described *G. diphtheriae* which was later isolated and described by Klebs and Loeffler and hence the name Klebs-Loeffler's bacillus.
31. In 1884 Gaffky isolated typhoid bacillus which was described by Eberth 4 years earlier.
32. Between 1884-86 Fraenkel and Weichsebaum demostrated the causative organism of lobar pneumonia.
33. Tetanus bacillus previously observed by Nicolarie (1884) was isolated by Kitasato in 1889.

34. Shiga isolated dysentery bacillus in 1898 which was named after him.
35. Lord Lister (1827-1912) is known as 'the father of antiseptic surgery'. He could realise that microorganisms so prevalent in the atmosphere might be responsible for postoperative inflammation and suppuration. In 1867, he introduced the antiseptic surgical technique in postoperative stage. Carbolic acid was used as spray on the wound or during operation.
36. Loeffler and Frosch (1898) first demonstrated that the foot and mouth disease of cattle was caused by a filtrable virus. The causal agent which was invisible under the microscope passed through bacterial filters.
37. Bacteriophage is the virus of bacteria. Haffkine in 1896 discovered self-sterilisation of water of river Yamuna but that property was lost when the water was boiled.
38. Twort (1915) while working on vaccine lymph first discovered glossy, transparent patches occurring in the white colonies of Staphylococcus on an agar plate.
39. In 1778, Edward Jenner began the study of immunity in smallpox. He came to know from the milkmaid who supplied him milk that they were immune to smallpox, but due to close contact with cow they were infected with mild doses of cowpox virus which was not virulent as that of smallpox. In 1978, he practised a method of immunisation by vaccinia against variola.
40. Haffkine (1898) discovered plague vaccine in India as prophylactic measure against plague.
41. In 1902, Portier and Richet carried out the first systemic study of anaphylaxis.
42. Roux and Yersin (1888) demonstrated toxin in the filtrate of the broth culture of the diphtheria bacillus and attributed symptoms to the action of the soluble toxin produced by bacillus.
43. Knowledge of agglutination was utilised in 1896 by Widal and his collaborators in the diagnosis of typhoid fever to detect antibodies in patient and the test is known as Widal test.
44. In 1898, Bordet utilised the reaction of specific agglutination of RBC with antiserum. This helped Landsteiner (1990) to find out agglutination reaction in the determination of blood groups.
45. In 1906 Wassermann, Neisser and Bruck established the serodiagnosis of syphilis and the test is known as Wassermann reaction.
46. In 1936 it was found by many observers that prontosil was converted into sulphonamide in the body which was the active agent responsible for its action against streptococci.
47. Hata (1910) discovered salvarson, the first successful chemotherapeutic agent and administered it in case of syphilis.
48. In 1838, a German gynaecologist Dr FA Wilde published writings containing revolutionary ideas on contraception and pleaded that women have every right to live healthy and useful life by adopting contraceptive methods.
49. Margret Sanger is great name in the history of contraception in the USA. A nurse by profession started a birth control movement in New York City in 1912 and published a periodical 'The Women Rebel' at her own risk. She established the first birth control clinic in Brooklyn in 1916 and the New York birth control clinic in 1923.
50. The first government sponsored birth control clinic in the world was opened at Mysore in 1930.
51. Condom is the oldest and most widely used male barrier method in the world. Dr. Condom a physician at the court of Charles II of England (1660-85 AD) is believed to have invented the condom
52. In 1909 R Richter, a German physician first introduced an intrauterine device for contraception.
53. In 1934 T Ota of Japan introduced intrauterine device made of gold or gold plated silver. The device was a ring with a small disc in the centre. The Ota ring was used extensively in Japan.

54. LL Doyle and TR Clewe in 1968 reported the use of hormones in IUD to increase their contraceptive efficiency.

55. "Vitamin B" was one of the first dietary essentials to be recognised, and the preparation from rice polishings by Funk in 1911, of a water soluble concentrate active in the cure of beriberi was an important contribution not only to the chemistry of Vit.B but to the establishment of the concept of deficiency disease.

56. The term water soluble vit. B was introduced by McCollum and Kennedy in 1916 to describe the substance essential for growth in rats and for prevention of beriberi.

57. In 1926, vitamin B_1 was isolated in crystalline form by Jansen and Donath and in the 1936 Williams determined its structure and synthesised in the same year.

58. Riboflavin was first identified in milk by Blyth in 1879 and was called lactochrome.

59. In 1913, long before Goldberger started his experiments to study pellagra Funk isolated nicotinic acid from rice polishings.

Warburg and his associates in 1935 obtained nicotinic acid amide from a coenzyme isolated from RBCs of the horse.

60. In 1936, Birch and Gyorgy gave the name vitamin B_6 and presented some of the details of its structure.

61. Pantothenic acid was first identified by Williams and associates in 1933 as a substance essential for the growth of yeast. Its name derived from Greek word signifying 'From every where' indicates its distribution in nature.

62. In 1916, Batemen observed that a high concentration of egg white in experimental diets was toxic. In 1927, Boas confirmed the fact that rats fed on a diet of raw egg white developed a syndrome characterised by neuromuscular disorder, severe dermatitis and loss of hair. She named it "Egg white injury" and she demonstrated that it could be prevented by cooking the protein.

63. In 1936, Kogl and Tonnis studying yeast growth factors isolated in crystalline form on essential factor from yolk of an egg and named 'biotin'.

64. Choline was identified chemically as a component of lecithin in 1862.

65. Lind (1757) in his exhaustive treatise on scurvy showed experimentally in human subjects that oranges and lemons in diet could prevent the disease.

66. King and Waugh in 1932 finally succeeded in isolating a crystalline compound from lemon juice and identified it as hexuronic acid and demonstrated its antiscorbutic acid.

67. Euler and associates (1929) and Moore (1929) demonstrated that the purified plant pigment carotene i.e. provitamin 'A' is a potent source of vitamin 'A'.

68. By 1920, the work of Mellanby and Huldschinsky had shown that addition of codliver oil or exposure to sunlight would prevent or treat rickets.

69. Dam and coworker in 1935, reported that spontaneous bleeding in chicken can be prevented by feeding an identified fat soluble and gave the name vitamin 'K'.

70. The existence of Vitamin 'E' was first demonstrated in 1922 by Evans and Bishop, who found that female rats required some unrecognised substance to sustain a normal pregnancy.

Later on vitamin 'E' was isolated by Evans and coworkers in 1936 from wheat germ oil.

71. Barbituric acid results from the condensation of malonic acid and urea. It was prepared in 1864 by Adolph Von Baeyer then a 29-year-old research assistant.

72. The first report on the treatment of mania with lithium was that of Cade(1949).

In 1950 chlorpromazine was synthesised in France. Its use by Delay and Deniker in 1952 marked the beginning of modern psychopharmacology.

The report on meprobamate by Berger in 1954 marked the beginning of antianxiety drugs.

73. Therapeutic application of whole root or *Rauwolfia serpentina* for the treatment of psychoses and hypertension were described in Indian Journal in 1931 by Sen and Bose. Little attention was paid till Vakil wrote the first report in a Western Medical Journal of its antihypertensive effect.

74. In 1803 a young German pharmacist Serturner isolated and described an opium alkaloid that he named morphine, after Morpheus the Greek God of dreams.

Robiquet isolated codeine in 1832 and papaverine by Merck in 1848.

75. In 1827 Leroux extracted salicin a bitter glycoside having antipyretic activity. On hydrolysis it gives glucose and saligenin. Piria in 1838 made salicylic acid from salicin.

The synthetic manufacture of this acid from phenol was accomplished in 1860 by Kolbe and Lautemann.

76. Paracetamol was first used in medicine by Von Mering in 1893. However it gained popularity in 1949 and was recognised as major active metabolite of acetanilide and phenacetin.

77. Colchicum was introduced for the therapy of acute gout by Von Strock in 1763. The alkaloid cholchicine was isolated from colchicum in 1820 by Pelletier and Caventou.

78. Anrep in 1880 studied pharmacological actions of cocaine and observed that the skin became insensitive to prick of pin when cocaine was infiltrated subcutaneously. He recommended its use as a local anaesthetics.

79. Procaine was synthesised by Einhorn in 1905 and introduced under the trade name of novobiocin. It is still used as local anaesthetics.

80. In 1864 Jobst and Hesse isolated physostigmine from calbar bean. Following year in 1865 Vee and Leven obtained the same alkaloid and named as eserine. In 1877 Laqueur used it in glaucoma.

81. Acetylcholine was first synthesised by Baeyer in 1867.

82. Pilocarpine is the chief alkaloid obtained from the leaflets of South American shrub pilocarpus. Natives were knowing that chewing of it causes salivation. It was isolated as pilocarpine by Weber in 1875 and actions were studied on pupil, salivary glands and sweat.

83. The active principle of suprarenal extract was named epinephrine by Abel in 1899.

84. Mein in 1831 isolated atropine in pure form. Preparations were known to ancient Hindus for many centuries.

85. Nicotine was first isolated from leaves of tobacco *Nicotina-tobacum* by Posselt and Reiman in 1828,

86. Lobeline is the chief constituent of Lobelia (Indian tobacco) and was first obtained in crystalline form by Wirland in 1915.

87. In 1927 Best, Dale, Dudley and Thorpe isolated histamine from liver and lung proving that this amine is a natural constituent of body. Name has been given histamine after the Greek word for tissue *(histos)*.

88. John Ferriar in 1799 was the first to ascribe to digitalis, as a drug having a primary action on heart and a diuretic effect of secondary importance.

89. Sulphnilamide was first prepared in 1908 by Gelmo in the course of investigations of azo dyes.

90. Gentamicin is a broad-spectrum antibiotic derived from the actinomycete *Micromonospora purpurea*. Drug was first described by Weinstein and co-workers in 1963 and isolated, purified by Rosselot and colleagues in 1964.

91. Kanamycin is an antibiotic produced by *Streptomyces kenamyceticus*. It was first isolated by Umezawa at the Japanese National Institute of Health in 1957.

92. In 1949, Waksman and Lechevalier isolated a soil organism *Streptomyces fradial* which produced a new antibiotic that a crude form contained an antifungal compound fradicin and antibacteria substance 'neomycin'.

93. The metabolic effect of PAS was found by Lehmann in 1946 to be associated with suppression of both growth and multiplication of tubercle bacilli. It increases O_2 consumption of bacilli.

94. In 1961, Thomas and co-workers found that ethambutol suppresses the growth of isoniazid and streptomycin-resistant tubercle bacilli.

95. Dutcher and colleagues in 1954, reported that Nystatin inhibits the growth of a variety of pathogenic and non-pathogenic yeasts and fungi but not bacteria.

96. Griseofulvin was first isolated from penicilliņ griseofulvin by Oxford and co-workers in 1939. It was ineffective against bacteria hence no further attention was paid. In 1946, Brian found that it causes shrinking and stunting of fungal hyphae. He named it griseofulvin.

97. In 1942, Goodman, Gilmann and Gongherty used nitrogen mustard in transplanted lymphosarcoma and launched the era of modern cancer chemotherapy.

98. In 1889, Brown-Sequard French physiologists prepared a testicular extract and administered himself and noticed that he gained vigour and capacity.

99. In 1880, on 6th November Alphonse Laveran' a French military surgeon, while working in Algiers discovered the parasite in an unstained preparation of a fresh blood. He noticed the amoeboid movement of the parasite and observed the flagellation of freshly drawn blood.

100. In 1983, Marchiafava found the ring forms of malaria using a derived blood film stained with methylene blue. In 1885 he transmitted the disease to man by inoculation of infected blood.

101. In 1855, Golgi demonstrated the course of development of quartan parasite (*P. malarie*) in the blood and in the following year the tertian parasite (*Vivax P.*). In 1886 Golgi separated the benign and quartan species associated with asexual schizogony with the malarial paroxysm.

102. In 1900, experiments undertaken by Manson finally proved beyond doubt the theory of mosquito transmission of Malaria. He allowed the mosquitoes infected in Rome with *Plasmodium vivax* to bite two persons in London, one of them was his son. Both of them developed the typical malarial fever.

103. In 1859, Lambin Prague found living amoeba in the stool of a child suffering from dysentery. In 1875, Losch in Leningrad discovered the amoeba in the stool of a Russian suffering from an attack of dysentery and named the organism as 'Amoeba Coli'.

104. In 1883, Robert Koch found the parasite in sections of ulcers of the large gut in man. In 1887, Kartulis found vegetative forms of amoeba and in 1893, Quincke and Ross discovered the cystic stage of the parasites.

105. Kala-azar was recognised as a clinical entity even before the discovery of the parasite. In Assam severe epidemics occurred, the severest one being in 1875. Rogers (1897) and Ross (1899) considered kala-azar to be a severe form of malaria. Giles (1892) reported the finding of hookworm in the stool of kala-azar patients and thought this to be the cause of the disease. The real cause of the disease was established when Leishman in May 1903 reported the finding of a parasite in the necropsy material of the splenic smear of a soldier who died in the England from a fever contracted at Dum Dum, Calcutta known as 'Dum Dum fever' i.e. kala-azar.

106. Angelo Dubini, an Italian physician in 1838 first discovered the parasite during autopsy of a Milanese woman. A relation to the *Ankylostoma duodenale* and anaemia was established after the fatal epidemic among the miners in Switzerland in 1880.

107. Guineaworm was the earliest helminth referred to in the old treatment. Hippocrates (460-377 BC) described beef tapeworm, i.e. *Taenia saginata* and recognised hydatid cyst. Aristotle (384-322 BC) mentioned the large roundworm and the guineaworm.

108. Calcified eggs of *Schistosoma haematobium* have been recovered from the kidneys of two mummies dating 3000 years back thereby demonstrating the existence of helminthic infection in the early days (Ruffer 1910).

109. Avicenna (980-1037 AD) the Persian physician was able to recognise four types of helminths :
   (i) Long worms i.e. beef tapeworm, *Taenia saginata*
   (ii) Flat worms (detached proglottides which were erroneously regarded by Avicenna as complete worm.
   (iii) Small worms (*Enterobious vermicularis*)
   (iv) Round worms (*Ascaris lumbricoides*)

110. Elephantiasis of Arabs caused by Bancroft's filaria was known to ancient Hindu physician (600 BC) as well as to Persian physician. In 1863, Demarquay in Paris found the larval form, i.e. *Microfilaria bancrofti* in the hydrocele fluid of a man from Havana.

   Wucherer (1866) in Brazil discovered the larval form in chylus urine.

   Bancroft (1876) in Australia found the adult female.

111. The first account of *Loa loa* was reported by Pigafetta (1589) in a book of Travels on the Congo. Mongin (1770) extracted the worm from the eye of a negress in St. Domingo, Manson (1891) demonstrated the microflaria in the blood.

   Loss (1940) made a careful observation about the morphology and lifecyle of this filaria.

112. Hippocrates (460-377 BC), Aretaeus (9-078 AD) and Galen (130-200 AD) were all clinically familiar with hydatid disease. Goeze (1782) first recognised the scolex (head) developing from the cyst wall to be taeniod cestode. Batsch (1786) named the parasite *Hydatigena granulosa*. Von Siebold (1852) recovered adult worms from the intestinal villi of dogs.

MEDICAL ABBREVIATIONS AND ACRONYMS

A&E	**accident and emergency department**
ABP	**arterial blood pressure**
ADLs	**activities of daily living**
ADM.	**admission**
AET.	**aetiology**
AI	**artificial insemination**
AIDS	**acquired immune deficiency syndrome**
ALG	**antilymphocyte globulin**
ALS	**antilymphocyte serum**
ARM	**artificial rupture of membranes (for delivery)**
BCG	**Bacille Calmette-Guerin (TB vaccine)**
BMI	**body mass index**
BMR	**basal metabolic rate**
BP	**blood pressure**
BPD	**bronchopulmonary dysplasia**
CA	**cancer**
CABG	**coronary artery bypass graft**
CAPD	**continuous ambulatory peritoneal dialysis**
CAT	**computerised axial tomography**
CCU	**coronary care unit**
CJD	**Creutzfeldt-Jakob disease**
CMV	**cytomegalovirus**
CNS	**central vervous system**
COAD	**chronic obstructive airways disease**
CPAP	**continuous positive airways pressure**
CPR	**cardiopulmonary resuscitation**
CSF	**cerebrospinal fluid; colony-stimulating factor**
CT	**computerized tomography**
CV	**cardiovascular**
CVA	**cardiovascular accident**
CVP	**central venous pressure**
CVS	**chorionic villus sampling**
CXR	**chest X-ray**
D&C	**dilation and curettage**
DHA	**district health authority**
DI	**donor insemination**
DIC	**disseminated intravascular coagulation**
DISCH.	**discharge**
DL	**danger list**
DMD	**Duchenne muscular dystrophy**
DNA	**deoxyribonucleic acid**
DOA	**dead on arrival**
DPT	**combined vaccine against diphtheria, whooping cough, and tetanus**
Dr	**doctor**
DRG	**diagnostic related group**
DTs	**delirium tremens**
DVT	**deep vein thrombosis**

ECG	electrocardiogram
ECT	electroconvulsive therapy
EEG	electroencephalograph
EMG	electromyograph
ENT	ear, nose, and throat
EPO	erythropoietin
ET	endotracheal tube
GH	growth hormone
GIFT	gamete intrafallopian transfer
GP	general practitioner
GVHD	graft-versus-host disease
HBIG	hepatitis B immunoglobulin
HCG	human chorionic gonadotrophin
HIV	human immunodeficiency virus
HLA	system human leucocyte antigen system
HRT	hormone replacement therapy
IBS	irritable bowel syndrome
ICD	international classification of diseases
ICP	intercranial pressure
ICU	intensive care unit
IHD	ischaemic heart disease
IMR	infant mortality rate
IMV	intermittent mandatory ventilation
IOP	intraocular pressure
IPPV	intermittent positive pressure ventilation
IQ	intelligence quotient
IUD	intrauterine device
IV	intravenous
IVP	intravenous pyelogram
IZS	insulin zinc suspension
K&M	kaolin and morphine
LBW	low birth weight
LP	lumbar puncture
LSD	lysergic acid diethylamide
MAB	monoclonal antibody
MAOI	monoamine oxidase inhibitor
MAP	mean arterial pressure
MBD	minimal brain dysfunction
MD	doctor of medicine
ME	myalgic encephalomyelitis
MHC	major histocompatibility complex
MI	myocardial infarction
MLD	minimum lethal dose
MMR	combined vaccine against measles, mumps, and German measles (rubella)
MND	motor neurone disease
MO	medical officer
MRI	magnetic resonance imaging
MRS	magnetic resonance spectroscopy

MRSA	methicillin-resistant Staphylococcus aureus
MS	multiple sclerosis
MSU	mid-stream urine specimen
NHS	National Health Service
NPO	nil per orem (nothing by mouth)
NTD	neural tube defect
O&G	obstetrics and gynaecology
OA	osteoarthritis
OD	overdose
OP	outpatient
ORT	Oral rehydration therapy
OT	occupational therapy
PAED	paediatrics
PATH	pathology
PCOD	polycystic ovary disease
PE	pleural effusion
PET	positron-emission tomography
PICU	paediatric intensive care unit
PID	pelvic inflammatory disease
PIH	pregnancy-induced hypertension
PKU	phenylketonuria
PM	postmortem
PMT	premenstrual tension
PO	per orem (by mouth)
PoP	plaster of Paris
PRE-MED	premedication
PRE-OP	preoperative
PTA	post-traumatic amnesisa
QA	quality assurance
QALY	quality adjusted life years
RA	rheumatoid arthritis
RDS	respiratory distress syndrome
REM	sleep rapid eye movement sleep
RES	reticuloendothelial system
RHA	regional health authority
RMO	resident medical officer
RN	registered nurse
RNA	ribonucleic acid
RQ	respiratory quotient
RSI	repetitive strain injury
RSV	respiratory syncytial virus
Rx	treatment/prescription
SAD	seasonal affective disorder
SAH	subarachnoid haemorrhage
SIDS	sudden infant death syndrome
SLE	systemic lupus erythematosus
STD	sexually transmitted disease
TAB	Combined vaccine against typhoid, paratyphoid A, and paratyphoid B

TB	tuberculosis
TENS	transcutaneous electrical nerve stimulation
TIA	transient ischaemic attack
TPA	tissue plasminogen activator (heart drug)
TPR	temperature, pulse, and respiration
TS	Tourette's syndrome
TSH	thyroid-stimulating hormone
Tx	transfusion, transplant
URTI	upper respiratory tract infection
UTI	urinary tract infection
VA	visual acuity
VD	venereal disease
VF	ventrinular fibrillation
WHO	World Health Organisation

MEDICAL PREFIXES AND SUFFIXES

a-(an-)	lacking
ab-	away from
andr(o)-	male
angi(o)-	blood or lymph vessel
anti(i)-	against, counteracting
ante-	before
arthr(o)-	joint
aut(o)-	self
bi-	twice, two
brachi(o)-	arm
brachy-	shortness
brady-	slowness
bronch(o)	bronchial tube
carcin(o)-	cancer
cardi(o)-	heart
cerebr(o)-	brain
cholecyst-	gall bladder
circum-	surrounding
colp(o)-	vagina
contra-	against
crani(o)-	skull
cry(o)-	cold
crypt-	hidden, concealed
cyst(o)-	bladder
cyt(o)-	cell
dent-	tooth
derm-	skin
di-	double
dys-	difficult, painful, abnormal
end(o)-	within, inner
enter(o)-	intestine
epi-	above, upon
ex(o)-	outside, outer
prefix	meaning
extra-	outside, beyond
gastr(o)-	stomach
gyn-	female
haem-	blood
hepat(o)-	liver
hist(o)-	tissue
hyper-	above
hypno-	sleep
hypo-	below
hyster(o)-	uterus
immuno-	immunity
infra-	below
intra-	within

laryng(o)-	larynx
mal-	abnormal, diseased
mast-	breast
muco-	mucus
my(o)-	muscle
necro-	death
neo-	new
nephr(o)-	kidney
neur(o)-	nerve
oculo-	eye
olig(o)-	deficiency, few
ophthalm(o)-	eye
oro-	mouth
ortho-	straight, normal
osteo-	bone
ot(o)-	ear
paed-	children
path(o)	disease
peri-	around, enclosing
pharmac(o)-	drugs
phleb(o)-	vein
phot(o)-	light
pneumon-	lung
prefix-	meaning
poly-	many, excessive
post-	after
pre- (pro-)	before
ren-	kidney
retro-	behind
rhin-	nose
sclero-	thickening
ser(o)-	serum
spondyl-	vertebra, spine
supra-	above
syn-	together, union
tachy-	fast
therm(o)-	heat, temperature
trache(o)-	trachea
uni-	one
urin-	urine, urinary system
utero-	uterus
vaso-	vessel
vesico-	bladder
-aemia	condition of blood
-algia	pain
-ase	enzyme
-blast	formative cell
-cele	tumour, swelling

-centesis	puncture
-cide	destructive, killing
-coccus	spherical bacterium
-cyte	cell
-derm	skin
-dynia	pain
-ectasis	dilation, extension
-ectomy	surgical removal of
-facient	making, causing
-fuge	expelling
-genesis	origin, development
-genic	causing, produced by
-iasis	diseased condition
-iatric	practice of healing
-itis-	inflammation of
-kinesis	movement
-lysis	breaking down, dissolution
-malacia	softening
-megaly	enlargement
-oid	likliness, resemblance
-oma	tumour
-opia	eye defect
-osis	disease, condition
-ostomy	surgical opening or outlet
-otomy	surgical incision into an organ or part
-pathy	disease
-penia	lack of, deficiency
-pexy	surgical fixation
-phage	ingesting
-philia	affinity for, morbid attraction
-phobia	fear
-plasty	reconstructive surgery
-plegia	paralysis
-pnoea	condition of breathing
-poiesis	formation
-ptosis	prolapse
-scopy	visual examination
-statis	stagnation, stoppage of flow
-uria	condition of urine

PERIOD OF INCUBATION/COMMUNICABILITY

When	*Incubation period*	*Period of communicability*
Influenza	1 to 3 days	About 1 week from onset
Dysentery (bacillary)	1 to 7 days	Till bacilli are present in stool
Typhoid	5 days	Until stool and urine are negative
Cholera	3 days	Until stool and urine are negative usually 7 to 14 days
Smallpox	7 to 17 days	Until scabs and crusts disappear
Mumps	2 to 3 weeks	Until the swelling subsides
Polio	7 to 14 days	From 7 to 21 days
Scabies	1 to 2 days	Till it cures
Measles	1 to 3 days	About 1 week from onset
Infective hepatitis	15 to 50 days	Unknown
Amoebiasis	3 to 4 weeks	Till cyst passes in stool
Tetanus	7 to 10 days	Not known
TB (lungs)	3 months to years	Positive cases

SCHEDULE OF IMMUNISATION

When	*What*	*Why*
16 to 39 weeks of pregnancy	2 doses of TT	Given to mother to protect both mother and the newborn from tetanus.
6 weeks to 9 months	3 injections of DPT and 3 doses of polio drops at an interval of one month	To protect the child from diphtheria, pertussis (whooping cough), tetanus and poliomyelitis
Birth to 9 months	One injection of BCG	To protect the child from tuberculosis
9 to 12 months	One injection of measles vaccine	To protect the child from measles
18 to 24 months	Booster doses of polio and DPT	To protect the child from diphtheria, (whooping cough) Tetanus and poliomyelitis
5 to 6 years	Two doses each of DPT and Typhoid	To protect the child from diphtheria, Tetanus and typhoid fever
10 years	Two doses of TT and Typhoid	To protect from tetanus and typhoid
16 years	TT and Typhoid	To protect from tetanus and typhoid

THE MUSCLES OF THE EXTREMITIES

Name	*Origin*	*Insertion*	*Action*
Muscles joining the upper limbs to the trunk			
Pectoralis major (medial and lateral pectoral)	Medial half of clavicle; sternum; costal cartilages; aponeuroses of external abdominal oblique	Lateral lip of intertubercular sulcus (bicipital groove)	Flexes and adducts arm; rotates arm medially
Pectoralis minor (medial pectoral)	Second, third, and fourth ribs or third, fourth, fifth ribs	Coracoid process	Draws shoulder downward; when scapula is fixed, it elevates the ribs
Serratus anterior (long thoracic) Latissimus dorsi (thoracodorsal)	Crest of ilium; spinous processes of lower thoracic, lumbar, and sacral vertebrae; part of this origin is by a tough aponeurotic sheet called the lumbodorsal fascia	Medial lip of intertubercular sulcus (bicipital groove)	Extends and adducts arm; rotates arm medially
Trapezius (spinal accessory and third and fourth cervical)	External occipital protuberance; superior nuchal line; spinous processes of cervical and thoracic vertebrae; the origin from the cervial spines is via an elastic ligament called the ligamentum nuchae	Lateral third of clavicle, acromial process and spine of scapula	Draw the scapula medially and backward; rotate, scapula; the upper fibers of the two muscles working together extend the head
Levator scapulae (third and fourth cervical)	Transverse process of first four cervical vertebrae	Vertebral border of scapula	Elevates scapula
Rhomboideus major (dorsal scapular)	Spinous processes of T_2-T_5	Lower half of vertebral border of scapula	Adducts scapula
Rhomboideus minor (dorsal scapular)	Spinous processes of C_7 and T_1	Vertebral border of scapula	Adducts scapula

Contd.

Name	*Origin*	*Insertion*	*Action*
Muscles of the shoulder			
Deltoid (axillary)	Lateral one-third of clavicle; acromial process and spine of scapula	Middle of lateral surface of the humerus.	Abducts arm; anterior fibres also flex arm; posterior fibres also extend arm
Teres major (lower subscapular)	Inferior angle of scapula	Medial lip of intertubercular sulcus	Extends and adducts arm; rotates arm medially
Tares minor (axillary)	Axillary border of scapula	Greater tubercle of humerus	Rotates arm laterally; draws head of humerus to glenoid cavity of scapula
Infraspinatus (suprascapular)	Infraspinous fossa of scapula	Greater tubercle of humerus	Rotates arm laterally; draws head of humerus to glenoid cavity of scapula
Supraspinatus (suprascapular)	Supraspinous fossa of scapula	Greater tubercle of humerous	Abducts arm; draws head of humerus toward glenoid cavity of scapula
Subscapularis (subscapular)	Subscapular fossa	Lesser tubercle of humerus	Rotates humerus medially; draws head of humerus to glenoid cavity of humerus
Muscles of the arm			
Biceps brachii (musculocutaneous)	Coracoid process (for short head); supraglenoid tubercle (for long head)	Radial tuberosity; deep fascia of forearm	Flexes and supinates forearm
Brachialis (musculocuta-eous and radial)	Anterior aspect of humerus	Coronoid process	Flexes forearm
Coracobrachialis (musculocutaneous)	Coracoid process	Medial aspect of humerus	Flexes and adducts arm

Contd.

Name	*Origin*	*Insertion*	*Action*
Triceps brachii (radial)	Humerus (lateral and medial head); infraglenoid tubercle (long head)	Olecranon process	Extends forearm; extends arm (long head)
Muscles of the forearm			
Pronator teres (medial)	Medial epicondyle; ulna	Radius	Pronates and flexes forearm
Flexor carpi radialis (median)	Medial epicondyle	Carpi and metacarpi on thumb side of hand	Flexes hand
Palmaris longus (median)	Medial epicondyle	Palmar aponeurosis (a thick sheet of tough fascia in palm of hand)	Flexes hand
Flexor carpi ulnaris (ulnar)	Medial epicondyle; ulna radius	Carpi and metacarpi on little finger side of hand	Flexes hand
Flexor digitorus sublimis (median)	Medial epicondyle; ulna; radius	Middle phalanx of each finger except thumb	Flexes finger and hand
Flexor digitorum profundus (median and ulnar)	Ulna	Distal phalanx of each finger except thumb	Flexes fingers and hand
Flexor pollicis longus (median)	Radius	Distal phalanx of thumb	Flexes thumb and hand
Pronator quadratus (median)	Distal end of ulna	Distal end of radius	Pronates forearm
Supinator (radial)	Lateral epicondyle; ulna	Radius	Supinates forearm
Brachioradialis (radial)	Ridge above lateral epicondyle	Radius	Flexes forearm
Extensor carpi radialis longus (radial)	Ridge above lateral epicondyle	Base of second metacarpus	Extends hand

Contd.

Name	*Origin*	*Insertion*	*Action*
Extensor carpi radialis brevis (radial)	Lateral epicondyle	Base of third metacarpus	Extends hand
Extensor carpi ulnaris (radial)	Lateral epicondyle; ulna	Base of fifth metacarpus	Extends hand
Extensor digitorum communis (radial)	Lateral epicondyle	Phalanges of each finger except thumb	Extends wrist and fingers
Extensor indicis proprius (radial)	Ulna	Phalanges of index finger	Extends index finger
Extensor pollicis longus (radial)	Ulna	Distal phalanx of thumb	Extends thumb
Extensor pollicis brevis (radial)	Radius	Proximal phalanx of thumb	Extends thumb
Abductor pollicis longus (radial)	Radius; ulna	First metacarpus	Abducts and extends thumb
Muscle of the hand			
Opponens pollicis (median)	Carpi on thumb side of hand	First metacarpus	Deepens palm
Flexor pollicis brevis (median)	Carpi on thumb side	Proximal phalanx of thumb	Flexes thumb
Adductor pollicis (ulnar)	Carpi on thumb side; third metacarpus	Proximal phalanx of thumb	Adducts thumb
Lumbricals (median and ulnar)	Tendon of flexor digitorum profundus	Proximal phalanx of each finger except thumb	Flex fingers at metacarpo-phalangeal joints; extend fingers at interphalangeal joints

Contd.

Name	*Origin*	*Insertion*	*Action*
Interossei (ulnar)	Shaft of metacarpi	Proximal phalanx of each finger except thumb	Four dorsal interossei abduct fingers; three volar interossei adduct fingers
Abductor digiti minimi (ulnar)	Carpi on little finger side hand	Proximal phalanx of little finger	Abducts little finger
Flexor digiti guinti brevis (ulnar)	Carpi on little finger side	Proximal phalanx of little finger	Flexes little finger
Opponens digiti minimi (ulnar)	Carpi on little finger side	Fifth metacarpus	Deepens palm
Muscles of the thigh & buttocks			
Psoas major (branches from lumbar plexus)	Bodies and intervertebral discs of lumbar vertebrae	Lesser trochanter	Flexes thigh and trunk
Illiacus (femoral)	Iliac fossa	Lesser trochanter	Flexes thigh and trunk
Gluteus maximus (inferior gluteal)	Dorsal surfaces of ilium, sacrum, and coccyx	Gluteal tuberosity and fascia lata of thigh	Extends thigh
Gluteus medius (superior gluteal)	Ilium	Greater trochanter	Abducts thigh
Gluteus minimus (superior sciatic plexus)	Ilium	Greater trochanter	Abducts thigh
Piriformis (branches from gluteal)	Sacrum	Greater trochanter	Abducts thigh
Tensor fasciae latae (superior gluteal)	Ilium	Iliotibial tract	Abducts thigh
Sartorius (female)	Anterior superior iliac spine	Proximal end of tibia (medial side)	Flexes hip and knee joints; rotates femur laterally

Contd.

Name	*Origin*	*Insertion*	*Action*
Quadriceps femoris (femoral);		Via patellar tendon into tibial tuberosity	Extends leg; flexes thigh (by rectus femoris only)
Vastus lateralis	Femur		
Vastus medialis	Femur		
Vastus intermedius	Femur		
Rectus femoris	Anterior inferior iliac spine		
Adductor magnus (obturator and sciatic)	Pubis and ischium	Femur	Adducts thigh
Adductor (obturator)	Pubis	Femur	Adducts thigh
Adductor longus (obturator)	Pubis	Femur	Adducts thigh
Gracilis (obturator)	Pubis	Medial condyle of tibia	Adducts thigh; flexes leg
Pectineus (femoral and sometimes also obturator)	Pubis	Femur	Flexes and adducts thigh
Biceps femoris (sciatic)	Ischial tuberosity; femur	Head of fibula	Flexes leg and extends thigh
Semimembranosus (sciatic)	Ischial tuberosity	Back of medial condyle of tibia	Flexes leg and extends thigh
Semitendinosus (sciatic)	Ischail tuberosity	Back of medial condyle of tibia	Flexes leg and extends thigh
Muscles of the leg			
Tibialis anterior (deep peroneal)	Tibia	First cuneiform; first metatarsus	Dorsiflexes and inverts foot
Extensor hallucis longus (deep peroneal)	Fibula	Distal phalanx of big toe	Extends big toe; dorsiflexes

Contd.

Name	Origin	Insertion	Action
Extensor digitorum longus (deep peroneal)	Fibula; tibia	Distal phalanges of toes 2-5	Dorsiflexes foot; inverts foot
Peroneus longus (superficial peroneal)	Fibula	First cuneiform and first metatarsus	Everts and plantar flexes foot
Peroneus brevis (superficial peroneal)	Fibula	Fifth metatarsus	Everts and plantar flexes foot
Gastrocnemius	Medial and lateral condyles of femur	Via Achilles tendon into calcaneus	Plantar flexes foot; flexes leg
Soleus (tibial)	Tibia; fibula	Via Achilles tendon into calcaneus	Plantar flexes foot
Popliteus (tibial)	Lateral condyle of femur	Proximal end of tibia	Flexes leg
Plantaris (tibial)	Lateral condyle of femur	Via long thin tendon into calcaneus	Plantar flexes foot; flexes leg
Tibialis posterior (tibia)	Tibia; fibula	Navicular	Inverts foot; supports longitudinal and transverse arches of foot
Flexor hallucis longus (tibial)	Fibula	Distal phalanx of big toe	Flexes big toe; plantar flexes foot
Flexor digitorum longus (tibial)	Tibia	Distal phalanx of each toe except big toe	Flexes toes; plantar flexes foot
Muscles of the foot			
Extensor digitorum brevis (deep peroneal)	Dorsal surface of calcaneus	Phalanges of each toe	Extends toes
Flexor digitorum brevis	Plantar surface of calcaneus	Phalanges of each toe except big toe	Flexes toes

Contd.

Name	*Origin*	*Insertion*	*Action*
Abductor hallucis	Calcaneus	Proximal phalanx of big toe	Abducts and flexes big toe
Abductor hallucis	Tarsi and metatarsi	Proximal phalanx of big toe	Abducts and flexes big toe
Flexor hallucis brevis	Tarsi	Prodimal phalanx of big toe	Flexes big toe
Abductor digiti quinti	Calcaneus	Proximal phalanx of fifth toe	Flexes and abducts little toe
Flexor digiti quinti brevis	Tarsi and metatarsi	Proximal phalanx of fifth toe	Flexes little toe
Quadratus plantae	Calcaneus	Tendon of flexor digitorum longus	Assists long flexor tendon in flexing toes
Lumbricals	Tendons of flexor digitorum longus	Proximal phalanx of each toe except big toe	Flex toes
Interossei	Shaft of metatarsi	Proximal phalanx of each toe except big toe	Four dorsal interossei abduct the toes; three plantar interossei adduct the toes (the axis of the foot is considered to extend through the second toe)
Muscles of the face			
Platysma	Tela subcutanea of upper part of chest	Skin and facia of lower jaw	Depresses skin of lower jaw, as in expression of sadness, fright, or suffering
Orbicularis oris	This muscle forms a ring around the mouth like a sphincter		All fibres working together close the mouth; separate parts of this muscle working alone have other actions
Quadratus labii superioris; or levator labii superioris	Bones and fascia of the face, just below the eye	Skin and fascia of upper lip	Elevates upper lip

Contd

Name	Origin	Insertion	Action
Quadratus labii inferioris, or depressor labii inferioris	Mandible	Skin and fascia of corner of	Draws down and everts lower lip
Zygomaticus	Zygomatic bone	Skin and fascia of corner of mouth	Raises corner of mouth
Triangularis	Mandible	Skin and fascia of corner of mouth	Depresses corner of mouth
Risorius	Tela subcutanea over parotid gland	Skin and fascia at corner of mouth	Draws corner of mouth laterally
Buccinator (main muscular mass of the cheek)	From a line in the cheek that extends from behind the last upper tooth to behind the last lower tooth	Skin and fascia at cornr of mouth; orbicularis oris; mucous membrane at corner of mouth	Draws corner of mouth laterally; used in chewing, swallowing, and whistling
Mentalis	Mandible just below the teeth	Skin and fascia at tip of lower jaw (mental protuberance)	Draws up the skin of the chin; trembles in a child about to cry
Orbicularis oculi	This muscle forms a ring about the eye like a sphincter. This muscle consists of vertical fibres in the tela subcutanea of the forehead		Closes eye Wrinkles brow
Muscles of masticaton			
Temporal (mandibular)	Bones at the side of the skull	Coronoid process of mandible	Elevates jaw
Masseter (mandibular)	Zygomatic arch	Outer surface of angle, body, and ramus of mandible	Elevates jaw
Lateral pterygoid (mandibular)	Great wing and pterygoid plate of sphenoid bone	Head and neck of mandible; capsule of mandibular joint	Working alone, it draws jaw to opposite side; working with mate, it depresses jaw
Medial pterygoid (mandibular)	Pterygoid plates of sphenoid	Inner surface of angle, body, and ramus of mandible	Elevates jaw

Contd.

Name	*Origin*	*Insertion*	*Action*
Mylohyoid (mandibular)	This muscle forms the floor of the mouth : it stretches as a gentle sling from one side of the mandible to the other; its posterior fibres are connected to the hyoid bone; a raphe (fibrous band) usually runs down the midline to the hyoid bone		Elevates hyoid bone and tongue
Digastric (anterior belly; mandibular; posterior belly; facial	The digastric consists of two bellies, end to end, separated by an intermediate tendon; the posterior belly takes origin from the mastoid region of the temporal bone; the intermediate tendon is bound to the hyoid bone, and the anterior belly is inserted into the mandible		Elevates hyoid bone and depresses jaw
Muscles of the neck			
Sternocleidomastoid (accessory)	Sternum and clavicle	Mastoid process	Working alone, rotates head toward opposite side; working with mate, flexes head; when head is fixed, elevates sternum, as in forced respirations
Scalenus anterior, scalenus medius, scalenus posterior	Transverse processes of cervical vertebrae	First and second ribs	Bends head to sides; fixes neck and upper ribs
Muscles of the back			
Sacrospinalis (erector spinae)	Bones of back (iliac crest, vertebrae, ribs)	Bones of back higher up (ribs, vertebrae, and skull)	Extends trunk; extends head
Muscles of the back			
Sacrospinalis (erector spinae)	Bones of back (iliac crest, vertebrae, ribs)	Bones of back higher up (ribs, vertebrae, and skull)	Extends trunk; extends head
Muscles of the thorax			
External intercostals (intercostal)	Rib above	Rib below	Elevate ribs; increase chest volume

Contd.

Name	*Origin*	*Insertion*	*Action*
Internal intercostals (intercostal)	Rib above	Rib above	Depresses ribs; decreases chest volume
Transversus thoracis (intercostal)	Inner surface of lower third of sternum	Inner surface of costal cartilages and anterior extremities of lower three or four true ribs	Depresses ribs; decreases chest volume
Diaphragm (phrenic)	From circumference of thoracic outlet	Central tendon	Draws central tendon down; increases volume of chest; decreases pressure in chest; increases pressure in abdomen; decreases volume in abdomen
Muscles of the abdomen			
Rectus abdominis (intercostal)	Pubic portion of innominate bone	Bottom of sternum; costal cartilages of ribs 5, 6-7	Flexes, trunk; compresses abdominal contents
External abdominal oblique (intercostal)	Lower eight ribs	Anterior half of iliac crest; linea alba via an aponeurosis	Compresses abdominal contents; assists in flexing trunk
Internal abdominal oblique (intercostal)	Lateral half of inguinal ligament; anterior half of iliac crest; lumbosacral fascia	Costal cartilages of lower three ribs; linea alba via an aponeurosis, pubis via falx inguinalis	Compresses abdominal tents; assists in flexing trunk
Transversus abdominis, or transversalis (intercostal)	Lateral part of inguinal ligament; crest of ilium; lumbosacral fascia; costal cartilages of lower six ribs	Linea alba via an aponeurosis; pubis via falx inguinalis	Compresses abdominal contents

Contd.

Name	***Origin***	***Insertion***	***Action***
Quadratus lumborum (T_{12} and L_1)	Iliac crest	Lowest rib; tips of transverse process of lumbar vertebrae	Lowers last rib; bends trunk laterally toward side of muscle
Muscles at the pelvis			
Levator ani (branches from pudendal)	Forms a hammock-like floor for the pelvis; it arises from the anterolateral and lateral wall of the pelvis minor and meets its mate of the other side at the midline		Supports and slightly raises the pelvic contents

TOXIC EFFECT OF DRUGS

Drugs that may cause ototoxicity

Streptomycin
Gentamicin
Kanamycin
Neomycin
Viomycin
Polymylxin sulphate

Drugs that may cause bone marrow depression

Chloramphenicol
Sulphonamides
Anticancer drugs
Phenylbutazone
Carbimazole
Rifampicin
Ibuprofen
Analgin (Novelgin; Metamizol)
Isonex (Isoniazid)
Thiabendazole
Griseofulvin

Drugs that may cause mental depression

Propranolol
Phenothiazines
Methyldopa
Prednisolone
Reserpine
Codeine
Morphine
Antihistaminics
Withdrawal of amphetamine

Neurological symptoms and causative drugs

Peripheral neuropathy	• Thalidomide • Nitrofurantoin • Isoniazid • Imipramine
Acute muscle weakness	• Diuretics—potassium loss • Neomycin—muscle blocking effect • Penicillamine myasthenic syndrome
Chronic muscle weakness	• Steroids • Chloroquine
Epileptic seizures	• Anticonvulsants (High dose) • Sedatives specially meprobamates • Phenothiazines (High dose) • Amphetamines • Cycloserine (precipitates seizures)

Headache	• Indomethacin • Monoamine oxidase (MAD) inhibitors • Excessive ergotamine • Birth control pill • Vit. A excess
Depression	• Birth control pills • Reserpine
Confusion and hypomania	• Antiparkinsonian drugs • Steroids • Excessive penicillin • Lithium carbonate
Parkinsonism	• Reserpine (Metoclopromide) • Phenothiazine (Butyrophenones) • Tricyclic antidepressants
Dystonic reaction	• Phenothiazines • L-Dopa • Metaclopramide
Visual disturbance	• Tricyclic antidepressant • Streptomycin • Chloramphenicol • Isoniazid • Chloroquine • Ethambutol • Birth control pill

UNION OF BONES AND EPIPHYSES

by 1½ year	the anterior, fontanelles should be closed.
„ 4-5 year	the greater tubercle fuses with head of humerus.
„ 9 year	the ilium, pubes, and ischium should meet in the acetabulum, rami of ischium and pubis fuse.
„ 18 year	these three should be united but still separable on maceration.
„ 15 year	the coracoid should be united to the scapula.
„ 16 year	the olecranon should be united to the ulna.
„ 16-17years	the head of the radius and the lower end of the humerus should be joined to their respective shafts.
„ 17-18 years	the internal epicondyle should be united to the humerus.
„ 18-20 years	the head of the femur should have joined the diaphysis.

UNITS AND CONSTANTS

Energy

1 Electron volt (eV) = 1.602 x 10^{-12} erg
1 Kiloelecron volt (keV) = 1.602 x 10^{-9} erg
1 Million electron volts (MeV) = 1.602 x 10^{-6} erg
1 joule (J) = 10^{-7} ergs
1 watt (W) = 10^{-7} ergs/s = 1 J/s
1 rad =1 x 10^{-2} J/kg = 100 ergs/s
1 gray (Gy) = 100 rad = 1 J/kg
1 sievert (Sv) = 100 rem =1 J/kg
1 horsepower (HP) = 746 W
1 calorie (cal) = 4.184 J

Charge

1 electronic charge = 4.8 x 10^{-10} electrostatic unit = 1.6 x 10^{-19} C
1 Coulomb (C) = 6.28 x 10^{18} charges
1 ampere (A) = 1 C/s

Mass and Energy

1 atomic mass unit (amu) = 1.66 x 10^{-24} g = 1/12 the atomic weight of ^{12}C
1 electron rest mass = 0.511 MeV
1 proton rest mass = 938.78 MeV
1 neutron rest mass = 939.07 MeV
1 pound = 453.6 g

Length

1 micrometer, or micron (mm) = 10^{-6} m = 10^{4} A
1 nanometer (nm) = 10^{-9} m
1 Angstrom (A) = 10^{-8} cm
1 fermi (F) = 10^{-13} cm
1 inch = 2.54 cm

Activity

1 curie (Ci) = 3.7 x 10^{10} disintegrations per second (dps) = 2.22 x 10^{12} disintegration per minute (dpm)
1 millicurie = 3.7 x 10^{7} dps = 2.22 x 10^{9} dpm
1 microcurie (mCi) = 3.7 x 10^{4} dps = 2.22 x 10^{6} dpm
1 becquerel (Bq) = 1 dps = 2.703 x 10^{-11} Ci
1 Kilobecquerel (kBq) = 10^{6} dps = 2.703 x 10^{5} Ci
1 megabecquerel (MBq) = 10^{6} dps = 2.703 x 10^{-5} Ci
1 gigabecquerel (GBq) = 10^{9} dps = 2.703 x 10^{-2} Ci
1 terebecquerel (TBq) = 10^{12} dps = 27.03 Ci

Constants

Avogadro' number = 6.02 x 10^{23} atoms/g.atom = 6.02 x 10^{23} molecules/ g. mole
Planck' constant (h) = 6.625 x 10^{-27} erg. s/cycle
Velocity of light = 3 x 10^{10} cm/sec
p = 3.1416
e = 2.7183

WEIGHT FOR HEIGHT IN MALES

Height cm	*Weight kg*	*Overweight limit (+2%)*	*Underweight limit (–20%)*
148	47.5	57.0	38.0
152	49.0	59.0	39.0
156	51.5	62.0	41.0
160	53.5	64.0	43.0
164	56.0	67.0	45.0
172	62.0	74.6	49.5
176	65.6	78.5	52.4
180	68.5	82.0	55.5
184	72.0	86.5	57.5

WEIGHT FOR HEIGHT IN FEMALES

Height cm	*Weight kg*	*Overweight limit (+20%)*	*Underweight limit (–20%)*
148	46.5	56.0	37.0
152	48.5	58.0	39.0
156	50.0	60.5	40.5
160	52.5	63.0	42.0
164	55.0	66.0	44.0
168	58.0	69.5	46.5
172	60.5	72.5	48.5
176	64.0	77.0	51.0
180	67.0	80.5	53.5

Section-3

Causes of Common Signs & Symptoms

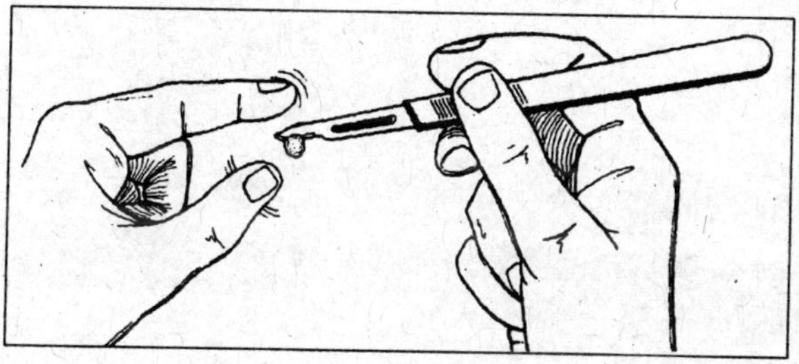

CONTENTS

Page No.

Causes of :

ABDOMINAL REFLEXES

Absent reflexes

- lesions of local reflex arc of T_{10} T_{12}
- pyramidal lesion (upper motor neuron) lesion
- marked Obesity and obdominal distention
- multiparous women
- typhoid perforation

Exaggerated

- psychoneurosis
- sensitive individual

ABDOMINAL RIGIDITY

Generalised

- perforation of hollow organs
- peritonitis

Localised

- intestinal strangulation
- appendicitis
- volvulus
- acute cholecystitis

In females

- ruptured ectopic gestation
- twisted ovarian cyst
- perforation of uterus
- acute salpingitis

ACUTE ATAXIA

Infections

- cerebellar abscess
- pyemia
- pyogenic meningitis
- toxic encephalopathy

Trauma

- birth Trauma
- cerebellar hemorrhage
- brainstem hemorrhage
- cervical nerve injury

Drugs and chemicals

- alcohol ingestion
- lead
- phenytoin
- piperazine

Tumors

- medulloblastoma
- cystic astrocytoma
- hemangioblastoma
- pontine glioma
- leukemia
- neuroblastoma

Other diseases

- posterior fossa tumor
- bacterial meningitis
- cerebellar hemorrhage
- hydrocephalous

ANKYLOSIS

Due to fibrous union of articulating bones

- tuberculous arthritis
- low grade pyogenic arthritis
- rheumatoid arthritis

Due to bony union

- bony callus
- suppurative arthritis
- tuberculous arthritis
- late rheumatoid arthritis

Abnormal bony mass

- excessive callus
- myositis ossificans
- ankylosing spondylitis

ARTHRITIS—TERMINAL INTERPHALANGEAL JOINT

Common Causes

- Osteoarthritis
- Gout
- Psoriatic arthritis

Uncommon Causes

- Juvenile chronic polyarthritis
- Sarcoidosis
- Septic arthritis
- Rheumatoid arthritis

ARTHRITIS IN CHILDREN

Bacterial infection

Rheumatic fever

Stills disease

Blood dyscrasia

- hemophilia
- sickle cell disease
- leukema
- bone marrow tumors

ARTHRITIS WITH SPONDYLITIS

Ankylosing spondylitis
Reiter's syndrome
Psoriatic arthritis
Arthritis with Crohn's disease

ATAXIA

Sensory ataxia

It is an incoordination of movements which occurs in limbs as a result of sensory loss.

- polyneuritis
- diphtheria
- diabetes
- alcoholism
- arsenical poisoning

Cerebellar ataxia

- head injuries
- disseminated sclerosis
- thrombosis of inferior cerebellar artery
- gliomata
- secondary growth

Ataxia due to drugs

- barbiturate poisoning
- carbon monoxide poisoning
- hypoglycemia

Hysterical

BACK PAIN

Congenital

- transitional vertebrae
- spondylosis
- spondylolisthesis
- short leg syndrome

Trauma

- damage to soft tissues/ligaments
- fracture of vertebra
- prolapse of disc

Inflammation

- ankylosing spondylitis
- sacroilitis
- osteomyelitis

Degenerative

- spondylosis
- ankylosis hyperostosis

BAD TASTE

- Ageing changes
- Poor oral hygiene
- Dental caries
- Periodontal disease
- Diabetes
- Medication
- Uremia
- Intraoral malignancies
- Acute necrotizing ulcerative gingivitis

BILATERAL PAROTID AND SUB-MANDIBULAR SWELLING

- Endemic parotitis
- Sjogren's syndrome
- Mikulicz's disease
- Tuberculosis
- Metabolic sialdenosis

BLEEDING GUMS

Systemic diseases

- Scurvy
- Thrombocytopenia
- Platelet dysfunction
- Acute leukemia
- Bleeding diathesis

Local conditions

- Injury
- Pyorrhea
- Receding gums
- Local lesions
  - Epulis
  - Epithelioma
  - Stomatitis
  - Papilloma

BONE SCLEROSIS

Paget's disease
Uremic osteodystrophy
Primary hyperparathyroidism
Cretinism

BREATH ODORS

Metabolic lesions

Diabetic ketoacidosis

- Uremia
- Hepatic failure

Drugs

- Alcohol
- Paraldehyde
- Cyanide poisoning
- Arsenic poisoning

Infections

- Chronic sinusitis
- Chronic dentooral sepsis
- Lung abscess
- Gangrene of lung

Food

- Onion/garlic consumption

BROWN LESIONS ON LIPS

- Nevus
- Labial melanotic macule
- Melanoma
- Albright's syndrome
- Addison's disease
- Hemochromatosis
- Kaposi's sarcoma

BURNING SENSATIONS IN TONGUE

- Idiopathic burning tongue
- Psychosis
- Neurosis
- Geographic tongue
- Xerostomia condition
- Anemia
- Achlorhydria
- Vitamin B deficiency
- Multiple sclerosis

CALCULUS FORMATION

Hypercalciuria

- Increased saturaton of calcium oxalate and calcium phosphate
- Spontaneous precipitation of calcium salts

Hyperuricosuria

- Increased saturation of monosodium urate
- Urate-induced crystallization

Hypocitraturia-renal tubular acidosis

- Increased saturation of calcium salts

Noncalcareous calculi

- Low urinary pH
- Gout
- Idiopathic
- Malignant tumors
- cystinuria
- Increased phosphate dissociation

CARPAL TUNNEL SYNDROME

Idiopathic
Complicating
  myxoedema
  acromegaly
  arthritis of wrist joint
  intermittent trauma

CEREBRAL PALSY

Prenatal causes
  developmental abnormalities
  intrauterine infections
  intrauterine radiation exposure
  toxemia of pregnancy
  multiple pregnancies
Intranatal
  anemia
  prematurity
Postnatal
  anoxia
  head injury
Infection
  —bacterial meningitis
  —cerebral abscess
  —viral encephalitis

CERVICAL LYMPHADENOPATHY

Infective
  gram positive
    Staphylococcus aureus
    Streptococcus
  gram negative
    E.coli
    pseudomonas
    proteus
  mycobacteria

Mycobacterium tuberculosis
atypical mycobacteria
viral
herpes zoster
infectious mononucleosis
Hyperplastic lymphadenopathy
Neoplastic
hodgkin's lymphoma
non-Hodgkin's lymphoma
giant lymph node hyperplasia
leukaemia
Saccoidosis

CHEST PAIN

Muscle
trauma
contusion
Bone
rib fracture
osteitis
costochondritis
Nerves
neuritis
toxemia
radiculitis
Pleural causes
pleurisy
pneumonia
cystic fibrosis
empyema
pneumothorax
subphrenic abscess
Oesophageal
foreign body
oesophagitis
achalasia
Cardiovascular
angina
aortic/pulmonary stenosis
pericarditis
myocarditis

CLAUDICATION

Arterial occulusion
atheroma
coarctation
venous occlusion
disc lesion
arthritis of hip and knee joint
hypothyroidism
congestive cardiac failure
anaemia
chronic inflammation
– tuberculosis
– Syphilis
carcinomatosis
collagen disease

COMA

Drug overdose
alcohol
barbit urates
morphine
Diffuse intracranial disorders
meningitis
encephalitis
subarachnoid hemorrhage
head injury
cerebral malaria
Severe infection
typhoid
cholera
Metabolic
anoxia
diabetic ketosis
hypoglycemia
kidney failure
hypthermia
With focal sign
(a) Brain stem lesion
infarction
postive hemorrhage
cerebellar hemorrhage
(b) Supratentorial
cerebral hemorrhage
subdural hematoma
extradural hematoma
brain tumor
(c) Diffuse intracranial disorder

CONFUSIONAL STATE

Cerebral
Cerebral infarction
thrombosis

embolism
hemorrhage
Transient cerebral inschemia
cerebral hypoxia
cerebral neoplasm
subdual hematoma
Toxic
infection
uremia
dehydration
diabetes mellitis

CRAMPS

Over exertion
Over use of certain muscles
Metaboilc
rickets in infants
hypokalemia
alkalosis
uremia
salt deficiency
diabetes mellitus
vitamin B deficiency
Toxic
alcholic neuritis
high fever
enteric fever
electrolyte imbalance
Circulation
Impaired arterial blood supply to legs
intermittent claudication
Specific muscle disease
Pain on exertion
muscle cramps

DELAYED MILESTONES

Bladder control delayed
delayed maturation of nervous system
mental abnormality
neglectful toilet training
Organic lesions
spina bifida
ureterocele
Speech delayed
familial
idiopathic
mental subnormality
deafness
poor environment
— tongue tie
Late smiling
lack of stimulation by mother
mental abnormality
delayed maturation
visual defect
Late walking
delayed motor maturation
mental subnormality
poor environment
hypotonia

DELAYED TOOTH ERUPTION

- Cysts
- Odontomas
- Maldevelopment
- Tumor
- Sclerosed bone
- Adontia
- Cleidocranial dysostosis
- Hypothyroidism

DELAYED UNION FRACTURE

Related to trauma
wide displacement of bone fragments
loss of bone substance
rupture of nutrient vessels
wide displacements of fragments
soft tissue interposition
estensive damage to surrounding tissue
compound fracture
foreign body in the wound
Related to treatment
inadequate reduction
excessive traction
intramedullary nailing damaging blood supply
General factors
hyperparathyroidism
rickets
anemia
diabetes mellitus
tuberculosis

DIFFUSE FACIAL SWELLING

- Cellulitis
- Emphysema
- Angioneurotic edema
- Cushing's syndrome
- Facial hemiartrophy
- Fibrous dysplasia

DISORDER OF TASTE

Loss or reduction of taste

- Damage to chorda tympanii
- Damage to VII nucleus (taste of 2/3 anterior tongue is affected)
- Lesions of lingual nerve
- Lesions of glossopharyngeal nerve
- Tongue—coated/glossitis

Distorted taste

- Post burn
- Drugs
    - Pencillamine
    - Griseofulvin
    - Lincomycin
    - Diuretics
- Metabolic disorder
    - Hypovitaminosis
    - Hypothyroidism
    - Adrenal cortical insufficiency
- Dyspepsia
- Psychosis

Foul taste in mouth

Local

- Caries
- Gingivitis
- Stomatitis
- Epithelioma
- Gumma in mouth

Gastrointestinal

- Gastric carcinoma
- Gastritis
- Pyloric stenosis

Pulmonary

- Bronchiectasis
- Lung abscess
- Tuberculous cavity

DRUG INDUCED MYOPATHY

Drugs :

heroin
alcohol
clofibrate
corticosteroid
phenytoin
chloroquine

DRUGS CAUSING LYMPHADENOPATHY

- Penicillin
- Hydantoin
- Streptomycin
- Sulfonamide
- INH
- Viomycin
- Heparin
- Phenylbutazone
- Phenacetin
- Iron dextran
- Antitoxins
- Follicular hormone

DRY MOUTH

- Local inflammation
- Infection and fibrosis of salivary gland
- Autoimmune disease
- Chemotherapy
- Postradiation changes
- Psychosis

FACIAL NERVE PARALYSIS

Supranuclear Lesions—lesion of lower part of motor cortex

- Cerebrovascular accidents
- Thrombosis
- Embolism
- Hemorrhage
- Tumor/infection
- Glioma
- Abscess
- Encephalitis
- Metastatic disease
- Multiple sclerosis

Lesions of brainstem

- Vascular insufficiency
- Head injury
- Infection
  - Poliomyelitis
  - Encephalitis
- Tumor
  - Pontine glioma
- Multiple sclerosis

Lesion of nerve trunk-infranuclear

- Head injury
- Cerebell opontine angle tumor/cyst
  - Acoustic neuroma
  - Meningioma
  - Arachnoidal cyst
  - Dermoid
- Granulomatous disease
  - Tuberculosis
  - Sarcoidosis
  - Syphilis

Intratemporal lesion

- Bell's palsy
- Fracture of temporal bone
- Acute otitis media
- Carcinoma middle ear

Extracranial lesions

- Tumors
  - Carcinoma of parotid
  - Metastatic disease
- Nerve injury during forceps delivery

Lesions any where along the nerve

- Congenital agenesis
- Diabetes mellitus
- Alcoholism
- Beriberi
- Polyneuritis cranialis

FACIAL PALSY

Newborn babies
- pressure in utero against facial nerve
- injury by forcep

Older Children
- bell's palsy
- mastoiditis
- polimyelitis
- cerebral tumor
- infectious mononucleosis

FEVER

Infective causes

- upper respiratory tract
  - common cold
  - tonsillitis
  - cervical lymphadenitis
  - otitis media
- CNS
  - acute bacterial meningitis
  - viral meningoencephalitis
- oral cavity
  - alveolar abscess
  - mumps
  - caries
- pulmonary
  - acute tracheobronchitis
  - bronchitis
  - pneumonia
  - TB
- cutaneous
  - cellulitis
  - viral xanthema
- musculoskeletal
  - spetic arthritis
  - osteomyelitis

FLUSHING OF FACE

- Alcohol
  - More in mongoloides
  - Severe after disulfiram
  - Chlorpropamide
- Menopause
- Drugs
  - Nitrites
  - Morphine injection
  - Nicotinic acid
  - Calcium channel blockers
  - TRH injection
- Neoplasia
  - Carcinoid syndrome
  - Pancreatic tumors
  - Medullary cancer thyroid
- Neurological
  - Psychological
  - Blushing
  - Anxiety
  - Parkinsonism

Tendonitis of rotator cuff
Shoulder injuries
Bursitis
Degenerative joint disease
Diabetes mellitus
Chronic pulmonary disease
Reflex sympathetic dystrophy

GAIT ABNORMALITIES—UNILATERAL

Stoppage gait
- lateral popliteal nerve palsy

Spastic gait
- hemiplegia

Limping gait
- shortening of one limb

Staggering gait
- unilateral cerebellar disease

Hysterial forward gait
Waddling gait
- dislocation of hip

GENERALISED STIFFNESS

Unaccustomed exercise
Systemic infection, e.g., influenza
Scleroderma
Hypothyroidism
Neuromuscular diseases
- cervical spondylosis with myelopathy
- tetanus
- myotonia

Other diseases
- rheumatoid arthritis
- generalised osteoarthritis
- serum sickness.

HALITOSIS

- Poor hygiene
- Periodontal disease
- Third molar opercula
- Decayed tooth
- Oral cancer
- Tobacco chewing
- Sinus infection
- Tonsillitis
- Diabetes
- Uremia

HEADACHE

Vasculature
- distension of scalp vessels
- arteritis
- aneurysm
- hypertension

Infections disease
- Viral infection
- bacterial septicemia
- infectious fevers
- sinusitis

Central nervous system disease
- neoplasm
- stroke
- meningitis
- neuralgia
- subdural hematoma

Eyes
- refractive error
- glaucoma

Cervical arthritis

HEADACHE DUE TO INFECTIONS

- Bacterial origin
  - Pneumonia
  - Meningitis
  - Encephalitis
  - Typhoid
- Protozoal origin
  - Malaria
- Viral Origin
  - Poliomyelitis
  - Dengue
  - Rabies
  - Post-herpetic

HYPERMOTILE JOINTS

Martan's syndrome
Homocytinuria
Osteogenesis imperfecta
Charcoat's arthropathy

HYPERTENSION

Essential hypertension
Secondary hypertension
- renal causes

— renal artery stenosis
— nephritis
— pyelonephritis
— polycystic disease
— diabetic kidney
— amyloidosis
endocrinal causes
— pheochromocytoma
— Crohn's syndrome
— Cushing's syndrome
in pregnancy
— pre-eclamptic toxemia
due to contraceptive pills
coarctation of aorta

HYPOGLYCAEMIA

Reactive

Induced by glucose
- postgastrectomy
- functional
- diabetes mellitus
- pancreatic beta cell tumour

Induced by galactose, fructose and leucine

HYPOTHERMIA

Accidental
Environmental exposure
Cold water immersion
Metabolic disorders
Hypoglycemia
Hypothyroidism
Adrenal insufficiency
Hypopituitarism
Diabetic ketoacidosis
Uremia
Drugs
- ethanol
- barbiturates
- phenothiazines
- general anesthesia

Acute illness
- congestive cardiac failure
- sepsis
- respiratory failure

Central nervous disorder
- brain tumor
- head injury, hypothalamic lesions
- spinal cord transection

INFECTIVE ARTHRITIS

Gonococcal arthritis
Meningococcal arthritis
Osteomyelitis
Acute hip synovitis
- virus
- mumps
- chicken pox
- infective hepatitis

JOINT CREPTIUS

Osteoarthrosis
Late rheumatoid arthritis
Tenosynovitis
Fracture
Skull
- hydrocephalus
- craniotabes
- severe rickets

JOINT PAIN

Inflammatory
- rheumatoid arthritis
- post viral arthritis
- septic
  - pyogenic
  - tubeculosis
- Degenerative changes
  - osteoarthrosis
  - chondromalacea
  - osteochondritis
- Metabolic disorder
  - gout
  - pseudogout
- Neoplasm
  - sarcoma
  - osteoclastoma
- Synovium
  - synovitis
  - synovial chondromatosis

Trauma
- dislocation
- fracture
- meniscus injury
- synovial contusion
- tendon rupture

Periarticular structures
- bursitis
- capsulitis
- tendinits

Systemic disease
- sarcoidosis
- carcinomatosis
- hypertrophic pulmonary osteoarthropathy
- leukemia

SWOLLEN JOINTS

Trauma
- simple
- internal derangement
- osteochondritis
- hemophilia

Infections
- acute bacterial arthritis
- viral infections
- chronic fungal arthritis

Rheumatic disorders
- juvenile rheumatoid arthritis
- scleroderma
- dermatomyositis
- ankylosing spondylitis

Postinfections
- viral infections
- hepatitis B

KNEE INSTABILITY

Ligamentous instability
- traumatic rupture

Patellar instability
- congenital dislocation
- acute dislocation
- recurrent dislocation

Paralytic instability
- after poliomyelitis

KYPHOSCOLIOSIS

Idiopathic
- skeletal
- osteomalacia
- rheumatoid arthritis

Congenital
- spina bifida
- hemivertebrae

Neurological
- neurofibroma
- syringomyelia
- poliomyelitis
- cerebral palsy

Chest disorders
- firbosis of lungs
- tubeculsosis

KYPHOSIS

Diffuse kyphosis
- scheurmann's disease
- rickets
- osteitis deformans
- rheumatoid arthritis
- ankylosing spondylitis
- senile kyphosis

Angular kyphosis
- tuberculsosis of vertebral body
- crush fracture of vertebrae
- metastasis
- hydatid disease of vertebra

LIMPING

Limp with fever
- periostitis
- septic arthritis
- collagen disease
- leukemia
- osteomyelitis

Soft tissue
- abscess/cellulitis
- lymphadenitis
- thrombophlebitis

Limp with trauma
- fracture
- hemoarthrosis
- sprain
- dislocation
- intervertebral disc herniation
- slipped capital femoral epiphysis
- tendinitis/bursitis

Acute limping
- aute osteomyelitis
- acute suppurative arthritis
- cellulitis
- acute rheumatic fever

leukemia
neuroblastoma

LOCALISED LYMPHADENOPATHY

Infection
- bacterial
  - —streptococcal
  - —staphylococcal
  - —tularemia
  - —symphilis
  - —tuberculosis
  - —viral
  - —herpes zoster
- protozoal
  - — leishmaniasis
- malignancy
  - —metastatic carcinoma
  - —lymphoma
  - —chronic myelogenous leukaemia
- local Inflammation
  - —reaction to antigen
  - —chronic skin trauma

LOOSE BODIES–JOINTS

Arising from synovial fluid
- hemarthrosis
- fibrinous loose body fibrous loose body
- tuberculosis of joint

Intraticular cartilage
- torn meniscus
- chipped off articular cartilage

Osteocartilaginous cartilage
- torn meniscus
- chipped off articular cartilage

Osteocartilaginous loose bodies
- chip fracture from articular surface
- displaced epiphysis

Degenerative disorders
- osteoarthrosis
- osteochondritis dissecans

Others
- detached osteophytes
- foreign body

LOSS OF CONSCIOUSNESS

Concussion
Midbrain compression
Brainstem compression
Cerebral infections
Hypoxia
Hypoglycemia
Epilepsy
Hypothalamic lesions

LOSS OF WEIGHT

Marked loss of weight suggests
- tuberculosis
- malignancy
- hyperthyroidism
- diabetes mellitus

Gradual loss of weight suggests
- malabsorption syndrome
- chronic infections
- alcoholism
- rheumatoid arthritis
- hemiplegia
- congestive cardiac failure

LOWER LIMB-PAIN

Congenital lesions
- dislocations
- subluxation
- transient synovitis of hip or knee

Slipped capital femoral epiphysis

Deformities
- genu valgum
- pes planus
- hypervitaminosis A
- baker's cyst

Avascular necrosis of bone
- legg-Calve Perthes' disease
- osgood-Schlatter's disease
- calcaneal apophysitis
- osteochondritis dissecans

Trauma
- fracture
- luxation/subluxation
- soft tissue injury
- traumatic synovitis

Infections
- osteomyelitis
- septic arthritis
- osteitis
- cellulitis

Vascular lesions
- thrombophlebitis
- hemophilia
- peripheral vascular insufficiency

Others
- rheumatoid fever
- rheumatic fever
- tumors
  - osteoid osteoma
  - bone cyst
  - osteosarcoma
  - ewing's
  - giant cell tumor

LYMPHADENOPATHY

Infective
- pyogenic bacteria
  - Staphylococcus aureus
  - Steptococcus pyogenes
  - mycobacterium tuberculosis
  - salmonella infection
- viral
  - infectious mononucleosis
- fungal
  - histoplasmosis
- neoplastic
  - Hodgkin's disease
  - non-Hodgkin's lymphoma
  - neuroblastoma
  - acute lymphocytic leukemia
- hemopoietic
  - sickle cell anemia
  - thalassemia
  - congenital hemolytic anemia

MONOARTICULAR JOINT DISEASE

Inflammatory arthritis
Osteo arthrosis
Infection
Trauma and meniscular tears

MONOPLEGIA

Sudden onset
- cerebrovascular accident
- poliomyelitis
- disseminated sclerosis
- encephalitis
- brachial/sacral plexus injury

Gradual onset
- primary/secondary cerebral neoplasm
- subdural haematoma
- spinal tumour
- paralytic brachial neuritis
- motor neurone disease

MUSCLE CRAMPS

Physiological muscle cramps
- Over exertion
  - Swimming
  - Strenuous exercise
- Professional cramps
  - Writers' cramp
  - Typists
  - Painters
- Late pregnancy

Pathological
- Hypocalcemia
- Rickets
- Prolonged lactation
- Parathyroid injury
- Hyponatremia
- Hypokalemia
- Heat cramps
- Urecemia
- Hemodialysis

Neuromuscular disorder
- Multiple sclerosis
- Nerve root irritation
- Toxic polyneuropathy
- Parkinson's syndrome

Other causes
- Vitamin B deficiency
- Tentanus
- Alkalosis
- Diabetes mellitus
- Gout
- Toxic cramps
  - Alcohol
  - Ergot
  - Lead
- High fever
- Idiopathic

MUSCLE PAIN AT REST

Tension headache
Low back pain
Fibrositis
Muscle cramps
Painful neuropathies
- alcohol
- arsenic
- polyarteritis nodosa

Myalgia

MUSCLE WEAKNESS

Congenital
- myasthenia gravis
- catalepsy/narcolepsy
- muscular dystrophies

Cardiovascular
- syncope

Neurological
- epilepsy
- raised intracranial pressure

Metabolic
- alcohol
- thyrotoxicosis
- cushing's disease

Malignancy
Polymyositis

MYOSITIS

Connective tissue disorder
- Rheumatic arthritis
- Fibrositis
- Polymyositis
- Scleroderma

Dermatological disorder
- Scleroderma
- Seborrholic dermatits
- Exfoliative dermatitus

Neuromuscular
- Myasthenia gravis
- Polyneuritis
- Progressive muscular dystrophy
- Polymyositis

MYOPATHY DUE TO TRAUMA

Physical
- direct injury
- surgical operation
- post severe exercise
- ischemia
- heat
- cold

NEUROPATHIC ARTHRITIS

Diabetes mellitus
Syringomyelia
Leprosy
Degenerative spinal disease (Fredvich's ataxia)
Tabes dorsalis
Aroneal muscular dystrophies

NEUROPATHIC FOOT

Neuropathy associated with systemic diseases
- Diabetes mellitus
- Uremia
- Amyloidosis

Neuropathy associated with nutritional disturbances
- Alcoholism
- Pernicious anemia

Neuropathy associated with infectious disease
- Leprosy
- Syphilis
- Poliomyelitis

Neuropathy on a vascular basis
- Cerebrovascular accident
- Spinal cord infarction
- Diabetic mononeuropathy Arteritis
- Peripheral vascular disease

Hereditary motor and sensory neuropathy
- Roussy-Levy syndrome
- Charcot-Marie-Tooth disease

Herediatry sensory and autonomic neuropathy
- Herediatry sensory neuropathy
- Congenital sensory neuropathy
- Dysautonomia (Riley-Day syndrome)

Cerebellar degeneration
- Friedreich's ataxia

Motor neuron disease
- Amyotrophic lateral sclerosis

Diseases of the spinal cord

Spina bifida
Syringomyelia
Trauma
Spinal cord injury
Peripheral nerve injury
Spinal root trauma
Compressive neuropathy
Spinal cord tumor
Peripheral nerve compression
Toxic neuropathy
Lead poisoining
Other causes
Cerebral palsy

NON-UNION OF FRACTURE

Poor vascularity
neck of femur
scaphoid
talus
Excess of soft tissue destruction
at the time of injury
during open reduction
Inadequate immobilisation
Soft tissue interposition between fragments
Infection
Over destruction of fracture
Deficiency states

OBESITY

Psychological factors
environmental influence
emotional response
parentral influence
Enocrine disorders
hypothyroidism
cushing's syndrome
corticosteroid therapy
pituitary dwarfism
General causes
delayed satiety
excessive caloric intake
limited calorie expenditure

OEDEMA

Generalised edema
Congestive cardiac failure
nephrosis
cirrhosis
gross anemia/hypoproteinemia
actue glomerulonephritis
Local oedema
hypersensitivity
inflammation
obstruction of venous /lymphatic flow

ORAL FETOR

- Oral cavity
  - Stomatitis
  - Abscess of tongue
  - Pemphigus
  - Erythema multiforme
  - Gingivitis
  - Dental caries
  - Pyorrhea
  - Periodontal disease
- Oral pharynx
  - Prolonged fasting
  - Acute tonsillitis
  - Pharyngitis
  - Xerostomia
  - Peritonsillar abscess
- Halitosis
  - Purulent bronchitis
  - Bronchiectasis
  - Pheumonias
  - Lung abscess
  - Pulmonary gangrene
- GIT
  - Hiatal hernia
  - Esophagitis
  - Ulcerative tumors of esophagus
- Other causes
  - Diabetes mellitus
  - Vitamin B_1 preparations
  - Arsenic

OSTEOMALACIA AND RICKETS

Nutritional vitamin D deficiency
premature infants
young children growing rapidly
pregnant women
Disorder of Vitamin D metabolism
chronic renal disease
long term anticonvalsant therapy

OSTEOMALACIA

Vitamin D deficiency
  dietary deficiency
  insufficient sun exposure
  malabsorption
Disordered vitamin D metabolism
  chronic renal failure
  anticonvulsant therapy
  chronic liver disease
Chronic acidosis
Phosphate depletion
Vitamin D resistant rickets
Osteopetrosis
Hypophosphatasia
Fluorsis

OSTEOMYELITIS

Spread by hematogenous route

- Bacteremia
- Septicemia
- Pyemia
- Boil/abscess or an occult focus

Contiguous spread

- Ischemic ulcers
- Diabetic ulcers
- Neuropathic ulcers

Direct inoculation

- Traumatic tissue necrosis
- Foreign body in wound
- Prosthetic joint
- Hematoma

OSTEOSCLEROSIS

Congenital
  pyknodysostosis
  axial osteomalacia
  hypoparathyroidism
Acquired
  flurosis
  plumbism
  carcinoma prostate
  leukaemia
  acromegaly

OSTEOPOROSIS

Endocrinal oseoporosis
  hyperparathyroidism
  hyperthyroidism
  cushing's syndrome
  acromegaly
  diabetes mellitus
Drug induced
  chronic alcoholism
  long term corticosteroid therapy
  chronic heparin therapy
Nutritional deficiency
  calcium deficiency
  vitamin C deficiency
  malnutirition
Primary osteoporosis
  postmenopausal
After ooporectomy
Nutritional causes
  calcium deficiency
  protein deficiency
  scurvy
  alcohol consumption
Endocrinal causes
  hyperadrenocorticalism
    cushing's syndrome
    corticosteroid therapy
  hypogonadism
  acromegaly
  thyrotoxicosis
Inherited
  osteogenesis imperfecta
Immobilization
  idiopathic
  juvenile
  postmenopausal
  senile
  pregnancy

OSTEOPOROSIS-ADULT

Primary
  post menopausal
  old age
  post oophorectomy
Secondary
  Diltary deficiency of calcium
  chronic liver disease

Endocrine
- hyperparathyroidism
- cushing's syndrome
- hypergonadism

Metabolic
- vitamin C deficiency
- pregency

Drugs
- Corticosteroid

Immobilization

Rheumatoid arthritis

Osteoporosis -Childhood

Osteogenesis imperfecta

Cyanotic heart disease

Immobilization

Acquired metabolic
- thyrotoxicosis
- cushing's syndroma
- scurvy
- lack of calcium intake

Neoplasm
- leukemia
- primary/seconary malignancy

PAIN IN UPPER LIMB

Neurological causes
- cervical root syndrome

PAIN MUSCLES ON EXERTION

Muscle ischemia

Cauda equina

Muscular dystrophy

Motor neuron disease

PAINFUL HIP

Avascular necrosis

Osteochondritis of epiphysis

Pigmented epiphysis·

Fracture

PARAPLEGIA

Acute paraplegia
- traumatic
- acute viral transverse myelitis
- prolapsed intervertebral disc
- meningovascular syphilis

Gradual onset paraplegia
- motor neurone disease
- lathyrism
- disseminated sclerosis
- subacute combined degeneration
- pellagra
- compression myelitis
- arachnoiditis
- syringomyelia

PATHOLOGICAL FRACTURE

Metabolic
- steroids
- paget's disease
- hyperparathyroidism
- scurvy

Degenerative, i.e. osteoporosis

Congenital, i.e., osteogenesis imperfecta

Neoplastic disease

Development disorder
- osteogenesis imperfecta
- arachnodactyly
- osteopetrosis

Nutritional
- rickets
- osteomalacia

Endocrine disorder
- hyperparathyroidism
- Cushing's syndrome
- hypogonadism

Cystic disorders
- solitary bone cyst
- aneurysmal bone cyst
- fibrous dysplasia

Bone tumors
- benign primary
  - chondroma, hemangioma
- Malignant
  - multiple myeloma, osteoclastoma
- secondaries
  - from lung, breast, prostate and kidney

PERIPHERAL NEUROPATHY

Metabolic
- diabetes mellitus
- chronic uraemia

Vitamin deficiency

subacute combined degeneration
pellagra
b-complex deficiency (alcoholism, beri beri)

Drugs and chemicals
isoniazide
nitrofuratoin
heavy metals

Infections
diphtheria
tetanus
leprosy

Miscellaneous
collagen vascular disease
malignancyo
sarcoidosis

POSITIVE `LE' CELLS IN BLOOD

Systemic lupus erythematosus
Rheumatoid arthritis
Occasionally other collagen diseases
Active chronic lupoid hepatitis
Malaria
Drugs
Hydralazine
Procainamide

POSITIVE RHEUMATOID FACTOR

Rheumatoid arthritis (80%)
Connective tissue disease, i.e., scleroderma
Chronic infections
syphilis
leprosy, pulmonary tuberculosis

After drugs
procainamide
isoniazid

Other diseases
biliary diseases
acute/Chronic hepatitis
sarcoidosis
lymphoma

PROXIMAL MUSCLE WEAKNESS OF LEG

Osteoarthrosis of hip/knee
Lumbar spondylosis
Diabetic amyotrophy
Motor neurone disease
Muscle disease with metabolic myopathy

RAISED ESR

Slow rising of ESR
pregnancy after 4 month
aneamia
acute myocardial infarction
—rheumatoid arhthritis
—carcinomatosis
—pulmonary tubeculosis
—acute gout
—burns
—acute infections
—after fracture and operations

Rapid rise in ESR
kala-azar
multiple myeloma
leukaemia
haemolytic anamia
chronic renal diseases
sarcoidosis

REFLEXES

Exaggerated
upper motor neurone lesions
tetanus
strychnine poisoning Hysteria
fright

Absent
myopathies
myasthenic syndromes
herpes zoster
tabes dorsalis
subacute combined degeneration
anterior nerve root tumor

REFLEXES—DIMINISHED

Transient
shock
massive hemorrhage
cerebral concussion
deep anaesthesia
diabetic ketoacidosis
hyperkalemia

Persistent
muscle disease

—dermatomyositis
—myotonia congenita
—periodic paralysis

Spinal cord disorder
—spinal compression
—syringomyelia
—hematomyelia
—acute poliomyelitis
—thrombosis

afferent pathway disease
—tabes dorsalis
—polyneuropathy
—motor neuron disease
—beriberi

SALIVARY GLAND PAIN

- Drug induced
  - Antihypertensive drugs
  - Cytotoxic drugs
  - Vinca alkaloids
- Common causes
  - Mumps
  - Stones
- Rare causes
  - Acute sialadenitis
  - Recurrent sialadenitis
  - Malignant tumors

SHOCK

Hypovolaemia

External fluid loss

haemorrhage
vomiting
diarrhoea
diabetes mellitus
burns

Internal Fluid Loss

Fractures
ascites
intestinal obstruction
haemothorax

Cardiogenic
myocardial infarction
arrhythmia
severe congestive heart failure

Neuropathic
drug induced, is ganglion blocking agents
anaesthesia
spinal cord injury

SHOULDER PAIN

Fracture/contusion
Bursitis
Bicipital tendinitis
Osteoarthritis
Infectious arthritis
Rheumatoid arthritis
Shoulder hand syndrome
Neoplasm
Myalgia
Fibrositis
Sychogenic pain
Referred pain
diaphragmatic irritation
apical lung cancer
cervical radiculopathy
Angina pectoris

SPINAL CORD COMPRESSION

Extradural
metastasis to spine
lymphoma, myeloma
disc vertebral collapse
tuberculosis, abscess
haematoma

Intradural extremedullary
meningioma
neurofibroma
arachnoid cyst

Intramedullary
glioma
syringo/haematomyelia

STIFF ACUTE NECK

Trauma
fracture of clavicle
hematoma
muscle injury

Inflammation
meningitis
cervical adenitis
retropharyngeal abscess
hysteria
tumors of nerves

STIFF NECK

Exposure to cold
Strain
Inflammtion of neck muscles
Meningitis
Rye neck torticolis
Acute thyroiditis

STOMATITIS

- Aphthous ulcers
- Debilitation
- Smoking
- Alcoholism
- Infection
  - Viral— Herpes simplex
    - Herpangina
    - Hand foot and mouth disease
  - Bacterial— Pyorrhea
    - Vincent's angina
    - TB
  - Fungal—Candida
- Systemic diseases
  - Leukemia
  - Neutropenia
  - Crohn's disease
  - Vit B_{12} deficiency
- Skin diseases
  - Pemphigus vulgaris
  - Lichen planus
- Drugs
  - Cytotoxic drugs
  - Mercury, bismuth
  - Antibiotics
- Leukoplakia
- Neoplasm
- Allergy
- Cheek biting dentures

SUDDEN DEATH

Acute myocardial infarction
Left ventrcular failure
Pulmonary embolism
Cerebral haemorrhage
Poisoning
Foreign bodies in trachea
IV injections in bypersensitive patients

TEMPERATURE OF HAND

Increased
- arterial aneurysm
- fever
- hypermetabolite states
- pontine hemorrhage
- gout
- diabetes mellitus
- environmental heat
- arteriosclerosis

Decreased
- shock
- hypothyroidism
- arterial occlusion
- raynaud's disease
- neurasthenia
- dermatomyositis

TENDERNESS OF CHEST

Inflammation of the skin
Myalgia chest
Intercostal neuritis
Herpes zoster
Pleural effusion
Pericarditis

TENDERNESS OF SPINE

Inflammatory
- pott's spine
- typhoid spine

Degenerative
- spondylosis
- osteochondritis

Neoplastic
- secondary deposits

Traumatic
- fracture
- dislocation
- disc herniation
- spondylolisthesis

Metabolic disorder
- osteoporosis
- osteomalacia
- hyperparathyroidism

THICKENED NERVES

Leprosy
Neurofibroma
Diabetes
Sarcoidosis
Amyloidosis
Idiopathic hypertrophic neuropathy

EXCESSIVE THIRST

Extreme Thirst with polyuria

- Diabetes mellitus
- Diabetes insipidus
- Chronic renal failure
- Potassium depletion
- Hypothalamic diseases
  - Tuberculosis
  - Sarcoidosis

Extreme thirst without polyuria

- Febrile state
- Excessive fluid loss
- Severe hemorrhage
- Hematemesis
  - Hemoptysis
  - Tubal rupture
  - Duodenal ulcer
- Drugs-Beladonna alkaloids

TRIGEMINAL NERVE PARALYSIS

Lesions of nerve trunk
Acoustic neuroma
Meningioma
Lesions of pons,medulla and cervical cord
Vascular lesions
Tumors
Syringo bulbia
Multiple sclerosis
At trigeminal ganglion
Tumors of ganglion
Fracture of base of skull
Herpes zoster infection
At retrosphenoidal space
Aneurysm of internal carotid artery
Cavernous sinus thrombosis
Steroid responsive granuloma
At sphenoidal fissure
Aneurysm
Invasive tumor
At apex of petrous bone
Apical petrositis
Tumors of petrons bone
Thrombophlebitis

TRISMUS

- *Inflammation in TMJ region*
  - Periostitis
  - Sialadenitis
  - Otitis externa
  - Malignant otitis externa
- *Muscle spasm/trauma*
  - Epilepsy
  - Fracture of zygoma
  - Mandibular fracture
  - TMJ dislocation
- *Tumours*
  - Benign tumor involving TMJ
  - Malignant tumor involving TMJ
  - Postradiation scarring
- *Inflammation of teeth and mandible*
  - Unerupted dentition
  - Stomatitis
  - Pulpitis
  - Osteomyelitis
  - Osteoarthritis
  - Chronic rheumatoid arthritis

VITAMIN B_{12} DEFICIENCY

Nutritional
extremely poor diet for a long time
Gastric causes of malabsorption
acquired pernicious anaemia
destruction lesion of stomach
partial and total gastrectomy
congenital intrinsic factor deficiency
Intestinal causes of malabsorption
chronic tropical sprue
jejunal diverticulosis
ileo-colic fistula
ileal resection
crohn's disease
fish tapeworm infestation

WASTING OF INTRINSIC HAND MUSCLES

Anterior horn cell
- polyneuritis
- syringomyelia
- motor neurone disease
- thrombosis of anterior spinal artery

Peripheral nerve
- radiculitis
- cervical spondylitis
- trauma
- polyneuritis
- carpal tunnel syndrome

Muscle
- dystrophia myotonica

Trophic disorders
- arthritis

WASTING OF MUSCLES

Systemic wasting
- tuberculosis
- malignancy
- thyrotoxicosis

Vertebral lesion
- craniovertebral anomalies
- vertebral metastasis

Anterior horn cell
- poliomyelitis
- peroneal muscular atrophy
- disseminated sclerosis

Disuse atrophy
- therapeutic immobilisation
- rheumatoid arthritis
- post paralytic

WHITE LESIONS OF LIPS

- Candidosis
- Squamous cell papilloma
- Verruca vulgaris
- Condylomata
- Lichen planus
- Actinic cheilosis
- Squamous cell carcinoma
- Cigarette smoker's lip
- Focal epithelial hyperplasia

XEROSTOMIA

- Local inflammation
- Fibrosis of salivary glands
- Drugs
  - Atropine
  - Other cholinergic drugs
  - Antihistamines
  - Tranquilizers
- Autoimmune diseases
- Postradiation changes
- Chemotherapy
- Psychosis

Section-4
Differenting Tables

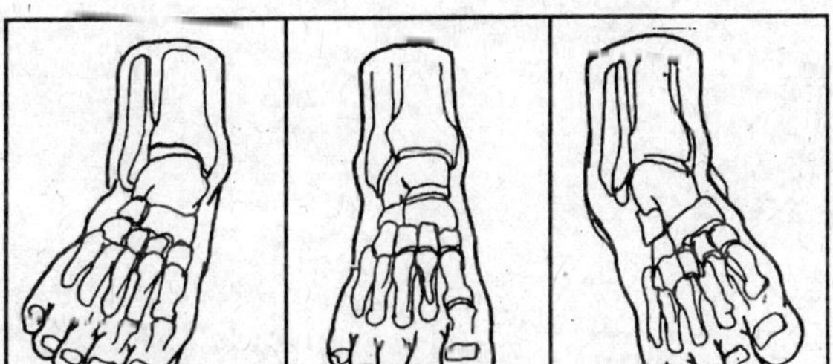

CONTENTS

ARTHRITIS

Osteoarthritis	*Gout*	*Frozen shoulder*
After 40 years often familial	25-40 years Hereditary	20-60 years males more affected
Insidious onset chronic joint changes	Attacks with sudden onset often during night	Usually sudden lucid intervals of mouth
Usually one or two	Usually single Big toe	Single asymmetrical
Asymmetrical knee, hips	Big toe Joints of hands	More of bursitis than arthritis
Aggravated by physical exertion effusion is rare	Moderate to severe agonising Swelling +	Stiffness, swelling due to effusion
Swelling not present	Not present	Present
Absent	Only in chronic stage	Absent
Wrinkling	Deep red, tense warm	Red and warm over bursal site
Locking of osteophytes	Absent	Absent
Voluntary restriction to avoid pain and limping	Very painful therefore restricted	Restricted pain and tenderness
Narrowing of joint space Osteoporosis Osteophytes No true ankylosis	Punched-out areas Gouty tophi Lipping Osteophytes	Areas of calcification

ARTHRITIS

	Rheumatoid arthritis	*Ankylosing spondylitis*	*Rheumatic arthritis*
Age	20-45 years	15-25 years, Sometimes hereditary	2-15 years
Onset	Insidious relapses	Insidious progressive	Rapid onset self-limiting
Number of joints involved	Multiple	Severe spinal joints	Multiple but migratory
Type of joints	Proximal interpharyngeal knee	Spinal joints sacroiliac and cervical joints	Knee bilateral peripheral joints rarely involved
Pain	Mild to severe relieved by rest	Mild to severe agonising Effusion +	Usually severe Swelling +
Muscle spasm	Present	Present	Natural splinting
Muscle atrophy	Marked in later stage	Present in later stage	Absent
Skin	Smooth & shing	Smooth	Red due to inflammation
Deformities	Flexion deformities fibrous ankylosis	Local kyphosis	Absent
Movements	Restriction in early stage tenderness stiffness absence of movements	Restriction from pain & stiffness progressive	Restriction due to pain, tenderness, swelling Natural splinting
X-ray	Osteoporosis joints space narrow. Bony ankylosis	Narrowing of joint space. Patchy areas of decalcification	Soft tissue swelling No specific changes of joints

ASSESSMENT OF GESTATIONAL AGE

Characteristic	*Gestational age in weeks*			
	28-30 weeks	32-34 weeks	36-38 weeks	40+ weeks
Breast nodule development	Absent	Absent	3-5 mm	7 mm+
Sole creases	Absent	Single anterior crease	2-3 creases	Many creases
Ear lobe	No cartilage	No cartilage	Pliable, some cartilage present	Stiff
Male genitalia	Testis unpalpable small, smoot scrotum	Testis in inguinal canal; small, smooth scrotum	Testis often descended : some scrotal rugae	Testis descended : scrotum fully rugose
Female genitalia	Prominent labia minora, labia majora flat	Prominent labia minora, labia majora flat	Labia majora almost cover labia minora, few rugae	Labia majora completely cover labia minora, marked rugae
Posture	Hypotonia	Some flexor tone at hips and knees	Some flexor tone at hips, knees and elbows	Marked flexor tone all joints
Scarf sign	Elbow past midline	Elbow past midline	Elbow reaches midline	Elbow does not reach midline
Toe to ear	Usual	Usual	Difficult	Impossible

BONE PAIN

Condition	*Nature of pain*	*Aggravated by*	*Worseningof pain at night*	*Swelling*	*Fracture*	*Bending of bone*	*Serum calcium level*
Paget's disease	deep aching	weight lifting	no	no	yes	yes	elevated
Hyperparathyroidism	vague	none	no	no	yes	yes	elevated
Osteomyelitis	localised	touch or movement	no	yes	no	no	normal
Osteomalacia	persistent	walking	no	no	no	no	decreased
Multiple myeloma	constant	none	no	no	yes	no	elevated
Acute leukaemia	generalised	none	no	no	no	no	elevated
Syphilis	deep pain	none	yes	yes	no	no	normal
Yaws	deep pain	none	no	yes	no	yes	normal

BRADYCARDIA					
	Sinus bradycardia	*Partial heart block (high grade)*	*Complete heart block*	*Sino-atrial block*	*Junctional rhythm*
Incidence	Fairly common	Common	Common	Very rare	Very rare
Heart rate	40-60	40 or less	40 or less (except congenital, in children or due to digitalis)	About 40	About 50-60
Associated condition	Athlete heart, increased intracranial tension, jaundice, myxoedema	Coronary disease, rheumatic fever or diphtheria, digitalis	Same as partial heart block beta-blocking agents, coronary disease, diphtheria	Increased vagal tone, digitalis,	Digitalis intoxication
Jugular venous pulsations	Normal 'a' waves preceding carotid impulse	Atrial waves more than ventricular rate	Position of 'a' wave continually changes with periodic cannon waves	No waves during pause in heart sounds	Cannon waves may be seen
Effect of exercise, atropine or emotion	Increase in rate	Abrupt slowing	No change or slight increase	May disappear	No change
Carotid sinus pressure	Further slowing especially if sensitive carotid sinus	Further slowing	No effect	Further slowing	May result in atrial standstill with persistent ventricular action
Heart sounds	Constant	No irregular change, atrial sounds may be heare	Changing intensity of Ist heart sound. Cannon sounds may be heard. Atrial sounds may be audible	Constant	Ist sound may be intensified due to simultaneous atrial and ventricular contraction

BURNS

	1st degree	*2nd degree*	*3rd degree*
Colour	Pink or red blanches on pressure	Pink, red mottled blanches on pressure	White brown, charred May show red mottling but does not blanch.
Blisters	Absent	Weeping base	Usually absent
Sensation to pin prick	Present	Present	Absent
Surface of wound	uniform	Elevated above normal skin	Depressed below normal skin
Healing	Without scarring	Minimal scarring	Granulation tissue

CARDIOVASCULAR CONDITIONS WITH CYANOSIS

	Oedema	*Blood Pressure*	*Visible Pulsation*	*Pulse*	*Apical impulse*	*Mumur*	*Other*
Persistent ductus arteriosus	—	low diastolic	supra sternal notch	Collapsing	—	machinery like	—
Fallot's tetralogy	—	—	—	—	absent	harsh systolic	soft second heart sound
Pulmonary stenosis	—	—	—	—	—	loud systolic	splitting second sound
Mitral stenosis	yes	low	low	low collapsing or irregular	tapping	diastolic crescendo	opening snap after second sound
Cardiac failure	yes	normal or high	external jugular	rapid and feeble	—	systolic	diminished pulmonary sound
Myocardial infarction	—	low or high	—	thready	diffuse	soft systolic blowing	diastolic gallop rhythm & third & fourth heart sound
Atrial septal defect	—	—	right ventricular	—	—	mid-diastolic	splitting second heart sound
Ventricular septal defect	—	—		—	—	pan-systolic	third heart sound at apex

CAUSES OF COLLAPSE

Causes	*Associated features*
Hypoglycaemia	Diabetic using medication Poor carbohydrate loading and intake High alcohol intake prior to event
Hyponattraemia	Ultra-endurance event Large amounts of plain water
Hypothermia	Slow athlete in endurance event Cold wind (change of weather)
Drug toxicity	Athlete using social or performance enhancing drug (e.g. cocaine, amphetamines)
Ischaemic heart disease/arrhythmia	Previous history of cardiac disease Family history High-risk factor profile
Stroke	Older athlete Hypertensive athlete
convulsions/coma	Epilepsy Head injury
Head injury	Contact sport

CENTRAL AND PERIPHERAL CYANOSIS

Point	*Central*	*Peripheral*
Initial site of appearance	Warm surface like tongue, inner surface of lips and conjunctiva	Depends upon the causes. It may appear earliest at the tip of nose, ear lobule, etc. Increase of low cardiac output and peripheral vasoconstriction.
Distribution of cyanosis	All over the body though the distribution will be more in the warm surface.	Localised or generalised skin surface but never present in warm surface.
Effect of application warm and cold	Warm-increased cold-increased.	Warm-increased cold-decreased.
Surface skin temp	Cyanosed part is warm due to increased blood flow.	Cyanosed part is cold due to less blood flow.
Pulse volume	High volume	Low volume
Clubbing	Present	Absent
Effect of O_2 inhalation	Cyanosis may be diminished	Usually no improvement.
Reduced haemoglobin concentration of arterial blood	Increased	Normal

CEREBROSPINAL FLUID IN VARIOUS DISEASES

Disease condition	*Physical characteristics*	*Cytology*	*Protein (g /l)*	*Glucose (mmol/l)*	*Tests for syphilis*	*Stained deposit*	*Culture*
Normal	Clear and colourless	0-5 cell/ml	0.1-0.5	2.5-4.2	Negative	No organisms	Sterile
Meningitis Bacterial	Yellowish and turbid	Polymorphs 200-2000- Lymphocytes 5-50	0.5-2.0	< 2.0	Negative	Bacteria	Positive
Tuberculous	Colourless sometimes viscous	Polymorphs 0-1000 Lymphocytes 100-300	> 0.5	< 2.0	Negative	Tubercle bacilli in films in some cases	Positive by special methods
Viral (includes poliomyelitis)	Usually clear	10-100 mixed cells at first, becoming lymphocytic in 36 hours	0.1-0.6 Poliomyelitis 0.3-0.2 remaining high 6-8 weeks	2.5-4.2	Negative	No organisms	Sterile
Multiple sclerosis	Clear and colourless	Rarely 5-15 lymphocytes	0.1-0.6 weeks. higher	2.5-4.2	Negative	No organisms	Sterile
Syphillis, GPI	Clear and Colourless	5-100 lymphocytes	0.4-1.0	2.5-4.2	Positive	No organisms	Sterile
Tabes	Clear and colourless	5-100 lymphocytes	0.3-0.6	2.5-4.2	20% negative by reagin tests	No organisms	Sterile
Meningeal	Clear and slightly turbid	10-50 poly-morphs 50-500 lymphocytes	0.5-2.0	May be slightly low	Positive	No organisms	Sterile

* CSF glucose is usually about half the blood glucose. Simultaneous blood and CSF glucose estimations should always be performed.

CHANCRE AND CHANCROID

	Chancre	*Chancroid*
Aetiology	Syphilis	A disease itself
Organism	*T. Pallidum*	*H. ducreyi*
Description	• Painless papule which rapidly erodes	Redish, ulcer, bleeds easily, painful
	• Edge feels cartilaginous • Induration	Superficial ulcer with ragged edges Base is covered with nectrotic exudate
Location	Penis cervix/labia/anus	Preputial orifice, prepuce, frenulum in women
Treatment	Pencillin G	Trimethoprim
	Tetracycline	Erythromycin

CHEST PAIN

Characteristic	*Chest wall pain*	*Nerve root pain*	*Angina*
Cause	Local trauma intercostal neuralgia	Osteoarthritis vertebral disease	Coronary artery disease, hypertension
Pain	Any part of chest	Dermatome	retrosternal neck or jaw
Radiation of pain	No particular radiation	Radiate from one part of radiotome to another	Mostly left arm occasionally neck/back
Quality of pain	Dull/sharp pricking pain	Sharp and fleeting chronic deep-seated dull pain	Squeezing, constricting griping, choking
Duration	Continuous/intermittent	Intermittent dull deep seated	1-3 minutes
	Local pressure increases pain	Increases by bending, coughing, sneezing	Effort emotion activity increases
Relieved by	Local application of warmth	Strong analgesic	Rest nitrites
Symptoms	Musculoskeletal pain elsewhere	Paresthesia in spinal segmental distribution	Feeling of impending death
Physical examination	Local tenderness Local swelling	Pain may be reproduced by pressure	± Hypertension
Investigation	Disease of rib or fracture on X-ray	Vertebral pathology ±	On ECG, ST and T wave abnormalities SGOT ++

CHEST PAIN

Myocardial	*Pericardial*	*Pleural pain*	*Oesophageal pain*
CAD, hypertension obesity	Tuberculous rheumatic	Tuberculous pneumonia malignancy	Oesophagitis, hiatus hernia, peptic ulcer
Retrosternal	Ant. chest epigastrium Left shoulder	At the site of pleurisy may be referred to shoulder	Retrosternal
Lasts more than half an hour	Sharp needs opiods	Inflammatory pain	Behind sternum upwards
Crushing, constricting, choking	Sharp cutting piercing	Sharp stabbing	Dullache, palpitation
Continuous for hours then fading	continuous fluctuating day to day	Intermittent	Variable dullache may be periodic
Unaccustomed exercise	Deep inspiration change in position	Pressure at the site of location, coughing	Swallowing
Not relieved by rest, relieved by morphine	Some relief by analgesics	Restriction of movements of chest wall	Upright position antacids
Sweating, weakness, pallor	Dyspnoea	Fever, cough, dyspnoea cough, fever	Dysphagia, excessive salivation haematemesis
Shock, BP falls	Pericardial rub	Tenderness hyperpalgesia pleural rub	Sour mouth acidity
on ECG, disturbance of rhythm and conduction	Typical contour of pericardial effusion	X-ray shows extent of pleural effusion	Barium swallow reveals hiatus hernia, oesophageal pathology

CHILDHOOD T.B. / ADULT T.B.

Childhood TB	*Adult Type*
• Since the infection has occurred for the first time tissues have no allergy to tuberculoprotein initially.	Tissues have already acquired allergy and immunity by prior infection in childhood.
• In this allergy plays significant role of pathogenesis of various lesions, i.e. oedema, necrosis and capillary haemorrhage.	In adult type tubercle bacilli plays major roll and not allergy.
• There is well-marked enlargement of mediastinal lymph node.	No significant hilar or regional lymphadenopathy.
• Tubercle bacilli spread by lymphatic and haematogenous route so extrapulmonary TB poses great danger.	Disease is localised to one organ due to prior immunity.
• Disease may run an acute course—younger the child more severe the degree of malnutrition. It is more severe in first 2-3 years.	Condition is usually chronic and runs a protracted course.
• Majority of deaths are due to extrapulmonary TB specially meningitis and miliary TB.	Cause of death is due to chronic TB not responding well to drugs.
• Healing is by calcification.	Healing is by fibrosis.

CHRONIC BRONCHITIS

	Chronic bronchitis	*Emphysema*	*Bronchial asthma*
Family History	Nil	±	+
H/o allergy	—	—	+
Duration	A few years	Few years	Many years
Early symptom	Morning cough, sputum	Persistent breathlessness	Paroxysmal breathlessness
Sputum	Copious, purulent	Scanty mucoid	Scanty
Dyspnoea	Intermittent	Progressive severe	Intermittent
Central cyanosis	Common	Absent	Present during attack
Clubbing	May be present	Usually absent	Absent
Wheeze	+	Absent	Common
Rhonchi	Sonorus/sibilinat	Absent	Wheezing rhonchi
Rt. ventricle hypertrophy	Frequently presents	Usually absent	Absent
WBC	often leucocytosis	No change	Eosinophilia
Moist sounds	Present	Absent	May be present
FEV_1	Low	Very low	Low during attack
PaO_2	Low	Normal	Low during attack
$PaCO_2$	Normal or high	Normal or low	Normal
Total lung capacity	Normal	Increased	Normal
ECG	Rt. axis deviation	Low voltage	Normal

CHRONIC RENAL DISEASE AND PREGNANCY

Renal disease	*Effects*
Chronic glomerulonephritis and focal glomerular sclerosis	There may be an increased incidence of high blood pressure late in gestation, but usually no adverse effect if renal function is preserved and hypertension absent before gestation; some disagree, believing that coagulation changes in pregnancy exacerbate these diseases, especially IgA nephropathy. FGS, and membranoproliferative glomerulonephritis.
Systemic lupus erythematosus	Expect more problems than most glomerular diseases, but prognosis most favourable if disease is in remission ≥ 6 mo before conception.
Periarteritis nodosa and scleroderma	Fetal prognosis is poor; associated with maternal deaths; reactivation of quiescent sclerodrma can occur during pregnancy and postpartum; therapeutic abortion should be considered.
Diabetic nephropathy	Pregnancy does not accelerate functional loss; increased frequency of covert bacteriuria; high incidence of heavy proteinuria and hypertension late in gestation.
Chronic pyelonephritis (infectious tubulointerstitial disease)	Bacteriuria in pregnancy may lead to acute exacerbations, but otherwise well tolerated.
Polycystic disease	There is controversy concerning whether functional impairment, often minimal in child-bearing years, is accelerated by pregnancy (we believe most are not)
Urolithiasis	Ureteral dilation and stasis do not seem to affect natural history, but infections can be more frequent; stents have been successfully placed during gestation.
Previous urologic surgery	Depending on indication other urogenital tract malformations may be present; urinary infections increase, and functional decrements have been observed; caesarean section may be necessary to avoid disruption of the continence mechanism if sphincters or neourethras are present.

COLITIS

	Amoebic colitis	*Ulcerative colitis*	*Crohn's disease*	*Ischaemic colitis*
Onset	Abrupt	Gradual	Gradual	Abrupt
Symptoms	Diarrhoea Streaks of blood	Rectal bleeding and diarrhoea	Diarrhoea with little or no bleeding	Sudden pain Rectal bleeding
Perianal inflammation	None	Occasionally	Common at times	None
Proctoscopy	Diffuse or isolated ulcer	Diffuse with friability	Normal, or focal discrete ulcers or diffuse	Usually normal
X-ray distribution	Sigmoid or caecum	Distal continuous segment	Rt side most frequent often discontinuous and asymmetric	Segmental splenic flexure often
Ileal involvement	Normal	Normal or dilated	Sometime normal often narrowed	Occasionally involved
Pathological findings	Submucosal and mucosal	Diffuse involvement of mucosa	Involvement of mucosa muscularis and serosa with deep fissure	Mucosa or transmural
None	None	None	Common	None

CONTACT LENS

Criteria	*Hard*	*Semisoft*	*Soft*
Dust problem	Present	Present	Absent
Normal wearing period	8+hours	18+hours	14+hours
Life of lens	4-5 years	3-4 years	2 years
Astigmatism correction	Possible	Possible	Not possible
Myopia control	Possible	Possible	Not possible
Adaptation	1-2 months	1-2 weeks	1-2 days
Comfort	Uncomfortable	comfortable	comfortable
Size of lens in relation to cornea	Slightly large	Quite large	Fully covering

CONVULSIONS OR COMA OR BOTH

Disorder	Headache	Tremor	Neck Tremor	Muscle cramp or twitching	Paresis	Con-vulsions	Coma
Viral encephalitis	yes	yes	yes	—	present	yes	yes
Bacterial meningitis	intense	—	yes	yes	present	yes	intense
Subarachnoid haemorrhage	severe	—	yes (late)	—	—	yes	severe
Brain abscess	yes	—	mild	—	slight	—	yes
Stroke	yes	—	yes	—	—	yes	yes
Intracranial neoplasms	yes	yes	—	—	present	—	yes
Respiratory acidosis	yes	yes	—	yes	—	yes	yes
Tetanus	—	—	yes	yes	—	—	—
Chronic renal failure	yes	—	—	yes	—	—	yes
Cerebral malaria	yes	—	—	—	present	yes	yes
Toxaemia of pregnancy	severe	—	—	yes	—	yes	severe

CORTICAL AND SUBCORTICAL DEMENTIA

Neurological sign	*Cortical*	*Subcortical*
Motor		
Speech	Normal	Dysarthria
Posture	Normal, upright	Flexed
Gait	Normal	Abnormal
Motor system	Normal	Slow movements, rigidity tremors ataxia
Mental system		
Language	Aphasia	No aphasia
Memory	Difficulty in learning new things	Difficulty in retrieving learned material
Cognition	Severely disturbed, aphasia	Impaired problem solving
Mood	May be depressed	Often depressed
Personality	Unconcerned	Apathetic
• Neurotransmitters involved	Acetylcholine	Dopamine
• Common disease	Alzheimer's disease	Parkinson's disease Progressive supranuclear palsy

DERMATOME

Segment	*Action*	*Muscle*	*Nerve*
C3	Abduction of shoulder	Deltoid	Axillary
C6	Flexion of supinated forearm	Biceps	Musculocutaneous
C7	Extension of forearm	Triceps	Radial
C8	Flexion of tip of ring and little fingers	Flexor digitorum profundus	Median
T1	Abduction of fingers	Dorsal interossei	Ulnar
L1	Flexion of hip	Iliopsoas	Nerve to iliopsoas
L2	Adduction of hip	Adductor magnus	Obturater
L3	Extension of knee	Quadriceps	Femoal
L4	Dorsiflexion of foot	Tibialis anterior	Nerve to tibialis anterior
L5	Dorsiflexion of big toe	Extensor hallucis longus	Nerve to hallucis longus
S1	Plantar flexion of foot	Gastrocnemius soleus	Posterior tibial
S2	Flexion of knee	Hamstrings	Sciatica
S3	Extension of hip	Gluteus maximus	Inferior gluteal

DYSPNOEA IN ADULTS

Condition	*Cough*	*Chest pain*	*Wheezing*	*Cyanosis*	*Haemolysis or bloody sputum*	*Chest sounds*	*Chest X-ray findings*
Persistent bronchitis	yes	yes	yes	yes	yes	hyperresonant percussion note; diminished vocal fremitus; rhonchi	no changes or prominent linear shadows with propgressive alterations in lung markings.
Bronchiectasis	yes	.....	yes	yes	yes	weak breath sounds; diminished vocal fremitus, rhonchi, coarse crepitations.	patchy consolidations ; increased bronchovascular markings.
Pneumonia	yes	yes	.....	yes	yes	impaired percussion note; crepitations; absent/ diminished breath sounds.	consolidation in the lobe or in patchy distribution.
Pleural effusion	yes	yes	.....	yes	.....	stony dull percussion; diminished/absent breath sounds and vocal fremitus; reduced vocal resonance.	homogeneous opacity; displaced mediastnum; obscured costophrenic angles; fluid in pleural spaces.
Pneumothorax	yes	yes	.....	yes	.....	absent/diminished vocal fremitus and breath sounds; hyperresonance	sharp edge of collapsed lung; translucency with no lung marking; mediastinal displacement
Pulmonary emphysema	yes	.....	yes	yes	.....	diffuse hyperresonance; scattered wheezes and rhonchi; diminished vocal fremitus	hypertranslucency of lung fields; widened intercoastal spaces; increased antero-posterior diameter of chest.

Contd.

Condition	*Cough*	*Chest Pain*	*Wheezing*	*Cyanosis*	*Haemolysis or bloody sputum*	*Chest sounds*	*Chest x-ray findings*
Pulmonary tuberculosis	yes	yes	yes	.....	yes	slightly increased percussion note at upper chest; weakened breath sounds	calcified and enlarged lymph nodes; consolidation with fibrosis.
Bronchial asthma	yes	.....	yes haps	per- sent	.....	hyperresonant percussion note; diminished vocal fremitus; high-pitched rhonchi.	nothing or increased bronchovascular markings.
Adult respiratory distress syndrome	yes	.....	.....	yes	.....	diminished breath sounds; coarse crepitations.	diffuse bilateral alveolar infiltration; later, snow-storm appearance.
Pulmonary eosinophilia	yes	yes	.....	.....	yes	hyperresonance, rhonchi and crepitations.	localised or diffuse opacity
Diffuse fibrosing alveolitis	yes	.....	.....	.....	.....	prominent breath sounds; crackling crepitations.	diffuse opacities; high diaphragm; later, honey comb appearance
Silicosis	yes	.....	yes	.....	yes	hyperresonant or dull percussion note; rhonchi.	nodular opacities; interstitial fibrosis; egg-shell opacities.
Cor pulmonale	yes	yes	yes	yes	yes	crepitant rales over lung base; diminished breath sounds.	enlargement of right ventricle & pulmonary artery; increased bronchovascular markings.

Contd.

Condition	*Cough*	*Chest Pain*	*Whee-zing*	*Cya-nosis*	*Haemo-lysis or bloody sputum*	*Chest sounds*	*Chest x-ray findings*
Cardiac failure	yes	.....	yes	yes	yes	accentuated pulmonary second sound; basal crepi-tations; some times rhonchi.	enlargement of right ventricle & pulmonary artery; increased bronchovascular markings.
Myocardial infarction	.....	yes	.....	yes	.....	soft systolic blowing murmur; presystolic or systolic gallop rhythm.	notching or enlarged cardiac shadow; pulmonary oedema.
Mitral stenosis	yes	.....	.....	.....	yes	accentuated first sound; doubling of first sound; Graham Steel's murmur.	straightening of left cardiac border; double contour of right border.
Mitral regurgitation	yes	.....	.....	.....	yes	high-pitched blowing decrescendo diastolic murmur; Dureziez murmur.	enlargement of left atrium and left ventricle.
Aortic stenosis	.....	yes	.....	.....	.....	gallop rhythm, loud systolic murmur at aortic area; diminished/absent second aortic sound	calcified aortic cusps and left ventricular enlargement.
Aortic regurgitation	.....	yes	.....	.....	.....	Austin Flint murmur; Cole-Cecil murmur; blowing decrescendo diastolic murmur.	aortic dilatation and left ventricular enlargement.

EFFORT ANGINA / ACUTE MYOCARDIAL INFARCTION

Point	*Effort angina*	*Acute myocardial infarction*
A. History		
Precipitating factors	Exercise, emotional upset, etc. But it never occurs at rest.	It may occur at rest without any provocation or may be opted by some factors
Severity	Severe	Very severe
Duration	½ to 3 minutes	Many hours
Relieved by	Rest or nitroglycerine tab	Only by deep sedation and opiods
Dyspnoea	Absent	Present
Symptoms of shock, cold extremities, excess sweating, etc.	Swealing present	Present
Fever	Absent	Present 24-48 hours after the attack.
Recurrent attacks of pain in the past.	Present	Absent
B. Physical Examination		
Attitude of the patient during attack	Motionless, stops walking	Restless, tossing over the bed for relief of pain

Contd.

Point	*Effort angina*	*Acute myocardial infarction*
Orthopnoea	Absent	Present
Cyanosis	Absent	Present
Pulse	Normal	Arrhythmias, pulsus alternans, extremely low vol. pulse due to shock present.
B.P.	Normal or slightly elevated.	Falls
Examination of heart	Normal or evidence of underlying factors present	Cardiac enlargement gallop rhythm, soft systolic murmur, pericardial rub, etc.
Exam. of lung	Normal	Basal crepitations
Embolic manifestations	Absent	Present
C. Investigations :		
ECG	Depression of ST segment and inversion of T wave	Elevation of ST segment, depression of T wave and presence of abnormal Q wave
Leucocytosis	Absent	Present
SGOT and SGPT, CPK level	Normal	Elevated

EPISODIC THORACIC PAIN	
Angina pectoris	Substernal visceral discomfort or distress, provoked by effort, emotion, eating and occasionally, by lying down. Relieved by rest and nitroglycerine.
Pleural pain	Precipitated by breathing or coughing; usually described as sharp. Associated physical and radiographic findigs of pleurisy.
Pain of pulmonary hypertension	Not closely related to activity or relieved by rest. Associated signs and symptoms of pulmonary hypertension and pulmonary disease.
Esophageal pain	Burning and substernal, with occasional radiation to the shoulder. Nocturnal occurrence (when lying flat). Relief with food or antacids.
Peptic ulcer	Nearly always intradiaphragmatic and epigastric. Nocturnal occurrence and daytime attacks relieved by food. Not worsened by activity.
Biliary disease	Usually under right scapula, prolonged in duration. Biliary disease is more important as triggering mechanism for angina than as a mimic.
Cervical disc	History of injury is common, provoked by activity only insofar as neck movement is involved. Persists after activity is discontinued. Local palpation and movement may produce pain.
Arthritis-bursitis	Usually of long (hours) duration. Local tenderness or pain with movement.
Neurocirculatory Asthenia (vasoregulatory asthenia)	Prolonged aches in various chest locations (often with arm radiation) likely to come at the end of an active day. Lethargy and fatigue, sighing respiration.
Hyperventilation	Tingling in circumoral area or hands; anxiety. Usually marked complaints of breathlessness without evidence of lung disease.
Chest wall	Provoked by movement, especially twisting, bending, etc. Usually long-tasting and often associated with local tenderness.
Psychoneurosis	Virtually always after anxiety; poorly described complaints, intramammary location of pain.

FEATURES OF VAGINAL INFECTIONS

Symptom	*Normal*	*Moniliasis*	*Gardnerella vaginitis*	*Trichomoniasis*
Discharge	Scant, varies with menstrual cycle	White, often thick	Profuse—yellow or green	Profuse, usually yellow or green, often frothy
Itch	Absent	May be absent	Present	Present
Odour	Absent	Present, may be the only feature	Fishy, worse after intercourse	Present, fishy odour
Inflammation	Absent	Absent / Present		Present, may have urinary symptoms
Tests that can be performed in the surgery				
pH	< 4.5	< 4.5	> 4.5	> 4.5
KOH (10%) Whiff test	Negative	Negative	Positive	May be positive
Wet film or Gram stain of a light vaginal swab				
Polymorphs	Few	Increased	Increased	Few
Specific features	Nil	Mycelia and spores (in KOH prep)	Mobile trichomonas seen in saline prep	'Clue cells'
Lactobacilli	Predominant	Predominant	Reduced	Reduced
Other organisms	Few	Few	Increased	Increased
Further investigations				
Fluorescent microscopy	Absent	Absent	Absent	Positive
Acridine orange culture		Sabouraud's medium	(Rarely indicated)	Feinberg-Whittington medium (rarely indicated)

FEVER IN ADULT

Abscess	*Malaria*	*Urinary tract infaction*	*Puerperal sepsis*	*Acute nephritis*
Symptoms	***Symptoms***	***Symptoms***	***Symptoms***	***Symptoms***
Acute onset of painful swelling in skin: It may be chronic as well. Tubercular abscess is one such example	Fever	Fever	Lower abdominal pain and fever within 4 weeks of child birth of children	Recent sore throat
	Body weakness Headache Mental contusion Diarrhoea	Pain on passing urine Frequency Incontinence in old patient		Sudden onset blood in urine
			Vomiting	Headaches
	Mild joint pains	Abdominal pain	Vaginal discharge	Swelling of eyes of face
Signs	***Signs***	***Signs***	***Signs***	***Signs***
Fever	Fever	Fever	Fever	Fever
Hot tender swelling	No signs of skin, chest ENT or urine infection	In old people mental confusion or incontinence may be the only signs	Tenderness in lower abdomen Rebound tenderness	Oedema of eyes or face Raised BP
Lymph gland enlargement	Anaemia Spleen Jaundice (no bile in urine) Malarial parasites in blood film	Urine cloudy, smells bad, slight protein	Discharge of bad smelling lochia Tender on vaginal examination Urine normal	Urine cloudy or pink and contains protein and red blood cells

Other conditions which can cause fever include : rheumatic fever, sickle cell crises, pneumonia, acute bronchitis, TB, hepatitis, appendicitis, peritonitis, septic abortion, meningitis, typhoid, septicaemia, kala-azar.

HAEMOPTYSIS AND HAEMATEMESIS

Points	*Haemoptysis*	*Haematemesis*
1. Preceding symptoms	Trickling sensation in the throat.	Nausea along with discomfort in the epigastrium Vomiting
2. Attended symptoms	Cough	Absent; may be present if material is aspirated.
3. Colour of blood	Dark red or bright red	Bright red of coffee gound depending upon the duration of the stay of blood in the stomach and on the gastric acid secretion capacity.
4. Particle mixed with	Commonly blood is mixed with sputum.	Blood may be mixed up with food particles, has taken just prior to vomiting of blood.
5. Reaction of blood	Alkaline	Acidic, but may be alkaline
6. Amount of blood	Usually scanty but may be massive	Usually massive.
7. Duration of blood	After the initial bout of bleeding the patient continues expectorating small amount of blood for a few days.	Usually bleeding is continuous or stops after a few bout depending on cause and extent of damage.
8. Melena	Uncommon	Invariably present after 24 to 72 hours.
9. Exam. of resp. and cardiovascular system	Abnormal physical findings are excepted to be present like mitral diastolic murmur, crepitation at the apex of lungs, leathery creptitation at the apex of lungs, leathery creptitation at base of the left lung.	Usually nothing found.
10. Exam. of GI system	No abnormality	Tenderness over the epigastrium ascites, splenomegaly etc.
11. Other associated symptoms	Dyspnoea, chest pain, cough, fetid expectoration etc.	Pain in the epigastrium, jaundice, bulging of abdomen, dysphagia
12. Chest X-ray	May reveal abnormality in the cardiac shadow or in the lung	Normal
13. Barium meal X-ray of oesophagus, stomach and duodenum	Normal	Oesophageal varix, peptic ulcer, gastric growth may be present.

HEAD-FACIAL PAIN

Headache	*Common migraine*		*Cluster*	*Psychogenic*	*Neurogenic*	*Atypical facial pain*
Quality	Throbbing	Throbbing	Borning sharp	Dull pressure	Lancinating	Dull
Duration	6-48 hr.	2-12 hr.	15-120 min.	Often unremitting	15-60 seconds	Often unremitting
Location	Unilateral	Unilateral	Orbital area	Diffuse bilateral	5th nerve	Uni or bilateral
Sporadic	Often several	Sporadic	Bunched cluster	Constant	Many times	May be constant
Associated symptoms	Nausea, vomitting, malaise, photophobia	Visual prodroma, vomitting, malaise, photophobia	Tearing, facial flushing, nasal stiffness, Horner's syndromes	Depression, anxiety	Identification trigger zone	Often associated with depression and psychosis

HEAT ILLNESS

Classification	*Mild*	*Moderate*	*Severe*
Type	• Heat cramps • Heat syncope	• Heat exhaustion	• Heat stroke
Symptoms	• Muscle cramps,especially calf and quadriceps • Fainting episode (at end of activity)	• Headache, exhaustion weakness, nausea, vomiting, confusion, ataxia	• Impaired consciousness
Signs	• Muscle tightness or spasm • Postural hypotension • Increased pulse	• Increased sweating • Decressed blood pressure • Increased heart rate • May need assisted respiration	• Decreased blood pressure • Increased heart rate • Often hot, dry skin (may be cold, sweaty)
Treatment	• Rest, ice • Massage • Oral glucose -electrolyte solution • Remove from sunlight • Lie down • Elevate legs and pelvis • Cool with ice/bath • Oral fluids	• As for mild • May need intravenous fluids	• Medical emergency : take to hospital • Rapid cooling • Intravenous fluids
Complications	No complications generally in in the absence of risk factors.	• Progression to heat stroke	• Neurological • Cardiovascular • Gastrointestinal • Renal • Disseminated intravascular coagulation • Rhabdomyolysis

HYPOTHERMIA

The clinical features of hypothermia vary depending on the degree of reduction in core temperature.

1. Mild : 35-36°C (95-97°F)
   - cold extremities
   - shivering
   - tachycardia
   - tachypnoea
   - urinary urgency
   - slight unco-ordination

---

2. Moderate : 32-34°C (90-93°F)
   - increased unco-ordination and clumsiness
   - fatigue
   - reduced shivering
   - slurred speech and amnesia
   - weakness and drowsiness
   - apathy, poor judgement
   - dehydration

---

3. Severe : <32°C (<90°F)
   - total cessation of shivering
   - inappropriate behaviour
   - reduced level of consciousness
   - muscle rigidity
   - hypotension and bradycardia
   - pulmonary oedema
   - cardiac arrhythmias

INDIRECT / DIRECT HERNIA

	Indirect	*Direct*
Site	Usually unilateral	Usually bilateral
Extent	May be incomplete/complete	Usually incomplete
Entrance and exit	Through deep inguinal ring may be through superficial inguinal ring.	Through floor of Hesselbach's triangle. Rarely through superficial inguinal ring
Shape of swelling	Usually pyriform shape with borad base below and narrow end above	Usually globular with broad base above
Reducibility	Gradually reduces after manipulation	Usually reduces at ease on lying down
Direction of reduction	Reduces upwards then laterally	Reduces up and backwards
Deep ring occlusion after reduction	Positive	Negative
Release of occlusion followed on coughing	Swelling appears first in middle of inguinal region and turns down to neck of scrotum	Swelling reappears
Obstruction/ Strangulation	Common	Rare

INTRACEREBRAL HAEMORRHAGE / SUBARACHNOID HAEMORRHAGE

Points	*Intracerebral*	*Subarachnoid*
Age	Elderly age	Young age
Past history	Uncontrolled malignant hypertension	Similar attack
Onset	Sudden severe headache, unconsciousness	Sudden with severe occipital headache may not be followed by unconsciousness.
BP	High of malignant type	Normal or high.
Coma	Progressively deepens in degree	Unconscious but no coma
Neck rigidity	Absent	Present due to meningeal irritation.
Hemiplegia present	Present	Absent
Cranial nerve paralysis	Absent	May be present
Fundus	Hypertensive changes exudate, narrowing of retinal arteries, papilloedema	Subhyaloid haemorrhage looking like half moon.
Recovery	Nil	Usual

IRREGULAR TACHYCARDIA

Characteristics	*Multiple ectopic beats*	*Atrial fibrillation*	*Atrial flutter (with varying block)*	*Sinus arrhythmia (with tachycardia)*
Associated condition	Idiopathic, ischaemic heart disease, digitalis toxicity, etc.	Rheumatic heart disease, thyro-toxicosis, ischaemic or hypertensive heart disease, or none	Same as in A. fibration	Normal heart, Common in children
Rate at apex	Usually less than 120	More than 120	About 160	Less than 140
Effect of exercise	Disappear	Rhythm becomes more irregular	May become regular	Disappears
Pulse apex deficit	May be present	Marked	None	None
Heart sounds	Occasionally only Ist sound heard	Vary in intensity	Variation of Ist heart sound	Normal
Other features	Long pauses preceded by pre-mature beats. Irregular cannon waves in jugular pulse	Pauses without preceding premature beats. More often permanent	Jugular pulse shows flutter waves. More often paroxysmal	Rhythm becomes regular if breath is held

LOOSE MOTIONS

	Cholera	*Acute gastro-enteritis*	*Food Poisoning*	*Bacillary dysentery*	*Algid malaria*	*Amoebic dysentery*	*Acute arsenic poisoning*
History	Epidemic	Sporadic	Group of people	Fever	Chill, High fever	Pain in abdomen before motion	Arsenic consumption
Abdominal symptoms	Effortless diarrhoea, vomiting	Vomiting and diarrhoea	Nausea loose motion	Pain abdomen tenesmus	Vomiting & diarrhoea	Colics mucus with stool	Pain abdomen, burning and vomiting
Vomitus	Whey water like	Bile stained	Bile stained	Less frequent	Bile stained	Vomiting not common	Blood may be present
Stool	Rice watery	Faecal matter bile pigment present	Blood +	Blood with mucous flakes	May be bilious	Microscopic bleeding not present	Blood may be
Abdomen	No pain	Griping pain	Griping and dull pain	Tenesmus more	No tenderness	Tenderness over sigmoid, caecum	Agonising pain
Temperature	Subnormal	Raised	Raised	High	Rectal 104°F	Normal	No fever
Anuria	Common	+	Not common	+	Early	Not occurs	Late
Stool examination	*V. cholerae* may be found	Pus cells	Not much of pus cells	Pus cells ++ RBCs Macrophages	M.P. on slide can be seen	*E. histolytica* found	Nothing particular

LOWER AND UPPER MOTOR NEURON LESION

	Lower	*Upper*
Wasting	Present	Absent
Tone	Tone decreased	Increased
Fasciculation	Present	Absent
Weakness	Segmental	Clumsiness, pyramidal pattern
Tendon reflex	Decreased/absent	Increased
Clonus	Absent	Present
Superficial reflexes	Present	Absent
Plantar (Reflex (Toe)	Plantar flexion of big toe	Dorsiflexion of big toe
(Foot)	Flexor plantar reflex	Extensor plantar reflex

MALIGNANT PERITONITIS / CIRRHOSIS LIVER

Age	*Malignant peritonitis*	*Cirrhosis liver*
Age	Old age	Any age
Duration	Short	Prolonged
Virchow's gland	May be palpable	Never palpable
Umbilicus	Nodular	Not nodular
Spleen	Not prominent	Palpable
Abdominal	Not prominent	Prominent
Liver	Enlarged hard coarsely nodular	Prominent
Degree of ascites	Usually moderate	Huge
Ascites	Malignant cells present, haemorrhagic	Colourless and transudative

MICROCYTIC HYPOCHROMIC ANAEMIA

Cause	*Marrow iron*	*S. Ferritin*	*Tr. Saturation*	*FEP : Hb*
Anaemia of chronic	Present	N	N	↑
Thalassaemia	Present↑	N↑	N↑	N
Sideroblastic anaemia	Ring sideroblast	↑	N↑	N
Iron deficiency anaemia	↓Absent	<12 mg/dl	<16 %	N
Copper deficiency	Present	N	N	N

MURMUR / PERICARDIAL RUB

Murmur	*Pericardial rub*
Quality of the sound is variable	Rubbery or leathery in quality
Systolic or diastolic or both in timing	Biphasic always
Maintains a constant relation with the heart sound	Relation with the heart sound is variable
Site of maximum intensity depends on site of production	Over the rth I.O.S. at Lt. parasternal region
Selective propagation may be present	Absent
Pressure of the stethoscope does not alter	Accentuates the intensity
Pain over the precordium is absent	Present
Fleeting nature not present	Fleeting nature may be present

NAIL DISCOLOURATION

	Onset	*Course*	*Nail colouration*	*Associated signs and Symptoms*
Cirrhosis	Insidious	Usually	White opacification of nail bed except for distal portion	Anorexia, weakness, splenomegaly liver size variable, ascites. Intermittent ankle oedema
Anaemia	Acute or insidious	variable	Nail bed appears pale with severe anaemia	Headache, vertigo, faintness, irritiability palpitation, dyspnoea systolic murmur, tachycardia
Chronic renal failure	Insidious	Progressive	Proximal portion is white	Polyuria, nocturia, oliguria and anuria, anoxia, hypertension, muscle twitching, cramps, numbness
Congestive cardiac failure	Insidious	Progressive	Lunale may be red	Fatigability, dyspnoea, orthopnoea nocturnal dyspnoea, cough, haemoptysis cardiomegaly, tachycardia
Vitamin B_{12} deficiency	Gradual	Usually resolves with therapy	Black pigmentation at nail bed	Fatigue palpation, dyspnoea, liver +, spleen ++, peripheral oedema may be present
Wilson's disease	insidious	variable	Blue brown discolouration	Tremors, incoordination, difficulty with speech and handwriting, dysphagia, rigidity
Arsenic intoxication	variable	variable	White bands in nail bed	vomiting, diarrhoea, abdominal pain, neuropathy, confusion
Chloroquin intoxication	variable	variable	Blue brown discolouration	Lens opacities, photophobia and bull's eye appearance of retina.

OEDEMA

	Ventricular failure	Nephritis type I	Nephrotic Syndrome
Onset	Oedema of feet precedes	Face, hands and scrotum	Face, hands and scrotum
Ascites	May occur late, severe	Occasional mild degree	Occasional may be recurring extensive
Liver	Enlarged, tender pulsatile	Not enlarged	Not enlarged
Spleen	Typically not enlarged	Not enlarged	Not enlarged
Heart	Enlarged murmurs gallop rhythm arrhythmias	Not enlarged Functional systolic murmur	Usually normal size
Blood pressure	May be elevated	Usually elevated	Normal
Diagnostic features	Heart size+exertional dyspnoea Enlargement of neck veins Oedema of dependent parts	Oedema in lower eyelids BP + RBC, albumin and cast in urine	Ascites oedema of face Heart size and BP normal Massive albuminuria No RBC in urine Hypoprotenaemia Transudate ascites

OEDEMA

Hepatic cirrhosis	*Hypoproteinaemia*	*Filarial*	*Hookworm*
Oedema of feet follows ascites	Generalised oedema starting at feet	swelling of feet spreading upwards	Oedema of feet
Usually present more often extensive	May be present mild or moderate degree	Not usual unless chylous	Not present
Enlargement during early stage later shrinks	Not enlarged	Not enlarged	Not enlarged
Usually 4-6 fingers enlarged	Not enlarged	Not enlarged	in severe anaemia enlarged
Normal size Systolic murmur	Normal may be mild + functional systolic murmur	Not affected	Not enlarged Functional systolic murmur
May be low	Not affected	Not affected	in severe anaemia low
Ascites then oedema Liver enlarged firm andnodular later shrinks Enlarged spleen Haematemesis	Low serum proteins Peripheral neuritis No heart or kidney disease High protein diets helps	Non-pitting oedema Presence of microfilaria in night sample Diethyl carbonate	Mild to moderate anaemia Eosinophilia Ova in stool Fatigue lethargy lassitude

	Prerenal failure	*Acute tubular necrusis*
History	Vomiting, diarrhoea, other causes of dehydration	Dehydration, ischaemic insult, ingestion of nephrotoxin; no specific history in 50% of cases.
Physical examination	Decreased blood pressure, increased pulse rate, poor skin turgor	May have signs of dehydration, but physical examination often normal
Urinalysis	Concentrated urine, few formed elements in sediment, but many hyaline casts.	Isosthenuria; setliment contains renal tubular cells and pigmented casts, but may be normal
Urinary sodium	< 20 mEq/l; most <10 mEq/l	≥25, usually >60mEq/l
Urine-plasma (U/P) ratios	High	Low
Osmolality	Often > 1.5	< 1.1
Urea	> 20	> 3
Creatinine	> 40	< 15
Fractional sodium excretion	< 1%	> 1%

ORGANIC CONFUSIONAL STATE / PSYCHIATRIC STATE

Organic state	*Psychiatric state (Functional)*
• Disoriented	Oriented
• Recent memory impaired	Recent memory retained
• Clouding of consciousness	Alert
• Usually no previous psychological history	May have previous psychological history
• Evidence of organic disease	No organic disease
• Non-specific clinical features such as neurological signs	Positive evidence for schizophrenia, mania or depression
• Older age group	Younger age group

PAIN ABDOMEN

Location of pain	*Location of organ*	*Common pathology*
• Epigastric	Stomach	Gastritis, peptic ulcer, cancer
• Substernal	Oesophagus	Oesophagitis, hiatus harnia, stricture malignancy
• Periumbilical	• 3rd part of duodenum • Jejunum and ileum	Duodenitis, tuberculosis Lymphoma, subacute obstruction
• Right hypochondrium	Liver	Hepatitis, cirrhosis, fatty liver, hepatic congestion
• Left hypochondrium	Tail of pancreas Spleen	Chronic pancreatitis malignancy Splenomegaly

POISONING

Poison	*Sign and symptoms*	*Treatment*
Hydrocyanic acid, cyanides	Syncope, dizziness, tachycardia Flushing Smell of bitter almonds	Gastric lavage, emetics. Inhale amylnitrate. 10 ml 3% sodium nitrite slowly, repeat every five minutes O_2 therapy
Methyl alcohol spiritis	Headache, dizziness, depression of CNS Nausea, vomiting dyspnoea, cyanosis, coma	Gastric lavage with bicarbonated water Treat acidosisbicarbonates by mouth 5 gm every 30 minutes In case of delirium—Nembutal 100 mg I.V. In case of cerebral oedema—Hypertonic glucose I.V.
Coal gas	Headache, psychic disturbance vomiting loss of consciousness Pink discolouration of mucus and skin Nervous disorder	Fresh air Oxygen therapy Antibiotics Treat shock and cerebral oedema 50 ml 50% glucose I.V.
Barbiturates	Comatose sleep slow respiration, cyanosis ± bronchopneumonia	Gastric lavage Humid oxygen Antibiotics Treat shock and cerebral oedema 50 ml 50% glucose I.V.
Phenol	Nausea, vomiting, diarrhoea Stuporous agitation, collapse, cyanosis Local corrosions	Gastric lavage. Lot of milk + water, charcoal Saline purgatives Ringer lactate I.V., analeptics
Mercurials	Metallic taste Severe abdominal pain, vomiting collapse anuria	Gastric lavage with milk Don't give emetics BAL Treat anuria

PYOGENIC / TUBERCULAR LUNG ABSCESS

	Pyogenic abscess	*Tubercular abscess*
Onset	Sudden	Gradual
Haemoptysis	Not common	Common
Fetid expectoration	Common with short duration	Not common
Clubbing	Usually common	Not common
Site	Usually on the base of right lung	Usually on the apex of right lung
Blood	Polymorphonuclear leucocytosis	Leucopenia
Sputum	Growth of pyogenic organism	Tubercular bacilli present
Chest X-ray	Wall ragged but smooth in chronic cases	Wall always smooth
Histopathology	Surrounding lung tissue normal	Surrounding tissue may show tubercular lesion

REFLEXES

	Afferent nerve	Efferent nerve	Centre
Superficial			
Corneal	Trigeminal	Facial	Pons
Pharyngeal	Glossopharyngeal	Vagus	Medulla oblongata
Upper abdominal	Thoracic 7-8-9-10	$T_{7\text{-}8\text{-}9\text{-}10}$	$T_{7\text{-}8\text{-}9\text{-}10}$
Lower abdominal	Thoracic T10-11-12	$T_{10\text{-}11\text{-}12}$	$T_{10\text{-}11\text{-}12}$
Cremasteric	Femoral	genitofemoral	L_1
Plantar	Tibial	Tibial	Sacral 1,2
Anal	Pudendal	Pudendal	Sacral 4-5
Deep reflexes			
Jaw	Trigeminal	Trigeminal	Pons
Biceps	Musculocutaneous	Musculocutaneous	C_5-C_6
Triceps	Radial	Radial	C_6-C_7
Supinator	Radial	Radial	C6-7-8
Wrist (flexion)	Median	Median	Cervical 6-7-8
Wrist (extension)	Radial	Radial	Cervical 7,8
Achilles	Tibial	tibial	Sacral 1,2
Visceral			
Light	Optic	Oculomotor	Midbrain
Accommodation	Optic	Oculomotor	Occipital cortex
Ciliospinal	Some, sensory nerve	Cervical sympathetic	Thoracic 1,2
Carotid sinus	Glossopharyngeal	Vagus	Medulla oblongata
Bulbo-cavernous	Pudendal	Pelvic autonomic	Sacral 2,3,4
Bladder and rectal	Pudendal	Pudendal and automatic	Sacral 2,3,4

REGULAR TACHYCARDIA

	Sinus tachycardia	*Supraventricular tachycardia*	*Ventricular tachycardia*	*Atrial flutter with 2:1 block*
Onset and termination	Gradual	Sudden	Sudden	May be sudden
Heart disease	Absent	Often absent	Usually present	Usually present
Heart rate	Rarely more than 160	160 or more	160 or more	Usually 150
Jugular venous pulse :				
(a) Rate compared to ventricular rate	Same	Same	Difficult to distinguish	Ventricular rate half of rate of flutter waves
(b) Cannon waves	Absent	Regular cannon waves may be seen	Irregular cannon waves	Regular cannon waves may be observed
Ist heart sound	Constant	Constant	Variable intensity	Constant
Carotid sinus pressure	Gradual slowing with gradual return to previous rate on release of pressure	No change or abrupt reversion to normal	No change	Abrupt slowing for few beats only

RETARDED INTRAUTERINE GROWTH : Biophysical profile scoring

Biophysical parameters	*Normal (score = 2)*	*Abnormal (score = 0)*
Fetal breathing movements in 30 minutes observation	One episode of > 30 seconds	Absence of fetal breathing > 30 seconds
Gross fetal movement in 30 minutes observation	Al least three discrete body/limb movement	Up to two episodes body/limb movements
Fetal tone	Active extension/flexion of limb(s) or trunk Opening or closing of hand	Slow extension/flexion or absent fetal movement
Reactive fetal heart rate in 30 minutes	At least 2 episodes of acceleration of > 15 bpm associated with fetal movement	Fewer than two accelerations or < 15 bpm
Amniotic fluid volume	At least one pocket > 2 cm in two perpendicular planes	< 2 cm fluid pocket in two perpendicular planes

RODS AND CONES

	Rods	*Cones*
Situated in central part of fovea	Absent	Present
Most of macula	Present—less than cones	More than rods
Intensity of illumination	For low intensity	For bright light
Type of vision	For peripheral vision	For central visions detection of colours
Number	130 million	7 million
Outer segment	700 membranous discs, contains rodopsin	1000 membranous disc at fovea
Inner segment	Striated rootless extending into fibres	Segment is thicker than in rods
Fibre	10-100 end foot synapse with one bipolar neuron	One end foot synapses with dendrites of several bipolar neurons

SECONDARY DYSMENORRHOEA

	Endometriosis	*Endometritis*
Location	Pelvic	Pelvic
Pattern	Recurrent with menses	Acute episode begins with menses. Pain may extend to involve whole of abdomen
Associated finding	Irregular menses Infertility Discharge ±	Fever Elevated WBC Elevated ESR Purulent discharge
Pelvic examination	Mild tenderness on involved area Thickening, beading of rectovaginal septum May be chocolate ovarian cyst No vaginal discharge	Tenderness over uterine area Purulent cervical discharge

SPECTACLE / CONTACT LENS

Criteric	*Spectacles*	*Contact lens*
Night Vision	Good	Disturbances due to halos around light
Day vision	Good	Better
Myopia control	Not possible	Possible
Astigmatism correction	Good	Better
Rain	Wetting present	Absent
Injury	Rare	Rare
Corneal abrasion	No	Possible
Marks on nose	Present	Absent
Cosmetic value	Not advisable	Advisable
Cost	Less	More

SYMPATHETIC / PARASYMPATHETIC

Sympathetic	*Parasympathetic*
• Postganglionic neurons in sympathetic trunk or plexus	Peripheral postganglionic neurons.
• Produces mass response	Discrete vegetative response
• Accelerates heart, increases blood pressure	Produces localised effects.
• Constriction of cutaneous arteries thus causing increase of blood supply to heart, muscle and brain	Slows the heart
• Slows down peristalsis, contraction of sphincters	Increases peristalsis, relaxes sphincters
• Preganglionic transmitter is acetylcholine	Increases glandular and peristaltic activities of gut.
• Postganglionic transmitter is noradrenaline	Acetylcholine
• Thoracolumbar outflow (T_1–L_2)	Postganglionic transmitter is acetylcholine. Craniosacral outflow sacral— S_2-S_4 cranial— 3rd, 7th, 9th and 10th cranial nerves

TACHYCARDIAS

	Atrial rate	*Ventricular rate*	*Clinical setting*	*Electrocardiographic features*
Sinus tachycardia	100-160 In children may be above 200	Same	Exercise, leve, emotion, anaemia, thyrotoxicosis, etc.	P-wave amplitude normal or increased. PR interval normal Usually appears and subsides gradually.
Atrial tachycardia	140-220	Same	No organic heart disese, RHD, CHD, ASHD, HCVD, thyrotoxicosis, drugs, pericarditis	Usually precisely regular P-wave precedes each QRS. P-wave configuration abnormal. QRS may show aberrancy simulating ventricular tachycardia. Rhythm appears and subsides abruptly.
Atrial tachycardia with AV block	140-200	Often a fixed fraction of the atrial rate	Digitalis, ASHD, RHD	RR interval usually two or three times atrial rate but variability may occur if degree of AV block is variable. Differs from atrial flutter by slower atrial rate and isoelectric baseline between P-waves.
Multifocal atrial tachycardia	> 100	Same	Severe underlying disease, often pulmonary	Variable PP, variable PR, multiform P-wave morphology.

Contd.

	Atrial rate	*Ventricular rate*	*Clinical setting*	*Electrocardiographic features*
Atrial flutter	220-320	Usually a fixed fraction of the atrial rate	RHD, ASHD, pulmonary embolus, pericarditis, thyrotoxicosis, CHD. digitalis	P or F waves occur with great regularity and result in a typical saw-tooth or picket fence undulation in leads II, AVF, V1 and V2
Atrial fibrilitation	320-500	40-300	RHD, ASHD, pericarditis, thyrotoxicosis, CHD digitalis pulmonary embolus	Totally irregular RR interval. Baseline may have fine or coarse fibrilatory waves. In some instances no evidence of atrial activity discernible and the diagnosis rests upon the grossly irregular ventricular response.
Wolff-Parkinson-White Syndome	60-100	60-100	No organic heart disease, CHD, RHD	Short PR interval due to early onset of QRS as a delta wave. Total QRS duration prolonged. P to S interval normal. May simulate posterior infarction or right-ventricular hypertrophy.
AV Junctional Tachycardia	140-220	140-220	Digitalis, ASHD, RHD CHD, no organic heart disease	Regular R-wave interval P-wave inverted in leads. II, III and upright in AVR P-waves may occur before, with, or after the QRS waves. AV Dissociation results in separate atrial and ventricular rates. QRS as in normal sinus rhythm.

Contd.

Contd.

	Atrial rate	*Ventricular rate*	*Clinical setting*	*Electrocardiographic features*
Accelerated junctional rhythm	60-100	60-130	Digitalis	Same as above except slower rate QRS as in normal sinus rhythm.
Accelerated ventricular rhythm	80-130	80-130	Acute myocardial infarction	Same as above. Rate often very close to sinus rate
Ventricular tachycardia	50-140	140-280	Acute myocardial infarction, anoxia, electric shock, digitalis, trauma, no organic heart disease appear	Borad, bizarre, slightly irregular QRS complexes. Independent and slower P-wave rate can sometimes be determined. Fusion beats may appear
Ventricular flutter and fibriliation	250-500	300 or greater	Acute myocardial infarction anoxia, electric, shocks, digitalis, trauma, quinidine	Disorganized, grossly irregular wave pattern.

TESTIS

Undescended	*Ectopic*
• Arrested descent of testis which lies in normal path of its descent.	The testis deviates from its normal path of descent.
• Undescended testis is poorly developed.	Usually well developed.
• Scrotum is not developed.	Scrotum is usually developed.
• Length of cord is usually short.	Length of the cord is adequate.
• Undescended testis lies deep in inguinal canal.	It lies superficial to inguinal canal
• Spermatogenesis becomes poor.	Spermatogenesis normal.
• On pressure the testis disappears upwards, backwards and laterally.	No effect on pressure.

TRANSUDATE / EXUDATE

	Transudate	*Exudate*
Colour	Colourless and clear	Straw red and milky
Coagulum	Absent	Present
Specific gravity	Less than 1018	More than 1018
Protein	Less than 2 gm %	More than 4 gm %
Cells	No inflammatory cells Endothelial cells present	Lymphocytes and polymorphs inflammatory cells
Culture	Sterile	Growth of organism

TYPHOID PERFORATION / TYPHOID HAEMORRHAGE

Typhoid	*Haemorrhage*	*Typhoid perforation*
Pathology	The haemorrhage is due to tearing or rupture of intestine	When ulcer is deep and penetrates the muscle coat result is perforation
Prognosis	Good	Bad
Symptom	Sudden with a sinking sensation accompanied by sudden fall of temperature	Sudden with a sense of giving way within
Stool	Melena or passage of blood per rectum	Absolute constipation
Urine	Oliguria	May be increased in frequency
Attitude	Restless	Dorsal decubitus with hip flexed
Abdomen	Except hurried peristalsis sound no other abnormality is detected	Rigidity in right iliac fossa
PR	Finger may be stained with anemia with stool	Nothing special
Blood	Normocytic normochromic anemic with leucocytosis	Marked leucocytosis with increased neutrophils

VITILIGO / TINEA

	Vitiligo	*Tinea*
Aetiology	Autoimmune	Fungal infection
Incidence	1%	Common
Pathology	Destruction on melanocyte	Decreased melanosomes in stratum corneum
Age	Young adults	Young adults
Description	Macular depigmented areas Absence of melanin	Small hypopigmented macules
Associated conditions	Graves disease Pernicious anaemia Diabetes mellitus Addison's disease	Unhyiegenic Inmates Excessive Sweating
Therapy	Trioxsalen with sun exposure	Selenium sulphide Sulphur ointment Salicylic acid

Section-5
Food and Nutrition

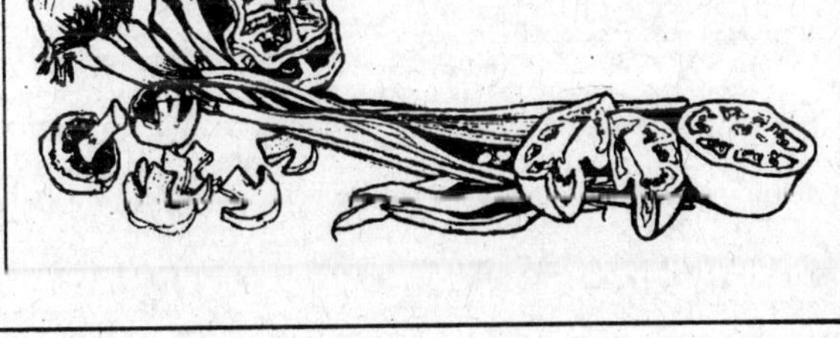

CONTENTS

NUTRIENT DEFICIENCY

Area of Examination	Sign/symptom	Potential nutrient deficiency
Hair	Alopecia	Zinc, essential fatty acids
	Easy pluckability	Protein, essential fatty acids
	Lacklustre	Protein, zinc
	"Corkscrew" hair	Vitamin C, vitamin A
	Decreased pigmentation	Protein, copper
Eyes	Xerosis of conjunctiva	Vitamin A
	Corneal vascularisation	Riboflavin
	Keratomalacia	Vitamin A
	Bitot's spots	Vitamin A
Gastrointestinal tract	Nausea, vomiting	Pyridoxine
	Diarrhoea	Zinc, niacin
	Stomatititis	Pyridoxine, riboflavin, iron
	Cheilosis	Pyridoxine, iron
	Glossitis	Pyridoxine, zinc, niacin, folate, vitamin B_{12}
	Magenta tongue	Riboflavin
	Swollen, bleeding gums	Vitamin C
	Fissured tongue	Niacin
	Hepatomegaly	Protein
Skin	Dry and scaling	Vitamin A, essential fatty acids, zinc
	Petechiae, ecchymoses	Vitamin C, vitamin K
	Follicular hyperkeratosis	Vitamin A, essential fatty acids
	Nasolabial seborrhea	Niacin, pyridoxine, riboflavin
	Bilateral dermatitis	Niacin, zinc
Extremities	Subcutaneous fat loss	Kilocalories
	Muscle wastage	Kilocalories, protein
	Oedema	Protein
	Osteomalacia, bone pain, rickets	Vitamin D
	Arthralgia	Vitamin C
Haematologic	Anaemia	Vitamin B_{12}, iron, folate, copper, vitamin E, vitamin K
	Leucopenia, neutropenia	Copper
	Low prothrombin, prolonged clotting time	Vitamin K
Neurologic	Disorientation	Niacin, thiamin
	Confabulation	Thiamin
	Neuropathy	Thiamin, pyridoxine, chromium
	Paraesthesia	Thiamin, pyridoxine, vitamin B_{12}
Cardiovascular	Congestive heart failure, cardiomegaly, tachycardia	Thiamin
	Cardiomyopathy	Selenium

TRACE ELEMENTS

Element	*Metabolism*	*Physiologic Function*	*Clinical Application*	*Requirements*	*Food Sources*
Iron (Fe)	Absorption according to body need; aided by vitamin C Haeme and nonhaeme forms Excretion from tissue in minute quantities body conserves then reuses Absorbed as iodides, taken up by thyroid	Haemoglobin formation Cellular oxidation of glucose Myoglobin in muscle Antibody production Drug detoxification Carotene conversion to vitamin A Collagen synthesis	Growing children Pregnancy demands increases Deficiency–anaemia	Men : 10 mg Women : 15 mg Pregnancy : 30 mg Lactation : 15 mg Children : 10.15 mg	Liver Meats Egg yolk Whole grains Enriched bread and cereal Dark green vegetables Legumes, nuts
Iodine (I)	Gland under control of thyroid stimulating hormone (TSH) Excretion by kidney Transported with plasma proteins	Synthesis of thyroxine, the thyroid hormone, which regulates cell oxidation BMR regulation Essential enzyme constituent	Deficiency–endemic colloid goitre; cretinism Hypothyroidism Hyperthyroidism Wound healing	Men : 150 mg Women : 150 mg Infants : 35-45 mg Children : 70-150 mg Men : 15 mg	Iodised salt Seafood
Zinc (Zn)	Excretion largely intestinal Stored in liver, muscle, bone, and organs	Combined with insulin for storage of the hormone Immune system leucocytes	Taste and smell acuity Retarded sexual and physical development	Women : 12 mg Children : 10-15 mg Infants : 5 mg	Meat Seafood, especially oysters Egg Milk Whole grains Legumes

Contd....

Element	*Metabolism*	*Physiologic Function*	*Clinical Application*	*Requirements*	*Food Sources*
Copper (Cu)	Stored in muscle, bone, liver, heart, kidney, and central nervous system Iron twin	Associated with iron in Energy production Haemoglobin synthesis Absorption and transport of iron	TPN deficiency Anaemia	Adults : 1.5-3.0 mg Children : 1.0-2.5 mg (estimated)	Liver Seafood Whole grains Legumes, nuts
Manganese (Mn)	Absorption limited Excretion mainly by intestine	Activates reactions in : Urea formation Protein metabolism Glucose oxidation Lipoprotein clearance and synthesis of fatty acids. Associated with glucose	Clinical deficiency in protein-energy malnutrition Inhalation toxicity in miners	Adults 2.5 mg (estimated) Children : 1-5 mg	Cereals, whole grain Soyabeans Legumes, nuts Tea Vegetables Fruits
Chromium (Cr)	Improves faulty uptake of glucose by body tissues as part of glucose tolerance factor.	metabolism; raises abnormally low fasting blood sugar levels. Constituent of vitamin	Possible link with cardiovascular disorders and diabetes	Adults : 50-200 mg mg (estimated) Children : 20-200 mg	Whole grains, cereal products
Cobalt (Co)	Absorbed chiefly as constituent of vitamin B_{12}	B_{12}; essential factor in red blood cell formation	Deficiency associated with deficiency of Vitamin B_{12}– pernicious anemia	Unknown	Supplied by preformed vitamin B_{12}

Contd....

Element	*Metabolism*	*Physiologic Function*	*Clinical Application*	*Requirements*	*Food Sources*
Selenium (Se)	Active as cofactor in cell oxidation enzyme systems	Associated with vitamin E as antioxidant; protects lipid in cell membrane	Keshan disease, heart muscle failure TPN deficiency	Men : 70 mg Women : 55 mg Children : 20 mg	Seafoods Kidney Liver Meats Whole grains
Molyb-denum (Mo)	Minute traces in the body	Constituent of specific enzymes involved in purine conversion to uric acid Aldehyde oxidation		Adult 75-250 mg (estimated)	Organ meats Milk Whole grains Leafy vegetables Legumes
Fluorine (Fl)	Deposited in bones and teeth	Associated with dental health	Small amount prevents dental caries Excess causes endemic dental fluorosis	Adults 1.5-4 mg (estimated) Children 0.5-2.5 mg	Fluoridated water (1 ppm Fl)

VITAMIN-DRUG INTERACTION

Vitamin	*Drugs with which vitamin interacts*
A	Corticosteroid, mineral oil, neomycin, bleomycin, benzpyrene
D	Cholestyramine, anticonvulsants, glutethimide, oxygen, bleomycin
E	Mineral oil, oxygen, cholestyramine
K	Oral anticogulants, salicylates, antibiotics, cephalosporins.
B_1	Oral contraceptive, thio-semicarbazone
B_2	Oral contraceptive, boric acid, galactoflavin
B_6	Levadopa, isoniazid, penicillamine, cycloserine
Niacin	Isoniazid, benzerazide, carbidopa
B_{12}	Potassium chloride, colchicine, neomycin, biguanides, phenformin
Folic acid	Anticonvulsants, barbiturates, cholestyramine
Pantothenic acid	Thio-semicarbazone
Vit. C	Oral contraceptive, salicylates, corticosteroids, calcitonin, alcohol

FOOD VALUES / 100 GRAM

Foods	Protein (g)	Fat (g)	Cal (mg)	Iron (mg)	Vit. C (mg)	Vit. A (IU)	Calories
Rice							
Raw milled	6.8	0.5	10	3.1	0	0	345
Par boiled	6.4	0.4	9	4.0	0	0	346
Flakes	6.6	1.2	20	20.0	0	0	346
Puffed	7.5	0.1	20	7.6	0	0	325
Wheat							
Whole flour	12.1	1.7	48	11.5	0	29	341
Flour refined	11.0	0.9	23	2.5	0	25	348
Suji	10.4	0.8	16	1.6	0	–	348
Bread white	7.8	0.7	11	1.1	0	0	245
Millets							
Bajra	11.6	5.0	42	5.0	0	132	361
Jowar	10.4	1.9	25	5.8	0	47	349
Maize	11.1	3.6	10	2.0	0	90	342
Ragi	7.3	1.3	344	6.4	0	42	328
Dals							
Bengal gram	20.8	5.5	56	9.1	1	129	372
Black gram	24.0	1.4	154	9.1	0	38	347
Green gram	24.5	1.2	75	8.5	0	49	348
Red gram	22.3	1.7	73	5.8	0	132	335
Whole dal							
Bengal gram,	17.1	5.3	202	10.2	3	189	360
Green gram,	24.0	1.3	127	7.3	3	92	334
Lentil (*Masur*)	25.0	0.7	69	4.8	3	294	343
Peas dry	19.7	1.1	75	5.1	0	39	315
Rajmah	22.9	1.3	260	5.8	0	–	346
Moth beans	23.6	1.1	202	9.5	0	9	330
Soya bean	43.2	19.5	240	11.5	0	426	432
Nut/seeds							
Groundnut	25.3	40.1	90	2.8	0	37	567
Til	18.3	43.0	1450	10.5	0	60	563
Poppy seeds	21.7	19	1584	–	–	–	408
Cashew nut	21.2	47	50	5.0	–	–	596
Almond	20.8	59	230	4.5	–	–	655
Dry coconut	6.8	62	40	2.7	7	–	662
Milk/other products							
Cow milk	3.2	4.1	120	0.2	2	174	67
Buffalo milk	4.3	8.8	210	0.2	1	160	117
Goat milk	3.3	4.5	170	0.3	1	182	72
Curd	3.1	4.0	149	0.2	1	102	60
Butter milk	0.8	1.1	30	0.8	–	0	30

Foods	Protein (g)	Fat (g)	Cal (mg)	Iron (mg)	Vit. C (mg)	Vit. A (IU)	Calories
Cheese	24.1	25.1	790	2.1	–	–	348
Khoya	14.6	31.2	650	5.8	–	–	421
Whole milk powder	25.8	26.7	950	0.6	1400	–	496
Skimmed milk powder	38.0	0.1	1370	1.4	5	0	357
Egg and Meat							
Egg hen	13.3	13.3	60	2.1	0	600	173
Mutton	18.5	13.3	150	2.5	–	0	194
Goat meat	21.4	3.6	12	–	–	–	118
Chicken	26.0	0.6	25	–	–	–	109
Beef	22.6	2.6	10	0.8	0	0	114
Pork	18.7	4.4	30	2.2	0	0	114
Liver Sheep	19.3	7.5	10	6.3	0	0	150
Fish							
Pomfrets	17.0	1.3	200	0.9	–	–	87
Hilsa	21.8	19.4	180	2.1	24	–	273
Prawn fresh	19.1	1.0	323	5.3	–	–	89
Fish fresh high fat	11.2	5.8	240	2.3	–	–	138
Fish dry	5.5	2.7	315	3.5	–	–	255
Crab	8.9	1.1	1370	21.2	–	–	59
Green Leafy Vegetables							
Amranth	4.0	0.5	397	25.5	99	5520	45
Bathua	3.7	0.4	150	4.2	35	1700	30
Cabbage	1.8	0.1	39	0.8	124	1200	27
Colocasia green leaves	3.9	1.5	227	10.0	12	10270	56
Coriander	3.3	0.6	184	18.5	135	6918	44
Drumstick leaves	6.7	1.7	440	7.0	220	6780	92
Methi	4.4	0.9	395	16.5	52	2300	49
Lettuce	2.1	0.3	50	2.4	10	990	21
Raddish leaves	3.8	0.4	265	3.6	81	5300	28
Palak	2.0	0.7	73	10.9	28	5580	26
Beet root	1.7	0.1	18	1.0	10	0	43
Carrot	0.9	0.2	80	2.2	3	1890	48
Raddish	0.7	0.1	35	0.4	15	0	17
Onion	1.2	0.1	47	0.7	2	0	50
Potato	1.6	0.1	10	0.7	17	0	97
Colocasia	3.0	0.1	40	1.7	0	–	97
Yam	1.2	0.1	50	0.6	0	260	79

Foods	Protein (g)	Fat (g)	Cal (mg)	Iron (mg)	Vit. C (mg)	Vit. A (IU)	Calo-ries
Other Vegetables							
Drumstick	2.5	0.1	30	5.3	120	110	26
Capsicum	1.2	0.3	10	1.0	137	420	24
Karela	1.6	0.2	20	1.8	88	125	25
Beans french	1.7	0.1	50	1.7	24	130	26
Beans cluster	3.2	0.4	130	4.5	49	200	60
Peas	7.2	0.3	20	1.5	9	80	93
Fruits							
Amla	0.5	0.1	50	1.2	600	9	58
Guava	0.9	0.3	10	1.4	212	0	51
Grape	0.7	0.1	20	0.2	31	0	32
Lemon	1.0	0.9	70	2.3	39	0	57
Musambi	0.8	0.3	40	0.7	50	0	43
Orange	0.7	0.2	26	0.3	30	1104	65
Orange juice	0.2	0.1	5	0.7	64	15	48
Lichi	1.1	0.2	10	0.7	31	0	61
Melon	0.3	0.2	32	1.4	26	170	17
Papaya	0.6	0.1	17	0.5	57	665	32
Pineapple	0.4	0.1	20	1.2	39	+	46
Sitaphal	1.6	0.4	17	1.5	37	0	104
Tomato	0.9	0.2	48	0.4	27	350	20
Apple	0.2	0.5	10	1.0	1	0	59
Bael fruit	1.8	0.3	85	0.6	3	55	137
Banana	1.2	0.3	17	0.9	7	78	116
Cherris	1.1	0.5	24	1.3	7	–	64
Figs	1.3	0.2	80	1.0	5	162	37
Mango	0.6	0.4	14	1.3	16	2740	74
Chiku	0.7	0.1	28	2.0	6	95	98
Fats & Oils							
Butter	–	81.0	–	–	–	960	730
Ghee (cow)	–	100.0	–	–	–	600	900
Ghee (buffalo)	100.0	–	–	–	–	240	900
Vanaspati	–	100.0	–	–	–	750	900
Refined oil	–	100.0	–	–	–	750	900
Miscellaneous							
Dates	2.5	0.4	120	7.3	3	25	317
Coriander seeds	14.1	16.1	630	18.0	0	940	288
Methi	26.2	5.8	160	14.1	0	95	335
Chillles green	2.9	0.6	30	1.2	111	175	29
Betel leaves	3.1	0.8	230	7.0	5	5760	44
Fish liver oil	–	100		–	–	–	900
Honey	0.3	0	5	0.9	4	–	320
Jaggery	0.4	0.1	80	11.4	–	165	383
Mushroom	4.6	0.8	6	1.5	12	0	43
Papad	18.8	0.3	80	17.2	–	–	288
Sago	0.2	0.2	10	1.3	–	–	351
Sugarcane juice	0.1	0.2	10	1.1	–	–	39

SHOWING APPROXIMATE VALUES

Food	*Quantity*	*Wt (g)*	*Calories*	*Proteins*	*Fats (g)*
Chapatis	2	57	193	5	5.5
Rice	1 plate	100	110	6	0.2
Pulse	1 cup	150	284	16	9
Omlette	1	39	77	5.8	5.7
Bread	2 slice	46	120	4.0	1.0
Biscuits	2	16	64	1.6	2.0
Milk	1 cup	703	300	9.0	6.0
Banana	1 piece	100	99	1.2	0.2
Apple	1 one	66	42	0.2	0.3
Butter	Table spoon	14	126	0.1	14
Sugar	1 teaspoon	5	20	–	–
Groundnut	1 ounce	30	165	8	14

EXPENDITURE OF CALORIES/HOUR

Activity	*Calories*	*Activity*	*Calories*
Dressing	33	Mental work	7-10
Sitting at rest	15	Sawing wood	420
Standing	20	Cycling	180-300
Running	500-900	Climbing	200-900
Sewing	25-30	Wrestling	980
Reading	20	Rifle cleaning	50
Sweeping	110	Brick laying	240
Knitting	31	Scrubbing floor	260

IMPORTANT SOURCES OF PROTEINS MG/100 G

Food	**Protein**	**Food**	**Protein**
Wheat	11.8	Egg hen	13.3
Rice	7.0	Fish	21.5
Maize	11.1	Mutton	18.3
Bengal gram	17.1	Cow milk	3.5
Lentil	25.1	Human milk	1.2
Peas dried	19.7	Groundnut	26.7
Green gram dal	24.0	Almond	20
Soya bean	42.0	Gengelly seeds	18.2

IMPORTANT SOURCES OF FAT

Food	**Percentage Fat**	**Percentage Food**	**Percentage Fat**
Ghee	100	Soya bean	19.5
Butter	81	Cow's milk	3.5
Almond	58	Egg	13.3
Cashewnut	46	Mutton	13.3
Groundnut	40	Fish	3.2

IMPORTANT SOURCES OF CHOLESTEROL MG/100 GRAM			
Food	***Cholesterol***	***Food***	***Cholesterol***
Butter	280	Egg white	0
Cheese	145	Egg yolk	1330
Cream	140	Chicken	40
Milk	11	Liver	250
Egg Hen	498	Fish	50

IMPORTANT SOURCES OF IRON MG/100 GM			
Food	***mg Iron***	***Food***	***mg Iron***
Bajra	8.8	Jaggery	11.4
Wheat whole	5.3	Betel leaves	5.7
Bengal gram	8.9	Coriander	1.0
Peas dry	4.4	Meithee	16.9
Soya bean	11.3	Mint	15.6
Bitter gourd	9.4	Tomato	2.4
Egg	2.1	Mutton	2.5

NUTRITIVE VALUE, CITRUS FRUITS (By ICMR)

(Per 100 g)

Nutrients	*Grape-fruit*	*Lemon*	*Lemon (sweet)*	*Lime sweet (Malta)*	*Lime sweet (Musambi)*	*Orange*	*Orange juice*
Calories (K cal)	32	57	35	36	43	48	9
Protein (gm)	0.7	1.0	0.7	0.7	0.8	0.7	0.2
Fat (gm)	0.1	0.9	0.3	0.2	0.3	0.1	0.1
Carbohydrates (gm)	7.0	11.1	7.3	7.8	9.3	10.9	1.9
Calcium (mg)	20	70	30	30	40	26	5
Iron (mg)	0.2	2.3	0.7	1.0	0.7	0.3	0.7
Carotene (mg)	—	0	0	0	0	1104	15
Vitamin C (mg)	31 (Juice)	39 (Juice)	45	54	50	30	64

TOTAL FIBRE CONTENT OF COMMON FOODS (g/100 g)

High (< 10)	***Medium*** (1 to 10)	***Low*** (< 1)	***Nil***
Wheat	Rice	Refined	Sugar
Jowar	Most vegetable	and processed	Fats/oils
Bajra	Most fruits	foods	Milk
Ragi	Coconut		All types of meat
Maize	Sesame (til)		
Legumes			
Dals (Pulses)			
Fenugreek			

Daily requirement of fibre is 6 g/day

APPROXIMATE NUTRIENT VALUE OF COMMON COOKED FOODS

Item	No. of serving	Weight of cooked preparation (g)	Energy (Kcal)	Fat (g)	Protein (g)
I. Cereal preparations					
Rice	1 K	100	110	0.1	2
Idli	1	60	75	0.1	2
Plain dosa	1	40	125	3	3
Masala dosa	1	100	200	6	4
Phulka	1	35	80	0	3
Paratha	1	50	150	4	4
Upma	1 K	130	200	9	5
Sevian upma	1 K	80	130	4	3
Bread toasted	2 slices	50	170	1	4
Poha (Awal)	1 K	100	200	9	2
Dalia	1 K	140	165	7	5
Khichri	1 K	100	210	7	4
Puri	1	25	80	3	2
II. Pulse preparations					
Plain *dal*	1 K	140	170	4	10
Sambar	1 K	160	81	2	4
Chhole/Sundal	1 K	150	115	5	7
III. Vegetable preparations					
With gravy	1 K	130	130	7	3
Dry	1 K	100	115	7	2
Bajara baigan	1 K	170	230	20	3
Vegetable *kofta*	1 K	145	220	14	4
IV. Fried snacks					
Bhaji	1	7	35	3	0.5
Samosa	1	65	210	12	2
Kachori	1	45	200	12	3
Potato *vada*	1	40	100	5	3
Sago *vada*	1	30	100	6	1
IV. Fried snacks					
Masala *vada*	1	20	56	2	2
Vada	1	20	65	3	3
Dahi vada	1	80	170	9	5
Vegetable cutlet	1	30	70	5	1
V. Chutneys					
Coconut/groundnuts/ Coriander	1 tbsp	25	64	5	3
Tomato	1 tbsp	50	10	0.3	0.3

Contd....

Item	No. of serving	Weight of cooked preparation (g)	Energy (Kcal)	Fat (g)	Protein (g)
VI. Non-vegetarian preparations					
Boiled egg	1	50	86	7.0	7.0
Omlette	1	65	155	14.0	7.0
Fried egg	1	50	155	14.0	7.0
Mutton curry	1 K	145	240	18	10
Chicken curry	1 K	125	260	15	26
Fish (fried)	2 pieces	85	220	12	18
VII. Bakery products					
Biscuits	2	40	220	14	3
Cake	1	40	220	13	3
Vegetable	1	60	170	10	3
VIII. Sweets					
Laddu, burfi, etc.	1	60	250	15	8
Halwa (Suji)	1 K	130	430	20	3
Doubleka meetha	1 K	105	280	18	4
Custard/puddings	1 K	110	180	6	5
Chikki	2	60	300	12	8
Jam/Jelly	1 tsp	7	20	0.04	0.04

K = Katori = Approximate 125 g

BALANCED DIET FOR DIFFERENT SEX AND AGE GROUPS

Food Item	Adult Man			Adult Woman			Children		Boys	Girls
	Sedentary work	*Moderate work*	*Heavy work*	*Sedentary work*	*Moderate work*	*Heavy work*	*1-3 yrs*	*4-6 yrs*	*10-12 yrs*	*10-12 yrs*
Cereals	460	520	670	410	440	575	175	270	420	380
Pulses	40	50	60	40	45	50	35	35	45	45
Leafy vegetables	40	40	40	100	100	50	40	50	50	50
Other vegetables	60	70	80	40	40	100	20	50	50	50
Roots and tubers	50	60	80	50	50	60	10	30	30	30
Milk	150	200	250	100	150	200	300	250	250	250
Oil and fat	40	45	65	20	25	40	15	25	40	35
Sugar or jaggery	30	55	55	20	20	40	30	40	45	45

SUGGESTED SUBSTITUTION FOR NON-VEGETARIANS

Food item which can be deleted from non-vegetarian diet	*Substitution that can be suggested for deleted item or items*
5% of pulses (20-30 g)	1. One egg or 30 g of meat or fish 2. Addition 5 g of fat or oil
10% of pulses (40-60 g)	1. Two eggs or 50 g of meat or fish or one egg+30 g of meat or fish. 2. 10 g of fat or oil.

ADDITIONAL ALLOWANCES DURING PREGNANCY AND LACTATION

Food items	*During pregnancy*	*Calories (Kcal)*	*During lactation*	*Calories (Kcal)*
Cereal	35 g	118	60 g	203
Pulses	15 g	52	30 g	105
Milk	100 g	83	100 g	83
Fat	—	—	+ 10 g	90
Sugar	10 g	40	10 g	40
Total		293		521

FATTY ACID COMPOSITION AND CHOLESTEROL CONTENT OF ANIMAL FOODS
*(g/100 g Edible Portion)

Item	*Fat g/100 g*	*Saturated fatty acids g/100 g*	*Choles-terol mg/100 g*
Butter	80	50	250
Ghee	100	65	300
Milk (cow)	4	2	14
Milk (buffalo)	8	4	16
Milk (skimmed)	0.1	–	2
Milk (condensed)	10	6	40
Cream	13	8	40
Cheese	25	15	100
Egg (whole)	11	4	400
Egg yolk	30	9	1120
Chicken without skin	4	1	60
Chicken with skin	18	6	100
Beef	16	8	70
Mutton	13	7	65
Pork	35	13	90
Organ meats			
Brain	6	2	2000
Heart	5	2	150
Kidney	2	1	370
Liver	9	3	300
Fresh water and sea foods			
Prawns/shrimps	2	0.3	150
Fish (lean)	1.5	0.4	45
Fish (fatty)	6	2.5	45

* Values vary depending on the feed of the animals

* One whole egg or yolk of one egg contains 210 mg cholesterol

FOOD GUIDE FOR A HEALTHY HEART

Foods	***Prefer***	***Limit***	***Avoid***
Cereals bajra, wheat, rice, maize, millet, ragi,	Wheat, rice with maida maize, jowar	White bread, biscuits	Cakes,pastries, ragi, *naan roti,* noodles
Pulses	Whole and sprouted	—	—
Vegetables	Green leafy vegetables and other vegetables	Roots and tubers	Fried vegeta-bles, banana chips, canned vegetables
Fruits	Fresh fruits		Dried fruits, canned fruits in syrup.
Dairy products	Low fat milk, Buttermilk skimmed milk	Whole milk, Milk powders	Cheese, butter *khoa*, condensed milk, mlik cream
Eggs	Egg white	—	Egg yolk
Animal foods	Fish	Chicken	prawns, shrimps, all types of meat
Fat	More than one type of vegetable oil	Total fat intake	Oily dishes, butter, ghee, coconut oil, fried foods
Sugar	Sugar, jaggery	Sugar in any home-made beverages	Sweets like chocolates icecreams
Nuts and oilseeds		All nuts and oilseeds	
Beverages	Fresh fruit juice light tea	coffee, cola, soft drinks	Alcohol
Salt	Foods in natural state	Too much salt in preparations	Pickles, *papads,* sauces, salt biscuits, fried crispies

SALADS AND CALORIES

Item	*No (Medium size)*	*Weight (g)*	*K cal*
Beetroot	1	65	30
Cabbage	1	250	70
Carrot	1	40	20
Cucumber	1	90	12
Lettuce	6 bundles	100	20
Onion	1	50	25
Radish	1	60	10
Tomato	1	50	10
Turnip	1	100	30

FRUITS AND CALORIES

Item	*No./ Quantity*	*Weight (g)*	*K cal*
Apple	1	100	65
Banana	1	80	90
Grapes	30	100	70
Guava	1	100	50
Jackfruit	4 pieces	100	90
Mango	1	250	180
Musambi/orange	1	100	40
Papaya	1 piece	250	80
Pineapple	1 piece	100	50
Sapota	1	80	80
Custard apple	1	130	130
Watermelon/muskmelon	1 piece	100	15

DIET AND DISEASES

PEPTIC ULCER

The patient of peptic ulcer should avoid

- Excessively sour, salty or spicy foods
- Coarse food such as raw vegetables, fruits with seeds and skin.
- Excessively hot drink/food
- Smoking, alcoholic beverage and aspirin should usually be avoided.
- Meat should consist of small servings. Try to eat about the same amount at each meal.
- Peptic ulcer is one disease where proper dietary management is equally or more rewarding than pure drug therapy.

Proteins

Normal protein requirement of 1 g/kg body weight, i.e. about 60 gm should be given. Milk protiens will not irritate gastric mucosa. Meat soup increases acidity.

Fats

Fat like butter, ghee, cheese and cream are helpful whereas fats of fried food articles are difficult to digest and may increase the symptoms.

Calories

Sufficient calories are to be given and vitamin 'C' may be helpful in healing the ulcer.

Lenhart's diet (after bleeding)

1st day	2 eggs + 200 ml of milk
2nd day	3 eggs + 300 ml of milk

Leube's diet

Breakfast	One piece bread (50 g)
Prelunch	300 ml of milk
Lunch	Mashed potato (50 g) Toasted bread (50 g) Butter (20 ml)
Evening	300 ml of milk Biscuit (50 g) Butter (20 g)
Night	300 ml of milk

Diet Sheet

Early morning	Milk 1 cup + 1 teaspoonful of sugar
Breakfast	Bread—2 slices with 10 g of butter Milk one cup+ one TSF sugar
Lunch	Fulka—3 small soft with ghee. Rice one medium bowl, well-cooked dal—3/4 bowl, vegetable—3/4 bowl, (No *tadka* or *zeera*, etc.)
4 P.M.	Milk 300 ml
6 P.M.	Suji porridge Suji 20 g Milk 1 cup sugar 2 TSF

Dinner	Fulka—3 small Rice—1 medium bowl, well-cooked dal—3/4 bowl, soft bland vegetable—3/4 bowl
Bed time	Milk—1 cup + 1 TSF sugar

DIABETES MELLITUS

The following food articles should be avoided

- Sweet drinks and carbonated drinks
- Dried and canned fruits
- Cakes, pastries, cream, and alcohol drinks
- Sugar, potatoes

Diabetes primarily affects the utilisation of carbohydrates in the diet. Insulin which is manufactured in the pancreas is required mainly to convert glucose circulating in the blood into glycogen a form in which it is stored in the muscles of the body. If insulin is insufficient glucose will build up in the blood and urine. A diabetic should know how to adjust his or her diet in order to keep his or her urine free of sugar.

Carbohydrate

Less than 250 g should be consumed. But drastic reduction of carbohydrate is forbidden as it might result in excessive metabolism of fat resulting in ketoacidosis.

Calories

Total calories should be adequate for the growing children and underweight persons. For the obese patients it, is necessary to reduce calories. They should consume more of green leafy vegetables which are filling in capacity, low in calorific value and contain less than 3% carbohydrate.

Proteins

1 g/kg of body weight, cheese is a good source of protein.Low consumption of fats will keep the cholesterol level low. High doses of B complex vitamin (B_2) will avoid the development of diabetic neuritis.

Potassium helps in release of insulin from pancreas.

Sweetening Agents

There are two chief sweetening agents. One is saccharine in liquid, tablet or granule form and another is sorbitol. Saccharine is a coal tar derivative 300 to 500 times sweeter than glucose and does not have any calorific value; of the sugars fructose is the sweetest (173) then sucrose (100), glucose (74) and lactose (60). Sugar free can be used by those obese diabetics who have a craving for sweets. One tablet provides only 0.4 calorie which is sufficient to sweeten one cup of tea.

Sorbitol is hydrogenated glucose and is converted into fructose in the body and hence does not cause glycosuria. Tonics of diabetics contain sorbitol.

Diet Sheet

Bed tea	Coffee/tea 1 cup
Breakfast	Tea 1 cup 2 toasts with little butter
Lunch	*Fulka*—2 (two) Rice—1 medium bowl, Dal—¾th medium bowl Leafy vegetables—1 bowl, oil for cooking—1½ TSF

Diet will provide 2300 calories and 65 gm of proteins.

After-noon	Light tea without sugar
Evening	Fruit / one normal size
Dinner	Fulka—2 small, Rice—1 medium bowl or 2 more vegetables—1 medium bowl
Bedtime	Glass toned milk without sugar
Approximate calories	1500
Carbohydrate below	230 g

INFECTIVE HEPATITIS

Proteins

Excessive intake of protein is harmful because of protein break down products may accumulate leading to coma. With mild hepatitis 60 to 80 g of proteins are permitted.

Fats

May be limited up to 30 g daily

Carbohydrates

Large quantities of oral carbohydrates are given because

- They constitute the major source of calories.
- They minimise the endogenous proteins breakdown.

If vomiting/nausea persists intravenous glucose should be given.

For mild jaundice 2000 calories and in severe jaundice 1600 to 2000 calories are recommended.

Vitamin B complex and vitamin C are helpful. Sufficient quantities of sodium chloride and potassium chloride to have electrolyte balance may be consumed.

Diet Sheet

Early morning	• Light tea—1 cup with 10 g sugar
Breakfast	• Fruit juice—150 ml + 15 g sugar Jam—2 tablespoon.
10 AM	• Sugar cane juice—1 glass
Lunch	Rice—2 medium bowl, Thin Dal ½ medium bowl, butter milk 1 cup+sugar.
4 PM	• Light tea + 2 TSF sugar, Banana 1 medium size.
Dinner	*Fulka*—2 medium size, mixed fruits 250 g well-cooked vegetable 1 bowl.

CHOLECYSTITIS

Food to be avoided are

- Pastries, cheese, fried potato chips.
- Fatty meat, fried eggs
- Cabbage, cauliflower, cucumber, peas and beans
- Nuts, popcorn and dry fruits
- Pickles, condiments and spices.

Proteins

One gm/kg body weight is permitted, very high protein intake may increase biliary cholesterol.

Fats

Restricted fat diet.

Calories

Minimum carbohydrates to maintain the calories. High carbohydrates will increase the biliary cholesterol. Fat soluble vitamins may be given.

Diet Sheet

Early morning	• Light tea—1 cup with sugar
Breakfast	• Toned milk without sugar, Toast 2 with little jam
Lunch	• Rice—1 medium bowl, Fulka—4 small thin, Thin dal—¾th medium bowl, Thin butter milk
	• Egg—one, cooked french beans and carrots, oil or cooking—1½ spoon.
4 PM	• Light Tea—1 cup with 1 TSF sugar. Biscuits 3 to 4
Dinner	• Fulka—4 small cooked mixed vegetable—1 bowl, Dal—¾th bowl, Orange-1
Bed time	• Milk—1 cup without sugar and cream

ISCHAEMIC HEART DISEASE

Proteins

1 g/kg of body weight in normal weight patient.

Fats

Saturated fats are to be avoided such as:

- Animal fats—beef, meat, pork
- Fats procured from dairy products such as cream, butter, ghee.
- Hydrogenated vegetable oils.
- Unsaturated fats such as kardi oil, sunflower oil, etc. can be used.

Carbohydrates

These are responsible for endogenous synthesis of cholesterol and triglycerides. Reduction in sugar intake decreases serum triglycerides.

Calories

Reduction of calories will reduce the weight.

Vitamin C is required for capillary stability. Nicotinic acid reduces lipids in blood, hence both are useful.

Adequate potassium and calcium in blood are required to prevent arrhythmias. Salt restriction is necessary in hypertension of heart failure.

Smoking is hazadous as it produces myocardial oxygen deficiency, increases beta and prebeta lipoproteins and enhances atherosclerosis.

Diet Sheet

Bed tea	• Light tea without sugar
Breakfast	• Milk one cup without sugar or cream.
Lunch	• Fulka 4 small size without ghee.
	• Rice one medium bowl, Salad.
	• Cooked vegetables 3/4th bowls. Oil for cooking—1½ TSF.
4 P.M.	• Light tea without sugar and milk.
	• Sweat lime and papaya.
	• Fulka—2 medium size
	• Pulses 3/4th medium bowl.
	• Salad

Diet will provide about—2000 calories and 35 g fat.

	• Curd—¾ the medium bowl.
Dinner	• Oil for cooking 1½ TSF.
	Cooked vegetables ¾th medium bowl

HYPERTENSION

- Pickles, pastries, salted biscuits, eggs, tinned food should be avoided.
- Drugs which retain sodium as aspirin, phenylbutazone, cortcosteroid should be avoided.
- Extra salt and baking powder should be avoided.

Protein

In mild hypertension 50 to 60 g of proteins are sufficient. In severe hypertension 40 g of proteins should be the limit.

Fats

Forty to Fifty gm of fats are permitted. High intake will cause atherosclerosis, which can cause and aggravate hypertension.

Carbohydrates

It should be the major part to provide calories.

Calories

In obese person low calories will help.

Sodium must be restricted in majority of the hypertensives because sodium has a water retaining property which aggravates the hypertension.

In some cases of low renin hypertension salt restrictions may be harmful as it may perpetuate the vicious circle of hypertension.

ACUTE GLOMERULONEPHRITIS

During severe oliguria, pulses, vegetable soups, pickles,meat and eggs are to be excluded.

Fluid intake should be equal to 500 ml more than the previous days's urine output.

Protein

In severe oliguria protein intake is to be restricted. When urine output is 500 to 800 ml protein intake of 0.5 to 0.75 gm per kg of body weight is allowed. If urine output is normal then there is no need of putting protein restriction.

Fats

About 40 to 55 g is usual because its excretion does not depend on kidney function.

Calories

No restriction

Vitamins and carbohydrates are to be supplied in normal quantity.

Sodium restriction is necessary so long there is oedema, oliguria or hypertension. Potassium is also restricted in oliguria (green leafy vegetables)

Diet Sheet

Bed tea	• Tea 1 cup with 2 TSF sugar
Breakfast	• Milk (150 gm) + TSF sugar, Bread 2 slices with 10 gm of butter.
Lunch	• Rice 1 1/2 medium bowl, Fulka 2 small size,
	vegetable 3/4th medium bowl.
	Curd 3/4th medium bowl.

Diet will provide about 1500 calories, 30 gm fat and 50 gm

Evening tea	•	Tea 1 cup with 2 TSF sugar a few potato chips.
Dinner	•	Rice 1 1/2 bowl, Fulka 2, Dal 1 bowl, Vegetable 3/4 bowl. Curd 3/4 bowl.
Bed time	•	1 cup milk with 1 TSF sugar.

NEPHROTIC SYNDROME

Following foods may be restricted.

Sodium rich butter, salted biscuits, preserved fish, *papad* and pickles.

High protein diet 2 to 3 gm/kg body weight per day is advised as there is massive loss of protein in urine. Groundnut, soya bean, skimmed milk can be frequently used. They can be added to wheat flour. Casilan contains 99% protein and only 0.1% sodium. Carbohydrates, calories and vitamins requirement remain the same as that of normal man.

When oedema subsides sodium restriction is not necessary.

Diet Sheet

Bed Tea	Light tea with 2 TSF sugar + 50 ml milk.
Breakfast	Milk one glass with 2 TSF sugar. Bread 2 slices with 10 gm butter, Egg 1 fried or omelette.
Lunch	Chapaties 2 medium size, Rice 1 medium bowl, Dal 1 medium bowl. Curd 1 medium bowl.
Evening	Roasted ground nut 30 gm, chana 30 gm, Milk one glass + 2 TSF protinex.
Dinner	Chapati 3 with ghee, Matar Paneer 3/4th bowl or Egg 2 as egg curry etc. Dal 3/4th bowl, sweet dish 100 gm.
Bed time	Milk one glass + 2 TSF sugar

RENAL FAILURE

Following foods should be restricted.

- Sodium is restricted if there is hypertension, oedema and oliguria.
- Salted biscuits, butter, meat, papad, pickles are not permitted
- Potassium is restricted.

Proteins

With an established disease 40 g of proteins are permitted.

Half of it should be first class proteins. Usually protein restriction is advocated when blood urea is above 80 mg%. Protein restriction usually varies from 0.3 to 0.5 g/kg.

Carbohydrates

They help to reduce endogenous protein breakdown and constitute main source of calories. Protein free preparations are allowed in plenty.

Calories

2000 to 2500 calories per day.

Diet provides about 1600 calories, 35 g fats.

Diet Sheet

Bed tea	Light tea with 1 TSF sugar
Breakfast	Milk 1 cup with 2 TSF sugar, Bread toast 2 slices with 10 gm of butter.
Lunch	Fulka 4 or 2 medium bowl of rice, Thin dal 3/4th bowl. Well-cooked mixed vegetables 1 bowl, Curd 1/2 medium bowl.
Evening tea	Light tea + 2 TSF sugar, Potato chips, one apple.
Dinner	Rice+*Moong Dal khichdi* 3 bowl with a TSF ghee, *Raita-Dahi*, 1 medium bowl well cooked vegetable, Ice cream 1 small cup.
Bed time	1 cup milk + 1 TSF sugar.

UNDERWEIGHT

Following should be encouraged

- Sweetened fruit juices
- Milk and its products. Cheese, butter and sweets
- Bread, jam and jelly
- Dried nuts and fruits
- Meat and eggs

Proteins

1.2 to 1.5 g/kg or more

Fats

These are encouraged to increase weight. These should not be taken in the beginning of food otherwise they will decrease the appetite. Large quantities may produce diarrhoea, flatulence and gastrointestinal upsets.

Carbohydrates

Potatoes, sweet potatoes, biscuits and sweets should be consumed in good quantity. Banana is a good source of calories.

Calories

Total calories consumed should be more than the required to put on weight.

Green leafy vegetables should not be consumed in sufficient quantities because these are not good source of calories but may fill up the stomach. Fluids should not be taken before and during meals. Sufficient vitamins are to be consumed.

Diet Sheet

Bed tea	Light tea 1 cup with sugar 2 TSF.
Breakfast	Milk one cup with sugar 1 TSF, Bread 2 slices butter 10 gm, Cheese 25 or one egg.
Lunch	Fulka 4 small with ghee, Rice one medium bowl, *Dal* one medium bowl, Curd 3/4th bowl + 1 TSF sugar

Diet provides about 2100 calories, 50 g proteins.

Evening	Preparation of 50 g, groundnut, fruit juice 1 glass, Banana 1
Dinner	Fulka 2 small with ghee, Fried rice 2 bowl. Curd 1/2 bowl. Dal fry 3/4th Bowl, Mixed vegetable 1 bowl, Ice cream/sweet 50 gm.
Bedtime	Milk one glass.

CONSTIPATION

Proteins

Normal 1 g/kg body weight.

Fats

Ghee and oils are beneficial and act as lubricant to the bowel and stimulate the bile flow for appropriate digestion.

Carbohydrates

Fruits like banana, figs, cucumber with skin and ladies finger are preferred. Cellulose stimulates peristalsis by forming a bulk and facilitate evacuation.

Yeast which is rich in B complex helps to regulate the bowels.

Liberal fluid intake and warm milk intake at bedtime are helpful.

DIARRHOEA

Food to be avoided are:

- Deep fry, spicy articles
- Sweets, dry fruits
- Chutney, pickles
- Salad and cellulose containing food.

Proteins

Protein rich substance like skimmed milk, white of an egg, butter milk are helpful. If diarrhoea is due to milk allergy, milk is to be avoided.

Fats

Fats will not be absorbed when there is intestinal hurry. They may aggravate the diarrhoea and are best avoided.

Carbohydrates

Easily digested carbohydrates, soft vegetables not with much of cellulose can be given.

As chronic diarrhoea may result in malnourishment high calories may be provided. Diarrhoea may result in loss of fluids and electrolytes. They must be replenished orally or in emergency intravenously.

Salted biscuits, fruit juices and oral electrolyte solutions will be helpful.

FLATULENCE

Food to be avoided are:

- Meat, egg
- Cabbage and cauliflower.
- High carbohydrates.

Proteins

Protein putrefaction in the gastroinstinal tract is the most common cause of flatulence.

Diet provides 2600 calories + 95 g proteins.

Fats

Fried fatty foods stay long in stomach, delayed emptying makes the patient feel uncomfortable.

Carbohydrates

Sweets, potatoes, turnip are to be avoided.

Calories

Obese patients generally do develop gases, hence low calorie diet will be helpful.

FEVER

Fever and rest means staying in bed with little physical activity and therefore little need for calories yet to build up the wasted tissue extra proteins are required, i.e. high protein and low calorie diet is required. Hence 70 g of proteins and 1800 calories will be sufficient.

Proteins can be in concentrated forms such as egg, curds and milk.

Fried foods and foods with high fibres should be avoided.

Plenty of fluids and minerals should be consumed.

GOUT

Person should avoid following foods because these are rich in purine content.

- Vegetarian food—beans, cauliflower, pulses, lentils, spinach, apple, mushrooms.
- Non-vegetarian food—liver, kidney, fish, meat proteins about 60 gram are enough preferably of vegetable origin.

Fats are to be restricted because they cause urate retention and obesity.

Carbohydrates should form the main part of the diet specially during attack of gout. Carbohydrates can spare proteins which reduce endogenous protein breakdown.

Low calorie diet will be helpful.

Increased intake of fluid produces increased urine output which will facilitate excretion of uric acid in urine alcohol and acute attack.

A few cups of tea and coffee are permitted as they contain methyl purines which are not converted to uric acid.

PROTEIN ENERGY MALNUTRITION

Proteins—20% of total calories should be provided from proteins, i.e. about 3 to 3.5 g per kg of expected body weight or about 45 to 55 gm of proteins per day. Sufficient quantity of protein is necessary to prevent or treat protein energy malnutrition. Better quality of protein can be got from milk, skimmed milk and pulses. Soya bean is better source of proteins as well as calories.

Fats—It should provide minimum 15- to 0% of total calories.

Calories—Daily requirement is 90 to 100 calories per kg of expected body weight.

National Institute of Nutrition, Hyderabad has formulated a rich mixture as follows.

Whole wheat roasted	40 gm
Bengal gram	16 gm
Groundnut	10 gm
Jaggery	20 gm
Total	86 gm
Total energy	330 kcal
Protein	11.3

Additional banana, egg will help in maintaining good health.

Diet will provide 1800 calories, 40 of proteins.

1000 Calories Diet Chart

Vegetarian

Morning	Tea—1 cup with milk 2 TSF and sugar 1 teaspoonful
Breakfast	Skimmed milk—1 cup or tea prepared out of it. Toast—1
Lunch	Vegetable soup—1 cup, Thin dal—¾ bowl Vegetable salad-radish, tomato, salad leaves, cucumber, etc. with salt and pepper. Cooked vegetables—pumpkin, French beans, brinjals, etc. except potato, peas, sweet potatoes, etc. No rice, jam, murubba, sweets, sweet meats, dry fruit, nuts, soft drinks.
Afternoon	Simple tea
Dinner	Tomato soup—1 cup, skimmed milk curd ½ bowl cooked vegetables, 2 chapatis, or bread 1 slice, Thin dal ¾ bowl.

Instead of sugar one can use saccharine in any quantity.

1000 Calories Diet Chart

Non-Vegetarian

Morning	Tea—1 cup with milk—2 TSF, sugar—1 teaspoon.
Breakfast	Egg—1 half boiled poached or scrumbled in milk, Toast—1.
Lunch	Meat soup—1 Cup, Boiled fish or roast mutton moderate quantity. vegetable salad/radish, tomato, salad leaves, cucumber, etc. Cooked vegetables, pumpkin, french beans except potato, Chapatis—2 or bread-slice. No rice, jam
Evening	Tea as of morning
Dinner	Chicken soup—1 cup Chicken roast—moderate quantity, Cooked vegetables, Bread—1 slice.

Section-6
(Laboratory Findings)

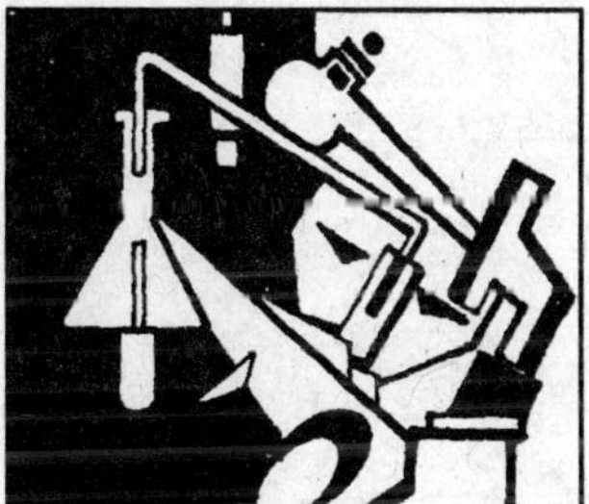

[illegible]

Chemical formula [illegible] indicate the composition [illegible]

[illegible]

CONTENTS

BLOOD VALUES

WBC

Normal values of WBC

5000 -10,000/cu mm

Granulocytes

Neutrophils	60-70%
Eosinophils	0.1-4%
Basophils	0.5-1%

Leucocytosis

Upto 20,000 is considered 'slight'
30,000 is moderate
50,000 is high.

Causes of leucocytosis

- Infections
- Haemorrhage
- Toxins as in uraemia, coma
- After drugs — Chloroform, adrenalin
- Serum sickness
- After steroids

Causes of leucopenia (cells below 4000)

- Viral infection
- Hypersplenism
- Bone marrow depression is due to

  Drugs
  Barbiturates
  Antibiotics
  Antihistamines
  Cancer chemotherapy
  Heavy metals
  Radiation
  Agranulocytosis
  Alcoholism
  Diabetes

Interfering factors

- There is an early morning low level and late afternoon high peak.
- In infants and newborn count is (10,000-20,000).
- Food, exercise, emotions and pain will increase the count.
- Menstruation, pregnancy will increase the count.
- Fever, anaesthesia, prolonged cold bath will cause an increase in values.

NEUTROPHILIA

(i) Conditions causing neutrophilia.

- Parasitic and bacterial infections.
- Diabetes, uraemia, gout.
- Haemorrhage.

(ii) An increase in mature cells is known as shift to right.
- In haemolysis.
- With drugs such as digitalis, ACTH, sulponamides.
- Burns, myocardial infarction, pus formation, after surgery.
- Allergy.

Comparison between neutrophils and total WBC.

- Increase in percentage of neutrophils represents severity of infection. Total WBC indicates patient's power of resistance.
- If leucocyte count and percentage of neutrophils increase proportionately, there is a moderate infection with good resistance offered by the patient.
- If neutrophil count is increased to a greater extent than the total count there is either a loss of resistance or severe infection.

Causes of neutropenia (decreased per cent)

- Acute viral infection, influenza, measles, mumps.
- Anaemia, agranulocytosis.
- Toxic agents.
- Thyrotoxicosis.

Interfering factors

- Children respond to infection with a greater degree of neutrophilic leucocytosis.
- Steroids do not allow neutrophils to increase.

EOSINOPHIL

Normal value

1 to 4 per cent of total leucocytes.

Eosinophilia It is an increase of circulating eosinophils greater than five per cent or more than 500 in absolute count.

- As response to hyper immune, allergic and degenerative reaction.
- Parasitic diseases.
- Lung and bone cancer.
- Hodgkin's disease.

Eosinopenia (decrease in eosinophil count)

- Infectious mononucleosis.
- Hypersplenism.
- Congestive heart failure.
- Drugs, ACTH, thyroxine.
- Pyogenic infection

Interfering factors

- Normal eosinophil count is lowest in morning, then rises from noon until after midnight.
- Stressful situations such as burns, SLE, electric shock and labour will decrease count.
- ACTH causes disappearance of eosinophils from blood.

RED BLOOD CELLS

Normal values

Men 4.2 to 5.4 million / cu mm

Women 3.6 to 5 million / cu mm

Decreased values

- Anaemia
- Diseases of bone marrow
  Hodgkin's disease
  Leukaemia
  Multiple myeloma
- Haemolytic and pernicious anaemia
- Rheumatic fever
- Subacute infective endocarditis

Increased values

- Polycythemia vera
- Severe diarrhoea
- Dehydration
- Actute poisoning

Interfering factors

- In lying position count is lower
- Extreme exercise and excitement produces higher count
- In newborn count is higher
- Higher the altitude greater the increase in RBC
- Gentamicin results in increased count

ESR

Normal values

Westergren Method	Men	0-15 mm per hour
	Women	0-20 mm per hour

ESR not raised

- Influenza
- Chronic focal dental infection
- Ectopic pregnancy
- Psychogenic disease

ESR raised

- Anaemia
- Acute myocardial infarction
- Pulmonary tuberculosis
- Acute gout
- Burns
- Acute infections

ESR very rapid increase

- Rheumatoid arthritis
- Leukaemia
- Chronic renal disease
- Sarcoidosis

Decreased values found in

- Polycythemia vera
- Congestive cardiac failure

Varied values found in

- **Acute disease** The change in rate may lag behind the temperature elevation and leucocytosis for 6 to 24 hrs reaching a peak after several days.

- **Convalescence** The increased rate tends to persist longer than the temperature or the leucocytosis.
- **Unruptured acute appendicitis** Even when suppurative or gangrenous, the rate is normal but if abscess or peritonitis develops the rate increases rapidly.
- In myocardial infarction ESR increases while in angina, rate is not increased.
- In rheumatic and acute gouty arthritis, the rate is significantly increased while in osteoarthritis rate is slightly raised. In neuritis, myositis rate is within normal limits.

ESR in prognosis and treatment

- In fevers, a rising ESR suggests progress of the disease.
- In rheumatic fever it is a specially sensitive index of persistent rheumatic infection.
- In coronary thrombosis repeated determination serves as a guide of healing.
- Factors leading to reduced rate
  High blood sugar
  High albumin level
- Drugs decreasing levels
  Ethambutol.
  Salicylates.
  ACTH

SERUM CHOLESTEROL

Normal values

150 to 250 mg per cent

Increased levels

- Cardiovascular disease and atherosclerosis
- Obstructive jaundice
- Nephrosis
- Uncontrolled diabetes
- Nephrotic syndrome

Decreased levels

- Malabsorption
- Liver disorders
- Anaemia
- Stress
- After antibiotic therapy

Interfering factors

- Cholesterol is increased in pregnancy
- Oestrogen decreases plasma cholesterol and oophorectomy increases it

HIGH DENSITY LIPOPROTEIN

Normal values

- Men 45 mg/100 ml
- Women 55 mg/100 ml
- Increased values are associated with chronic liver disorders.
- Decreased levels are associated with increased risk for coronary heart disease.
- Long distance runners have higher levels of HDL.

Interfering factors

- Decreased HDL is associated with smokers.
- Increased HDL is associated with moderate intake of alcohol.
- Recent weight gain and loss can interfere results.
  Ratio of HDL-LDL should be minimum 1:4.

VLDL AND LDL

Normal values

VLDL cholesterol—25 to 50 per cent.

VLDL is a major carrier of triglycerides (60-70 per cent Triglyceride, 10 to 15 per cent cholesterol) degradation of VLDL leads to major source of LDL.

TRIGLYCERIDES

Normal values

40–150 mg per cent in the blood.

Triglycerides produce energy for the body. Excess triglycerides are stored in adipose tissue.

Increased levels

- Liver disease
- Nephrotic syndrome
- Hypothyroidism
- Poorly controlled diabetes
- Myocardial infarction

Decreased levels

- Malabsorption

Interfering factors

- Transient increase will occur after heavy meal or alcohol consumption
- Increased values seen in pregnancy and with oral
  contraceptive therapy

GLUCOSE TOLERANCE TEST

Fasting blood sugar

Normal value—70-100 mg per 100 ml

Elevated blood sugar

- Acute myocardial infarction
- Diabetes
- Pituitary adenoma
- Pancreatitis
- Chronic liver disease

Lower glucose level

- Overdose of insulin
- Bacterial septicaemia
- Carcinoma of pancreas

Two hour postprandial blood sugar

Normal value—Less than 140 mg/100 ml

Increased levels

- Diabetes

- Malnutrition
- Acromegaly
- Myocardial infarction
- Pregnancy

Lower levels

- Anterior pituitary insufficiency
- Addison's disease
- Steatorrhoea

Oral glucose tolerance test

Fasting blood sugar 110 mg. per cent

2 hours after— 140 mg per cent

Indications of test

- Family history of diabetes
- Obesity
- Unexplained episodes of hypoglycaemia
- History of recurrent infections
- History of delivery of large fetus, still birth.

Diabetic curve

- Fasting blood sugar—above 120 mg.
- A value above 180 mg is recorded at some time during test.
- Blood sugar does not return to normal within two hours.
- Positive urine test for sugar

Lag curve

- Normal fasting blood glucose level.
- Blood sugar rises above 180 mg during test.
- After two hours blood sugar level falls at or below normal fasting level.
- Urine sample may be positive

SERUM BILIRUBIN

Normal—0.8 mg %, range 0.2 to 0.8 mg %

Increased levels

- Hepatocellular jaundice results from injury or disease of parenchymal cells of liver.
- Viral hepatitis.
- Cirrhosis of liver.
- Drug — chlorpromazine.
- Obstructive jaundice due to obstruction of common bile duct. It causes high conjugated bilirubin due to its regurgitaion.
- Haemolytic jaundice.
- Erythroblastosis fetalis
- Pernicious anaemia.
- Transfusion reaction.

Interfering factors

- A high fat diet may cause decreased bilirubin levels.
- One hour exposure of specimen to sunlight will decrease the bilirubin content.

Lab Investigation	*Haemolytic*	*Obstructive*	*Hepatocellular*
Serum bilirubin	Indirect	Direct	Biphasic
Urine bilirubin	Absent	Present	Present
Urine urobilinogen	Increased	Absent or decreased	Increased
Stool colour	Dark colour	Clay colour	Pale
Flocculation turbidity test	Negative	Negative	Positive
Serum alkaline phophatase	Normal	Increased	Slightly increased
Serum cholesterol	Normal	Increased	Decreased

BLOOD UREA NITROGEN (BUN)

Normal values—25-40 mg per cent

Increased level

- Impaired renal function
- Shock
- Dehydration
- Diabetes
- Acute myocardial infarction
- Chronic gout
- Excessive protein intake

Decreased BUN

- Liver failure
- Malnutrition
- Nephrotic syndrome
- Over hydration

Interfering factors

- Combination of low protein and high carbohydrates causes decreased BUN level
- Increased BUN values normally occur in late pregnancy and infancy.
- Excessive IV fluids can lower BUN levels

URIC ACID

Normal values 4 to 7 mg per cent

It is commonly increased in gout but amount of increase is not directly related to the severity of the disease.

Increased levels found in

- Leukaemia
- Metastatic cancer
- Starvation
- Shock
- Chemotherapy for cancer
- Excessive radiation
- Diabetic ketosis

Interfering factors

- Stress will cause increased levels
- Prolonged low dose of salicylates, vitamin C, ethambutol, methyldopa increase levels.
- ACTH, phenothiazenes decrease uric acid levels

URINE ANALYSIS

SPECIFIC GRAVITY

Normal values

1.003-1.025 (usually between)

1.025-1030 + (concentrated urine)

Specific gravity varies universally with urine excretion (decrease in volume, increase in specific gravity). In following conditions relationship is affected

- Diabetes—increased volume, increased specific gravity.
- Hypertension—normal volume, decreased specific gravity.
- Early renal disease—increased volume, decreased specific gravity

Low specific gravity (1.001-1.010)

- Diabetes insipidus
- Glomerulonephritis
- Severe renal damage

Increased specific gravity

- Diabetes mellitus, nephrosis
- Fever, vomiting and other conditions of excessive water loss, dehydration.

Interfering factors

- Specific gravity is highest in the morning specimen.
- Specific gravity is increased in fever, vomiting and diarrhoea.
- Cold and freezed urin e will have higher specific gravity.

COLOUR OF URINE

- Yellow is the normal colour of urine.
- Straw coloured urine is normal and indicates a low specific gravity under 1.010
- Amber coloured urine is normal and indicates concentrated urine with specific gravity of 1.010.
- Colourless urine is seen in
  Large fluid intake
  Untreated diabetes mellitus
  Alcohol ingestion
  Diuretic therapy
- An orange coloured urine is seen in
  Concentrated urine
  Restricted fluid intake
- Yellow foam may be due to biliverdin bile pigment.
- Red colour may be due to haemoglobinuria.
- Brown black colour is due to haemoglobin, lysol poisoning or melanin.
- Smoky colour may be due to red blood cells.

Interfering factors

- Colour of normal urine darkens on standing. This is due to the oxidation of urobilinogen to urobilin.
- Beets will turn urine red.
- Rhubarb can cause colour to be brown.
- Amidopyrine may change colour to orange.
- Pyridium can change colour from orange to red.
- Sulphonamides can change the colour to rust yellow.
- Dilantin will turn urine to red brown.

- Phenolic drug may turn urine to dark brown.
- Methylene blue will change colour from blue to green.
- Iron salts will result in dark coloured urine.

ODOUR

- Aromatic odour of fresh urine is due to volatile acids.
- The sweet smell of acetone in diabetic ketosis.
- Heavily infected urine has an unpleasant odour.
- Some food, i.e. *Asparagus* produces characteristic odours.
- Urine on standing for long time due to ammonia produces pungent odour which is formed by bacterial activity and decomposition of urea in specimen.

pH

Average range—4.6-8

Urine becomes increasingly acidic as the amount of sodium and excess acid retained by the body increases. Alkaline urine, usually contains bicarbonates and carbonic acid buffer.

- Streptomycin, neomycin and kanamycin are effective in genitourinary tract infection provided the urine is alkaline.
- Urine should be kept acidic in the treatment of urinary tract infection.

Acidic urine

- Found in alkalosis, uncontrolled diabetes, pulmonary emphysema, diarrhoea and starvation.
- Found in respiratory diseases.

Alkaline urine

- Found in urinary tract infection, pyloric obstruction, renal tubular acidosis.

Interfering factors

- On standing urine will become alkaline because CO will diffuse into the air.
- High protein diet causes highly acidic urine.
- Ammonium chloride produces acidic urine.
- Sodium bicarbonate produces alkaline urine.

TURBIDITY

Fresh urine is clear.

- Pathological urine is turbid or cloudy.
- UTI may also result in turbid urine.
- Presence of WBCs or bacteria may result in turbid urine.

Interfering factors

- After ingestion, food urates and phosphates may produce cloudiness.
- Vaginal contamination from female patients.
- Greasy cloudiness may be caused by large amount of fat.

HAEMATURIA

To identify blood cells, urine is centrifuged and sediment examined microscopically. It may be one of the early indications of blood in urine.

- Haemoglobinuria is found in
  Extensive burn and crush injuries

Febrile intoxication

Malaria.

Snake bite.

- Haemolytic anaemias.
- Coumarin and aspirin may cause it.
- High doses of Vitamin C may cause false-negative result.
- False-positive result may be due to bromides, oxidizing agents.

Interfering factors

- Pregnancy and lactation may cause a false-positive test.
- Stress, excitement, testing after heavy meal may cause false-positive test
- Vit C in very large doses may cause false-negative test.

PROTEIN

Normal values—Nil

- Proteinuria occurs in following renal disease
  - Nephritis
  - Nephrosis
  - Polycystic kidney
  - Kidney stones
  - Tuberculosis
- Proteinuria may occur in following non-renal disease
  - Fever
  - Trauma
  - Toxaemia
  - Convulsive disorder
  - Hyperthyroidism

Interfering factors

Functional, mild and transitory protein in urine is due to

- Violent exercise
- Severe emotional stress
- Cold bath

Increased protein in urine occurs

- After eating large amount of protein
- In pregnancy
- In orthostatic proteinuria

- Alkaline urine can give a false low protein value
- Drugs which can give false-positive test for protein include
  - Massive doses of penicillin
  - Chlorpromazine
  - Sulphamethoxazole

Clinical implications

- Heavy proteinuria (4 gm per 24 hour)
  - Glomerulonephritis
  - Amyloid disease
  - Nephrotic syndrome
- Moderate proteinuria (0.5 to 4 g per 24 hour)
  - Nephrosclerosis

- Pyelonephritis
- Diabetes
- Kidney stones
- Minimal proteinuria (less than 500 mg)
  - Polycystic kidney
  - Renal tubular disease

SUGAR

Normal—Nil

Clinical implications

- Increased glucose is found in diabetes mellitus, brain injury, myocardial infarction, etc.

MICROSCOPIC EXAMINATION

Red Cells and Red Cell Cast

Normal Values

1 or 2/low power field

0-1/high power field

RED CELL CASTS

- It indicates acute inflammatory or vascular disorders in the glomeruli

  It may be due to

  Renal infarction

  Collagen disease

  Acute glomerulonephritis

RED CELLS

- Increased red cells occur in

  Pyelonephritis

  Renal stones

  Cystitis

  Tuberculosis
- RBCs in excess of WBCs indicate bleeding into the urinary tract

  Aspirin ingestion

  Trauma
- Increased numbers of RBCs can be found following violent exercise, passage of stones and catheterisation

WHITE CELLS AND CAST

Normal Values

WBCs 0–4/ high powered field

WBCs casts—Negative

Clinical implications

- Large number of white cells indicate bacterial infection in urinary tract.
- If infection is in kidney WBC tends to be associated with cellular and granular casts.
- It indicates renal parenchymal infection.
- It is associated with

  Pyelonephritis

  Acute glomerulonephritis

EPITHELIAL CELLS AND CAST

Normal

(Occasional renal epithelial cell found)

Clinical implications

- It indicates damage to glomerular capillary membrane
- Hyaline casts may be seen temporarily
  - Fever
  - Postural strain
  - Emotional exercise
- In nephrotic syndrome large number of hyaline casts appear with heavy proteinuria and fine granular casts
- May be found in alkaline pH.

GRANULAR CASTS

Normal values

(Occasional granular casts are found)

These are found in

Acute tubular necrosis
Severe glomerulonephritis
Pyelonephritis
Chronic lead poisoning

CELLS FOUND IN URINE

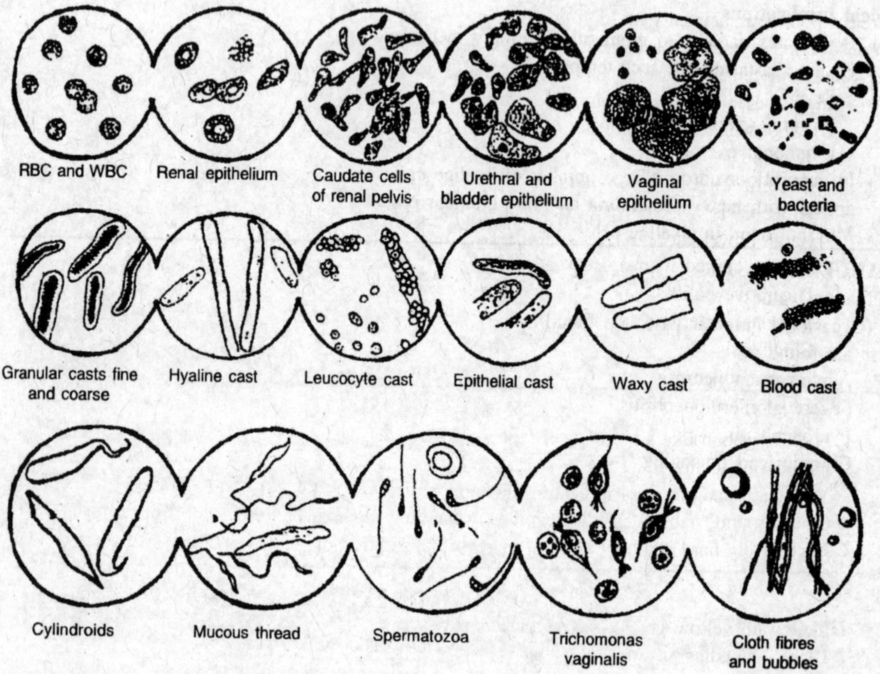

CRYSTALS FOUND IN ACID URINE 400 ×

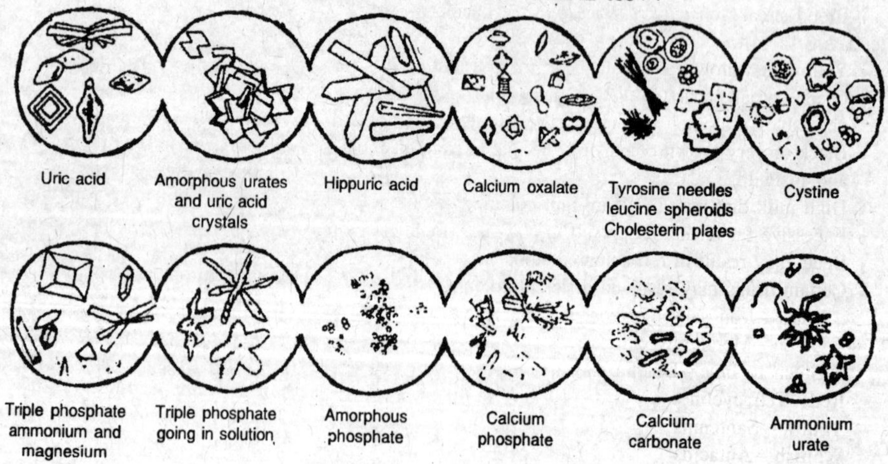

STOOL EXAMINATION

CONSISTENCY

Greasy stool is associated with high fat content.
In obstruction of common bile duct, stool gives a putty-like appearance. It is due to presence of unabsorbed fat. Sprue and celiac disease appearance of stool resembles aluminium paint due to fatty acid.

- In cystic fibrosis there is greasy, butter stool.
- Diarrhoea mixed with mucus and blood is seen in
  - Typhoid
  - Cholera
  - Amoebiasis
  - Large bowel cancer
- Diarrhoea mixed with mucus and pus
  - Ulcerative colitis
  - Regional enteritis
  - Shigellosis
  - Salmonellosis

SHAPE AND SIZE

- Narrow ribbon-like stool suggests the possibility of spastic bowel, rectal narrowing or a partial obstruction.
- Very large calibre stool indicates dilatation of viscus
- Small, round, habitual stools accompany habitual moderate constipation.
- Excessively hard stools are due to increased absorption of fluids.

COLOUR OF STOOL

- Yellow to yellow green—severe diarrhoea
- Black—bleeding in upper GI tract
- Tar or clay coloured—pancreatic insufficiency
- Red—bleeding from lower GI tract
- Blood streaks on outer surface indicate haemorrhoids

Interfering factors

- Yellow to yellow green colour occurs in breastfed infants.
- Green colour occurs in diets high in chlorophyll rich vegetables. Calomel drug can also cause it.
- Black or very brown colour may be due to iron, charcoal and bismuth.
- High milk diet may result in light coloured stool
- Excessive fat intake may result in clay-like stool
- Beets may result in red coloured stool
- Certain drugs may result in different colours
  - Black—Iron salts, charcoal
  - Green—Mercurous chloride
  - Green to blue—Diathiazenes
  - Red—Tetracyclines
  - Yellow—Santenins
  - Whitish—Antacids
  - Orange—Phenazopyridine

BLOOD IN STOOL

Normal Values—Nil

- A dark red to black tarry appearance of stool is indicative of loss of 0.50 ml to 0.75 ml of blood from upper GI tract
- Gross or occult blood in stool indicates non-specific ulcerative colitis.

Interfering factors

- Meat in the diet contains haemoglobin and enzymes that can give false-positive test.
- Vitamin C more than 500 mg daily may result in false negative test.
- Drugs that may cause false-positive test for occult blood are
  - Bromides
  - Colchicine
  - Oxidising agents

MUCUS IN STOOL

- Translucent gelatinous mucus clinging to the surface of stool occurs in
  - Mucous colitis
  - Emotionally disturbed patient
  - Excessive straining at stool
  - Bloody mucus clinging to stool is due to drugs,
  - Inflammation or neoplasm of rectal canal
- Mucus with pus and blood is associated with
  - Ulcerative colitis
  - Bacillary dysentery
  - Acute diverticulitis
  - Intestinal tuberculosis

LEUCOCYTES IN STOOL

- Complete absence of leucocytes is associated with
  - Cholera
  - Non-specific diarrhoea
  - Viral diarrhoea
- Primary mononuclear leucocytes appear in
  - Shigellosis
  - Salmonellosis
  - Ulcerative colitis
- Large amounts of pus accompany
  - Chronic ulcerative colitis
  - Chronic bacillary dysentery
  - Localised abscess.

CEREBROSPINAL FLUID

Normal CSF values in Adults

Volume	90-150 ml clear
Pressure	75-150 mm
Specific gravity	1.006-1.008
Glucose	45-85 mg/dl
Lactic acid	24 mg/dl
AG ratio	8:1
Chloride	118-132 mEq/Liter
Urea nitrogen	6-16 mg/dl
Cholesterol	0.2-0.6 mg/dl
Bilirubin	Nil
Uric acid	0.5-4.5 mg/dl

Colour changes in CSF

Appearance	*Condition*
Opalescent, slightly yellow with delicate clot	TB Meningitis
Opalescent to purulent, slightly yellow with coarse clot	Acute pyogenic meningitis
Slightly yellow clear or	Acute anterior poliomyelitis
opalescent with delicate clot Xanthochromic	Toxoplasmosis
Bloody purulent	Tumour of brain/cord

- **CSF glucose**
    - Normal values—45-85 mg/dl

Decreased levels

- Pyogenic, tuberculous and fungal infections
- Lymphomas with meningeal spread
- Leukaemia
- Hypoglycaemia
- Mumps, meningoencephalitis

Increased level

- **Diabetes**
- **CSF chloride**

Normal—118-132 MEq/litre

Decreased level

Tuberculous meningitis

Bacterical meningitis

- **CSF lactic acid**

Normal—24 mg/dl

Increased level

- Bacterial meningitis
- Hydrocephalus
- Brain abscess
- Cerebral ischaemia
- Traumatic brain injury
- Low arterial PO_2
- Cerebral infarct
- Low BP
- Respiratory alkalosis
- Idiopathic seizures

- **CSF total cell count**

  Normal values—0-5 cu/mm

Increased (300-500 with predominantly monocytic clear cell)

Viral infections
Syphilis of CNS
Tuberculous meningitis
Multiple sclerosis
Encephalopathy
Sarcoidosis
Polyneuritis
Periarteritis

Increased neutrophils

- Bacterial meningitis
- Early viral meningoencephalitis
- Mycotic meningitis
- Osteomyelitis of skull
- Subdural empyema
- Metastatic tumour

- **CSF PRESSURE**

  Normal 75-150 mm H_2O lateral decubitus.

Increased level

- Intracranial tumours
- Purulent or tuberculous meningitis
- Low-grade inflammatory processes
- Encephalitis

Decreased pressure

- Diabetic coma
- Obstructing tumour of spinal cord

- **PROTEINS IN CSF**

  Normal 15-45 mg/dl

Increased level

- Purulent meningitis
- Tuberculous meningitis
- Aseptic meningitis
- Brain abscess
- Subarachnoid haemorrhage
- Poliomyelitis
- Syphilis

RHEUMATOID FACTOR

Normal values Negative (<1:20)

Positive test

Early rheumatoid arthritis
Lupus erythematosus
Endocarditis
Tuberculosis
Syphilis
Sarcoid

- Cancer
- Viral infections

FREE THYROXINE T_4

Normal value—1-2.3 ng/dl

Increased levels

- Graves' disease
- Thyrotoxicosis
- Cirrhosis of liver

Decreased levels

- Primary hypothyroidism
- Secondary hypothyroidism
- Thyrotoxicosis due to T_3

TRI-IODOTHYRONINE T_3

Normal values—110-230 mg/100 ml

Increased values

- Hyperthyroidism
- T_3 thyrotoxicosis
- Acute thyroiditis

Decreased values

- Hypothyroidism
- Starvation
- Acute illness

MAJOR CHANGES ASSOCIATED WITH THE AGING PROCESS

Hormone	*Effect of aging*
Pituitary hormones	
Growth hormone	
24-h secretion	Decreased
Response to GHRH	Decreased
Response to repetitive GHRH	Restored
Response to repetitive	Unchanged
Prolactin	Mild increase
TSH	
Basal	Normal
Response to TRH	Decreasd (males)
ACTH	
Basal	Normal
Response to CRF	Mild increase
β-endorphin	Blunting of circadian rhythm
Gonadotrophins	
Males	Inappropriately low (LH) and increased (FSH)
Females	Increased
Thyroid hormones	
Thyroxine	Normal
Tri-iodothyronine	Mild decrease
Adrenal hormones	
Cortisol, basal	Normal
Dexamethasone suppression	Less efficient
Aldosterone	Decreased
Dehydroepiandrosterone sulphate	Decreased
Epinephrine	Unchanged
Calcitropic hormones	
PTH	Increased
Calcitonin	Decreased
25 (OH) Vitamin D	Decreased
1,25 (OH)2 Vitamin D	Normal or decreased

Contd.....

Hormone		Effect of aging
Pancreatic hormones		
	Insulin	Increased
	Amylin	Increased
	Glucagon	Unchanged
	Pancreatic polypeptide	Increased
Sex hormones :		
Males	Testosterone	Normal or decreased
	Bioavailable testosterone	Decreased
	Dehydrotestosterone	Decreased
	Sex hormone binding globulin	Normal or increased
	Oestradiol	Normal
Females	Oestradiol	Decreased
	Oestrone	Decreased
	Androstenedione	Decreased
	Testosterone	Decreased
Miscellaneous		
	Norepinephrine	Increased
	Renin	Decreased
	Gastric inhibitory polypetide	Unchanged
	Cholecystokinin	Increased
	Vasoactive intestinal peptide	Increased; loss of circadian rhythm
	Atrial natriuretic factor	Increased
	Arginine vasopressin	Increased